Pediatric Critical Care Medicine

EDITORS

■ ANTHONY D. SLONIM, MD, DrPH, FCCM

Executive Director, Center for Clinical Effectiveness
Attending Physician, Critical Care Medicine
Children's National Medical Center
Associate Professor and Vice Chairman of Pediatrics
The George Washington University School of Medicine
Washington, DC

■ MURRAY M. POLLACK, MD, MBA, FCCM

Executive Director, Center for Hospital-Based Specialities
Division Chief, Critical Care Medicine
Children's National Medical Center
Professor of Pediatrics
The George Washington University School of Medicine
Washington, DC

SECTION EDITORS

Michael J. Bell, MD
John T. Berger III, MD
Joseph A. Carcillo Jr, MD
Heidi J. Dalton, MD, FCCM
Jonathan S. Evans, MD
Mark J. Heulitt, MD, FAARC, FCCP
Richard A. Jonas, MD

Paul Kaplowitz, MD, PhD
Naomi L. C. Luban, MD
Robert E. Lynch, MD, PhD, FCCM
JoAnne Natale, MD, PhD
Daniel A. Notterman, MD, FCCM
David M. Steinhorn, MD
Edward C. Wong, MD

Lippincott Williams & Wilkins
a Wolters Kluwer business
Philadelphia · Baltimore · New York · London
Buenos Aires · Hong Kong · Sydney · Tokyo

Acquisitions Editor: Anne Sydor/Brian Brown
Managing Editor: Nicole Dernoski/Fran Murphy
Developmental Editor: Molly Connors, Dovetail Content Solutions
Project Manager: Nicole Walz
Senior Manufacturing Manager: Ben Rivera
Senior Marketing Manager: Angela Panetta
Design Coordinator: Terry Mallon
Cover Designer: Joseph DePinho
Production Services: Laserwords Private Limited
Printer: Edwards Brothers

© 2006 by Lippincott Williams & Wilkins, a Wolters Kluwer business
530 Walnut Street
Philadelphia, PA 19106
WWW.LWW.COM

Library of Congress Cataloging-in-Publication Data

Pediatric critical care medicine / [edited by] Anthony D. Slonim, Murray
  M. Pollack. —1st ed.
    p. ; cm.
  Includes bibliographical references and index.
  ISBN 0-7817-9469-2
  1. Pediatric intensive care.   I. Slonim, Anthony D.   II. Pollack, Murray
M.
  [DNLM: 1. Critical Care—Child. 2. Critical Care—Infant. WS 366
P3684 2006]
  RJ370.P28 2006
  618.92'0028—dc22
                                                          2005032133

Care has been taken to confirm the accuracy of the information presented and to describe generally accepted practices. However, the authors, editors, and publisher are not responsible for errors or omissions or for any consequences from application of the information in this book and make no warranty, expressed or implied, with respect to the currency, completeness, or accuracy of the contents of the publication. Application of this information in a particular situation remains the professional responsibility of the practitioner.

The authors, editors, and publisher have exerted every effort to ensure that drug selection and dosage set forth in this text are in accordance with current recommendations and practice at the time of publication. However, in view of ongoing research, changes in government regulations, and the constant flow of information relating to drug therapy and drug reactions, the reader is urged to check the package insert for each drug for any change in indications and dosage and for added warnings and precautions. This is particularly important when the recommended agent is a new or infrequently employed drug.

Some drugs and medical devices presented in this publication have Food and Drug Administration (FDA) clearance for limited use in restricted research settings. It is the responsibility of health care providers to ascertain the FDA status of each drug or device planned for use in their clinical practice.

The publishers have made every effort to trace copyright holders for borrowed material. If they have inadvertently overlooked any, they will be pleased to make the necessary arrangements at the first opportunity.

To purchase additional copies of this book, call our customer service department at (800) 638-3030 or fax orders to (301) 223-2320. International customers should call (301) 223-2300. Lippincott Williams & Wilkins customer service representatives are available from 8:30 am to 6:30 pm, EST, Monday through Friday, for telephone access. Visit Lippincott Williams & Wilkins on the Internet: http://www.lww.com.

10 9 8 7 6 5 4 3 2

This work is dedicated to my family, friends, colleagues, and patients, all of whom have had a material impact on my development as a physician.

A.D.S

This work is dedicated to my wife, Mona, who exemplifies persistence and courage; my children Seth and Haley, who make me want to be a better physician; and the Critical Care Division at CNMC who teach me every day about clinical excellence and the values of being a physician.

M.M.P

Contents

List of Contributors

LISA P. ABRAMSON, MD
Pediatric Surgery Fellow, Division of Pediatric Surgery, Children's Memorial Hospital, Chicago, Illinois

MELVIN C. ALMODOVAR, MD
Assistant Professor, Department of Pediatrics, University of Colorado Health and Science Center; Director of Cardiac Intensive Care, The Children's Hospital Heart Institute, The Children's Hospital Denver, Denver, Colorado

ORAL ALPAN, MD
Director, Center for Allergy, Asthma, and Immune Disorders, South Riding, Virginia

BASEM ZAFER ALSAATI, MD
Assistant Professor, Department of Pediatrics, Queen's University; Attending Physician, Department of Pediatrics, Kingston General Hospital, Kingston, Ontario, Canada

ANNE L. ANGIOLILLO, MD
Associate Professor, Department of Pediatrics, The George Washington University School of Medicine; Attending Physician, Division of Hematology and Oncology, Center for Cancer and Blood Disorders, Children's National Medical Center, Washington, DC

AUDREY AUSTIN, MD
Assistant Professor, Department of Pediatrics, The George Washington University School of Medicine and Health Sciences; Endocrinologist, Department of Pediatrics, Children's National Medical Center, Washington, DC

RUBA K. AZZAM, MD
Assistant Professor, Department of Pediatric Gastroenterology and Hepatology, The University of Chicago, Comer Children's Hospital, Chicago, Illinois

CINDY SUTTON BARRETT, MD
Senior Fellow in Pediatric Critical Care, Pediatric Critical Care Fellow, Department of Pediatric Critical Care, Duke University Medical Center, Durham, North Carolina

MICHAEL J. BELL, MD
Associate Professor of Pediatrics and Critical Care Medicine, Department of Pediatrics, Division of Critical Care Medicine, The George Washington University School of Medicine; Director, Neurocritical Care, Department of Pediatrics, Division of Critical Care Medicine, Children's National Medical Center, Washington, DC

CRAIG WILLIAM BELSHA, MD
Associate Professor, Department of Pediatrics, St. Louis University; Director, Hypertension Program, Division of Pediatric Nephrology, SSM Cardinal Glennon Children's Hospital, St. Louis, Missouri

ROBERT A. BERG, MD
Associate Dean for Clinical Affairs, Professor, Department of Pediatrics, The University of Arizona College of Medicine; Pediatric Intensivist, Department of Pediatrics, University Medical Center and Tucson Medical Center, Tucson, Arizona

JOHN T. BERGER III, MD
Assistant Professor, Department of Pediatrics, The George Washington University School of Medicine; Director, Cardiac Intensive Care, Department of Critical Care Medicine and Cardiology, Children's National Medical Center, Washington, DC

DOUGLAS L. BLOWEY, MD
Associate Professor, Departments of Pediatric Nephrology and Clinical Pharmacology, University of Missouri—Kansas City School of Medicine, Children's Mercy Hospitals and Clinics, Kansas City, Missouri

ANDREW M. BONWIT, MD
Assistant Professor, Department of Pediatrics, The George Washington University School of Medicine; Attending Pediatrician, Children's National Medical Center, Washington, DC

RONALD A. BRONICKI, MD
Assistant Clinical Professor, Department of Pediatrics, Harbor—University of California Los Angeles Medical Center, University of California Los Angeles School of Medicine; Attending Physician, Cardiac Intensive Care, Children's Hospital of Orange County, Orange, California

DEREK A. BRUCE, MB, CHB
Professor of Neurosurgery and Pediatrics, Department of Neurosurgery, The George Washington University School of Medicine; Attending Neurosurgeon, Departments of Neuroscience and Behavioral Medicine, Children's National Medical Center, Washington, DC

JOSEPH M. CAMPOS, PhD
Professor, Departments of Pediatrics, Pathology, and Microbiology/Tropical Medicine, The George Washington University Medical Center; Director, Microbiology Laboratory and Laboratory Informatics, Department of Laboratory Medicine, Children's National Medical Center, Washington, DC

JOSEPH A. CARCILLO, MD
Associate Professor, Department of Critical Care Medicine, University of Pittsburgh, Center for Clinical Pharmacology; Associate Director, Pediatric Intensive Care Unit, Department of Critical Care Medicine, Children's Hospital of Pittsburgh, Pittsburgh, Pennsylvania

PAUL A. CHECCHIA, MD
Assistant Professor of Critical Care and Cardiology, Department of Pediatrics, Washington University School of Medicine; Chief, Pediatric Cardiac Critical Care Service, Co-director, Pediatric Intensive Care Unit, St. Louis Children's Hospital, St. Louis, Missouri

IRA M. CHEIFETZ, MD, FCCM, FAARC
Division Chief, Critical Care Medicine, Associate Professor, Department of Pediatrics, Duke University School of Medicine, Duke University Medical Center; Medical Director, Pediatric Intensive Care Unit, Medical Director, Pediatric Respiratory Care and ECMO, Department of Pediatrics, Duke Children's Hospital, Duke University Medical Center, Durham, North Carolina

THOMAS J. CHOLIS III, MD
Clinical Instructor, Department of Pediatrics, The George Washington University School of Medicine, Children's National Medical Center, Washington, DC

STEVEN A. CONRAD, MD, PhD, FCCM
Professor, Departments of Medicine, Pediatrics, Emergency Medicine, and Anesthesiology, Louisiana State University Health Sciences Center; Director, Critical Care Service, and Extracorporeal Life Support Program, Louisiana State University Hospital, Shreveport, Louisiana

CHRISTIANE O. CORRIVEAU, MD
Assistant Professor, Department of Pediatrics, The George Washington University Medical Center; Director, Departmental Education and Fellowship Training, Divison of Critical Care Medicine, Children's National Medical Center, Washington, DC

RUSSELL R. CROSS, MD, MSBME
Assistant Professor, Department of Pediatrics, The George Washington University School of Medicine; Attending Physician, Department of Pediatric Cardiology, Children's National Medical Center, Washington, DC

HEIDI J. DALTON, MD, FCCM
Professor, Department of Pediatrics, The George Washington University School of Medicine and Health Sciences; Director, Pediatric Intensive Care Unit and Pediatric ECMO, Department of Critical Care Medicine, Children's National Medical Center, Washington, DC

K. ALEX DANESHMAND, DO
Pediatric Intensive Care Fellow, Department of Pediatric Critical Care Medicine, University of Florida; Pediatric Intensive Care Fellow, Department of Pediatric Critical Care Medicine, Shands Children's Hospital, Gainesville, Florida

EMILY L. DOBYNS, MD
Associate Professor, Section of Critical Care Medicine, Department of Pediatrics, University of Colorado Denver Health Sciences Center; Medical Director, Pediatric Critical Care Unit, Department of Pediatric Critical Care Medicine, The Children's Hospital, Denver, Colorado

ANNE F. EDER, MD, PhD
Executive Medical Officer, Biomedical Headquarters, American Red Cross, Washington, DC

EILEEN ELLIS, MD
Professor, Department of Pediatrics, University of Arkansas for Medical Sciences, Little Rock, Arkansas; Professor, Department of Pediatrics, Arkansas Children's Hospital, Little Rock, Arkansas

JONATHAN S. EVANS, MD
Staff Physician, Division of Pediatric Gastroenterology and Nutrition, Nemours Children's Clinic, Jacksonville, Florida

JAMES B. FINK, MS, RRT, FAARC
Fellow, Respiratory Science, Department of Scientific Affairs, Aerogen, Inc., Mountain View, California

JULIA C. FINKEL, MD
Associate Professor, Departments of Anesthesiology and Pediatrics, The George Washington Universtiy School of Medicine; Director, Anesthesia Pain Management Service, Children's National Medical Center, Washington, DC

RICHARD T. FISER, MD
Associate Professor, Departments of Pediatric Critical Care and Cardiology, University of Arkansas for Medical Sciences—College of Medicine, Little Rock, Arkansas; Medical Director, ECMO, Arkansas Children's Hospital, Little Rock, Arkansas

JAMES D. FORTENBERRY, MD, FCCM, FAA
Clinical Associate Professor, Department of Pediatrics, Emory University School of Medicine; Division Director, Department of Critical Care Medicine, ECMO, Children's Healthcare of Atlanta, Atlanta, Georgia

WILLIAM DAVIS GAILLARD, MD
Professor, Departments of Neurology and Pediatrics, The George Washington University School of Medicine; Director, Comprehensive Pediatric Epilepsy Program, Department of Neurology, Children's National Medical Center, Washington, DC

DONALD E. GEORGE, MD

Academic Affiliate, Department of Pediatrics, University of Florida School of Medicine; C-Clinical Associate Professor, Pediatric Gastroenterology, Nemours Children's Clinic, Jacksonville, Florida

CYNTHIA L. GIBSON, MD

Clinical Instructor, Department of Pediatrics, The George Washington University School of Medicine and Health Sciences; Pediatric Critical Care Fellow, Department of Pediatric Critical Care Medicine, Children's National Medical Center, Washington, DC

STUART L. GOLDSTEIN, MD

Associate Professor, Department of Pediatrics, Baylor College of Medicine; Medical Director, Renal Dialysis Unit, Texas Children's Hospital, Houston, Texas

SYLVIA GÖTHBERG, MD, PhD

Department of Pediatric Anesthesiology and Intensive Care, The Queen Silvia Children's Hospital, Göteborg, Sweden

EVA NOZIK GRAYCK, MD

Associate Professor, Department of Pediatrics, University of Colorado at Denver and Health Science Center; Attending Physician, Pediatric Intensive Care Unit, Department of Pediatrics, Denver Children's Hospital, Denver, Colorado

YONG Y. HAN, MD

Assistant Professor, Pediatrics and Communicable Diseases, University of Michigan Medical School, Ann Arbor, Michigan

NAZEEH HANNA, MD

Associate Professor, Department of Pediatrics, University of Medicine and Dentistry of New Jersey—Robert Wood Johnson Medical School; Medical Director and Co-Chief, Division of Neonatology, Department of Pediatrics, University of Medicine and Dentistry of New Jersey—Robert Wood Johnson University Hospital, New Brunswick, New Jersey

DIANE E. HECK, PhD

Professor, Department of Pharmacology and Toxicology, Rutgers University, Piscataway, New Jersey

MARK J. HEULITT, MD, FAARC, FCCP

Professor, Departments of Pediatrics, Physiology, and Biophysics, University of Arkansas for Medical Sciences, College of Medicine; Director, Applied Respiratory Physiology Laboratory, Arkansas Children's Hospital Research Institute; Pediatric Intensivist, Pediatric Critical Care Medicine, Associate Medical Director Respiratory Care Services, Arkansas Children's Hospital, Little Rock, Arkansas

ANGELA A. HSU, MD

Adjunct Instructor, Department of Pediatrics, The George Washington University Medical Center; Pediatric Critical Care Fellow, Department of Critical Care Medicine, Children's National Medical Center, Washington, DC

JENNIFER HURST, RN, BSN

Infection Control Nurse Coordinator, Department of Epidemiology, Children's National Medical Center, Washington, DC

REBECCA N. ICHORD, MD

Assistant Professor, Departments of Neurology and Pediatrics, Pediatric Stroke Program, Universtiy of Pennsylvania School of Medicine; Director, Pediatric Stroke Program, Department of Neurology, Children's Hospital of Philadelphia, Philadelphia, Pennsylvania

MOHAMMAD ILYAS, MD

Assistant Professor, Department of Pediatrics, University of Arkansas for Medical sciences; Staff Pediatric Nephrologist, Department of Pediatric Nephrology, Arkansas Children's Hospital, Little Rock, Arkansas

D. DUNBAR IVY, MD

Associate Professor, Chief and Selby's Chair of Pediatric Cardiology, Department of Pediatrics, University of Colorado; Chief and Selby's Chair of Pediatric Cardiology B,100, Pediatric Cardiology, The Children's Hospital, Denver, Colorado

YEWANDE J. JOHNSON, MD

Assistant Professor, Departments of Anesthesiology and Pediatrics, The George Washington University Medical Center; Attending Staff, Department of Anesthesiology, Children's National Medical Center, Washington, DC

RICHARD A. JONAS, MD

Professor, Department of Surgery, The George Washington University School of Medicine; Chief, Cardiac Surgery, Co-Director Children's National Heart Institute, Children's National Medical Center, Washington, DC

ALOK KALIA, MD

Associate Professor of Pediatrics, Director, Division of Pediatric Nephrology, University of Texas Medical Branch, Galveston, Texas

NAYNESH R. KAMANI, MD

Professor, Department of Pediatrics and Microbiology, Immunology, and Tropical Medicine, The George Washington University School of Medicine; Chief, Division of Stem Cell Transplantation and Immunology, Children's National Medical Center, Washington, DC

PAUL KAPLOWITZ, MD, PhD

Professor, Department of Pediatrics, The George Washington University School of Medicine, Washington, DC

MARSHA KAY, MD

Staff Physician, Department of Pediatric Gastroenterology and Nutrition, Cleveland Clinic Foundation, Cleveland, Ohio

KAREN E. KING, MD

Assistant Professor, Departments of Pathology and Oncology, The Johns Hopkins University School of Medicine; Director, Hemiparesis and Transfusion Support Service, Associate Director, Transfusion Medicine, Department of Pathology, The Johns Hopkins Hospital, Baltimore, Maryland

ANTHONY YUN LEE, MD

Adjunct Instructor, Department of Pediatrics, The George Washington University School of Medicine; Fellow, Department of Critical Care Medicine, Children's National Medical Center, Washington, DC

LYNNE L. LEVITSKY, MD

Associate Professor, Department of Pediatrics, Harvard Medical School; Chief, Pediatric Endocrine Unit, Pediatric Services, Massachusetts General Hospital, Boston, Massachusetts

JOHN C. LIN, MD

Adjunct Assistant Professor, Division of Pediatric Critical Care Medicine, Children's Hospital of Pittsburgh, Pittsburgh, Pennsylvania; Staff Pediatric Intensivist, San Antonio Military Pediatric Consortium, Wilford Hall Medical Center, Lackland Air Force Base, Texas

NAOMI L. C. LUBAN, MD

Professor, Department of Pediatrics and Pathology, The George Washington University School of Medicine and Health Sciences; Chairman, Laboratory Medicine and Pathology, Director, Transfusion Medicine, Vice Chairman, Academic Affairs, Department of Laboratory Medicine, Children's National Medical Center, Washington, DC

ROBERT E. LYNCH, MD, PhD, FCCM

Professor and Director Pediatric Critical Care, Department of Pediatrics, St. Louis University; Medical Director, Pediatric Intensive Care Unit, SSM Cardinal Glennon Children's Hospital, St. Louis, Missouri

JAMES D. MARSHALL, MD, FAAP

Pediatric Intensivist, Medical Director of Clinical Research, Department of Pediatric Intensive Care, Cook Children's Medical Center, Fort Worth, Texas

JEFFEREY P. MOAK, MD

Professor, Department of Pediatrics, The George Washington University School of Medicine; Director, Electrophysiology and Pacing, Department of Cardiology, Children's National Medical Center, Washington, DC

FRANZISKA MOHR, MD, MRCPCH

Fellow, Departments of Pediatric Gastroenterology and Nutrition, Cleveland Clinic Foundation, Cleveland, Ohio

VINAY NADKARNI, MD, MSC

Associate Professor, Departments of Anesthesia and Pediatrics, University of Pennsylvania; Director, Pediatric Critical Care Fellowship Program, Department of Anesthesia and Critical Care Medicine, The Children's Hospital of Philadelphia, Philadelphia, Pennsylvania

SUMATI NAMBIAR, MD, MPH

Clinical Assistant Professor, Division of Pediatrics, The George Washington University School of Medicine and Health Sciences, Children's National Medical Center, Washington, DC; Center for Drug Evaluation and Research, US Food and Drug Administration, Rockville, Maryland

JOANNE E. NATALE, MD, PhD

Assistant Professor, Departments of Pediatrics, Genetics and Neurosciences, The George Washington University School of Medicine; Attending Physician, Department of Pediatric Critical Care Medicine, Children's National Medical Center, Washington, DC

DAVID P. NELSON, MD, PhD

Associate Professor, Department of Pediatrics, The Lillie Frank Abercrombie Section of Cardiology, Baylor College of Medicine; Director, Cardiovascular Intensive Care Unit, Texas Children's Hospital, Houston, Texas

DANIEL A. NOTTERMAN, MD, FCCM

University Professor and Chair, Department of Pediatrics and Molecular Genetics, The University of Medicine and Dentistry of New Jersey—Robert Wood Johnson Medical School; Physician-In-Chief, The Bristol-Myers Squibb Children's Hospital at Robert Wood Johnson University Hospital, New Brunswick, New Jersey

NATAN NOVISKI, MD

Associate Professor, Department of Pediatrics, Harvard Medical School; Chief, Department of Pediatric Critical Care Medicine, Massachusetts General Hospital, Boston, Massachusetts

SUSAN B. NUNEZ, MD

Assistant Professor, Department of Pediatrics, The George Washington University Medical Center; Faculty, Departments of Endocrinology and Diabetes, Children's National Medical Center, Washington, DC

GEORGE OFORI-AMANFO, MD

Assistant Professor of Clinical Pediatrics, Department of Pediatrics, Columbia University College of Physicians and Surgeons; Assistant Attending Pediatrician, Department of Pediatrics, Morgan Stanley Children's Hospital of New York, New York, New York

REGINA OKHUYSEN-CAWLEY, MD

Assistant Professor, Department of Pediatric Critical Care Medicine, University of Arkansas for Medical Sciences College of Medicine, Little Rock, Arkansas

RICHARD ANDREW ORR, MD

Professor, Department of Critical Care Medicine, University of Pittsburgh; Associate Director, Department of Pediatric Critical Care, Children's Hospital Pittsburgh, Pittsburgh, Pennsylvania

PAUL OUELLET, PHDC, RRT, FCCM

Associate Professor, Department of Surgery, Université de Sherbrooke; Clinical specialist, Intensive Care Unit, Regional Health Authority Four, Sherbrooke, Quebec, Canada

ROGER J. PACKER, MD

Professor, Departments of Neurology and Pediatrics, The George Washington University School of Medicine; Executive Director Neurosciences and Behavioral Medicine, Chairman, Department of Neurology, Children's National Medical Center, Washington, DC

MATTHEW L. PADEN, MD

Pediatric Critical Care Fellow, Department of Pediatrics, Emory University; Pediatric Critical Care Fellow, Department of Pediatric Critical Care, Children's Healthcare of Atlanta, Atlanta, Georgia

EVELIO D. PEREZ-ALBUERNE, MD, PhD

Assistant Professor, Department of Pediatrics, The George Washington University School of Medicine; Attending Physician, Division of Stem Cell Transplantation and Immunology, Children's National Medical Center, Washington, DC

VICTOR M. PINEIRO-CARRERO, MD, FAAP

Associate Professor, Department of Pediatrics, Uniformed Services University, Bethesda, Maryland; Chief, Division of Gastroenterology, Nemours Children's Clinic, Orlando, Florida

JEFFERSON PEDRO PIVA, MD, PhD

Associate Professor, Department of Pediatrics, Medical School Pontificia Universidade Católica do RS; Associate Director, Pediatric Intensive Care Unit, Department of Pediatrics, Hospital São Lucas da Pontificia Universidade Católica do RS, Porto Alegre (RS), Brazil

MURRAY M. POLLACK, MD, MBA, FCCM

Executive Director, Center for Hospital-Based Specialities, Division Chief, Critical Care Medicine, Children's National Medical Center, Professor of Pediatrics, The George Washington University School of Medicine, Washington, DC

RAJANI PRABHAKARAN, MD

Clinical and Research Fellow, Department of Pediatric Endocrinology, Massachusetts General Hospital for Children, Harvard Medical School, Boston, Massachusetts

PARTHAK PRODHAN, MD

Assistant Professor, Department of Pediatrics, College of Medicine, University of Arkansas Medical Sciences, Arkansas Children's Hospital, Little Rock, Arkansas

J. CARTER RALPHE, MD

Assistant Professor, Department of Pediatrics, University of Pittsburgh; Assistant Professor, Department of Pediatric Cardiology, Children's Hospital of Pittsburgh, Pittsburgh, Pennsylvania

ASRAR RASHID, MRCPCH

Attending Consultant, Pediatric Intensive Care, Queens Medical Center Nottingham, University Hospital NHS Trust, Nottingham, United Kingdom

LAURA T. RUSSO, RD, CSP, LDN

Critical Care Dietitian, Department of Clinical Nutrition, Children's Memorial Hospital, Chicago, Illinois

LETICIA MANNING RYAN, MD

Adjunct Instructor, Department of Pediatrics, The George Washington University School of Medicine and Health Sciences; Fellow, Division of Pediatric Emergency Medicine, Children's National Medical Center, Washington, DC

RONALD C. SANDERS JR, MD, MS

Assistant Professor, Department of Pediatrics, University of Florida; Medical Director of Pediatric Respiratory Care Services, Department of Pediatrics, Shands Children's Hospital, Gainesville, Florida

MIGUEL SAPS, MD

Assistant Professor, Department of Pediatrics, Division of Pediatrics, Gastroenterology, Hepatology, and Nutrition, Children's Memorial Hospital, Northwestern University, Feinberg School of Medicine, Chicago, Illinois

STEVEN M. SCHWARTZ, MD

Associate Professor, Department of Pediatrics, University of Toronto School of Medicine; Head, Division of Cardiac Critical Care Medicine, Department of Critical Care Medicine, The Hospital For Sick Children, Toronto, Ontario, Canada

ADITI SHARANGPANI, MD

Assistant Professor, Department of Pediatrics, The George Washington University School of Medicine; Attending Physician, Critical Care Medicine, Children's National Medical Center, Washington, DC

AMITA SHARMA, MD, FAAP

Instructor, Department of Pediatrics, Harvard Medical School; Assistant Pediatrician, Department of Pediatrics, Massachusetts General Hospital, Boston, Massachusetts

NALINI SINGH MD, MPH

Professor, Departments of Pediatrics, Epidemiology and International Health, The George Washington University School of Medicine and Public Health; Chief, Division of Infectious Diseases, Director of Hospital Epidemiology, Children's National Medical Center, Washington, DC

ANTHONY D. SLONIM, MD, DrPH, FCCM

Executive Director, Center for Clinical Effectiveness, Attending Physician, Critical Care Medicine, Children's National Medical Center, Associate Professor and Vice Chairman of Pediatrics, The George Washington University School of Medicine, Washington, DC

SOPHIA R. SMITH, MD

Assistant Professor, Department of Pediatrics, The George Washington University School of Medicine and Health Sciences; Pediatric Intensivist, Medical Director Respiratory Care, Department of Pediatric Critical Care Medicine, Children's National Medical Center, Washington, DC

MARK D. SORRENTINO, MD, MS

Clinical Assistant Professor, Department of Pediatrics, The George Washington University School of Medicine; Attending Physician, Department of Critical Care Medicine, Children's National Medical Center, Washington, DC

HANS M. L. SPIEGEL, MD

Assistant Professor, Departments of Pediatrics and Tropical Medicine, The George Washington University School of Medicine; Director Special Immunology Service, Department of Infectious Diseases, Children's National Medical Center, Washington, DC

CHRISTOPHER F. SPURNEY, MD

Assistant Professor, Department of Pediatrics, The George Washington University School of Medicine and Health Sciences; Assistant Professor of Pediatrics, Division of Cardiology, Children's National Medical Center, Washington, DC

DAVID M. STEINHORN, MD

Associate Professor, Department of Pediatrics, Northwestern University, Feinberg School of Medicine; Attending Physician, Pulmonary and Critical Care, Children's Memorial Hospital, Chicago, Illinois

W. TAIT STEVENS, MD

Clinical Instructor, Department of Pathology and Laboratory Medicine, Loma Linda University School of Medicine; Resident Physician, Clinical Laboratory, Loma Linda University Medical Center, Loma Linda, California

DAVID C. STOCKWELL, MD

Assistant Professor, Department of Pediatric Critical Care, The George Washington University School of Medicine; Attending Physician, Department of Critical Care Medicine, Children's National Medical Center, Washington, DC

RICCARDO A. SUPERINA, MD

Professor, Department of Surgery, Northwestern University, Feinberg School of Medicine; Director, Transplant Surgery, Children's Memorial Hospital, Chicago, Illinois

STEPHEN J. TEACH, MD, MPH

Associate Professor, Department of Pediatrics, The George Washington University School of Medicine and Health Sciences; Associate Chief, Division of Emergency Medicine, Children's National Medical Center, Washington, DC

NEAL J. THOMAS, MD, MSC

Associate Professor, Department of Pediatrics and Health Evaluation Sciences, Division of Pediatric Critical Care Medicine, Penn State Children's Hospital, The Pennsylvania State University College of Medicine, Hershey, Pennsylvania

CYNTHIA J. TIFFT, MD, PhD

Associate Professor, Department of Pediatrics, The George Washington University School of Medicine and Health Sciences; Chief, Division of Genetics and Metabolism, Center for Hospital-Based Specialties, Children's National Medical Center, Washington, DC

I. DAVID TODRES, MD, FCCM

Professor, Department of Pediatrics, Harvard Medical School; Chief, Ethics Unit, Department of Pediatrics, Massachusetts General Hospital—ACC 731, Boston, Massachusetts

WILLIAM T. TSAI, MD

Assistant Professor, Department of Pediatrics, The George Washington University; Attending Physician, Children's National Medical Center, Critical Care and Emergency Medicine, Washington, DC

TAMMY NORIKO TSUCHIDA, MD, PhD

Assistant Professor, Departments of Neurology and Pediatrics, The George Washington University School of Medicine; Assistant Professor, Department of Neurology, Children's National Medical Center, Washington, DC

WENDY TURENNE, MS
Statistician, Center for Clinical Effectiveness, Children's National Medical Center, Washington, DC

JOHN N. VAN DEN ANKER, MD, PhD
Professor, Departments of Pediatrics, Pharmacology, and Physiology, The George Washington University School of Medicine and Health Sciences; Chief, Division of Pediatric Clinical Pharmacology, Department of Pediatrics, Children's National Medical Center, Washington, DC; Professor, Department of Pediatrics, Erasmus MC—Sophia Children's Hospital, Rotterdam, The Netherlands

BARRY WEINBERGER, MD
Associate Professor, Department of Pediatrics, University of Medicine and Dentistry of New Jersey—Robert Wood Johnson Medical School; Co-Chief, Division of Neonatology, Department of Pediatrics, Robert Wood Johnson University Hospital, New Brunswick, New Jersey

STEVEN L. WEINSTEIN, MD
Professor, Departments of Neurology and Pediatrics, The George Washington University School of Medicine; Vice Chairman, Department of Neurology, Children's National Medical Center, Washington, DC

DOUGLAS F. WILLSON, MD
Associate Professor, Departments of Pediatrics and Anesthesia, Medical Director, Pediatric Intensive Care Unit, University of Virginia Children's Hospital, Charlottesville, Virginia

EDWARD C. WONG, MD
Assistant Professor, Departments of Pediatrics and Pathology, The George Washington University School of Medicine and Health Sciences; Associate Director of Hematology, Director of Hematology, Departments of Pediatrics and Pathology, Children's National Medical Center, Washington, DC

ELLEN G. WOOD, MD
Professor, Department of Pediatrics, St. Louis University; Director, Division of Pediatric Nephrology, Department of Pediatrics, Cardinal Glennon Children's Hospital, St. Louis, Missouri

ANGELA T. WRATNEY, MD, MHSC
Assistant Professor, Department of Pediatrics, The George Washington University School of Medicine and Health Sciences; Attending, Department of Critical Care Medicine, Children's National Medical Center, Washington, DC

M. NILUFER YALINDAG-OZTURK, MD
Attending Physician, Department of Critical Care, Children's National Medical Center, Washington, DC

GUY YOUNG, MD
Assistant Professor, Department of Pediatrics, David Geffen School of Medicine at University of California Los Angeles; Attending Hematologist, Department of Hematology, Children's Hospital of Orange County, Orange, California

DINA J. ZAND, MD
Assistant Professor, Department of Pediatrics, The George Washington University Medical Center; Attending Physician Department of Genetics and Metabolism, Children's National Medical Center, Washington, DC

Preface

Pediatric Critical Care Medicine was conceived as a core text-book and reference text that would provide the foundation for physiologically based clinical practice. We believe that it will provide trainees and practicing physicians with the concepts relevant to caring for the acutely ill or injured children. Our intention was to create a textbook that carefully integrates core principles with clinical practice. The content both provides adequate preparation for the subspecialty certification examination and is a readily available reference for the clinical care of the critically ill child. Although the information provided is the most recently available, the book does not focus on "hot topics," late-breaking information, or niche content because these days this information can be found more readily through electronic resources.

We believe that we have created a book for the various stages of a pediatric intensivist's practice. The book addresses the physiologically based concepts that need to be learned by new trainees, provides reference for a particular clinical question, and is substantive enough in its scope to provide a thorough review for the more experienced clinician, refreshing his or her knowledge or preparing for recertification. The organizational philosophy of *Pediatric Critical Care Medicine* mirrors the mental processes that intensive care physicians use in patient care. Intensive care medicine begins with a core knowledge base focused on organ system physiology. Clinicians apply their knowledge of physiologic systems to patient care issues. Life support, as well as other therapies for organ system dysfunction, disease, and failure, depends on a strong understanding of organ system functioning under a variety of conditions. Knowledge about clinical issues is applied to this foundation of physiologic knowledge. As a result, a large part of the text centers on chapters that contain organ system physiology.

Importantly, we relied heavily on our section editors for their expertise in developing the physiology sections and recruiting authors with expertise in the clinical areas. This approach provided the appropriate integration of physiologic materials without duplication and defined the knowledge base that authors of clinical sections could depend on to write their clinical chapters, which were purposely designed to be relatively short and concise and only detail the clinical issues and any unique pathophysiology.

Anthony D. Slonim, MD, DrPH, FCCM
Murray M. Pollack, MD, MBA, FCCM

Acknowledgments

We would like to extend our heartfelt thanks to those who made this project possible. We relied heavily on our section editors to provide us with guidance regarding content, both physiologic and clinical, and to undertake the day-to-day management of their sections. The demands and timelines we imposed for this effort were unreasonable, but everyone performed in an exemplary manner that was professional, collaborative, and goal-directed. Their efforts are truly appreciated, and this text is as much their work as it is ours. They, along with the contributors, have provided a product of which we are proud.

Our thanks to Molly Connors from Dovetail Content Solutions who can manage a project like no one else we have ever seen. Her organizing capabilities and attention to detail kept us on track throughout the entire effort. Our team at Lippincott Williams & Wilkins has been an important resource that carried us through each of the phases of the work from design through production and marketing. Special thanks to Anne Sydor, who was a confidante, coach, and calming influence. She allowed us the opportunity to convert a vision into a reality.

In our office, Yolanda Jones has been supportive of our effort and keeping us on the task with meetings, e-mails, and organization. Lastly, a special thanks to our colleagues at the Children's National Medical Center who have put up with us in our efforts to bring this work from conception to fruition in less than 1 year.

Physiology and Pathophysiology

The Cell

Barry Weinberger   Nazeeh Hanna   Diane E. Heck   Daniel A. Notterman

The maintenance of health ultimately depends on the optimal functioning of the cells that make up the tissues and organs of the body. Therefore, a background in the structural morphology of cells, as well as the molecular mechanisms that regulate their activity, is essential for understanding disease processes and therapeutics. Although somatic cells differentiate into a wide variety of specialized forms that are structurally and functionally distinct, the fundamental organization of cells into nucleus, cytoplasm, membrane, and cytoplasmic organelles remains identifiable.

THE CELL MEMBRANE

All eukaryotic cells are contained within a membrane composed of lipids (phospholipids and cholesterol), protein, and oligosaccharides covalently linked to some of the lipids and proteins. The cell membrane functions as a selective barrier, regulating the passage of a specific molecule on the basis of charge and size. Although lipophilic molecules are most likely to pass passively through the membrane lipid bilayer, the membrane is a metabolically active organelle. Proteins within the membrane function as channels, permitting both passive and active transport of essential ions and other molecules. The carbohydrate moieties of glycoproteins and glycolipids that project from the external surface of the plasma membrane are important components of receptors that mediate cell activation, adhesion, response to hormones, and many other cell functions in response to environmental stimuli. Integration of the proteins within the lipid bilayer is the result of hydrophobic interactions between the lipids and nonpolar amino acids present in the outer folds of membrane proteins. These integral proteins are not bound rigidly in place but rather "float" in the lipid membrane; they may aggregate, or "cap," at specific sites on the cell, providing polarity in response

to ligand binding or to movement of actin-containing intracellular microfilaments. However, unlike earlier views of the plasma membrane as a "fluid mosaic,"[1] in which integral membrane proteins were thought to float and diffuse freely through a sea of homogeneous lipids, a more contemporary view of the plasma membrane is that proteins are much more heterogeneously distributed and can be found clustered within specialized microdomains, called *lipid rafts*. These lipid rafts are thought to form by the aggregation of glycosphingolipids and sphingomyelin in the Golgi apparatus (held together by transient and weak molecular interactions) and are then delivered to the plasma membrane as concentrated units.[2] The characterization and function of the cell membrane and of cell-surface receptors and ion channels will be discussed in greater detail.

THE CYTOPLASM

The cell cytoplasm is a highly organized structure rather than simply the medium supporting the large organelles. The cytoplasmic matrix contains a complex network of microtubules, microfilaments, and intermediate filaments, collectively referred to as the *cytoskeleton*. The cytoskeleton is essential in maintaining cell shape, membrane integrity, and essential spatial relationships, as well as in promoting cell motility and deformability in specific cell types. Microtubules are essential for cell and chromosomal division during mitosis; antimitotic alkaloids such as vinblastine are used therapeutically to arrest tumor cell proliferation. Kartagener syndrome, characterized by chronic respiratory infection and male infertility, is caused by a specific defect in the synthesis of dynein, leading to immotile cilia and flagella on epithelial and other specialized cells. Other major cytoplasmic structures with known functions include the ribosomes, endoplasmic reticulum (ER), and Golgi complex (apparatus). Ribosomes, composed of ribosomal RNA and proteins, are the sites where messenger RNA molecules derived from nuclear DNA gene templates are translated into proteins. Polyribosomes (polysomes), which are chains of ribosomes held together by a strand of messenger RNA, are observed during the assembly of amino acids into proteins—either free in the cytoplasm for intracellular proteins or bound to the ER for exported or membrane-bound proteins. The ER is a primarily membranous structure that occupies the cytoplasm and is the site of lipid and carbohydrate synthesis and the initial post-translational modifications of cellular proteins. The ER segregates newly synthesized proteins for export or intracellular utilization and is the site of limited proteolysis of the signal sequence of newly synthesized proteins, glycosylation of glycoproteins, and assembly of multichain proteins. Rough ER is defined by the presence of polyribosomes and is involved primarily in protein synthesis and export, whereas smooth ER is associated with a variety of specialized functional capabilities. For example, smooth ER in muscle cells and polymorphonuclear leukocytes is involved in the sequestration and mobilization of intracellular Ca^{2+} that regulate contraction and motility. Post-translational enzymatic modifications of proteins synthesized in the rough ER are completed, and membrane-packaged proteins processed, in the Golgi complex. The Golgi complex also appears to be the site where membranes are recycled and processed for distribution. It consists of several curved, disk-shaped, membranous cisternae arranged in a stack. A distinct polarity exists across the cisternal stack, consistent with the sequential processing of proteins on passage through this organelle.

Several other cytoplasmic structures are less prominent in size and morphology but are known to play key roles in specific diseases. Lysosomes are membrane-limited vesicles that contain a large variety of hydrolytic enzymes, the main function of which is intracytoplasmic digestion. Although present in all cells, lysosomes are most abundant in phagocytic cells, including polymorphonuclear leukocytes. Lysosomal enzymes are synthesized and segregated in the rough ER and subsequently transferred to the Golgi complex, where the enzymes are glycosylated and packaged as lysosomes. Phosphorylation of one or more mannose residues at the 6′ position by a phosphotransferase in the Golgi complex appears to distinguish lysosomal enzymes from secretory proteins. Deficiency or mutation in expression of lysosomal enzymes leads to specific diseases in the pediatric age-group, including Hurler (α-L-iduronidase) and Tay-Sachs (hexosaminidase A).

Peroxisomes are spherical membrane-bound organelles containing D- and L-amino oxidases, hydroxyacid oxidase, and catalase, which protect the cell from oxidative injury by metabolizing hydrogen peroxide to oxygen and water. Peroxisomes also contain enzymes that preferentially catalyze the β-oxidation of very long chain fatty acids (VL-CFA). Other functions of peroxisomes include catabolism of purines and polyamines, production of etherlike phospholipids, and gluconeogenesis. Peroxisomal defects are characterized primarily by abnormal accumulation of VL-CFA, with deleterious effects on membrane structure and function, as well as on brain myelination. Zellweger syndrome, which is the most severe condition in this group, is a neuronal migration defect presenting with hypotonia and neurologic abnormalities in the neonatal period, developmental delay, and pediatric mortality. It is associated with defects in the *PEX7* gene and with defective mitochondrial β-oxidation and formation of acetyl-CoA from short-chain fatty acids. Cholesterol biosynthesis from acetate is preserved, resulting in a relative deficiency in docosahexanoic acid (DHA), which plays an important role in the structure of cell membranes, particularly of neuronal tissues and retinal photoreceptor cells. This suggests that the DHA deficiency observed in patients with Zellweger syndrome contributes to the clinical symptomatology of this syndrome (demyelination, psychomotor retardation, and retinopathy). Therefore, supplementation of DHA might result in at least some clinical improvement in patients with Zellweger syndrome. Because peroxisomal β-oxidation is an essential step in the biosynthesis of DHA, studies of patients with a deficiency of a single β-oxidation enzyme could shed more light on the role of DHA in the pathology of peroxisomal fatty acid oxidation disorders.

THE NUCLEUS

The nucleus is the most prominent single structure in cells. It is membrane-bound but functions in continuity with surrounding structures. On the classical histologic level, the nucleus comprises the nuclear envelope, chromatin, nucleolus, and nuclear matrix. The nuclear membrane consists of two parallel membranes separated by a narrow space called the *perinuclear cisterna*. Nuclear pores, with an average diameter of 70 nm, consist of eight subunits and are spanned by a single-layer diaphragm of protein. Nuclear pores are permeable to mRNA and many cytoplasmic proteins. Most of the nucleus is occupied by chromatin, which is composed of coiled strands of DNA bound to histone proteins. The basic structural unit of chromatin is the nucleosome, consisting of approximately 150 base pairs of DNA wrapped 1.7 times around a protein octamer containing two copies each of histones H2A, H2B, H3, and H4. Each chromosome consists of a single huge nucleosomal fiber, constantly undergoing a dynamic process of folding and unfolding. The nucleolus is a spherical intranuclear structure that is particularly rich in ribosomal RNA and protein. Ribosomal RNA is transcribed from "nucleolar organizer DNA" in the nucleolus. Proteins, synthesized in the cytoplasm, become associated with ribosomal RNA in the nucleolus, and ribosomal subunits then migrate to the cytoplasm. The nuclear matrix constitutes the remaining nuclear contents, including the fibrillar nucleoskeleton and the fibrous lamina of the nuclear envelope.

Nuclear "anatomy" provides a window to the crucial issue of how the expression of specific genes is regulated. The complex and dynamic organization of DNA and protein in chromatin, as well as the permeability of the nuclear membrane to cytoplasmic proteins, suggests that proteins regulate gene activity. The best-studied level of gene regulation is that of the individual gene, involving cis-acting elements, such as promoters, enhancers, and silencers, and trans-acting factors, including DNA-binding transcription factors, cofactors, chromatin-remodeling systems, and RNA polymerases.[3] Transcription factors bind to DNA in a sequence-specific manner and mark a gene for activation through recruitment of coactivator or corepressor proteins. Coactivator proteins often directly modify histones in ways that allow greater access to the DNA. Examples of these are p300 and CREB-binding protein (CBP), histone acetyltransferases (HATs) that interact with a wide variety of transcription factors to support transcription of targeted genes.[4] A considerable number of post-translational modifications of core histones have been identified; histone acetylation and phosphorylation are rapidly reversible, consistent with a dynamic role in cell signaling. A further level of regulatory control of gene transcription occurs at the larger nuclear level. Chromatin is in a highly folded state that brings together loci that are far apart on the linear genome or on separate chromosomes. It is likely that the regulation of genome function can also occur in *trans*. For example, regulatory elements that control expression of one allele may functionally interact with the promoter of the allele on the homologous chromosome.[3] The activation of nuclear transcription factors by signal-transduction pathways in the cytoplasm and cell membrane will be discussed in the subsequent text.

MITOCHONDRIA

Mitochondria regulate cellular energy production, oxidative stress, and cell death and signaling pathways. The metabolism of fatty acids and sugars to molecular oxygen and carbon dioxide is completed in these organelles, which occupy a significant fraction of the cytosol of virtually all mammalian cells. Mitochondria are generally elongated cylinders with diameters of approximately 0.5 to 1.0 μm. They contain an outer membrane and an interior that is densely packed with an additional membrane and an array of enzymes. The extensive intraorganelle membrane system provides scaffolding, localizing the enzyme complexes of respiration and facilitating chemiosmosis, a process by which the energy released during oxidation of sugars is used to generate an electrochemical proton gradient. Ultimately, the energy stored in this gradient is converted back into chemical energy as the universal cellular energy currency of adenosine triphosphate (ATP).

Maternal Inheritance

In 1910, Mereschowsky hypothesized that mitochondria may have arisen from a symbiotic relation between precursor cells. Later, in the 1970s, Lynn Margolis postulated that mitochondria were, in fact, the remnants of once free-living species and that eukaryotes were derived from interacting communities of bacterial precursors. Newer studies present novel alternatives to this route, often based on the geologic compartmentalization of species in the deep crevices of the Precambrian oceans; however, a symbiotic origin for mitochondria and energy-producing organelles is well established. Considering this view of the origin of mitochondria, it is hardly surprising that mitochondria contain their own genetic material in the form of DNA. Mitochondria carry out their own DNA replication, transcription, and even limited protein synthesis. However, many constituents of mitochondria are synthesized by extramitochondrial cellular systems and are encoded in the nuclear genome, as a result of extensive shuttling of genomic material between the organelle and the cell nucleus during evolution. Genetic studies of several diseases associated with death during infancy have led to the observation that in some instances the inheritance of genetic diseases does not conform to Mendelian patterns, suggesting a rather direct inheritance through the maternal line. This is consistent with inheritance of traits through the mitochondrial DNA. In higher animals, ova contribute much more cytoplasm, and consequently far more mitochondria, than sperm. In fact, in some animals, including humans, the sperm contribute virtually no cytoplasm or mitochondria. Furthermore, the number of mitochondria contained in an egg is not fixed, and the number of mitochondria, as well as the genetic makeup of each mitochondrion, is subject to variation. The resultant patterns of mitochondrial, or "maternal," inheritance can be complex and can reflect mutations accumulated through many generations in some, but not all, of a cell's mitochondria. This phenomenon, termed *heteroplasia*, can result in some surprising patterns of inheritance. Therefore, mothers who are asymptomatic or minimally symptomatic can have offspring who are severely affected, or vice versa. Mitochondrial-inherited conditions may vary from benign to acute, depending on the assortment of mitochondria received by the offspring, even between twins who are identical with regard to inheritance of nuclear DNA. In humans, the mitochondrial genome has been sequenced, and, surprisingly, the genetic material appears to be almost completely used to encode RNA and proteins. Fewer tRNA sequences are used in mitochondrial protein synthesis, and the codon–anticodon pairing is somewhat relaxed, allowing for broader but somewhat less accurate protein synthesis. Human mitochondrial transcripts do not contain introns, but they are extensively processed and, similar to bacteria, distinct proteins may arise through differential cleavage of the same transcript.

Within the mitochondria, the outer membrane serves not only to separate the organelle from the intracellular confines but also to form the outer barrier of the intermembrane space. Whereas proteins within the outer membrane form numerous aqueous and solute channels, rendering it permeable to most agents with a mass less than 10,000 Da, the inner membrane is highly impermeable. The specific and limited protein concentrations and the high concentration of cardiolipin within the inner membrane are largely responsible for the unique impermeability of this structure. The inner membrane is convoluted and highly folded; the infoldings of this structure are referred to as *cristae*. The cristae form a contiguous matrix that is populated by protein complexes that synthesize ATP, regulate the transport of ions and metabolites, and catalyze the oxidation reactions of the respiratory chain (see Fig. 1.1).

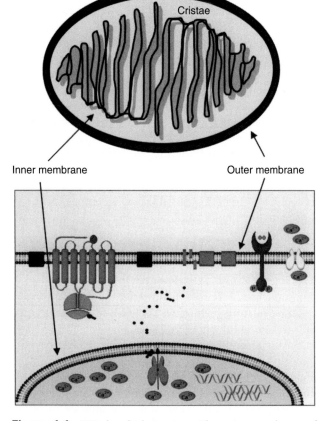

Figure 1.1 Mitochondrial structure. The outer membrane of mitochondria contains numerous aqueous and solute channels. The impermeable inner membrane, which is folded into cristae, tightly regulates the passage of Ca^{2+} and other ions, and contains the mitochondrial DNA. Protein complexes that synthesize adenosine triphosphate (ATP) and catalyze the oxidation reactions of the respiratory chain are aligned at the inner membrane.

Mitochondria in Energy Metabolism

A brief overview of the role of mitochondria in energy metabolism begins with the generation of stored energy in the form of acetyl-CoA. This energetic intermediate is formed in the matrix space of mammalian mitochondria, where the pyruvate produced during glycolysis and the oxidized fatty acids are reduced to acetyl-CoA by enzyme complexes localized in the matrix.

Formation of Acetyl-CoA

Pyruvate is actively transported into mitochondria, where pyruvate dehydrogenases convert it into acetyl-CoA. Alternatively, this energetic intermediate can be produced through the oxidation of fatty acids that have been transported into the outer and inner mitochondrial membranes. In fatty acid oxidations, each completed cycle of reactions consumes one molecule of ATP to reduce the long carbon chains by two carbons, generating one molecule each of adenosine monophosphate (AMP), acetyl-CoA, nicotinamide adenine dinucleotide (reduced form) (NADH), and flavin adenine dinucleotide ($FADH_2$). The resulting acetyl-CoA then enters the citric acid cycle (Krebs cycle), in which its oxidation produces NADH and $FADH_2$ for the respiratory chain.

The Citric Acid Cycle

During the citric acid cycle, closely linked enzymatic reactions catalyzed by matrix-bound proteins convert the carbons of acetyl-CoA into carbon dioxide, generating high-energy electrons that are ultimately used in the production of three additional molecules of NADH and one of $FADH_2$. The reaction cycle also produces another molecule of ATP through a direct phosphorylation, similar to ATP generation during glycolysis. These reactions begin with the formation of citric acid through the condensation of one molecule of acetyl-CoA with one molecule of oxaloacetate. Then, in seven subsequent reactions, two carbon atoms are oxidized to carbon dioxide and oxaloacetate is regenerated.

Bioenergetics

In a complex process, the high-energy electrons generated during these oxidation reactions are efficiently harnessed and stored as ATP. The biochemistry of this process was first established by Peter Mitchell in his "chemiosmotic hypothesis." This theory, now the cornerstone of bioenergetics, is based on the coupling of a stepwise reduction in the energy of excited electrons to the generation of a proton gradient across the inner mitochondrial membrane. The release of this gradient is used to drive the synthesis of ATP from adenosine diphosphate (ADP) by a membrane-bound ATP synthetase. The concept of synthesis by energetically coupled reactions rather than direct catalysis was so revolutionary that Mitchell was not only initially discredited but also stripped of his position in the Zoology Department of Edinburgh University. After more than 17 years of controversy, Mitchell was exonerated and in 1978 was awarded the Nobel Prize in chemistry for this discovery.

In Mitchell's theory, the energy released by the passage of electrons along a chain of enzyme complexes is effectively stored as a proton gradient across the inner mitochondrial membrane. The pH significantly drops within the matrix space as a voltage gradient is generated by the displacement of protons. The combination of these two forces subsequently constitutes an electrochemical proton gradient. This protomotive force can be measured and is approximately 220 mV in respiring mitochondria. The pH gradient generated during respiration is approximately -1. The proteins of the ATP synthetase complex catalyze the formation of ATP from ADP as the protons flow back down the gradient. However, this is not the only process powered by Mitchell's electromotive force. ADP and other charged molecules are actively transported across the impervious inner membrane to supply the substrates required for ATP generation. Often, this process is coupled to the cotransport of another charged species down, rather than up, its energy gradient, thereby rendering transport less costly in terms of energy and also facilitating additional physiologic processes. The protomotive force also serves to facilitate the pumping of calcium out of the cytosol. Subsequent release of sequestered calcium back into the cytosol triggers signaling pathways providing energy for responses to an array of stimuli. The speed and efficiency of oxidative phosphorylation keeps the cytosolic ATP pool highly charged. Many biosynthetic enzymes use ATP hydrolysis to provide energy for catalysis, thereby producing a constant requirement for respiration and further driving energetic processes. However, when mitochondrial activity is halted, cellular ATP stores are quickly depleted and viability is compromised.

There are three protein complexes in the respiratory chain that efficiently convert the electrons from NADH into a proton gradient. Complex 1, the NADH dehydrogenase complex, acts as the initial electron acceptor, receiving electrons from NADH and passing them to ubiquinone. This small lipid carrier molecule travels about ten times more quickly than the larger enzyme complexes within the lipid bilayer. It is speculated that random collisions between carrier molecules and protein complexes within the mitochondrial membranes account for the rate of electron transfer. Complex 2 (bc complex), the next receptor, contains eight distinct polypeptide chains including two cytochromes. This complex transfers electrons from ubiquinone to cytochrome c. Finally, cytochrome c passes the significantly less excited electron to the cytochrome oxidase complex, complex 3. The seven polypeptide chains of cytochrome oxidase span the inner membrane. In another complex series of reactions, cytochrome c accepts four electrons in single-electron transfer events, which ultimately reduce molecular oxygen into two molecules of water. The affinity of each protein complex of the respiratory chain for

electrons defines its redox potential. This electron pressure gradient can be measured and it drops from approximately -300 to -700 mV, releasing approximately 25 kcal of free energy along the chain. The energy conversion mechanism requires that each respiratory complex translocate hydrogen ions in the same direction across the inner mitochondrial membrane. This vectorial organization of the protein complexes is a key feature of the mitochondrial driving of ATP synthesis.

Regulation of Mitochondrial Respiration

Precise regulation of respiration is vital to numerous cellular processes; to integrate these needs, mammalian cells have developed an elaborate system of feedback controls. Although the flow of electrons through the respiratory chain strictly regulates ATP formation, the rates of NADH formation and degradation, availability of other cellular reducing equivalents, glucose and glycogen stores, and oxygen tension also control mitochondrial respiration. Indeed, poorly regulated respiration resulting in energy depletion often precedes cell death. In a chemically induced model of Parkinson disease, the reactive mediator formed from MPTP, MPP1, inhibits complex 1, poisoning the mitochondrial electron transport chain, depleting cellular ATP, and enhancing the formation of superoxide. Interaction of superoxide with nitric oxide results in the formation of DNA-damaging peroxynitrite, which, in turn, leads to DNA damage, which activates production of poly(ADP-ribose). Activation of the enzyme that forms this cellular mediator, poly(ADP-ribose) polymerase, then depletes nicotinamide adenine dinucleotide (NAD) by poly-ADP-ribosylation of nuclear proteins, and ATP stores are even further depleted in an effort to resynthesize NAD, leading to cell death by energy depletion.

Mitochondria respond to agents that uncouple ATP production from electron transport by increasing both electron transport and oxygen uptake. When agents such as the toxin dinitrophenol collapse the electron gradient generated during respiration, the process runs at the maximal rate that the availability of substrates will allow. In contrast, when an abnormally large electron gradient is formed across the inner membrane, electron flow can actually reverse. Clearly, the sensitivity of the electron transport chain to its own activity is the primary regulator of mitochondrial respiration. Interestingly, innate uncoupling mechanisms exist in brown fat. In response to specific stimuli, these specialized fat cells can dissipate energy in the form of heat. This mechanism serves such diverse processes in mammals as permitting seals to dive in the ice-cold polar oceans, reviving hibernating bears, and protecting the organs in newborns.[5]

Although it has long been recognized that oxygen deprivation results in inhibition of respiration, the mechanisms by which oxygen availability regulates oxidative phosphorylation and the resulting cellular damage is poorly understood. Recent studies have revealed that oxygen availability controls respiratory activity through the actions of another gaseous mediator, nitric oxide, a key regulator of the activity of the terminal mitochondrial complex. In these studies, it was noted that the affinity of cytochrome oxidase for nitric oxide varies with oxygen tension. When oxygen is freely available, the enzyme's affinity for nitric oxide is low and the gas has little apparent effect on mitochondrial respiration. However, when oxygen levels are low, nitric oxide binds and reduces the activity of cytochrome oxidase. This mechanism appears to be the primary mechanism by which the rate of energy generation by the electron transport chain is matched to the availability of oxygen. Indeed, when nitric oxide production is inhibited, electron transport continues even under hypoxic conditions. In these circumstances, the electrons flowing through the chain are transferred to inappropriate acceptors, resulting in reactive species and cellular damage. In experimental animals, restoring intracellular nitric oxide limits the resultant pathology. These and similar findings have significant implications for the potential development of new therapies to limit hypoxic injury.

Mitochondrial Functions in Immunity and Cellular Defense

Phylogenetic analysis of the heat shock family of proteins has led to the identification of a mitochondrial heat shock protein, Hsp60. This protein is present in the mitochondrial matrix in eukaryotes and participates in the folding processes of newly imported proteins, preventing aggregation of stress-denatured polypeptides in challenged mitochondria. In mitochondria, newly imported proteins are found complexed with Hsp60 when ATP levels are low. Hsp60-complexed proteins are loosely folded and highly protease-sensitive. When ATP levels return to normal, the accumulated unfolded protein is released from Hsp60 in a protease-resistant, fully folded conformation. In this manner, mitochondrial Hsp60 facilitates protein folding and assembly in an ATP-dependent manner by interacting directly with the unfolded protein.

In mycobacterial infections, blood-borne reactivity to heat shock proteins is found. During infection, Hsp60 released from the mitochondria of infected cells serves to stimulate immune cells. In this manner, Hsp60 has been found to act as an immunodominant target of the antibody and T-cell response in both mice and humans. Hsp60-specific antibodies also have been detected in patients with tuberculosis and leprosy, indicating that mitochondrial release of the protein modulates immune responses to these infections. Immune responses to Hsp60 are also frequently found in other microbial infections. For example, in a murine model of yersiniosis, direct involvement of Hsp60-specific T cells in the antipathogenic immune response

has been demonstrated. Similarly, in infants, levels of antibodies against Hsp60 have been found to increase after vaccination with a trivalent vaccine against tetanus, diphtheria, and pertussis. These findings further suggest that priming of the immune system to mitochondrial Hsp60 is a common phenomenon, occurring at an early stage of life.

Pediatric Disorders of Mitochondrial Metabolism

Disorders of mitochondrial metabolism are of particular interest to critical care physicians because defects in energy generation and metabolism often lead to multiple organ system dysfunction. Concurrent with increasing understanding of the complex and multiple roles of mitochondria in cells, several diseases that present in childhood are now known to be related to specific defects in mitochondrial metabolism. For example, Alpers syndrome (diffuse degeneration of cerebral gray matter with hepatic cirrhosis) is usually characterized by a clinical triad of psychomotor retardation, intractable epilepsy, and liver failure in infants and young children. Definitive diagnosis is shown by postmortem examination of the brain and liver. Cases with specific disturbances in pyruvate metabolism and NADH oxidation have been described. For example, Naviaux et al.[6] found global reduction in the respiratory chain complex 1, 2/3, and 4 activity and deficiency of mitochondrial DNA polymerase γ activity in a patient with mtDNA depletion and Alpers syndrome.

Amyotrophic Lateral Sclerosis

Amyotrophic lateral sclerosis (ALS, Lou Gehrig disease) is thought to result from missense mutations in the gene for SOD1, an enzyme normally localized in the intermembrane space of mitochondria. Matsumoto and Fridovich[7] proposed that mutant forms of SOD1 bind and inactivate heat shock proteins, which normally protect cells from apoptosis. Functional deficiency in the activity of heat shock proteins causes mitochondrial swelling and vacuolization, leading to the gradual death of motor neurons.

Childhood Parkinson Disease

Childhood Parkinson disease (autosomal recessive juvenile parkinsonism) is caused by a mutation in the *PARK2* gene. This gene encodes the protein parkin, which is a ubiquitin–protein ligase involved in protein degradation. In juvenile parkinsonism, mutation in the *PARK2* gene is linked to the death of dopaminergic neurons. Yao et al.[8] showed both *in vitro* and *in vivo* that nitrosative stress leads to S-nitrosylation of wild-type parkin and, initially, to a dramatic increase followed by a decrease in the E3 ligase–ubiquitin–proteasome degradative pathway. The initial increase in the E3 ubiquitin ligase activity of parkin leads to autoubiquitination of parkin and subsequent inhibition of its activity, which would impair ubiquitination and clearance of parkin substrates. Yao et al.

concluded that these findings may provide a molecular link between the free radical toxicity and protein accumulation in sporadic Parkinson disease.[8]

Peripheral Myelin Protein–22 Disorders (Charcot-Marie-Tooth Disease)

Peripheral myelin protein (PMP) duplication xenografts show proximal axonal enlargement with an increase in neurofilament and mitochondria density, suggesting an impairment of axonal transport. Distally, there is a decrease in myelin thickness with evidence of axonal loss, axonal degeneration and regeneration, and onion bulb formation. Sahenk et al.[9] concluded that PMP-22 mutations in Schwann cells cause perturbations in the normal axonal cytoskeletal organization that underlie the pathogenesis of these hereditary disorders.

Adrenoleukodystrophy

The *ABCD1* gene expresses a half-transporter, which is located in the peroxisome. When mutated, ABCD1 results in adrenoleukodystrophy with an elevation in very long chain fatty acids. ABCD1 is one of four related peroxisomal transporters that are found in the human genome; the others include ABCD2 (601081), ABCD3 (170995), and ABCD4 (603214). These genes are highly conserved in evolution, and two homologous genes, *PXA1* and *PXA2*, are present in the yeast genome. The *PXA2* gene has been demonstrated to transport long-chain fatty acids.[10] A defective *PXA1* gene in the plant *Arabidopsis thaliana* results in defective import of fatty acids into peroxisomes. Ultimately, this results in profound deficiency in mitochondrial and peroxisomal β-oxidation and accumulation of long-chain fatty acids.

Leigh Syndrome

Leigh syndrome (deficiency of cytochrome c oxidase) is characterized by an early onset progressive neurodegenerative disorder with a characteristic neuropathology consisting of focal, bilateral lesions in one or more areas of the central nervous system (CNS), including the brain stem, thalamus, basal ganglia, cerebellum, and spinal cord. The lesions are characterized by demyelination, gliosis, necrosis, spongiosis, or capillary proliferation. Clinical symptoms depend on the areas of the CNS that are involved. The most common underlying cause is a defect in oxidative phosphorylation.

Other Mitochondrial Disorders

Olivopontocerebellar atrophy/autosomal dominant cerebellar ataxia (spinocerebellar ataxia) manifests as neurotoxicity, resulting in progressive cerebellar ataxia with pigmentary macular degeneration. It is mediated by accumulation of mutant ataxin-7, a mitochondrial carrier protein. Alterations in solute transport mediated by ataxin-7 result in programmed cell death initiated by mitochondria-derived apoptosis-inducing factor (AIF). Another disorder,

systemic carnitine deficiency, causes generalized mitochondrial abnormality in the muscle system, especially in the heart. ATP-P_i exchange activity of the heart mitochondria is greatly decreased. Other mitochondrial myopathies are associated with defects in mitochondrial DNA, leading to (i) defects in substrate utilization, as in the deficiency of carnitine and carnitine palmitoyltransferase, and defects in various components of the pyruvate dehydrogenase complex; (ii) defects in the coupling of mitochondrial respiration to phosphorylation, as in Luft disease, and mitochondrial ATPase deficiency; and (iii) deficiencies in components of mitochondrial respiratory chain, such as nonheme iron protein, cytochrome oxidase, cytochrome b deficiency, or NADH-CoQ reductase. Friedrich ataxia presents as excessive mitochondrial iron accumulation and oxidative damage as a result of loss of the iron metabolism regulatory protein YFH1. Cytochrome c oxidase deficiency is clinically heterogeneous, ranging from isolated myopathy to severe multisystem disease, with onset from infancy to adulthood.

CELL SIGNALING

The evolution of multicellular organisms has been highly dependent on the ability of cells to communicate with each other and with the environment. Cell signaling plays an important role in cellular growth, survival, and apoptosis. For example, cell function and growth require the induction of protein expression in response to stimuli that originate outside the cell. To accomplish this, external signals are passed through specific intracellular pathways to regulate the expression of specific genes. Although the field of biochemistry has traditionally been focused on enzymology and structural proteins, it is now recognized that many cellular proteins function primarily to modulate such signals. These range from cell-surface receptors that mediate cell-to-cell signals to a wide array of second messenger and transducer proteins that convert activated receptors into intracellular biochemical/electrical signals. Studies of signaling pathways have traditionally focused on delineating immediate upstream and downstream interactions and then organizing these interactions into linear cascades that relay and regulate information from cell-surface receptors to cellular effectors such as metabolic enzymes, channels, or transcription factors.[11] In recent years, it has become apparent that these signals are not linear pathways emanating from individual receptors but, rather, a network of interconnected signaling pathways that integrates signals from a variety of extracellular and intracellular sources.[12] For a cell to convert an extracellular signal into a specific cellular response (signal-transduction pathway), several key elements are needed:[13] a ligand, a specific receptor binding the ligand, the propagation of the signal within the cell, and, finally, a cellular response by producing specific proteins. If any of these key elements becomes abnormal or nonfunctional, the cellular process is altered, potentially causing disease. Therefore, understanding specific pathways is essential in understanding the pathogenesis of diseases. In this review, we will illustrate different signaling pathways with special emphasis on those related to cardiac muscle function in humans.

Signaling Molecules (Ligands)

Extracellular signaling can be classified into three patterns on the basis of how close the target cell is to the signal releasing cell: (a) endocrine signaling, by which the signaling molecules (hormones) are carried by the blood stream to act on target cells distant from their site of synthesis; (b) paracrine signaling, in which the target cell is located close to the signal-releasing cell; and, finally, (c) autocrine signaling, by which cells respond to substances that they themselves release. Signaling molecules can act in two or even three types of cell-to-cell signaling. For example, epinephrine can function both as a neurotransmitter (paracrine signaling) and as a systemic hormone (endocrine signaling).[14-18]

There are several chemical classes of signaling molecules:

- *Small hydrophilic molecules* derived from amino acids, such as neurotransmitters, epinephrine, acetylcholine, dopamine, serine, and histamine.
- *Small hydrophobic molecules* derived from cholesterol, such as steroid hormones, estrogens, progestins, and thyroid hormone.
- *Gases* such as nitric oxide and photons (light).
- *Peptides and proteins*, which constitute one of the major types of ligands in human cell signaling and include classical proteins such as insulin, glucagon, and growth hormone.
- Other types of peptides and proteins ligands include the following:
  - Mitogens or growth factors such as epidural growth factor, platelet-derived growth factor (PDGF), and neuron GF.
  - Neuropeptides such as endorphins, enkephalins, oxytocin, and vasopressin.
  - Immune system peptides such as cytokines, chemokines, and immunoglobulins.
  - Adhesion molecules such as integrins and selectins.

Receptors

The cellular responses to a particular extracellular signaling molecule (ligand) depend on its binding to a specific receptor protein located on the surface of a target cell or in its nucleus or cytosol. Binding of a ligand to its receptor causes conformational changes in the receptor that initiate a sequence of reactions leading to specific cellular responses. The response of a cell to a specific molecule depends on the type of receptors it possesses and on the intracellular reactions initiated by the binding of the signaling molecule to that receptor. These receptors have both binding specificity (defines the ligands that bind and activate the receptor) and effector specificity (defines the effector enzymes that will be activated). Different receptor types and subtypes may have similar binding specificity but different effector specificity, allowing a single molecule to have diverse effects. Different cell types may have different sets of receptors for the same ligand, each of which induces a different response. Conversely, the same receptor may occur on various cell types, and binding of the same ligand may trigger a different response in each type of cell.[14-18] There are two main types of receptors—intracellular receptors and cell-surface receptors.

Intracellular Receptors

Intracellular receptors bind hydrophobic or small lipophilic molecules that diffuse across the plasma membrane and interact with receptors in the cytosol or nucleus. The resulting ligand–receptor complexes bind to transcription-control regions in the DNA, thereby affecting expression of specific genes. Lipophilic molecules that bind to intracellular receptors include steroids (cortisol, progesterone, estradiol, and testosterone), thyroxine, and retinoic acid.

Hydrophobic molecules such as nitric oxide can also diffuse freely across cell membranes and have been shown to play important roles in cell signaling. Because nitric oxide is consumed rapidly, it acts in a paracrine or even autocrine fashion, affecting only cells near its point of synthesis.[19] The signaling functions of nitric oxide begin with its binding to protein receptors in the cell. This binding triggers an allosteric change in the protein, which, in turn, triggers the formation of a "second messenger" within the cell. The most common protein target for nitric oxide seems to be guanylyl cyclase, the enzyme that generates the second messenger cyclic GMP (cGMP), which regulates several enzymes and ion channels.[20,21] In smooth muscles, an important action of cGMP is to induce muscle relaxation. As the prototypical endothelium-derived relaxing factor, nitric oxide is a primary determinant of blood vessel tone and thrombogenicity.[22] The discovery of the modulation of cardiac contractility with nitric oxide has fueled considerable interest and hope in the possibility of reversing cardiac dysfunction with nitric oxide synthase (NOS) inhibitors.[12] Nitric oxide is produced from virtually all cell types composing the myocardium and regulates cardiac function through both vascular-dependent and vascular-independent effects.[23-26] The former include regulation of coronary vessel tone, thrombogenicity, and proliferative and inflammatory properties, as well as cellular cross-talk, supporting angiogenesis. The latter comprise the direct effects of nitric oxide on several aspects of cardiomyocyte contractility, from the fine regulation of excitation–contraction (EC) coupling to modulation of (presynaptic and postsynaptic) autonomic signaling and mitochondrial respiration.[27–29] Loss of tight molecular regulation of the nitric oxide synthesis, such as with excessive nitric oxide delivery from inflammatory cells (or cytokine-stimulated cardiomyocytes), may result in profound cellular disturbances leading to cardiovascular failure.[30] Future therapeutic manipulations of cardiac nitric oxide synthesis will necessarily draw on additional characterization of the cellular and molecular determinants for the net effect of this molecule on cardiac and vascular biology.[22]

Cell-Surface Receptors

Receptors on the cell surface generally bind water-soluble signaling molecules that cannot diffuse across the plasma membrane. However, some lipid-soluble molecules, such as eicosanoids, also bind to cell-surface receptors.

The major classes of cell-surface receptors are as follows:

1. G protein–coupled receptors.
2. Ion channel receptors.
3. Tyrosine-kinase receptors.

Signaling by G Protein–Coupled Receptors

G protein–coupled receptors (GPCRs) represent the most diverse group of proteins involved in transmembrane signaling pathways.[31] In vertebrates, this family contains 1,000 to 2,000 members (>1% of the genome) including >1,000 coding for odorant and pheromone receptors. GPCRs have transmembrane domains with an external N terminus and internal C terminus. Intracellular loops mediate binding to G proteins. GPCRs are stimulated by various ligands, including neuromediators, glycoproteinic hormones, peptides, biogenic amines, nucleotides, lipids, calcium ions, and sensory substances (taste, odor, and light). G proteins contain three subunits: α, β, and γ (see Fig. 1.2). G protein functions as a switch that is on or off, depending on which of two guanine nucleotides, GDP or GTP, is attached. When GDP is bound, the G protein is inactive; when GTP is bound, the G protein is active. When a hormone or other ligand binds to the associated GPCRs, conformational changes takes place in the receptor that will trigger an allosteric change in $G\alpha$, causing GDP to dissociate and be replaced by GTP. GTP activates $G\alpha$, causing it to dissociate from $\beta\gamma$ subunits (which remain linked as a dimer).[13,14,19] The separated α or $\beta\gamma$ subunits bind to specific effector membrane proteins (e.g., adenylyl cyclase, phospholipases C and A2, cGMP phosphodiesterase and some ionic channels). Activation of effector proteins induces variations in the intracellular second messenger, which, in turn, initiate a series of intracellular events triggering the cell to produce the appropriate gene products in response to the initial signal at the cell surface.

Multiple mechanisms exist to control the signaling and density of GPCRs. On agonist binding and receptor activation, a series of reactions contribute to the desensitization of

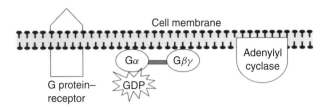

A Inactive G protein

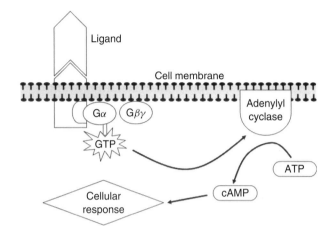

B Activated G protein

Figure 1.2 Signaling by G protein–coupled receptors. Ligand binding induces a conformational change in the G protein–receptor, causing dissociation of GDP from the $G\alpha$ subunit and phosphorylation to GTP. GTP causes dissociation of the $G\alpha$, from the $\beta\gamma$ subunit. These protein subunits can bind to and activate effector proteins, including adenylyl cyclase. Activation of effector proteins activates second messengers, inducing cellular responses.

GPCRs.[32] For example, the GPCRs may be phosphorylated by protein kinases and consequently uncoupled from G proteins. The molecular events underlying desensitization generally start with agonist-induced receptor phosphorylation by a G protein–coupled receptor kinase (GRK).[33] The phosphorylated GPCR possesses an increased affinity for a cytosolic protein of the arrestin family. This complex (phosphorylated receptor/arrestin) prevents the further coupling of that receptor to its G protein, reducing the capacity of second-messenger synthesis.

Seven mammalian genes encoding GRKs (1 to 7) have been cloned to date.[34–36] On the basis of sequence and functional similarities, the GRK family has been divided into three subfamilies:[37] (a) the rhodopsin kinase subfamily (GRK1 and 7), (b) the β-adrenergic receptor kinase subfamily (GRK2 and 3), and (c) the GRK4 subfamily (GRK4, 5 and 6). GRKs have a key role in GPCR desensitization; because these receptors are involved in so many vital functions, it seems likely that disorders affecting GRK-mediated regulation of GPCR would contribute to different diseases.

In human chronic heart failure, the combined effects of enhanced expression of GRK2 and the resulting reduced activity of β_1-receptors have been implicated in the diminished response to β-receptor agonists and the loss of cardiac contractility.[38–40] β_1-Receptor number and levels were decreased by approximately 50% in failing hearts, whereas these levels were unaltered for β_2-receptors. By contrast, GRK2 levels and enzymatic activity were increased two- or threefold in failing human hearts compared with nonfailing controls.[39] It was hypothesized that increased GRK2 activity may reduce the effectiveness of the β-adrenergic receptors in patients with heart diseases and that GRK2 inhibition may offer a novel therapeutic target in congestive heart failure.[39,41]

Signaling by Ion Channel Receptors

Ion channels are membrane proteins that allow ions to pass through. On the basis of their selectivity to specific ions, they can be divided into calcium channel, potassium channel, sodium channel, and so on. The calcium channel is more permeable to calcium ions than other types of ions, the potassium channel selects potassium ions over other ions, and so on. Ion channels may also be classified according to their gating mechanisms. In a voltage-gated ion channel, the gate opening depends on the membrane voltage, whereas in a ligand-gated ion channel, the opening depends on the binding of small molecules (ligands). Ligand binding changes the conformation of the receptor so that specific ions flow through it; the resultant ion movements alter the electric potential across the cell membrane.[4] The acetylcholine receptor at the nerve–muscle junction is an example. Ion channels are essential to a wide range of physiologic functions, including neuronal signaling, muscle contraction, cardiac pacemaking, hormone secretion, and cell proliferation.[42] Several human neurologic disorders such as epilepsy, migraine headache, deafness, episodic ataxia, periodic paralysis, malignant hyperthermia, and generalized myotonia can be caused by mutations in genes for ion channels.[43] Many of the so-called channel diseases are episodic disorders the principal symptoms of which occur intermittently in individuals who otherwise may be healthy and active.

To meet changing hemodynamic demands placed on the heart, EC coupling is constantly modulated by multiple signaling pathways.[44] The most important regulator of cardiac function on a beat-to-beat basis is the autonomic nervous system. Release of catecholamines from the autonomic nervous system activates adrenoceptors. Cardiac β-adrenergic receptors are the primary targets for sympathetic neurotransmitters (e.g., norepinephrine) and adrenal hormones (e.g., epinephrine). Stimulation of the β-adrenergic receptors signaling pathway increases the chronotropic (heart rate), inotropic (strength of contraction during systole), and lusitropic (rate and extent of relaxation during diastole) states of the heart. At the cellular level, stimulation of β-adrenergic receptors modulates the cAMP-dependent protein kinase A (PKA) signaling pathway, altering the

phosphorylation of a number of target proteins. These include sarcolemmal and transverse tubule L-type calcium (Ca^{2+}) channels, which conduct the trigger Ca^{2+} currents that initiate EC coupling, the sarcoplasmic reticulum (SR) ryanodine receptor (RyR)–sensitive Ca^{2+}-release channels, and sarcolemmal potassium (K^+) channels responsible for the slowly activating outward current.[45–49]

Cardiac K^+ channels determine the resting membrane potential, the heart rate, the shape and duration of the action potential and are important targets for the actions of neurotransmitters, hormones, drugs, and toxins known to modulate cardiac function.[50–52] K^+-channel blockers prolong the cardiac action potential duration and refractoriness without slowing impulse conduction, that is, they exhibit Class III antiarrhythmic actions, being effective in preventing/suppressing re-entrant arrhythmias. Unfortunately, drugs that delay the repolarization prolong the QT interval of the electrocardiogram and represent a major cause of acquired long QT syndrome (LQTS).[53–55] In mammalian cardiac cells, K^+ channels can be categorized as voltage-gated and ligand-gated channels.[51–53] The configuration and duration of the cardiac action potentials vary considerably among species and different cardiac regions (atria vs. ventricle), and specific areas within those regions (epicardium vs. endocardium). This heterogeneity mainly reflects differences in the type and/or expression patterns of the K^+ channels that participate in the genesis of the cardiac action potential. Moreover, the expression and properties of K^+ channels are not static but are influenced by heart rate, neurohumoral state, pharmacologic agents, cardiovascular diseases (cardiac hypertrophy and failure, myocardial infarction), and arrhythmias (atrial fibrillation [AF]).[56–58]

Signaling by Tyrosine-Kinase Receptors

Tyrosine phosphorylation is one of the key covalent modifications that occur in multicellular organisms during cellular signaling. The enzymes that carry out this modification are the protein tyrosine kinases (PTKs), which catalyze the transfer of phosphate groups from ATP to the amino acid tyrosine on a substrate protein.[13,14,59] Tyrosine-kinase receptors are membrane receptors that attach phosphates to protein tyrosines. There are two main classes of PTKs: receptor PTKs and cellular, or nonreceptor, PTKs. These enzymes are involved in cellular signaling pathways and regulate key cell functions such as proliferation, differentiation, antiapoptotic signaling, and neurite outgrowth.[60]

The receptor tyrosine kinases (RTKs) are transmembrane proteins that span the plasma membrane and are a major type of cell-surface receptors (see Fig. 1.3). RTKs have an extracellular domain containing a ligand-binding site, a single hydrophobic transmembrane α helix, and a cytosolic domain that includes a region with PTK activity.[61] In the absence of specific signal molecules, tyrosine-kinase receptors exist as single polypeptides in the plasma membrane. Activation of the kinase is achieved by ligand binding to the extracellular domain, which induces

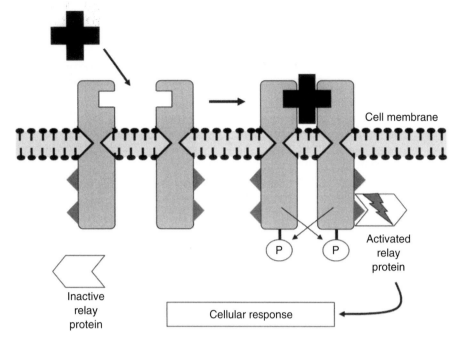

Figure 1.3 Activation of receptor tyrosine kinases (RTK). Ligand binding causes two RTK polypeptide subunits to aggregate, forming a dimer. This activates each subunit of the dimeric receptor, leading to phosphorylation of tyrosine residues near the catalytic site in the other subunit. The resulting phosphotyrosine residues serve as docking sites for proteins involved in RTK-mediated signal transduction.

Cell membrane

Inactive
relay
protein

P   P

Activated
relay
protein

Cellular response

dimerization of the receptors and activation of one or more cytosolic PTKs.

Binding of a ligand to two adjacent tyrosine-kinase receptors causes receptor activation in two steps. First, the ligand binding causes two receptor polypeptides to aggregate, forming a dimer, and second, this aggregation activates the tyrosine-kinase parts of both polypeptides, each of which then adds phosphates to the tyrosines on the tail of the other RTK polypeptide, a process termed *autophosphorylation*. The resulting phosphotyrosines serve as docking sites for other proteins involved in RTK-mediated signal transduction. Each such protein (called *relay proteins*) binds to a specific phosphorylated tyrosine, undergoing a structural change that activates the relay protein (the protein may or may not be phosphorylated by the tyrosine kinase). Signaling proteins that bind to the intracellular domain of receptor tyrosine kinases in a phosphotyrosine-dependent manner include RasGAP, PI3-kinase, phospholipase C (PLC), phosphotyrosine phosphatase SHP and adaptor proteins such as Shc, Grb2, and Crk. Many of these proteins are also tyrosine kinases (the human genome encodes 90 different tyrosine kinases). In this way, a cascade of expanding phosphorylations occurs within the cytosol. Some of these cytosolic tyrosine kinases act directly on gene transcription by entering the nucleus and transferring their phosphate to transcription factors, thereby activating them. Others act indirectly through the production of second messengers. One tyrosine-kinase receptor dimer may activate ten or more different intracellular proteins simultaneously, triggering many different transduction pathways and cellular responses. The ability of a single ligand-binding event to trigger so many pathways is a key difference between these receptors and G protein–linked receptors. Some

ligands that trigger RTKs include insulin; PDGF; vascular endothelial growth factor (VEGF); epidermal growth factor (EGF); fibroblast growth factor (FGF), a mutation in its receptor causes achondroplasia—the most common type of dwarfism; and macrophage–colony-stimulating factor (M-CSF).[14]

In contrast to receptor PTKs, cellular PTKs are located in the cytoplasm and nucleus, or are anchored to the inner leaflet of the plasma membrane. They are grouped into eight families: SRC, JAK, ABL, FAK, FPS, CSK, SYK, and BTK. Each family consists of several members. With the exception of homologous kinase domains (Src Homology 1, or SH1 domains) and some protein–protein interaction domains (SH2 and SH3 domains) they have little in common, structurally. Of those cellular PTKs whose functions are known, many, such as SRC, are involved in cell growth. In contrast, FPS PTKs are involved in differentiation, ABL PTKs are involved in growth inhibition, and FAK activity is associated with cell adhesion. Some members of the cytokine receptor pathway interact with JAKs, which phosphorylate the transcription factors, STATs. Still other PTKs activate pathways whose components and functions remain to be determined.[62–67]

RTK signaling pathways have a wide spectrum of functions including regulation of cell proliferation and differentiation, promotion of cell survival, and modulation of cellular metabolism. Because PTKs are critical components of cellular signaling pathways, their catalytic activity is strictly regulated. Given the importance of PTKs in signaling pathways that lead to cell proliferation, it is not surprising that numerous RTKs have been implicated in the onset/progression of different diseases. Unregulated activation of these enzymes, through mechanisms such as point mutations or overexpression, can lead to inappropriate expression of receptors that trigger cell division leading to various forms of cancer, as well as benign proliferative conditions.[60] Indeed, more than 70% of the known oncogenes and proto-oncogenes involved in cancer code for PTKs.[68,69] Some RTKs have been identified in studies on human cancers associated with mutant forms of growth-factor receptors, which send a proliferative signal to cells even in the absence of growth factor. One such mutant receptor, encoded at the *neu* locus, contributes to the uncontrolled proliferation of certain human breast cancers. The importance of PTKs in health and disease is further underscored by the existence of aberrations in PTK signaling occurring in inflammatory diseases, diabetes, and cardiac diseases.[70]

Experimental and clinical data suggest that the loss of membrane RTK activity in cardiac myocytes results in increased frequency of apoptotic cell death and progression of heart failure. Her2/neu and Her4 are membrane RTKs implicated in both hypertrophic and survival signaling pathways in cardiomyocytes.[71,72] They also play an important role in cardiac development, because targeted disruption of Her2/neu, Her4, or their ligands, neuregulins, results in premature death by cardiac malformations.[73] Studies have demonstrated that inhibitory antibodies to Her2/neu (Herceptin), used to treat patients with breast cancer, were found to induce heart failure.[74,75]

Propagation of the Signal within the Cell

Most signal molecules will bind to a specific receptor on the plasma membrane. This receptor–ligand communication will trigger the first step in the signal-transduction pathway that mediates the sensing and processing of stimuli. The transduction cascade will be propagated within the cells by molecules that are often activated by phosphorylation. This information is passed on from one relay molecule to the other (phosphorylation cascade) until the protein that produces the final cellular response is activated. Phosphorylation of proteins is a common cellular mechanism that regulates protein activity and is usually mediated by a protein kinase enzyme that transfers phosphate groups from ATP to a protein. Cytoplasmic protein kinases phosphorylate their substrates on specific serine, threonine, and tyrosine residues in proteins. Such serine/threonine kinases are widely involved in signaling pathways in humans. Many of the relay molecules in signal-transduction pathways are protein kinases, and they often act on each other.

To terminate a cellular response to an extracellular signal, the cell must have mechanisms for quenching the signal-transduction pathway when the initial signal is no longer present. Activated protein kinase molecules are inactivated by the removal of the phosphate group by protein phosphatases. Signaling processes that are not terminated

properly may lead to uncontrolled cell growth and other abnormal cellular responses.

Mitogen-Activated Protein Kinases

Mitogen-activated protein kinase (MAPK) cascades are among the most thoroughly studied of signal-transduction systems and have been shown to participate in a diverse array of cellular programs, including cell differentiation, cell movement, cell division, and cell death. Three major groups of MAPKs exist: the p38 Map kinase family, the extracellular signal-regulated kinase (Erk) family, and the c-Jun NH$_2$-terminal kinase (JNK) family.[76] The p38 Map kinase family is composed of four different isoforms (p38α, p38β, p38γ, and p38δ) that share significant structural homology, whereas the JNK kinase group includes three members, JNK1, JNK2, and JNK3.[76–81] The Erk family of kinases includes the classic Erk1 and Erk2; however, other kinases (Erk3–8) have been identified and share some structure homology with Erk1 and 2 but have distinct functions.[82,83]

As shown in Figure 1.4, MAPKs are typically organized in a three-kinase architecture consisting of a MAPK, a MAPK activator (MEK, MKK, or MAPK kinase [MAPKK]), and a MEK activator (MEK kinase [MEKK] or MAPK kinase kinase [MAPKKK]). In order for the different MAPK to be activated by various stimuli, there is a requirement for dual phosphorylation on threonine (Thr) and tyrosine (Tyr) residues present in specific motifs for each kinase group. Transmission of signals is achieved by sequential phosphorylation and activation of the components specific to the cascade in the following general path:

Stimulus > MAPKKK > MAPKK > MAPK > Response

Activation of the MAPKKKs or MAPKKs occurs downstream from small G proteins such as Ras for the Erk pathway and members of the Rho family of proteins (Rac1, Cdc42, RhoA, and RhoB) for the p38 and JNK pathways.[76]

The activation of different MAPK signaling cascades by various stimuli is required for induction of various important cellular biologic responses. Biologic activity of cytokines and growth factors can be mediated through MAPK pathways. Such biologic activities vary with the specific family of MAPKs activated and the distinct stimulus inducing such activation. The Ras/Erk pathway mediates primarily cell growth and survival signals, but the stress-activated p38 and JNK kinase pathways mediate mainly proapoptotic and growth inhibitory signals, as well as proinflammatory responses.[76] However, activation of the p38 pathway may also induce antiapoptotic, proliferative, and cell survival signals under certain conditions, depending on the tissue and specific isoform involved.

A key question in studies of such cascades is how ubiquitously activated enzymes generate specific and biologically appropriate cellular responses. Cells are simultaneously exposed to multiple extracellular signals, so each cell must integrate these inputs to choose an appropriate response.

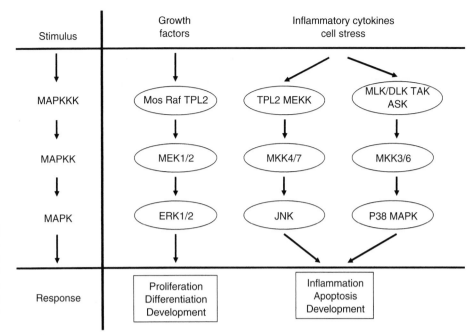

Figure 1.4 Schematic overview of mitogen-activated protein (MAP) kinase pathways. MAP kinase cascades are triggered by specific extracellular signals, leading to characteristic cellular responses involved in regulating cell growth, differentiation, inflammation, and stress responses.

Therefore, activation of the MAPK cascade can lead to contrasting physiologic responses depending on the cell type, suggesting that signal specificity is also determined by regulatory mechanisms other than the selective activation of a MAPK module.[84–86] It was postulated that events that define MAPKs specificity involve physical interactions of the MAPKs with other proteins.[87,88] Because MAPK pathways form a cascade of kinases, each downstream kinase serves as a substrate for the upstream activator. Therefore, direct enzyme–substrate interactions play a critical role in the transmission of signals and offer a potential platform for generating specificity. For example, different studies have shown that members of the Raf family specifically bind to and activate MEKs[89,90] but not MKKs in the stress pathways.[91] The interaction of MEKs with Raf is dependent on a proline-rich sequence unique to MEKs and not found in other MKKs. Deletion of this proline-rich sequence ablates the ability of MEK to bind to Raf and greatly diminishes the ability of Raf to activate MEK.[92]

These results indicate that Raf family members can interact differentially with different substrates. Additionally, much of this specificity is also a consequence of quantitative differences in protein–protein affinities and can be lost when the partners are overexpressed. Therefore, it appears that despite the extensive MAPK networks and the multiple MAPK members involved, specificity for MAPK responses relies upon distinct interactions of different effector proteins with specific domains within the structure of MAPKs.

Second Messengers

Second-messenger molecules are important in generating and amplifying signals. They are often free to diffuse to other compartments of the cell, such as the nucleus, where they can influence gene expression and other processes. The signals may be amplified significantly in the generation of second messengers. Enzymes or membrane channels are almost always activated in second-messenger generation; each activated macromolecule can lead to the generation of many second messengers within the cell. Therefore, a low concentration of signal in the environment, even as little as a single molecule, can yield a large intracellular signal and response. The use of common second messengers in multiple signaling pathways creates both opportunities and potential problems. Input from several signaling pathways, often called *cross talk*, may affect the concentrations of common second messengers. Cross talk permits more finely tuned regulation of cell activity than would the action of individual independent pathways. However, inappropriate cross talk can cause second messengers to be misinterpreted. The two most widely used second messengers are cAMP and Ca^{2+}. A large variety of relay proteins are sensitive to the cytosolic concentration of one or the other of these second messengers.

Cyclic Adenosine Monophosphate

The cAMP is a component of many G protein–signaling pathways. The signal molecule—the "first messenger"—activates a G protein–linked receptor, which activates a specific G protein. In turn, the G protein activates adenylyl cyclase, which catalyzes the conversion of ATP to cAMP. The immediate effect of cAMP is usually the activation of a serine/threonine kinase called PKA. The activated kinase then phosphorylates various other proteins, depending on the cell type.

The cAMP is involved in the pathogenesis of different disease processes such as bacterial infection. Vibrio cholerae

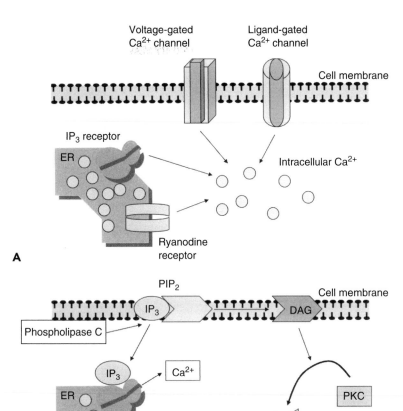

Figure 1.5 Calcium as a second messenger. **A:** The flux of Ca^{2+} into the cytosol from the extracellular space is regulated by voltage-gated or ligand-gated plasma membrane Ca^{2+} channels. Ca^{2+} release from intracellular stores is controlled by IP_3-activated or ryanodine-activated Ca^{2+} channels in the endoplasmic reticulum (ER). **B:** Phospholipase C cleaves phosphatidylinositol bisphosphate (PIP_2), generating two molecules: Diacylglycerol (DAG), which activates protein kinase C, and IP_3, which binds to IP_3-activated channels in the endoplasmic reticulum (ER), resulting in the release of Ca^{2+} into the cytosol.

bacteria can colonize the lining of the small intestine and produce toxins that modify the G protein on the cell membrane involved in regulating salt and water secretion. Because the modified G protein is unable to hydrolyze the active GTP to GDP, it continuously stimulates adenylyl cyclase to make cAMP. The resulting high concentration of cAMP causes the intestinal cells to secrete large amounts of water and salts into the intestines. An infected person develops profuse diarrhea.

Calcium Ions and Inositol Triphosphate

Many signal molecules induce responses in their target cells by signal-transduction pathways that increase the cytosolic concentration of Ca^{2+}. Ca^{2+} is more widely used than cAMP as a second messenger. Ca^{2+} is actively transported out of the cytosol by a variety of protein pumps. Pumps in the plasma membrane move Ca^{2+} into the extracellular fluid, and pumps in the ER membrane move Ca^{2+} into the lumen of the ER. Consequently, the Ca^{2+} concentration in the cytosol (usually in the micromolar range), is usually much lower than in the extracellular fluid (millimolar range) and ER. Because the cytosolic calcium level is low, a small change in absolute numbers of ions represents a relatively large percentage change in Ca^{2+} concentration.

The flux of Ca^{2+} into the cytosol, where they serve as intracellular messengers, is regulated by two distinct families of Ca^{2+}-channel proteins (see Fig. 1.5). These are the plasma membrane Ca^{2+} channels (voltage-gated Ca^{2+} channels or ligand-gated channels), which control Ca^{2+} entry from the extracellular space, and the intracellular Ca^{2+} release channels, which allow Ca^{2+} to enter the cytosol from intracellular stores. The intracellular channels include the large Ca^{2+} channels (RyRs) that participate in cardiac and skeletal muscle EC coupling, and smaller inositol 1,4,5-trisphosphate (IP_3)–activated Ca^{2+} channels.[93,94] Diacylglycerol (DAG) and IP_3 are membrane lipids that can be converted into intracellular second messengers. The two most important messengers of this type are produced from phosphatidylinositol bisphosphate (PIP_2). This lipid component is cleaved by PLC, an enzyme activated by certain G proteins and by Ca^{2+}. PLC splits the PIP_2 into two smaller molecules, each of which acts as a second messenger. One of these messengers is DAG, a molecule that remains within the membrane and activates protein kinase C, which phosphorylates substrate proteins in both the plasma membrane and elsewhere. The other messenger is IP_3, a molecule that leaves the cell membrane and diffuses within the cytosol. IP_3 binds to IP_3 receptors, the channels

TABLE 1.1
SECOND MESSENGER–DEPENDENT PROTEIN KINASES

Second Messenger	Protein Kinase
Cyclic AMP	Cyclic AMP–dependent protein kinase
Cyclic GMP	Cyclic GMP–dependent protein kinase
$4(Ca^{2+})$-calmodulin complex	Ca^{2+}/calmodulin-dependent protein kinase
Ca^{2+} and 1,2-diacylglycerol	Protein kinase C

AMP, adenosine monophosphate; GMP, guanylic acid.

that release calcium from the ER. In some cases, Ca^{2+} activate a signal-transduction protein directly, but often they function by means of calmodulin, a Ca^{2+}-activated switch protein that mediates many of the signal functions of Ca^{2+}. Binding of Ca^{2+} to calmodulin will cause it to wrap around a target domain of specific proteins, causing conformational changes that alter the activity of that protein. The proteins most frequently regulated by calmodulin are protein kinases and phosphatases—the most common relay proteins in signaling pathways. In cardiac myocytes, protein kinases regulate numerous biologic processes, including the regulation of contraction, ion transport, fuel metabolism, and growth. Binding of the regulatory molecule to its membrane receptor often changes the intracellular level of one of the second messengers (see Table 1.1), which then modulates the activity of protein kinase.

There are two distinct Ca^{2+} cycles that participate in cell signaling, both of which control the entry and removal of Ca^{2+} from the cytosol.[94] The first is the extracellular cycle, in which Ca^{2+} enters and leaves the cytosol by crossing the plasma membrane from the extracellular space. A second Ca^{2+} cycle is seen in more specialized cells, such as adult cardiac myocytes, in which Ca^{2+} is pumped into and out of limited stores contained within an intracellular membrane system. In cardiac myocytes, the family of plasma membrane Ca^{2+} channels includes L-type channels, which respond to membrane depolarization by generating a signal that opens the intracellular Ca^{2+} release channels. Ca^{2+} entry through L-type Ca^{2+} channels in the sinoatrial (SA) node contributes to pacemaker activity, whereas L-type Ca^{2+} channels in the atrioventricular (AV) node are essential for AV conduction. The T-type Ca^{2+} channels, another member of the family of plasma membrane Ca^{2+} channels, participate in pharmacomechanical coupling in smooth muscles. Opening of these channels in response to membrane depolarization contributes to SA node pacemaker currents, but their role in the working cells of the atria and ventricle is less clear. Like the IP_3-activated intracellular Ca^{2+} release channels, T-type plasma membrane channels

may regulate cell growth. Because most of the familiar Ca^{2+} channel–blocking agents currently used in cardiology, such as nifedipine, verapamil, and diltiazem, are selective for L-type Ca^{2+} channels, the recent development of drugs that selectively block T-type Ca^{2+} channels offers promise of new approaches to cardiovascular therapy.

Several signaling pathways have been implicated in hypertrophic responses in cardiomyocytes.[95–97] Much work has focused on the control of transcription in cardiomyocytes, especially in neonatal cells. It has been recognized that Erk (classical MAP kinase; Ras/Raf/MEK/Erk) and phosphatidylinositol 3-kinase (PI3K) pathways are involved in the pathogenesis of cardiac hypertrophy. Cardiac hypertrophy involves increased heart size caused by increased cardiomyocyte size. Initially, it is an adaptive response to increased workload or to defects in the efficiency of the contractile machinery. However, in the longer term, it contributes to the development of heart failure and sudden death. Increased protein synthesis is a key feature of cardiac hypertrophy and likely underlies the increased cell and organ size observed under this condition.[98]

Animal studies have shown that cardiac-specific expression of an activated form of MEK1 leads to development of concentric hypertrophy involving thickened septal and left ventricular walls.[99] In fact, activation of MEK/Erk signaling appears to be sufficient to induce hypertrophy *in vivo*. Interestingly, overexpression of Ras gives rise to a different phenotype, characterized by pathologic ventricular remodeling.[100] This may reflect its ability to activate additional signaling pathways. In addition, targeted overexpression of constitutively active PI3K in the heart results in increased organ size whereas expression of a dominant-negative mutant decreases it.[101] Interestingly, the increased heart size was associated with a similar increase in myocyte size, indicating true hypertrophy.

Cellular Response to Signals

Often the final stage of cell signaling involves the transduced signal functioning as a transcription factor. Such a transcription factor will regulate several different genes, triggering a specific cellular response and controlling various cellular activities. As reviewed previously, many classes of receptors bind their ligands and activate protein kinases inside the cell. Activation frequently leads to a protein kinase cascade, resulting in the rapid amplification of extracellular signals. Signaling pathways with a large number of steps have two important benefits: They amplify the signal dramatically and contribute to the specificity of response. Cells can have similar receptors, but they produce very different responses to the same ligand. The response produced depends on the availability of targets. One cell may have target proteins that lead to cell cycle arrest, whereas another may have target proteins that induce apoptosis, following DNA damage. Different cells respond distinctly to similar signals because they differ in one or more of the proteins that handle and respond to the signal.

Apoptosis/Cell Death

Cells die continually during the life of multicellular organisms, but the integrity of the organism depends on the ability to either regulate the turnover of cells or limit the injury to surrounding cells that can occur when senescent cells release their contents. The problem of controlling the rate and processes surrounding cell death is particularly acute in settings of critical trauma or infection, when cascades of tissue injury can compound long- and short-term sequelae. The process of apoptosis is an energy-dependent, tightly regulated physiologic process of programmed cell death in both normal and pathologic tissues. Apoptotic cells display characteristic morphology, including membrane blebbing, nuclear condensation, and degradation of DNA into large fragments of uniform length. Moreover, expression of surface proteins, such as annexins, on the surface of apoptotic cells serves to mark these cells for ingestion and removal by phagocytes. Sequential waves of programmed cell death are necessary for normal development during embryogenesis, tissue remodeling following injury or ischemia, and tissue homeostasis throughout life. In contrast to apoptosis, cell necrosis is a passive form of cell death that is induced mainly by nonphysiologic agents that damage the cell membrane, leading to autophagy of the cell. Necrosis is uncontrolled and the release of proteases and reactive oxygen and nitrogen species from necrotic cells can cause considerable damage to surrounding tissues.

The classical pathways of apoptosis are mediated by a family of aspartyl-specific cysteine proteases known as *caspases*. These enzymes are the key mediators of apoptosis, cleaving their substrates at specific aspartate residues. The expression of caspases is tightly regulated during fetal and neonatal development and in response to environmental stimuli. Moreover, specific caspase inhibitors have been developed that may contribute to future therapeutics designed to preserve cells in the CNS and elsewhere. On the basis of their specific functions in apoptosis, caspases are divided into "initiators" (caspases-2, -8, -9, -10) and "effectors" (caspases-3, -6, -7). The effector caspases degrade multiple substrates, including structural and regulatory proteins in the cell nucleus, cytoplasm, and cytoskeleton.[102]

Several distinct pathways regulate caspase activity (see Fig. 1.6). The best defined is the receptor mediated-pathway, which is initiated by the binding of ligands to death receptors of the tumor necrosis factor (TNF)/nerve growth-factor (NGF) receptor family. These receptors contain a "death domain"—a conserved segment of approximately 80 amino acids—on their intracellular terminals. On activation, the death domain engages and activates the apoptotic cascade. The Fas receptor is the best characterized of this group. Binding of Fas by its ligand, or by activating antibodies, leads to recruitment of the adaptor protein Fas-associated death domain protein (FADD) and the initiator caspase-8.[103] Alternatively, caspases may be activated by the nuclear protein p53, which regulates the expression of many apoptosis-related genes. p53 is activated by a variety of cellular stress signals, including DNA damage, oncogene activation, and cellular hypoxia.

Caspases may be activated in a receptor-independent manner by a variety of stimuli, and it is clear that mitochondria are key effectors in this "intrinsic" pathway. During apoptosis, mitochondrial membrane permeability

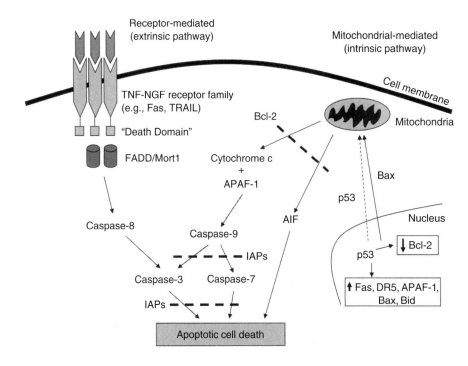

Figure 1.6 Caspase-mediated apoptosis. The cascade of caspase activation, leading to apoptosis, is initiated by the binding of ligands to receptors of the TNF–nerve growth factor (NGF) family ("extrinsic pathway") or by release of cytochrome c from mitochondria ("intrinsic pathway"). The intrinsic pathway is tightly regulated by the relative expression of proapoptotic (e.g., Bax) and antiapoptotic (e.g., Bcl-2) proteins of the Bcl-2 family, as well as activity of the proapoptotic nuclear p53 protein. "Inhibitor of apoptosis proteins" (IAP) block the activity of the downstream caspases-3 and caspases-7, which directly mediate processes leading to cell death.

increases and caspase-dependent and caspase-independent factors are released into the cytosol. Cytochrome c release from mitochondria is an important mechanism for the activation of caspase-3 and the initiation of cell apoptosis in response to intrinsic stimuli, including oxidative and nitrosative stress.[104] Cytochrome c combines with the scaffold protein Apaf-1, procaspase-9, and ATP to generate a 700 to 1,400 kDa supramolecular complex, called an *apoptosome*. Caspase-9 is activated on formation of the apoptosome, which then triggers the downstream caspases-3 and caspases-7 that lead to apoptotic cell death. Understandably, mitochondrial activity and integrity are tightly regulated within the cell, in large part through interactions with a family of proteins known as the Bcl-2 family. Although they all contain Bcl-2 homology (BH) domains that allow for interaction with other pro- and antiapoptotic proteins, these proteins have divergent localizations and roles. Bcl-1, Bcl-xl, and Mcl-1 protect cells from potentially death-inducing stimuli and are localized at the mitochondrial membrane. Bax, Bak, and Bok proteins, which are found on the membrane and in the cytosol, promote apoptosis by oligimerizing and inserting into the mitochondrial membrane, leading to disruption of the membrane and release of cytochrome c and other mitochondrial contents. Another group of Bcl-2 family proteins, the BH3-only proteins (e.g., Bad), serves a super-regulatory role by binding and inactivating antiapoptotic Bcl-2 family proteins, facilitating Bax/Bad-induced apoptosis.

Mitochondria have also been implicated in apoptotic pathways that are not dependent on downstream caspase activity. Indeed, numerous studies have indicated that apoptosis proceeds even in the presence of broad-spectrum caspase inhibitors. Pathogenic conditions, such as ischemia/reperfusion, neurodegeneration, and liver diseases are associated with instability of mitochondrial membranes as a result of cell hypoxia, increased oxidative load, or deficiency of glycolytic substrates. Subsequently, mitochondrial outer membrane permeabilization induces cell death by release of both caspase-activating molecules (e.g., cytochrome c–mediated apoptosome formation) and caspase-independent effectors. Caspase-independent pathways of apoptosis are not completely understood. One likely pathway involves AIF. This protein is released from the mitochondrial intermembrane space during programmed cell death and translocates, under regulation by Bcl-2, from the mitochondria to the cytosol and nucleus. In the cytosol, AIF induces production of reactive oxygen species, accelerating cell stress and apoptosis. In the nucleus, it is thought to act directly, triggering chromatin condensation and DNA degradation.[105]

Signaling Events in Tissue Injury

Mechanisms of Ventilator-Induced Lung Injury

Ventilation-induced lung injury is a major source of morbidity and mortality associated with pediatric and neonatal intensive care, and strategies to prevent it constitute major advances in practice during the last decade. For example, bronchopulmonary dysplasia (BPD) in premature infants following treatment of respiratory distress syndrome using supplemental oxygen and mechanical ventilation is characterized by injury to pulmonary tissues, leading to fibrosis and asymmetric aeration. Similar pathology is occasionally seen following positive pressure ventilation in pediatric patients. Although chronic lung injury is precipitated by oxygen toxicity, barotrauma, and volutrauma to the lung, it is now evident that inflammation is the common end pathway mediating cell injury.[106]

The intracellular signaling mechanisms by which increased intraluminal pressure and shear stress induce inflammation in the lung have been referred to as *mechanotransduction*. The mechanisms of mechanotransduction are diverse. Activities of several transcription factors, including AP-1, NF-κB, Sp-1, and Egr-1 are known to be increased during mechanical ventilation. These lead to increased transcription of genes encoding vasoactive mediators (prostacyclin, nitric oxide), adhesion molecules, monocytes chemoattractant protein-1, cytokines (IL-1, IL-6), and growth factors (PDGF and TGF-β) in endothelial cells.[107] Moreover, excessive peak ventilatory pressures can lead to stress failure of plasma membranes in the lung parenchyma. This leads to necrosis of pulmonary epithelial cells, with the release of preformed reactive oxygen intermediates and other inflammation-inducing cytoplasmic contents. Stress failure of endothelial and epithelial barriers also leads to the loss of compartmentalization. Hemorrhage and accumulation of leukocytes in the lung can contribute to epithelial injury and respiratory failure. Dissection of air into the interstitium of the lung or pulmonary interstitial emphysema is a radiographically evident indicator of excessive ventilatory pressures and incipient chronic lung injury. Consistent with clinical experience, the Acute Respiratory Distress Syndrome Network reported that specific ventilation strategies have a major effect on the degree of subsequent lung injury.[107] Strategies associated with inadequate end expiratory pressure and high inspiratory pressure trigger excessive mechanotransduction and are associated with long-term lung injury. Numerous studies support the concept of "gentle ventilation" and maintenance of optimal lung volumes during ventilation. High-frequency jet and oscillator ventilations have been shown to reduce lung injury in premature infants and to be associated with reduced quantities of inflammatory mediators in bronchoalveolar lavage (BAL) fluid.[108]

Neutrophil-mediated inflammation plays a direct role in the etiology of ventilator-induced lung injury. For example, in chronic lung disease in premature newborns, increased expression of cytokines, reactive oxygen intermediates, and other mediators leads to acute inflammation and accumulation of activated neutrophils in the lung. BAL neutrophil counts peak on the fourth day of life and then decline rapidly to normal by the end of the first week in infants who recover from BPD. In contrast, BAL neutrophil counts decline much more slowly in infants who go on to develop BPD.[109] Activated neutrophils in the lung generate oxygen radicals, secretory hydrolases, elastase, and arachidonic acid metabolites that are damaging to tissue and can cause the development of chronic lung disease. Another point of interest is that the depletion of neutrophils has been associated with decreased lung injury caused by hyperoxia and oxygen free radical products.[110] Conversely, defects in neutrophil apoptosis result in neutrophil accumulation and have been shown to contribute to the pathology in sepsis and in acute respiratory distress syndrome. Apoptosis in lung neutrophils is decreased following lung hemorrhage or endotoxemia, tissue hypoxia, or elevated extracellular calcium.[111] Moreover, clearance of neutrophils by apoptosis is decreased in the systemic inflammatory reaction syndrome and in children with recurrent respiratory infections.[112] These findings indicate that dysregulation of neutrophil apoptosis may account, in large part, for the severity of inflammatory diseases observed in newborns and children.

Several lines of evidence suggest that apoptosis, in contrast to necrosis, provides a clearance mechanism for neutrophils that limits tissue injury and promotes resolution, rather than persistence of inflammation.[113,114] First, neutrophils undergoing apoptosis or programmed cell death become isolated from the inflammatory milieu, unable to degranulate or to up-regulate activation-associated ligand receptors such as ICAM-1.[115,116] Second, phagocytosis of apoptotic neutrophils by macrophages prevents the release of proinflammatory cytokines by neutrophils.[113] In contrast, neutrophil necrosis occurs in the absence of activated macrophages, resulting in the release of cytotoxic products, including neutrophil elastase and myeloperoxidase.[117] Third, uptake of large numbers of apoptotic neutrophils by macrophages does not activate these cells to secrete proinflammatory mediators such as granule enzymes, thromboxane, and chemokines.[118] This is in sharp contrast to the activation of macrophages observed, following the uptake of opsonized nonapoptotic neutrophils. The mechanisms by which macrophages recognize apoptotic neutrophils are unclear, but they are thought to involve vitronectin and thrombospondin receptors on neutrophils, as well as phosphatidylserine residues exposed on the surface of apoptotic cells.[119,120] The process of neutrophil apoptosis followed by clearance by alveolar macrophages (AM) has been shown to be important in the resolution of oleic acid-induced acute lung injury in rats.[121] Similarly, histologic evidence indicates that neutrophils undergo apoptosis and are subsequently phagocytosed by macrophages in the lung during mechanical ventilation.[122]

Given the evidence that neutrophil apoptosis represents a mechanism for safely removing these cells and restoring normal homeostasis, it is reasonable to expect that this process is tightly regulated. The physiologic half-life of neutrophils in the circulation is approximately 6 hours, indicating that these cells have a high rate of constitutive apoptosis. This can be altered by a wide range of factors that can be deranged in the setting of BPD. For example, the activities of the inflammatory cytokines IL-1, IL-6, and IL-8 are increased in BAL fluid in BPD, whereas those of IL-1 receptor antagonist and the anti-inflammatory cytokine IL-10 are decreased.[110,123–125] Levels of transforming growth factor (TGF-β) are also increased in BPD. This cytokine is present at sites of chronic inflammation, mediates neutrophil chemotaxis and activation, and promotes fibrosis in the lung. Most inflammatory cytokines (e.g., IL-1, IL-6, IL-8), as well as some soluble stimuli, including bacterial lipopolysaccharide (LPS), inhibit neutrophil apoptosis in parallel with the enhancement of neutrophil function.[126,127] Conversely, the constitutive rate of neutrophil apoptosis is accelerated by Fas ligand[128] or IL-10.[129,130] Although TGF-β has been implicated in intercellular induction of apoptosis in some cell types,[131,132] its role in the control of apoptosis in neutrophils is not known.

At the intracellular level, signals mediating apoptosis are modulated by pro- and antiapoptotic cytoplasmic proteins. Expression of these proteins is known to be regulated during the maturation of cultured myelocytes. Whereas mature neutrophils express proapoptotic proteins like Bax, Bad, and Bak,[133,134] antiapoptotic proteins, including Bcl-2, Bcl-xl, and Mcl-1, are expressed in decreasing quantities during cell maturation.[133–136] This is consistent with the short life of mature neutrophils in the circulation. Regulation of apoptosis in inflammatory neutrophils has also been shown to occur through alterations in the expression of caspase proteins. Caspase activity is instrumental in mediating apoptosis in response to several signals. For example, LPS inhibits spontaneous and anti-Fas antibody-induced neutrophil apoptosis, in part, by decreasing expression of intracellular caspases.[137]

Apoptosis of neutrophils is also closely linked to signals mediating neutrophil activation. In general, proinflammatory cytokines are antiapoptotic (e.g., IL-6, IL-1, and IL-8), whereas anti-inflammatory cytokines (e.g., IL-10) are proapoptotic. Coregulation of neutrophil activation and cell survival is physiologically important as it may allow for prolonged survival of neutrophils that are required to fight pathogens, as well as the removal of senescent or dysfunctional neutrophils. For example, the proinflammatory cytokine IL-8 delays spontaneous and TNFα-induced apoptosis in human neutrophils.[138] However, physiologic activation, *per se*, does not appear to be solely responsible for suppression of neutrophil apoptosis. There are several intracellular signaling pathways that mediate cellular responses to receptor binding. These include phosphoinositide 3-kinases (PI3-K), p38 mitogen-activated protein (MAP) kinase, and nuclear factor-κB (NF-κB).[139,140] PI3-K catalyzes the phosphorylation of the serine/threonine protein kinase Akt (also known as *protein kinase B*). Akt has been shown to play a role in cytokine-mediated cell survival, and several mechanisms have been proposed. This enzyme inhibits proteases that specifically cleave the poly(ADP-ribose) polymerase and inactivates the proapoptotic protein, Bad, by phosphorylation, thereby promoting survival. In addition, Akt directly and indirectly causes phosphorylation and degradation of the inhibitor protein-κB (I-κB), leading to increased activity of NF-κB.[141]

NF-κB is a transcription factor known to regulate the expression of genes involved in leukocyte activation, as well as of the genes that modulate cell death.[140] NF-κB activation has been shown to play an important role in inhibiting neutrophil apoptosis.[142,143] For example, NF-κB-mediated induction of TNF receptor-associated factors (TRAF) and inhibitor of apoptosis proteins (c-IAP) proteins leads to the suppression of caspase-8 activation and reduced apoptosis.[144] In models of acute lung injury caused either by hemorrhage or endotoxemia, NF-κB activation is increased in the lung but not in peripheral blood neutrophils, and apoptosis is diminished in lung neutrophils.[140] Cells derived from NF-κB RelA (p65) knockout mice exhibit enhanced sensitivity to TNF-induced cell death.[145] Moreover, IL-10 promotes apoptosis and the resolution of LPS-induced neutrophilia in the lung *in vivo*,[111] in part, by suppressing NF-κB activation.[146] However, NF-κB can, under some circumstances, contribute to cell death. For example, in conjunction with AP-1, NF-κB can induce Fas ligand expression in T cells.[145] The role of p38 MAP kinase in neutrophil apoptosis has been similarly controversial. This pathway has been reported to mediate stress- and LPS-induced neutrophil apoptosis.[147,148] However, it has also been implicated in hypoxia-induced suppression of neutrophil apoptosis,[149] and has been reported to be either instrumental or not involved in spontaneous neutrophil apoptosis.[139,150] NF-κB and p38 MAP kinase activation appear to be the primary determinants of lung inflammation and injury, but the mechanisms mediating these actions are not completely understood.

Lipid Mediators in Health and Disease

The process of inflammation is essential for host defense but requires tight regulation in order to avoid injury to surrounding tissues by reactive intermediates and enzymes produced by activated leukocytes. The range of chemical mediators regulating this process includes cytokines and chemokines, gases such as nitric oxide and carbon monoxide, reactive oxygen species, and nucleotides such as adenosine and inosine monophosphate. Recently, endogenous lipid mediators have emerged as key regulators of inflammation. Specifically, bioactive metabolites of arachidonic acid or eicosanoids are expressed in many cell types and have diverse effects on neutrophil and monocytes activity. Therefore, leukotrienes and many prostaglandins are proinflammatory, and lipoxins decrease inflammation. Similarly, leukotrienes generally induce vasoconstriction and smooth muscle contraction, whereas prostacyclins

induce vasodilation. Arachidonic acid, the precursor to eicosanoids, is the most precisely regulated fatty acid in cellular phospholipids. The release and oxygenation of arachidonic acid are critical events in regulating key processes in host defense, inflammation, and hemodynamics. The pattern of control of arachidonate is determined by synthesis, transfer between lipids, release, and metabolism. Unesterified arachidonic acid released from cell membranes through activity of phospholipase A_2 may be reacylated into phospholipids or triglyceride, providing a mechanism for remodeling the fatty acid composition of different cellular pools of lipid. However, most of it is metabolized by cyclooxygenases into prostaglandins, by lipoxygenases into leukotrienes, lipoxins, and hydroxyeicosa-tetraenoic acids (HETEs), or oxidized by P-450 enzymes into eicosatrienoic acids.[151]

Lipoxins are derived through a double lipoxygenation of arachidonic acid by both 5-lipoxygenase, expressed in myeloid cells, and 12,15-lipoxygenase from platelets, epithelial cells, and monocytes.[152] The major isomers, LXA4 and LXB4, are of particular interest because they are thought to act as endogenous braking signals in inflammation. Specifically, these metabolites inhibit neutrophil chemotaxis, suppress calcium mobilization, and promote neutrophil apoptosis. Lipoxins may also antagonize the proinflammatory effects of TNF-α, down-regulate the induction of many other genes regulated by NF-κB, protect enterocyte integrity, and inhibit cytokine production.[151] It has been suggested that a physiologic switch from the generation of inflammatory eicosanoids from intracellular arachidonic acid to production of lipoxins is a primary mechanism by which the process of inflammation is modulated. Moreover, aspirin acetylation of cyclooxygenase 2 promotes the generation of a series of 15-epimers of LXA4, known as *aspirin-triggered lipoxins* (ATL). These metabolites may account for some of the bioactivity profile of aspirin and possibly other nonsteroidal anti-inflammatory drugs (NSAIDs).

The intracellular mechanisms by which arachidonic acid derivatives signal and modulate the inflammatory response have been a subject of intense study. Proximate events, such as alterations in thiol generation, kinase signaling, and mitochondrial activity have been described.[153] However, a paradigm shift in the physiology and pharmacology of intracellular lipid signaling has occurred as a result of studies describing the role of peroxisome proliferator-activated receptors (PPARs). PPARs are ligand-activated nuclear transcription factors that function as regulators of lipid and lipoprotein metabolism and glucose homeostasis, and influence cellular proliferation, differentiation, and apoptosis.[154] In response to ligands, PPARs heterodimerize with the retinoic X receptor (RXR) and bind to PPAR response elements (PPRE) located in the promoter region of target genes, which consist of a direct repeat of the nuclear receptor hexameric AGGTCA recognition sequence separated by one or two intervening nucleotides.[155] PPARs regulate the expression of genes associated with lipid homeostasis, degradation of fatty acids and their derivatives, and inflammation. As such, PPARs act as lipid sensors by translating changes in lipid mediator and fatty acid balance in the local metabolism into tissue-specific effects that are generally anti-inflammatory. For example, PPARs induce macrophage apoptosis.[156] PPARs interfere with the AP-1, STAT, and NF-κB signaling pathways by preventing the binding of these transcription factors to their target sequences, and block intracellular signaling by the c-Jun and p65 pathways.[157] As a result, PPARs agonists decrease expression of the inflammatory cytokines IL-2, IL-6, IL-8, and TNF-α, as well as of leukocyte metalloproteases.

PPAR-α and PPAR-γ have distinct tissue distributions and physiologic roles. Activation of PPAR-α, which is present in the liver, kidney, heart, muscle, and mononuclear cells, inhibits vascular cell proliferation, migration, and inflammatory gene expression.[158] PPAR-α has been shown to bind to and induce degradation of leukotriene B4, limiting the duration of LTB4-induced inflammation.[159] In addition, PPAR-α signals proliferation and suppresses apoptosis in hepatic cells, possibly through p38 MAP kinase signaling.[160] PPAR-γ is also widely expressed in adipose, monocytic cells, and other tissues. It exhibits anti-inflammatory activity by inhibiting cytokine production, increasing CD36 expression, and enhancing phagocytosis of apoptotic neutrophils, which is essential in the resolution of inflammation. PPAR-γ agonists inhibit expression of inducible nitric oxide synthase, gelatinase B, and scavenger receptor A genes.[161,162] Expression of PPAR-γ is decreased by inflammatory cytokines, including IL-1α, IL-1β, and IL-6, and is increased in monocytes by IL-4, an anti-inflammatory cytokine.[163]

The physiologic roles of PPARs have been elucidated by determining natural ligands for these transcription factors. PPAR-α is activated by lipoxygenase-derived arachidonic acid metabolites, such as 8S-HETE and LTB4. PPAR-γ agonists include cyclooxygenase and lipoxygenase-derived mediators, including 15-deoxyprostaglandin J2 and 15-HETE.[154] Activation of PPARs by these mediators suggests that lipid-induced inflammation is modulated by a negative feedback system. Anti-inflammatory activity signaled and mediated by the activation of PPARs is presumably distinct from, but concurrent with, the phenomenon of increased production of lipoxins relative to inflammatory eicosanoids during the resolution phase of inflammation. Pharmacologic interest in PPARs has been driven by the recognition that several classes of synthetic pharmaceutics exert their effects, in part, by activating PPAR-α and/or PPAR-γ. Fibrates, a class of first-line drugs used in the treatment of hypertriglyceridemia and hyperlipidemia, are potent synthetic ligands for PPAR-α. The antidiabetic glitazones, currently used in the treatment of insulin insensitivity, are synthetic high-affinity ligands for PPAR-γ.

In addition, NSAIDs, including indomethacin and ibuprofen, are activators of PPAR-γ in the micromolar range,[162] suggesting that anti-inflammatory effects of high-dose NSAIDs are related to PPAR activation rather than to cyclooxygenase inhibition, which occurs at much lower serum concentrations. Metabolism of arachidonic acid and trafficking of intracellular lipids are tightly regulated signaling processes that are essential for initiation, maintenance, and resolution of inflammation. Inappropriate inflammation is a key component in the pathophysiology of both acute and chronic conditions, including atherosclerosis, acute respiratory distress syndrome, and bronchopulmonary dysplasia. The effects of widely used drugs are likely related to anti-inflammatory and antilipogenic actions mediated by PPARs, and the rational use of specific PPARs agonists will likely lead to new approaches and therapies for common neonatal and pediatric conditions.

Regulation of Vascular Tone

Classic studies of agonist and antagonist binding kinetics, tissue distribution, and clinical potency have led to the differentiation of autonomic receptor subtypes, including muscarinic and nicotinic cholinoceptors, α- and β-adrenoceptors, and dopaminergic receptors. Further subcategories of receptors have been defined, based on sensitivity to specific antagonists. The site-specific activity of endogenous and exogenous ligands for these receptors is determined by the anatomy and neurotransmitter chemistry of the autonomic nervous system. Almost all efferent preganglionic fibers leaving the CNS and all parasympathetic postganglionic fibers are cholinergic. The terminals of these neurons are characterized by large numbers of membrane-bound vesicles, which contain acetylcholine that is secreted into the synaptic space. After release from the presynaptic terminal, acetylcholine molecules may bind to and activate cholinoceptors, and excess acetylcholine is degraded by acetylcholinesterase. The physiologic effect of cholinergic activation then depends on the tissue-specific type and density of the receptor. Binding of muscarinic M_1 receptors, which are localized primarily in the CNS and other neural tissues, results in the formation of IP_3 and DAG, as well as in increased intracellular calcium. Muscarinic M_2 receptors are localized to myocardium and smooth muscle and act by opening potassium channels and inhibiting activity of adenylyl cyclase. Muscarinic M_3 receptors, which mediate secretion from exocrine glands, are also found on smooth muscle and endothelial cells and act similarly to M_1 cholinoceptors. In contrast, nicotinic cholinoceptors are localized primarily in postganglionic neurons (N_N) and skeletal muscle (N_M) and act primarily by opening membrane Na^+ and K^+ channels, resulting in membrane depolarization.

Adrenergic receptors are important in the regulation of smooth muscle tone, including the maintenance of vascular tone and tissue perfusion, and pulmonary constriction.

α Adrenoceptors are localized primarily in smooth muscles, and activation is associated with vasoconstriction. α-Receptors are also found in some presynaptic nerve terminals, platelets, and lipocytes. β_1-Receptors, found in the heart, lipocytes, and brain cells, are best known for pharmacologic effects in increasing cardiac inotropy and chronotropy. β_2-Receptors mediate cardiac chronotropy and smooth muscle relaxation; β_2-agonists are therapeutically indicated for tocolysis and bronchodilation.

The biology of adrenergic receptors is of particular importance in intensive care medicine because adrenergic agonists, including catecholamines, are frequently used clinically for the maintenance of vascular tone. Pharmacologic manipulation of the cardiovascular system is usually aimed at increasing the inotropic state of the myocardium or altering the tone of the systemic vascular system so as to result in improved perfusion. The final common mediator for both processes is the concentration of calcium in the cytosol. The pathway by which pharmacologic agents affect this parameter is a function of their specific cell-surface receptors. Catecholamines modify cellular physiology by interacting with a specific adrenergic receptor. The classic paradigm of α and β adrenergic receptors can be further broken down into several subtypes of α_1-, α_2-, and β-receptors.[164] Adrenergic receptors mediate their effects through G proteins and as such are classified as G protein–coupled receptors. The adrenergic receptor itself contains seven membrane spanning α-helical domains, an extracellular N-terminal segment, and a cytosolic C-terminal segment. The action resulting from a ligand binding to a particular adrenergic receptor is a function of the specific type of subunits compromising the G protein–receptor complex.

Adrenergic receptors are typically coupled to one of three types of G proteins: G_s, G_i, or G_q. G_s proteins produce an increase in adenylate cyclase activity, whereas G_i proteins promote a decrease in adenylate cyclase activity. G_q protein receptors stimulate PLC to generate DAG and IP3. The nature of the G protein is usually a function of the type of α subunit (α_s, α_l, α_q, and $\alpha_{12/13}$).[165] In the example of the G_s protein, ligand binding to the coupled receptor causes a conformational change in the G protein, resulting in GDP disassociating from the $G_{s\alpha}$ subunit and GTP binding to the α subunit. This GTP-G α complex then disassociates from the $G_{\beta\gamma}$ subunit and binds to adenylate cyclase, leading to an increase in activity of this enzyme. Adenylate cyclase catalyzes the conversion of ATP to cAMP, thereby increasing cellular levels of cAMP. G_i proteins have a different α subunit; when the $G_{i\alpha}$ GTP complex binds to adenylate cyclase, the enzyme is inactivated. By inhibiting this enzyme, G_i-coupled receptor agonists produce a decrease in the cellular concentration of cAMP. The specific cellular response that follows an alteration in the concentration of cAMP depends on the specialized function of the target cell. Typically, an increase in concentration of cAMP leads to activation of a cAMP-dependent protein kinase. These kinases then phosphorylate and activate other structures and enzymes.

Myocardial β_1-adrenergic receptors are associated with G_s. When this receptor type is engaged by an agonist agent, the result is enhanced activity of adenylate cyclase and a rise in the concentration of cAMP, leading to the activation of PKA. PKA in turn phosphorylates voltage-dependent calcium channels, increasing the fraction of channels that can be open and the probability that these channels are open, producing an increase in intracellular calcium concentration.[166] Calcium then binds to troponin C, allowing for actin–myosin cross bridge formation and sarcomere contraction. Also, PKA phosphorylates phospholamban, relieving the disinhibitory effect of the unphosphorylated form on calcium channels in the Sr. The accumulation of calcium by the SR is therefore enhanced, increasing the rate of sarcomere relaxation (lusitropy) and subsequently increasing the amount of calcium available for the next contraction. This increase leads to both enhanced contractility and active diastolic relaxation.

α_1 Adrenergic receptors mediate vascular smooth muscle contraction. Although α-receptors may have inotropic effects less than those of β-adrenergic receptors, they do have significant effects in the myocardium. Interestingly, in heart failure, down-regulation of β-receptors has been noted, whereas α-receptors are preserved.[167] The α_1-receptor is coupled to the family of $G_{q/11}$ proteins, which act independently of cAMP. Signal transduction across this receptor is initiated by the activation of PLC, which hydrolyzes phosphatidylinositol 4,5-biphosphate (PIP$_2$) to IP$_3$ and 1,2-diacylglycerol (1,2DG). IP$_3$ binds to specific receptors on the SR, causing a release of calcium into the cytosol and promotes movement of extracellular calcium into the cell. 1,2DG with calcium activates protein kinase C, which regulates movement of calcium into the cytosol. As a result, in vascular smooth muscles, medium light chain kinase is activated and it phosphorylates myosin light chain 2, leading to smooth muscle contraction.[168] It has also been shown that a similar mechanism underlies the inotropic effect of the α_1-receptor in the myocardium.[169] The α_1-receptors also activate calcium influx through voltage dependent and independent calcium channels; α-receptors also promote the activation of MAP kinases, which are key regulators of cell growth. Dopaminergic receptors in effector tissues, such as smooth muscle of the renal vascular bed, cause vasodilation by activating adenylyl cyclase and increasing cellular cAMP. D2, D3, and D4 dopaminergic receptors in the CNS act by inhibiting adenylyl cyclase.

Agents other than catecholamines also serve to regulate vascular tone through receptor-mediated mechanisms. Arginine vasopressin (AVP) is a noncatecholamine, nonpeptide hormone synthesized in the supraoptic and paraventricular nuclei of the hypothalamus. There are three subtypes of vasopressin receptors, known as V_1, V_2, and

V_3 (or V_{1b}). V_2 receptors are present in the renal collecting duct, whereas V_1 receptors are located in the vascular bed, kidney, bladder, spleen, and hepatocytes, among other tissues. AVP is released in response to small increases in plasma osmolality or large decreases in blood pressure or blood volume. The plasma osmolality threshold for release of AVP is 280 mOsm per kg; beyond this threshold, there is a steep linear relation between serum osmolality and AVP levels. Changes of at least 20% in blood volume are needed to effect a change in AVP levels, although levels may then increase by 20- to 30-fold.[170] Hypovolemia also shifts the response curve for AVP to osmolar changes to the left and increases the slope of the curve. Vasopressin can produce vasoconstriction through V_1 receptors in the vascular bed, but it also activates V_1 receptors in the CNS, including receptors in the area postrema.[171]

Intracellular Signaling in Traumatic and Hypoxic Brain Injury

Neuronal and glial cell death occurs by apoptosis or necrosis. Apoptotic and necrotic cells have both been identified in the brain following traumatic or hypoxic injury, and degenerating oligodendrocytes and astrocytes have been observed within white matter tracts. Although necrotic cell death is, by definition, a noncontrolled response to diverse insults, the process of apoptosis in brain tissue is tightly regulated. As in the lung and other tissues, shifts in the relative expression of survival-promoting proteins (Bcl-2, Bcl-xL, p42/44 MAP kinase) and death-inducing proteins (Bax, p53, caspases) are likely to determine the rate of neuronal cell apoptosis.[172] Expression of these proteins is generally affected by two categories of signals in the cell and the microenvironment following injury. First, CNS injury triggers oxidative stress due to generation of reactive oxygen species. These free radicals act on nuclear DNA, resulting in increased strand breaks and induction of poly(ADP-ribose) polymerase-1 (PARP-1), a repair enzyme. In the presence of extensive DNA damage, PARP-1 activation can lead to depletion of cellular nicotinamide adenine dinucleotide phosphate (NADPH) pools, resulting in cell death by necrosis. Inhibition of PARP-1 has been shown to preserve intracellular energy stores and activate caspase-9, resulting in a shift to controlled apoptotic cell death.[173] Cell survival may also be increased by PARP-1 inhibition, but this is at the potential cost of the preservation of cells with significant DNA damage.

The second broad mechanism of neuronal cell injury following trauma or hypoxia is by alterations in the activity of membrane-selective ion pumps. The process by which synaptic overactivity leads to the excessive release of glutamate, a major neurotransmitter, is known as *excitotoxicity*. Glutamate activates postsynaptic cell membrane receptors, which lead to the opening of membrane channel pores, leading to influx or efflux of ions. One such channel is the brain Na^+/Ca^{2+} exchanger, of which three isoforms—NCX1, NCX2, and NCX3—have been identified in the brain.[174] Under normal conditions, these and other ion-specific channels tightly maintain intracellular Na^+ and Ca^{2+} homeostasis. However, the influx of cations, particularly Ca^{2+}, during excitotoxicity activates intracellular Ca^{2+}-dependent signaling cascades that lead to neuronal cell death by mechanisms that have not been well defined.[175]

Neuronal Cell Response to Hypoxia

Patterns of brain injury in the developing brain differ in specific and consistent ways from the hypoxic brain injury in adult patients and older children. In the immature brain, ischemia superimposed on hypoxia is required for injury, so the neonatal brain, in particular, is quite resistant to damage in the face of transient hypoxic periods such as those that occur during labor and delivery. Tissue injury also tends to evolve over hours to days after a neurotoxic cascade is triggered by hypoxic ischemia in the immature brain; imaging studies are often negative or nonspecific immediately after significant neuronal insults. The typical locations that are vulnerable to injury also differ in the neonatal period. In older childhood and adulthood, infarcts often occur in cortical watershed regions. In contrast, the basal ganglia and periventricular white matter motor tracts are particularly vulnerable in the immature brain; damage in these regions is associated with characteristic extrapyramidal palsies and spastic diplegia, respectively.[176]

Mechanisms of neuronal cell death are also qualitatively and quantitatively different in the immature CNS. As described previously, hypoxic-ischemic neuronal degeneration is mediated by two distinct pathways: excitotoxicity and neuronal apoptosis. The initial response to hypoxia/ischemia is excitotoxicity, and developmental changes in the distribution of glutamate-containing neurotransmitter circuits probably account, in part, for the specific vulnerability of specific regions of the brain to injury. Consistent with this, N-methyl D-aspartate NMDA receptors are known to be up-regulated in these areas, and rapid bulk movement of Ca^{2+} into neuronal cells has been documented in response to hypoxia in these cells.[177] After the initial burst of excitotoxic cell death, apoptosis appears to be responsible for the continuation and extension of characteristic patterns of brain injury. Because neurons, during the developmental period of synaptogenesis, are programmed to undergo apoptosis if they fail to achieve normal connectivity, the excitotoxic death of neurons that would normally provide synaptic input may account for the subsequent wave of apoptotic cell death.[178] Moreover, animal studies have shown that apoptotic mechanisms, as well as expression of proapoptotic proteins, are more vigorous in immature brain cells than in adults. At the molecular level, nuclear translocation of AIF, cytochrome c release, caspase-3 expression, and caspase activation are all increased several-fold in the brains of immature mice with experimental unilateral hypoxia/ischemia.[179] The influx of Ca^{2+} associated with the response to hypoxia-ischemia and with NMDA receptor activity may also induce expression of proapoptotic proteins of the Bcl-2 family, which are critical regulators of apoptosis in response to diverse stimuli.[180] Consistent with this, apoptosis was identified in over 50% of degenerating cells in several regions of the hypoxic-ischemic 7-day-old rat brain, compared with a ratio of only 1:6 of apoptosis to necrosis in an adult middle cerebral ischemia model.[181] The prominence of apoptosis in neurodegeneration in the immature brain suggests that it will be important to understand these processes to develop neuroprotective strategies. A combination of NMDA antagonists and caspase inhibitors may provide a longer therapeutic window than either alone.

Molecular and Cellular Basis of Pulmonary Hypertension

The cellular and molecular bases of pulmonary hypertension have been elucidated by recent advances in the understanding of mechanisms by which nitric oxide mediates vasodilation. In 1999, inhaled nitric oxide was approved for open-label use in the United States for term and near-term infants with persistent pulmonary hypertension. Nitric oxide has a very short half-life in gaseous or liquid media, and is inactivated on contact with hemoglobin. Therefore, the vasodilatory effects of this agent in the lung are localized there; no significant systemic vasoactivity or hypotension has been reported. Nitric oxide is known to increase the activity of soluble guanylyl cyclase, most likely by interaction with the heme moiety in the enzyme.[182] Guanylyl cyclase catalyzes the formation of cGMP, which acts directly on cell proteins as a second messenger. Regulation of cellular events by cGMP is accomplished by the interaction of the molecule with specific classes of target proteins, such as cyclic nucleotide-regulated protein kinases. cGMP-regulated protein kinases, or G kinases, are soluble or membrane-bound enzymes,[183] which are critical initiators of many intracellular signaling pathways. Effects mediated through activation of guanylyl cyclase and cGMP account, in part, for nitric oxide–mediated vasodilation, and the vasodilator actions of nitric oxide donors are blocked by inhibitors of soluble guanylyl cyclase.[184] Activation of G-kinases by cGMP may lower intracellular Ca^{2+} by phosphorylating and activating Ca^{2+}-ATPase or components associated with the transporter.[185] Because increased intracellular Ca^{2+} is required in the steps leading to the contraction-producing phosphorylation of myosin light chain, cGMP-mediated alteration of intracellular Ca^{2+} currents is one way by which nitric oxide mediates smooth muscle relaxation and vasodilation.[186]

Increased cGMP is also related to phosphorylation and activation of calcium-gated potassium channels in vascular smooth muscle cells. K^+-channel activation by nitric oxide is inhibited by blockade of G-kinases, and the activating effect of nitric oxide on K^+ channels in pulmonary artery smooth muscle cells can be simulated by pharmacologic activation of G-kinases.[187] It appears that cGMP-dependent activation of Ca^{2+}-activated K^+ channels is another mechanism by which nitric oxide mediates vasodilation. Treatment with iberiotoxin, an inhibitor of these channels, can reverse the relaxing effect of nitric oxide donors on lung smooth muscle cells. Interestingly, chronic hypoxia has been shown to reduce nitric oxide–mediated and cGMP-mediated activation of the Ca^{2+}-dependent K^+ channels, by decreasing phosphorylation of the channel.[188] This finding may underlie the phenomena of hypoxic vasoconstriction and of refractory pulmonary hypertension in newborns following *in utero* hypoxia. Nitric oxide can also activate K^+ channels directly, in the absence of cGMP or G-kinases, suggesting that the direct effect of nitric oxide on the K^+ channels is most likely a result of chemical modification of intracellular sulfhydryl groups.

Several other mechanisms have been described pertaining to cGMP-dependent or -independent alterations in vascular smooth muscle tone by nitric oxide. For example, exposure to nitric oxide down-regulates the number and binding activity of receptors for angiotensin II, a potent vasoconstrictor that is involved in the physiologic regulation of systemic and pulmonary blood pressure. Treatment of smooth muscle cells with nitric oxide donors also increases heme oxygenase (HO-1) mRNA transcription (three- to sixfold) and protein levels in a concentration and time-dependent manner. HO-1-mediated production of carbon monoxide is increased following exposure to endogenous or exogenous nitric oxide. Carbon monoxide, as a cellular mediator, induces guanylate cyclase and increased intracellular levels of cGMP, thereby providing a novel secondary mechanism by which nitric oxide can exert its effects.

Endothelin (ET-1) is an important mediator of endothelium-dependent regulation of vascular smooth muscle tone. Chronic treatment of vascular smooth muscle cells with endogenous or exogenous nitric oxide in culture produces a time- and dose-dependent increase in the number of endothelin receptors and in the affinity of the receptors for ET-1.[189] This effect can be mimicked by administration of cGMP or cAMP analogues. A physiologic balance between ET-1 activity and nitric oxide activity may be necessary in the maintenance of physiologic vasomotor tone in the lungs.

Tissue Response to Hypoxia

Oxygen sensing is important for the homeostasis and survival of mammalian cells. Physiologic studies have defined macroscopic, whole organism mechanisms by which the body regulates oxygen intake and delivery to tissues. For example, chemoreceptors in the heart and carotid circulation affect cardiac output and respiration, respectively. Vasoconstriction or dilation of specific vascular beds appears to be tightly regulated by the release of nitric oxide from stable circulating metabolites, such as protein nitrosothiols.[190] Therefore, alterations in the oxygen content of the blood or of perfusion to specific organs results in broad variations in the availability of oxygen to cells under physiologic and pathophysiologic conditions. Some tissues exhibit site-specific responses to hypoxia. For example, hypoxia induces a proinflammatory response in endothelial cells, manifested by increased production of cytokines, chemokines, tissue factor, and plasminogen activator inhibitor-1.[191] Activation of the transcription factor early growth response-1 (Egr-1) by hypoxia contributes to vascular remodeling that ultimately can lead to redistribution of blood flow and oxygen delivery. Exposure to hypoxia also induces expression of TGF-β2, a cytokine with potent regulatory effects on vascular inflammatory responses. In the retina and vitreous of the eye, alternate periods of hyper- and hypoxia lead to up-regulation of VEGF, an endothelial cell-specific mitogen that contributes to the onset of neovascular diseases, including retinopathy in premature babies. Hypoxia also directly reduces apoptosis of neutrophils and other leukocytes, allowing for their survival under relatively hypoxic conditions in tissue during inflammation.[192]

Because the response to hypoxia is so central to survival, it is now recognized that oxygen sensing involves universal cellular signaling pathways that trigger specific and nonspecific responses in all tissues. These include Smad proteins and EPAS-1/hypoxia-inducible factor 2.[193] The best described oxygen sensing pathway is regulation by the α dimers of the hypoxia-inducible factor (HIF) transcriptional complex. More than 40 HIF-1 target genes have been identified, encoding genes that play important roles in angiogenesis, vascular remodeling (including VEGF), erythropoiesis, glucose transport, glycolysis, iron transport, cell proliferation, and survival. The regulation of HIF-1α subunits occurs at both protein and transcriptional levels through the action of prolyl and asparaginyl hydroxylase enzymes. Under normoxic conditions, HIF-1α is maintained at very low levels by action of these enzymes. Reduction of hydroxylase activity by hypoxia results in increased protein stability and transcriptional activity of the HIF complex. HIF activation has been shown to be central in the antiapoptotic effects of hypoxia on neutrophils, probably through induction of NF-κB activity in these cells.[192]

Intracellular Signaling in Liver Injury

Liver injury in pediatric intensive care occurs most often in the setting of either toxic drug injury or hypoperfusion secondary to hemodynamic instability, with resulting tissue hypoxia. Liver toxicity from any cause appears to occur through two common pathways: inflammation and free radical injury/lipid peroxidation. Defining the specific contributions of these mechanisms in generating injury is important in devising strategies to prevent or treat liver

damage. Inflammation, it appears, makes the larger contribution to these disease processes. Sepsis/endotoxemia, ischemia-reperfusion injury, and certain drug-induced liver toxicities (including acetaminophen) are all characterized by systemic and local inflammation with recruitment of macrophages (Kupffer cells) into the hepatic vasculature,[194] either directly or through the activation of the complement. Activated Kupffer cells produce large amounts of inflammatory mediators, including TNF-α, IL-1, and complement factor C5a. These activate additional Kupffer cells and also attract and activate circulating neutrophils. Adhesion molecules on both neutrophils and endothelial cells are up-regulated, resulting in neutrophilia and extravasation of these cells into the parenchyma. Proteases and reactive intermediates generated by Kupffer cells and neutrophils can exacerbate or generate damage to hepatic tissue.

Postischemic oxidant stress during reperfusion can lead to cell death directly by lipid peroxidation. Oxidant stress-induced cell killing involves oxidation of pyridine nucleotides and accumulation of calcium in mitochondria, ultimately leading to loss of integrity of the cell and mitochondrial membranes. Reactive oxygen can also promote reperfusion injury through stimulation of the transcription factors, NF-κB and AP-1.[195] However, it appears that inflammation is the primary mechanism of hypoxia-reperfusion liver injury. Postischemic oxidant stress can enhance the expression of genes such as *TNF-α*, nitric oxide synthase, heme oxygenase-1, chemokines, and adhesion molecules. Kupffer cells and neutrophils release abundant reactive oxygen intermediates into tissues during hypoxia-reperfusion stress, and it has been demonstrated *in vivo* that these inflammatory cells can kill hepatocytes by reactive oxygen species. Release of both superoxide anion and nitric oxide by Kupffer cells may lead to formation of peroxynitrite, a highly reactive intermediate that contributes to peroxidation of lipid membranes. As reperfusion injury progresses, neutrophils are recruited into the liver vasculature, in which activation of β_2 integrins by chemotactic factors and up-regulation of ICAM-1 on endothelial cells leads to adherence, extravasation, and accumulation of these cells. Indeed, after the ongoing insult, liver damage can be attributed directly to release of proteases by activated neutrophils. Reactive oxygen intermediates may exert their effects on tissue, in part, by inhibition of the activity of antiproteases. Therefore, inflammation can be viewed as a common pathway to hepatocellular injury caused by hypoxia and reperfusion, as well as by infection or by drug toxicity.

The common endpoint of hepatocellular injury is cell death by either necrosis or apoptosis. Some groups have reported that apoptosis is the primary means of hepatocyte removal after injury. Consistent with this idea, it is known that bile acid–induced liver failure during cholestasis is associated with widespread hepatocellular apoptosis, induced, in large part, by the activation of cell-surface Fas receptors. Because several of the pathways of apoptosis are understood, a predominance of apoptotic cell death in the liver would suggest therapeutic interventions that might preserve liver tissue regardless of the initial insult. However, the role of apoptosis in hepatocellular death has been controversial. Some groups have shown that >90% of cells die by necrosis during ischemia-reperfusion, a mechanism that is less compatible with pharmacologic prevention.[196] The final step in the pathogenesis of liver damage is the induction of fibrogenic cytokines, such as TGF-β and IL-6, which lead to the common endpoint of liver cirrhosis.

In this chapter, we have demonstrated that physiology and pathophysiology in pediatric critical care are best understood at the cellular level. Increasing knowledge of cell structure and function has increased the apparent complexity of these processes. However, common patterns are evident in the mechanisms of signaling and of regulating cell survival in response to infection, hypoxia, or tissue injury. The tools of molecular biology (e.g., monoclonal antibodies, genomic, and proteomic analysis) have improved dramatically in recent years. Major advances in the practice of critical care medicine in the future are most likely to originate in the cell biology laboratory.

REFERENCES

1. Singer SJ, Nicolson GL. The fluid mosaic model of the structure of cell membranes. *Science.* 1972;175:720–731.
2. Van Meer G, Burger KN. Sphingolipid trafficking—sorted out? *Trends Cell Biol.* 1992;2:332–337.
3. Van Driel R, Fransz PF, Verschure PJ. The eukaryotic genome: A system regulated at different hierarchical levels. *J Cell Sci.* 2003;116:4067–4075.
4. Spiegelman BM, Heinrich R. Biological control through regulated transcriptional activators. *Cell.* 2004;119:157–167.
5. Boyer BB, Barnes BM, Lowell BB, et al. Differential regulation of uncoupling protein gene homologues in multiple tissues of hibernating ground squirrels. *Am J Physiol.* 1998; 275:R1232–R1238.
6. Naviaux RK, Nyhan WL, Barshop BA, et al. Mitochondrial DNA polymerase gamma deficiency and mtDNA depletion in a child with Alpers' syndrome. *Ann Neurol.* 1999;45:54–58.
7. Okado-Matsumoto A, Fridovich I. Amyotrophic lateral sclerosis: A proposed mechanism. *Proc Natl Acad Sci U S A.* 2002;99:9010–9014.
8. Yao D, Gu Z, Nakamura T, et al. Nitrosative stress linked to sporadic Parkinson's disease: S-nitrosylation of parkin regulates its E3 ubiquitin ligase activity. *Proc Natl Acad Sci U S A.* 2004;101:10810–10814.
9. Sahenk Z, Chen L, Mendell JR. Effects of PMP22 duplication and deletions on the axonal cytoskeleton. *Ann Neurol.* 1999;45:16–24.
10. Verleur N, Hettema EH, van Roermund CW, et al. Transport of activated fatty acids by the peroxisomal ATP-binding-cassette transporter Pxa2 in a semi-intact yeast cell system. *Eur J Biochem.* 1997;249:657–661.
11. Weng G, Bhalla US, Iyengar R. Complexity in biological signaling systems. *Science.* 1999;284:92–96.
12. Jordan JD, Landau EM, Iyengar R. Signaling networks: The origins of cellular multitasking. *Cell.* 2000;103:193–200.
13. Campbell N, Reece J. *Biology,* 6th ed. Menlo Park, CA: Benjamin/Cummings Publishing Company; 2002.
14. Lodish H, Berk A, Matsudaira P, et al. *Molecular Cell Biology,* 4th ed: W. H. Freeman and Company; 2000.
15. Baulieu EE, Kelly PA. *Hormones: From molecules to disease.* London: Chapman & Hall; 1990.
16. Barritt GJ. *Communication within animal cells.* Oxford: Oxford Science Publications; 1992.
17. Wallis M, Howell SL, Taylor KW, eds. *The biochemistry of polypeptide hormones.* New York: John Wiley and Sons; 1986.
18. Wilson JD, Foster DW, Kronenberg HM, et al. *Williams textbook of endocrinology,* 9th ed Philadelphia, PA: WB Saunders; 1998.
19. Kimball JW. Kimball's Biology Pages http://users.rcn.com/jkimball.ma.ultranet/BiologyPages, October 2004.
20. Russwurm M, Koesling D. Guanylyl cyclase: NO hits its target. *Biochem Soc Symp.* 2004;71:51–63.
21. Alderton WK, Cooper CE, Knowles RG. Nitric oxide synthases: Structure, function and inhibition. *Biochem J.* 2001; 357: 593–615.
22. Massion PB, Feron O, Dessy C, et al. Nitric oxide and cardiac function: Ten years after, and continuing. *Circ Res.* 2003;93(5): 388–398. Review.
23. Kelly RA, Balligand JL, Smith TW. Nitric oxide and cardiac function. *Circ Res.* 1996;79:363–380.
24. Shah AM, MacCarthy PA. Paracrine and autocrine effects of nitric oxide on myocardial function. *Pharmacol Ther.* 2000;86: 49–86.
25. Brutsaert DL. Cardiac endothelial-myocardial signaling: Its role in cardiac growth, contractile performance, and rhythmicity. *Physiol Rev.* 2003;83:59–115.
26. Casadei B, Sears CE. Nitric-oxide-mediated regulation of cardiac contractility and stretch responses. *Prog Biophys Mol Biol.* 2003;82:67–80.
27. Moncada S, Erusalimsky JD. Does nitric oxide modulate mitochondrial energy generation and apoptosis? *Nat Rev Mol Cell Biol.* 2002;3:214–220.
28. Trochu JN, Bouhour JB, Kaley G, et al. Role of endothelium-derived nitric oxide in the regulation of cardiac oxygen metabolism: Implications in health and disease. *Circ Res.* 2000; 87:1108–1117.
29. Massion PB, Balligand JL. Modulation of cardiac contraction, relaxation and rate by the endothelial nitric oxide synthase (eNOS): Lessons from genetically modified mice. *J Physiol.* 2003;546:63–75.
30. Mungrue IN, Gros R, You X, et al. Cardiomyocyte overexpression of iNOS in mice results in peroxynitrite generation, heart block, and sudden death. *J Clin Invest.* 2002;109:735–743.
31. Kostenis E, Conklin BR, Wess J. Molecular basis of receptor/G protein coupling selectivity studied by coexpression of wild type and mutant m2 muscarinic receptors with mutant G alpha(q) subunits. *Biochemistry.* 1997;36(6):1487–1495.
32. Hausdorff WP, Caron MG, Lefkowitz RJ. Turning off the signal: Desensitization of beta-adrenergic receptor function. *FASEB J.* 1990;4(11):2881–2889. Review. Erratum in: *FASEB J* 1990;4(12):3049.
33. Krupnick JG, Benovic JL. The role of receptor kinases and arrestins in G protein–coupled receptor regulation. *Annu Rev Pharmacol Toxicol.* 1998;38:289–319. Review.
34. Weiss ER, Raman D, Shirakawa S, et al. The cloning of GRK7, a candidate cone opsin kinase, from cone- and rod-dominant mammalian retinas. *Mol Vis.* 1998;4:27.
35. Pitcher JA, Freedman NJ, Lefkowitz RJ. G protein–coupled receptor kinases. *Annu Rev Biochem.* 1998;67:653–692. Review
36. Palczewski K. GTP-binding-protein-coupled receptor kinases-two mechanistic models. *Eur J Biochem.* 1997;248(2):261–269. Review.
37. Premont RT, Inglese J, Lefkowitz RJ. Protein kinases that phosphorylate activated G protein–coupled receptors. *FASEB J.* 1995;9(2):175–182. Review.
38. Jaber M, Koch WJ, Rockman H, et al. Essential role of beta-adrenergic receptor kinase 1 in cardiac development and function. *Proc Natl Acad Sci U S A.* 1996;93(23):12974–12979.
39. Thierry Métayé, Hélène Gibelin, Rémy Perdrisot, et al. Pathophysiological roles of G protein–coupled receptor kinases. *Cell Signal.* 2005;17(8):917–928.

40. Ungerer M, Bohm M, Elce JS, et al. Altered expression of beta-adrenergic receptor kinase and beta 1-adrenergic receptors in the failing human heart. *Circulation*. 1993;87(2):454–463.

41. Rockman HA, Chien KR, Choi D-J, et al. Expression of a β-adrenergic receptor kinase 1 inhibitor prevents the development of myocardial failure in gene-targeted mice. *Proc Natl Acad Sci U S A*. 1998;95(12):7000–7005.

42. Doyle JL, Stubbs L. Ataxia, arrhythmia and ion-channel gene defects. *Trends Genet*. 1998;14(3):92–98. Review.

43. Cooper EC, Jan LY. Ion channel genes and human neurological disease: Recent progress, prospects, and challenges. *Proc Natl Acad Sci U S A*. 1999;96(9):4759–4766. Review.

44. Hulme JT, Scheuer T, Catterall WA. Regulation of cardiac ion channels by signaling complexes: Role of modified leucine zipper motifs. *J Mol Cell Cardiol*. 2004;37(3):625–631. Review.

45. Reuter H. Calcium channel modulation by neurotransmitters, enzymes and drugs. *Nature*. 1983;**301**:569–574.

46. Catterall WA. Structure and regulation of voltage-gated calcium channels. *Annu Rev Cell Dev Biol*. 2000;16:521–555.

47. Tsien RW, Bean BP, Hess P, et al. Mechanisms of calcium channel modulation by beta-adrenergic agents and dihydropyridine calcium agonists. *J Mol Cell Cardiol*. 1986;18:691–710.

48. Marks AR. Ryanodine receptors, FKBP12, and heart failure. *Front Biosci*. 2002;7:d970–d977.

49. Clancy CE, Kass RS. Defective cardiac ion channels: From mutations to clinical syndromes. *J Clin Invest*. 2002;110:1075–1077.

50. Snyders DJ. Structure and function of cardiac potassium channels. *Cardiovasc Res*. 1999;42:377–390.

51. Coetzee W, Amarillo Y, Chiu J, et al. Molecular diversity of K$^+$ channels. *Ann N Y Acad Sci*. 1999;868:233–285.

52. Nerbonne JM. Molecular basis of functional voltage-gated K$^+$ channel diversity in the mammalian myocardium. *J Physiol*. 2000;525:285–298.

53. Roden DM, Balser JR, George AL Jr, et al. Cardiac ion channels. *Annu Rev Physiol*. 2002;64:431–475.

54. Tamargo J. Drug-induced torsade de pointes: From molecular biology to bedside. *Jpn J Pharmacol*. 2000;83:1–19.

55. Clancy CE, Kurokawa J, Tateyama M, et al. K$^+$ channel structure–activity relationships and mechanisms of drug-induced QT prolongation. *Annu Rev Pharmacol Toxicol*. 2003;43:441–461.

56. Näbauer M, Kääb S. Potassium channel downregulation in heart failure. *Cardiovasc Res*. 1998;37:324–334.

57. Pinto JM, Boyden PA. Electrical remodeling in ischemia and infarction. *Cardiovasc Res*. 1999;42:284–297.

58. Tomaselli GF, Marbán E. Electrophysiological remodeling in hypertrophy and heart failure. *Cardiovasc Res*. 1999;42:270–283.

59. Fantl WJ, Johnson DE, Williams LT. Signalling by receptor tyrosine kinases. *Annu Rev Biochem*. 1993;62:453–481. Review. No abstract available

60. Hubbard SR, Till JH. Protein tyrosine kinase structure and function. *Annu Rev Biochem*. 2000;69:373–398. Review.

61. Hubbard SR. Protein tyrosine kinases: Autoregulation and small-molecule inhibition. *Curr Opin Struct Biol*. 2002;12(6):735–741. Review.

62. Hanke JH, Gardner PJ, Dow RL, et al. Discovery of a novel, potent, and Src family-selective tyrosine kinase inhibitor. *J Biol Chem*. 1996;271:695–701.

63. Kovalenko M, Gazit A, Bohmer A, et al. Selective platelet derived growth factor receptor kinase blockers reverse sis-transformation. *Cancer Res*. 1994;54:6106–6114.

64. Levitzki A. Protein tyrosine kinase inhibitors as therapeutic agents. *Pharmacol Ther*. 1999;82:231–239.

65. Levitzki A, Gazit A. Tyrosine kinase inhibition: An approach to drug development. *Science*. 1995;257:1782–1788.

66. Mohammadi BK, McMahon G, Sun L, et al. Structures of the tyrosine kinase domain of fibroblast growth factor receptor complex with inhibitors. *Science*. 1997;276:955–960.

67. Osherov N, Levitzki A. Epidermal growth factor dependent activation of Src family kinases. *Eur J Biochem*. 1994;225:1047–1053.

68. Rodrigues GA, Park M. Oncogenic activation of tyrosine kinases. *Curr Opin Genet Dev*. 1994;4(1):15–24.

69. Hunter T. Oncoprotein networks. *Cell*. 1997;88(3):333–346.

70. Levitzki A, Gazit A. Tyrosine kinase inhibition: An approach to drug development. *Science*. 1995;267(5205):1782–1788.

71. Zhao YY, Sawyer DR, Baliga RR, et al. Neuregulins promote survival and growth of cardiac myocytes. Persistence of ErbB2 and ErbB4 expression in neonatal and adult ventricular myocytes. *J Biol Chem*. 1998;273:10261–10269.

72. Rohrbach S, Yan X, Weinberg EO, et al. Neuregulin in cardiac hypertrophy in rats with aortic stenosis. Differential expression of erbB2 and erbB4 receptors. *Circulation*. 1999;100:407–412.

73. Lee KF, Simon H, Chen H, et al. Requirement for neuregulin receptor erbB2 in neural and cardiac development. *Nature*. 1995;378:394–398.

74. Ewer MS, Gibbs HR, Swafford J, et al. Cardiotoxicity in patients receiving transtuzamab (Herceptin): Primary toxicity, synergistic or sequential stress, or surveillance artifact? *Semin Oncol*. 1999;26:96–101.

75. Uray IP, Connelly JH, Thomazy V, et al. Left ventricular unloading alters receptor tyrosine kinase expression in the failing human heart. *J Heart Lung Transplant*. 2002;21(7):771–782.

76. Platanias LC. Map kinase signaling pathways and hematologic malignancies. *Blood*. 2003;101(12):4667–4679. Epub 2003 Mar 6. Review.

77. Dong C, Davis RJ, Flavell RA. MAP kinases in the immune response. *Annu Rev Immunol*. 2002;20:55–72.

78. Robinson MJ, Cobb MH. Mitogen-activated protein kinase pathways. *Curr Opin Cell Biol*. 1997;9:180–186.

79. Li Z, Jiang Y, Ulevitch RJ, et al. The primary structure of p38 γ: A new member of the p38 group of MAP kinases. *Biochem Biophys Res Commun* 1996;228:334–340.

80. Chang L, Karin M. Mammalian MAP kinase signaling cascades. *Nature*. 2001;410:37–40.

81. Derijard B, Hibi M, Wu IH, et al. JNK1: A protein kinase stimulated by UV light and Ha-Ras that binds and phosphorylates the c-Jun activation domain. *Cell*. 1994;76:1025–1037.

82. Abe MK, Kuo W, Hershenson MB, et al. Extracellular signal-regulated kinase 7 (ERK7), a novel ERK with a C-terminal domain that regulates its activity, its cellular localization, and cell growth. *Mol Cell Biol*. 1999;19:1301–1312.

83. Zhou G, Bao ZQ, Dixon JE. Components of a new human protein kinase signal transduction pathway. *J Biol Chem*. 1995;270:12665–12669.

84. Schaeffer HJ, Weber MJ. Mitogen-activated protein kinases: Specific messages from ubiquitous messengers. *Mol Cell Biol*. 1999;19(4):2435–2444.

85. Marshall CJ. Specificity of receptor tyrosine kinase signaling: Transient versus sustained extracellular signal-regulated kinase activation. *Cell*. 1995;80:179–185.

86. Smith A, Ramos-Morales F, Ashworth A, et al. A role for JNK/SAPK in proliferation, but not apoptosis, of IL-3-dependent cells. *Curr Biol*. 1997;7:893–896.

87. Weston CR, Lambright DG, Davis RJ. Map kinase signaling specificity. *Science*. 2002;296:2345–2347.

88. Enslen H, Davis RJ. Regulation of MAP kinases by docking domains. *Biol Cell*. 2001;93:5–14.

89. Dent P, Haser W, Haystead TA, et al. Activation of mitogen-activated protein kinase kinase by v-Raf in NIH 3T3 cells and in vitro. *Science*. 1992;257:1404–1407.

90. Kyriakis JM, App H, Zhang XF, et al. Raf-1 activates MAP kinase-kinase. *Nature*. 1992;358:417–421.

91. Minden A, Lin A, McMahon M, et al. Differential activation of ERK and JNK mitogen-activated protein kinases by Raf-1 and MEKK. *Science*. 1994;266:1719–1723.

92. Catling AD, Schaeffer HJ, Reuter CW, et al. A proline-rich sequence unique to MEK1 and MEK2 is required for Raf binding and regulates MEK function. *Mol Cell Biol*. 1995;15:5214–5225.

93. Arnold M. Katz calcium channel diversity in the cardiovascular system August. *J Am Coll Cardiol*. 1996;28(2):522–529.

94. Ehrlich BE, Watras J. Inositol 1,4,5-trisphosphate activates a channel from smooth muscle sarcoplasmic reticulum. *Nature*. 1988;336:583–586.

95. Christopher G. Proud. Ras, PI3-kinase and mTOR signaling in cardiac hypertrophy. *Cardiovasc Res*. 2004;63(3):403–413.

96. Frey N, Olson EN. Cardiac hypertrophy: The good, the bad, and the ugly. *Annu Rev Physiol.* 2003;65:45–79.

97. Molkentin JD, Dorn GW. Cytoplasmic signaling pathways that regulate cardiac hypertrophy. *Annu Rev Physiol.* 2001; 63:391–426.

98. Hannan RD, Jenkins A, Jenkins AK, et al. Cardiac hypertrophy: A matter of translation. *Clin Exp Pharmacol Physiol.* 2003; 30:517–527.

99. Bueno OF, De Windt LJ, Tymitz KM, et al. TheK1-ERK1/2 signaling pathway promotes compensated cardiac hypertrophy in transgenic mice. *EMBO J.* 2000;19:6341–6350.

100. Hunter JJ, Tanaka N, Rockman HA, et al. Ventricular expression of a MLC-2v-ras fusion gene induces cardiac hypertrophy and selective diastolic dysfunction in transgenic mice. *J Biol Chem.* 1995;270:23173–23178.

101. Shioi T, Kang PM, Douglas PS, et al. The conserved phosphoinositide 3-kinase pathway determines heart size in mice. *EMBO J.* 2000;19:2537–2548.

102. Philchenkov A. Caspases: Potential targets for regulating cell death. *J Cell Mol Med.* 2004;8:432–444.

103. Abraham MC, Shaham S. Death without caspases, caspases without death. *Trends Cell Biol.* 2004;14:184–193.

104. Boyd CS, Cadenas E. Nitric oxide and cell signaling pathways in mitochondrial-dependent apoptosis. *Biol Chem.* 2002;383:411–423.

105. Lorenzo HK, Santos SA. Mitochondrial effectors in caspase-independent cell death. *FEBS Lett.* 2004;557:14–20.

106. Pierce MR, Bancalari E. The role of inflammation in the pathogenesis of bronchopulmonary dysplasia. *Pediatr Pulmonol.* 1995;19:371–378.

107. Uhlig S. Ventilation-induced lung injury and mechanotransduction: Stretching it too far? *Am J Physiol Lung Cell Mol Physiol.* 2002;282:L892–L896.

108. Donn SM, Sinha SK. Can mechanical ventilation strategies reduce chronic lung disease? *Semin Neonatol.* 2003;8:441–448.

109. Ogden BE, Murphy SA, Saunders GC, et al. Neonatal lung neutrophils and elastase/proteinase inhibitor imbalance. *Am Rev Respir Dis.* 1984;130:817–821.

110. Pierce MR, Bancalari E. The role of inflammation in the pathogenesis of bronchopulmonary dysplasia. *Pediatr Pulmonol.* 1995;19:371–378.

111. Parsey MV, Kaneko D, Shenkar R, et al. Neutrophil apoptosis in the lung after hemorrhage or endotoxemia: Apoptosis and migration are independent of interleukin-1. *Chest.* 1999;116: 67S–68S.

112. Pryjma J, Kaszuba-Zwoinska J, Pawlik J, et al. Alveolar macrophages of children suffering from recurrent infections of respiratory tract are less efficient in eliminating apoptotic neutrophils. *Pediatr Pulmonol.* 1999;27:167–173.

113. Savill J. Apoptosis in resolution of inflammation. *J Leukoc Biol.* 1997;61:375–380.

114. Haslett C. Granulocyte apoptosis and its role in the resolution and control of lung inflammation. *Am J Respir Crit Care Med.* 1999;160:S5–S11.

115. Whyte MK, Meagher LC, MacDermot J, et al. Impairment of function in aging neutrophils is associated with apoptosis. *J Immunol.* 1993;150:5124–5134.

116. Dransfield I, Buckle AM, Savill JS, et al. Neutrophil apoptosis is associated with a reduction in CD16 (Fc gamma RIII) expression. *J Immunol.* 1994;153:1254–1263.

117. Haslett C, Savill JS, Whyte MK, et al. Granulocyte apoptosis and the control of inflammation. *Philos Trans R Soc Lond B Biol Sci.* 1994;345:327–333.

118. Meagher LC, Savill JS, Baker A, et al. Phagocytosis of apoptotic neutrophils does not induce macrophage release of thromboxane B2. *J Leukoc Biol.* 1992;52:269–273.

119. Savill J, Hogg N, Ren Y, et al. Thrombospondin cooperates with CD36 and the vitronectin receptor in macrophage recognition of neutrophils undergoing apoptosis. *J Clin Invest.* 1992;90:1513–1522.

120. Fadok VA, Savill JS, Haslett C, et al. Different populations of macrophages use either the vitronectin receptor or the phosphatidylserine receptor to recognize and remove apoptotic cells. *J Immunol.* 1992;149:4029–4035.

121. Hussain N, Wu F, Zhu L, et al. Neutrophil apoptosis during the development and resolution of oleic acid-induced acute lung injury in the rat. *Am J Respir Cell Mol Biol.* 1998;19: 867–874.

122. Grigg JM, Savill JS, Sarraf C, et al. Neutrophil apoptosis and clearance from neonatal lungs. *Lancet.* 1991;338:720–722.

123. Rindfleisch MS, Hasday JD, Taciak V, et al. Potential role of interleukin-1 in the development of bronchopulmonary dysplasia. *J Interferon Cytokine Res.* 1996;16:365–373.

124. Kotecha S. Cytokines in chronic lung disease of prematurity. *Eur J Pediatr.* 1996;155:S14–S17.

125. Bagchi A, Viscardi RM, Taciak V, et al. Increased activity of interleukin-6 but not tumor necrosis factor-in lung lavage of premature infants is associated with the development of bronchopulmonary dysplasia. *Pediatr Res.* 1994;36: 244–252.

126. Lee A, Whyte MK, Haslett C. Inhibition of apoptosis and prolongation of neutrophil functional longevity by inflammatory mediators. *J Leukoc Biol.* 1993;54:283–288.

127. Daffern PJ, Jagels MA, Hugli TE. Multiple epithelial cell-derived factors enhance neutrophil survival. Regulation by glucocorticoids and tumor necrosis factor-alpha. *Am J Respir Cell Mol Biol.* 1999;21:259–267.

128. Kasahara Y, Iwai K, Yachie A, et al. Involvement of reactive oxygen intermediates in spontaneous and CD95 (Fas/APO-1)-mediated apoptosis of neutrophils. *Blood.* 1997;89:1748–1753.

129. Cox G. IL-10 enhances resolution of pulmonary inflammation in vivo by promoting apoptosis of neutrophils. *Am J Physiol.* 1996;271:L566–571.

130. Liles WC, Kiener PA, Ledbetter JA, et al. Differential expression of Fas (CD95) and Fas ligand on normal human phagocytes: Implications for the regulation of apoptosis in neutrophils. *J Exp Med.* 1996;184:429–440.

131. Wahl SM, Costa GL, Mizel DE, et al. Role of transforming growth factor-in the pathophysiology of chronic inflammation. *J Periodontol.* 1993;64:450–455.

132. Haufel T, Dorfmann S, Hanusch J, et al. Three distinct roles for TGF-during intercellular induction of apoptosis: A review. *Anticancer Res.* 1999;19:105–112.

133. Weinmann P, Gaehtgens P, Walzog B. Bcl-Xl- and Bax-alpha-mediated regulation of apoptosis of human neutrophils via caspase-3. *Blood.* 1999;93:3106–3115.

134. Ohta K, Iwai K, Kasahara Y, et al. Immunoblot analysis of cellular expression of Bcl-2 family proteins, Bcl-2, Bax, Bcl-X and Mcl-1, in human peripheral blood and lymphoid tissues. *Int Immunol.* 1995;7:1817–1825.

135. Santos-Beneit AM, Mollinedo F. Expression of genes involved in initiation, regulation, and execution of apoptosis in human neutrophils and during neutrophil differentiation of HL-60 cells. *J Leukoc Biol.* 2000;67:712–724.

136. Leuenroth SJ, Grutkoski PS, Ayala A, et al. The loss of Mcl-1 expression in human polymorphonuclear leukocytes promotes apoptosis. *J Leukoc Biol.* 2000;68:158–166.

137. Watson RW, Rotstein OD, Parodo J, et al. Impaired apoptotic death signaling in inflammatory lung neutrophils is associated with decreased expression of interleukin-1 converting enzyme family proteases (caspases). *Surgery.* 1997;122:163–171.

138. Klein JB, Rane MJ, Scherzer JA, et al. Granulocyte-macrophage colony-stimulating factor delays neutrophil constitutive apoptosis through phosphoinositide 3-kinase and extracellular signal-regulated kinase pathways. *J Immunol.* 2000;164:4286–4291.

139. Aoshiba K, Yasui S, Hayashi M, et al. Role of p38-mitogen-activated protein kinase in spontaneous apoptosis of human neutrophils. *J Immunol.* 1999;162:1692–1700.

140. Abraham E. NF-κB activation. *Crit Care Med.* 2000;28: N100–N104.

141. Marte BM, Downward J. PKB/Akt: Connecting phosphoinositide 3-kinase to cell survival and beyond. *Trends Biochem Sci.* 1997;22:355–358.

142. Ward C, Chilvers ER, Lawson MF, et al. NF-κB activation is a critical regulator of human granulocyte apoptosis in vitro. *J Biol Chem.* 1999;274:4309–4318.

143. Nolan B, Collette H, Baker S, et al. Inhibition of neutrophil apoptosis after severe trauma is NF-κB-dependent. *J Trauma.* 2000;48:599–604.

144. Wang CY, Mayo MW, Korneluk RG, et al. NF-κB antiapoptosis: Induction of TRAF1 and TRAF2 and c-IAP1 and c-IAP2 to suppress caspase-8 activation. *Science.* 1998;281:1680–1683.

145. Webster GA, Perkins ND. Transcriptional cross talk between NF-kappaB and p53. *Mol Cell Biol.* 1999;19:3485–3495.

146. Yoshidome H, Kato A, Edwards MJ, et al. Interleukin-10 inhibits pulmonary NF-kappaB activation and lung injury induced by hepatic ischemia-reperfusion. *Am J Physiol.* 1999;277:L919–923.

147. Nolan B, Duffy A, Paquin L, et al. Mitogen-activated protein kinases signal inhibition of apoptosis in lipopolysaccharide-stimulated neutrophils. *Surgery.* 1999;126:406–412.

148. Frasch SC, Nick JA, Fadok VA, et al. p38 mitogen-activated protein kinase-dependent and -independent intracellular signal transduction pathways leading to apoptosis in human neutrophils. *J Biol Chem.* 1998;273:8389–8397.

149. Leuenroth SJ, Grutkoski PS, Ayala A, et al. Suppression of PMN apoptosis by hypoxia is dependent on Mcl-1 and MAPK activity. *Surgery.* 2000;128:171–177.

150. Pongracz J, Webb P, Wang K, et al. Spontaneous neutrophil apoptosis involves caspase 3-mediated activation of protein kinase C-delta. *J Biol Chem.* 1999;274:37329–37334.

151. Goh J, Godson C, Brady HR, et al. Lipoxins: Pro-resolution lipid mediators in intestinal inflammation. *Gastroenterology.* 2003;124:1043–1054.

152. Serhan CN, Hamberg M, Samuelsson B. Lipoxins: Novel series of biologically active compounds formed from arachidonic acid in human leukocytes. *Proc Natl Acad Sci U S A.* 1984;81:5335–5339.

153. Serhan CN, Levy B. Novel pathways and endogenous mediators in anti-inflammation and resolution. *Chem Immunol Allergy.* 2003;83:115–145.

154. Chinetti G, Fruchart JC, Staels B. Peroxisome proliferator-activated receptors (PPARs): Nuclear receptors at the crossroads between lipid metabolism and inflammation. *Inflamm Res.* 2000;49:497–505.

155. Ijpenberg A, Jeannin E, Wahli W, et al. Polarity and specific sequence requirements of peroxisome proliferator-activated receptor (PPAR)/retinoid X receptor heterodimer binding to DNA. *J Biol Chem.* 1997;272:20108–20117.

156. Chinetti G, Griglio S, Antonucci M, et al. Activation of proliferator-activated receptors α and γ induces apoptosis of human monocytes-derived macrophages. *J Biol Chem.* 1998;273:26673–25580.

157. Delerive P, DeBosscher K, Besnard S, et al. PPARα negatively regulates the vascular wall inflammatory gene response by negative cross-talk with transcription factors NF-κB and AP-1. *J Biol Chem.* 1999;274:32048–32054.

158. Bishop-Bailey D, Wray J. Peroxisome proliferator-activated receptors: A critical review on endogenous pathways for ligand generation. *Prostaglandins Other Lipid Mediat.* 2003;71:1–22.

159. Devchand PR, Keller H, Peters JM, et al. The PPARα-leukotriene B4 pathway to inflammatory control. *Nature.* 1996;384:39–43.

160. Roberts RA, James NH, Woodyatt NJ, et al. Evidence for the suppression of apoptosis by the peroxisome proliferator activated receptor-α (PPAR-α). *Carcinogenesis.* 1998;19:43–48.

161. Ricote M, Li AC, Willson TM, et al. The peroxisome proliferator-activated receptor-γ is a negative regulator of macrophage activation. *Nature.* 1998;391:79–82.

162. Jiang C, Ting AT, Seed B. PPAR-γ agonists inhibit production of monocyte inflammatory cytokines. *Nature.* 1998;391:82–86.

163. Huang JT, Welch JS, Ricote M, et al. Interleukin 4-dependent production of PPAR-γ ligands in macrophages by 12/15-lipoxygenase. *Nature.* 1999;400:378–382.

164. Guimaraes S, Moura D. Vascular adrenoceptors: An update. *Pharmacol Rev.* 2001;53:319.

165. Steinberg SF. The molecular basis for distinct beta-adrenergic receptor subtype actions in cardiomyocytes. *Circ Res.* 1999;85:1101.

166. Kamp TJ, Hell JW. Regulation of cardiac L-type calcium channels by protein kinase and protein kinase C. *Circ Res.* 2000;87:1095.

167. Michelotti GA, Price DT, Schwinn DA. Alpha 1-adrenergic receptor regulation: Basic science and clinical implications. *Pharmacol Ther.* 2000;88:281.

168. Somlyo AP, Somlyo AV. Signal transduction and regulation in smooth muscle. *Nature.* 1994;372:231.

169. Anderson GO, Qvigstad E, Schiander I, et al. AR induced positive inotropic response in heart is dependent on myosin light chain phosphorylation. *Am J Physiol Heart Circ Physiol.* 2002;283:H1471.

170. Jackson E. Vasopressin and other agents affecting the renal conservation of water. In: Hardman JG, Limbird LE, eds. *Goodman & Gilman's the pharmacologic basis of therapeutics.* New York: McGraw-Hill; 2001.

171. Notterman D, Kelly M, Sturgill M. Pharmacology of the cardiovascular system. In: Fuhrman B, Zimmerman J, eds. *Pediatric critical care,* 3rd ed. St. Louis: Mosby; 2005.

172. Raghupathi R. Cell death mechanisms following traumatic brain injury. *Brain Pathol.* 2004;14:215–222.

173. Cole K, Perez-Polo JR. Neuronal trauma model: In search of Thanatos. *Int J Dev Neurosci.* 2004;22:485–496.

174. Annunziato L, Pignataro G, Di Renzo GF. Pharmacology of brain Na+/Ca2+ exchanger: From molecular biology to therapeutic perspectives. *Pharmacol Rev.* 2004;56:633–654.

175. Sattler R, Tymianski M. Molecular mechanisms of calcium-dependent excitotoxicity. *J Mol Med.* 2000;78:3–13.

176. Johnston MV, Trescher WH, Ishida A, et al. Neurobiology of hypoxic-ischemic injury in the developing brain. *Pediatr Res.* 2001;49:734–741.

177. Johnston MV, Nakajima W, Hagberg H. Mechanisms of hypoxic neurodegeneration in the developing brain. *Neuroscientist.* 2002;8:212–220.

178. Young C, Tenkova T, Dikranian K, et al. Excitotoxic versus apoptotic mechanisms of neuronal cell death in perinatal hypoxia/ischemia. *Curr Mol Med.* 2004;4:77–85.

179. Zhu C, Wang X, Xu F, et al. The influence of age on apoptotic and other mechanisms of cell death after cerebral hypoxia-ischemia. *Cell Death Differ.* 2005;12:162–176.

180. Delivoria-Papadopoulos M, Mishra OP. Nuclear mechanisms of hypoxic cerebral injury in the newborn. *Clin Perinatol.* 2004;31:91–105.

181. Li Y, Sharov VJ, Jiang N, et al. Intact, injured, necrotic, and apoptotic cells after focal cerebral ischemia in the rat. *J Neurol Sci.* 1998;156:119–132.

182. Murad F. Regulation of cytosolic guanylyl cyclase by nitric oxide: The NO-cyclic GMP signal transduction system. *Adv Pharmacol.* 1994;26:19–33.

183. Lincoln TM, Cornwell TL. Intracellular cyclic GMP receptor proteins. *FASEB J.* 1993;7:328–338.

184. Moro MA, Russel RJ, Cellek S, et al. cGMP mediates the vascular and platelet actions of nitric oxide: Confirmation using and inhibitor of soluble guanylyl cyclase. *Proc Natl Acad Sci U S A.* 1996;93:1480–1485.

185. Schmidt HW, Lohman SM, Walter U. The nitric oxide and cGMP signal transduction system: Regulation and mechanism of action. *Biochim Biophys Acta.* 1993;1178:153–175.

186. Murad F. Cyclic guanosine monophosphate as a mediator of vasodilation. *J Clin Invest.* 1986;78:1–5.

187. Hampl V, Huang JM, Weir EK, et al. Activation of the cGMP-dependent protein kinase mimics the stimulatory effect of nitric oxide and cGMP on calcium-gated potassium channels. *Physiol Res.* 1995;44:39–44.

188. Peng W, Hoidal JR, Karwande SV, et al. Effect of chronic hypoxia on K+ channels: Regulation in human pulmonary vascular smooth muscle cells. *Am J Physiol.* 1997;272:C1271–C1278.

189. Redmond EM, Cahill PA, Hodges R, et al. Regulation of endothelin receptors by nitric oxide in cultured rat vascular smooth muscle cells. *J Cell Physiol.* 1996;166:469–479.

190. Shvedova AA, Tyurina YY, Gorbunov NV, et al. tert-Butyl hydroperoxide/hemoglobin-induced oxidative stress and damage to vascular smooth muscle cells: Different effects of nitric oxide and nitrosothiols. *Biochem Pharmacol.* 1999;57:989–1001.

191. Akman HO, Zhang H, Siddiqui MAQ, et al. Response to hypoxia involves transforming growth factor-β2 and Smad proteins in human endothelial cells. *Blood.* 2001;98:3324–3331.

192. Walmsley SR, Print C, Farahi N, et al. Hypoxia-induced neutrophil survival is mediated by HIF–1α dependent NF–kB activity. *J Exp Med.* 2005;201:105–115.

193. Fink MP. Research: Advances in cell biology relevant to critical illness. *Curr Opin Crit Care.* 2004;10:279–291.

194. Jaeschke H, Gores GJ, Cederbaum AI, et al. Mechanisms of hepatotoxicity. *Toxicol Sci.* 2002;65:166–176.

195. Fan C, Zwacka RM, Engelhardt JF. Therapeutic approaches for ischemia/reperfusion injury in the liver. *J Mol Med.* 1999;77:577–592.

196. Jaeschke H. Molecular mechanisms of hepatic ischemia-reperfusion injury a preconditioning. *Am J Physiol Gastrointest Liver Physiol.* 2003;284:G15–G26.

Endocrinology and Metabolism

Murray M. Pollack   *Paul Kaplowitz*

The modern concepts of stress response were initiated in the late 1920s in Glasgow, Scotland, by a young chemist, David Cuthbertson. When studying long bone fractures, he noted that the body lost urea, nitrogen, potassium, phosphorus, sulfur, and creatinine in amounts much greater than bed rest alone. This observation initiated the focus on a generalized reaction of the body associated with systemic breakdown of lean tissue, particularly skeletal muscle. Cuthbertson's studies were replicated and extended to involve stress hormones. His studies initiated a long history of investigations involving the relationships of stress, metabolism, and the hormonal milieu. Glucocorticoids were studied in World War II in combat casualties. In the 1950s, Hume and Egdahl demonstrated an intact neurologic system was important in the stress response. Subsequently, Hume demonstrated the importance of the hypothalamic–pituitary axis, and Goodall found that increased catecholamine secretion was associated with burns. Therefore, by the time of the "modern era" of critical care, the foundations of the systemic metabolic and neuroendocrine responses to injury and illness were secured.[1] Today we realize that there is a relatively tight relation between the hormonal milieu that defines the severity of the stress response and the catabolism of critical illness that results in morbidity and mortality (see Table 2.1).

There have been many observations that lead to our belief that modifications of the neurohumeral response to injury and illness could improve outcome. Epidural anesthesia and spinal anesthesia have been used for decades with the suggestion that there was a benefit to neuraxial blockade over general anesthesia, an observation recently confirmed using meta-analysis.[3] Hypothermia during operations increases the stress response and is associated with increased wound infections and catabolism. β-Blockage in acutely burned children reduces catabolism and improves protein balance.[4] Attenuating the stress response in infants undergoing cardiac surgery by administering deep opioid anesthesia with reductions in the stress hormones—cortisol, catecholamines, and glucagons—was associated with a reduction in sepsis, metabolic acidosis, disseminated intravascular coagulation, and death.[5]

This chapter focuses on the two avenues of critical care endocrinology. First, the physiology of the major stress hormones is discussed as a background to understanding the stress response. Second, the stress response and its consequences are considered.

HORMONES MOST RELEVANT TO PEDIATRIC CRITICAL ILLNESS

A critically ill child will respond to illness with adaptive (and sometimes maladaptive) changes, which affect every organ system. This section considers the normal physiology of the hormones that are most involved in this response.

Insulin

Insulin is a polypeptide hormone of molecular weight 6,000 kDa that is made in the pancreatic β cells in response to the influx of carbohydrates and amino acids following ingestion of a meal. Its release is modulated by a variety of gut factors and hormones, which are also released in response to a meal, as well as the autonomic nervous system. Insulin is synthesized as a single polypeptide chain precursor called *proinsulin*, which is cleaved within the β cell to remove a 31 amino-acid fragment called *C-peptide*, leaving a molecule with both an A-chain and a B-chain linked by two sulfhydryl bonds. Insulin acts on a variety of tissues but primarily on muscle, adipocytes,

TABLE 2.1

CORRELATION OF THE STRESS INDICES IN ADULTS

Stress Level	Urinary Nitrogen Excretion (g/d)	Plasma Lactate (mmol/L)	Plasma Glucose (mg/dL)	Oxygen Consumption (mL/min/m^2)
Low	<10	<1.5	<150	<140
Medium	10–20	1.5–3.0	150–250	140–180
High	>20	>3.0	>250	>180

The stress level is correlated to metabolic indices of critical illness.[2]
From Cerra FB. Multiple organ failure syndrome. In: Bihari DJ, Cerra FB, eds. *Multiple organ failure.* Fullerton, CA: Society of Critical Care Medicine; 1989:1–24.

and liver cells, by binding to a specific heterodimeric receptor of molecular weight 125,000 kDa. This binding event initiates a cascade of intracellular events, some of which modulate gene expression and protein synthesis (see Table 2.2). However, the most important acute effect is the translocation of the glucose transporter glut-4 to the cell surface where it acts to facilitate the uptake of glucose into skeletal muscle and adipose tissue. There are also glucose transporters in red blood cells, brain, kidney, and liver, but these are not hormonally regulated. After a meal, the amount of insulin secreted is normally just adequate to promote the uptake of excess extracellular glucose into adipose and muscle cells, which can store the glucose for use as an energy source during periods of fasting, thereby maintaining blood glucose levels in a narrow range of 70 to 120 mg per dL. Insulin has additional metabolic actions, which include inhibition of proteolysis and lipolysis and hepatic glucose production—all actions that are appropriate following a meal.

Glucagon

Whereas insulin is considered the hormone of feasting, glucagon, a 28–amino acid product of the α cells of the pancreatic islets, is the hormone of fasting. Its release is suppressed following carbohydrate intake and is stimulated during periods of starvation, stress, and exercise. It binds to specific receptors on hepatocytes and initiates a cascade of events involving stimulation of adenyl cyclase and increased production of cyclic adenosine monophosphate (cAMP), which leads to hepatic glycogen breakdown and glucose release. It also promotes gluconeogenesis from amino acids and stimulates the breakdown of triglycerides into free fatty acids to provide another source of energy when carbohydrate stores in the form of liver glycogen are depleted. Therefore, whereas insulin is primarily anabolic, the net effect of glucagons is catabolic, and high levels of glucagons during stress and critical illness are a major contributing factor to the insulin resistance typically seen in these situations (Table 2.2)

Glucocorticoids

Cortisol, the main steroid hormone secreted by the adrenal cortex, is a critical hormone in maintaining normal glucose homeostasis and in mediating the response to stress. Its principle effect on energy balance is to decrease insulin-stimulated glucose metabolism and to increase hepatic glucose production and protein breakdown (Table 2.2). Therefore, like glucagon, it has a catabolic counterinsulin effect, leading to hyperglycemia, unless there is a sufficient increase in insulin secretion to overcome the insulin resistance. The primary regulator of cortisol production is adrenocorticotropic hormone (ACTH or corticotropin), a 39–amino acid peptide produced in the anterior pituitary gland as part of a larger precursor molecule called *pro-opiomelanocortin* (POMC), a 241–amino acid protein, which, when cleaved, yields melanocyte-stimulating hormone (MSH) and the endogenous opioid peptide β-endorphin. ACTH acts on cells in the adrenal cortex through cAMP to stimulate the uptake of low-density lipoprotein (LDL) cholesterol from the blood and to facilitate transport of cholesterol into the mitochondria, thereby increasing the pool of cholesterol available for action by the side chain cleavage enzyme, the first step in the biosynthesis of cortisol. These actions occur within minutes and mediate the acute effect of ACTH on cortisol production, whereas the more chronic effects of ACTH are mediated by increased transcription of genes needed for the other steroidogenic enzymes involved in cortisol biosynthesis.

The main regulator of ACTH secretion is corticotropin-releasing factor (CRF), a 41–amino acid peptide produced in the neurons of the paraventricular nucleus of the hypothalamus. The same neurons that produce CRF also produce the antidiuretic hormone arginine vasopressin (AVP), and both CRF and AVP stimulate production of ACTH, although by different intracellular mechanisms. As will be discussed in a later section of this chapter, the combined actions of CRF and AVP, as well as the cytokines and catecholaminergic neurons of the medulla and pons, interact in a complex manner to orchestrate both the hormonal and behavioral response to stress, whereas

	TABLE 2.2	

EFFECTS OF VARIOUS HORMONES INVOLVED IN METABOLIC REGULATION ON BLOOD GLUCOSE

Hormone	Effects on Metabolism	Net Effect on Blood Glucose
Insulin	■ Stimulates cell uptake of glucose Inhibits hepatic glucose release Inhibits fat breakdown and proteolysis	Decrease
Glucagon	■ Stimulates glycogen breakdown Increases gluconeogenesis	Increase
Growth hormone	■ Decreases insulin-stimulated glucose utilization Increases hepatic glucose release Stimulates lipolysis Stimulates protein synthesis	Increase
Cortisol	■ Decreases insulin-stimulated glucose utilization Increases hepatic glucose output Increases proteolysis	Increase
Epinephrine	■ Decreases insulin-stimulated glucose utilization Increases hepatic glucose release	Increase

the increase in glucocorticoid release from the adrenals has a feedback inhibitory action on multiple parts of this system to keep the stress response from spinning out of control.

The daily rate of cortisol production in healthy children has been a source of controversy. Although earlier studies from 1966 to 1980 estimated the rate at 12 mg/m^2/day, a more recent study using a stable isotope-dilution technique in 33 healthy children aged 8 to 17 years found the average rate to be only 7 mg/m^2/day.[6] Patients in the intensive care unit (ICU) setting frequently receive doses of cortisol (as Solucortef) or prednisolone (Solumedrol, which is at least five times as potent as cortisol) at daily doses that are well over an order of magnitude higher than the daily production rate. As discussed later, this may be appropriate for severely stressed patients (e.g., after multiple trauma) but is probably excessive in the mild to moderately stressed children who may be unable to increase their cortisol production and who will do fine with three to five times the daily requirement of cortisol (i.e., 25 to 40 mg/m^2/day).

It is difficult to accurately assess the adequacy of glucocorticoid secretion, particularly in critically ill patients. Serum cortisol levels are highest at 8 AM (6 to 22 μg per dL), the peak of the normal diurnal variation, but levels are far lower at 4 PM (4 to 11 μg per dL) and at 11 PM (<5 μg per dL). Measuring urinary free cortisol in a 24-hour sample is useful in documenting glucocorticoid excess but not deficiency, and it is very difficult to collect a 24-hour sample in a critically ill patient. In the ICU, the diurnal variation of serum cortisol may be masked by the effects of acute stress, but a single level of >20 μg per dL is generally considered indicative of an intact pituitary–adrenal axis. However, it is not clear that levels in the 7 to 20 μg per dL range are diagnostic of adrenal insufficiency, particularly in patients whose illness has persisted for days. Rather than relying on random cortisol levels, one can assess adrenal responsiveness to ACTH by giving a single IV dose of cosyntropin (Cortrosyn) (a synthetic peptide made up of the first 24 amino acids of ACTH) at 15 μg per kg for children younger than 2 years and 250 μg for children older than 2 years. Serum cortisol is measured at baseline and 30 to 60 minutes later.[7] This is an excellent test for diagnosing primary adrenal insufficiency, but the response may be normal (defined by some as a cortisol level of >20 μg per dL) in patients with partial ACTH deficiency. One pediatric study defined adrenal dysfunction in the pediatric ICU as a random cortisol of <7 μg per dL or a post-ACTH level of <18 μg per dL, and reported that four of 13 patients with a PRISM score of >10 μg per dL and hemodynamic instability met this criteria.[8] However, there is no way of determining if the cutoffs chosen by the authors actually identify those children who would benefit from steroid replacement therapy. If there is suspicion of primary adrenal insufficiency (e.g., there is hyponatremia and hyperkalemia), a serum ACTH level should be determined; if it is clearly elevated, it confirms a diagnosis of primary adrenal insufficiency, which is much less common than secondary adrenal insufficiency but is more likely to be permanent.

The relative anti-inflammatory potencies of the various steroids available to physicians are sometimes confusing. The relative potencies are shown in Table 2.3.[9]

TABLE 2.3

RELATIVE ANTI-INFLAMMATORY POTENCY OF CORTICOSTEROIDS

Substance	Source	Systemic Anti-inflammatory Potency
Cortisol	Natural	1
Prednisone	Synthetic	4
Methylprednisolone	Synthetic	5
Dexamethasone	Synthetic	30

The Renin–Angiotensin–Aldosterone System

Renin is a 340–amino acid protease enzyme produced primarily in the juxtaglomerular cells of the kidney, which is released in response to decreased blood pressure, sodium depletion, vasodilatory drugs, and β-adrenergic stimulation. It acts specifically on a large glycosylated protein in the circulation called *angiotensinogen* to release a 10–amino acid peptide called *angiotensin I*. This peptide is biologically inactive until a converting enzyme found in the lungs and blood vessels cleaves off the two carboxy-terminal amino acids to form angiotensin II. The enzyme that does this can be inhibited by drugs such as captropril, which are useful in the treatment of hypertension associated with elevated renin levels.

Angiotensin II has two activities, both of which result in increased blood pressure. Within seconds, it stimulates arteriolar vasoconstriction, and within minutes, it stimulates the synthesis and release of the potent mineralocorticoid hormone aldosterone from the glomerulosa cells of the adrenal cortex. Aldosterone acts at the level of the renal tubules to promote exchange of sodium ions for potassium ions. This action helps to maintain intravascular volume and blood pressure during the volume loss, which occurs during hemorrhage and during states of volume depletion caused by third space losses. It should be noted that ACTH is not a clinically important mediator of aldosterone production. This is an important clinical distinction because patients with adrenal insufficiency caused by central nervous system (CNS) injury resulting in decreased ACTH secretion will generally have normal function of the renin–angiotensin–aldosterone system, whereas patients with primary adrenal insufficiency (usually caused by autoimmune destruction) will have a deficiency of both cortisol and aldosterone production and will require both glucocorticoid and mineralocorticoid replacement.

Catecholamines

In the adrenal medulla and the sympathetic nervous system, the amino acid tyrosine can be converted to DOPA, then to dopamine, and subsequently to norepinephrine. The final step in this pathway, the conversion of norepinephrine to epinephrine, only occurs in the adrenal medulla. The regulation of sympathetic nervous system activity is under the influence of centers in the brain and spinal cord. Norepinephrine effects are predominantly mediated through the α-receptors, through a calcium-mediated mechanism that results in vasoconstriction and intestinal smooth muscle relaxation. Epinephrine affects both the α- and the β-receptors, the latter involving cAMP as the second messenger, which mediate cardiac stimulation and vasodilation. Important indirect effects relevant to the response to acute stress include the increase in hepatic glucose output by glycogenolysis in both liver and skeletal muscle, the inhibition of insulin secretion, and the decrease in insulin-stimulated glucose metabolism (Table 2.2). There is also a redistribution of blood flow so that glucose released from the liver is distributed to the tissues with the greatest need. It is clear that catecholamine release in response to acute stress is a critical part of the adaptive response in that it rapidly mobilizes energy stores and increases cardiac output and muscle performance. It is less clear how these effects are modulated in the intensive care setting as acute stress becomes more chronic.

The only clinical syndrome that the intensivist might encounter that specifically involves altered catecholamine production is the *pheochromocytoma*, a rare tumor that can arise in the adrenal medulla or less often in the abdominal sympathetic chain. A family history of multiple endocrine neoplasia 2B should create a high level of suspicion. There are marked elevations of both epinephrine and norepinephrine, with the secretion of norepinephrine usually predominating. Hypertension is typically the most dramatic finding with systolic blood pressure levels as high as 200 mm Hg, and it can be either sustained or paroxysmal. At times of increased catecholamine release, patients experience headaches, sweating, palpitations, flushing, and emotional lability. The most reliable diagnostic test is the analysis of a 24-hour urine sample for the two active catecholamines and their metabolites, metanephrine, normetanephrine, and vanillylmandelic acid (VMA). Measuring plasma levels is less reliable because they may overlap with those of healthy patients during asymptomatic periods.

The Growth Hormone–Insulinlike Growth Factor Axis

Human growth hormone (GH) is a 191–amino acid protein, which is secreted by the anterior pituitary gland. Its effect on childhood growth is primarily mediated by the increased production of insulinlike growth factor (IGF-1), both in the liver and in target tissues such as the chondrocytes of the growth plates. IGF-1 is a 70–amino acid peptide, which is homologous to proinsulin (its C-peptide region is part of the molecule and not cleaved during processing) but primarily acts through a distinct IGF-1 receptor, which is homologous to the insulin receptor. IGF-1 circulates largely bound to a high-molecular-weight ternary complex with two GH-dependent proteins, IGF-binding protein-3 (IGFBP-3) and an acid-labile subunit (ALS). This complex substantially prolongs the biologic half-life of IGF-1 and results in relatively stable circulating levels over 24 hours, unlike the pulsatile variation in GH levels. Therefore, measuring IGF-1 is a good screening test for GH deficiency and is a far more meaningful way of assessing endogenous GH production than a random GH level measurement. Insulinlike growth factor-2 (IGF-2) is another GH-dependent growth factor, which has 60% homology with IGF-1 but interacts with different receptors. Compared with IGF-1, its role in human physiology is not well understood, and serum measurements provide little useful clinical information.

Secretion of GH is under dual control by the hypothalamus. It is stimulated by growth hormone–releasing hormone (GHRH) and inhibited by somatostatin. The recently discovered gut peptide, ghrelin, also referred to as a *GH-releasing peptide*, also stimulates GH release although it acts on a somatotroph receptor, which is distinct from that which GHRH binds to. The secretion of GH is highly pulsatile, with an average of five to eight distinct pulses per day and with very low trough levels between pulses. There is increasing evidence that the pulsatile nature of GH secretion is more important for its metabolic effects than for the total amount of GH secreted. There are many other factors that modulate GH secretion, one of the most important being the feedback inhibition caused by IGF-1 at both the hypothalamic and pituitary levels (see Fig. 2.1).

Thyroid Hormones

Thyroid hormones are produced in the thyroid gland under the influence of thyroid-stimulating hormone (TSH), which binds to the thyroid follicular cells and activates adenyl cyclase. The release of TSH from the pituitary is stimulated by the hypothalamic tripeptide thyrotropin-releasing hormone (TRH), and the release of TRH is modulated by environmental temperature through peripheral and hypothalamic temperature sensors. Circulating levels of thyroid hormones exert feedback inhibition on both the hypothalamus and the pituitary to maintain circulating thyroid hormone levels in the normal range (see Fig. 2.2).

The most abundant thyroid hormone is L-thyroxine (T_4), which circulates at concentrations of 5 to 12 μg per dL, but only 0.03% of this is free and available to cells and tissues, the rest being bound to serum proteins, mostly thyroid-binding globulin (TBG). The extensive binding of T_4 to binding proteins is responsible for its long half-life and the absence of rapid fluctuation in levels over the course of a day. Therefore, thyroid status can be assessed from a single blood sample, and if the patient is taking thyroid hormone, the time of the sample relative to the last dose is not critical.

T_4 can be monodeiodinated, mostly peripherally, to triiodothyronine (T_3), which is more active than T_4 but circulates at much lower concentrations (80 to 200 ng per dL). However, a greater proportion of T_3 (0.03%) is in the free form. T_4 can also be metabolized to reverse T_3 (rT_3), which is completely inactive. Under normal circumstances, T_3 and rT_3 are produced at similar rates, but in pathologic situations, including critical illness, the metabolism of T_4 can be shifted largely to rT_3. The affinity of T_3 for thyroid hormone receptors is approximately 10-fold greater than that of T_4, so it is believed that despite lower circulating

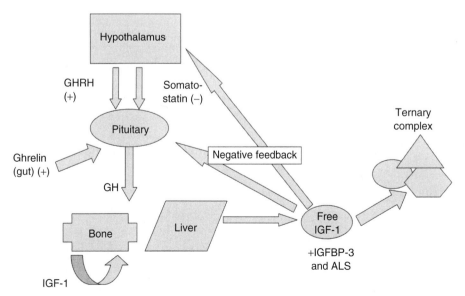

Figure 2.1 The growth hormone–IGF axis. GHRH, growth hormone-releasing hormone; GH, growth hormone; IGF-1, insulinlike growth factor-1; IGF-BP-3, insulinlike growth factor binding protein-3; ALS, acid labile subunit. Growth hormone is under dual control by the hypothalamic hormones GHRH and somatostatin. Under the influence of GH, cartilage produces IGF-1, which stimulates its own growth, but the source of circulating IGF-1 is mainly production by the liver. IGF-1 circulates largely as a complex with IGF-BP3 and ALS to prolong its half life in blood, but free IGF-1 exerts feedback inhibition on GH secretion at both the hypothalamic and pituitary levels.

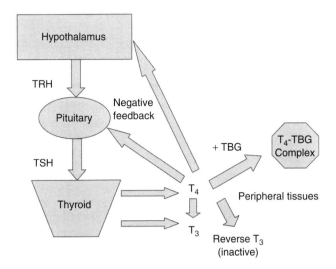

Figure 2.2 The hypothalamic–pituitary–thyroid axis. TRH, thyrotropin-releasing hormone; TSH, thyroid-stimulating hormone; TBG, thyroid-binding globulin.

levels, most of the biologic action of thyroid hormones can be attributed to T_3. However, assays of T_3 are a less reliable reflection of thyroid status than are total or free T_4 levels because mildly elevated T_3 levels can be seen in euthyroid patients with normal TSH, and T_3 can be in the low–normal range in patients who are clearly hypothyroid.

Thyroid hormones are required for healthy childhood growth through effects on GH secretion and through a direct effect on bone metabolism and growth. They are essential for normal brain development in the first 2 to 3 years of life, by stimulating neuronal cell migration, dendritic arborization, and myelinogenesis. They also regulate oxygen consumption, increase amino acid and lipid metabolism and water and ion transport, and stimulate thermogenesis through their effect on brown adipose tissue. Their ability to stimulate adrenergic receptor binding is most likely responsible for their effect on heart rate, most notably the tachycardia usually seen in patients with hyperthyroidism.

Hormones Regulating Calcium Metabolism

The concentration of extracellular calcium ions is very closely regulated, because of the critical role of calcium in maintaining normal cardiac and skeletal muscle contractility. Ca^{2+} enters cells through specialized transmembrane protein channels, which are found in neurons; cardiac, skeletal and smooth muscles; several endocrine glands; white blood cells; and platelets (where they play a critical role in the clotting system). Approximately 98% of total body calcium is present in crystalline form (complexed with phosphate) in the skeleton, 1% is in recently deposited bone, which is metabolically active, and only 1% is found in the vascular, intracellular, and extracellular spaces, where it mediates its biologic effects. Approximately 40% of the

total serum calcium is bound to albumin and globulin; 10% is chelated with a variety of anions including citrate, lactate, and phosphate; and 50% is the biologically active Ca^{2+}. The two major factors that affect calcium binding are the level of serum albumin and pH. Patients with low serum albumin level typically have a low total serum calcium level but a normal ionized serum calcium level. For every gram per deciliter reduction in albumin, the protein-bound fraction of calcium is reduced by approximately 0.8 mg per dL. Because low albumin level is common in critically ill patients, it is accepted that measurement of Ca^{2+} is a more accurate reflection of calcium status than total calcium. Acid pH decreases binding of calcium to albumin, increasing Ca^{2+} levels, whereas alkalosis does the opposite.

Regulation of serum calcium primarily involves the parathyroid hormone (PTH) and vitamin D (see Fig. 2.3). PTH, an 84–amino acid protein, is secreted by the primary cells of the parathyroid gland in a manner inversely related to the serum Ca^{2+} level; this is mediated by a calcium-sensing receptor on the surface of the parathyroid cells. PTH secretion is also stimulated by high phosphate levels and inhibited by low phosphate levels, which may explain the hypersecretion of PTH in patients with chronic renal failure who usually have hyperphosphatemia. PTH has important actions on both the bone and the kidney. It binds to receptors on the surface of osteoclasts, and, by means of a cAMP-mediated mechanism, leads to release of calcium and phosphate from bone mineral into the extracellular fluid. In the kidney, PTH increases urinary loss of phosphate and promotes tubular reabsorption of calcium. It also stimulates the conversion of 25-hydroxyvitamin D to the highly active metabolite, 1,25-dihydroxyvitamin D (calcitriol), which promotes intestinal absorption of both calcium and phosphate. The overall effect of PTH is to raise serum calcium and lower serum phosphate levels. The other calcium-regulating hormone, calcitonin, is a 32–amino acid protein made in the C cells of the thyroid gland in response to rising Ca^{2+} levels. It rapidly decreases the bone resorptive action of osteoclasts and promotes urinary calcium excretion, the opposite of the effects of PTH.

Hypocalcemia is seen in the pediatric intensive care setting both in patients with primary disorders of the PTH–vitamin D system, and as a consequence of critical illness. For patients in the first year of life with hypocalcemic seizures, making the correct diagnosis quickly is vital because infusions of calcium salts will increase serum Ca^{2+} levels only transiently and hypocalcemia will recur unless the underlying problem is addressed. Hypoparathyroidism should be suspected if severe hypocalcemia (total calcium level <7 mg per dL) occurs in the first weeks of life and is accompanied by an elevated serum phosphate level (9 to 12 mg per dL). If there is coexisting congenital heart disease, a diagnosis of DiGeorge syndrome should be considered. It has been estimated that 70% of patients with apparent isolated hypoparathyroidism have a

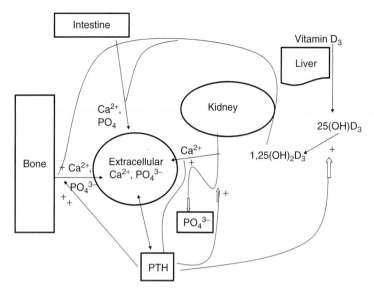

Figure 2.3 Regulation of calcium and phosphate metabolism by vitamin D and PTH (parathyroid hormone). Vitamin D is metabolized in the liver to 25-hydroxyvitamin D (25(OH) D_3), which is activated in the kidney in the presence of PTH to 1,25 dihydroxyvitamin D (1,25(OH)$_2$ D_3). This vitamin hormone raises or maintains serum calcium by increasing Ca^{2+} absorption from the gut and mobilization of calcium from the bone. PTH secretion is stimulated by both low Ca^{2+} and by elevated phosphate; it helps to lower phosphate by increasing urinary phosphate excretion, while decreasing urinary Ca^{2+} excretion. (From Brown EM, Physiology of calcium metabolism. In: Becker KL, ed. *Principles and practice of endocrinology and metabolism.* 3rd ed. Philadelphia, PA: Lippincott Williams & Wilkins; 2001:480.)

deletion at chromosome 22q11.2, the deletion associated with DiGeorge syndrome, even in the absence of other clinical features of DiGeorge syndrome.[10] A less common cause of congenital hypoparathyroidism is an activating mutation in the calcium-sensing receptor, such that PTH secretion remains suppressed even in the presence of low to normal Ca^{2+} levels. Measurement of intact serum PTH levels at the time of hypocalcemia will confirm the diagnosis. A more common but poorly understood situation is the 6- to 10-day-old healthy infant presenting with a hypocalcemic seizure, an elevated serum phosphate level, and a PTH level in the normal range. Curiously, in these infants, the hypocalcemia resolves rapidly in response to therapy and does not recur when therapy is withdrawn weeks or months later. Whether this is a result of phosphate overload, transient hypoparathyroidism, maternal vitamin D deficiency, or maternal hyperparathyroidism (easily ruled out by checking the maternal serum calcium) is not clear.

When severe hypocalcemia with or without seizures is found in a child between 4 months and 18 months of age, the diagnosis of vitamin D deficiency should be suspected. The setting for this once rare condition is almost always breast-feeding in a dark-skinned child who is not receiving supplemental vitamins.[11] Laboratory tests are the key to making this diagnosis. Phosphate levels will be normal to mildly elevated (usually not >7 mg per dL), and alkaline phosphatase levels, which are normal in hypoparathyroidism, are almost always elevated, typically in the 600 to 1,500 U per L range (normal for age 450). The level of 25-hydroxyvitamin D is invariably low to unmeasurable in this patient and the PTH level is quite high because the hypocalcemia produces a state of secondary hyperparathyroidism. Levels of 1,25-dihydroxyvitamin D can be low, normal, or high and are therefore of no diagnostic value. Because PTH and vitamin D levels usually

take days for testing, the alkaline phosphatase evaluation done as part of the comprehensive metabolic profile is extremely helpful in making an early diagnosis. The results of key blood tests in the diagnosis of hypocalcemia are summarized in Table 2.4.

Treatment of hypocalcemia always involves providing extra calcium initially; in the patient who is convulsing or is markedly hypocalcemic (total calcium <6 mg per dL or Ca^{2+} <0.7 mmol per L), a slow infusion of calcium gluconate or calcium chloride can be given while monitoring the heart rhythm. However, repeated IV boluses of calcium are counterproductive because they do not produce a sustained rise in serum calcium level and may delay the correction of the underlying problem. The next step is starting oral calcium (CaCO$_3$ is recommended because it contains 40% elemental calcium) at a dosage of 50 to 75 mg of elemental calcium/kg/day, divided into four doses. However, extra oral calcium will be ineffective unless vitamin D is provided to allow the gut to absorb it. For infants with hypoparathyroidism, one needs to provide the active metabolite 1,25-dihydroxyvitamin D, which the kidney is unable to produce, at an initial dosage of 0.25 to 0.5 μg per day. Those with vitamin D deficiency will be able to convert ordinary vitamin D (calciferol) to 1,25-dihydroxyvitamin D, so calciferol (initial dosage 2,000 units per day) is the treatment of choice, although many prefer to give calcitriol for a few days until calcium levels start to rise, because of its more rapid biologic action.

Hypocalcemia developing in children in the intensive care setting can be caused by impairment of PTH release due to hypomagnesemia, burns, sepsis, and drugs such as aminoglycosides. A study of the ionized hypocalcemia seen in ten children with burns of at least 30% of total body surface area found that PTH levels were uniformly low or low-normal, and that, in addition, there was resistance

TABLE 2.4
BLOOD TESTS USEFUL IN DIAGNOSIS OF HYPOCALCEMIA

	Phosphate	Alkaline Phosphatase	Parathyroid Hormone	25-Hydroxy Vitamin D
Hypoparathyroidism	Elevated	Normal	Low	Normal
Vitamin D deficiency	Low to slightly elevated	Elevated	Elevated	Low
Transient hypocalcemia during infancy	Elevated	Normal	Normal	Low-normal to normal

to the action of infused PTH.[12] Hypomagnesemia was found as well, and magnesium depletion was felt to have a possible role in the low calcium and PTH levels. Hypocalcemia can also be a result of respiratory alkalosis or bicarbonate infusions, which increase binding of calcium ions to serum proteins or hyperphosphatemia (most often caused by renal failure), which can chelate calcium ions in the blood and reduce both total and Ca^{2+}. In prolonged critical illness, adults were vitamin D–deficient and the current recommended vitamin D dose did not normalize vitamin D status.[13] Providing extra IV or oral calcium and treating the underlying problem usually resolves the problem without the need for vitamin D therapy.

Hypercalcemia is not commonly encountered in the pediatric intensive care setting, but calcium levels of >15 mg per dL can constitute a life-threatening emergency as a result of its deleterious effects on the heart, CNS, and kidneys. Hyperparathyroidism in children is extremely rare and will be accompanied by a very low serum phosphate level and a PTH level inappropriate for the degree of hypercalcemia; a family history of multiple endocrine neoplasia should increase the suspicion of PTH excess. Patients with certain malignancies may produce parathyroid hormone–related protein (PTH–RP), which, because of its similarity to PTH, can mobilize excess calcium from bone; specific assays for PTH-RP are available. Hypercalcemia can also be caused by increased absorption of calcium from the gut, most often, due to vitamin D intoxication. This can be seen in patients started on calciferol or calcitriol for treatment of hypocalcemia if calcium levels are not monitored on a regular basis and dosage of vitamin D adjusted accordingly. Hypercalcemia caused by increased gut absorption can also be a result of sarcoidosis, which has been associated with increased ectopic production of 1,25-dihydroxyvitamin D.

Arginine Vasopressin and Water Balance

Regulation of water balance and normal extracellular fluid tonicity is largely under the control of the antidiuretic hormone AVP. AVP, a 9–amino acid peptide with a disulfide ring, is produced in the hypothalamic paraventricular and supraoptic nuclei as part of a 164–amino acid protein called *preprovasopressin*, which is sequentially processed to produce the active peptide. It is carried by axonal transport to the posterior pituitary, where it is released into the systemic circulation. The primary function of AVP is to regulate water and solute excretion by the kidney. Plasma tonicity changes by as little as 1% change the volume of hypothalamic osmoreceptor cells and subsequently stimulate the neurons of the supraoptic and paraventricular nuclei. Glucose and urea, under normal physiologic conditions, readily traverse neuron membranes and do not affect the release of AVP. The change in tonicity is proportionate to the amount of AVP secreted from the axon terminals of the posterior pituitary. Once the osmolality exceeds 280 to 290 mOsm per kg, the secretion rate is very steep. After release into the circulation, AVP binds to V_2 receptors located on collecting duct principle cells in the kidney, enabling free water reabsorption across the apical membrane of the collecting duct, and decreasing plasma osmolality. It also increases NaCl reabsorption in the thick ascending loop of Henle, which maintains the hypertonicity of the medullary interstitium. Plasma concentrations of AVP correlate to tonicity (see Table 2.5). Therefore, graded increases in vasopressin secretion and action help the kidneys to regulate water balance over a wide range of physiologic conditions, conserving water when there is excessive water loss or volume depletion and allowing a brisk diuresis under conditions of water overload.

In the intensive care setting, there are two common situations in which vasopressin production or action is altered: (a) diabetes insipidus (DI), in which the lack of vasopressin results in abnormally high urinary water losses, resulting in hypernatremia if not detected and treated promptly, and (b) the syndrome of inappropriate antidiuretic hormone secretion, in which there is a failure to turn off vasopressin secretion in the presence of volume expansion and hyponatremia. Both of these conditions are discussed in Chapter 11.

TABLE 2.5

RELATION BETWEEN PLASMA TONICITY, URINE OSMOLALITY, AND ARGININE VASOPRESSIN CONCENTRATIONS

Plasma Tonicity	Urine Osmolality (mOsm/kg Water)	AVP (pg/mL)
Hypertonic	1,200	>5.0
Hypotonic	50	Undetectable
Isotonic	600	0.5–2.5

Modified from Lee CR, Watkins ML, Patterson JH, et al. Vasopressin: A new target for the treatment of heart failure. *Am Heart J.* 2003;146: 9–18.[14]

THE STRESS RESPONSE

Hypothalamic–Pituitary–Adrenal Axis

The body's response to stress involves activation of the regulatory centers in the CNS with resulting activation of the hypothalamic–pituitary–adrenal (HPA) axis and the autonomic nervous system. This stimulates other endocrine systems and interacts with the inflammatory system. Although this system is responsive to many stimuli including circadian, neurosensory, and limbic signals, it is the response to immune-mediated inflammatory reactants such as tumor necrosis factor-α (TNF-α), interleukin-1 (IL-1), and IL-6 that trigger the stress response of critical illness.[15] Because of such effects, these substances have been called *tissue corticotropin-releasing factors*.

The CNS is not immune to the inflammatory response and this availability to the inflammatory response is responsible for the activation of the HPA axis. Activated monocytes, lymphocytes, and macrophages can cross the blood–brain barrier and secrete their inflammatory mediators including cytokines, leukotrienes, and prostaglandins. Microglia, which are embryologically related to macrophages, are activated by toxins, antigens, and cell injury products and can also secrete cytokines and inflammatory mediators. Glia cells that secrete IL-1 and neurons that contain IL-1 are present in the hypothalamus. Endothelial and smooth muscle cells of the CNS blood vessels can also secrete cytokines and interleukins.[16] Therefore, the CNS is both simulated by the inflammatory response, and is capable of producing cytokines.

The HPA axis is composed of the central components in the hypothalamus and brain stem and the peripheral components, principally the pituitary–adrenal axis, the adrenomedullary response, and systemic sympathetic nervous systems (see Fig. 2.4).[17] The central components of the HPA axis are the paraventricular nuclei in the hypothalamus and the locus caeruleus in the brain stem. Both are stimulated by cholinergic and serotonergic neurotransmitters and

inhibited by γ-aminobutyric acid (GABA), benzodiazepine, and peptides from the arcuate nucleus POMC. The paraventricular nucleus releases corticotropin-releasing hormone (CRH) and AVP. CRH and the noradrenergic neurons from the locus caeruleus stimulate each other; CRH stimulates the secretion of norepinephrine through specific receptors, and norepinephrine stimulates the secretion of CRH primarily by α_1-noradrenergic receptors. Autoregulatory ultrashort negative-feedback loops from collateral fibers exist for both CRH and norepinephrine, inhibiting presynaptic CRH and noradrenergic receptors. Additionally, CRH stimulates the secretion of ACTH from the anterior pituitary. Therefore, CRH is a major, central regulator of the stress response. Although AVP acts synergistically with CRH to stimulate pituitary (ACTH) release, corticotropin is the key regulator of glucocorticoid secretion by the adrenal gland.

Each of the paraventricular nuclei has three areas involved in the stress response. The medial division secretes CRH into the hypophysial portal system, the intermediate group secretes AVP also into the hypophysial portal system, and a lateral group innervates the noradrenergic neurons of the stress response areas in the brain stem. Neurons from the paraventricular area also innervate POMC-containing neurons in the arcuate nucleus of the hypothalamus and innervate pain-control areas of the hindbrain and spinal cord. These latter innervations account for the secretion of opioids, which enhance analgesia commonly associated with the stress response.

Recently, the HPA axis was found to undergo a biphasic change during critical illness.[18] In the first few days, high cortisol concentrations appear to be induced by augmented ACTH release, which is driven by cytokines and by the noradrenergic tone. During this phase, basal cortisol levels are lower and the response to CRH is impaired in nonsurvivors compared to survivors.[19] In the second phase, ACTH level is relatively low, yet cortisol level remains high. This discrepancy between the low ACTH and high cortisol concentrations suggests that cortisol release is stimulated through alternative pathways, postulated by some to involve endothelin, atrial natriuretic hormone, and the splanchnic nerve stimulation. This second phase is discussed in the subsequent text as the chronic phase of the stress response.

Because almost all components of the immune response are inhibited by cortisol, the hypercortisolism elicited by disease or trauma can be interpreted as an attempt by the organism to modify the inflammatory response, protecting itself against possible endogenous over-responses. Also, it has been suggested that acute cortisol-induced hyperglycemia and catabolism (see subsequent text) provide available energy and postpone anabolism. In contrast, prolonged hypercortisolism is often interpreted as a negative consequence of stress as it leads to immune suppression, impaired healing, hyperglycemia, and myopathy.

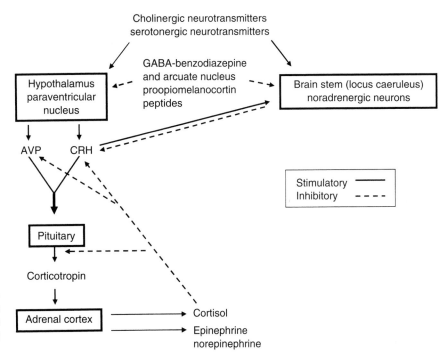

Figure 2.4 The hypothalamic–pituitary–adrenal axis. PTH, parathyroid hormone; GABA, γ-aminobutyric acid; AVP, arginine vasopressin; CRH, corticotropin-releasing hormone.

Neuroendocrine–Inflammatory Interactions

A very complex set of neuroendocrine–inflammatory interactions are central to the stress response (see Fig. 2.5). There are many aspects to these interactions. For example, immune cells contain receptors for classical hormones (see Table 2.6), and most endocrine cells are affected by cytokines. Immune cells may also synthesize classical hormones including ACTH, β-endorphin, GH, prolactin, vasoactive intestinal polypeptide (VIP), and substance P.

Perhaps the most important interactions occur in the hypothalamus. IL-1, IL-6 and TNF-α are both synthesized in the hypothalamus and enter the CNS through the blood stream. IL-1 is particularly abundant in the paraventricular nuclei, a central aspect of the HPA axis. Although cytokines (especially, IL-1, IL-6, TNF) directly stimulate the HPA axis, immune cells can also directly produce CRH and AVP, affecting the release of ACTH from the anterior pituitary, and altering the systemic concentrations of CRH and AVP.

TABLE 2.6

ENDOCRINE RECEPTORS FOUND ON IMMUNE CELLS

Corticosteriods
  Insulin
  Glucagon
  Prolactin
  Growth hormone
  Estradiol
  Testosterone
  β-Adrenergic agonists
  Endorphins
  Enkephalins
  Substance P
  Somatostatin
  Vasoactive intestinal peptide

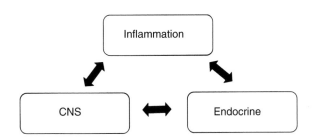

Figure 2.5 The neuroendocrine–inflammatory response. CNS, central nervous system.

Table 2.7 lists many of the multiple controlling influences that cytokines have on the endocrine system.

The link between the immune and neuroendocrine processes provides explanations for the response of the pituitary and adrenal glands to infection and inflammation, including alterations in pituitary–thyroid and pituitary–gonadal function that occur in patients with nonendocrine disease.[21] The activation of cytokines in the CNS can lead to profound changes in neural function, ranging from mild behavioral changes to the destruction of neurons, as well as the direct effects the HPA axis, as discussed in the preceding text.

TABLE 2.7
SOME OF THE DIRECT EFFECTS OF CYTOKINES ON ENDOCRINE CELLS

Effect on Endocrine System	Cytokine
Stimulates CRH release	IL-1, IL-2, IL-6, IL-8, TNF
Stimulates AVP	IL-1β, IL-2, IL-6, IFN-α
Stimulates somatostatin	IL-1, TNF-α
Inhibits TRH	IL-1, TNF
Stimulates ACTH	IL-1, IL-2, IL-6, TNF-α, IFN-γ
Stimulates glucagons	IL-1, TNF-α
Inhibits thyroid hormone	IL-1, TNF-α
Stimulates corticosteroids	IL-1, IL-2, IL-6, TNF-α, IFN-α

CRH, corticotropin-releasing hormone; IL, interleukin; TNF, tumor necrosis factor; AVP, arginine vasopressin; IFN, interferon; TRH, thyrotropin-releasing hormone; ACTH, adrenocorticotropic hormone. Modified from Zaloga GP, Bhatt B, Marik P. Critical illness and systemic inflammation. In: Becker KL, ed. *Principles and practice of endocrinology and metabolism.* 3rd ed. Philadelphia, PA: Lippincott Williams & Wilkins; 2001:2077–2087.[20]

Glucocorticoids and the Hypothalamic–Pituitary–Adrenal Axis

Glucocorticoids are the best known substances involved in the HPA that modify the immune response. Glucocorticoids inhibit many functions of leukocytes and immune accessory cells including suppression of immune activation, and inhibition of the production of cytokines and other inflammatory mediators, and they cause resistance to cytokines. As such, they are the major hormones responsible for inhibiting the toxicity caused by the inflammatory response. For example, glucocorticoids suppress the production of IL-6 and IL-1β by decreasing both the transcription rates of the genes and the stability of their messenger RNA.

Critical illness increases serum cortisol concentrations with loss of circadian rhythm. Although in the past, it was estimated that cortisol production tripled during stress, more recent studies indicate an average sixfold increase in urinary free cortisol with severe bacterial infection and abdominal surgery, a 10-fold increase after cardiothoracic surgery, and a 20-fold increase after a motor vehicle injury.[22] Serum cortisol concentrations are a good measure of stress and correlate inversely with the outcome from critical illness including head trauma and systemic injury. It is generally believed that the pituitary–adrenal axis in critical illness cannot be inhibited by exogenous steroid administration. The competency of the HPA was recently tested in patients with severe sepsis using CRH administration.[23] Patients who died had a reduced response, implying that HPA axis suppression is important in critical illness outcome. The metabolic response to critical illness (see subsequent text) is also tightly integrated into the physiology of glucocorticoids.[24]

Glucocorticoids are also central to the metabolic response to critical illness (see subsequent text). They stimulate gluconeogenesis in the liver, kidney, and skeletal muscle; inhibit glucose uptake; and facilitate the release of catecholamines. Glucocorticoids stimulate glucagon secretion and inhibit both the release and action of insulin. Therefore, the normal balance of anabolism (insulin-dependent) and catabolism (glucagon-dependent) favors catabolism. The hypercortisolism of acute illness has several teleological explanations. Because most components of the immune response are inhibited by cortisol, the hypercortisolism of critical illness may be an effort at self-protection by reducing the inflammatory cascade. In contrast, prolonged hypercortisolism leads to immune suppression, impaired healing, steroid diabetes, and myopathy.

Other hormones from the HPA axis are important in immune mediation. ACTH and β-endorphin have immune potentiating and proinflammatory properties. CRH and AVP have proinflammatory effects. For example, inflammatory sites may contain large amounts of CRH, with concentrations reaching as high as in the hypophysial portal system. In these inflammatory sites, the CRH is found mostly within immune cells and the inflammatory exudate. CRH, its messenger RNA, or both are present in circulating white cells and in cells of the thymus and spleen. And, neutralizing antibodies against CRH reduce inflammation in a similar amount as neutralization of TNF-α.

Catecholamines

Catecholamines are also central to the inflammatory cascade. Catecholamines are released from the nerve terminals of the sympathetic nervous system (norepinephrine), and adrenal medulla (epinephrine), with approximately five times more epinephrine being produced than norepinephrine. Both are stimulated by cytokines such as TNF-α and IL-1 and have a major role in the control of inflammation through the stimulation of IL-6, which inhibits the cytokines such as TNF-α and IL-1, and participates in the induction of the production of acute-phase reactants. Catecholamines have direct consequences on the metabolic response to injury as well, which in many ways mirror the effects of glucocorticoids. Catecholamines augment hepatic gluconeogenesis and glycogenolysis, increase lipolysis, inhibit insulin secretion and decrease tissue sensitivity to insulin, and promote GH and glucagons activity and secretion.

Inflammation is also influenced by afferent sensory fibers and postganglionic sympathetic neurons of the peripheral nervous system. The sensory fibers not only signal the CNS but also secrete proinflammatory or anti-inflammatory neuropeptides, such as substance P or somatostatin, into the inflammatory site. The postganglionic sympathetic neurons, which are peripheral extensions of the central stress system, also secrete proinflammatory and anti-inflammatory substances locally.

Prolactin and Sex Steroids

Prolactin is increased during acute stress. Prolactin receptors are present on human T and B lymphocytes, and T lymphocytes depend on prolactin for maintenance of immune competence. Cyclosporine has a common binding site on T cells with prolactin, indicating that part of its immunosuppressive effect could be caused by the blocking of the prolactin receptor.

Severe inflammatory illness also alters sex hormones and gonadal function, inducing anovulation and amenorrhea in women and decreased spermatogenesis and decreased plasma concentrations of testosterone in men. Cytokines transported by the blood or produced within the gonadal tissues are partially responsible. Presumably, the HPA axis is also mainly involved. Under normal circumstances, low plasma concentrations of testosterone or estrogen would lead to increased secretion of gonadotropins through decreased negative feedback on the hypothalamic–pituitary axis, but this response is inhibited during critical illness.

Dehydroepiandrosterone sulfate is the most abundant steroid secreted by the adult adrenal cortex under pituitary control and is decreased in severe illness. Dehydroepiandrosterone is a strong stimulus to the immune response and antagonizes the effect of glucocorticoids on T cell function. In one study of sepsis, survivors and nonsurvivors showed profound differences in dehydroepiandrosterone sulfate and dehydroepiandrosterone levels during early sepsis with dehydroepiandrosterone sulfate being lower in early sepsis in nonsurvivors compared with survivors.[25] Testosterone is the most important endogenous anabolic steroid. Catabolic states such as starvation and critical illness are associated with reduced testosterone.

Arginine Vasopressin

AVP is involved in a number of physiologic activities important to the intensivist. Through the activation of its V_{1a}, V_{1b}, and V_2 receptors (see Table 2.8), AVP has been demonstrated to play an important role in various physiologic functions, including secretion of anterior pituitary hormones, body water regulation as discussed earlier in this chapter, vascular tone regulation, and cardiovascular contractility. V_{1a} receptors are located on both vascular smooth muscle cells and cardiac myocytes, and modulate blood vessel vasoconstriction and myocardial function. V_2 receptors are located on renal collecting duct principle cells, which are coupled to water channels and regulate volume status through stimulation of free water and urea reabsorption. V_{1b} receptors are located in the anterior pituitary and are responsible for ACTH and β-endorphin release.

AVP regulates vascular tone by V_{1a} receptors located on vascular smooth muscle cells. When cardiopulmonary and sinoaortic baroreceptors detect reductions or increases in blood pressure, AVP release is stimulated or suppressed,

TABLE 2.8

ARGININE VASOPRESSIN RECEPTORS PERTINENT TO CRITICAL ILLNESS

Receptor Subtypes	Site of Action	Effects
V_{1a}	Vascular smooth muscle	Vasoconstriction
	Adrenal cortex	Glycogenolysis
	Platelets	Platelet aggregation
	Lymphocytes and monocytes	Coagulation factor release
V_{1b}	Anterior pituitary	ACTH and β-endorphin release
V_2	Renal collecting duct	Free water reabsorption

ACTH, adrenocorticotropic hormone.
Modified from Van den Berghe G, Van Roosbroeck D, Vanhove P, et al. Bone turnover in prolonged critical illness: Effect of vitamin D. *J Clin Endocrinol Metab.* 2003;88:4623–4632.

respectively. The release of AVP in response to changes in volume or pressure is less sensitive than release in response to osmoreceptors, and an 8% to 15% reduction in blood volume or pressure is needed to stimulate the release of AVP. However, once AVP is stimulated, the increase in response to baroreceptors is logarithmic, and the levels of AVP achieved are markedly above those achieved by osmotic stimulation. Hypovolemia-induced secretion of AVP overrides osmolar responses, and plasma levels may reach 10- to 1,000-fold higher than normal. AVP is a potent stimulator of arteriole vasoconstriction with increases in systemic vascular resistance. In healthy individuals, however, physiologic increases in AVP release do not usually produce significant increases in blood pressure, as AVP also potentiates the sinoaortic baroreceptor reflex in response to elevated systemic vascular resistance by V_2 receptor stimulation. This results in lowered heart rate and cardiac output and maintains constant blood pressure. Therefore, in normal individuals, AVP release increases systemic vascular resistance without increasing blood pressure by stimulation of both V_{1a} and V_2 receptors. Blood pressure changes become detectable only with supraphysiologic concentrations of AVP, and V_{1a}-activated increases in systemic vascular resistance (SVR) are out of proportion to the V_2 potentiation of the baroreceptor reflex.

AVP has been associated with both positive and negative cardiac inotropic effects in animal studies. Supraphysiologic AVP concentrations can reduce cardiac contractility and coronary blood flow secondary to V_{1a}-mediated coronary vasoconstriction. However, if coronary perfusion is maintained, AVP has a positive inotropic effect at physiologic ranges. Therefore, in healthy individuals, small, transient increases in cardiac contractility most likely occur when AVP concentrations rise within the normal physiologic range, with reductions in contractility only observed when supraphysiologic concentrations are attained. Animal studies also suggest that AVP can induce myocardial hypertrophy by enhancing cell growth without affecting cell division.

In critical illness, AVP synthesis is activated by both the systemic nervous system and the renin–angiotensin–aldosterone system, as well as by the mechanisms previously discussed. Stimulation of the baroreceptor reflex stimulates the systemic nervous system, which stimulates the supraoptic and paraventricular nuclei to synthesize and release AVP. Vasoconstrictors including angiotensin II and endothelin-1 also stimulate the release of AVP.

The use of AVP infusion as a vasoconstrictor in critical conditions including sepsis[26] and cardiac arrest is increasing.[27] There are some excellent reasons to consider this approach. First, the vascular beds of the splanchnic circulation, muscles, and skin—all vasodilatory sites in vasodilatory septic shock—have a high concentration of V_{1a}. Vasoconstriction of these sites would theoretically alter some of the pathophysiology of the hypotension. Second, although the effects of AVP are not usually as pronounced as those of catecholamines or other vasoconstrictors, AVP is synergistic with the pressor hormones, norepinephrine and angiotensin II. All three hormones have intracellular signaling that involves an increase in the cytosolic calcium concentration. Third, AVP may be advantageous in preserving renal function even when it acts as a pressor because it constricts the efferent renal arteriole as it increases blood pressure but has less effect on the afferent arteriole. Therefore, glomerular filtration pressure increases without constricting afferent arteriole flow. This is postulated to help preserve renal function because renal blood flow is not affected by the infusion. Fourth, a theoretical advantage that may help in treating vasodilatation is the observation that AVP decreases the synthesis of smooth muscle nitric oxide by inhibiting inducible nitric oxide synthase and inhibiting cyclic guanosine monophosphate (cGMP) signaling by nitric oxide, attenuating the arterial vasodilatation and pressor resistance during sepsis.

Studies show that AVP concentrations are elevated in early septic shock (200 to 300 pg per mL), but with continued shock levels decline. Even after a few hours, the neurohypophysial stores of vasopressin may become depleted and plasma concentrations may fall to approximately 30 pg per mL. Most patients decrease their levels to the normal range between 24 and 48 hours.[28] This has been called *relative vasopressin deficiency* because, in the presence of hypotension, AVP would be expected to be elevated. One potential mechanism for this relative AVP deficiency would be the depletion of pituitary stores, possibly in conjunction with impaired synthesis.

The decision to use AVP as a pressor agent, however, must involve consideration of several additional physiologic properties. First, AVP infusions can constrict the coronary arteries and cause myocardial infarction. Second, unlike dopamine and epinephrine, AVP is a direct vasoconstrictor, potentially increasing afterload without augmenting cardiac performance. Third, because AVP is a very potent venoconstrictor that decreases splanchnic compliance, excessive fluid that is administered may be distributed more centrally, including in the lung, leading to noncardiogenic pulmonary edema. Dosages of AVP >0.04 units per minute have been associated with myocardial ischemia and are not generally recommended.

Growth Hormone

GH has anabolic, lipolytic, and immune-stimulating properties. Normally, GH has peaks and troughs in which the levels may be undetectable. As discussed earlier, many of the actions of GH are mediated by IGF-1, a peptide produced in the liver and bound to specific binding proteins, particularly, IGFBP-3. In critical illness, GH is increased, whereas IGF-1 and IGFBF-3 are decreased. The decreased IGF-1 has been interpreted as GH resistance. This may be a result of cytokines inhibiting the GH–IGF-1 relation. The reduced IGFBP-3 levels may be a result of protease activity. There is limited specific knowledge of the GH–IGF relation in children. Recent evidence from children with meningococcal sepsis suggests that the relations are similar to adult studies, GH and IGFBP-1 levels were higher and IGF-1 levels were lower in those who died than in those who survived, and that PRISM scores correlated with levels of IGFBPs.[29] In critically ill patients, serum IGF-1 values correlate well with conventional nutritional indices, such as nitrogen balance, emphasizing the anabolic nature of GH. GH increases protein synthesis, decreases protein breakdown, and increases lypolysis—actions that are mediated through IGF-1. GH stimulates T lymphocytes directly and stimulates neutrophils through IGF-1.

In recent years, the effects of critical illness on GH secretion and GH action have been carefully studied, as has been the possibility of using GH as a therapeutic agent in intensive care patients. The direct actions of GH are generally opposed to the actions of insulin. Therefore, GH causes impairment of insulin-stimulated glucose uptake, increased hepatic glucose production, and stimulates lipolysis. These effects are in some ways similar to those of cortisol, but while cortisol is catabolic and causes protein degradation, GH is anabolic and stimulates protein synthesis. The fact that GH and cortisol have similar effects on glucose metabolism has two important implications. First, deficiencies of both, such as seen in children with multiple pituitary deficiencies, put the child at high risk for hypoglycemia if there is a moderate to prolonged interruption of energy intake. Second, stresses that increase levels of both (as well as of glucagon) can increase the risk of hyperglycemia because of insulin resistance.

The question as to what changes in the GH–IGF-1 axis have been observed in critical illness has been addressed in detail by the review of Van den Berghe.[30] During the initial period after an acute stress, GH levels become elevated but the normal temporal profile is altered, such that both the peaks of GH and the trough levels are elevated. However, levels of IGF-1 and the GH-dependent IGFBP-3 are decreased, which implies a state of peripheral resistance to GH. This combination of hormonal changes allows for the lipolytic and counterinsulin actions of GH, whereas because of low IGF-1, the growth-promoting effects of GH are minimized. This would appear to be beneficial because it would direct essential substrates toward survival instead of anabolic pathways in critically ill patients. With more prolonged critical illness, however, a different picture emerges, such that the amount of GH released in pulses is decreased with a high number of very small pulses, whereas the nonpulsatile secretion of GH remains high. Furthermore, the levels of the GH-dependent factors IGF-1 and IGFBP-3 are further suppressed, creating a catabolic situation that could explain the wasting seen in the chronic phase of critical illness. The reasons for low GH secretion during this chronic phase have been explored, and GH-secreting cells have been found to retain full responsiveness to GH-releasing peptides like ghrelin and some responsiveness to GHRH. This suggests that the fall in GH secretion is not because of an inability of the pituitary to make and secrete GH, or to an excess of somatostatin, but more likely because of a decrease in endogenous production of GHRH and/or GH-releasing peptides.

The finding of low levels of GH during the chronic phase of critical illness has raised the question of whether giving GH to such patients may have a beneficial effect on survival and could decrease the length of stay in intensive care. It had been previously shown that the administration of GH can attenuate the catabolic response to injury, surgery, and sepsis. For example, GH has been found to speed up healing and improve nitrogen balance in patients with burns, provided that adequate nutritional support is given.[10] In 1999, Takala et al. reported the results of two prospective, multicenter, double-blind, randomized, placebo-controlled trials involving 247 Finnish patients and 285 patients in other European countries who had been in an ICU for 5 to 7 days and who were expected to require intensive care for at least 10 days.[11] The patients received either GH at a mean daily dose of 0.10 mg per kg body weight (two to three times standard replacement doses used in treating GH deficiency) or placebo until discharge from intensive care or for a maximum of 21 days. In-hospital mortality rate was higher in the patients who received GH than in those who did not ($p < 0.001$ for both studies). In the Finnish study, the mortality rate was 39% in the GH group, as compared with 20% in the placebo group. The respective rates in the multinational study were 44% and 18%. Among those who survived, length of stay in intensive care and in the hospital, and the duration of mechanical ventilation were prolonged in the GH group. The excessive mortality in those patients receiving GH was related to infections and development of multiple organ failure. Although the mechanism for this deleterious effect is not well understood, at the present time, administration of GH to critically ill patients is not recommended.

Thyroid Hormones

Thyroid hormones also are altered in critical illness, and the thyroid response to critical illness may be a reflection of the severity of the illness. Within a few hours of a severe stress such as trauma or surgery, serum levels of T_3 decrease and levels of T_4 and TSH briefly rise, most likely as a result of decreased peripheral conversion of T_4 to T_3 with an increase in conversion of T_4 to rT_3. However, patients who have been in ICUs for several weeks typically have both low T_3 and low T_4 levels, with low or low-normal TSH. This is often referred to as the *euthyroid-sick syndrome*. There may also be a more rapid turnover of these hormones, possibly because of the hypermetabolic state. One interpretation of these changes is that they represent a physiologic response to reduced energy expenditure, similar to changes seen in starvation, and therefore no treatment is indicated. However, some believe that critical illness results in the inability of hypothalamic TRH secretion to maintain TSH and thyroid hormone production and that replacement therapy would be beneficial. It is thought that inflammation and sepsis inhibit TSH secretion, in part, through the action of cytokines on the hypothalamus and the inhibition of the TSH response to TRH by TNF-α. Other medications, such as glucocorticoids, may suppress pituitary TSH release and inhibit T_4 to T_3 conversion. Recent evidence from tissue specimens obtained immediately postmortem illustrate change in tissue deiodinase activities, particularly when there was decreased tissue perfusion and these findings correlate with the altered circulating thyroid hormone levels.[31]

Low TSH levels, both in their absolute reduction and the duration of the reduction, are associated with a poor prognosis, whereas a recovery of levels is generally thought to be a good sign. Similarly, low T_4 levels are also associated with a poor prognosis.

Reduced T_3 may have important effects. T_3 has inotropic, lusitropic, and afterload-reducing effects. Normal concentrations of T_3 are required for protein synthesis, for normal muscle metabolism, and for GH secretion and responsiveness. Therefore, reduced T_3 may be important to the catabolic phase of critical illness.

Dopamine in Critical Illness

Dopamine is such a commonly used vasoactive agent in pediatric critical care that its neuroendocrine-inflammatory effects deserve comment. Dopamine suppresses the circulating concentrations of all anterior pituitary-dependent hormones, except cortisol.[32] This pattern of pituitary suppression resembles chronic stress. Therefore, dopamine infusions have been postulated to favor the catabolic, immunocompromised state by inhibiting anabolic hormones (GH, IGF), inhibiting immune stimulating hormones (prolactin), and not affecting hypercortisolism. Membrane-bound dopamine receptors are present in the anterior pituitary and hypothalamic median eminence. These areas are both "outside" the blood–brain barrier. In healthy subjects, dopamine suppresses prolactin, TSH, and luteinizing hormone. Dopamine infusion induces an impairment of T-lymphocyte proliferative response, which has been attributed to prolonged hypoprolactinemia. Dopamine infusion reduces pulsatile GH secretion, without effecting insulin and cortisol concentrations, and prolonged dopamine infusion was associated with low concentrations of IGF-1. This may contribute to catabolism and to the failure of nutritional support to induce anabolism. Dopamine infusion suppresses serum concentrations of dehydroepiandrosterone sulfate. The observation that dopamine suppresses circulating concentrations of dehydroepiandrosterone sulfate without affecting the hypercortisolism suggests a differential regulation of adrenal androgen and cortisol metabolism in critical illness.

In the newborn, dopamine infusion also suppresses the physiologic hyperprolactinemia. In preterm infants, hypoprolactinemia has been associated with poor outcome, possibly through the additional effects of prolactin on surfactant synthesis, whole body water regulation, and gastrointestinal maturation. Dopamine also inhibits GH secretion in the newborn.

METABOLIC PATHWAYS FOR THE INTENSIVIST

Metabolism must fulfill the basic needs of energy storage and retrieval, energy production, and breakdown and synthesis of the substances necessary for each of the separate organ systems and their functions. Hormonal signals integrate and coordinate the metabolic activities of the different tissues and bring about the optimal allocation of fuels and precursors. Metabolism is controlled in three ways. First, allosteric enzymes change their catalytic activity in response to stimulatory or inhibitory modulators. Second, hormones coordinate metabolic responses. Third, the concentration of enzymes in cells may change in response to a variety of stimuli.

Glucose is the body's major cellular fuel and is stored as glycogen. Storing glucose as glycogen allows the cell to store energy with minimal osmolar effects. Glycolysis is the almost universal pathway of glucose metabolism, and in some cells such as erythrocytes, the renal medulla,

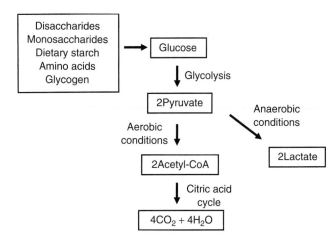

Figure 2.6 Glycolysis results in the formation of pyruvate, which is converted to acetyl-CoA under aerobic conditions and lactate under anaerobic condition.

and the brain, it is the major source of energy. There are ten steps of the breakdown of a 6-carbon sugar into two 3-carbon pyruvates (see Fig. 2.6). Pyruvate is anaerobically converted to lactate, or aerobically to acetyl-CoA, which enters the citric acid cycle (Krebs cycle) to be metabolized to carbon dioxide and water.

Glucose catabolism is regulated differently in different tissues. For example, in muscles, glucose is used for muscle activity, whereas in the liver, it is more involved in whole-body homeostasis. The hormonal milieu will also affect the metabolism of glucose. For example, in muscles, epinephrine alters the allosteric enzymes, phosphorylase-a (active form) and phosphorylase-b (inactive form), to favor glucose metabolism. In the liver, glucagon alters the same

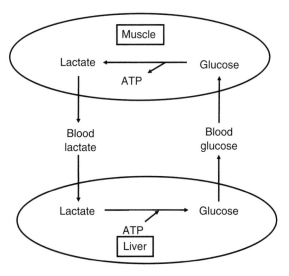

Figure 2.7 The Cori cycle. Lactate is shuttled to the liver for production of glucose, which is returned to the muscle for energy. ATP, adenosine triphosphate.

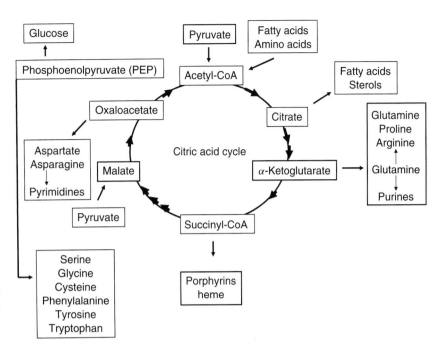

Figure 2.8 Citric acid cycle. The major intermediates of the citric acid cycle are shown, as are the important synthetic derivatives of the cycle.

enzyme, which eventually results in the release of glucose into the circulation.

Metabolic "cooperation" occurs between the skeletal muscle and the liver, and may be especially important during hypermetabolic critical illness. An example of this cooperation is the Cori cycle (see Fig. 2.7), in which glucose is utilized in the muscle, producing lactate. Lactate is shuttled to the liver and glucose is produced from the lactate.

The citric acid cycle is central to energy generation (see Fig. 2.8). Pyruvate, fatty acids, and amino acids that enter the citric acid cycle are predominantly converted to acetyl-CoA, the most common entry point in the citric acid cycle. The citric acid cycle is the most important energy-yielding process. Overall, one molecule of glucose aerobically metabolized will result in 38 molecules of adenosine triphosphate (ATP) formed (see Table 2.9). Most of the body's ATP production is from the citric acid cycle. Although the citric acid cycle is critical for energy generation, it is also important in generating many substances for the body's homeostasis (Fig. 2.8). Intermediate metabolites in the cycle can be shunted to

TABLE 2.9

ENERGY PRODUCTION FROM THE AEROBIC OXIDATION OF A MOLECULE OF GLUCOSE BY GLYCOLYSIS, THE PYRUVATE DEHYDROGENASE REACTION, AND THE CITRIC ACID CYCLE

Reaction	Number of ATP Formed
Glucose → glucose-6-phosphate	−1
Fructose-6-phosphate → fructose-1,6-bisphosphate	−1
2Glyceraldehyde-3-phosphate → 2(1,3-bisphosphoglycerate)	6
2(1,3-Bisphosphoglycerate) → 2(3-phosphoglycerate)	2
2Phosphoenolpyruvate → 2pyruvate	2
2Pyruvate → 2acetyl-CoA	6
2Isocitrate → 2α-ketoglutarate	6
2α-Ketoglutarate → 2succinyl-CoA	6
2Succinyl-CoA → 2succinate	2
2Succinate → 2fumarate	4
2Malate → 2oxaloacetate	6
Total	**38**

ATP, adenosine triphosphate.

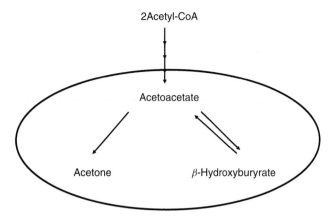

Figure 2.9   Ketone bodies.

produce other important substances. For example, citrate is used to produce fatty acids and sterols, α-ketoglutarate produces glutamine, succinyl-CoA produces porphyrins and heme, and oxaloacetate is important in producing many amino acids.

Fatty acids are oxidized in the mitochondria. β-Oxidation is the first step and removes the two successive carbon units in the form of acetyl-CoA, which enters the citric acid cycle. Therefore, the 16-carbon fatty acid palmitic acid results in eight acetyl-CoA molecules. Palmitoyl-CoA oxidation to carbon dioxide and water through the citric acid cycle results in 131 molecules of ATP.

Acetyl-CoA formed in the oxidation of fatty acids may enter the citric acid cycle or may be converted to ketone bodies (see Fig. 2.9). Acetoacetate is produced from acetyl-CoA, which is then converted to β-hydroxybutyrate, or acetone. Overproduction of ketone bodies is especially important in starvation and diabetes (see Fig. 2.10). During starvation, gluconeogenesis depletes the citric acid cycle of intermediates (especially oxaloacetate), diverting acetyl-CoA to ketone body production. In diabetes, hepatic

gluconeogenesis and fatty acid oxidation in the liver and muscle result in an increase in ketones as a result of the inability of the citric acid cycle to utilize the acetyl-CoA. In particular, acetyl-CoA is converted to acetoacetate. The brain can adapt to the use of acetoacetate or β-hydroxybutyrate instead of glucose during starvation. Acetone is exhaled.

Amino acids also contribute to energy metabolism under three circumstances. First, during normal protein turnover, some of the amino acids released undergo oxidative degradation if they are not needed for protein synthesis. Second, if a diet has excess of amino acids, they will be utilized for energy as they cannot be stored. Third and most important to the intensivist, amino acids are used for energy during starvation or critical illness when carbohydrates are either unavailable or the hormonal milieu favors protein oxidative degradation. Importantly, not only are the amino acids metabolized but they also provide three and four carbon units that can be converted to glucose by gluconeogenesis.

There are 20 different catabolic pathways for amino acids, and taken together, this degradation normally consumes 10% to 15% of the body's energy production. Therefore, the use of amino acids as fuels during critical illness is not as efficient as the use of carbohydrates or fat. The 20 different pathways yield only five products, and all can enter the citric acid cycle for energy production or can be diverted to gluconeogenesis or ketogenesis. Although much of this happens in the liver, the three branched-chain amino acids, leucine, isoleucine, and valine, are oxidized primarily in the muscle, adipose, kidney, and brain.

As each amino acid has an amino group, every degradation pathway contains a key step in which the amino group is transferred to another substance or ammonia is formed (see Fig. 2.11). In general, amino groups from the amino acids are transferred to α-ketoglutarate to form glutamate. The amino acids therefore are converted to α-ketoacids that

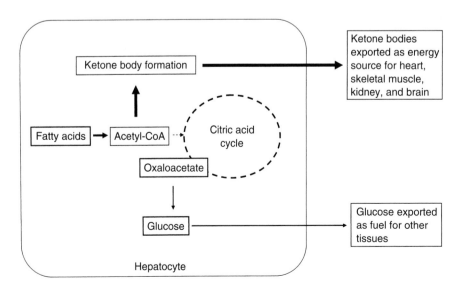

Figure 2.10   Ketone body production during starvation or diabetes.

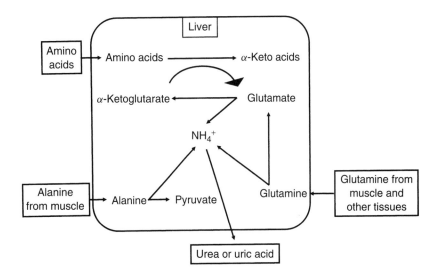

Figure 2.11 Amino acid metabolism.

can enter the energy production process. The amino group from glutamate is removed in the mitochondria to form ammonia and reform α-ketoglutarate. Amino groups are also transported from other tissues and muscles as glutamine, accounting for its relatively high concentration in blood compared to that of other amino acids. The amino groups are removed from glutamine, forming glutamate, which is available to form α-ketoglutarate and ammonia. In muscles, excess amino groups are generally transferred to pyruvate to form alanine, which is transported to the liver. When the amino group is removed from alanine, the pyruvate is free to enter the citric acid cycle. In the glucose–alanine cycle, alanine serves as a carrier of ammonia and provides the carbon skeleton of pyruvate from muscle to the liver. The ammonia is excreted, and the pyruvate is used to produce glucose, which is returned to the muscle.

Urea is formed in the liver by the urea cycle. The urea cycle combines two amino groups and bicarbonate to form one molecule of urea. It is an energy-consuming process, requiring three molecules of ATP.

METABOLIC RESPONSE TO CRITICAL ILLNESS

The metabolic response to critical illness often results in nutritional depletions secondary, in large part, to the metabolic pathways controlled by the neuroendocrine response to critical illness discussed in the preceding text. The series of events initiated by HPA axis results in events that, in large part, determine the severity of illness and the primary and secondary outcomes from critical illness. The metabolic response has been best characterized for trauma and burns because they are distinct events and the extent of illness can be relatively well characterized by the extent of body surface burned, the trauma score, or the number of organ systems involved in the injury. Table 2.10 illustrates the classical metabolic response to critical illness.

During the resuscitation phase when active fluid resuscitation is ongoing and tissue perfusion is reduced, there is a general reduction in metabolic rate and oxygen consumption. Lipolysis is present and glucose production is enhanced, providing free fatty acids and glucose to vital organs. Nitrogen loss is minimal. The early resuscitative phase is characterized by normal to mild increases in insulin and other stress hormones.

After the resuscitation, the hypermetabolic/catabolic phase of the illness starts. The etiology of the hypermetabolism is often unclear and has sometimes been referred to as a dichotomy of *push versus pull*.[33] Metabolism may be "pushed" to higher levels by the neuroendocrine milieu discussed previously or pulled to increased levels by the local inflammatory response of the infection or "organ of repair" if there is injury. This phase can last several weeks. The control of the catabolic phase of acute illness is incompletely understood but certainly involves both the HPA axis and proinflammatory hormones including TNF and IL-6. The catabolic phase either resolves as the critical illness resolves or evolves into the phase of prolonged ICU illness, the wasting syndrome (see subsequent text). Importantly, GH therapy for the acute phase of critical illness may increase mortality and is not recommended.[34,35]

In the classic hypermetabolic phase, metabolic rate and oxygen consumption are increased. The respiratory quotient (RQ) in disorders such as the systemic inflammatory response syndrome (SIRS) is often 0.8 to 0.85, reflecting a mixed energy supply of about a third carbohydrates, a third fats, and a third proteins. Compared to starvation, there is a reduction in the proportional use of glucose as an energy source, whereas there is a net loss of cellular protein from increased hepatic synthesis, primarily of acute-phase reactants, and increase in protein breakdown. The amount of this protein synthesis does not match the impressive catabolism. Table 2.11 displays the general neuroendocrine response to critical illness with the effect of each change on protein catabolism. Therefore, there is an obligate net

TABLE 2.10

CLASSIC METABOLIC RESPONSES AFTER SEVERE INJURY[a]

	Ebb Phase (Initial 24–36 h)	Flow Phase (Initial Weeks After Resuscitation)	Convalescence
Body temperature	Often reduced	Increased	Normalized
Cardiac output	Reduced	Increased	Normalized
Oxygen consumption	Reduced	Increased	Normalized
Body nitrogen loss	Reduced	Increased	Normalized
Endogenous glucose production (glycogenolysis, gluconeogenesis)	Increased	Increased	Normalized
Glucose uptake by tissues (especially spleen, liver, and immune cells)	Increased	Increased	Normalized
Lipolysis	Increased	Increased	Normalized
Plasma-free fatty acids	Increased	Increased	Normalized
Plasma lactate	Normal	Increased	Normalized
Plasma glucose	Increased	Increased	Normalized
Plasma insulin	Reduced	Increased	Normalized
Counter-regulatory hormones	Increased	Increased	Normalized
Insulin resistance	Yes	Yes	No

[a]Responses vary as a function of the nature, timing and severity of illness, nutrient provision, drug administration, and other factors.
Modified from Ziegler TR. Fuel, metabolism, and nutrient delivery in critical illness. In: Becker KL, ed. *Principles and practice of endocrinology and metabolism.* 3rd ed. Philadelphia, PA: Lippincott Williams & Wilkins; 2001:2104.[32]

TABLE 2.11

FACTORS AFFECTING PROTEIN SYNTHESIS AND PROTEIN DEGRADATION IN MUSCLE

Factor	Synthesis	Degradation
Insulin	Increased	Decreased
Growth hormone	Increased	No effect
Thyroid hormone	Increased	Increased
Glucocorticoids	Decreased	Increased
Prostaglandin E$_2$	No effect	Increased
β-Adrenergic stimulation	No effect	Decreased
Glucose	No effect	Decreased
Amino acids	Increased	Decreased
Ketones	No effect	Decreased
Free fatty acids	Increased	Decreased
Starvation	Decreased	Increased
Fever	No effect	Increased
Trauma	No effect	Increased

Adapted from Mitch WE, Clark AS. Muscle protein turnover in uremia. *Kidney Int.* 1983;24:S2.[36]

loss of protein as reflected in the urinary nitrogen, which may reach >20 g of nitrogen per day in adults. The protein catabolism is also correlated with the metabolic rate and oxygen consumption (Table 2.1).

Glucose homeostasis is altered in critical illness[37] (see Fig. 2.12). Overall, the hormonal response described in the preceding text in which glucagons, epinephrine, and cortisol oppose and overwhelm the action of insulin, leads to lipolysis, and proteolysis. This increases gluconeogenic precursors such as alanine and lactate. The degree of hyperglycemia is often out of proportion to the amount of insulin believed by many to be a result of insulin resistance. Therefore, hyperglycemia is fostered by both overproduction and reduced utilization of glucose.

Severe injury and infection are associated with a different peripheral glucose uptake and utilization response than either the normal response to hyper- and hypoglycemia or starvation. Glucose is transported into cells by binding to carrier proteins that increase its lipid solubility. A sodium–glucose cotransporter actively transports glucose across the cell membrane in conjunction with sodium in the small intestine and proximal tubule of the kidney. Passive transport occurs by carrier proteins of which three glucose transporter isoforms are most important. GLUT1 is responsible for basal glucose uptake and can be found in many tissues. GLUT2 is expressed predominantly in the liver, kidney, small intestines, and pancreatic β cells. GLUT4 is found only where glucose uptake is mediated by insulin; tissues with the most insulin sensitivity are muscle, fat, and heart. Noninsulin-mediated glucose uptake (NIMGU) occurs in both insulin-sensitive and insulin-insensitive tissues. Following a meal, approximately 80% of whole body glucose uptake is by NIMGU.

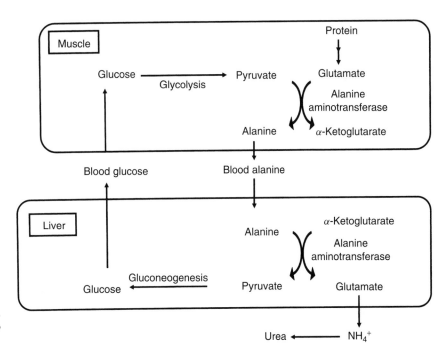

Figure 2.12 The glucose–alanine cycle. Alanine formed from pyruvate is shunted to the liver for the production of glucose.

Normally, an increase in blood glucose would stimulate insulin secretion from the pancreas, which mediates peripheral glucose uptake and inhibition of gluconeogenesis. When insulin is bound to the cell receptor, carrier proteins migrate to the cell membrane and general carrier protein activity is increased; counter-regulatory proteins such as catecholamines and glucagon inhibit this activity. Stress increases cellular uptake of glucose, predominantly through NIMGU processes involving the GLUT1 carrier protein, especially in muscles. This is probably mediated by cytokines. For example, TNF can increase glucose uptake in many tissues.[38]

Once taken up by the cell, glucose is either metabolized to pyruvate by glycolysis or stored as glycogen as described in the preceding text. During stress, glycolysis is favored over glycogen synthesis as glycogen formation in the liver and muscle actually appears to be inhibited during the acute stress phase (see Fig. 2.13). Increased glycolytic activity seems to be secondary to the augmented glucose uptake, and ATP turnover and AMP production, which stimulate phosphofructokinase, the rate-limiting enzyme of glycolysis.

Pyruvate (Fig. 2.13) can be oxidized by the citric acid cycle to carbon dioxide and water, converted to lactate, transaminated to alanine, and recycled to glucose by oxaloacetate. The conversion of pyruvate to lactate is most often attributed to tissue hypoperfusion and persistent hyperlactatemia is not uncommon in patients who have been resuscitated from severe injury or infection, especially septic shock. However, the etiology of the hyperlactatemia in many patients may not be hypoperfusion or anaerobic metabolism. In general, the degree of hyperlactatemia correlates with other measures of hypermetabolism such as urinary nitrogen loss and oxygen consumption, but not necessarily with the extent of the hypoperfusion. "Stress hyperlactatemia" is often accompanied by a normal lactate to pyruvate ratio (10:1 to 15:1) suggesting that the increased lactate is a result of an equilibration process driven by increased pyruvate. A likely explanation for the hyperlactatemia for many patients is that the stress response promotes increased glucose uptake, which stimulates glycolysis, producing lactate and pyruvate by a mass–action effect. Increased lactate could also be a result of alterations in the use of pyruvate. For example, evidence for reduced pyruvate dehydrogenate activity suggests that pyruvate may serve less as a substrate for oxidation or lipogenesis and more as a substrate for lactate, alanine, and gluconeogenesis.

Gluconeogenesis is increased during stress. Glucagon, cortisol, and epinephrine, all part of the hormonal milieu of the stress response, stimulate gluconeogenesis, whereas insulin inhibits gluconeogenesis. Figure 2.14 illustrates the conversion of lactate and alanine to glucose. Lactate is recycled to glucose by the Cori cycle (see preceding text) and alanine is recycled to glucose in the glucose–alanine cycle. In the illustration, muscle produces an excess of both alanine and lactate, which are converted in the liver by the Cori and glucose–alanine cycles to glucose, which reenters the circulation for those tissues that have an obligate glucose requirement. Although the figure shows the alanine as coming from muscle, only 30% of it comes from muscle, with the remainder being supplied by *de novo* synthesis. Alanine also serves as a method to transport ammonia to the liver in a nontoxic form.

Hyperglycemia is commonly seen during the acute stress response; approximately 50% of critically ill adults have hyperglycemia. Until recently, hyperglycemia was generally

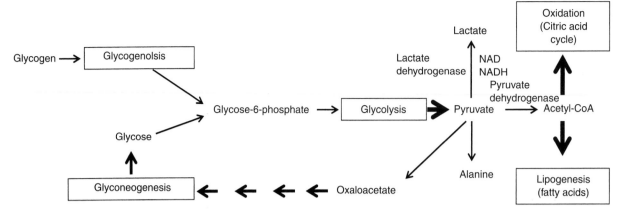

Figure 2.13 The predominant glucose pathways during acute stress. NAD, nicotinamide adenine dinucleotide; NADH, nicotinamide adenine dinucleotide (reduced form).

viewed as an adaptive mechanism to insure adequate glucose delivery. The etiology of hyperglycemia has been attributed to peripheral insulin resistance characterized by impaired insulin-mediated glucose uptake despite normal or increased insulin levels. Insulin resistance is clearly present in the skeletal muscle but may also be present in other tissues including fat, liver, and heart. The mechanism probably involves a defect in the postreceptor binding processes. Additionally, the hormonal milieu of increased counter-regulatory hormones of catecholamines, glucagons, GH, and cortisol decreases the activity of glucose transporter proteins; it increases gluconeogenesis and decreases glycogen synthesis. Cytokines such as IL-1, IL 6, and TNF have also been postulated to be the direct and indirect mediators of insulin resistance.

More recently, the potential for tighter glucose control contributing to improved outcomes in the ICU setting has been emphasized. Among several studies that show increased glucose levels correlated with increased mortality is one that was undertaken in a pediatric intensive care unit

(PICU). It was found that although the degree of blood glucose elevation that was detected on the first day did not correlate with increased mortality, the highest blood glucose level documented within 10 days of finding an elevated blood glucose level was a fairly strong predictor of mortality.[39] This suggests that persistent rather than acute hyperglycemia may increase the risk of poor outcomes in the critical care setting. The strongest evidence for the deleterious effect of hyperglycemia was provided by the landmark study of Van den Berghe et al.[40] They looked at the effect of intensive IV insulin therapy in 1,548 mechanically ventilated surgical ICU patients. One group of randomly assigned patients was given insulin by algorithm to maintain blood glucose concentrations between 80 and 110 mg per dL, whereas the control group got IV insulin only when the blood glucose exceeded 200 mg per dL, with a target range of 180 to 200 mg per dL. The intensive insulin therapy group had an ICU mortality rate of 4.6%, compared to 8% for the conventional group, a reduction of 43%. Perhaps even more important, the mortality reduction

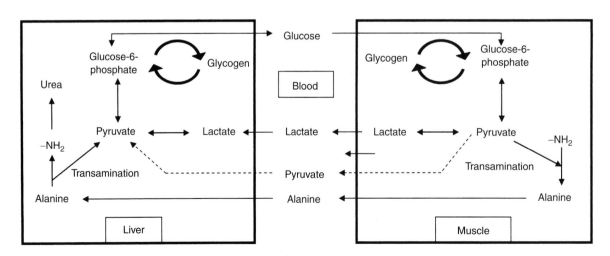

Figure 2.14 The Cori cycle and glucose–alanine cycle in critical illness.

was most dramatic in those requiring ICU care for >5 days when the mortality reduction was from 20.2% to 10.6%. The intensive insulin group also achieved reductions in hospital mortality, duration of mechanical ventilation, and duration of ICU stay. Further analysis of this study and other studies showed clearly that the control of blood glucose rather than the insulin dose *per se* was the factor associated with improved outcomes.[41] The mechanism for mortality and morbidity reduction currently remains speculative.[42]

Exogenous administration of protein can improve synthesis and thereby set targets for nutritional support. Unfortunately, as organ dysfunction worsens, hepatic synthesis decreases significantly and is associated with an adverse outcome.

Table 2.10 illustrates the general hormonal changes characteristically seen in critical illness.

Amino acids become an important energy source and are derived from skeletal muscle, connective tissue, and intestinal viscera, leading to impressive loss of lean body mass, a condition termed *autocannibalism*. The branched-chain amino acids (e.g., leucine, isoleucine, and valine) are favored in the peripheral oxidation that occurs.[43] Importantly, glutamine and alanine are preferred amino acids and they are derived primarily from muscle breakdown. They are used as a primary fuel and for gluconeogenesis. Glutamine, in particular, is a fuel substrate for gut mucosa and immune cells.

Protein metabolism is affected in many types of critical illness. Protein catabolism is relatively unaffected by administering exogenous amino acids. The result of protein catabolism is increased gluconeogenic amino acids and urea production.

The control of the hypermetabolic state is unknown. Healthy adults infused with glucagons, hydrocortisone, and epinephrine show an increased nitrogen loss, insulin resistance, and increased metabolic rate.[44] Cytokines may be involved in the control of the metabolic processes as well.

ACUTE VERSUS PROLONGED CRITICAL ILLNESS

Led by the work of Van den Berghe, we have recently begun to better conceptualize the neuroendocrine response to critical illness in the acute phase and the prolonged phase.[45] The acute phase is that conceptualized by Cuthbertson's "ebb" and "flow," with the ebb phase being characterized by reduction in metabolism and tissue perfusion and direction of nutrients and flow to vital organs, and the flow phase with its hypermetabolism fueled by lipolysis, gluconeogenesis, and catabolism providing the substrates for inflammation and healing. Without nutritional support and a cessation of the hypermetabolism, the catabolism will consume sufficient protein stores to be incompatible with life. Therefore, the syndrome is characterized by an

TABLE 2.12

ENDOCRINE RESPONSES IN ACUTE VERSUS PROLONGED CRITICAL ILLNESS[a]

	Acute (Initial 7–10 d)	Prolonged (>10 d)
Cortisol	↑↑	↑
Adrenal androgens	↓	↓
Aldosterone	↑	NL to ↓
Glucagon	↑↑	↑
Insulin	NL to ↓	↑
Catecholamines	↑↑	↑
Triiodothyronine (total)	↓↓	↓
Thyroxine (total)	NL to ↑	NL to ↓
IGF-1	↓	↓
IGFBP-3	↓	↓
Testosterone	↓	↓
Cytokines (TNF, IL-1, IL-6)	↑	NL

[a]Responses vary as a function of the nature, timing, and severity of illness underlying nutritional status, drug administration, and other factors. Alterations in growth hormone and thyroid-stimulating hormone pulse amplitude and/or pulse number also may occur.
↑, increased blood levels; ↓, decreased blood levels; NL, generally normal blood levels; IGF, insulinlike growth factor; IGFBP, IGF-binding protein; TNF, tumor necrosis factor; IL, interleukin.
Modified from Ziegler TR. Fuel, metabolism, and nutrient delivery in critical illness. In: Becker KL, ed. *Principles and practice of endocrinology and metabolism.* 3rd ed. Philadelphia, PA: Lippincott Williams & Wilkins; 2001:2104.[32]

actively secreting anterior pituitary and a lack of activity of anabolic hormones at the periphery.

Prolonged critical illness presents a different profile. Table 2.12 contrasts the acute versus the prolonged hormonal profiles. The wasting syndrome seen predominantly in adult patients is characterized by continued loss of protein despite adequate nutritional support. Protein is lost by increased degradation and lack of synthesis even while fat is accumulating in adipose tissue and in other organs. Unlike the flow phase of acute illness, this syndrome is characterized by immune paralysis. There is a limited ability of the immune system to respond to challenge. As the syndrome continues, there is atrophy of muscles with weakness and the secondary consequences of prolonged mechanical ventilation and bed rest, atrophy of intestinal mucosa and intestinal muscles with the prolonged need for parenteral alimentation, and fatty infiltration of the liver with interruption of hepatic metabolic processes. And this response results not from the stimulus of critical illness or the severity but from the duration of critical illness. Although the set of changes in the prolonged critical illness syndrome have not been elucidated, it seems to be most consistent with dysfunction of the HPA axis. There is a uniformly reduced pulsatile activity of anterior pituitary hormones, resulting in reduced hormones except for cortisol levels that are believed to be maintained from nonpituitary mechanisms.

In prolonged critical illness, ACTH level is low, whereas cortisol is elevated, indicating that cortisol may be driven by other mechanisms. The etiology of the low ACTH is not known. The level of immune stimulant dehydroepiandrosterone sulfate, which has stimulatory effects on helper T cells, is also low. Aldosterone level is also low, although plasma renin is often elevated. It has been postulated that this represents a shift from mineralocorticoid and adrenal androgen pathways toward the glucocorticoid pathway, and is directed by "peripheral drive."

In prolonged critical illness, there are markedly different physiologies in the relation between hypothalamic control and peripheral endocrine physiology. In the acute phase, GH is increased, and IGF-1 and IGFBP-3 are decreased. GH is released in very high peaks, and the troughs are also elevated. Since serum concentrations of free fatty acids and glucose are elevated and insulin levels are also increased, GH may still be an effective controller of this response, stimulating lipolysis, gluconeogenesis, and through insulin antagonism. During prolonged critical illness, GH is released in lower peaks, with interpulse levels still being elevated. GH and IGF-1 are positively correlated instead of the negative correlation of the acute phase.

The thyroid axis in acute and chronic critical illness is also different. In acute illness, TSH is relatively normal, although T_3 is decreased within the first day (proportionate to severity of illness), possibly because of reduced T_4 to T_3 conversion, and increased breakdown. rT_3 level is elevated, in part because of the reduced rT_3 degradation. The relatively low TSH in the presence of low T_3 (low T_3 syndrome) implies a hypothalamic–pituitary axis dysfunction. Perhaps it is an adaptation to the catabolic state. In contrast to the acute phase, TSH pulse levels are reduced but TSH is positively correlated to T_3 levels, implying there is a central hypothyroidism.

Prolactin level is elevated in acute stress, perhaps because of its immune stimulatory properties. In prolonged critical illness, it is reduced.

THE ENDOCRINE SYSTEM AND OTHER DISEASES AND CONDITIONS

Because hormones affect all systems of the body, they both contribute to and are affected by diseases of various organ systems. Although most of these interactions do not involve critical illness, some of the interactions are important to both understand and treat conditions encountered in the ICU. Many of these endocrine disorders are more likely to affect adults but are occasionally important to children in PICUs, especially during adolescence. Table 2.13 summarizes some of the associations of organ system dysfunction and endocrine abnormalities.

TABLE 2.13

SELECTED ORGAN SYSTEM DYSFUNCTIONS RELATED TO ENDOCRINE DISORDERS

Organ Dysfunction	Associated Hormonal Abnormality
Central nervous system dysfunction (confusion, delirium, psychosis, depression, organic brain syndrome, etc.)	Hyperparathyroidism, hypoparathyroidism, hypercortisolism, increased CRH
Lung maturation	Corticosteroids, thyroid hormones, insulin
Upper airway obstruction (e.g., macroglossia, laryngeal spasm)	Growth hormone excess, hypoparathyroidism
Central sleep apnea	Hypothyroidism
Heart failure	Hypothyroidism
Hypertension	Hyperthyroidism, Cushing syndrome, pheochromocytoma
Muscle weakness (including dysphagia with aspiration)	Hyperthyroidism, hypothyroidism, steroid excess, hyperaldosteronism, elevated calcium, hypophosphatemia

CRH, corticotropin-releasing hormone.

CNS mood disorders, if severe, can result in ICU illness. Psychosis, dementia, depression, and organic brain syndromes occasionally are components of ICU illnesses and may be caused by a variety of endocrine disorders. Hypothyroidism, hyperparathyroidism, hypoparathyroidism, Cushing disease, and Cushing syndrome are examples of endocrinopathies that can cause severe mood disorders resulting in, or contributing to, critical illness.

The respiratory system is affected both prenatally and postnatally. Corticosteroids, thyroid hormones, estrogen, and perhaps insulin, all affect lung development *in utero*. Endocrine disorders involving GH excess may cause macroglossia, and hypocalcemia can result in laryngeal tetany, both conditions causing upper airway obstruction. Diseases of the lung such as pneumonia and metastatic tumors may be associated with syndrome of inappropriate secretion of antidiuretic hormone (SIADH). Hypothyroidism also may cause sleep apnea. Disorders such as acromegaly may cause abnormalities of the chest but are very unlikely to present during childhood or adolescence.

Endocrine disorders,[46] especially thyroid disorders,[47] have many cardiac effects. Hypothyroidism is associated with decreased levels of catecholamines, down-regulation of the β-adrenergic receptors, and rarely heart failure from decreased heart rate, stroke volume, cardiac output, and blood volume. Hyperthyroidism is associated with up-regulation of the β-adrenergic receptors, tachycardia,

TABLE 2.14

ELECTROCARDIOGRAPHIC ABNORMALITIES ASSOCIATED WITH THYROID DISORDERS

Sinus tachycardia, atrial fibrillation, notched P waves, first-degree heart block	Hyperthyroidism
Sinus bradycardia, decreased P wave amplitude, prolonged QT interval, prolonged QRS, ventricular arrhythmias	Hypothyroidism

and increased contractility. Both hyperthyroidism and hypothyroidism are associated with electrocardiographic abnormalities (see Table 2.14). Hypertension is associated with hyperthyroidism, conditions of steroid excess, conditions associated with hyperparathyroidism, and pheochromocytoma.

Liver disease has an especially important influence on hormones because of synthesis and degradation. If liver function is sufficiently disturbed to alter its synthetic and metabolic functions, the effects on hormones may be clinically significant. This is especially true of GH and thyroid hormones. GH effects are mediated, in part, through IGF-1, which is produced in the liver, and one of GHs primary sites of degradation is the liver. Binding proteins for thyroid hormone as synthesized in the liver and

these binding proteins will determine the amount of free thyroid hormone present in the plasma. Liver disease is also associated with increased T_4, decreased T_3 from decreased conversion of T_4 to T_3, increased rT_3, and increased thyroid binding globulin. Usually, patients with liver disease are clinically euthyroid and the TSH is usually normal or only slightly elevated. The association of these thyroid hormone abnormalities with liver disease (e.g., T_3, T_3/T_4 ratio) has been proposed as a way to follow the severity of liver disease.

Perhaps the most profound organ affected by a diversity of hormones is the kidney. Table 2.15 illustrates the kidney's response to nonrenal hormones. There are many important effects in the maintenance of water and electrolyte homeostasis secondary to the interaction of the renal and endocrine systems.

The kidney is also an important site of hormone metabolism that may be altered or lost with acute or chronic renal failure. In renal failure, there may be increasing hormonal levels and increasing hormonal effects. Renal metabolism of hormones occurs at the glomerulus for some small, relatively simple hormones, hydrolysis by the brush border membrane, hydrolysis or other degradation by the proximal tubular cells after internalization, and by the peritubular circulation. Local hormonal metabolism at the glomerulus occurs for angiotensin, bradykinin, and calcitonin; this is a minor, although potentially

TABLE 2.15

KIDNEY RESPONSES TO NONRENAL HORMONES

Hormone	Glomerular-Filtration Rate	Renal Blood Flow	Urinary Sodium Excretion	Urinary Potassium Excretion	Urinary Calcium Excretion
Mineralocorticoids	NC	NC	↓	↑	NC or ↑
Glucocorticoids	↑	↑	±	↑	↑
Antidiuretic hormone	NC	NC	NC or ↑	?↑	NC or ↑
Parathyroid hormone	NC or ↓	NC or ↑	↑	↑	↓
Calcitonin	NC	NC	↑	↑	↑
Insulin	NC	NC	↓	↓	↑
Glucagon	↑	↑	↑	↑	↑
Estrogen	NC	NC	↓	NC	↓
Progesterone	↑	↑	↑	±	—
Thyroid hormone	↑	↑	NC or ↑	NC	↑
Prolactin	NC or ↑	NC or ↑	↓	↓	↑
α-Adrenergic agonists	↓	↓	↓	—	? ↑
β-Adrenergic agonists	NC	↑	NC or ↑	? ↓	—
Growth hormone	NC or ↑	±	↓	↓	↑
Atrial natriuretic hormone	↑	NC	↑	↑	? ↑

NC, no change; ↓, decrease; ±, variable; ?, questionable; ↑, increase.
From Kimmel PL, Rivera A, Khatri P. Effects of nonrenal hormones on the normal kidney. In: Becker KL, ed. *Principles and practice of endocrinology and metabolism*. 3rd ed. Philadelphia, PA: Lippincott Williams & Wilkins; 2001:1886.[48]

TABLE 2.16
EFFECTS OF CHEMOTHERAPY ON ENDOCRINE FUNCTION

Chemotherapeutic Agents	Endocrine Function
Hypothalamus–Pituitary	
L-asparaginase[a]	↓ TSH release
Vincristine (animal data)	↓ GH release
Cyclophosphamide; vincristine; vinblastine; melphalan; cisplatin	SIADH
Thyroid	
L-asparaginase	↓ TBG levels
5-Fluorouracil; mitotane	↑ TBG levels
BVP (bleomycin, vinblastine, cisplatin) chemotherapy	↓ Thyroid hormone clearance (? through ↓ deiodinase activity)
Vinblastine (animal data)	↓ Thyroidal hormone secretion
[131]I-containing radiopharmaceuticals; aminoglutethimide; vincristine, carmustine (or lomustine), procarbazine	↑ TSH; ↓ T_3, T_4
Cisplatin, vinblastine; busulfan, cyclophosphamide	↑ TSH; normal T_3, T_4
Parathyroid	
Vinblastine, L-asparaginase (animal data); multidrug chemotherapy for acute leukemia	↓ PTH secretion
Pancreas	
Vincristine, L-asparaginase; streptozocin; plicamycin; mitomycin C; 5-fluorouracil	↓ Insulin secretion
Cyclophosphamide	Autoimmune diabetes
Dacarbazine, mitomycin, doxorubicin, cisplatin, GM-CSF[a]	↑ Insulin secretion, ↓ insulin action
L-asparaginase[a]	↑ Glucagon secretion
Adrenal	
5-Fluorouracil; 5-fluorodeoxyuridine	↓ *In vitro* steroidogenesis
Mitotane; aminoglutethimide	↓ Cortisol, ± ↓ aldosterone
Renal	
Cisplatin; multidrug chemotherapy for ALL, AML[a]	↓ 1,25-dihydroxyvitamin D, ↓ Ca, ↓ Mg
Ifosfamide; streptozocin	Nephrogenic DI

[a]concomitant corticosteroid administration.

↓, decreased; ↑, increased; TSH, thyroid-stimulating hormone; GH, growth hormone; SIADH, syndrome of inappropriate secretion of antidiuretic hormone; TBG, thyroxine-binding globulin; T_3, triiodothyronine; T_4, thyroxine; PTH, parathyroid hormone; GM-CSF, granulocyte-macrophage colony-stimulating factor; ALL, acute lymphoblastic leukemia; AML, acute myeloblastic leukemia; DI, diabetes insipidus; ATRA, all-*trans* retinoic acid.

Modified from Bajorunas DR. Endocrine consequences of cancer therapy. Effects of nonrenal hormones on the normal kidney. In: Becker KL, ed. *Principles and practice of endocrinology and metabolism.* 3rd ed. Philadelphia, PA: Lippincott Williams & Wilkins; 2001:2058.[49]

significant, contribution to the metabolic clearance rate of the hormones. Larger and more complex hormones such as insulin, parathyroid hormone, and GH that are filtered can be internalized by the proximal tubular cells after binding to the receptor megalin. From 25% to over 50% of GH is metabolized in the kidney, most of it through filtration and uptake by the proximal tubular cells. There is also some uptake and metabolism of GH by the peritubular blood vessels. After filtration, over 99% of GH is taken up by the proximal tubular cells. Therefore, in renal failure, plasma GH levels are elevated and the half-life is prolonged by up to 50%. AVP is filtered and removed by both brush border membrane hydrolysis and uptake by the proximal tubular cells. Up to 66% of the metabolic clearance of AVP is by the kidney. The kidney also accounts for 24% of the metabolic clearance of glucagons, predominantly by proximal tubular degradation and a small amount of removal by the peritubular circulation. Similar to GH, insulin, once filtered, is almost completely reabsorbed and degraded, and there is also some absorption by the peritubular circulation. Approximately 33% of insulin is normally degraded in the kidney. The major role of the kidney in the elimination of many other hormones including steroids, and aldosterone is the elimination of the inactive metabolites from hepatic degradation.

Shock has been associated with many endocrinologic complications. Pituitary necrosis may present with partial or complete panhypopituitarism of sudden onset. Pancreatitis with necrosis and adrenal hemorrhage has also occurred with shock.

Cancer and chemotherapy result in complex physiologic changes including changes in the hormonal milieu. Many of the aspects of the stress response are applicable to these patients, especially when they become acutely ill with sepsis or other disorders. In particular, chemotherapeutic regimens are well known to alter the hormonal milieu (see Table 2.16).

Infections can cause endocrine complications pertinent to the intensivist. Bilateral adrenal hemorrhage (Waterhouse-Friedrichsen syndrome) occurs predominantly with infections from *Neisseria meningitides, Haemophilus influenzae, Staphylococcus pyogenes,* and *Staphylococcus pneumoniae.* Hypothalamic–pituitary infections are rare but may occur secondary to pneumococcal, streptococcal, listerial, or tuberculous meningitis. Acute infections of the thyroid, pancreas, adrenal, and gonads have been reported. Human immunodeficiency virus is associated with hypothalamic-pituitary dysfunction, SIADH, hypothyroidism, pneumocystis carinii thyroiditis, and both increased insulin sensitivity and insulin resistance.

REFERENCES

1. Wilmore DW. From Cuthbertson to fast-track surgery: 70 years of progress in reducing stress in surgical patients. *Ann Surg.* 2002;236:643–648.
2. Cerra FB. Multiple organ failure syndrome. In: Bihari DJ, Cerra FB, eds. *Multiple organ failure.* Fullerton, CA: Society of Critical Care Medicine; 1989:1–24.
3. Rogers A, Walker N, Schug S, et al. Reduction of postoperative mortality and morbidity with epidural or spinal anesthesia: Results from overview of randomized trials. *Br Med J.* 2000;321:1493–1504.
4. Herndon DN, Hart DW, Wolf SE, et al. Reversal of catabolism by β-blockade after severe burns. *N Engl J Med.* 2001;345:1223–1229.
5. Anand KJS, Hickey PR. Halothane-morphine compared with high-dose sufentanil for anesthesia and postoperative analgesia in neonatal cardiac surgery. *N Engl J Med.* 1992;326:1–9.
6. Lashansky G, Saenger P, Fishman K, et al. Normative data for adrenal steroidogenesis in a healthy pediatric population: Age and sex-related changes after ACTH stimulation. *J Clin Endocrinol Metab.* 1991;73:674.
7. Cassorla F, Linder BL, Esteban NV, et al. The cortisol production rate in children: Implications for therapy. *Endocrinologist.* 1991;1:98–101.
8. Menon K, Clarson C. Adrenal function in pediatric critical illness. *Pediatr Crit Care Med.* 2002;3:112–116.
9. Burchard K. A review of the adrenal cortex and severe inflammation: Quest of the euthyroid state. *J Trauma.* 2001;51:800–814.
10. Adachi M, Tachibana K, Masuno M, et al. Clinical characterization of children with hypoparathyroidism due to 22q11.2 deletions. *J Pediatr.* 1998;157:33.
11. Kreiter SR, Schwartz RP, Kirkman HN Jr, et al. Nutritional rickets in African American breast-fed infants. *J Pediatr.* 2000;137:153–157.
12. Klein GL, Nicolai M, Langman CB, et al. Dysregulation of calcium homeostasis after severe burn injury in children: Possible role of magnesium depletion. *J Pediatr.* 1997;131:246–251.
13. Van den Berghe G, Van Roosbroeck D, Vanhove P, et al. Bone turnover in prolonged critical illness: Effect of vitamin D. *J Clin Endocrinol Metab.* 2003;88:4623–4632.
14. Lee CR, Watkins ML, Patterson JH, et al. Vasopressin: A new target for the treatment of heart failure. *Am Heart J.* 2003;146:9–18.
15. Akira S, Hirano T, Taga T, et al. Biology of multifunctional cytokines: IL 6 and related molecules (IL 1 and TNF). *FASEB J.* 1990;4:2860–2867.
16. Reichlin S. Mechanisms of disease: Neuroendocrine-immune interactions. *N Engl J Med.* 1993;329:1246–1253.
17. Chrousos GP. The hypothalamic-pituitary-adrenal axis and immune-mediated inflammation. *N Engl J Med.* 1995;332:1351–1363.
18. Van den Berghe G, de Zegher F. Anterior pituitary function during critical illness and dopamine treatment. *Crit Care Med.* 1996;24:1580–1590.
19. Schoroeder S, Wichers M, Klingmuller D, et al. The hypothalamic-adrenal axis of patients with severe sepsis: Altered response to corticotropin-releasing hormone. *Crit Care Med.* 2001;29:310–316.
20. Zaloga GP, Bhatt B, Marik P. Critical illness and systemic inflammation. In: Becker KL, ed. *Principles and practice of endocrinology and metabolism.* 3rd ed. Philadelphia, PA: Lippincott Williams & Wilkins; 2001:2077–2087.
21. Reichlin S. Mechanisms of disease: Neuroendocrine-immune interactions. *N Engl J Med.* 1993;29:1246–1253.
22. Levine A, Cohen D, Zadik Z. Urinary cortisol values in children under stress. *J Pediatr.* 1994;125:853–857.
23. Shroeder S, Wichers M, Dlingmuller D, et al. The hypothalamic-pituitary-adrenal axis of patients with severe sepsis: Altered response to corticotropin-releasing hormone. *Crit Care Med.* 2001;29:310–316.
24. Alafifi AA, Van den Berghe G, Snider RH. Endocrine markers and mediators in critical illness. In: Becker KL, ed. *Principles and practice of endocrinology and metabolism.* 3rd ed. Philadelphia, PA: Lippincott Williams & Wilkins; 2001:2077–2087.
25. Marx C MD, Petros S MD, Bornstein SR MD, et al. Adrenocortical hormones in survivors and nonsurvivors of severe sepsis: Diverse time course of dehydroepiandrosterone, dehydroepiandrosterone-sulfate, and cortisol. *Crit Care Med.* 2003;31:1382–1388.
26. Dellinger RP, Carlet JM, Masur H, et al. Surviving sepsis campaign guidelines for management of severe sepsis and septic shock. *Crit Care Med.* 2004;32:858–873.
27. Wenzel V, Krismer AC, Arntz HR, et al. A comparison of vasopressin and epinephrine for out-of-hospital cardiopulmonary resuscitation. *N Engl J Med.* 2004;350(2):105–113.
28. Sharshar T, Blanchard A, Paillard M, et al. Circulating vasopressin levels in septic shock. *Crit Care Med.* 2003;31:1752–1758.
29. De Groof F, Joosten KFM, Janssen JAMJL, et al. Acute stress response in children with meningococcal sepsis: Important differences in the growth hormone/insulin-like growth factor I axis between nonsurvivors and survivors. *J Clin Endocrinol Metab.* 2002;87:3118–3124.
30. Van den Berghe G. Endocrine evaluation of patients with critical illness. *Endocrinol Metab Clin North Am.* 2003;32:385–410.
31. Peeters RP, Wouters PJ, Kaptein E, et al. Reduced activation and increased inactivation of thyroid hormone in tissues of critically Ill patients. *J Clin Endocrinol Metab.* 2003;88(7):3202–3211.
32. Ziegler TR. Fuel, metabolism, and nutrient delivery in critical illness. In: Becker KL, ed. *Principles and practice of endocrinology and metabolism.* 3rd ed. Philadelphia, PA: Lippincott Williams & Wilkins; 2001:2104.
33. Stoner HB. Metabolism after trauma and in sepsis. *Circ Shock.* 1986;19:75–87.

34. Takala J, Ruokonen D, Webster NR, et al. Increased mortality associated with growth hormone treatment in critically in adults. *N Engl J Med.* 1999;341:785–792.

35. Demling R. Growth hormone therapy in critically ill patients. *N Engl J Med.* 1999;341:837–839.

36. Mitch WE, Clark AS. Muscle protein turnover in uremia. *Kidney Int.* 1983;24:S2.

37. Robinson LE, van Soeren MH. Insulin resistance and hyperglycemia in critical illness: Role of insulin in glycemic control. *AACN Clin Issues Adv Pract Acute Crit Care.* 2004;15:45–62.

38. Mizock B. Alterations in carbohydrate metabolism during stress; a review of the literature. *Am J Med.* 1995;98:75–84.

39. Faustino EV, Apkon M. Persistent hyperglycemia in critically ill children. *J Pediatr.* 2005;146:30–34.

40. Van den Berghe G, Wouters P, Weekers F, et al. Intensive insulin therapy in critically ill patients. *N Engl J Med.* 2001;345:1359–1367.

41. Van den Berghe G, Wouters PJ, Bouillon R, et al. Outcome benefit of intensive insulin therapy in the critically ill: Insulin dose versus glycemic control. *Crit Care Med.* 2003;31:359–366.

42. Van den Berghe G. How does blood glucose control with insulin save lives in intensive care? *J Clin Invest.* 2004;114(9):1187–1195.

43. Ziegler TR. Fuel, metabolism and nutrient delivery in critical illness. In: Becker KL, ed. *Principles and practice of endocrinology and metabolism.* 3rd ed. Philadelphia, PA: Lippincott Williams & Wilkins; 2001:2102–2108.

44. Bessey PQ, Lowe KA. Early hormonal changes affect the catabolic response to trauma. *Ann Surg.* 1993;218:476.

45. Van den Berghe G. Neuroendocrine response to acute versus prolonged critical illness. In: Becker KL, ed. *Principles and practice of endocrinology and metabolism.* 3rd ed. Philadelphia, PA: Lippincott Williams & Wilkins; 2001:2094–2102.

46. Schrier RW, Abraham WT. Mechanism of disease: Hormones and hemodynamics in heart failure. *N Engl J Med.* 1999;341:577–585.

47. Lein I, Ojamaa K. Mechanisms of disease: Thyroid hormone and the cardiovascular system. *N Engl J Med.* 2001;344:501–509.

48. Kimmel PL, Rivera A, Khatri P. Effects of nonrenal hormones on the normal kidney. In: Becker KL, ed. *Principles and practice of endocrinology and metabolism.* 3rd ed. Philadelphia, PA: Lippincott Williams & Wilkins; 2001:1886.

49. Bajorunas DR. Endocrine consequences of cancer therapy. Effects of nonrenal hormones on the normal kidney. In: Becker KL, ed. *Principles and practice of endocrinology and metabolism.* 3rd ed. Philadelphia, PA: Lippincott Williams & Wilkins; 2001:2058.

Immunology, Inflammation, and Infectious Diseases

Anthony D. Slonim   Nalini Singh

The study of immunity, inflammation, and infectious diseases is important to the pediatric intensivist. It represents the mechanisms by which the host—in this case, the critically ill child—defends itself against and responds to disease caused by environmental elements. This section deals with the mechanisms of host defense that traverse different organ systems and provides both generic and specific responses to external insults.

Host defense involves interactions between the host, the pathogen, and the environment. It helps determine the extent and outcome of a broad group of clinical diseases (see Fig. 3.1). Chapter 3.1 provides the structural and functional components of host defense. Chapter 3.2 describes the host's response to generic external insults. Inflammation is essential in that it provides protection by coordinating the destruction and removal of the offending agent and helps in repair. Chapter 3.3 considers the role of the pathogen and the environment in disease causation and provides the intensivist with opportunities to assist

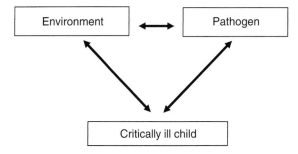

Figure 3.1 The interrelationship between the critically ill child, the environment, and the pathogens.

the critically ill child in compensating and correcting these problems. Together, these three components—each of which could form a textbook on its own—provide an integrated system for protecting the child against disease caused by the environment.

Immunology

Anthony D. Slonim

The immune system is an essential defense mechanism against environmental insults. The intensivist needs to understand the importance of immune mechanisms in protecting the critically ill child against disease and of the autoimmune or immunopathologic states that arise from its dysregulation. For example, children with burns lose their epithelium, a major protective barrier that serves as the first line of defense against infection. Children who develop cancer may initially have had problems with immune surveillance that initiated the cancer, but they are also at risk of immunosuppression from the disease-modifying therapies used to treat their cancer. Many immunodeficiency syndromes, including primary and secondary syndromes, as well as allergic responses, are immune-mediated.

The constituents of this system that provide the host with defense from environmental invasion are considered in the first section. These constituents are grouped into barriers to infection, and cellular and soluble (humoral) components of the immune system. The second section addresses the host's responses to invasion by discussing the innate and acquired immune responses. The distinction between the two types of immune responses is in some ways artificial, and considerable "cross-talk" occurs between the different elements. Finally, the immune mechanisms underlying allergic, rheumatologic, and autoimmune diseases are considered.

BARRIERS TO INFECTION

The host has numerous nonspecific host defense mechanisms, which provide a very important first line of defense against environmental insults. These are broadly categorized into anatomic barriers, mechanical mechanisms, and chemical and antimicrobial substances, and they represent the foundation of the hierarchical approach to protecting the host from invasion by foreign elements.

The skin is an important "organ" providing a keratinized epidermal surface, which prevents the entry of microorganisms, and a dermis, which contains many cellular elements of the immune response (e.g., dendritic cells) that are able to process antigens, produce cytokines, and eliminate organisms that gain entry beyond the epidermis.

Cell-surface modifications provide additional defense against infection. These include cells with hair and cilia (e.g., in the nares and in the respiratory tract) that capture microorganisms at the portal of entry. Cells of the inner membranes produce mucus that traps the microorganisms and prevents their adherence to cells. A mucosal defense system buttresses these membranes should a pathogen gain entry.

Secretions in the membranes possess antimicrobial activity. Alterations in the chemical and physical properties of these secretions, such as the acidity, sodium content, or temperature, and the synthesis of antimicrobial proteins, such as defensins, lysozymes, and immunoglobulin A (IgA), provide an additional level of support.

Mechanical mechanisms such as coughing or sneezing and, most importantly, normal physiologic functions such as saliva production, normal urine flow, and tearing help prevent the intrusion of the body by microorganisms. Finally, the host is enriched by normal bacterial colonization, which is important in preventing the overgrowth of more pathogenic microbes.

Intensivists need to be mindful of the disruptions that pathogenic microbes can create in these very important immunologic barriers. Intravascular and urinary catheters, inhalational therapy, intracerebral shunts, surgery, and other invasive procedures are all necessary to sustain the critically ill child, but they impinge on these very important anatomic barriers to infection. Similarly, indiscriminate use of antimicrobial agents may disrupt the normal flora and may lead to the emergence of resistant pathogenic organisms that can readily gain access to an already compromised host.

CELLULAR COMPONENTS OF THE IMMUNE SYSTEM

Functions of the Cellular Components

The cellular components of the immune system are involved in both innate and acquired immunologic responses. The cellular components primarily perform three functions: phagocytosis, antigen presentation, and mediator secretion. In reality, different cell types often perform more than one function.

Phagocytosis

Phagocytosis is an important function of innate immunity. It provides the body with a mechanism to subdue and eliminate invading pathogens. This function is carried out by specialized immune cells that can localize to the site of inflammation, perpetuate the immune response, and, as their name implies, engulf and digest invading organisms. The cells with phagocytic ability consist primarily of neutrophils, monocytes, and macrophages. Some authors also include eosinophils in this classification.

Antigen Presentation

Endogenous proteins are continuously being recycled within cells. Similarly, exogenous proteins or antigens continually make their way into cells, and their degradation products can be recycled and used by the cell for rebuilding. However, some of these exogenous antigens, particularly those from viruses or intracellular bacteria, are potentially dangerous to the cells, and if not controlled by the immune response, they can lead to the cells' destruction. In a series of steps, these proteins are unfolded, exposed to enzymes, degraded, and broken down into amino acids and short peptides for reuse (see Fig. 3.1.1). These peptides are transported by molecules called transporters associated with antigen processing (TAP) to the endoplasmic reticulum, where they are bound (depending on the cell type) to class I or class II molecules of the human leucocyte antigen (HLA) system. They then make their way to the cell surface and facilitate the display of antigenic material to other cells, primarily CD4 and CD8 cells of the T-cell system (Fig. 3.1.1). Each cell surface has several hundred thousand antigens that are available for presentation. These antigens are one method the body has to discriminate self from non-self. If non-self antigens are detected, an immune response is initiated and propagated.

Human Leucocyte Antigen Complex

The HLA complex is critical to the function of antigen presentation (Fig. 3.1.1). It is located on the short arm of chromosome 6 in humans. The complex contains approximately 200 genes; more than 20% of these genes code for leucocyte antigens that are important in differentiating self from non-self in the immune system. The genes of the complex are divided into "classes," which are named 1, 2, and 3 and have different structures and functions.

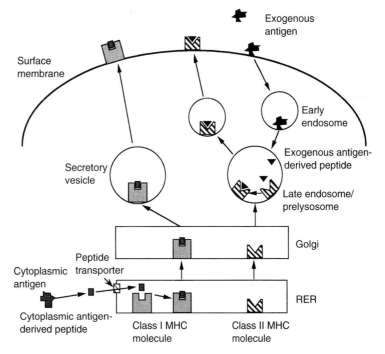

Figure 3.1.1 Pathways of antigen processing. Exogenous antigen enters the cell by endocytosis and is transported from early endosomes into late endosome or prelysosomes, where it is fragmented and where the resulting peptides (exogenous antigen-derived peptides) may be loaded into class II major histocompatibility complex (MHC) molecules. The latter have been transported from the rough endoplasmic reticulum (RER) through the Golgi apparatus to the peptide-containing vesicles. Class II MHC molecules/exogenous antigen-derived peptide complexes are then transported to the cell surface, where they may be recognized by T-cell receptor (TCR) expressed on CD4$^+$ T cells. Cytoplasmic antigens are degraded in the cytoplasm and then they enter the RER through a peptide transporter. In the RER, cytoplasmic antigen-derived peptides are loaded into class I MHC molecules that move through the Golgi apparatus into secretory vesicles and are then expressed on the cell surface where they may be recognized by CD8$^+$ T cells. (From Paul WE, Development and function of lymphocytes. In: Gallin JI, Goldstein I, Snyderman R, eds. *Inflammation.* New York: Raven; 1992:776.)

Class I genes are contained within all nucleated cells of the body and are coded by three loci, HLA-A, HLA-B, and HLA-C, which when taken together are known as the *class A* or *classic* genes that are expressed differently depending on the cell type. The class I molecules encoded by these genes consist of an α chain and a β chain. The β chain is encoded by a gene called the β_2-*microglobulin gene* on chromosome 15 and is noncovalently bound to the α chain. These molecules are transmembrane glycoproteins that present antigens to T cells and, through their recognition, initiate an immune response. Class I molecules present an antigen to the cytotoxic T (T_C) cells (CD8), whose receptors recognize the antigen to be foreign and engage and destroy the foreign cells.

Class II genes are limited in their expression to B and T cells, macrophages, dendritic cells, and epithelial cells. These class II genes have their loci on chromosome 6 in the HLA-D region. The class II molecules also consist of an α and a β chain. Like class I molecules, class II molecules also have a transmembrane component that allows the presentation of antigens. Class II molecules, however, present the antigen to T helper (T_H) (CD4) cells, which are then able to produce interferon-γ (IFN-γ) for additional immune modulation.

Class III genes are somewhat different in that they code for complement components C2, C4, and factor B. These genes are located between the classic and HLA-D regions. There are also the nonclassical major histocompatibility complex (MHC) molecules that are located on chromosome 6. These molecules have a role in the recognition of some cells as self and thereby prevent the attack of these cells by natural killer (NK) cells.

Mediator Secretion

Cytokines are protein mediators that are produced by cells in many different forms. They have a role in intercellular messaging, the induction and continuation of the inflammatory response, and the regulation of immune responses. Included in this group are the interleukins, the tumor necrosis factors (TNFs), and the colony-stimulating factors (CSFs). Because their role in inflammation is pivotal, they are discussed more fully in Chapter 3.2.

The Cellular Components

Neutrophils

Neutrophils are the most common leucocytes in the blood, originating from the hematopoietic stem cell in the bone marrow and developing under the influence of granulocyte colony-stimulating factor (G-CSF) (see Fig. 3.1.2). They constitute approximately 60% of the normal leucocytes. Half of them circulate in the bloodstream, while the remainder attach to the blood vessel wall in the marginating pool. They circulate until they are activated to respond to a source of inflammation. Neutrophils and immature

neutrophils (band forms) are stimulated to leave the marrow by stress, infection, IL-1, and TNF. Band forms are less common (<5% of leucocytes) and less proficient than mature neutrophils at microbial killing, perhaps because of the lack of fully developed granules and because of the relatively ineffective mechanisms for oxygen-independent killing (see Chapter 3.2).

Neutrophils are the primary cells involved in innate immunity, and they can quickly (within 6 to 12 hours) and efficiently respond to an inciting trigger. Triggers for neutrophil activation include complement fragments, nonself proteins, and cytokines. The neutrophil has cell surface receptors to allow for their "activation." Once activated, the internal machinery of these cells is upregulated and additional cell surface receptors are displayed. These systems are highly complex and an in-depth analysis is beyond the scope of this discussion. Nonetheless, their role in phagocytosis, mediator production, and microbial killing is critical to the inflammatory response, and a more detailed discussion of these functions can be found in Chapter 3.2.

Eosinophils

Eosinophils constitute only 1% to 3% of the leucocytes and function primarily in allergic disorders, hypersensitivity syndromes, vasculitic syndromes, parasitic and helminthic infections, and malignancies. Some authors will exclude eosinophils from the classification of phagocytes because rather than truly engulfing an organism, they expel the contents of their granules into the extracellular space where the organism resides. Most granules in eosinophils are specific granules that contain major basic protein, eosinophil cationic protein, lysosomal enzymes, eosinophil-derived neurotoxin, and peroxidase. The minority of granules are primary granules that contain Charcot-Leyden crystal (CLC) protein and eosinophil peroxidase. CLCs, by their presence in end organs, may assist with the diagnosis of eosinophil-mediated diseases (see Fig. 3.1.3). Eosinophils also possess the capability for a respiratory burst and for using reactive oxygen species. These mechanisms may be important both for microbial killing and in tissue-related damage caused by eosinophils.

Eosinophils originate in the bone marrow and are released under the influence of IL-3, IL-5, and granulocyte-macrophage colony-stimulating factor (GM-CSF) (Fig. 3.1.2; see Table 3.1.1). Eosinophils can enter the tissues, where they may persist for some time. These cells become activated, roll, adhere to the endothelial cells through adhesion molecules, and then migrate to the tissues, responding to chemoattractant factors such as eosinophil chemotactic factors (eotaxins) and regulated on activation, normal T expressed and secreted (RANTES) in a process similar to that in neutrophils and described in more detail in Chapter 3.2. Immunoglobulin E (IgE) is a major component of the response to allergy, hypersensitivity, and parasitic syndromes. It engages with receptors on mast

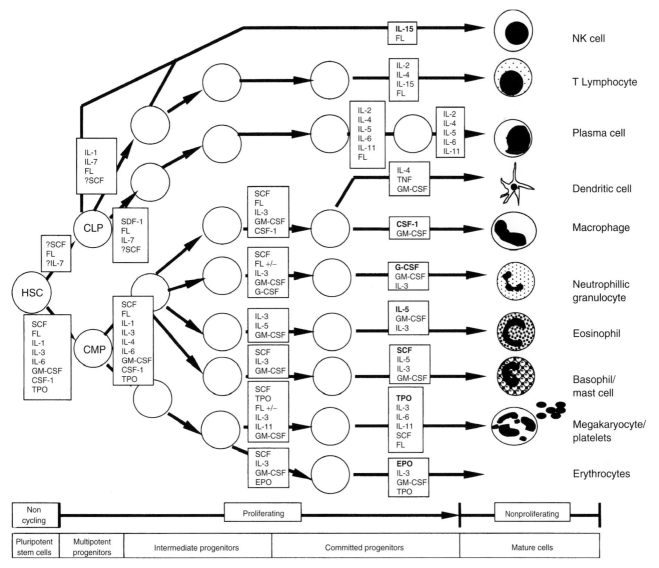

Figure 3.1.2 Hematopoietic cells, indicating the points of *in vivo* and *in vitro* regulation by hematopoietic cytokines. Note that some cytokines, such as granulocyte-macrophage colony-stimulating factor (GM-CSF), may not regulate steady state hematopoiesis but may be used to regulate hematopoiesis pharmacologically. Cytokines primarily regulating the proliferation and differentiation of committed progenitors of individual lineages are in bold. CLP, common lymphoid stem cell; CMP, common myeloid stem cell; HSC, hematopoietic stem cell; TNF, tumor necrosis factor; IL, interleukin; FL, Fl+3/Flk-2- ligand; EPO, eosinophil peroxidase; SCF, stem cell factor; TPO, thrombo-poietin. (From Austin KF, Frank MM, Atkinson JP, et al. *Samter's immunologic diseases.* 6th ed. Philadelphia, PA: Lippincott Williams & Wilkins; 2001:176.)

cells, basophils, and eosinophils, leading to degranulation. The substances released during degranulation lead to additional eosinophil recruitment to the sites of these reactions.

Basophils

Basophils develop in the bone marrow and are released under the influence of IL-3, IL-5, and GM-CSF, as are eosinophils (Fig. 3.1.2). Eosinophils and basophils originate from a common progenitor cell in the bone marrow (Fig. 3.1.2). Basophils account for <1% of leucocytes

in the circulation and enter the tissues in response to allergic triggers in a process that is similar to that in neutrophils and eosinophils. Once in the tissues, basophils contribute to the manifestations of allergy and asthma by secreting a number of products contained in their granules (see Table 3.1.2). Histamine is the most important preformed product contained within basophil granules and is available immediately upon degranulation to exert its effects (Table 3.1.2). These products function in both immediate and delayed hypersensitivity reactions. Basophils possess receptors for IgE and produce IL-4 and

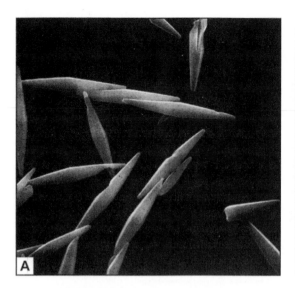
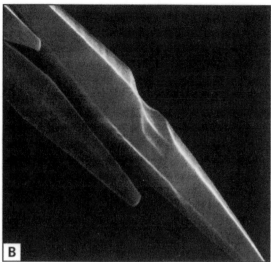

Figure 3.1.3 Electron photomicrograph of Charcot-Leyden crystals (CLCs). CLCs are composed of the enzyme lysophospholipase. These electron photomicrographs demonstrate the unique shape of CLCs (**A**, magnification × 400; **B**, magnification × 4,000). These unique hexagonal bipyramidal crystals can be found in the sputum of patients with asthma, in the stool of patients with eosinophilic gastroenteritis, and in the urine of patients with drug-induced interstitial nephritis. The presence of CLCs should be pursued when eosinophil-mediated diseases are suspected because, in many instances, the eosinophils have undergone lysis and cannot be detected in biologic specimens. (From Moy JN. The eosinophil. In: Lieberman PL, Blaiss MS eds. *Atlas of allergic diseases.* Philadelphia, PA: Lippincott Williams & Wilkins and Current Medicine; 2002:45.)

TABLE 3.1.1
REGULATION OF EOSINOPHILOPOIESIS AND EOSINOPHIL FUNCTION

Regulatory Factors	Source	Function
IL-5	T$_H$2 cells, mast cells	Stimulate bone marrow production of eosinophils Promote chemotaxis Prolong survival Enhance production and secretion of mediators
IL-3	T cells, thymic epithelial cells	Synergistic with IL-5 for bone marrow production
GM-CSF	Macrophages, respiratory epithelial cells, T cells	Synergistic with IL-5 for production and secretion of mediators
Eotaxin	Endothelium, epithelium, monocytes, T cells	Most potent eosinophil chemoattractant
RANTES	Endothelium, epithelium, platelets, T cells	Eosinophil chemoattractant
TGF	Monocytes, T cells	Suppress eosinophil differentiation
TGF-β	Adrenal glands	Induce apoptosis of eosinophils

Eosinophils are constantly under the tight control of many biologic compounds. The major substances that regulate eosinophil production and function are shown here. Corticosteroids are very effective in the treatment of eosinophil-mediated diseases because they induce apoptosis and inhibit cytokine production. IL, interleukin; GM-CSF, granulocyte-macrophage colony-stimulating factor; RANTES, regulated on activation, normal T expressed and secreted; TGF, transforming growth factor.
From Moy JN. The eosinophil. In: Lieberman PL, Blaiss MS eds. *Atlas of allergic diseases.* Philadelphia, PA: Lippincott Williams & Wilkins and Current Medicine; 2002:45.

TABLE 3.1.2
MEDIATORS CONTAINED WITHIN MAST CELLS AND BASOPHILS

	Mast Cell	Basophils
Mediators preformed		
	Histamine	Histamine
	Tryptase	Charcot-Leyden crystals
	Chymase	Major basic protein
	Chondroitin sulfate	Chondroitin sulfate
	Carboxypeptidase A	Cathepsin G
	Cathepsin G	Tryptase
	Acid hydrolase	
	Heparin	
Newly synthesized lipids		
	LTC_4, A_4, B_4, D_4, E_4	LTC_4, D_4, E_4
	PAF	PAF
	PGD_2	
Cytokines		
	IL-3, -4, -5, -6, -8, -10, -13, -16	IL-4, -5, -6, -8, -10, -12, -13
	TNF-α	TNF-α
	MIP-1α	MIP-1α
	GM-CSF	
	β-FGF	RANTES
	SCF	
	TGF-β	
	VEGF, VPF	
	RANTES	
	MCP	

LTC, leucotriene C4; PAF, platelet activating factor; PGD, prostaglandin D; IL, interleukin; TNF, tumor necrosis factor; MIP, macrophage inflammatory protein; GM-CSF, granulocyte-macrophage colony-stimulating factor; FGF, fibroblast growth factor; SCF, stem cell factor; TGF, transforming growth factor; VEGF, vascular endothelial growth factor; VPF, vascular permeability factor; RANTES, regulated on activation, normal T expressed and secreted; MCP, monocyte chemotactic proteins.
From Grant JA, Leonard PA. In: Mast cell- and basophil-derived mediators. Lieberman PL, Blass MS. *Atlas of allergic diseases*, Philadelphia, PA: Lippincott Williams & Wilkins and Current Medicine; 2002:32.

IL-13, both of which serve to assist with inciting IgE reactions. Basophils also possess receptors for other elements of the immune system, including complement components, lipid mediators, and cytokines, that provide for their role in the late phase of allergy with T_H2 lymphocytes and eosinophils.

Mast Cells

Mast cells originate from the bone marrow and circulate to sites that interface with the environment, such as the skin and gastrointestinal tract (Fig. 3.1.2). These cells have a role in allergic responses, parasitic infections, innate immunity, and acquired immunity. Like basophils, mast cells also contain a number of important preformed mediators in their granules (Table 3.1.2). When activated, either through nonspecific mechanisms or through their IgE receptors, they degranulate and cause an immediate response that includes vascular reaction, exudation, and leucocyte recruitment (immediate type hypersensitivity). Histamine release from the mast cell can further up-regulate leucocyte recruitment and rolling. Mast cells are capable of phagocytosis, oxygen-dependent and -independent killing,

and antigen presentation to T cells in the presence of class I or II HLA molecules.

Monocytes and Macrophages

Mononuclear phagocytes (monocytes) and macrophages comprise the mononuclear phagocytic (MNP) system and perform the functions of phagocytosis, antigen presentation, and mediator secretion. They arise from the granulocyte-macrophage colony-forming unit in the bone marrow under the influence of IL-3, GM-CSF, and macrophage CSF (Fig. 3.1.2). Once differentiated into monocytes, they circulate within the vascular space, with most of them marginating on vessel walls. After a few days, monocytes migrate into the tissues, becoming tissue macrophages. Some of these cells are unique because they reside in tissues such as in the liver (Kupffer cells), lung (alveolar macrophages), brain (microglia), and bone (osteoclasts) and perform a number of specialized functions.

Monocytes and macrophages are phagocytic and contain a number of enzymes in their granules to assist with tissue digestion and microbial killing during the inflammatory response. During maturation, monocytes increase in size and exhibit a corresponding increase in the number of lysosomal granules. Macrophages enter an inflammatory site approximately 24 hours after the initiation of inflammation in response to the macrophage chemotactic factor produced by monocytes and neutrophils. IFNs produced by NK and T cells also increase macrophage activation.

After activation, monocytes transit into the tissues by binding with adhesion molecules (L-selectin on the monocyte interacts with E- and P-selectins on endothelial cells). However, this may take up to a week to be completed. The processes of rolling, migrating, and then taking up residence in the inflamed tissue replacing the neutrophils occur next and are akin to those described for neutrophils in Chapter 3.2. Macrophages, however, are capable of dividing in the acidic environment of inflammation, whereas neutrophils cannot. It is in the tissues that phagocytosis usually takes place.

The MNP system is robust in the number of cell surface markers for Igs, cytokines, growth factors, and other hormones that can assist with binding these inflammatory mediators and further influencing inflammation. Macrophages can take up proteins, hydrolyze them using acid hydrolases, complex these antigens with the major histocompatibility determinants, and send them back to the cell surface for presentation to the T cells (Fig. 3.1.1). IL-1, produced by the macrophage, helps regulate the interactions between the macrophage and the T cell.

Proinflammatory cytokines such as IL-1, IL-6, IL-8, and IL-12 are produced by macrophages to propagate the inflammatory response. The macrophage has an important regulatory role and also responds to cytokines that have anti-inflammatory effects. For example, IL-10 can inhibit macrophage inflammatory protein 1α (MIP 1α) production and can affect antigen presentation by MHC class II molecules. Macrophages are capable of a respiratory burst and can use reactive oxygen species for the intracellular killing of microorganisms, as described in the section on neutrophils. They are also important in phagocytosing apoptotic cells and can act as scavengers for these inflammatory by-products. Tissue remodeling and wound healing–macrophages are helpful in debriding the devitalized tissue, secreting enzymes, and promoting the synthesis of tissue factors responsible for repair.

Dendritic Cells

Dendritic cells arise from hematopoietic cells in the bone marrow and also evolve from monocytes (Fig. 3.1.2). They are less phagocytic than other components of the MNP system but have sophisticated antigen-presenting abilities. These cells may either circulate or reside in tissues, particularly the lymphoid tissues (e.g., Langerhans cells in the skin), and are able to elaborate a variety of cytokines to assist in propagating the immune response.

Dendritic cells are extremely well equipped for the endocytosis of a variety of extracellular antigens. On activation, these cells prepare antigens for presentation to

T cells through MHC class II molecules. After preparation, these cells are sophisticated in sending the antigen to the cell surface for display to T_H cells (Fig. 3.1.1). Activated dendritic cells then progress to the lymph node, where they mediate the selection, activation, and expansion of specific T cells, thereby playing a role in networking the innate and acquired immune systems (see Fig. 3.1.4).

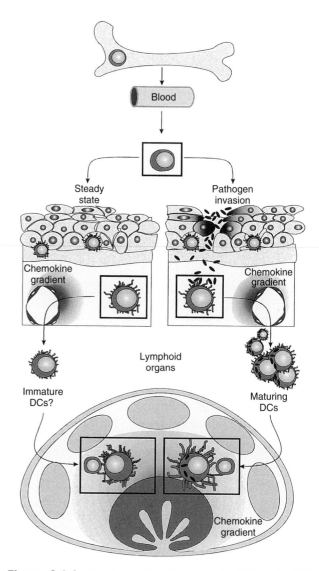

Figure 3.1.4 Developmental stages of dendritic cells (DCs) *in vivo*. The generation of DC precursors in the bone marrow, the recruitment of immature DCs in peripheral tissues, and the migration of DCs into the lymphoid organs are illustrated. The maturation of DCs into potent antigen-presenting cells (APCs) in case of infection of inflammation and their migration have been amply documented **(right)**, but there is also evidence that in the "steady state" (i.e., in the absence of a "danger signal") these immature DCs may migrate into the lymphoid organs while remaining at the immature stage **(left)**. The phenotype of the DC migrating in baseline condition is still unclear. The movement of maturing DCs and the "constitutive" migration of immature DCs have been shown to depend on chemokine gradients. (From Paul WE. *Fundamental immunology*. 5th ed. Philadelphia, PA: Lippincott Williams & Wilkins; 2003:456.)

Not only do these cells present antigens but they can also independently initiate a primary immune response (Fig. 3.1.4). Dendritic cells can interact with a number of different cell types, including B cells, T cells, and NK cells. It is through these interactions that they can facilitate the immune response.

B Lymphocytes

B lymphocytes undergo antigen-independent development arising from the hematopoietic stem cells of the bone marrow and fetal liver (see Fig. 3.1.5). They emerge in the second stage of their development, known as the *antigen-dependent stage*, which begins when they are stimulated by the antigen. This second stage occurs in the secondary lymphoid tissues of the spleen, lymph nodes, and gut-associated lymphoid tissue.

B lymphocytes contain cell surface receptors called *Igs*, which bind to the antigen presented by microorganisms and activate the B cells (see Fig. 3.1.6). Specific antigens react with a structurally similar antibody on the surface of B lymphocytes. Two different mechanisms lead

to B-cell activation. First, some antigen components become internalized in the B cell and are conjoined with MHC class II molecules before transportation to the cell surface as part of the T-cell receptor complex to engage T_H cells. Alternatively, multiple membrane Ig receptors become stimulated simultaneously and lead to intracellular messengers that can activate the B-cell response. Once activated, these cells undergo clonal expansion into plasma cells, creating antibodies with a similar shape to the antibody receptor on the B lymphocytes. After activation, the B lymphocytes divide into two different clones; one of these clones contains memory cells that lie dormant until rechallenged with the same antigen. This rechallenge is called *a secondary response* and is more robust than the primary response or first exposure to antigen. The second clone becomes antibody-producing plasma cells that are the effector arm of the B lymphocytes. These plasma cells produce antibodies, which are proteins that are specifically targeted against the antigen or can bind to these cells so that they are identified and destroyed by phagocytic cells in the circulation.

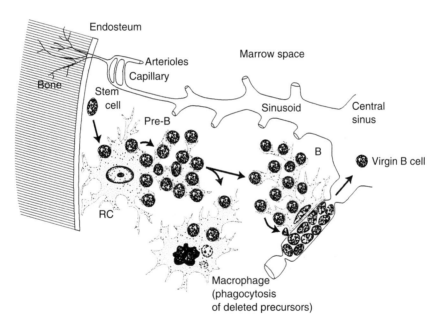

Figure 3.1.5 Organization of the bone marrow and B-cell development within this organ. Terminal bone marrow arterioles form capillary networks near the endosteum, marking the most peripheral portion of the marrow cavity. Hematopoietic stem cells appear to localize near the endosteum, probably nurtured by the growth factors produced in high concentration in this area. Proliferation and differentiation of cells along the B-lineage pathway depends on reticular stromal cells (RCs) that lie in the spaces surrounding the cells, undergoing progressive heavy-chain and light-chain rearrangement, ultimately resulting in the formation of virgin B cells that then enter the circulation. Generally, B-cell differentiation proceeds in a spatially organized fashion, with the most primitive B-cell precursors located near the endosteum and the differentiated virgin B cells emerging near the center of the marrow compartment. Once heavy-chain rearrangement is complete, a process of testing cells for successful *Ig* gene rearrangements is initiated, and cells that fail to generate productive rearrangements are removed by apoptosis and cleared by phagocytosis by bone marrow macrophages. (From Picker LJ, Siegelman MH. Lymphoid tissues and organs: In: Paul WE, ed. *Fundamental immunology.* 4th ed. Philadelphia, PA: Lippincott Williams & Wilkins; 1999;479–531.)

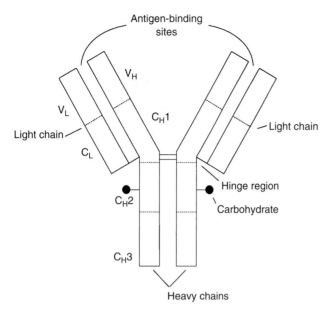

Figure 3.1.6 The structure of an immunoglobulin molecule. (From McClatchey KD. *Clinical laboratory medicine*, 2nd ed. Philadelphia, PA: Lippincott Williams & Wilkins; 2002.)

Immunoglobulins

Ig molecules are produced from activated B cells. These molecules are composed of two heavy chains and two light chains (Fig. 3.1.6). The heavy chains help identify the different classes (isotypes) of Ig molecules (Fig. 3.1.6). They are named *IgM, IgA, IgG, IgD,* and *IgE.* Several of these Igs also have subclasses, and two of the Igs exist as polymeric forms (IgA is a dimer and IgM is a pentamer). The polymeric forms are joined by a "J" region. Both the classes and subclasses of Ig have different functions. For example, IgE is of importance in allergic reactions and has an ability to react with eosinophils in propagating an allergic response. IgA is important for the immune function of secretions at mucosal surfaces. The Ig molecule also contains two types of light chains known as κ and λ, respectively.

The heavy and light chains of the molecules contain domains known as the *constant and variable regions* (represented by *C* and *V* in Fig. 3.1.6). The heavy chains have a single variable region and several constant regions; the light chains have a single variable region and a single constant region (Fig. 3.1.6). The constant region provides the Ig with its class-specific functions (Fc portion), whereas the variable region (also known as the *Fab region*) provides the site for antigen binding.

Immunoglobulin Classes

IgG is the Ig with the largest serum concentration. It contains four subclasses, labeled IgG1 to IgG4, which differ in their binding affinities for receptors. IgG is the major Ig produced in a secondary immune response. IgM is the Ig with the next highest serum level. It is the first Ig produced

by neonates. This is also the Ig that is responsible for the primary immune response because it has a very strong affinity for antigens. IgM is also important in mucosal immunity. IgM can bind IgG and create rheumatoid factor, which is important in some autoimmune rheumatologic diseases. IgA is the Ig present in most secretions, including tears, saliva, and serum. IgD is represented in small amounts but serves as an important receptor for antigens and is as important as IgM in this regard. IgE is important in activating mast cells, basophils, and eosinophils in allergic and parasitic reactions through an important receptor known as the *FcεRI.*

T Lymphocytes

T lymphocytes are a major component of the adaptive immune system. They arise from the bone marrow, migrate to and develop in the thymus along two different pathways (Fig. 3.1.2), and emerge as two different types of cells, classified on the basis of the T-cell receptors (TCR) present on their cell surface (see Fig. 3.1.7). The first type of T lymphocytes is called the $\alpha\beta$ *T cell* because its cell surface TCR molecule consists of two chains: an α and a β chain (Fig. 3.1.7). In contrast, the $\gamma\delta$ T cell expresses a (TCR) that consists of γ and δ chains. These two T-cell types are distinct in both their location and function. Both subtypes act as the corresponding units that recognize a myriad of antigens (similar to an Ig) and interact with other plasma proteins of the CD3 complex to facilitate intracellular signaling (Fig. 3.1.7).

$\alpha\beta$ T Cells

The $\alpha\beta$ T-cell group also contains either CD4 or CD8 receptors on their cell surface. The $\alpha\beta$ T cell recognizes protein antigens presented by either MHC class I or class II molecules but are only able to do so if they have CD4

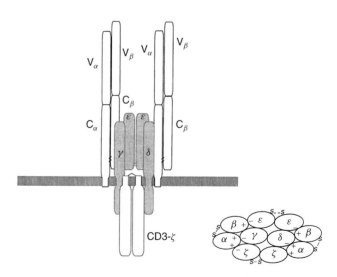

Figure 3.1.7 A schematized model of the $\beta\alpha$-CD-3 complex. (From Terhorst C, Spits H, Stall F, et al. T lymphocyte signal transduction. In: Hames BD, Glver DM, eds. *Molecular immunology.* 2nd ed. Oxford, UK: IRL Press; 1996:132–188.)

or CD8 expression. Their dependence on MHC molecule presentation has led to their designation as MHC-restricted cells. The ability to express CD4 or CD8 is derived from the development of the T cell in the thymus. CD4 cells are referred to as T_H cells and they assist with antibody production and the facilitation of the humoral arm of the immune response and with cell-mediated immunity. CD8 cells are referred to as T_C cells and act to destroy cells infected with foreign antigens such as viruses. These cells are activated after binding with the appropriate molecules. They then begin to send a series of internal signals to facilitate the cell's responses. These signals depend on costimulatory molecules such as CD28 and CD40, which also need to be activated for the responses to occur.

$\gamma\delta$ T Cells

The $\gamma\delta$ T cells represent <15% of the circulating lymphocytes and recognize nonprotein antigens. These lymphocytes are present in the intestines, mucous membranes, and skin. Most of these cells express neither CD4 nor CD8 surface markers, which allows them to directly recognize and function against foreign antigens without the need for antigen presentation by the MHC complex. This ability allows a readily available immune response against a number of viruses, bacteria, and protozoa without the need for antigen processing. These cells play an important role in immunity that is similar to NK cells, which do not require antigen presentation and processing to elicit an immune response.

Specific T-Cell Types

T Helper Cells. The T_H cell plays a central role in both cell- and humoral-mediated immunity. Two discrete classes of T_H cells have been identified and have been classified as T_H1 and T_H2, in part, on the basis of the cytokines they produce (see Fig. 3.1.8). T_H1 cells produce IL-2 and IFN-γ, which assist in promoting a T_C cell response (Fig. 3.1.8). T_H2 cells produce IL-4, IL-5, IL-6, IL-10, and IL-13, which assist with humoral B-cell activity (Fig. 3.1.8). T_H cells can also provide cytotoxic activity by releasing enzymes, when costimulated by CD8 cells. These cells differentiate on the basis of genetic, environmental, and stimulatory factors. The T_H1 cells play an important role in autoimmunity for a number of diseases, and the T_H2 cells are critical in the allergic response.

Cytotoxic T Cells. T_C cells are also important in the immune response and are primarily used to defend against intracellular microorganisms such as viruses and some bacteria. T_C cells express CD8 on their surface and respond to antigens presented to the TCR by MHC class I molecules. When stimulated, the T_C cell attacks, adheres to, and kills the affected cell through one of two mechanisms. In the first mechanism, the T_C cell releases granules with granzyme and perforin that are taken up by the infected cell through endocytosis. These enzymes produce pores in cell membranes or induce apoptosis by binding to caspases (see Fig. 3.1.9). The second mechanism involves the Fas ligand pathway, which becomes expressed on the T_C cell surface, and is then able to interact with the target cell Fas receptor (Fig. 3.1.9). T_C cells also have a major role in immune dysfunction, leading to autoimmunity from a variety of mechanisms including hypersensitivity reactions and graft versus host disease.

NK Cells. The NK cell constitutes <10% of the lymphocyte population and is a major link between the innate and acquired immune systems. These cells develop in the bone marrow under the influence of IL-15 (Fig. 3.1.2). They possess granules in their cytoplasm, which contain a number of enzymes including glycoproteins, acid phosphatase, β-glucuronidase, and arylsulfatase, and which have spontaneous cytotoxicity against intracellular bacteria, viruses, and tumor cells. The NK cells also exhibit a number of cell surface molecules that are able to identify antigenic determinants. NK cells secrete IFN-γ and TNF-α, which allows these cells to mediate adaptive immune responses of other cells.

A number of cytokines increase NK activity, including IL-2, IL-12, IL-15, and IFN-α, -β, and -γ. Interestingly, MHC class I molecules inhibit the function of NK cells and block their activity, which is important as a mechanism to prevent autoimmune destruction of somatic cells by NK cells. When somatic cells lose MHC class I molecules, this inhibitory function also disappears, as in some cancers; the NK cells are then directed toward these self-tissues. These determinants play a major role in differentiating self and they can recognize and destroy non-MHC–identified cells before an inflammatory reaction or the initiation of the acquired T- and B-cell responses. These cells are believed to play major roles in graft versus host disease, malignancy, and rejection.

Endothelial Cells and Platelets

Endothelial cells and platelets are also cell types that are important for the proper functioning of the immune system. The endothelial cells and platelets are metabolically active cells that can release cellular mediators and assist in controlling the movement of other cells. Endothelial cells are also important for the adherence and movement of cells to sites of inflammation, angiogenesis, and vasomotor tone. The biology of these two cell types is covered in depth in Chapter 4.

THE ORGANS

The Thymus

The thymus is derived from the third pharyngeal pouch and provides considerable assistance to the differentiation of T lymphocytes during the early years of life. The organ

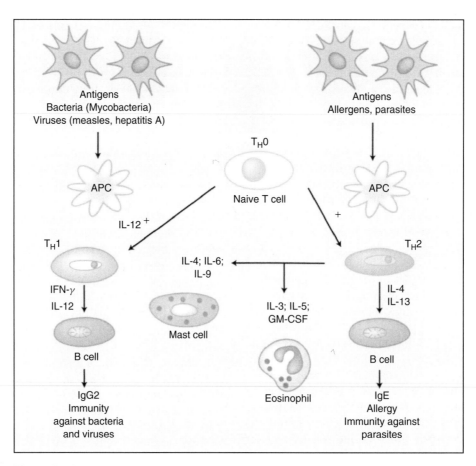

Figure 3.1.8   Immune response to antigens: the role of T helper (T$_H$) imbalance. T$_H$ lymphocytes are the principal cells orchestrating the immune responses in asthma and other allergic diseases. Antigen-presenting cells (APCs), such as dendritic cells uptake the antigens and present them to T$_H$ cells after processing them. Genetic predisposition and the nature of the antigen presented are thought to determine the direction of a naïve T$_H$ cell (T$_H$0) toward type 1 (T$_H$1) or type 2 (T$_H$2) lymphocytes. Some antigens (mycobacterium, measles virus, and hepatitis A virus) induce T$_H$-cells toward T$_H$1, whereas allergens and parasites induce a T$_H$2 immune response. Interleukin (IL)-4 and IL-13 are the principal cytokines produced by T$_H$2 cells. They stimulate the B lymphocytes to produce IgE. Other T$_H$2 cytokines stimulate the production and recruitment of mast cells and eosinophils. T$_H$1 cells produce interferon-γ and IL-12, which stimulate B cells toward IgG2 production, augmenting cell-mediated immunity. T$_H$1 cytokines also inhibit the T$_H$2 responses. In other words, in healthy subjects there is a balance between T$_H$1 and T$_H$2 response; in asthma, including nonatopic asthma, the balance is tipped toward T$_H$2. IFN, interferon; IL, interleukin; GM-CSF, granulocyte-macrophage colony-stimulating factor; IgE, immunoglobulin E. (From Gnanakumaran G, Holgate ST. Asthma in adults. In: Lieberman PL, Blaiss MS, eds. In: *Atlas of allergic diseases*. Philadelphia, PA: Lippincott Williams & Wilkins and Current Medicine; 2002:181.)

involutes, becoming practically nonexistent by the age of 3 years. T-cell development progresses from the subcapsular zone to the cortex and to the medulla and is monitored by the presence of T-cell surface molecules (see Fig. 3.1.10). In early development, T cells contain CD3-TCR, CD4, and CD8 surface molecules. With maturation, they lose one or more molecules and become "single positive," with either a CD4 or a CD8 marker. At this point, they depend on the MHC presentation of antigen.

As the thymocytes develop, they undergo a process known as *selection* (Fig. 3.1.10). Cells entering the cortex that are insufficiently able to differentiate self from non-self

will undergo apoptosis. This is known as *positive selection* (Fig. 3.1.10). Once in the medullary region, T cells with excessive affinity to self will undergo apoptosis in a process known as *negative selection* (Fig. 3.1.10). Cells that survive both positive and negative selection leave the thymus and enter the periphery as naïve T cells. When a stimulatory response from the antigen occurs, T cells bind to complexes of HLA molecules and foreign peptides and further differentiate on the basis of the HLA molecule engaged. The response is perpetuated because the stimulated T$_H$ cells produce cytokines that increase the expression of class II molecules.

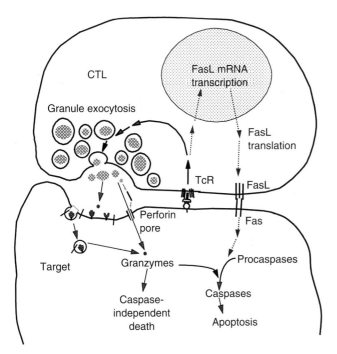

Figure 3.1.9 The two cytotoxic pathways used by cytotoxic T lymphocytes include a granule cytotoxic pathway on the left and a Fas ligand pathway on the right. CTL, cytotoxic T lymphocytes. (From Paul WE. *Fundamental immunology.* 5th ed. Philadelphia, PA: Lippincott Williams & Wilkins; 2003:1129.)

Lymph Nodes

The lymph nodes assist in the immune response to microorganisms in the tissues. Naïve lymphocytes, which have not been previously exposed to antigen, enter the lymph nodes through specialized capillaries known as *high endothelial venules* (HEV) and migrate, depending on their type, to different zones of the lymph node. The T cells exit the circulation in a process that is similar to that in neutrophils in that they bind to cell surface adhesion molecules that first allow the cells to slow, roll, adhere, and migrate into the tissue. T cells occupy the paracortex and B cells occupy the area under the capsule known as the *follicle*. The paracortex is also the location in which dendritic cells accumulate and are able to present the antigen from the periphery to the awaiting T cells. Once activated by the presentation of the antigen, clonal expansion of the lymphocyte begins. This activation allows the T and B cells to migrate toward each other, allowing the entire group of antigen-presenting cells and effector cells to be in one location within the lymph node. The T cells become effector cells, differentiate over 3 to 5 days, and, depending on the type of pathogen, emerge as T_H1, T_H2, or CD8 lymphocytes and migrate to the areas of inflammation, sending intercellular signals that upregulate selectins and assist in the inflammatory response. Other T cells differentiate into memory cells that either migrate to peripheral tissues or take up residence in peripheral

lymphatic organs and maintain immunologic memory. They are a component of the specific immune response and undergo clonal expansion on restimulation by a similar antigen. The germinal center is the location where memory B cells and plasma cell precursors are generated.

Spleen

The spleen is an important organ for immune function and consists of two types of tissues, referred to as the *red pulp* and the *white pulp*. The red pulp is lined by reticuloendothelial cells and contains sinuses filled with blood. The white pulp consists of the zones of lymphocytes. T cells tend to congregate around arterioles in the spleen in regions known as the *periarteriolar lymphocyte sheath* (PALS). B cells congregate in the periphery of the white pulp in the follicular zone surrounding the PALS. Immunologically, the spleen functions to respond to antigens, clear microorganisms and antigens from systemic infections in the circulation, produce cellular and humoral mediators of inflammation, and remove senescent or damaged blood cells.

Mucosa-Associated Lymphoid Tissues

The mucosa-associated lymphoid tissue (MALT) is a term applied to immune tissues distributed throughout a number of organs near mucosal surfaces. These tissues, because of their location near a portal of entry, maintain surveillance for infectious agents that have bypassed the barriers to infection and the epithelial membrane. The specific tissues associated with lymphoid activity include the gastrointestinal tract, known as the *gut-associated lymphoid tissues* (GALT); the bronchial tree, known as the *bronchus-associated lymphoid tissues* (BALT); and tissues within the skin known as the *intraepithelial lymphocytes*. These organs assist the body in localizing an immune response to a mucosal surface and prevent the impact of inflammation on the host's tissues. For the intensivist, this component of the immune response is less important than the more robust systemic immune responses that lead to inflammation in these tissues.

INNATE IMMUNITY

Innate immunity is a nonspecific, yet integrated, series of protective mechanisms that shields the host from the dangers of its environment. Despite its lack of specificity, the innate immune system is capable of distinguishing self from non-self. The response to non-self is exactly the same, regardless of how many times the host has been presented with the antigen. Innate immunity suffers from a lack of immunologic memory. The components of the innate immune system include the chemical, mechanical, and physical barriers to infection, which attempt to keep

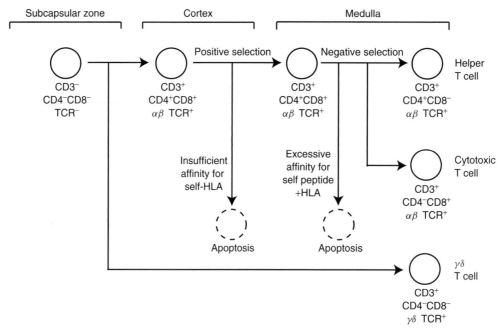

Figure 3.1.10 Compartmentalization of T-cell development in the thymus. Discrete populations of epithelial cells are present in the thymic subcapsular zone, cortex, and medulla, with each epithelial population supporting the stages of thymic development that occur in each compartment. The subcapsular epithelial cells support the expansion of the thymocyte pool from a committed T-cell precursor population. T-cell receptor (TCR) gene rearrangement is induced during the movement of cells from the subcapsular region to the cortex where double-positive cells are subjected to positive selection. Cells that fail positive selection are removed by apoptosis. Following positive selection, the developing thymocytes undergo negative selection on medullary epithelial cells that present a huge array of self-peptides. This is accompanied by transition to CD4+ or CD8+ single-positive cells. Again, failure of selection leads to death of the developing thymocyte by an apoptotic mechanism. A fraction of $\gamma\delta$ cells develops in the thymus, but the role of the defined thymic epithelial cell populations in differentiation of this lineage is not defined. HLA, human leucocyte antigen. (From Paul WE. *Fundamental immunology.* 5th ed. Philadelphia, PA: Lippincott Williams & Wilkins; 2003:426; Adapted from Chaplin DD. Overview of the immune response. *J Allergy Clin Immunol.* 2003;111:S442–459.)

foreign particles from gaining entry to the body. Once entry is gained, the mucosal lymphoid tissues, the cell surface modifications, and the natural defensins may subdue the organism, depending on the portal of entry.

Pathogen Recognition

The next phase of the innate immune system takes over if the barriers were breached by the offending agent. This begins with the recognition that a foreign pathogen has entered the body. The recognition of non-self by the immune system is required to activate the cells of the innate immune response and to begin the multiple cascades of reactions necessary to isolate and detoxify the intruding agent. Heterogeneous receptors present either on the surface of a neutrophil, monocyte, macrophage, or dendritic cell or circulate freely in the plasma, and are referred to as *pattern recognition receptors* (PRRs). PRRs are able to identify the characteristic structures of foreign material from a number of microorganisms (see Fig. 3.1.11). They do not bind to "self" tissues. When

activated, the PRRs are able to stimulate the release of cytokines, upregulate additional receptors, initiate the phagocytic response, and provide a variety of triggers to internal pathways (Fig. 3.1.11).

The structures that are bound on the microorganism are referred to as *pathogen-associated molecular patterns* (PAMPs) and are essential elements of a microorganism's pathogenicity. Examples of PAMPs include the lipopolysaccharide (LPS) of gram-negative bacteria and the peptidoglycan of the gram-positive bacterial cell wall. The PAMP of the microorganism binds to the PRR of the host cell in an interaction analogous to the receptor–ligand interaction that occurs in biochemical pathways.

One group of PRRs known as *toll-like receptors* (TLR) has emerged, with homology to receptors found in *Drosophila* (Fig. 3.1.11). It has been suggested that TLRs play a central role in the recognition of infectious pathogens by mammals. These TLRs consist of a variety of different receptors that are a fundamental and essential component of innate and adaptive immunity. One example of TLR activation is demonstrated by the LPS of the gram-negative

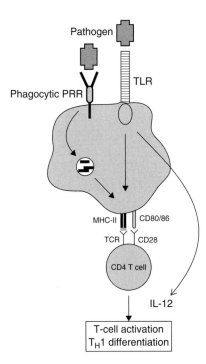

Pathogen

Phagocytic PRR

TLR

MHC-II   CD80/86

TCR   CD28

CD4 T cell

IL-12

T-cell activation
T_H1 differentiation

Figure 3.1.11 Innate immune recognition and control of adaptive immune responses. Recognition of pathogens or pathogen-associated molecular patterns (PAMPs) by pattern recognition receptors (PRRs) expressed on dendritic cells leads to dendritic cell maturation and activation of naïve T cells. Phagocytic PRRs internalize the pathogens into antigen-processing compartments, where pathogen-derived proteins are processed into antigenic peptides that are subsequently presented by MHC class II molecules on the cell surface. Therefore, expression of MHC-II/peptide complexes, induction of costimulatory molecules (CD80/CD86), and production of inflammatory cytokines (e.g., IL-12) are all induced by the Toll-like receptors (TLRs) upon stimulation by microbial ligands. TLR-induced IL-12 directs T-cell differentiation into T_H1 effector cells. The receptors involved in the recognition and initiation of T_H2 responses are currently unknown. IL, interleukin; MHC, major histocompatibility complex; TCR, T-cell receptor. (From Paul WE. *Fundamental immunology.* 5th ed. Philadelphia, PA: Lippincott Williams & Wilkins; 2003:513.)

bacteria, which can lead to septic shock. Once the TLR on the surface of a neutrophil recognizes the PAMP of LPS, a series of intracellular changes, known as *signal transduction*, occurs (Fig. 3.1.11). An adaptor protein associates with a protein kinase known as *IL-1R associated kinase* (IRAK). Through a series of phosphorylation steps, NFκB is released from its inhibitor and is translocated to the nucleus. NFκB then begins to modulate the immune response through the induction of immune response genes that govern the transcription of cytokines, the release of antimicrobial defenses, and the initiation of phagocytosis.

Activation of the Cellular Components of Innate Immunity

Once the PRR has identified a PAMP, the cellular components described in the preceding text become activated

to respond to the organism and to keep it localized. The neutrophil is a key component of innate immunity and is an early participant in inflammation. The macrophage is an important cell that can phagocytose microbial agents, summon other immune cells to their location, and prepare antigens for display to the arriving cells. The dendritic cells are all nonspecifically activated and can function to present antigens to the lymphoid tissue, where they start a specific immune response. In allergic reactions, the basophils, mast cells, and eosinophils are the dominant cell types (see allergic reactions). In addition, T-cell subsets, including the αβ T_H cells, γδ cells and NK cells, although usually considered components of the acquired immune response, will also respond as components of the innate immune response. T cells require two signals to become activated; one is the antigen binding to the appropriate MHC molecules and the other is a costimulatory factor. The PRR engaging with a PAMP will also initiate a signal that generates the adaptive immune response for antigen-specific immune responses.

Complement and Other Opsonins

In addition to the cellular components described so far, other entities are also active components of the innate immune response because they bind to invading pathogens, thus identifying them as foreign and enhancing their ability to be phagocytosed. These mechanisms are described more fully in Chapter 3.2. One of the most important elements that is operative here is complement. Complement, especially the alternative complement pathway, produces immunologically active substances that are opsonic for phagocytic cells. Complement also causes the release of inflammatory mediators from mast cells, and C5a acts as a neutrophil chemoattractant. The membrane attack complex of complement perforates cell membranes and destroys some invading microorganisms, particularly those of *Neisseria* spp.

Acute-phase proteins respond to a number of generic events like infection, inflammation, and injury. These substances are primarily produced in the liver and function as opsonins. They may be, in part, related to the constitutional symptoms, including fever, fatigue, and anorexia, experienced by some patients. Cytokines are soluble mediators that act as messengers both within and between the immune system and other systems of the body. Each of these systems is regulated through intricate pathways that prevent the overproduction and self-destruction that can occur with runaway immune responses.

ADAPTIVE IMMUNITY

The initiation of the adaptive immune response depends to a great extent on the important defense mechanisms discussed in the preceding text with respect to the innate immune response. The offending microorganism needs to breach the many barriers to infection that have been discussed so far. Once the epithelial membrane is bypassed, dendritic cells, macrophages, neutrophils, $\gamma\delta$ T cells, and MALT from the innate immune system can provide important intercellular messages and present antigens to T cells to enhance the effectiveness of the adaptive immune response. In addition, once a microorganism is successful in gaining entry, a PRR engages a PAMP, the innate immune response is activated, and a signal is also sent to the adaptive immune system to initiate a simultaneous response. Therefore, the antigen-specific response depends on the determination of a pathogen either by the nonspecific receptors of the innate immune system or by a specific identification by T or B cells of the cellular immune system, which is described in the next section (see Fig. 3.1.12).

The adaptive immune system relies on the recognition of a specific structural feature of a pathogenic organism. These distinctive antigens (epitopes) are recognized during the development of the immune system when exposure to non-self antigens induces immunologic memory through the clonal expansion of T and B cells. When T and B cells are first stimulated, they develop along two separate lines of differentiation. The first line is the effector cells that will bind antigens and assist in the immune response. The second line of development is the creation of memory cells that will record the specific antigenic exposure and improve

the ability of the immune system to respond more quickly and efficiently upon re-exposure or secondary response.

When dendritic cells are activated by antigens, they migrate to the spleen or to the local lymph nodes, where they present the antigens to naïve T cells, fostering their further differentiation. This differentiation is influenced by the presence of cytokines and MHC epitopes and is known as the T_H1/T_H2 paradigm. The naïve T cells will develop into T_H1 cells that produce IFN-γ and IL-2, which assist with further recruitment and activation of macrophages and T_C cells to assist with the immune response. Alternatively, the naïve T cells will develop into T_H2 cells that produce IL-4, IL-5, and IL-6, which induce B cells into an antibody-producing state. Antibodies produced by plasma cells are protective because they prevent the binding of the organism to the receptor in much the same manner that a receptor and ligand are reciprocally bound. The antibody also coats the offending pathogen, allowing it to be recognized and overcome by other cells of the immune system. This intercellular messaging assists in regulating the immune response by directing cellular development down a particular differentiation pathway and inhibiting the development of cells in the alternative pathway. Further differentiation is controlled by the MHC epitopes. If naïve T cells encounter a considerable amount of MHC 1 epitope, further differentiation along a CD8

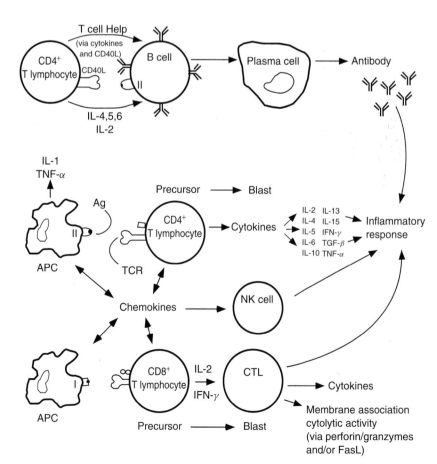

Figure 3.1.12 The cellular response of the adaptive immune system. IL, interleukin; TNF, tumor necrosis factor; APC, antigen-presenting cell; TCR, T-cell receptors; CTL, cytotoxic T lymphocytes; FasL, Fas ligand; NK cell, nature killer cell; IFN-γ, interferon-γ; TGF-β, transforming growth factor-β. (From Austin KF, Frank MM, Atkinson JP, et al. *Samter's immunologic diseases.* 6th ed. Philadelphia, PA: Lippincott Williams & Wilkins; 2001:196.)

cell line occurs. If MHC 1 is present in low concentration, B-cell expansion and further T_H-cell proliferation occur. The adaptive and innate immune systems have been presented here as discrete systems, but the reader must realize that these systems are highly regulated and interdependent in their ability to protect the body from pathogenic invasion.

ALLERGIC DISORDERS

The responses of the immune system to noninfectious antigens in the environment, such as food, medications, and insects, are termed *allergic reactions*. They are commonly considered synonymous with IgE-mediated immune reactions, although IgE is not an essential feature. These disorders are responses to often naturally occurring proteins. These antigens gain entry through many portals including the skin, gastrointestinal tract, or respiratory system. Hypersensitivity occurs when a tissue response becomes manifest. These diseases and the host's responses are important to the intensivist because the intensivist is often required to respond to the acute respiratory and hemodynamic manifestations of these reactions.

The patient who elicits an allergic response may be genetically or environmentally primed to respond to these antigens with an exaggerated T_H2 response (see Fig. 3.1.13). Microbial agents are recognized by the immune system and phagocytosed, resulting in an immune response that is mediated by T_H1 type cells. Allergens in sensitized individuals cause a T_H2 response (Fig. 3.1.13). This response may be caused by exposure to these antigens *in utero* or after birth. The response is characterized by the production of T_H2 cytokines, the production of IgE from B cells, the release of preformed mediators, and the recruitment of additional cells to the reaction site (see Table 3.1.3). In contrast, nonallergic individuals respond to allergens with

a T_H1 response and the production of IFN-γ and IgG. When allergic disorders are treated in individual patients, there is a shift from a T_H2 response back to a T_H1 response.

Once sensitized, antigen exposure initiates an allergic response that is classified in terms of phases (see Fig. 3.1.14).

An acute reaction occurs seconds to minutes after the exposure, a delayed or late reaction occurs several hours after the exposure, and a delayed or chronic reaction occurs days to years after the exposure (Fig. 3.1.14). A traditional classification schema by Gell and Coombs, which categorizes hypersensitivity reactions on the basis of the time course, pathophysiologic characteristics, and clinical characteristics, is of value to the clinicians (see Table 3.1.4). This approach specifies four types of hypersensitivity reactions from the immediate hypersensitivity reactions (Type I) that depend on the immediate release of preformed mediators from mast cells and basophils to the delayed type hypersensitivity reactions (Type IV) that rely on the T-cell system (Table 3.1.4). This overview of the pathophysiology of the immune response of allergic diseases is important to guide the pharmacologic therapy for these conditions (see Chapter 19).

AUTOIMMUNITY

Autoimmunity is a failure of the regulatory ability of the immune response to differentiate self from non-self. It occurs from a genetic predisposition but may also require a triggering event from the environment to incite the destruction of self-tissues (see Fig. 3.1.15). These triggers may be infectious (e.g., viral infection), drug-induced (e.g., procainamide), or caused by haptens that bind to and incite immunologic reactions (e.g., penicillin). Autoimmune phenomena may be localized to a particular organ or may be systemic. Their occurrence results from the abnormal activation of all the cells discussed at the

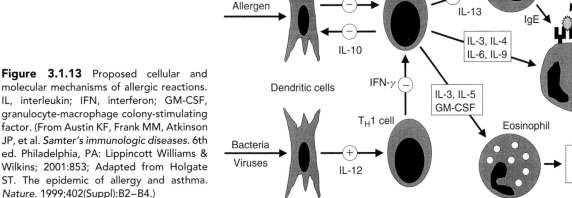

Figure 3.1.13 Proposed cellular and molecular mechanisms of allergic reactions. IL, interleukin; IFN, interferon; GM-CSF, granulocyte-macrophage colony-stimulating factor. (From Austin KF, Frank MM, Atkinson JP, et al. *Samter's immunologic diseases.* 6th ed. Philadelphia, PA: Lippincott Williams & Wilkins; 2001:853; Adapted from Holgate ST. The epidemic of allergy and asthma. *Nature.* 1999;402(Suppl):B2–B4.)

TABLE 3.1.3
MAJOR FEATURES OF ALLERGIC IMMUNE RESPONSES

1. Responses are elicited by certain groups of environmental allergens such as food, drugs, and proteins derived from pollens, insects (house dust mite), and animal dander
2. In susceptible individuals, allergens are presented to naïve T cells by dendritic cells residing in the mucosa of the skin, the GI tract, or the respiratory tract. For reasons that are not well understood, T cells of atopic individuals undergo differentiation to a T_H2 cytokine-producing pattern
3. Elaboration of T_H2 cytokines (IL-4, IL-5, IL-3, IL-9) initiates the allergic cascade through their combined ability to regulate IgE production, FcεRI expression, mast cell phenotype and development, and recruitment and activation of eosinophils
4. Under the control of T_H2 cell-derived signals (IL-4, IL-13, and CD40L), B cells undergo class switching to production of the IgE subclass
5. Upon re-exposure to the offending allergen, acute responses occurring within minutes of allergen exposure result from release of preformed mediators (histamine, tryptase) from FcεRI-bearing cells through the cross-linking of allergen and IgE on their surface. Cells activated during the acute phase also release cytokines and mediators, which perpetuate the T_H2-driven response
6. Late-phase responses result from the combined effects of inflammatory cells (eosinophils and T cells) recruited to the tissues within 6–24 h after the initial allergen exposure
7. Repeated allergen exposures in the context of an already inflamed tissue results in structural changes (remodeling), such as smooth muscle thickening, tissue fibrosis, and mucous cell hyperplasia

FcεRI, crystallized fragment ε receptor type I; GI, gastrointestinal; IgE, immunoglobulin E; IL, interleukin; T_H2, T helper cell type 2.
From Paul WE. *Fundamental immunology* 5th ed. Philadelphia, PA: Lippincott Williams & Wilkins; 2003;1441–1442.

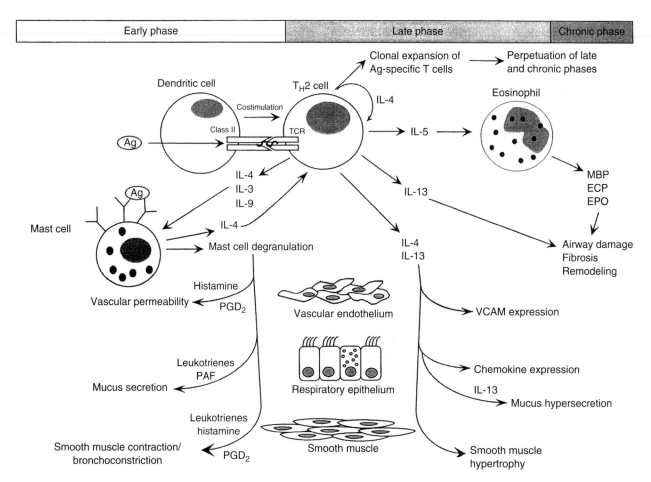

Figure 3.1.14 Overview of the acute, late, and chronic phases of the allergic response. IL, interleukin; MBP, major basic protein; ECP, eosinophil cationic protein; EPO, eosinophil peroxides; VCAM, vascular cellular adhesion molecules. (From Paul WE. *Fundamental immunology.* 5th ed. Philadelphia, PA: Lippincott Williams & Wilkins; 2003:1470.)

TABLE 3.1.4
THE GELL AND COOMBS CLASSIFICATION OF HYPERSENSITIVITY REACTIONS

Hypersensitivity Reaction	Type I	Type II	Type III	Type IV
Synonym	Anaphylaxis (immediate type)	Cytotoxic (antibody-dependent)	Immune complex–mediated	Cell-mediated (delayed hypersensitivity)
Immunomodulator	IgE	IgG, IgM	IgG, IgM	T cells
Chemical mediators	Vasoactive products of basophils and mast cells (e.g., histamine, bradykinin, slow-reacting substance of anaphylaxis arachidonate PGE_1 and PGE_2)	Complement—with either a combination of IgG or IgM antibodies with epitopes on cell surface or tissue or the adsorption of antigens or haptens to tissue or cell membrane, with subsequent attachment of antibodies to the adsorbed antigens	Generally occurs in the region of antigen excess. Virtually any antigen that induces a detectable antibody response will suffice. The antibodies involved are primarily precipitating IgG and IgM capable of fixing complement	Lymphokines and monokines
Time to onset	Seconds to minutes	1–24 h	2–72 h	Maximal at 2–4 d
Cellular level and above	Accumulation of neutrophils, eosinophils, smooth muscle contraction. Vasodilation, vascular leakage	Macrophages, NK, mast cell, vasodilation and vascular leakage	Accumulation of neutrophils, macrophages. Release of lysosomal enzymes	Lymphocytes and macrophage accumulation forming granulomas
Examples	Anaphylaxis, atopic dermatitis, urticaria, angioedema	Autoimmune hemolytic anemia, hemolytic disease of the newborn, transfusion reactions, Goodpasture syndrome, myasthenia gravis	SLE, serum sickness, poststreptococcal glomerulonephritis	Contact dermatitis, Hashimoto thyroiditis, organ allograft rejection

IgE, immunoglobulin E; IgG, immunoglobulin G; IgM, immunoglobulin M; PGE, prostaglandin E; NK, natural killer; SLE, systemic lupus erythematosus.

beginning of this chapter. There is still some controversy and ongoing research about the exact mechanisms of these clinical entities. Nonetheless, several classic mechanisms of autoimmunity do exist.

Tolerance

One explanation for autoimmunity implicates defects in "tolerance," a state of unresponsiveness to an antigen. This unresponsiveness to self-antigens prevents autoimmunity and occurs through an important selection process that begins in the thymus and is known as *central tolerance*. Those cells that are unable to adequately recognize MHC molecules will die, those with over-recognition for self-antigens (potentially autoimmune) will be selected out, and those cells with appropriate recognition will be released to peripheral locations such as the lymph nodes and spleen

to function as CD4 or CD8 lymphocytes (Fig. 3.1.10). Autoimmunity results from a failure of autoreactive T cells to undergo apoptosis. These T cells can be released to the peripheral circulation and may lie dormant in the peripheral organs until an environmental trigger allows them to work against self-antigens in these peripheral tissues. When normal immune cells with an ability to differentiate self have been released to the periphery, these cells are expected to continue to respond appropriately by not activating against self-tissues. This is known as *peripheral tolerance*. Occasionally, inappropriate activation signals may be provided to these peripheral lymphocytes in the presence of self-antigens that are presented by MHC molecules. This, in part, explains the genetic linkage between certain autoimmune diseases and alleles of the MHC. The result is that these lymphocytes become autoreactive instead of undergoing apoptosis. This is the

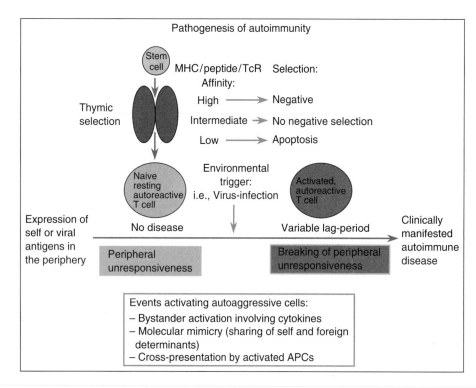

Figure 3.1.15 Potentially autoreactive lymphocytes can escape thymic negative selection and escape into the periphery. Such initially naïve cells can be activated by several mechanisms involving cytokines, inflammation, and possible external triggers such as viral infections. APCs, antigen-presenting cells; MHC, major histocompatibility complex. (From Paul WE. *Fundamental immunology.* 5th ed. Philadelphia, PA: Lippincott Williams & Wilkins; 2003:1405.)

mechanism behind acetylcholine receptors in myasthenia and behind type II collagen destruction in rheumatoid arthritis.

Tolerance can also occur with B cells. Many autoreactive B cells undergo clonal deletion or become anergic as they mature in the bone marrow. B cells recognize native antigen; therefore, there is no role for the MHC molecules in any of these processes. In the periphery, tolerance to self-antigens is built in by the T-cell population, which does not provide the help necessary for antibody production by self-reactive B cells. Therefore, when B cells react against self-antigens or when T cells begin to assist these self-reactive B cells, the B cells produce autoantibodies targeted against self-tissues, leading to damage.

Defects in tolerance may appear clinically as inflammatory reactions in multiple organs that occur episodically at times of disease flare-ups. These defects can occur from several different mechanisms. One mechanism relates to the highly specific ability of T and B cells to distinguish antigens. On occasion, a cross-reactive response against self-antigens occurs because a self-antigen is modified and no longer resembles the structure of self-tissues. An immune response is propagated against these antigens. A second mechanism involves the exposure to an antigen that cross-reacts with a normal self-antigen. This is known as *molecular mimicry*. A common example of this mechanism is demonstrated when poststreptococcal myocarditis proteins react with cardiac myocytes. Another method of avoiding tolerance is when foreign antigens attach themselves to cells and the cells are then recognized as foreign and have an immune response propagated against them.

Finally, tissue antigens that are exposed as a part of the injury and inflammation may lose their "self" identity and become the target of immunologic attack.

GELL AND COOMBS REVISITED

Table 3.1.4 presented the classification schema proposed by Gell and Coombs for hypersensitivity reactions. The Type I or immediate type hypersensitivity reactions are IgE-mediated. For the intensivist, the important example of this reaction is anaphylaxis with its resulting hemodynamic and respiratory compromise. The Type II reactions are antibody-dependent cytotoxic reactions that depend on IgG and IgM antibodies (Table 3.1.4). These antibodies bind to the membranes of the target organ and initiate an inflammatory response that includes the recruitment of immune cells including macrophages, serum components such as complement, and other mediators of inflammation through the activation of the coagulation cascade. The inflammatory response that ensues is responsible for the tissue damage. An example of this type of reaction is Goodpasture disease, in which these antibodies attack the glomerular basement membrane (Table 3.1.4). Type III responses are immune complexes that form from the binding of an antigen with an antibody. The antigens are heterogeneous, which accounts for the wide variety of diseases in which immune complexes are relevant. These immune complexes are particularly successful in activating the classical pathway of complement and propagating inflammatory responses. Systemic lupus erythematosus

(SLE) is a good example of a Type III immune response. Finally, a Type IV hypersensitivity reaction depends on a cellular reaction. Macrophages, lymphocytes, and the multitude of cellular products that they produce are responsible for this reaction (Table 3.1.4).

Additional autoantibodies may develop in systemic rheumatologic and immune diseases that cause damage through their role on target tissues. For the most part, these autoantibodies are IgG in origin. The identification of autoantibodies may assist in making a clinical diagnosis. For example, the identification of antibodies targeted at the double-stranded DNA is specific for SLE. However, these results must be interpreted cautiously because there is a considerable overlap in the diseases associated with some of these autoantibodies (e.g., antinuclear antibody [ANA]). On an organ system level, autoantibodies may either stimulate or inhibit the function of an organ. For example, in myasthenia gravis, an autoantibody against the acetylcholine receptor blocks the binding of acetylcholine molecules to the receptor on the postsynaptic junction and is responsible for the muscular weakness characteristic of this particular disease. Alternatively, in Graves disease, autoantibodies to the thyroid-stimulating hormone (TSH) receptor leads to unregulated stimulation of thyroid hormone and the clinical manifestations of hyperthyroidism.

CONCLUSION

This chapter on immunity was primarily concerned with the host's machinery for preventing and responding to invasion from external insults. The mechanical, cellular, and organ-specific mechanisms of host defense and their interactions in effecting a general immune response and specific responses as the foundation for both allergic and rheumatologic diseases in the critically ill child have been covered. Finally, the important principles of autoimmunity were discussed not only because of their relevance as a risk factor for infection in the critically ill child but also because of their relevance to the induction of immune suppression as a treatment strategy for a range of diseases often seen in the pediatric intensive care unit.

ACKNOWLEDGMENTS

Supported in part by grant KO-8 HS14009-01, Agency for Healthcare Research and Quality, Rockville, MD.

RECOMMENDED READINGS

1. Aird WC. Endothelium as an organ system. *Crit Care Med.* 2004;32:S271–S279.
2. Beutler B. Inferences, questions and possibilities in Toll-like receptor signaling. *Nature.* 2004;430:257–262.
3. Davidson A, Diamond B. Advances in immunology: Autoimmune disease. *N Engl J Med.* 2001;346:340–350.
4. Delves PJ, Roitt IM. The immune system: First of two parts. *N Engl J Med.* 2000;343:37–49.
5. Delves PJ, Roitt IM. The immune system: Second of two parts. *N Engl J Med.* 2000;343:108–116.
6. Firestein GS. Evolving concepts of rheumatoid arthritis. *Nature.* 2003;423:356–361.
7. Heinzel FP. Antibodies. In: Gallin JI, Snyderman R, Fearon DT et al., eds. *Inflammation.* Philadelphia, PA: Lippincott Williams & Wilkins; 1999.
8. Johnson RM, Brown EJ. Cell mediated immunity in host defense against infectious diseases. In: Gallin JI, Snyderman R, Fearon DT et al., eds. *Inflammation.* Philadelphia, PA: Lippincott Williams & Wilkins; 1999.
9. Kay AB. Advances in immunology: Allergy and allergic diseases (first of two parts). *N Engl J Med.* 2001;344:30–37.
10. Kay AB. Advances in immunology: Allergy and allergic diseases (second of two parts). *N Engl J Med.* 2001;344:109–113.
11. Klein J, Sato A. Advances in immunology: The HLA system (first of two parts). *N Engl J Med.* 2000;343:702–709.
12. Klein J, Sato A. Advances in immunology: The HLA system (second of two parts). *N Engl J Med.* 2000;343:782–786.
13. Medzhitov R, Janeway C. Advances in immunology: Innate immunity. *N Engl J Med.* 2000;343:338–344.
14. Uthaisangsook S, Noorbibi KD, Bahna SL, et al. Innate immunity and its role against infections. *Ann Allergy Asthma Immunol.* 2002;88:253–265.
15. Von Andrian UH, Mackay CR. Advances in immunology: T cell function and migration-two sides of the same coin. *N Engl J Med.* 2000;343:1020–1034.

Inflammation

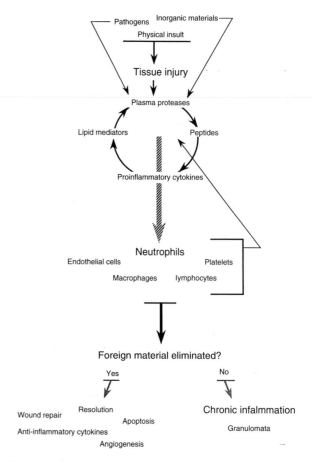

3.2

Anthony D. Slonim

This chapter focuses on inflammation, a complex process occurring in vascularized tissues. It is a nonspecific host response that depends on the interaction of cellular and soluble mediators from different pathways aimed at controlling and eliminating an offending agent and repairing the underlying tissues (see Fig. 3.2.1). Inflammation is a delicate balance between the beneficial effects of the host's innate immune response and the deleterious effects associated with ongoing inflammation and scar formation.

Inflammation manifests itself as either a local or a systemic phenomenon. Many syndromes in pediatric critical care are centered on this balance between inflammation and its control at the system level. Inflammation consists of three phases: initiation, amplification, and termination. Many stimuli can initiate the host response, including microbial products, endotoxemia, acute respiratory distress syndrome (ARDS), burns, and trauma. The response is then amplified by the effects of potent biologic mediators. Finally, inflammation is terminated after removal of the offending agent or when anti-inflammatory control products are produced. When inflammation fails to be contained at the local level, a syndrome known as the systemic inflammatory response syndrome (SIRS) may result.

Acute inflammation is usually initiated immediately after an insult, and it is self-limited, lasting 8 to 10 days. Its propagation is characterized by the infiltration of phagocytes, which are central to the inflammatory process (Fig. 3.2.1). However, this highly orchestrated process is also reliant on other cells and their products, the plasma protein systems, and the vascular and cellular responses induced by mediators that assist the organism in responding to the changes in the tissues. Chronic inflammation begins after the period of acute inflammation has been unsuccessful in terminating the inciting agent. In addition, chronic inflammation results from an inability to terminate the immune response, or, as occurs in some rheumatologic diseases, tissue damage may provide a stimulus for ongoing inflammation. Persistent inflammatory reactions

Figure 3.2.1 Molecular and cellular events of the inflammatory response. (From Paul WE. *Fundamental immunology.* 5th ed. Philadelphia, PA: Lippincott Williams & Wilkins; 2003:1152.)

are characterized by the infiltration of lymphocytes and macrophages. The simultaneous processes of continuous inflammation associated with ongoing healing and scar formation are discussed as major outcomes of chronic inflammation.

ACUTE INFLAMMATION

Historically, Celsus was credited with describing the four discrete clinical signs of local inflammation. They include dolor or pain, rubor or redness, tumor or swelling, and calor or heat. Subsequently, loss of function was added as a fifth classic sign. Since then, our understanding of the inflammatory response at the cellular level has improved dramatically. The inflammatory response has many stimuli, each of which initiates a similar cascade of pathophysiologic events. These stimuli may be mechanical, such as the insults associated with exposure to cold, heat, trauma, or surgery. The stimuli may be chemical, associated with insults such as ischemia, radiation, or toxins, or they may be infectious, such as those associated with a variety of microorganisms that adversely affect the host. Considerable interest in critical care currently resides with identifying genetic predispositions to these stimuli and with discovering the reasons why, in some patients, they elicit an overwhelming inflammatory response, whereas in others they do not.

Microcirculation Responses

Microcirculation is important for regulating the intravascular to extravascular flow of fluids in both health and in disease. A number of forces maintain this important balance of fluids. However, when activated by an inflammatory stimulus, these forces are altered because the goals of the microcirculation become focused on localizing, identifying, destroying, and removing the offending agent and on delivering cellular and soluble products to the site of inflammation. During inflammation, the microcirculation assists by isolating the inflammatory stimulus, thereby preventing the systemic spread of by-products. In addition, the microcirculation stimulates an immune response, combating the agent and promoting healing once the agent has been successfully overcome. Three microcirculation responses are described in acute inflammation.

First, the microcirculation undergoes brief vasoconstriction, followed by the vasodilation of arterioles and venules. This occurs immediately and is mediated by the effects of cell and plasma-derived mediators such as histamine, leukotrienes, nitric oxide, and bradykinin. The vasodilation augments the flow of blood at the site of inflammation and increases the hydrostatic pressure of the vasculature, leading to edema formation (see Fig. 3.2.2). The classic signs of inflammation include fluid congestion, edema, erythema, swelling, warmth, and a reduction in mobility. A second type of response occurs with direct injury to and necrosis of the endothelial cells, as occurs in burns. In this situation, the changes last for hours or days and the vasculature increases its permeability to fluids rich in proteins. Finally, a third type of endothelial damage leading to changes in vascular permeability can occur after hours or days in response to specific stimuli, as occurs in a Type IV (delayed) hypersensitivity reaction.

The fluid accumulating in the acute inflammatory process will assume different characteristics, depending on the fluid's source, its contents, and the mechanism and duration of its accumulation. Edema is the loss of fluids and electrolytes from the intravascular space into the interstitial and extravascular spaces of the body. Edema fluid is subcategorized as a transudate if the protein content is low or as an exudate if the protein content is high and if it contains inflammatory cells. The differential diagnosis will vary depending on the type of fluid accumulating in these different body spaces. Exudates are classified as serous, serosanguinous, fibrinous, purulent, membranous, and hemorrhagic, depending on the constituents.

Fluid loss to the tissues results in a slowing and stasis of the red blood cells remaining in the circulation. This stasis may be transient if the injury is mild. However, if prolonged, white blood cells (WBCs), particularly neutrophils, marginate along the endothelial surface, allowing for their adherence and migration to the site of inflammation. These WBCs can assist in mediating the inflammatory response through the release of inflammatory mediators and the ingestion of debris and cellular products. These cells may also be directly injurious to the endothelial cells and may lead to further leakage of fluid from the intravascular space. When inflammation is present, edema fluid may be reabsorbed through channels in the epithelium or in the lymph vessels. This fluid passes to the lymph nodes where it stimulates B lymphocytes to become antibody-producing plasma cells, or T lymphocytes to become T-effector cells, thereby propagating the inflammatory response.

Leucocyte Recruitment in Inflammation

The WBCs are an important group of cells involved in the cellular response to inflammation. Many types of WBCs are important, including neutrophils, basophils, mast cells, lymphocytes, monocytes, and macrophages, and each brings to the site of inflammation its own functional abilities. These WBCs become activated through many stimuli, including cytokines, antigen–antibody complexes, and bacterial products, with receptors on their cell walls. After activation, the WBCs upregulate a number of products that improve their ability to interact with the endothelial cell, also a very important cell in inflammation.

As inflammation continues, the activated WBCs need to become actively engaged at the site of injury (see Fig. 3.2.3). Once in the tissues, they can work directly on the foreign material. Through the production of cytokines, WBCs summon other cells to participate in the inflammatory reaction. These processes are outlined here for the neutrophil and include rolling, adhesion, migration, chemotaxis, and phagocytosis, but they also occur for eosinophils, basophils, and lymphocytes.

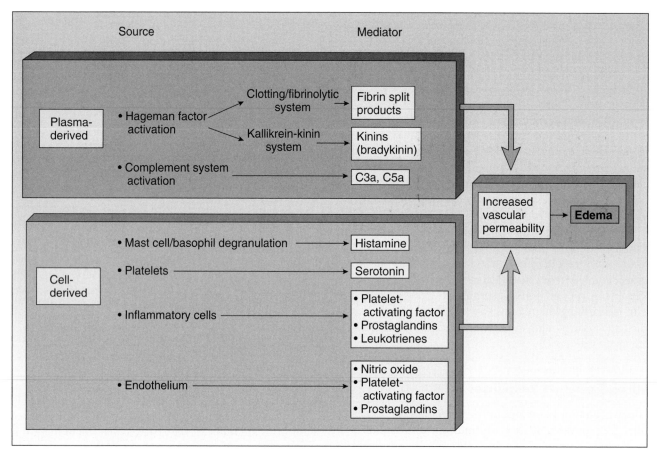

Figure 3.2.2 Vasoactive mediators of increased vascular permeability. (From Rubin E. *Essential pathology*. 3rd ed. Philadelphia, PA: Lippincott Williams & Wilkins; 2000:40.)

Rolling/Adhesion

While neutrophils are freely circulating, they make contact with the endothelial surface in a chaotic manner. Once activated by an inflammatory stimulus, endothelial cells engage reversibly with neutrophils in a process known as *rolling*, slowing their free flow through the circulation and allowing the chemoattractant properties of the expressed mediators to affect the neutrophil. Adhesive glycoproteins on the surface of the neutrophil and endothelial cells, called *selectins* and *integrins*, facilitate these interactions (Fig. 3.2.3). L-selectin, which is contained on the cell surface of leucocytes and includes neutrophils, exhibits

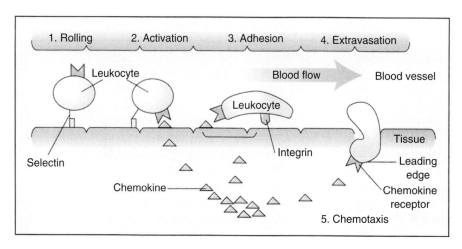

Figure 3.2.3 Processes of neutrophil response during inflammation. (From Ritter YS, Marshall GD. Chemokines and their receptors. In: Lieberman PL, Blaiss MS, eds. *Atlas of allergic diseases*. Philadelphia, PA: Lippincott Williams & Wilkins and Current Medicine; 2002:27.)

sialyl-Lewis^X, a glycoprotein that interacts with the E and P selectins of the endothelial cells. Interleukin 1 (IL-1), tumor necrosis factor (TNF), and histamine assist in the upregulation of the endothelial cell selectins. As the neutrophil approaches the site of inflammation, L selectin becomes less important on the neutrophil surface, and integrins, which are routinely expressed on the neutrophil's surface, become activated, preparing the neutrophil for adhesion and subsequent migration.

Migration

Adhesion is followed by diapedesis or migration through the retracting endothelial cells and basement membrane into the surrounding tissue (Fig. 3.2.3). This migration is mediated by intercellular adhesion molecule-1 (ICAM-1) present on the endothelium's cell surface. ICAM-1 becomes upregulated during inflammation in the presence of IL-1, TNF, and interferon-γ (IFN-γ) and associates with the integrins on the neutrophil surface. This interaction allows the neutrophil to stop, flatten, and migrate into the extravascular space of the postcapillary venule to the site of inflammation with the assistance of platelet-endothelial cell adhesion molecules 1 (PECAM-1). Once in the extravascular space, enzymes present in the neutrophil allow for its progression into the tissues toward the chemokine.

The granulocytes are the first cells attracted to the site of inflammation by cellular mediators. These substances include bacterial products, complement components, peptides, fibrin-degradation products, prostaglandins, and the membrane attack complex (MAC) of complement, all of which can contribute to a concentration gradient along which migration occurs. Neutrophil movement is mediated by the activity of intracellular actin and myosin filaments, which, through their interaction with calcium, form a gel, which, when extended into pseudopods, allows the neutrophil to migrate toward the inflammatory stimulus. Gelsolin breaks down the actin cross-linking to prevent cellular rigidity and allows it to move toward the site of inflammation. Once at the site of inflammation, the neutrophil upregulates other receptors including the Fc fragment of immunoglobulins and complement components to facilitate the innate immune response.

Phagocytosis

The neutrophils must engulf and internalize the foreign material to kill the cells in a process known as *phagocytosis*. The foreign material is recognized by receptors on the polymorphonuclear neutrophil (PMN) membrane, including the Fc portion of immunoglobulins and complement receptors; the intracellular signaling mechanism then begins the phagocytic process. The phagocyte is assisted in adhering to the cell membrane of the foreign material by opsonins produced through other parts of the inflammatory process. Pseudopodia are then extended through the actin–myosin–calcium mechanism as described earlier to engulf the particle in a phagosome. After fusion of the phagosome with enzyme-containing vesicles, phagolysosomes are created, which form the site of microbial killing, destruction, and digestion.

Microbial Killing

After phagocytosis, two mechanisms for microbial killing by the neutrophil have been elucidated—an oxygen-independent mechanism that capitalizes on the neutrophil's granules and an oxygen-dependent mechanism that requires significant amounts of energy to affect the killing. Granules are a very important structural characteristic of phagocytes—so important that neutrophils, eosinophils, and basophils are subcategorized as granulocytes because of the appearance of these prominent granules during microscopy. Each of these cells has granules that assist in carrying out their function. For example, several different types of granules form during neutrophil development and affect the ability of the neutrophil to neutralize a microorganism (see Table 3.2.1). Together, the granules form what is known as the *oxygen-independent method of killing*. Azurophil granules contain a number of hydrolytic enzymes and bactericidal proteins, including elastase, cathepsin G, hydrolases, defensins, and bactericidal permeability–increasing protein (BPI), which is structurally similar to serum lipopolysaccharide (LPS)–binding protein. Because of BPI, the azurophil granules have a role in combating infections with gram-negative bacteria. These products are antimicrobial in nature and help to fortify the innate immune system. Specific granules contain collagenase, lysozyme, cytochrome b_{588}, and lactoferrin. Importantly, specific granules contain a number of products that can be upregulated during an immune response. Lactoferrin, for example, can compete with the microorganism for iron, which is an essential growth factor. Gelatinase granules contain gelatinase predominantly, but they also contain cytochrome b_{588}. These granules are important in recruiting other neutrophils during inflammation and in repairing the tissues. Finally, secretory granules are rich in cell-surface receptors that can move easily to the surface of the neutrophil to participate actively in inflammation.

The second mechanism of killing is referred to as *oxidative killing* because it is highly dependent on oxygen for energy and on the formation of oxygen radicals for effective destruction of the microorganism (see Table 3.2.2). After phagocytosis, neutrophils rapidly consume oxygen in a "respiratory burst" to produce superoxide (O_2^-) and other active oxygen intermediates. The hexose monophosphate shunt provides nicotinomide adenine dinucleotide phosphate (reduced form) (NADPH), which is produced through the activity of glucose-6-phosphate dehydrogenase (G6PD). When catalyzed by NADPH oxidase in the presence of oxygen, NADPH produces $NADP^+$ and O_2^- .

TABLE 3.2.1
CONTENTS OF HUMAN NEUTROPHIL GRANULES

Type of Constituent	Azurophil (Primary) Granule	Specific (Secondary) Granule	Other
Antimicrobial enzyme	Lysozyme Myeloperoxidase	Lysozyme	
Antimicrobial peptides and proteins	Bactericidal/permeability-increasing protein	Lactoferrin	
		Cathelicidin/hCAP-18	
	Defensins Azurocidin/CAP37/heparin-binding protein		
Enzymes	Acid phosphatase β-Glucosaminidase α-Mannosidase	Cytochrome b_{558}	Cytochrome b_{558} β-Glucosaminidase α-Mannosidase
	Arylsulfatase α-Fucosidase Neutrophil serine protease PR3 (proteinase 3)	Gelatinase B/MMP9 Histaminase	Gelatinase B/MMP9
	Cathepsin G Cathepsin D	Heparinase	Cathepsin D
	Elastase/MMP-12 Phospholipase A Histonase Deoxyribonuclease 5'-Nucleotidase	Sialidase	
	Collagenase-2/MMP-8 β-Glycerophosphatase β-Glucuronidase	Collagenase-2/MMP-8	β-Glucuronidase
Receptors		iC3h fMLP	
Other	Glycosaminoglycans Chondroitin sulfate	Laminin Vitamin B_{12}-binding protein	Laminin
	Heparin sulfate		

CAP, cationic antimicrobial protein; MMPs, matrix metalloproteinases; fMLP, fMet-Leu-Phe receptor.
From Gorbach SL, Bartlett JG, Blacklow NR. *Infectious diseases*. 3rd ed. Philadelphia, PA: Lippincott Williams & Wilkins; 2003:21.

The superoxide anion is then converted by superoxide dismutase to hydrogen peroxide (H_2O_2). Hydrogen peroxide is more effective as a killing agent than O_2^-.

Additional oxidative killing mechanisms in the neutrophil include halides, hydroxyl radicals, and nitric oxide species. The enzyme myeloperoxidase (MPO) catalyzes a reaction between the halides (chloride, bromide, or iodide) and hydrogen peroxide to produce halogen-associated reactive species that are very powerful antimicrobial agents. The most common example of this group of compounds is hypochlorous acid (HOCL) (Table 3.2.2). Hydroxyl radical ($OH^\bullet$) is a potent oxidant formed when superoxide and hydrogen peroxide react in the presence of iron in what is known as the *Fenton reaction*. The $OH^\bullet$ is particularly harmful to host tissues and may be involved in ischemia-reperfusion injury. Finally, nitric oxide ($NO^\bullet$) is formed when NADPH reacts with L-arginine in the presence of oxygen. Citrulline, NADPH, and water are the by-products of this reaction, which is mediated by inducible nitric oxide synthase (iNOS). This reaction can be upregulated in neutrophils, monocytes, and macrophages. Nitric oxide functions as an intracellular messenger, but it can also combine with superoxide to produce a highly toxic peroxynitrite radical ($ONOO^\bullet$).

Plasma Factors

Three major plasma-derived systems assist in regulating and propagating the inflammatory response. Each of these systems is composed of a series of inactive enzymes or proenzymes that, when activated, initiate a cascade of events and activate the next component of the system. The

TABLE 3.2.2

REACTIONS INVOLVING REACTIVE OXYGEN METABOLITES PRODUCED BY PHAGOCYTIC CELLS

Reduction of molecular oxygen

$O_2 + e^- \rightarrow O_2^-$ Superoxide anion

Dismutation of O_2^-

$O_2^- + O_2^- + 2H^+ \rightarrow O_2 + H_2O_2$ Hydrogen peroxide

Haber-Weiss reaction

$H_2O_2 + O_2^- \rightarrow O_2 + OH^- + OH^\bullet$ Hydroxyl radical

Fenton reaction (iron-catalyzed)

$H_2O_2 + Fe^{2+} \rightarrow Fe^{3+} + OH^- + OH^\bullet$ Hydroxyl radical

Myeloperoxidase reaction

$H_2O_2 + Cl^- + H^+ \rightleftharpoons H_2O + HOCl$ Hypochlorous acid

From Rubin WE. *Essential pathology.* 3rd ed. Philadelphia, PA: Lippincott Williams & Wilkins; 2000:40.

three systems are the complement system, the coagulation system, and the kinin system (see Fig. 3.2.4). The Hageman factor (factor XII) is a protein synthesized by the liver, which plays a pivotal role in activation of these three systems. The coagulation system is detailed in Chapter 4, and only its relation to inflammation is discussed in this chapter. The complement system is important for ongoing immune surveillance and for modulating the different components of the innate immune system and inflammatory response. The kinin system is important in mediating the effects on the vasculature during inflammation.

The Coagulation System

Without excessively elaborating on the coagulation system and its two pathways, this section highlights the importance of the coagulation cascade in initiating and propagating the inflammatory response (Fig. 3.2.4). The coagulation system is a plasma protein system that becomes activated by a number of stimuli, including exposed basement membranes, bacterial and tissue products, plasma proteins from the complement and kinin systems, and cellular debris. The Hageman factor, once activated, can initiate the activity of the complement, kinin, and coagulation systems.

The Hageman factor activation initiates the clotting cascade (Chapter 4). In the clotting cascade, prothrombin is converted to thrombin, which activates fibrinogen to form fibrin monomers (Fig. 3.2.4). These fibrin monomers increase vascular permeability by enhancing the effect of

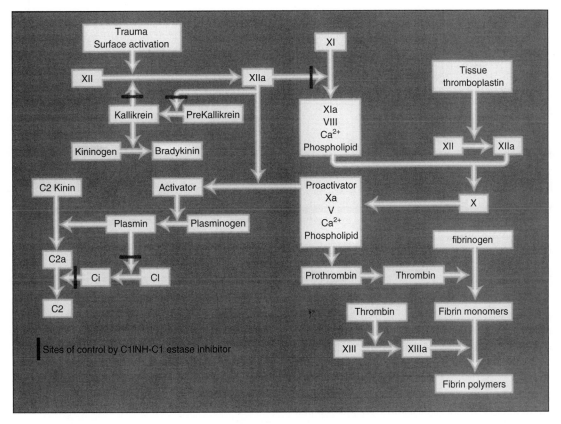

Figure 3.2.4 Interaction of clotting, fibrinolysis, kinin system, and complement pathways. (From Blaiss MS. The complement system. In: Lieberman PL. Blaiss MS. *Atlas of allergic diseases.* Philadelphia, PA: Lippincott Williams & Wilkins and Current Medicine; 2002:22.)

bradykinin. They are also chemotactic for neutrophils. Fibrin polymers form and assist in preventing hemorrhage, trapping bacteria within inflamed or injured tissue, and preventing the spread of infection and inflammation. This fibrin network also sets the stage for future repair and healing after the inflammatory response dissipates.

Simultaneously, the fibrinolytic system is being activated by the Hageman factor to counter-regulate clotting. The Hageman factor converts plasminogen to plasmin, which assists in fibrinolysis. Plasmin also activates the complement cascade (Fig. 3.2.4). Finally, the Hageman factor activates the conversion of prekallikrein to kallikrein in the kinin system.

The Complement System

Complement is a major component of the humoral immune system and is actively engaged in innate immune responses and inflammation. The complement system consists of more than 30 soluble proteins that can be found in plasma or attached to cell surfaces. These proteins are produced primarily in the liver and organized into three "pathways" that serve primarily to defend against bacterial infections and dispose of immune complexes and inflammatory debris. The pathways are referred to as the *classic pathway*, the *alternative pathway*, and the *mannan-binding lectin pathway*, each of which provides for the sequential activation of a series of proteins (see Fig. 3.2.5). Whereas many of the complement components facilitate the destruction of bacteria by PMNs, the MAC, which can be activated through any of the complement pathway mechanisms, is directly cytotoxic. The complement system is tightly integrated and regulated. However, system instability can result in autoimmune and rheumatologic diseases.

The Classic Pathway

The activation of the classic pathway of complement is initiated by circulating immunoglobulin M (IgM) and IgG antibodies that bind to antigen (Fig. 3.2.5). Because of its dependence on antibody, the classic pathway of complement is considered important in acquired immunity. These antigen–antibody complexes attach themselves through the Fc portions of the antibody to the C1 molecule, which circulates freely in the serum. The binding of antibody to C1 activates C1r, which subsequently activates C1s through protease activity. Activated C1s then works through a protease to cleave C2 into C2a and C2b and C4 into C4a and C4b. C4a simply dissipates, whereas C4b combines with C2a into a complex known as *C4b2a* (also known as *C3 convertase*), which is stabilized by C2b and is responsible for activating C3 repetitively to perpetuate the response (Fig. 3.2.5). C3 and its products, C3a and C3b, play pivotal roles in the remainder of the complement cascade. As C3 is activated, C3a, an important anaphylatoxin, is created, and C3b provides an important, although transient, binding site for bacteria and acts as an opsonin. C3b can interact

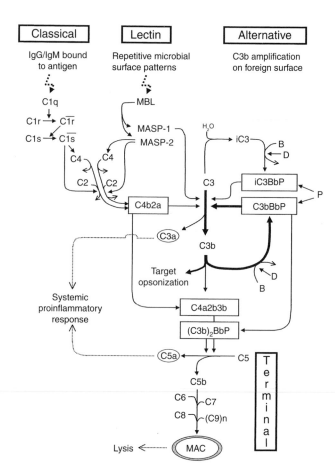

Figure 3.2.5 Overview of complement activation pathways. The C3 or C5 convertases of the pathways are *boxed*. The alternative pathway amplification loop of C3b generation is indicated by *thick arrows*. Note the systemic action of the anaphylatoxins in contrast to the effect of opsonization or lysis through a membrane attack complex that occurs on the target surface. MBL, mannose-binding lectin; MASP, MBL-associated serine proteases; MAC, membrane attack complex. (From Paul WE. *Fundamental immunology.* 5th ed. Philadelphia, PA: Lippincott Williams & Wilkins; 2003:1078.)

with either C4b2a of the classic system and form a complex known as *C4b2a3b* or *Bb* of the alternative pathway to create C3bBb, both of which have the ability to activate C5 into its components C5a and C5b. C5a is an anaphylatoxin and chemoattractant. C5b can combine with available C6 to begin the formation of the MAC, which is directly cytotoxic by inserting itself into the lipid bilayer of the cell membranes. Fulfillment of the MAC cytotoxicity is achieved by sequential inclusion of C7, C8, and C9 to the C5b6 complex. The complex creates a pore in the cell membrane and allows for the influx of water and, ultimately, lysis.

The Alternative Pathway

The alternative pathway does not require an antibody for its activation; rather, it can be activated directly through bacterial, viral, or yeast particles and other "non-self" cells (Fig. 3.2.5). Therefore, the alternative pathway is considered an important component of innate immunity. This pathway begins when factor B binds to C3b that is provided either through the classic pathway or the Mannose-binding lectin pathway. After factor B binds to C3b, it is susceptible to cleavage by factor D, which circulates in the plasma. Factor D cleaves B into Ba, which diffuses away, and into Bb, which binds to C3b and forms the C3bBb complex that binds and activates additional molecules of C3 to perpetuate the response. Properdin is also an important element here. It provides stability to the C3bBb complex, which, if excessive, leads to the autoimmune activation of complement. The C3bBb complex then activates C5, as in the classic pathway, resulting in the sequential formation of the MAC.

The Mannose-Binding–Lectin Pathway

The mannose-binding–lectin (MBL) pathway hinges on an MBL plasma protein that is similar in structure to C1, except that it is antibody-independent (Fig. 3.2.5). Rather, the MBL protein in turn binds to the exposed sugars on some microorganisms. This protein leads to the activation of three proteases termed *MBL-associated serine proteases 1–3* (MASPs). MASP 1 can activate MASP 2. MASPs 1 and 3 can directly activate C3, leading to C3a and C3b. MASP 2 can activate C2 and C4, which can proceed to activate C3 as described above for the classic pathway,. The MBL pathway provides a mechanism of activating complement before the antibody response occurs. Its deficiency is associated with susceptibility to a variety of infections, particularly, in the interval between the loss of maternal antibody and the acquisition of immune surveillance.

Control of Complement

Complement pathways must remain under strict control because their unopposed activation will lead to complement attack on "self" tissues. These control pathways occur through soluble or membrane-bound proteins that act to retard the critical elements of activation or to accelerate the decay of proteins in the pathway. C1 inhibitor (C1-INH), which is a serine protease inhibitor, provides tight control over C1s and C1r of the classic pathway and the MASPs of the MBL pathway. In addition, C1-INH provides a mechanism of common control over the clotting, fibrinolytic, and kinin pathways (Fig. 3.2.4). A number of other "downstream" inhibitors of the classic pathway include C4-binding protein and decay-accelerating factor. In the alternative pathway, C3 convertases will self-decay with time and prevent further propagation of this pathway. This process is accelerated by decay-accelerating factor and Factor H.

Kinin System

The kinin system is a plasma protein system that produces peptide products with wide-ranging effects on the microvasculature. This system is an essential component in the amplification of the inflammatory response. Prekallikreins are precursor molecules that are present in blood or tissues. As with the complement and coagulation plasma protease systems, prekallikreins are activated through the Hageman factor of the coagulation system described earlier and other chemical and enzymatic factors (see Fig. 3.2.6). The Hageman factor converts prekallikrein to kallikrein. Kallikreins are proteolytic enzymes that are contained either in the tissues or in the plasma. Kallikreins utilize kininogens as a substrate to produce kinins. Tissue kallikreins use low-molecular-weight kininogen to produce kallidin that may be converted to bradykinin by plasma aminopeptidase. Plasma kallikrein uses high-molecular-weight kininogen to produce bradykinin. Through the action of kininase 1, kallidin or bradykinin can also be converted to active kinin by-products.

Kinins have very short half-lives and are rapidly inactivated by plasma and tissue kininases. However, while active, they exhibit many effects that are important to inflammation, including the dilation of blood vessels, the induction of pain, contraction and relaxation of smooth muscle, increases in vascular permeability, and migration of leucocyte. They can stimulate tissues and inflammatory cells to generate mediators including prostanoids, cytokines, TNF, ILs, nitric oxide, and tachykinins.

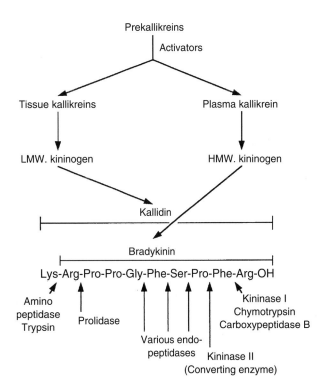

Figure 3.2.6 Formation and degradation of kinins. LMW, low molecular weight; HMW, high molecular weight. (From Regoli D. Polypeptides et antagonists. In: Giroud J-P, Mathé G, Meyniel G, eds. *Pharmacologie clinique: Bases de la thérapeutique.* 2nd ed. Paris: Expansion Scientifique Francaise; 1988:691.)

Cellular Products of Inflammation

The cells of the innate immune system produce several products that initiate the inflammatory response, recruit cells to participate in the inflammatory response, and remove debris that prepares the setting for repair and regeneration. Several classes of cellular products are discussed in this section, including the eicosanoids, which are lipid-derived mediators, and the cytokine families, which are protein-derived mediators and include the IFNs, ILs, TNFs, chemokines, and colony-stimulating growth factors (CSFs). The vasoactive amines, nitric oxide, acute-phase reactants, and neuropeptides are also briefly covered. All of these products act in a nonspecific manner to enhance the inflammatory response. Each of these products has effects that depend on the target cell to which it binds.

Eicosanoids

Eicosanoids are lipid-derived mediators formed rapidly by the oxidation of arachidonic acid (AA). They are very important in inflammation. AA is created when phospholipase A_2 (PLA$_2$) or phospholipase C acts on the phospholipids of the cell membranes. Chemical, infectious, or mechanical agents can activate this process. The process can also be inhibited by the administration of steroids (see Fig. 3.2.7).

Eicosanoids include four distinct products: prostaglandins, leukotrienes, thromboxanes, and lipoxins (Fig. 3.2.7).

Two separate pathways lead to these products. The first is called the *cyclooxygenase pathway*. In this pathway, AA is oxygenated to form cyclic intermediates that ultimately lead to prostaglandins and thromboxanes. The second is called the *lipoxygenase pathway* (Fig. 3.2.7). In this pathway, AA is oxygenated to form hydroperoxyeicosatetraenoic acid (HPETE). This HPETE is then converted to hydroxyeicosatetraenoic acid (HETE) and the leukotrienes and lipoxins.

Cyclooxygenase Pathway

Cyclooxygenase (COX-1) is a constitutively expressed enzyme found in most cells and is particularly helpful early in the inflammatory response. COX-2 is an inducible enzyme that becomes more important as inflammation progresses. Both enzymes catalyze the formation of prostaglandin H (PGH$_2$), which rapidly gets converted to the prostaglandins PGI$_2$ (prostacyclin), PGD$_2$, PGE$_2$, and PGF$_2$, and Thromboxane A$_2$ (TxA$_2$) (Fig. 3.2.7). Prostacyclin (PGI$_2$) is an important factor in vasodilation, bronchodilation, and inhibition of platelet aggregation. PGD$_2$, E$_2$, and F$_2$ cause vasodilation and edema formation. TxA$_2$ causes vasoconstriction, bronchoconstriction, and platelet aggregation. The prostaglandins effect change by binding to cell-surface receptors and activating intracellular signaling pathways.

Prostaglandin production is increased when inflammation is induced by any number of inciting stimuli. The production of the different prostaglandins depends on

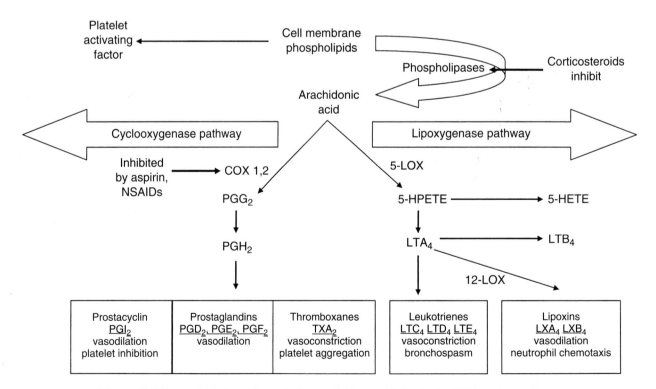

Figure 3.2.7 Arachidonic acid metabolism and Eicosanoid Synthesis. COX, cyclooxygenase; 5-LOX, 5-lipoxygenase; PG, prostaglandins; HPETE, hydroxyperoxyeicosatetraenoic acid; HETE, hydroxyeicosatetraenoic acid.

the types of cells located in the area of the inflammatory response. For example, TxA_2 is produced primarily by platelets. Nonsteroidal anti-inflammatory drugs (NSAIDs) are both analgesic and anti-inflammatory in their effects. This arises from their inhibition of the COX-1 and -2 enzymes (Fig. 3.2.7). COX-1 also functions protectively in the kidney and in the maintenance of the gastrointestinal mucosal lining. Newer NSAIDs that do not affect the COX-1 enzyme but are COX-2 specific are thought to be protective of the adverse effects on the stomach and kidney.

Lipoxygenase Pathway

5-Lipoxygenase (5-LOX) is the enzyme responsible for the conversion of AA to HPETE. HPETE gets converted to HETE, which is chemotactic (Fig. 3.2.7). The leukotriene precursor LTA_4 is formed from HETE. The next depends on the cell type. Neutrophils will convert LTA_4 to LTB_4, a powerful chemotactic agent that is especially important in inflammation. Other cell types convert the LTA_4 to LTC_4, LTD_4, and LTE_4, proinflammatory molecules that lead to vasoconstriction, bronchospasm, edema, and endothelial activation. When taken together, leukotrienes are known as the *slow-reacting substance of anaphylaxis* (SRS-A). Their effects are similar to those of histamine. However, whereas histamine is readily available, leukotrienes take longer because they require the induction of enzymes.

Lipoxins

Lipoxins are a class of proinflammatory products produced in the vascular lumen from the interactions between cells. In the presence of platelets, the LTA_4 of neutrophils will be converted by platelet 12-lipoxygenase to form lipoxin A_4 and B_4 (LXA_4 and LXB_4) (Fig. 3.2.7). In the presence of monocytes, 15(S)-HETE will be converted by 5-LOX to LXA_4 and LXB_4. Lipoxins can also be produced when aspirin is administered. COX-2 leads to the formation of 15(R)-HETE, which, in the presence of neutrophils, creates 15-epimeric lipoxins (15-epi-LXs). Lipoxins cause vasodilation, stimulate monocyte adhesion, and inhibit neutrophil chemotaxis.

Platelet Activating Factor

Platelet activating factor (PAF) is another phospholipid-derived proinflammatory mediator. PAF is formed by the action of PLA_2 on phosphatidylcholine. An acetyltransferase then completes the reaction to form PAF, which activates specific receptors that act through G proteins and the activation of adenyl cyclase. PAF has a number of effects that are useful in inflammation. First, it is considerably more potent than histamine in causing vasoconstriction and bronchoconstriction. Second, it is chemotactic for a number of cells including neutrophils, macrophages, and platelets. Finally, PAF can stimulate the production of other eicosanoids, platelet aggregation, and the activation and adhesion of leucocytes.

Cytokines

Cytokines are a family of proteins secreted by many cell types and act over short distances to assist in regulating the inflammatory response. The five different cytokine families are the IFNs, the ILs, the TNFs, the chemokines, and the CSFs (see Table 3.2.3). Each of these families is produced by different cell types and has a variety of biologic functions.

These proteins can be grouped broadly as proinflammatory, anti-inflammatory, or immunoregulatory proteins (see Table 3.2.4). The cytokines whose actions are primarily proinflammatory include IL-1, -6, -8, -12, -15, and -18, and TNF-α. Those with primarily anti-inflammatory activity include IL-4, -6, -10, -11, and -13. Finally, those cytokines with activity that assists in modulating the inflammatory response include IFN-γ, and IL-2, -4, -5, -7, and -11.

Interferons

The IFNs are one major family of cytokines that are protective against viral illness. Although they are not "antiviral" in their activity, they are produced by virus-infected cells and assist healthy neighboring cells in improving their resistance to viral invasion. They have been divided into two types, both of which have anti-inflammatory functions. Type I consists of IFN-γ, which is produced by leucocytes, and IFN-γ, which is produced by fibroblasts. IFN-γ is a type II IFN and is produced by T lymphocytes and natural killer (NK) cells and assists the host in protecting from viral agents and in increasing the inflammatory response. IFN-γ is important in activating macrophages, assisting major histocompatibility complex (MHC) Class I and II protein expression, thereby promoting antigen presentation and enhancing cell-mediated immunity.

Interleukins

The ILs are cytokines produced mainly by macrophages or lymphocytes in response to inflammation. These mediators assist other cells in responding to the inflammatory stimulus. Table 3.2.5 contains a synopsis of the IL functions. A few of the major ILs relevant to inflammation are discussed in this section.

Interleukin 1

Macrophages, monocytes, neutrophils and, other inflammatory cells produce IL-1 early in the course of inflammation. IL-1 often works with TNF and is a proinflammatory IL promoting the activation of other inflammatory cells (e.g., neutrophils). IL-1 upregulates the adhesive glycoprotein, ICAM-1, and assists in upregulating other proinflammatory proteins such as TNF, IL-6, IL-8, and the acute-phase reactants from the liver. IL-1 is associated with fever and the generation of acute-phase reactants from the liver. It initiates the immune response, recruits cells to the nidus of inflammation, removes debris, and promotes repair and regeneration. Inhibition of IL-1 in the setting of sepsis has not been successful in improving mortality.

TABLE 3.2.3

FAMILIES OF HUMAN CYTOKINES

Cytokine Family	Producing Cells	Functions	Role in Infectious Diseases
Interferons	Nonimmune (type I) and immune (type II)	Antiviral, antiproliferative	Used to treat several chronic viruses; direct antiviral effects
Interleukins	Cells of the immune system	Regulate immune cells—stimulate and inhibit proliferation of immune cells	Function as immune stimulators
Chemokines	Endothelial and epithelial cells	Attract neutrophils and macrophages	Initiate movement of immune cells, activate immune cells
TNF family	Endothelial, epithelial, and immune cells	Inflammatory; initiate vascular permeability and migration of cells	Antibodies to TNF and TNF family receptors decrease inflammation; inhibitors used in control of sepsis syndrome
Hematopoietic growth factors	Multiple cells	Stimulate growth and differentiation of bone marrow—derived cells	Enhance production of polys; "arm" macrophages; may be important in immune stimulation

TNF, tumor necrosis factor.
From Gorbach SL, Bartlett JG, Blacklow NR. *Infectious diseases.* 3rd ed. Philadelphia, PA: Lippincott Williams & Wilkins; 2003:65.

Interleukin 4

Although T cells also produce IL-4, the major activity of IL-4 is as a B-cell growth factor. It has the ability to induce antigen expression on B cells, to enhance the ability of B cells to produce IL-6 and TNF, and to activate macrophages. IL-4 assists in removing debris from the site of inflammation. It potentially has some antitumor effect against lymphomas.

Interleukin 6

IL-6 is an acute-phase IL that is primarily produced by macrophages in response to IL-1 and TNF or microbial cell products. It assists in the initiation of the host's response in inflammation, including the production of acute-phase proteins by the liver. IL-6 enhances the proliferation of hematopoietic stem cells through growth factor induction, increases the secretion of stress hormones, assists in immunoglobulin production, and assists in stimulating T and B cells. IL-6 is important in the inflammatory response for cellular recruitment, in the removal of debris, and in the promotion of repair.

Tumor Necrosis Factors

TNF-α and TNF-β are two well-known members of this class of proteins. TNF-α is produced by a number of cells and has a pivotal role in inflammation. Together with IL-1, it is a major constituent in the response to endotoxic shock and has myocardial depressant capability. As one of the major mediators, it assists the host in responding to microbial products by localizing the stimulus of infection and proliferating the inflammatory response. It can be cytotoxic to some cells, resulting in apoptosis, and can activate a variety of cellular activities, including cytokine production and cellular adhesion. TNF-α is also known as *cachectin* because of its effects in suppressing appetite and inducing weight loss in conditions such as infection and cancer. TNF-β is also referred to as *lymphotoxin* and is produced by the B-cell line of lymphocytes. It stimulates B-cell production and works against certain tumors.

Chemokines

Chemokines are a large group of proteins that are classified on the basis of their chemical structure as either C-X-C or C-C chemokines. The nomenclature derives from the separation of the two cysteines (represented diagrammatically as "C") in their chemical structure by an amino acid (C-X-C) or their adjacency (C-C). Chemokines are named by their structure, followed by L and the number of their gene

TABLE 3.2.4
CYTOKINE ACTIONS

Cytokine	Source	Major actions
Immunoregulatory		
IL-2	Activated T cells	T and B cells growth and differentiation; immunoglobulin secretion by B cells; NK-cell growth and activity; production of IFN-γ and TNF-β
IL-4	T_H2 cells	T and B-cell growth and differentiation
IL-5	T cells; mast cells, eosinophils	Differentiation of B cells and eosinophils; chemotaxis
IL-7	Bone marrow stromal cells	Pre–B- and pre–T-cell growth and maturation
IL-11	Bone marrow stromal cells	Megakaryocyte colony formation, myelopoiesis, erythropoiesis, lymphopoiesis
IFN-γ	Activated T cells	Antiviral activity; activates monocytes, macrophages, neutrophils; NK cells; T-cell cytotoxicity
Proinflammatory		
IL-1β	Macrophages; T and B cells; endothelial cells	Activates T, B, NK cells, neutrophils; induces proinflammatory cytokines, coagulation, fibrinolysis; mediates acute-phase response; downregulates IL-1RA; increases ACTH, endorphins, vasopressin, somatostatin release
TNF-α	Macrophages, activated T and B cells	—
IL-6	Many cells including macrophages, activated T and B cells, endothelial cells, smooth muscle cells, fibroblasts, mast cells, intestinal cells	Activates T and B cells, acute-phase proteins; activates phospholipase A$_2$
IL-8	Monocytes, macrophages, neutrophils, endothelial cells	Neutrophil and basophil chemotaxis; neutrophil activation
MCP-1, MCP-2, MCP-3	Monocytes, macrophages, fibroblasts, B cells, endothelial cells	Chemotactic for monocytes; release of lysosomal enzymes and superoxide anion; stimulates eosinophils and basophils
MIP-1	T and B cells	Chemotactic for monocytes; expression of β-1 integrins
RANTES	T cells, platelets, renal epithelium, mesangial cells	Chemotactic for monocytes, CD4 cells, eosinophils, basophils
Anti-inflammatory		
IL-1RA	Monocytes, macrophages	Inhibits IL-1α and IL-1β
IL-4	T_H2 cells	Induces IL-1RA, IL-10; inhibits antigen presentation; inhibits production of IL-1, TNF, IL-8
IL-6	Many cells, including macrophages, activated T and B cells, endothelial cells, smooth muscle cells, mast cells	Decreases TNF production; induces IL-1RA and sTNF-R55
IL-10	Activated T and B cells	Inhibits IFN, IL-1, IL-6, and TNF production; induces IL-1RA
IL-13	T_H2 cells	B-cell growth and differentiation; promotes IL-1ra production; inhibits IL-1, IL-6, IL-8, IL-10, TNF, IFN-γ production

IL, interleukin; NK, natural killer; TNF, tumor necrosis factor; T_H2, helper T-lymphocyte type 2; IFN, interferon; ACTH, adrenocorticotropic hormone; MCP, monocyte chemotactic protein; MIP, macrophage inflammatory protein; RANTES, regulation on activation, normal T-expressed and secreted; IL-1RA, interleukin-1 receptor antagonist.
From Becker KL. *Principles and practices of endocrinology and metabolism.* Philadelphia, PA: Lippincott Williams & Wilkins; 2001:2070.

(e.g., C-X-CL1 or C-CL1). The receptors for chemokines are labeled with an "R" (e.g., C-X-CR1 or C-CR1). The chemokines are proinflammatory proteins that can accentuate the functions of many different WBCs and they assist with migration and chemotaxis. C-X-C chemokines include IL-8 and epithelial-dermoid neutrophil attractant (ENA). They are produced by macrophages, endothelium, or neutrophils and are chemotactic for neutrophils. C-C chemokines include RANTES (regulated on activation, normal T cell expressed and secreted), which is chemotactic for CD4 cells. In addition, C-C chemokines include monocyte chemotactic protein-1 (MCP-1) and macrophage inflammatory proteins-1α and β (MIP-1α and β), which are chemotactic for lymphocytes, eosinophils, and monocytes.

TABLE 3.2.5
CYTOKINES AND INFECTIOUS DISEASES

Cytokine	Type	Cell Producing	Clinical Data	Potential Therapeutic Uses
IL-1	Inflammatory	Macrophages, monocytes, others	Associated with fever, acute-phase reactants	Inhibitors (IL-1RA) used in sepsis syndrome failed to improve mortality
IL-2	T-cell growth factor	T cells	Stimulates T-cell growth	Used to restore T cells in HIV-1
IL-3	Growth factor	T cells, NK cells, mast cells	Stimulates growth of platelets and macrophages	Not effective as in one study to prevent infections in BMT
IL-4	B-cell growth factor	T cells, mast cells	B-cell growth factor, stimulates IgG1, IgE	Potentiates T$_H$2 responses
IL-5	B-cell growth factor	T cells, mast cells	Stimulates B cells and differentiates eosinophils	Stimulates eosinophils
IL-6	T-cell growth factor	T cells	Responsible for fever and induction of acute phase	Stimulates T cells and B cells
IL-7	Pre–T- and Pre–B-cell growth factor	Marrow, thymus, some T cells		
IL-8	Chemokine	Macrophages, endothelial cells	Attracts neutrophils	Attracts and activates neutrophils; may be associated with inflammatory disease
IL-9	Mast cell activator	T cells	Activates mast cells	May affect intracellular parasites
IL-10	Inhibits T-cell growth	T$_H$2 cells and macrophages	Inhibits T$_H$1 cells	Could be used as an anti-inflammatory, anti–T-cell factor; inhibits HIV production in vitro
IL-11	Platelet growth factor	Fibroblasts	Stimulates megakaryocytes	Acts on mucous membranes to antagonize the effects of inflammatory cytokines; improves survival in animals
IL-12	T-cell and NK-cell activator	B cells and macrophages	Stimulates T$_H$1 responses	Stimulates IFN-γ release; could be used to stimulate T$_H$1 cells; has been used to treat hepatitis C

IL	Descriptor	Action	Source	Comments
IL-13	B-cell growth factor	Stimulates B cells to produce Ig	T cells	Stimulates Ig production; mouse studies suggest an inhibitor may prevent schistosome-induced responses
IL-14	B-cell growth factor	Stimulates B-cell memory	T cells	May stimulate neutrophil function *in vitro* activation of NK activity
IL-15	T-cell growth factor	Stimulates neutrophils	T cells, epithelial cells	May augment IL-2 activity
IL-16	T-cell growth factor	Stimulates T cells	T cells	May activate neutrophils; animal model of *Klebsiella pneumonia*
IL-17	Neutrophil growth and activation factor	Expression induces inflammatory cytokines	T cells	Members of the IL-17 family
IL-17C and IL-17F	Neutrophil growth and activation factor	Expression induces inflammatory cytokines	T cells	
IL-18		Stimulates production of IFN-γ by NK cells	T cells, NK cells	May activate NK cells to eliminate intracellular organisms; possible role in pneumonia
IL-19		Homologous to IL-10		Mouse models suggest a role in skin disease
IL-20		Homologous to IL-10		
IL-21		Related to IL-12 and IL-15	T cells, NK cells, B cells	
IL-22		Reported to be involved in IL-10 signaling		Inhibits IL-4 production by T_H2 cells
IL-23	T-cell activation factor	Combines with the p40 subunit of IL-12 to form a new factor that stimulates T cells to proliferate and produce IFN-γ	T cells	Could be used with IL-12 as a T-cell activator
IL-24	T_H T stimulant	Induces T_H1 cytokines in PBMCs	T cells and monocytes	IL-10 family member, formerly termed melanoma differentiation–associated gene
IL-25	T-cell produced growth factor	Induces T_H2 cytokines	T cells	IL-10 family member, formerly termed AK155
IL-26	IL-10 family		T_H2 cells and monocytes	

IL, interleukin; NK, natural killer; Ig, immunoglobulin; HIV-1, human immunodeficiency virus type 1; BMT, bone marrow transplants; IFN-γ, interferon-γ; PBMC, peripheral blood mononuclear cell.
From Gorbach SL, Bartlett JG, Blacklow NR. *Infectious diseases.* 3rd ed. Philadelphia, PA: Lippincott Williams & Wilkins; 2003:67.

They are also able to stimulate the production of other inflammatory mediators such as TNF, IL-1, and histamine. Chemokines play a major role in diseases in which there is an accentuated inflammatory component.

Colony Stimulating Factors

Growth factors are glycoproteins that can stimulate hematopoiesis and regulate the immune response. They are produced by many cell types, including T cells, macrophages, and endothelial cells. They function to encourage the production and activation of many different types of blood cells. Granulocyte-macrophage colony stimulating factor (GM-CSF), granulocyte colony stimulating factor (G-CSF), and IL-3 all have similar roles with different cell lines. Their use in patients with bone marrow suppression related to chemotherapy has been established.

Other Cellular Products

Acute-phase Proteins

Many plasma protein concentrations change during acute inflammation. The products of the plasma protease systems have been discussed earlier; however, a number of other acute-phase proteins are worthy of consideration (see Table 3.2.6). These "acute-phase reactants" are a heterogeneous group of proteins produced in the liver after stimulation by IL-6 and IL-1. Maximal circulating levels of these proteins are usually achieved in 10 to 40 hours of their production (see Fig. 3.2.8). However, not all proteins increase their concentration during acute inflammation; some have their rate of synthesis reduced during inflammation and are consumed during the inflammatory response. The groups that increase their concentration include the complement proteins, the coagulation and fibrinolytic proteins, the antiproteases, transport proteins, and a number of other proteins. Included among the proteins that increase in concentration during acute inflammation are fibrinogen, C-reactive protein, haptoglobin, serum amyloid protein A, α_1 antitrypsin, and ceruloplasmin (Table 3.2.6). Their value in acute inflammation depends on their function. For example, the iron-binding proteins, transferrin, haptoglobin, and hemopexin can bind free iron and prevent its uptake by invading microorganisms. These molecules are also able to salvage nutrients from dying cells and to provide a resource-conserving strategy for the organism under stress.

Heat Shock Proteins

Many of the same nonspecific stimuli that foster an inflammatory response at the tissue level also affect the patient at the cellular level. In a well-preserved biologic mechanism, these nonspecific stressors have the ability to "turn off" gene expression for some genes and "turn on" gene expression for other genes that encode for proteins

TABLE 3.2.6
HUMAN ACUTE-PHASE PROTEINS

Proteins Whose Plasma Concentrations Increase
Complement system
Factor B
Cl inhibitor
C4b-binding protein
Mannose-binding lectin
Coagulation and fibrinolytic system
Fibrinogen
Plasminogen
Tissue-plasminogen activator
Urokinase
Protein S
Vitronectin
Plasminogen activator inhibitor-1
Antiproteases
α_1-Protease inhibitor
α_1-Antichymotrypsin
Pancreatic secretory trypsin inhibitor
Inter-α-trypsin inhibitors
Transport proteins
Ceruloplasmin
Haptoglobin
Hemopexin
Participants in inflammatory responses
Secreted phospholipase A_2
Lipopolysaccharide-binding protein
Interleukin-1–receptor antagonist
Granulocyte colony-stimulating factor
Others
C-reactive protein
Serum amyloid A
α_1-Acid glycoprotein
Fibronectin
Ferritin
Angiotensinogen

Proteins Whose Plasma Concentrations Decrease
Albumin
Transferrin
Transthyretin
α_2-HS glycoprotein
α-Fetoprotein
Thyroxine-binding globulin
Insulinlike growth factor I
Factor XII

α_2-HS, α_2-Heremans-Schmid.
Adapted from Gabay C. Kushner I. Acute-phase proteins and other systemic responses to inflammation [published erratum in *N Engl J Med.* 1999;340:1376]. *N Engl J Med.* 1999;340:448;
From Becker KL. *Principles and practices of endocrinology and metabolism.* Philadelphia, PA: Lippincott Williams & Wilkins; 2001:2081.

useful during the stress response and important to immune function. There are several families of these stress proteins (heat shock proteins [HSPs]) that serve a variety of roles in cells. Mechanisms to ensure preferential activation and

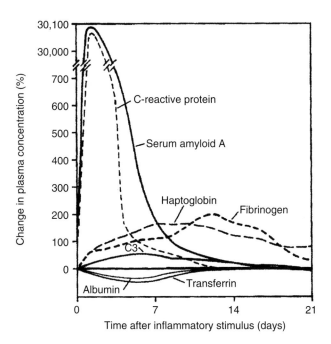

Figure 3.2.8 Secretion and time course of several acute-phase proteins after an inflammatory stimulus. C3, complement 3. (From Gabay C, Kushner I. Acute-phase proteins and other systemic responses to inflammation [published erratum in *N Engl J Med.* 1999;340:1376]. *N Engl J Med.* 1999;340:448.)

synthesis of these proteins are a necessary component of the stress response and are highly regulated at several levels through the stress response of the endocrine system and the production of catecholamines. There are two potential benefits for HSPs to human functioning during stress. The first is their ability to respond and recover from a sublethal cellular stressor such as heat or ischemia. This incites a phenomenon known as *tolerance*, in which the cell responds to subsequent similar stressors that would have been lethal but are now tolerated by the cell in a process known as *preconditioning*. The second benefit is cross-tolerance. Essentially, the stressor causing the insult to the cell does not have to be the same stressor that incited the initial cellular response. The cell develops "protective" responses across a range of stimuli.

Nitric Oxide

Nitric oxide is a soluble gas that has a number of far-reaching, yet short-lived effects that are important to inflammation. Nitric oxide is produced by many cells and exists in constitutive and inducible forms. The constitutive form exists in neuronal and endothelial cells and produces relatively low concentrations of nitric oxide that are heavily dependent on calcium concentration. Formerly known as *endothelial-derived relaxing factor* (EDRF), the vasodilatation and hypotension seen in systemic inflammatory systems are thought to be due to this molecule. The inducible form is present in many cells and is independent of the calcium concentration. LPS and the proinflammatory mediators including IL-1, TNF, and IFN induce it.

Nitric oxide is produced from L-arginine, oxygen, and NADPH in the setting of NOS. Nitric oxide has a number of functions in inflammation including its action as a microbial agent in oxygen-dependent killing (see earlier), its effects in initiating an inflammatory response through vasodilation, its diverse effects on blood cells, particularly its inhibition of neutrophil and platelet functioning, and its role as an intracellular messenger. Nitric oxide inhibitors including N-nitro-L-arginine methyl ester (L-NAME) and N-monomethyl-L-arginine (L-NMMA) inhibit NOS and have been used in attempts to reduce the production of nitric oxide as a treatment strategy. There have been mixed results.

Preformed Vasoactive Amines

Both seretonin and histamine are preformed mediators that are contained within WBC granules and can produce rapid effects on smooth muscle in the vasculature and airways. Histamine is contained within mast cells and is released in response to the anaphylatoxins of complement, cytokines (IL-1 and -8), and IgE-related antibodies. Histamine causes bronchoconstriction, increased vascular permeability, and vasodilation. It is inactivated by histaminase. Seretonin is contained within platelets and has a number of actions similar to histamine.

Other Compounds

A number of other compounds have become important as the understanding of inflammation in critical illness has improved. The levels of calcitonin precursors (CTpr) are elevated in severe inflammation in response to TNF and IL-1. Other neurokinins, including substance P and neurokinins A and B induce changes in inflammation such as edema formation, airway inflammation, and vascular changes. Their role in mediating the outcome of the critically ill child with sepsis has not yet been established, but each demonstrates an important linkage between inflammation and the endocrine system.

Regulation of Inflammation

The inflammatory response requires careful regulation to prevent the unopposed exposure of tissues to the destructive effects of these cellular products. Inflammation is necessary and very important in host defense; however, it can also cause excessive tissue destruction if not controlled. Released lysosomal products will continue to contribute to the ongoing inflammation including vascular permeability, chemotaxis, breakdown of connective tissue, and activation of complement and kinins until disabled.

Several mechanisms exist for regulating the inflammatory response. First, a number of scavengers exist for the free radicals and active oxygen species. Superoxide dismutase, catalase, and glutathione are examples. Neutrophils can also act as cellular "scavengers" through apoptotic mechanisms. However, when the phagocyte dies at the inflammatory site and releases its contents, further tissue damage is caused. α_1 Antitrypsin, produced by the liver, is helpful in inhibiting the enzymes released by the dead phagocyte. Second, a number of enzymes can also be successful in inactivating the effects of a number of cellular products. For example, histaminase is able to neutralize histamine and leukotrienes. As discussed earlier, antagonists exist for the plasma proteases of the kinin, complement, kallikrein, and plasmin systems. Third, there are also systems that are in "balance," with one ligand providing proinflammatory activity and the other providing anti-inflammatory activity. For example, H_1 receptors on the bronchial smooth muscle cells promote inflammation and increase chemotaxis. H_2 receptors inhibit inflammation by altering degranulation and by reducing the functions of leucocytes.

Outcomes of Inflammation

The outcomes of acute inflammation depend on the control of inflammation at the local level and on what tissues are involved. When acute inflammation spreads beyond the local nidus of stimulation, it causes many systemic effects, including fever, vital sign changes, increased WBC counts, and plasma proteins. The patient with signs of evolving inflammation may decompensate further and experience systemic inflammation, shock, multiorgan dysfunction, and potentially death. This is one mechanism for the SIRS described in more detail later in the book (Chapter 23). The patient may be able to overcome acute inflammation, particularly, if the underlying cause is treated early and aggressively.

The resolution of acute inflammation depends on the elimination of the inciting stimulus, and the removal of microbial products and tissue debris. Fluid balance gets restored and healing begins. Some tissues have an ability to regenerate after an inflammatory insult; others will form scars that are nonfunctional in that organ. Some inflammatory responses will not resolve completely, or the inflammatory response will continue, leading to chronic inflammation.

CHRONIC INFLAMMATION

Chronic inflammation occurs when the inflammatory response persists beyond 2 weeks. This may occur because the acute response was unsuccessful in eliminating the cause of inflammation, or because the appropriate resolution of the inflammatory response has not occurred. Chronic inflammation may also occur from numerous nonspecific insults, including trauma, cancer, and immune factors (autoimmune diseases).

Repair is the replacement of destroyed tissue with scar. Before repair can take place, the debris from acute inflammation must be removed. The steps include the replacement of destroyed tissue with collagen, epithelialization with scar tissue, and contraction of the scar to complete the reconstructive phases of inflammation. It is important to note that scarred tissues may result in organ dysfunction. For example, cell death is a very different phenomenon when it occurs in brain tissue as compared to other tissues. Inflammation in the meninges provides the potential for functional devastation if not diagnosed and treated early in its course. Scarring of the brain tissue may lead ultimately to a nidus for seizures or to a loss of function, depending on its location.

Cells of Chronic Inflammation

Chronic inflammation is characterized by an infiltration of macrophages, lymphocytes, and fibroblasts, which contributes to tissue repair and scarring, two hallmarks of chronic inflammation. Initially, acute inflammatory cells may still be present at the nidus of inflammation, but, with time, the enzymes they release become destructive to the connective tissue matrix and prevent healing. Macrophages are a source of enzymes and are mediators for chronic inflammation. The enzymes assist in clearing debris, and the mediators assist in attracting fibroblasts for repair. Fibroblasts are capable of forming new connective tissue.

Dendritic cells function exceptionally well as antigen-presenting cells during chronic inflammation. They are also able to migrate to lymph nodes and stimulate the T cells for an ongoing inflammatory response. T cells assist in regulating macrophage activity and in recruiting other cells through specific mediators. If the macrophages and lymphocytes are unsuccessful in eradicating the inflammatory nidus, the macrophages can differentiate and fuse into multinucleated giant cells that are phagocytic for larger particles. These altered immune responses may lead to granuloma formation in which the body attempts to isolate inflammatory stimuli. A number of low-grade yet persistent infections lead to granuloma formation; these include tuberculosis and infections caused by fungi and listeria. Noninfectious etiologies such as the deposition of antigen–antibody complexes, asbestos, talc, and surgical foreign bodies also exist.

CONCLUSION

Inflammation is the response of the innate immune system in vascularized tissues to a nonspecific insult. This chapter detailed the functions and responses of the tissues, the cells, and the multitude of chemical mediators that are operative in this process. This foundation can provide the clinician with important insights into the systemic effects of inflammation in clinical medicine and into the response of the body to insults such as infectious agents and trauma.

ACKNOWLEDGMENTS

Supported in part by grant KO-8 HS14009-01, Agency for Healthcare Research and Quality, Rockville, MD.

RECOMMENDED READINGS

1. Becker KL, Nylen ES, White B, et al. Procalcitonin and the calcitonin gene family of peptides in inflammation, infection and sepsis: A journey from calcitonin back to its precursors. *JCEM.* 2004;89:1512–1525.
2. Bulger E, Maier RV. Lipid mediators in the pathophysiology of critical illness. *Crit Care Med.* 2000;28:N27–N36.
3. Delves PJ, Roitt IM. The immune system. First of two parts. *NEJM.* 2000;343:37–49.
4. Dinarello CA, Wolff SM. Mechanisms of disease: The role of interleukin 1 in disease. *NEJM.* 1993;328:106–113.
5. Etzioni A. Adhesion molecules-their role in health and disease. *Ped Res.* 1996;39:191–198.
6. Funk CD. Prostaglandins and leukotrienes: Advances in eicosanoid biology. *Science.* 2001;294:1871–1875.
7. Jaye DL, Waites KB. Clinical applications of C-reactive protein in pediatrics. *Ped Inf Dis J.* 1997;16:735–747.
8. Menger MD, Vollmar B. Adhesion molecules as determinants of disease: From molecular biology to surgical research. *Br J Surg.* 1996;83:588–601.
9. Nathan C. Points of control in inflammation. *Nature.* 2002;420: 846–852.
10. Regoli DC. Chapter 170 Kinins. In: Becker KL, ed. *Principles and practices of endocrinology and metabolism.* 3rd ed. Philadelphia, PA: Lippincott Williams & Wilkins; 2001.
11. Robertson RP. Chapter 172 Prostaglandins, thromboxanes, and leukotrienes. In: Becker KL, ed. *Principles and practices of endocrinology and metabolism.* 3rd ed. Philadelphia, PA: Lippincott Williams & Wilkins; 2001.
12. Tracey KJ. The inflammatory reflex. *Nature.* 2002;420:853–859.
13. Walport MJ. Complement. First of two parts. *NEJM.* 2001;344: 1058–1066.
14. Walport MJ. Complement. Second of two parts. *NEJM.* 2001;344: 1140–1144.

Infectious Diseases

Anthony D. Slonim   Nalini Singh

Chapter 3.3 focuses on infectious diseases and the interactions between the environment, the host, and the pathogenic microorganism. The components of this section include important introductory concepts related to epidemiology, study design, and statistics, followed by specific attention to the diagnosis of infectious diseases in the clinical microbiology laboratory, the specific pathogens causing diseases of interest to the intensivist, and the antimicrobial armamentarium available to treat those infectious diseases in the pediatric intensive care unit PICU. The objective is to provide a foundation for understanding infectious diseases in the setting of the PICU.

FOUNDATIONS OF INFECTIOUS DISEASES IN THE PEDIATRIC INTENSIVE CARE UNIT

Anthony D. Slonim, Wendy Turenne, and Nalini Singh

EPIDEMIOLOGY

Epidemiology is the study of health and disease in patient populations. It is a discipline that consists of both robust content and methods. Through an analytic approach, risk factors associated with the occurrence of a particular disease can be determined. Understanding risk factors can assist in the development of preventive or therapeutic strategies. The fundamentals of epidemiology are important for the intensivist because they provide an approach that extends beyond providing care to a single critically ill child to a more thoughtful approach of providing care to a population of critically ill children being served by the PICU. In this way, epidemiology and the associated methods of biostatistics provide the intensivist with a fundamental understanding of evidence-based medicine, study design, and the ability to interpret studies published in the scientific literature, thereby improving the care for all critically ill children.

TYPES OF EPIDEMIOLOGIC STUDIES

There are three major types of epidemiologic studies: descriptive, analytic, and experimental. Descriptive epidemiology is concerned with the description of a disease's occurrence, patterns, and the factors associated with occurrence. It is not concerned with the elements of causation. Descriptive studies include population-based occurrence rates, case reports and series, and cross-sectional studies. Incidence data, which indicate the number of new disease occurrences in the population, and prevalence data, which indicate the number of existing disease occurrences at a given moment in time, are both helpful in describing population-based occurrences.

The case report and case series are additional types of descriptive studies that provide information on either a single patient or a group of patients with a given disease and the characteristics of those patients. These studies do not provide information about whether or not a particular characteristic poses an increased risk of disease occurrence. Importantly, the investigator can often manipulate the case definition and affect the number of patients included in this type of study.

A cross-sectional study investigates a population of patients at a given point in time. Cross-sectional studies should be contrasted to longitudinal studies, which study a patient or groups of patients over time. A cross-sectional study allows the investigator to identify that a particular risk factor and disease coexist, without providing information regarding the effect of that risk factor on disease occurrence.

A longitudinal study also provides information regarding disease occurrence.

Analytic epidemiology has as its central tenet the collection of data with the explicit purpose of analyzing those data to identify trends in disease occurrence and the factors associated with that occurrence. An analytic study is designed to answer a specific question and it considers the associated patient and geographic characteristics that affect the outcome. Analytic studies include case–control studies and cohort studies.

Case–control studies identify a group of patients with a disease or condition and a group of patients without the disease or condition and compares them for the exposure to risk factors associated with the disease of interest. These studies are conducted when the disease of interest is relatively rare and would require a large cohort for follow-up. Case–control studies are often retrospective; the disease already exists, and the identification of the risk factors that led up to the disease is of primary interest. It is important that the selection of cases and controls should be similar to each other except for the risk factor of interest. All the cases should be newly diagnosed (incident), with specific characteristics. The selection of controls is also important. Controls should be representative of the population and have the same opportunity for risk factor exposure as the cases. The selection of inadequate controls can introduce bias into the study. In designing case–control studies and establishing a relationship between a risk factor and a disease, it is important to consider the influence of "confounding variables," that is, factors known to be associated with both the exposure of interest and causally with the disease under study. Confounding factors are important to control because they may lead to spurious conclusions or biased relationships between the risk factors and the disease. Confounding factors can be controlled for in the study design through matching on a particular demographic characteristic, or in the analysis through the use of a regression analysis that can control simultaneously for several variables. The advantages of case–control studies are that they are rather inexpensive to conduct and the number of subjects can be small, as the study is initiated by the identification of cases (rare-disease event) that can be compared to a similar number of controls. These studies also can identify more than one risk factor.

Cohort studies investigate a group of patients based on exposure to a known risk factor and compare the development of disease in that group to that in a group of unexposed individuals. These studies are often, but not always, prospective in nature because the development of disease is observed at some point in the future. Prospective cohort studies are longitudinal because they observe a group of patients for the development of the outcome of interest. These studies allow for the measurement of incidence rates among those exposed and those not exposed and allow for the observation of many outcomes. The ratio of the incidence rate for patients exposed to a risk factor to the incidence rate for those not exposed is defined as a relative risk (RR). The disadvantages of such studies are that they usually take a long time and are expensive. In a longitudinal cohort study, the prolonged time frame leads to problems

	Disease present	Disease absent
Exposure present	A	B
Exposure absent	C	D

- Relative risk: $\dfrac{A/A + B}{C/C + D}$

- Attributable risk: $(A/A + B) - (C/C + D)$

- Odds ratio: $\dfrac{A/C}{B/D} = \dfrac{AD}{CB}$

	Disease present	Disease absent
Test positive	A	B
Test negative	C	D

- Sensitivity: $A/A + C$

- Specificity: $D/B + D$

- Positive predictive value: $A/A + B$

- Negative predictive value: $C/C + D$

- False-positive rate: $B/B + D$

- False-negative rate: $C/A + C$

- Accuracy: $A + D/A + B + C + D$

Figure 3.3.1 Common epidemiologic formulas.

of attrition or the loss of patient follow-up. In a retrospective cohort study, the participants with the disease are asked about potential risk factors that may have affected its occurrence. Such a study is subject to the problem of recall bias.

With case–control or cohort studies, if there is a positive association between the risk factor and the disease (see Fig. 3.3.1), those exposed will tend to develop the disease (group A), whereas those not exposed will tend not to develop it (group D). Before conducting a study, it is important to calculate the sample size necessary to achieve statistically meaningful results.

Experimental epidemiology uses the associated findings from an analytic study to determine the efficacy of a prevention or treatment strategy on the outcome of interest. Experimental studies are also known as *clinical trials* or *intervention studies* and have particular importance to the intensivist who is concerned with assessing the efficacy of a particular treatment. In these studies, the investigator assigns a treatment (exposure) to a patient based on some experimental schema and observes the patient for the clinical outcome of interest. Experimental studies are difficult and expensive to perform and often require large sample sizes. The experimental question needs to be specified, the control groups need to be appropriately selected, and the imposition of bias at multiple levels needs to be considered.

EPIDEMIOLOGIC ANALYSIS

The underlying premise of epidemiology is that disease occurrence has associated risk factors that do not occur by chance. Furthermore, if the risk factors can be identified, opportunities to prevent the occurrence of disease may be realized. The clinician in the PICU has a number of epidemiologic tools available to assist in understanding whether risk factors occur to a greater degree than by chance alone.

Disease Occurrence and Testing

A two-by-two table is often used as a method of comparing exposure and disease states (Fig. 3.3.1). The presence or absence of exposure each constitutes one of the two rows in the table and the presence or absence of disease each constitutes a column in the table. Analysis of this table provides the intensivist with a considerable amount of information about disease occurrence, associations, and diagnostic testing.

Risk is a measure of the probability of the occurrence of disease over time. The RR is a ratio of the probability of disease occurrence if the risk factor is present to the probability of the disease occurrence if the risk factor is absent (Fig. 3.3.1). Attributable risk is the absolute risk in the exposed compared to that in the unexposed. It is an estimate of excess risk and is calculated as the risk in the exposed minus the risk in the unexposed. In a case–control study, the occurrence of disease is not determined by

its natural occurrence in the population; rather, it is determined by the number of cases selected by the investigator. Therefore, risk cannot be ascertained. The odds ratio (OR) provides an estimate of the RR in case–control studies. The OR is the odds of having the disease if the exposure to the risk factor is present divided by the odds of having the disease if the exposure to the risk factor is absent. When the RR or OR is equal to 1, there is no greater probability of developing the disease whether the risk factor is present or absent. When the RR or OR is <1, there is a lower likelihood of developing the disease if the risk factor is present; if the RR or OR is >1, there is a greater likelihood of developing the disease if the risk factor is present.

A modification of the two-by-two table can be used for assessing the ability of a screening test to detect a particular disease entity when it is present or absent in a particular patient (Fig. 3.3.1). Recognizing that every diagnostic test or procedure presents some risks and benefits, the clinician attempts to appropriately apply tests and procedures that have the opportunity to maximize benefits in terms of diagnosis or treatment while minimizing risks. A variety of measures can be obtained by analysis of disease occurrence and test results.

The sensitivity of a test describes how well it identifies those patients with the disease, when the disease is actually present. The specificity of a test describes how well the test appropriately provides a negative result when the disease is absent in the patient (Fig. 3.3.1). For example, when a test returns a result with 85% sensitivity, it implies that 85% of the patients with a positive test will have the disease. A test with a specificity of 98% implies that a negative result indicates absence of the disease 98% of the time. A better relationship may be ascertained by using the positive and negative predictive values, which account for disease prevalence. The positive predictive value is the proportion of positive tests in diseased patients. The negative predictive value is the proportion of negative tests in nondiseased patients. The false-positive and false-negative rates describe the misclassification of patients based on erroneous test results. The false-positive rate describes the probability of having a positive test when the patient is disease free. The false-negative rate describes the probability of having a negative test when the patient actually has the disease. A test's accuracy can be defined as the proportion of test that provides the appropriate outcome.

Statistical Concepts

For many clinicians, engaging in an understanding of statistical concepts lacks a certain appeal and enthusiasm. However, it is important to be able to look at data and derive the appropriate information in a manner that is easily comprehended and allows for decision making.

Variables

Variables are traditionally separated into two types: dependent and independent. The dependent variable is the variable of primary interest and usually represents the experimental response or outcome under study. The independent variable represents the conditions under which the response is analyzed. There may be several predictors that influence the outcome under study. These predictors would be considered independent variables. Intervening or confounding variables also need to be considered in an experimental design. These are variables that may have a significant effect on the outcome of interest but may be unmeasured or inadequately controlled for in the experimental design, thereby creating bias and effect differences in the outcome under study.

Descriptive Statistics

Several important statistical concepts assist the clinician in understanding the central location of the data elements. The mean is the arithmetic average of the data. It is calculated by summing the data values and then, dividing by the number of data points. The mean is subject to considerable influence as a measure of centrality based on the number of extreme cases represented in the data. To overcome this limitation, the median, which represents the exact point at which 50% of the data elements are above and 50% below this central value, is determined. Another measure of central tendency is the mode, which is the data value that occurs most often in the distribution.

Once an estimate of location is accomplished, the user must become comfortable with the distribution of the data to assist in understanding the characteristics of the population. The range is the simplest conceptual measure of the distribution. It represents the difference between the highest and the lowest values of a variable and is highly dependent on the number of observations. The interquartile range is found by identifying the median in a data distribution, which achieves the separation of the data into two equal halves. The median of each half is then found so that the data are equally divided into four quartiles. The middle two quartiles of data represent the interquartile range. The variance assists in understanding the spread of observations across a distribution and is calculated as the sum of the squared differences from the mean divided by the number of data points. The square root of the variance is the standard deviation, which more appropriately represents the variation from the mean in a distribution of data points.

Inferential Statistics

The ability to study hypotheses is central to the performance of experimental studies. Of course, not all potential subjects are studied in an experiment, but based on the responses of a sample of study participants, insight into the responses of a population might be gained. This is known as *inference*. Two hypotheses are generally defined. The null hypothesis often considers the state in which the experimental approach has no effect on the outcome under study. The alternative hypothesis considers the state in which the experimental approach has a direct impact on the observed results, but the nature of that relationship is often vague and nonspecific.

Investigators are most concerned with identifying when a treatment has an effect on the outcome of interest, so statistical testing is done to disprove the null hypothesis. Of course, some error is involved. The Type I error is the probability of accepting a treatment effect (rejecting the null hypothesis) when one does not actually exist. The probability of this occurring is called α and is usually established as 0.05. Therefore, before accepting a treatment effect as nonrandom, investigators want to assure themselves that the probability of seeing that effect by mere chance, the *p*-value, is not greater than 5%. It is only able to test the significance of a single hypothesis; it tells nothing about the magnitude or the variability of an effect.

The magnitude of an effect is measured by obtaining a point estimate from a sample and then comparing it to the likelihood that it corresponds to what would occur in the actual population. A confidence interval (CI) is the interval around a point estimate that is likely to contain the true population value. The CI is calculated using $(1-\alpha)$, and is therefore usually defined at 95%. Therefore, 95 out of every 100 times the study is performed, that interval would contain the true population value. If the CI does not include the null point, the null hypothesis can be rejected. If the interval contains the null point, the null hypothesis cannot be rejected. Therefore, the CI can be used as a surrogate test of significance and is also useful to gauge the magnitude of the effect and the variability of the point estimate. A Type II error is called β, and it represents the acceptance of the null hypothesis (no treatment effect exists) when one actually does exist. The power of a statistical test is represented as $1-\beta$, and it represents the ability of the statistic to adequately discern a true difference.

Specific Statistical Tests

When only two variables are of interest, bivariate statistical tests are used to assess the relationship between the independent variable and the dependent one.

When both variables are categorical, and not continuous, statistical tests assess whether the two variables are independent of each other, in order to test the null hypothesis. A chi-square statistic tests whether the frequencies observed in a sample are different from those expected if the null hypothesis of no association is true. If they are different, the null hypothesis may be rejected.

When the dependent variable is continuous and the independent variable is categorical, *t* tests may be used. *t* Tests rely on the assumption of a normal (Gaussian) distribution and compare the means of two groups. For example, the *t* test could be used to determine if blood pressure in a group of patients in a treatment arm is higher or lower as compared to that in the control arm. When the distributions cannot be assumed to be normal, a nonparametric test is needed. These tests (e.g., Wilcoxon signed ranks test) use the differences from the median values in the samples to determine whether the two groups are different. Analysis of variance (ANOVA) tests compare the means of the dependent variable across more than two groups of an independent variable.

Correlations test the magnitude and nature of a relationship between two continuous variables. A correlation coefficient is most commonly used to demonstrate correlations. The correlation coefficient is a statistic that ranges from −1 to +1. A negative sign indicates that the two variables are related, but in an inverse manner. As one value increases, the other one decreases. A zero correlation or a number close to zero indicates that the two variables are not correlated whereas a number that is close to one indicates a perfect linear relationship between the two variables.

When more than two variables are of interest, multivariate statistical tests are used. Regression analysis assists in estimating the relationship between multiple independent variables and a dependent variable. If the relationship of interest is between independent variables and a continuous dependent variable, a linear regression model is performed. Often the assumption is made that this relationship is a straight line. The statistics estimated as a result of a regression model are the intercept (denoted as α) and slope (denoted as β) of that line. The intercept is the value of the dependent variable when the independent variables are all equal to zero. The slope is the number of units the dependent variable changes for every one-unit change in the independent variable. For regression models with multiple independent variables, a slope is estimated for each effect. If the relationship of interest is between independent variables and a categorical dependent variable, a logistic regression model is performed. The β parameters of a logistic regression model are often transformed and represented as the OR for ease of discussion and interpretation.

This subsection provides the appropriate context for the pediatric intensivist to understand the principles of epidemiologic tools. Subsequent chapters will more directly consider the role of the infectious agent, its diagnosis, prevention, control, and treatment in caring for the critically ill child who is infected or is at risk of becoming infected.

THE MICROBIAL AGENTS

Anthony Yun Lee and Anthony D. Slonim

The microbial agents causing disease in the critically ill child are highly variable and depend on many factors for their pathogenesis. The intensivist needs an understanding of the characteristics of the microbial agents, their pathogenesis, and the categories of disease they cause in the critically ill

child (see Table 3.3.1). Table 3.3.2 assists the intensivist in understanding the common bacterial agents associated with disease, categorized by the organ system involved. This section is intended to provide the intensivist with guidance related to the common microorganisms responsible for diseases encountered in a PICU practice.

BACTERIA

An elaborate classification schema exists for the categorization of bacterial organisms (Table 3.3.1). The Gram staining method still provides a useful tool to classify bacteria, based on the staining characteristics of their cell wall. Gram-positive organisms appear blue under light microscopy, whereas gram-negative organisms are decolorized and counterstained, thus appearing red under the microscope. This schema has been used for more than a century; some bacteria will not stain effectively and will require additional techniques to enhance their visibility.

Beyond the staining characteristics, bacteria are classified based on shape. Two common shapes are cocci, which appear ovoid, and bacilli, which are rod-shaped. The organization of the cells in pairs, chains, or clusters is also helpful in identifying the organism. Chemical procedures in the microbiology laboratory are also useful for further differentiation. The ability of a microorganism to use oxygen or sugar provides an insight into the etiology. For the intensivist, understanding the etiology allows appropriate selection of antimicrobial agent.

Gram-positive Organisms

The gram-positive cocci, particularly the *Staphylococcus* and *Streptococcus* sp., represent some organisms that are common and pathogenic in children (Table 3.3.1). Staphylococci are ubiquitous and are included as normal human skin flora. These organisms are catalase positive, aerobic or facultatively anaerobic, nonmotile, and occur in grapelike clusters or pairs. *Staphylococcus aureus* is the only coagulase-producing species and causes a broad-spectrum of human diseases including skin infections, abscesses, endocarditis, pneumonia, and toxic shock syndrome. *S. aureus* is a major pathogen in the development of nosocomial pneumonia and bacteremia.

The virulence of *S. aureus* is due to the production of a variety of substances, including hyaluronidase, hemolysins, enterotoxins, epidermolytic toxins, and toxic shock syndrome toxin type I (TSST-I). The clinical manifestations of *S. aureus* include skin and soft-tissue infections, abscess formation, wound infections, lymphadenitis, and thrombophlebitis. *S. aureus* pneumonia can occur either primarily or secondarily after a preceding viral respiratory illness such as influenza. Pleural effusion or pneumothoraces can occur with staphylococcal pneumonia.

TABLE 3.3.1

A CLASSIFICATION SCHEMA OF CLINICALLY SIGNIFICANT BACTERIAL INFECTIONS

Form		Characteristics	Species	Other Features, Toxins, Virulence Factors	Significant ICU Considerations
Coccus	Gram-positive	Aerobic Catalase-positive	Staphylococcus aureus	Coagulase-positive, Staphylococcus protein A, TSST-I, enterotoxins, leukocidin, α-hemolysin	Important nosocomial pathogens: wound and CSF shunt infections. Neonatal sepsis (S. epidermidis) and meningitis. Toxic shock syndrome (S. aureus), community-acquired and ventilator-associated pneumonia. Urinary tract infections (S. saprophyticus)
			Staphylococcus epidermidis	Biofilm production, bacteriocidins, δ-toxin	
			Staphylococcus saprophyticus	Urease, protein-hemagglutinin	
Coccus	Gram-positive	Aerobic Catalase-negative	Enterococcus faecalis	Group D; aggregation substance aids adhesion	Viridans group streptococci and Enterococcus are important pathogens in endocarditis, sepsis, meningitis, and urinary tract infections. Growing resistance of Enterococcus to vancomycin is an increasing problem in the intensive care setting. Toxic shock syndrome and necrotizing fasciitis are associated with S. pyogenes
			Enterococcus faecium	Group D; aggregation substance aids adhesion	
			Streptococcus milleri group	Viridans group streptococci adheres to oral mucosa and damaged cardiac valves	
			Streptococcus mitis group includes Streptococcus pneumoniae	Viridans group streptococci adheres to oral mucosa and damaged cardiac valves Polysaccharide capsule, neuraminidase, pneumolysin (Pneumococcus)	
			Streptococcus mutans group	Viridans group streptococci adheres to oral mucosa and damaged cardiac valves	
			Streptococcus pyogenes	Group A, β hemolytic. M-protein, streptolysin	
			Streptococcus agalactiae	Group B; adheres to epithelium, capsular polysaccharide	
Coccus	Gram-positive	Anaerobic	Peptostreptococcus spp.	Adherence factors, proteolytic toxins, capsular polysaccharide, lipopolysaccharide	Peritonitis usually after trauma, surgery, ventilator-associated pneumonia, bacteremia
Coccus	Gram-negative	Aerobic Catalase-positive oxidase-positive	Neisseria gonorrhoeae	Pili binding, utilizes iron from transferrin lipo-oligosaccharide on the cell surface acts as a virulence factor	Meningococcemia, meningitis, myocarditis, and pneumonia (N. meningitidis). Otitis media, sinusitis (M. catarrhalis)
			Neisseria meningitidis Moraxella catarrhalis	Lipo-oligosaccharide endotoxin Endotoxin	

(continued)

TABLE 3.3.1
(continued)

Form	Characteristics	Species	Other Features, Toxins, Virulence Factors	Significant ICU Considerations
Coccus Gram-negative	Anaerobic	Veillonella dispar Veillonella parvula		—
Bacilli Gram-positive	Aerobic Catalase (+) or (−)	Bacillus anthracis	Virulence factors include lethal toxin, edema toxin, poly-D-glutamic acid capsule	Lung disease (B. anthracis, M. tuberculosis, atypical mycobacteria, N. asteroides), airway obstruction (C. diphtheriae), meningitis (B. anthracis, L. monocytogenes, M. tuberculosis, N. asteroides), sepsis (L. monocytoses, Clostridium perfringens), GI disease (B. cereus, B. anthracis), hemorrhagic shock (anthrax), catheter-related bacteremia (atypical mycobacteria)
		Bacillus cereus	Emetic toxin and diarrheal toxin	
		Corynebacterium diphtheriae	Toxin-mediated tissue necrosis, patchy exudates formation, pseudomembrane	
		Erysipelothrix rhusiopathiae	Acquired by contamination of breaks in skin. Antiphagocytic capsule	
		Gardnerella vaginalis	Suspected to be secondary overgrowth when number of lactobacilli decrease (such as in bacterial vaginosis)	
		Listeria monocytogenes	Internalization into cell (internalins), listeriolysin O (hemolysin)	
		Mycobacterium avium-intracellulare complex	—	
		Mycobacterium kansasii		
		Mycobacterium leprae	Capable of surviving and multiplying in macrophages	
		Mycobacterium tuberculosis	Transmission by infected droplets. Acid-fast staining	
		Mycobacterium ulcerans	Mycolactone (toxin) inhibits TNF and IL-2, reducing inflammatory reaction growth is best at 30°C–33°C	
		Nocardia asteroides	Branching, beading filaments on Gram stain	
		Tropheryma whippelii	Oral ingestion of bacillus suspected; unlikely to be contagious; evidence of cell-mediated immunity in pathogenesis	
Bacilli Gram-positive	Anaerobic Non-spore forming	Actinomyces israelii	Colonizes oral cavity	Pneumonia, pleural effusions, peritonitis (usually following trauma or surgery)
		Lactobacillus acidophilus	—	
		Lactobacillus vaginalis		
		Peptostreptococcus	Normal flora of mouth, colon	
		Propionibacterium spp.	Adherence factors, proteolytic toxins, capsular polysaccharide, lipopolysaccharide	

				Organism	Toxins/Characteristics	Diseases
Bacilli	Gram-positive	Anaerobic	Spore forming	*Clostridium botulinum*	Heat-labile botulinum toxins A, B, E, and F, acts at neuromuscular junction to irreversibly block acetylcholine release	Neuromuscular disease (*C. botulinum*, *C. tetani*), nosocomial pathogen (*C. difficile*), necrotizing fasciitis (*C. perfringens*)
				Clostridium difficile	Toxins A and B	
				Clostridium perfringens	α-Toxin (most important), hyaluronidase, collagenase, fibrinolysin, leukocidin, deoxyribonuclease	
				Clostridium tetani	Tetanolysin and tetanospasmin (causes clinical features of tetanus) Tetanospasmin inhibits acetylcholine release from motor end plates of skeletal muscle	
Bacilli	Gram-negative	Aerobic	Oxidase (−)	Enterobacteriaceae *Citrobacter freundii*	Colonizes perineum and GI tract. Vertical transmission	Wound infections, nosocomial infections (*E. cloacae*, *P. stuartii*), necrotizing fasciitis (*E. cloacae*), urinary tract infections, sepsis and meningitis, pneumonia, enteritis
				Enterobacter cloacae	β-Lactamase producers, endotoxin, Shiga toxin	
				Escherichia coli	ETEC: secretory enterotoxins (LT, ST) EPEC: attaching and effacing lesion EHEC: Shigalike toxin EIEC: invades epithelial cells EAggEC: binds to HEp-2 cells	
				Klebsiella pneumoniae spp.	Upper respiratory tract colonization	
				Morganella morganii spp.	Splits urea, forms ammonium hydroxide, increases urinary pH	
				Proteus mirabilis	Splits urea, increases urinary pH, increases regeneration at higher pH	
				Providencia stuartii	*Klebsiella*-like hemagglutinin possibly helps adhere to indwelling catheters, prolonging bacteriuria. Urolithiasis is rare	
				Salmonella ser. typhi	Adherence to intestinal epithelium, choleralike enterotoxin	
				Serratia marcescens	Protease enhances vascular permeability, can degrade fibronectin and immunoglobulins. Adheres to bladder epithelial cells	
				Shigella dysenteriae	Invades M cells. Shiga toxin (exotoxin). Affects distal colon and rectosigmoid more severely	

(continued)

TABLE 3.3.1
(continued)

Form	Characteristics	Species	Other Features, Toxins, Virulence Factors	Significant ICU Considerations
		Yersinia enterocolitica	Affects intestinal lymphoid tissue; multiplies in Peyer patches and lymphoid follicles	
		Yersinia pestis	Endotoxin, virulent strains replicate in macrophages, increasing amount of endotoxin	
		Yersinia pseudotuberculosis	Affects intestinal lymphoid tissue; multiplies in Peyer patches and lymphoid follicles	
Bacilli	Oxidase (+), ferment sugars	Non-Enterobacteriaceae		Gastroenteritis, hypovolemic dehydration, skin infections (*A. hydrophila, P. multocida, V. vulnificus*), meningitis (*A. hydrophila, P. multocida, V. vulnificus*)
Gram-negative		*Aeromonas hydrophila*	α-Hemolysins and β-hemolysins, enterotoxin, cytotoxin	
Aerobic		*Pasteurella multocida* spp.	Antiphagocytic capsule	
		Vibrio cholerae	Enterotoxin CTX activates adenylate cyclase, leads to secretion of water and chloride by the intestinal crypt cells	
		Vibrio parahaemolyticus	Thermostable direct hemolysin causes intestinal cells to secrete chloride by increasing intracellular calcium concentration	
		Vibrio vulnificus	Collagenase, cytolysin, protease aids in spread within tissues. Polysaccharide capsule	
Bacilli	Catalase (+) oxidase variable nonfermentative	Non-Enterobacteriaceae		Bacteremia, sepsis, meningitis (usually after trauma or neurosurgical procedures), nosocomial infections (*Burkholderia cepacia, Achromobacter* spp., *P. aeruginosa, S. maltophilia*)
Gram-negative		*Acinetobacter baumannii*	No specific virulence factors identified	
Aerobic		*Achromobacter (Alcaligenes)* spp.	Increasing hospital pathogens, weakly virulent	
		B. cepacia	Resists nonoxidative killing by neutrophils; elastase, gelatinase	
		Pseudomonas aeruginosa	Endotoxin, enterotoxin, phospholipase C, exoenzyme S, exotoxin A, glycocalyx formation aids in adherence and impairing phagocytosis	

			Organism	Characteristics	Diseases
Bacilli	Gram-negative	Anaerobic	*Stenotrophomonas maltophilia*	Produces biofilm, adheres to plastic	
			Bacteroides fragilis group	Produces protease, elastase, fibrinolysin, DNase, RNase, weakly virulent	Bacteremia, sepsis, meningitis, necrotizing fasciitis (*B. fragilis*), Lemierre syndrome (*F. necrophorum*), ventilator-associated pneumonia (*B. fragilis, P. gingivalis, Prevotella* spp.)
				Adherence factors, proteolytic toxins, capsular polysaccharide, lipopolysaccharide	
			Fusobacterium necrophorum sp.	Complication of infections involving perimandibular region; adherence factors, proteolytic toxins, capsular polysaccharide, lipopolysaccharide	
			Porphyromonas gingivalis	Adherence factors, proteolytic toxins, capsular polysaccharide, lipopolysaccharide	
			Prevotella spp.	Adherence factors, proteolytic toxins, capsular polysaccharide, lipopolysaccharide	
Cocco-bacillus	Gram-negative	Aerobic	Fastidious	*Bartonella bacilliformis*	Parasitization of erythrocytes	
			Bartonella henselae	Activation of endothelial cells by activation of NFκB	Encephalitis/meningitis (*Brucella* sp., *C. brunetti, Ehrlichia* spp., *Haemophilus influenzae, R. prowazekii, S. moniliformis*). Pneumonia (*H. influenzae, B. pertussis, L. pneumophila, F. tularensis*), sepsis (*H. influenzae, C. jejuni*), seizures (*B. pertussis* in neonates), rash and sepsislike syndrome (*R. rickettsii, Ehrlichia* spp.)
			Bartonella quintana	Humans are only a reservoir; vector is body louse, *Pediculus humanus*	
			Bordetella pertussis	Fimbriae, pertussis toxin, heat-labile toxin, endotoxin, tracheal cytotoxin, *Bordetella* resistance to killing factor, filamentous hemagglutinin	
			Brucella spp.	Inhibit peroxidase-hydrogen peroxide-halide system	
			Calymmatobacterium granulomatis	Intracytoplasmic cysts, Donovan bodies	
			Campylobacter jejuni spp.	Incompletely understood mechanism. Possibly heat-labile enterotoxin or cytotoxin	
			Cardiobacterium hominis	One of HACEK organisms	
			Coxiella burnetii	Q Fever: Inhalation main route of infection. Resistant to heat and desiccation	
			Ehrlichia spp.	*Ehrlichiosis:* Incompletely understood. Lone Star tick primary vector of human monocytic ehrlichiosis	

(continued)

TABLE 3.3.1
(continued)

Form	Characteristics	Species	Other Features, Toxins, Virulence Factors	Significant ICU Considerations
		Francisella tularensis	Tularemia: Facultative intracellular parasite inducing humoral and cell-mediated response	
		Haemophilus ducreyi	Chancroid: Not well understood. Possibly related to pili, lipo-oligosaccharide, cytolethal distending toxin	
		H. influenzae	Capsular polysaccharide, lipopolysaccharide, outer membrane proteins, IgA protease	
		Haemophilus parainfluenzae	No specific virulence factors identified	
		Helicobacter pylori	Cytotoxin, catalase, lipopolysaccharide, Lewis oligosaccharide, urease	
		Kingella kingae	Pathogenesis not yet understood	
		Legionella pneumophila	Legionnaire disease: Pathogenesis unknown	
		Orientia tsutsugamushi	Tsutsugamushi disease: Similar to other rickettsia diseases	
		Rickettsia prowazekii	Louse-borne typhus: Similar to R. rickettsii	
		Rickettsia rickettsii	Rocky Mountain spotted fever: Unclear, thought to be toxic products from metabolism of rickettsia; multiplication in cells lining blood vessels causing vasculitis; competition of organism for substrates	
		Streptobacillus moniliformis	Rat-bite fever: Poorly understood pathophysiology	

Others	Chlamydia	Obligate intracellular organism, gram-negative envelope	*Chlamydia pneumoniae*	Exact mechanism of infection is unclear. Thought to be from inhaling infected respiratory secretions	Atypical pneumonia, associated with acute-chest syndrome (sickle cell disease)
			Chlamydia psittaci	Infection by inhalation of secretions, fecal dust of infected animals	
			Chlamydia trachomatis	Utilizes host ATP. Major outer membrane protein determines classification	
	Mycoplasma	Pleomorphic	*Mycoplasma pneumoniae*	Hydrogen peroxide generation, inhibition of catalase activity	Atypical pneumonia, sepsis, meningitis, encephalitis
			Ureaplasma urealyticum	Produces urease. Reservoir is genital tract of adults	
	Trepone-mataceae	Spiral-shaped	*Borrelia burgdorferi*	*Lyme disease:* Vector is *Ixodes scapularis* (dammini). Organism induces IL-1B, IL-6, TNF	Arrhythmias, heart block (*B. burgdorferi*), meningitis (*L. interrogans, T. pallidum*), aortitis, pulmonary arteritis (*T. pallidum*) cerebrovascular accident (*L. interrogans*), neurologic abnormalities (*B. burgdorferi, T. pallidum*)
			Borrelia recurrentis	*Relapsing fever:* Variable major protein (VMP) surface protein. Vector is human body louse	
			Leptospira interrogans	*Leptospirosis:* Transmission from infected animals. Virulence factors unknown	
			Treponema pallidum	*Syphilis:* Hyaluronidase, fibronectin coat from host helps protect against phagocytosis. Changes in the host cell-mediated immunity during primary and secondary syphilis	

CSF, cerebrospinal fluid; TSST-1, toxic shock staph toxin 1; TNF, tumor necrosis factor; IL, interleukin; ETEC, enterotoxigenic *E. coli*; LT, heat labile; ST, heat stable; EPEC, enteropathogenic *E. coli*; EHEC, enterohemorrhagic *E. coli*; EIEC, enteroinvasive *E. coli*; EAggEC, enteroaggregative *E. coli*; NFκB, nuclear factor kappa B; HACEK, hemophilus, actinobacillus, cardiobacterium, eikenella, kingella; TDH, thermostable direct hemolysin; OMP, outer membrane protein; MOMP, major outer membrane protein; ATP, adenosine triphosphate; IgA, immunoglobulin A.

TABLE 3.3.2

COMMON BACTERIAL PATHOGENS BY SYSTEMS OF INVOLVEMENT

	System	Organism	Manifestations
Community-acquired	Upper airway	*Streptococcus pneumoniae*	Otitis media, sinusitis, pharyngitis, epiglottitis
		H. influenzae	Otitis media, sinusitis, pharyngitis, uvulitis, epiglottitis
		Moraxella catarrhalis	Otitis media, sinusitis, pharyngitis
		Streptococcus pyogenes	Pharyngitis, tonsillitis, uvulitis, parapharyngeal abscess, cervical lymphadenitis
		Staphylococcus aureus	Sinusitis, lymphadenitis
		Mycobacterium spp.	Cervical lymphadenitis
	Lower airway	*Mycoplasma pneumoniae*	Acute bronchitis, bronchiolitis
		Streptococcus pneumoniae	Bacterial pneumonia
		H. influenzae	Bacterial pneumonia
		S. aureus	Bacterial pneumonia, lung abscess
		Legionella pneumophila	Atypical pneumonia
		Chlamydia trachomatis	Nonbacterial pneumonia (neonates)
	Systemic	*Streptococcus agalactiae*	Neonatal sepsis
		Escherichia coli	Neonatal sepsis
		Listeria monocytogenes	Neonatal sepsis
		S. pneumoniae	Sepsis/meningitis
		H. influenzae	Sepsis/meningitis
		Neisseria meningitidis	Sepsis/meningitis
		S. aureus	Toxic shock syndrome
	Cardiac	*Streptococcus pyogenes*	Rheumatic fever
		S. aureus	Pericarditis
		H. influenzae	Pericarditis
		Streptococcus viridans spp.	Subacute endocarditis
		S. aureus	Acute endocarditis
		Staphylococcus epidermidis	Prosthetic valve endocarditis
		Enterococcus spp.	Subacute endocarditis
	Central nervous system	*S. agalactiae*	Neonatal meningitis
		E. coli	Neonatal meningitis
		L. monocytogenes	Neonatal meningitis
		S. pneumoniae	Bacterial meningitis
		H. influenzae	Bacterial meningitis
		N. meningitidis	Bacterial meningitis
	GI tract	*E. coli*	Bacterial gastroenteritis, cholangitis, peritonitis
		Salmonella spp.	Bacterial gastroenteritis
		Shigella dysenteriae	Bacterial gastroenteritis
		Yersinia enterocolitica	Bacterial gastroenteritis
	Urinary tract	*E. coli*	Cystitis/pyelonephritis
		Klebsiella pneumoniae	Cystitis/pyelonephritis
		Enterobacter cloacae	Cystitis/pyelonephritis
		Staphylococcus saprophyticus	Cystitis/pyelonephritis
		Enterococcus spp.	Cystitis/pyelonephritis
	Musculoskeletal	*S. aureus*	Osteomyelitis, septic arthritis
		H. influenzae	Osteomyelitis, septic arthritis
		Salmonella spp.	Osteomyelitis (especially sickle cell disease)
Nosocomial	Bloodstream	*S. epidermidis*	Catheter-related infections
		S. aureus	Catheter-related infections
	Respiratory	*S. aureus*	Ventilator-associated pneumonia
		Pseudomonas aeruginosa	Ventilator-associated pneumonia
		K. pneumoniae	Nosocomial pneumonia
		E. cloacae	Nosocomial pneumonia
		Stenotrophomonas maltophilia	Nosocomial pneumonia
	GI tract	*Clostridium difficile*	Pseudomembranous colitis/antibiotic-associated colitis
	Urinary tract	*Enterococcus* spp.	Urinary tract infections
		E. cloacae	Urinary tract infections
		K. pneumoniae	Urinary tract infections
	Central nervous system	*S. epidermidis*	CSF shunt infections
		S. aureus	CSF shunt infections

GI, gastrointestinal; CSF, cerebrospinal fluid.

Bacteremia with *S. aureus* is seen in the presence of a primary source of entry, such as an invasive catheter or a skin infection. *S. aureus* is also important in septic arthritis, osteomyelitis, pericarditis, and acute endocarditis in those without preexisting heart disease. Epidermolytic toxin is associated with staphylococcal scalded skin syndrome, which manifests as acute desquamation or a diffuse erythroderma (Table 3.3.1).

Toxic shock syndrome (TSS) manifests as an initial period of fever, chills, myalgias, and gastrointestinal symptoms. Tachypnea, tachycardia, and erythroderma can develop. Capillary leak syndrome with the loss of peripheral vascular resistance can lead to hypotension and shock. Since about half of nonmenstrual TSS does not produce TSST-I, other enterotoxins are believed to play a role in the development of TSS.

Coagulase-negative staphylococci, such as *S. epidermidis*, are important pathogens in catheter-related nosocomial bloodstream infections (Table 3.3.1). The organism enters the bloodstream through breaks in the skin, such as by central lines or through the respiratory tract. Production of a biofilm of exopolysaccharide slime helps *S. epidermidis* to bind to prosthetic devices; various exotoxins are thought to contribute to its pathogenesis. Clinical manifestations of *S. epidermidis* include infections arising due to indwelling or prosthetic devices such as central lines, peritoneal dialysis catheters, hemodialysis shunts, cerebrospinal fluid (CSF) shunts, and prosthetic valves. *S. epidermidis* is also an important pathogen in neonatal sepsis (Table 3.3.1).

Catalase-negative, gram-positive cocci include the streptococcal species that are also important human pathogens. The streptococci have been differentiated by their ability to lyse sheep red blood cells either partially (α-hemolytic strep) or completely (β-hemolytic strep). A further characterization based on antigenic reactivity was performed by Lancefield, and represents an alphabetic grouping of similar organisms. Group A streptococci (*Streptococcus pyogenes*) form chains and induce β (clear) hemolysis on blood agar. Important virulence factors include M proteins (surface proteins), which are antiphagocytic, streptolysins O and S, and exotoxins (Table 3.3.1). The most common manifestations are tonsillitis, pharyngitis, and skin infections, such as impetigo and erysipelas. Important clinical considerations for the intensivist include TSS and necrotizing fasciitis. Complications of group A streptococcal infections include postinfectious glomerulonephritis, peritonsillar and parapharyngeal abscesses, empyema, and osteomyelitis.

Enterococci, including *Enterococcus faecalis* and *Enterococcus faecium*, are group D streptococci. They are normal gastrointestinal tract flora and are common causes of urinary tract infections, usually in the setting of an indwelling bladder catheter or structural abnormality. Neonatal sepsis and meningitis, septic arthritis, and endocarditis of both prosthetic and native valves are other possible manifestations. Invasive disease with *Enterococcus* is a particular concern among those with underlying gastrointestinal abnormalities. Vancomycin-resistant enterococci (VRE) is a growing problem in the intensive care unit (ICU) as a nosocomial pathogen. Environmental contamination with VRE is an important part of healthcare-associated acquisition. The development of multidrug resistance has led to important challenges in the treatment of invasive enterococcal disease, such as endocarditis (Table 3.3.1).

Viridans group streptococci, also known as α-hemolytic streptococci, are normal flora of the oral mucosa. They cause dental caries and gingival disease. Because they also colonize the female genital tract, *Viridans* group streptococci are important in causing chorioamnionitis and are associated with neonatal sepsis and meningitis (Table 3.3.1). Because of an ability to adhere to diseased endocardium, *Viridans* group streptococci remain the most frequent cause of subacute endocarditis.

Streptococcus pneumoniae (pneumococcus) remains a major cause of disease in all age-groups. *S. pneumoniae* is a gram-positive coccus that typically appears in pairs but may also form chains. Primary virulence factors include an antiphagocytic polysaccharide capsule and the ability to develop tolerance to β-lactam antibiotics. *S. pneumoniae* is a major cause of otitis media, sinusitis, mastoiditis, and community-acquired pneumonia. Pneumococcal pneumonia typically presents with an acute onset of fever, malaise, chest pain, and productive cough. With the development of antibiotics, mortality caused by pneumococcal pneumonia is low. The important clinical consideration for the intensivist is invasive disease caused by *S. pneumoniae*. *Pneumococcus* is the most common cause of bacteremia and bacterial meningitis in the United States. Fulminant sepsis occurs in up to 10% of those with *S. pneumoniae* bacteremia. The emergence of antimicrobial resistance, particularly to β-lactam drugs and macrolides, poses another clinical dilemma for the intensivist in the management of invasive disease.

Streptococcus agalactiae, also known as *group B. Streptococcus*, colonizes or asymptomatically infects the maternal genital tract and is the cause of perinatal infections. Manifestations include maternal postpartum endometritis and urinary tract infection, neonatal sepsis, pneumonia, and meningitis (Table 3.3.1). The incidence of serious neonatal infections has decreased since the institution of routine peripartum antibiotic prophylaxis.

Gram-positive Aerobic Bacilli

Anthrax is a disease caused by *Bacillus anthracis* that has recently regained interest because of its potential use as a biologic warfare agent. The organism is a spore-forming, nonmotile, aerobic rod. Transmission to humans occurs through contact with infected animal products. The specific virulence factors for anthrax include a poly-D-glutamic acid capsule, lethal toxin, and edema toxin (Table 3.3.1). The manifestations of anthrax are cutaneous disease, inhalational anthrax, meningitis, and gastrointestinal anthrax (see Fig. 3.3.2).

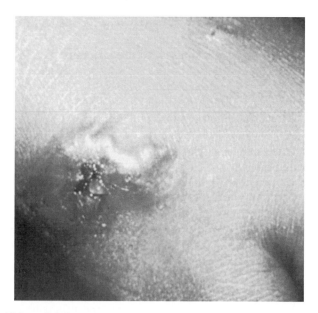

Figure 3.3.2 Early cutaneous lesion of anthrax on the thumb of a 6-year-old boy from Zimbabwe. (Courtesy of Wilhelm Kobuch, Toulouse, France. From Gorbach SL, Bartlett JG, Blacklow NR. *Infectious diseases*. 3rd ed. Philadelphia, PA: Lippincott Williams & Wilkins; 2003:1461.)

Cutaneous disease occurs after contact of injured skin with spores; papules form and evolve into a vesicle, eventually undergoing necrosis, leaving a black eschar. Inhalational anthrax begins as a nonspecific upper respiratory illness, progressing rapidly to fulminant respiratory failure after several days. Radiographically, the mediastinum is widened, with common occurrence of pleural effusions. Primary meningitis is more common in young adults who acquire *B. anthracis* through occupational exposures. Clinical manifestations of anthrax meningitis are similar to other forms of bacterial meningitis, with decreased CSF glucose and elevated protein. Gastrointestinal anthrax occurs after ingestion of meat that is contaminated by spores. Clinical manifestations include severe abdominal pain with fever, hematemesis or coffee-ground emesis, and ascites. Relevant intensive care issues include the development of hemorrhagic shock with the development of fluid and electrolyte imbalances (Table 3.3.1).

Listeria monocytogenes is a motile, non–spore-forming gram-positive rod that causes perinatal infections in humans (Table 3.3.2). The organism colonizes animals and humans, and the mode of transmission is incompletely understood. In the United States, most cases are caused by the ingestion of contaminated food products. Clinical disease includes neonatal sepsis, pneumonia, and meningitis (Table 3.3.1). Skin and pharyngeal lesions, resulting from disseminated macro- and microabscesses, may be seen. Late-onset of disease can be seen within the first 8 weeks of life.

Corynebacteria are club-shaped, nonmotile, non-spore-forming bacilli. *Corynebacterium diphtheriae* is the cause of diphtheria, which was a significant cause of morbidity and mortality in children before the development of antitoxin and vaccine. Transmission occurs through contact with infected droplets while talking, sneezing, or coughing. Infection occurs after *C. diphtheriae* enter the upper respiratory tract and remains on the mucosal surfaces. The diphtheria toxin causes local tissue necrosis with associated inflammation, eventually forming a fibrinous exudate that is difficult to remove. Clinically, diphtheria presents as a nonspecific upper respiratory infection, or as a crouplike illness. Laryngeal involvement with membrane formation can lead to respiratory tract obstruction, leading to respiratory failure. *Corynebacterium JK* plays an important role in causing catheter-related bloodstream infections.

Mycobacteria

Mycobacteria are pleomorphic, nonmobile, non–spore forming, and weakly gram-positive rods. Acid fastness refers to the ability of the organism to form extremely stable mycolate complexes with crystal violet, carbolfuchsin, rhodamine, and auramine dyes. The specific staining properties are used in the identification of mycobacteria. The organism is slow-growing, and is hydrophobic because of the high proportion of lipids in the cell wall.

Tuberculosis remains the predominant human pathogenic disease caused by mycobacteria. Originally identified by Koch in 1882, *Mycobacterium tuberculosis* currently causes significant morbidity and mortality. Manifestations of tuberculosis include a latent infection without any clinical signs or symptoms of infection and a positive tuberculin test (Table 3.3.1). Most primary lung infections begin with a single focus with subsequent lymphogenic spread. The primary focus, along with lymphangitis, and regional lymphadenitis make up the primary complex, originally described by Ghon.

The primary pulmonary manifestation of the primary complex is bronchial obstruction, which can cause atelectasis, postobstructive hyperaeration, and wheezing. Pleural effusions, either unilateral or bilateral may occur, but these are uncommon in children younger than 5 years. Progressive pulmonary tuberculosis occurs when the primary focus continues to enlarge into a nearby bronchus, forming a primary cavity, releasing large amounts of the organism to spread to other parts of the lung. Clinical manifestations include malaise, fever, weight loss, and cough.

Other manifestations of tuberculosis include myocarditis, pericarditis, and pericardial effusion (Table 3.3.1). The mycobacteria can spread to the central nervous system (CNS), causing tuberculous meningitis, brain abscesses, or tuberculomas. Bone and joint involvement can be seen in up to 5% of untreated primary infections. Vertebrae are the most commonly affected, and the infection can progress to severe destruction of the vertebral bodies (Pott disease). Mesenteric lymphadenitis, tuberculous peritonitis, regional lymphadenitis (scrofula), and renal tuberculosis are other sites of involvement.

Other mycobacteria that cause significant disease in humans include the *Mycobacterium avium-intracellulare complex* (MAI or MAC). This complex includes *Mycobacterium avium* and *M. intracellulare*, which cause disease in both immunocompetent and immunocompromised patients. Manifestations include lung disease, bacterial peritonitis in patients receiving peritoneal dialysis, and osteomyelitis. Atypical mycobacteria, including MAI and *M. scrofulaceum*, cause lymphadenitis of submandibular and cervical nodes. *M. kansasii* is another commonly found mycobacterial pathogen in humans, causing a chronic pneumonia primarily in adults. *M. chelonae* is a cause of mediastinitis and catheter-related bloodstream infections.

Anaerobic Organisms

The clinically significant gram-positive anaerobic bacteria include the Clostridia species and the Actinomycetes. Clostridia are spore-forming, gram-positive anaerobes that are ubiquitous and found in soil, intestinal tract, and decaying tissues. Disease manifestations are based on various toxins produced by Clostridia.

Clostridium tetani is the cause of tetanus, which continues to be a major contributor to mortality in developing nations. The exotoxin tetanospasmin produces tetanus. However, the exact mechanism of action of tetanospasmin as well as how the toxin is absorbed is not completely understood. The toxin exerts its effects on different parts of the nervous system by inhibiting acetylcholine release from skeletal muscle motor end plates, blocking inhibitory synapses in the spinal cord and similarly in the brain and the sympathetic nervous system. Skin wounds are usual sites of *C. tetani* infections.

Tetanus can be localized after an incubation of 3 to 21 days; patients can experience rigidity and pain near the site of entry. Localized disease has low mortality and typically resolves without sequelae. Generalized tetanus presents with trismus in approximately 50% of patients. Involvement of other muscle groups follows, with extreme pain associated with the spasms. Generalized seizures or tetanospasms may also occur. The causes of death with tetanus are unclear. With modern therapy and the availability of antitoxins, mortality can be reduced from as high as 70% to approximately 10% to 30%.

Clostridium botulinum is the cause of botulism. Botulinum toxin, a neurotoxin, is often regarded as the most lethal naturally occurring substance. Transmission of botulism in the United States occurs mostly through home-processed foods and from wounds. The toxin acts at the neuromuscular junction, blocking the release of acetylcholine. Botulism is manifested by a symmetric, descending, motor paralysis, initially involving the cranial nerves. Gastrointestinal symptoms and visual changes may be present. The most serious manifestation is respiratory muscle weakness, leading to respiratory compromise. Vital capacity and negative inspiratory force are sensitive indicators of respiratory status in critically ill adult patients.

Infant botulism, although also caused by *C. botulinum*, is a distinct disease from food-borne botulism. In infant botulism, the spores that are ingested colonize the colon, where the neurotoxin is produced. The clinical presentation varies, but typically includes poor feeding, constipation, and lethargy, with poor head control, hypotonia, and ptosis. Bulbar palsies will be present with infant botulism. The typical clinical course involves a worsening of the weakness to a nadir at 1 to 2 weeks, followed by another 1 to 3 weeks before any improvement is noted.

Clostridium perfringens produces multiple toxins, of which the α-toxin is the most clinically significant. The toxin causes muscle necrosis and gas within tissues, and is characterized by a lack of significant leukocyte infiltration at the site of infection. *C. perfringens* is a cause of gas gangrene, cellulites, and necrotizing fasciitis. Occasionally, neonatal sepsis and meningitis can be caused by *C. perfringens*.[1]

Pseudomembranous colitis is mostly caused by *Clostridium difficile*. *C. difficile* produces toxins A and B, of which toxin A causes the enterotoxic effects. Usually occurring after the use of antimicrobial drugs, classical manifestations include fever, abdominal cramps, and watery diarrhea that can become bloody or mucoid. Infection with *C. difficile* can range from a self-limited mild illness to severe toxicity and an acute-abdomen–like presentation. Environmental contamination is an important means of nosocomial spread of the organism (Table 3.3.2).

Peptostreptococci are normal flora of the mouth and colon (Table 3.3.1). They are frequent causes of dental caries and secondary peritonitis after trauma or surgery. Peptostreptococcus has also been isolated from patients with ventilator-associated pneumonia and aspiration pneumonia, usually mixed with aerobic organisms. *Propionibacterium acnes* is an anaerobic, gram-positive bacillus that is part of the normal skin flora. Clinical manifestations include cutaneous eruptions (acne vulgaris) and CSF shunt infections. Lactobacillus is part of the gastrointestinal and vaginal flora and may play a role in preventing overgrowth of flora. Lactobacillus has been used to treat gastrointestinal infections by recolonizing the intestine.

Actinomyces are also normal oral flora and a cause of human actinomycosis. They are non–spore forming, non-motile, gram-positive rods. Actinomycosis presents as a chronic infection involving the oral or cervicofacial region, abdomen, or lungs, with the disease occurring after disruption of the mucous membranes. An important clinical consideration for the intensivist is to take actinomycosis into account in the differential diagnosis of pneumonia and chronic pleural effusions in the immunocompromised patient.

Gram-negative Bacteria

Among the gram-negative cocci, the most clinically significant is the *Neisseria* sp. *Neisseria meningitidis* remains a significant cause of epidemic meningitis and sepsis.

N. meningitidis is a nonmotile, aerobic gram-negative coccus occurring in pairs. Disease in the United States occurs most commonly between November and March. Epidemic cases are seen more commonly in older children and adolescents. Pathogenesis of disease is through the effects of an outer membrane with lipo-oligosaccharide, which is a potent endotoxin (Table 3.3.1). Individuals at risk for developing meningococcal disease include those with late complement component deficiencies, properdin pathway deficiencies, and acquired complement deficiencies, such as systemic lupus erythematosus and nephrotic syndrome. Infection can be asymptomatic or can manifest as a rapidly progressing, fulminant sepsis or meningitis. A preceding nonspecific upper respiratory infection with a rash and fever can rapidly progress to purpura and shock. Meningitis presents with fever, stiff neck, and occasionally seizures, and can be complicated by hydrocephalus and subdural effusions. After receiving antibiotic therapy, some individuals may have a worsening clinical course, thought to result from the release of endotoxin from killed organisms. Meningococcal pneumonia, myocarditis, and pericarditis are other possible manifestations. Mortality in the United States from invasive disease approaches 20%. Worse prognosis is associated with the presence of hypotension, white blood cell count less than 10,000 per mm^3, erythrocyte sedimentation rate less than 10 mm per hour, petechiae for less than 12 hours prior to admission, and absence of meningitis. The development of a vaccine against *N. meningitidis* is an effective means of primary and secondary prevention in household contacts for serogroups A, C, Y, and W135. However, serogroup B is the most common cause of small outbreaks in industrialized nations, and no vaccine is currently available.

Neisseria gonorrhoeae is a nonmotile, aerobic, gram-negative coccus occurring in pairs. The highest infection rates occur in adolescents and present as urethritis, cervicitis, epididymitis, and tenosynovitis. The gonococcus can adhere to mucosal epithelium. A lipo-oligosaccharide capsule is important for its pathogenesis. Important clinical manifestations in the newborn include ophthalmia neonatorum and scalp abscesses following fetal monitoring devices. Septic arthritis is an uncommon, but reported, complication of perinatally acquired gonococcal infection.

Moraxella catarrhalis is a kidney-shaped, gram-negative coccus morphologically similar to *Neisseria*. *M. catarrhalis* is the normal flora of the upper respiratory tract and a common pathogen in diseases involving this region (Table 3.3.2). The primary virulence factor is the production of endotoxin (Table 3.3.1). These organisms are usually β-lactamase producers, which is clinically important when choosing antimicrobial therapy. *M. catarrhalis* is a cause of sinusitis, otitis media, bacterial tracheitis, and pneumonia. In immunocompromised patients, more severe infections, such as sepsis and meningitis, can be seen.

The gram-negative bacilli include an extensive range of significant human pathogens (Table 3.3.1). Among the most common are the enterobacteria, which include *Escherichia*, *Klebsiella*, *Shigella*, *Enterobacter*, *Salmonella*, *Serratia*, *Pseudomonas*, and *Vibrio* organisms. Virulence factors of the enterobacteria commonly involve the production of toxins that cause a large variety of diseases. Because enterobacteria are common habitants of the gastrointestinal tract, they are common causes of urinary tract infections, urosepsis, and perinatal infections (Table 3.3.2).

Escherichia coli is a common cause of neonatal sepsis and meningitis and one of the primary bacterial causes of diarrheal illness worldwide. Serious invasive disease with *E. coli* is of particular concern among patients with galactosemia. Although the overall incidence in neonatal sepsis associated with *E. coli* is decreasing, the rate of drug-resistant *E. coli* is on the rise. Enterotoxigenic *E. coli* is the most common cause of traveler's diarrhea, whereas enterohemorrhagic *E. coli* (i.e., O157:H7) causes hemorrhagic colitis, and is associated with hemolytic uremic syndrome (HUS) (Table 3.3.1). Fever is usually absent and pretreatment with trimethoprim-sulfamethoxazole has been implicated as a risk factor for the development of HUS.

The *Salmonella* sp. are nonencapsulated, motile, gram-negative bacilli. Included in this group are the serotypes *Typhi*, *Paratyphi*, and *Enteritidis*. Approximately 10^5 to 10^{10} organisms are required to cause disease in humans. Humans act as the reservoir for *S. ser. Typhi*, and disease occurs after contact with an infected individual. A specific virulence factor includes a choleralike enterotoxin (Table 3.3.1). *Salmonella* causes acute gastroenteritis and enteric fever (more commonly with *S. ser. Typhi*). Bacteremia, meningitis, and osteomyelitis are more commonly seen in immunocompromised patients and in patients with sickle-cell anemia.

Shigellae are nonencapsulated, nonlactose fermenting gram-negative bacilli that cause diarrheal illnesses (Table 3.3.2). Transmission is fecal–oral and is more commonly seen where individuals live in close proximity. Virulence is attributed to specific exotoxins (Shiga toxins) and enterotoxins. *S. dysenteriae* causes watery diarrhea, which may be severe and cause circulatory collapse. Seizures associated with *S. dysenteriae* can occur in up to 45% of cases and can be generalized or focal. Chronic diarrhea or recurring diarrhea can be seen in patients who are immunocompromised.

Citrobacter freundii is a straight, gram-negative bacillus found occasionally as intestinal flora. Vertical transmission plays a role in neonatal disease. In patients who are immunocompromised, selective colonization occurs, with antimicrobial drugs suppressing other organisms. Certain strains produce verotoxins, causing the manifestations of disease. *Citrobacter* sp. cause neonatal sepsis, meningitis, and diarrhea outbreaks. An increased risk of brain abscesses is seen with *Citrobacter* meningitis.

Proteus sp. are nonlactose fermenting, motile gram-negative rods found in sewage and soil. The organism splits urea, increasing pH through the formation of ammonium hydroxide, leading to increased risk of urolithiasis. *Proteus mirabilis* is a rare cause of neonatal sepsis, meningitis, urinary tract infections, and urolithiasis (Table 3.3.1). Other manifestations can include pneumonia, osteomyelitis, and brain abscesses, particularly in patients with sickle-cell anemia or who are immunocompromised.

Yersinia pestis is a nonmotile, pleomorphic, gram-negative rod that is the cause of plague. Humans are infected by the bite of an infected flea. Once the organism enters the skin, disease can remain localized or may enter the bloodstream, leading to disseminated infection. The amount of endotoxin determines the severity of the disease. Bubonic plague is manifested by a localized tender lymphadenopathy that may become suppurative (Table 3.3.1). In pneumonic plague, a fulminant disease with rapid progression of dyspnea and hemoptysis occurs that is usually fatal if not treated. Other clinical manifestations of plague include disseminated intravascular coagulation, a sepsislike syndrome, and, rarely, meningitis.

Enterobacteria also play an important role as nosocomial pathogens in causing bacteremia (Table 3.3.2). *Klebsiella pneumoniae* is a citrate-positive, oxidase-negative nonmotile gram-negative bacillus. A capsular polysaccharide is thought to be a virulence factor. *K. pneumoniae* is a cause of nosocomial infections of the respiratory tract, urinary tract, bloodstream, and biliary system. Lung disease caused by *K. pneumoniae* results typically from aspiration of the colonized organism from the upper respiratory tract. Pneumonia caused by *K. pneumoniae* can occur with the formation of lung abscesses, but the pathogen is otherwise similar to other causes of community-acquired disease. Urinary tract infection is commonly associated with indwelling bladder catheterization. *K. pneumoniae* bacteremia is seen in children who are immunocompromised.

Serratia marcescens is a catalase-positive, motile gram-negative bacillus that produces a red pigment. Specific virulence factors include a protease and hemolysin. Important considerations for the intensivist include the role of *S. marcescens* in nosocomial infections. *S. marcescens* is a cause of bloodstream infections associated with central venous catheters, urinary tract infections with bladder catheterization, nosocomial pneumonia, and meningitis.

Enterobacter sp. are facultatively anaerobic, motile gram-negative rods found in water, sewage, and soil. Clinically, *Enterobacter* is significant as an increasing nosocomial pathogen, and is seen in patients with chronic illnesses. Virulence is related to an endotoxin and an ability to develop resistance to cephalosporins and penicillins. Transmission is vertical in newborns, leading to neonatal sepsis, pneumonia, and meningitis (Table 3.3.1). Sepsis in patients who are immunocompromised is associated with central venous catheters; urinary tract infections are seen more often with indwelling bladder catheters. *Enterobacter* is also a cause of postsurgical wound infections and ventilator-associated pneumonia. An increasing amount of *Enterobacter* strains

producing extended-spectrum β-lactamases have been isolated, making antibiotic selection and treatment a challenge for the intensivist.

Among the non-Enterobacteriaceae are many clinically significant gram-negative organisms. *Pseudomonas* sp. are major causes of human disease in all age-groups. *Pseudomonas aeruginosa* is a motile, aerobic, non–spore forming nonlactose fermenting gram-negative rod. It is found in water and soil and is a cause of illness in patients who are immunocompromised. Specific virulence factors include an enterotoxin and an endotoxin (Table 3.3.1). Disease in healthy individuals may occur, typically as folliculitis and osteomyelitis following puncture wounds. *P. aeruginosa* is also a cause of otitis externa and eye infections. Of clinical relevance to the intensivist is the fact that *P. aeruginosa* causes neonatal sepsis, wound infections in patients with burns, urinary tract infections, and ventilator-associated pneumonia. Bacteremia and sepsis are seen more commonly in patients who are immunocompromised. *P. aeruginosa* is also commonly recovered from respiratory cultures of patients with cystic fibrosis.

Burkholderia cepacia (formerly *Pseudomonas cepacia*) is an obligate aerobic gram-negative bacillus. Recently, *B. cepacia* has become an important pathogen in nosocomial infections. It causes ventilator-associated pneumonia, wound infections, endocarditis, and meningitis. *B. cepacia* is a common pathogen in lung infections in cystic fibrosis and in other patients who are immunocompromised. A significant clinical dilemma is *B. cepacia*'s resistance to carboxypenicillins and aminoglycosides, making selection of antimicrobial therapy a challenge.

Aeromonas sp. are motile gram-negative bacilli found in water sources. *A. hydrophila* produces α and β hemolysin, enterotoxin, and various other enzymes that are important in its virulence. *Aeromonas* has been described as a cause of sepsis, wound infections, pneumonia, and meningitis in patients who are immunocompromised. *A. hydrophila* also causes gastroenteritis and has been associated with HUS.

Vibrio cholerae is the cause of cholera, a significant worldwide diarrheal illness. *V. cholerae* is a curved, motile, gram-negative rod. Transmission occurs in humans after ingestion of water or food that is contaminated with the organism. Disease occurs more commonly in warm months. Virulence is determined by the production of an enterotoxin CTX, which activates adenylate cyclase on the intestinal epithelial cell, causing secretion of chloride and water by intestinal crypt cells. This leads to the characteristic watery diarrhea by the secretion of isotonic fluid from the intestine. Cholera is characterized by massive volume loss, with associated electrolyte disturbances, vascular collapse, and shock (Table 3.3.1). *Vibrio vulnificus* is the primary cause of vibrio-related deaths in the United States. *V. vulnificus* is commonly transmitted to humans through contaminated seafood and is a cause of sepsis and wound infections. Those with underlying liver diseases, such as viral or alcoholic hepatitis and hemochromatosis, are at increased risk for serious infection with *V. vulnificus*.

Acinetobacter sp. are gram-negative organisms usually appearing as rods, but occasionally they are spherical. They are ubiquitous, and can be found in water, soil, and sewage. The exact virulence factors are yet to be identified. *Acinetobacter* is emerging as a common cause of nosocomial infections in immunosuppressed patients. Manifestations can include meningitis after trauma or a neurosurgical procedure, bacteremia, and pneumonia in mechanically ventilated patients or those requiring tracheostomy. Urinary tract infections can also be seen and are more common with indwelling bladder catheters (Table 3.3.1). A recent increase in resistant Acinetobacter infections has made treatment of significant disease a challenge for the intensivist.

Anaerobic Organisms

Clinically significant gram-negative anaerobic bacteria include *Bacteroides*, *Prevotella*, Veillonella, and *Fusobacterium* sp. Because anaerobic organisms represent a large proportion of gastrointestinal tract flora, they are common pathogens in secondary peritonitis and abdominal abscesses. Gram-negative anaerobic bacteria are also causes of ventilator-associated pneumonia, aspiration pneumonia, and chronic sinusitis. *Bacteroides fragilis* has been reported as a cause of CNS shunt infections. *Prevotella* sp. and *B. fragilis* are causes of bite wound infections. *Fusobacterium necrophorum* is associated with Lemierre syndrome, manifesting as septic thrombophlebitis of the jugular vein with metastatic abscesses.

Other Bacterial Agents

Chlamydia

Chlamydiae are interesting organisms, of which *Chlamydia pneumoniae* and *Chlamydia trachomatis* are the main human pathogens. They are obligate intracellular organisms with a gram-negative envelope and possess two distinct forms (infectious and reproductive). One of these forms, the elementary body, is taken into the host cell by endocytosis after infection. They, in turn, differentiate into the second form, the reticulate body, which, after 36 hours, will differentiate to elementary bodies. After 4 days, they are released within their inclusion, leaving the host cell intact.

C. trachomatis is a common sexually transmitted organism that is primarily asymptomatic. In newborns, *C. trachomatis* is acquired during birth and causes neonatal pneumonia and conjunctivitis (Table 3.3.1). Pneumonia usually presents between 4 and 12 weeks of age with cough and congestion associated with a lack of fever. Radiographically, hyperinflation can be seen; lung consolidation is uncommon. In older children, *C. trachomatis* infection is clinically significant as a marker of sexual abuse and does not cause a specific syndrome.

C. pneumoniae transmission is unclear, but is believed to be through infected respiratory secretions. Clinically,

C. pneumoniae causes mostly mild lung disease. However, infection with *C. pneumoniae* can be a significant pathogen in patients who are immunocompromised and has been seen as a causative agent of acute-chest syndrome in patients with sickle cell disease.

Haemophilus influenzae is a pleomorphic, gram-negative coccobacillus that are important pathogens of the human upper respiratory tract (Table 3.3.2). *H. influenzae Type b* is an encapsulated strain that is a significant cause of invasive disease, such as epiglottitis, sepsis, and meningitis (Table 3.3.1). Since the introduction of the *H. influenzae Type b* vaccine, there has been a decline in the incidence of invasive disease. Virulence factors include a polysaccharide capsule, outer membrane proteins, and lipopolysaccharides. Transmission is through infected respiratory secretions to the mucosa of the respiratory tract. In invasive disease, the bacteria spreads from the mucosa to the bloodstream and disseminates to other locations in the body. *H. influenzae Type b* is a cause of pneumonia, sepsis, epiglottitis, and meningitis. Other manifestations include cellulitis, septic arthritis, CNS shunt infections, pericarditis, and necrotizing fasciitis. Non–type-B strains are common pathogens in conjunctivitis, sinusitis, and otitis media. *H. influenzae* is also a cause of "culture-negative" endocarditis (see Fig. 3.3.3).

Legionella

Legionella pneumophila is the cause of Legionnaires disease, an uncommon finding in children. *L. pneumophila* is an aerobic, gram-negative bacillus and requires L-cysteine for

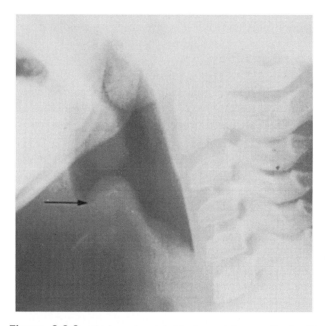

Figure 3.3.3 Thickened epiglottis (*arrow*) in a patient with epiglottitis. (Courtesy of Dr. A. Weber, *Massachusetts Eye and Ear Infirmary*, Boston, MA. From Gorbach SL, Bartlett JG, Blacklow NR. *Infectious diseases*. 3rd ed. Philadelphia, PA: Lippincott Williams & Wilkins; 2003:461.)

growth. The organism is ubiquitous in water environments. The exact pathogenesis of Legionnaires disease is unclear. Presentation is usually as an atypical pneumonia, often with high fever (Table 3.3.1). Complications include empyema and lung cavitations. Disease is more severe in patients who are immunocompromised; healthy patients mostly recover without sequelae.

Mycoplasma and Ureaplasma

Mycoplasma and *Ureaplasma* are ubiquitous, pleomorphic organisms lacking cell walls. They are the smallest of free-living microorganisms. *Mycoplasma* was originally considered a virus when first recovered in 1944. *Mycoplasma pneumoniae*, a common cause of atypical pneumonia, is slow-growing is able to grow in both anaerobic and aerobic conditions (Table 3.3.2). Transmission is through respiratory secretions of an infected person. The incubation period varies greatly to as much as 3 weeks and is thought to be related to the size of the inoculum.

Interestingly, different antibodies develop to *M. pneumoniae* infection and are commonly used to aid in diagnosis. Cold agglutinins are antibodies against erythrocyte I antigen and are found in up to 75% of patients with pneumonia due to *M. pneumoniae*. In addition, antibodies can be found to Wasserman cardiolipin antigen, smooth muscle, lung, liver, and brain.

Manifestations of *M. pneumoniae* infection include pneumonia with fever and cough (Table 3.3.1). The cough is initially nonproductive, with the presence of dry rales. Conjunctivitis and otitis media are other common findings. Radiographically, both lobar and interstitial involvement can be seen but findings commonly include diffuse, bilateral reticular infiltrates. In children and adolescents, pharyngitis and upper respiratory tract symptoms can be the only symptoms of *M. pneumoniae* infection. Other manifestations include croup, urticarial rash, Stevens-Johnson syndrome, hemolytic anemia, arthritis, encephalitis, polymyositis, and hepatitis. Rarely, myocarditis and pericarditis can be seen.

Ureaplasmas are distinct from *Mycoplasmas* in their ability produce urease. This ability to hydrolyze urea is helpful in the isolation of the organism in culture. In humans, *Ureaplasma urealyticum* colonizes the adult genital tract as a result of sexual contact. Infants become infected through the birth canal or *in utero* with ruptured membranes. *U. urealyticum* is associated with chorioamnionitis and low birth weight. Manifestations of infection include neonatal pneumonia, sepsis, and meningitis (Table 3.3.1). In adults, *U. urealyticum* is a common cause of nongonococcal urethritis.

Rickettsia

Rickettsial diseases are caused by organisms that possess characteristics of both viruses and bacteria. They require living cells to grow, but they also possess enzymes for protein synthesis and electron transport. Rickettsial diseases cause vasculitis of small blood vessels and fever, and are sensitive to broad-spectrum antibiotics early in the disease course.

Rickettsia rickettsii is the causative agent of Rocky Mountain spotted fever, the most common rickettsial disease in the United States (Table 3.3.1). The vectors of the disease are the dog tick, wood tick, or Lone Star tick. After a bite by an infected tick, the organisms replicate within the endothelial cells lining small blood vessels and eventually disseminate through the bloodstream. Classic manifestations include headache, high fevers, myalgias, and rash 2 to 8 days after the initial bite. The rash usually appears on day 2 or 3 on the ankles and wrists, involving the palms and soles, and continues up to the trunk (see Fig. 3.3.4). Initially, the erythematous blanching macules become maculopapular and petechial. Patients will appear toxic, with signs of meningoencephalitis. Other common findings include edema, arrhythmias, and congestive heart failure. Without treatment, mortality can approach 25%. Generally, recovery can be expected if antibiotics are initiated within the first week of the illness.

Ehrlichiosis was identified as a tick-borne disease in 1986, caused by various *Ehrlichia* sp. Human granulocytic ehrlichiosis (HGE) and human monocytic ehrlichiosis

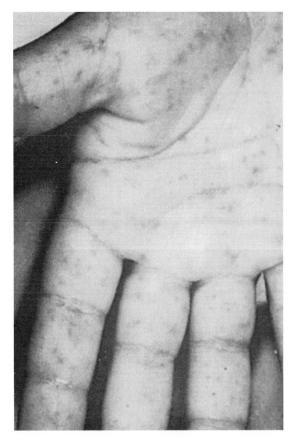

Figure 3.3.4 Petechial rash on the palm of a patient with Rocky Mountain spotted fever. (From Gorbach SL, Bartlett JG, Blacklow NR. *Infectious diseases.* 3rd ed. Philadelphia, PA: Lippincott Williams & Wilkins; 2003:1476.)

(HME) are two separate forms of the disease, but both are characterized by headache, fever, and leukopenia. The primary vector for HME is the Lone Star tick, in which the macrophage is the primary cell of involvement. For HGE, the vector is the deer tick or the black-legged tick, and the granulocyte is the main cell of involvement. The exact mechanism of the pathology is not completely understood. Classic clinical findings include fever, headache, myalgias, and anorexia (Table 3.3.1). Meningitis has been reported to occur. In children, a rash involving the extremities and trunk is common, but this is rare in adults. Other manifestations include thrombocytopenia and leukopenia, but these are usually mild. These differences involving the rash and hematologic abnormalities can help differentiate ehrlichiosis from Rocky Mountain spotted fever.

Spirochetes

Spirochetes are motile, slender, helix-shaped, heterotrophic bacteria of which only *Borrelia*, *Treponema*, and *Leptospira* cause significant diseases in humans. *Treponema pallidum*, the causative agent of syphilis, is transmitted by direct inoculation from an infected individual, with sexual contact being the most common mode of transmission. The infection is lifelong, originating with a chancre, a nontender, inflammatory lesion at the site of inoculation. Secondary disease occurs 2 to 10 weeks after the primary lesions and is manifested by lesions on the skin (particularly the palms and soles) and in the mucous membranes and the CNS. Tertiary disease occurs years after secondary syphilis, with the development of dermal lesions called *gummata*. If syphilis is not treated, those with early CNS manifestations can develop late neurosyphilis, which can include seizures, tabes dorsalis, dementia, or optic atrophy. In addition, cardiovascular complications, including aortitis and pulmonary arteritis, may develop in untreated patients (Table 3.3.1).

In congenital syphilis, the spirochetes are transmitted either by contact in the birth canal or transplacentally. Syphilis can be transmitted throughout the duration of a pregnancy. Early congenital syphilis findings include bony abnormalities, hepatosplenomegaly, hematologic abnormalities (thrombocytopenia, anemia, leukocytosis, or leukopenia), rhinitis (snuffles), rash, and CNS abnormalities (seizures, hydrocephalus). Late congenital syphilis findings include changes in dentition (Hutchinson teeth), skeletal changes (sabre shin, frontal bossing), saddle nose deformity, interstitial keratitis, and CNS abnormalities similar to early congenital disease (Table 3.3.1).

Lyme disease, another spirochete-related illness, was first recognized in 1975. The causative agent, identified as *Borrelia burgdorferi*, is transmitted to humans with the Ixodes genus of ticks as the likely vector. The organism is introduced into the bloodstream through deposited fecal material from the tick or through its saliva. Migration to the skin causes the characteristic rash of Lyme disease (see Fig. 3.3.5), or the spirochete can disseminate to distant sites through the bloodstream. The first stage of Lyme disease is characterized by localized erythema migrans at the site of the tick bite. Stage 2 of the disease can be characterized by arthralgias, headache, malaise, lymphadenopathy, and aseptic meningitis. Cardiac involvement including atrioventricular block, myocarditis, and pericarditis can be seen in up to 10% of untreated patients within several weeks of infection. Stage 3 disease includes late neurologic involvement such as fatigue and neuropsychiatric problems (more common in adults), and recurrent arthritis (Table 3.3.1).

Leptospirosis is a less common disease characterized by systemic vasculitis. The causative agent, various *Leptospira* sp. is transmitted to humans through contact with infected animals such as rodents, foxes, opossums, and cattle or by swimming in infected water. Infection is characterized by anicteric (most common) or icteric forms. Patients with anicteric leptospirosis experience chills, fever, headache, and malaise (septicemic phase), followed by a second phase (immune phase) of rash, fever, meningitis, and leptospiruria (Table 3.3.1). Icteric leptospirosis, or Weil syndrome, is characterized by jaundice. Total bilirubin

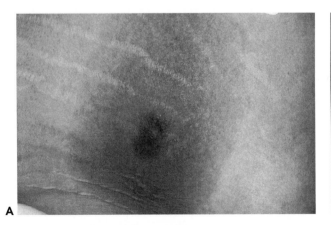
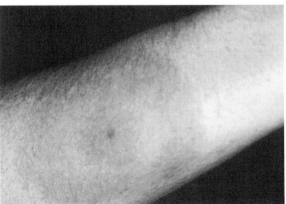

Figure 3.3.5   Examples of erythema migrans skin lesions. (From Gorbach SL, Bartlett JG, Blacklow NR. *Infectious diseases.* 3rd ed. Philadelphia, PA: Lippincott Williams & Wilkins; 2003:1817.)

concentration remains usually <20 mg per dL. Pruritus, hepatomegaly, hyponatremia, acalculous cholecystitis, proteinuria, nonspecific electrocardiographic changes, and rarely congestive heart failure and cerebrovascular accidents may be seen with Leptospirosis.

VIRUSES

The viral pathogens causing disease in the critically ill patient are extensive. Viruses are classified on the basis of the nucleic acid, either DNA or RNA (see Table 3.3.3). Further categorization is based on the capsid, the presence of an envelope, and the size and symmetry of the particle. DNA structure can be single or double-stranded, linear or circular. The capsid can be described as icosahedral or complex. RNA structure can also be single or double-stranded, linear or circular with an icosahedral or helical capsid. Typical of viral infections is the transmission into the host, replication with damage to cells, viral spread to other organs or cells, development of an immune response, and occasionally, persistence of the virus in the host. For the

intensivist, understanding the morphology and life cycle of the virus aids in directing therapeutic modalities.

DNA Viruses

Adenoviruses are common causes of illness in children. They are nonenveloped DNA viruses in the form of an icosahedron. Adenovirus causes up to 25% of respiratory illnesses in children. Transmission occurs through infected droplets. Common manifestations include upper respiratory infections, pharyngitis, tonsillitis, and conjunctivitis (Table 3.3.3). Occasionally, adenovirus is a cause of bronchiolitis and tracheitis. Severe pneumonia can also be seen, more commonly in neonates. Other manifestations include bronchiolitis obliterans, acute hemorrhagic cystitis, nephritis, gastroenteritis, hepatitis, appendicitis, pericarditis, myocarditis, and mesenteric lymphadenitis. Occasionally, meningitis and encephalitis may be seen with adenovirus.

Hepatitis B virus (HBV) is a member of the family named *hepadnavirus*. HBV is an enveloped DNA virus. Hepadnaviruses replicate like retroviruses by RNA reverse transcription. HBV infects hepatocytes preferentially, but

TABLE 3.3.3

COMMON VIRUSES OF INTEREST TO THE PEDIATRIC INTENSIVIST

Type of Virus	Virus Name	Manifestations
DNA viruses	Adenoviruses	Upper respiratory infections, pharyngitis, tonsillitis, bronchiolitis, tracheitis, and pneumonia. Meningitis and encephalitis can also be seen
	Hepatitis B virus	Hepatic disease with occasional extrahepatic manifestations including vasculitis. Important occupational health hazard through needlesticks. Chronic infection can lead to hepatocellular carcinoma
	Herpesviruses (includes HSV, varicella-zoster, cytomegalovirus, Epstein-Barr virus, human herpesviruses 6 and 7)	HSV 1, 2, and varicella-zoster virus can be latent. Encephalitis, meningitis, and neonatal sepsis can occur. Cytomegalovirus can cause congenital infections with the manifestations of jaundice, pneumonia, calcifications. This is an important pathogen for the immunosuppressed patient after bone marrow or solid-organ transplantation, or in patients with AIDS. Epstein-Barr virus causes infectious mononucleosis type syndrome but may also cause aplastic anemia, hemolytic anemia, and meningitis. Human herpesvirus 6 and 7 are important pathogens in immunosuppressed patients
	Poxviruses	Smallpox is an important biologic warfare agent
	Parvovirus B19	Causes hydrops fetalis, aplastic crisis, hepatitis, and myocarditis
RNA viruses	Hepatitis A virus	Asymptomatic or hepatitis with nausea, vomiting, and gastrointestinal pain
	Hepatitis C virus	Perinatal and transfusion-related transmission
	Hepatitis E virus	Gastroenteritis; liver failure in pregnant women
	Influenza virus	Febrile illness, cough, coryza, anorexia, pneumonia, and Reye syndrome if salicylate is used
	Respiratory syncytial virus	Bronchiolitis and pneumonia, important cause of nosocomial pneumonia in PICU. Primary prevention available for children with congenital heart disease and bronchopulmonary dysplasia
	Rotavirus	Gastroenteritis and dehydration

AIDS, acquired immunodeficiency syndrome; HSV, herpes simplex virus; PICU, pediatric intensive care unit.

immune responses play a significant role in liver damage. Transmission in humans occurs vertically, parenterally, or sexually. A significant occupational health concern is the high rate of transmission to healthcare workers through needlestick injuries (Table 3.3.3). Horizontal transmission can occur in regions where HBV is highly endemic. Hepatic disease is the primary manifestation; in adults, extrahepatic disease including vasculitis, polyarteritis nodosa, and mononeuritis occurs. The disease course includes chronic infection and an association with hepatocellular carcinoma. Hepatitis D virus (HDV) requires HBV to cause infection. HDV can be acquired as a coinfection with HBV. The extent of hepatic disease is similar to HBV and usually develops 2 months after initial exposure.

Herpesviruses include the families, herpes simplex virus (HSV) types 1 and 2, Epstein-Barr virus (EBV), cytomegalovirus (CMV), varicella-zoster virus (VZV), and human herpesviruses (HHV) 6, 7, and 8 (Table 3.3.3). HSV-1 and 2 and VZV have the unique characteristic of establishing latency in the sensory ganglia. Transmission is through genital or oral secretions. Replication occurs at the site of inoculation, usually the skin or mucous membranes. Manifestations include vulvovaginitis, gingivostomatitis, and conjunctivitis. Of importance to the intensivist is the role of HSV as a cause of encephalitis, meningitis, and neonatal sepsis. Diagnosis of HSV infections is by isolation of the organism in culture. Polymerase chain reaction assays to regions of HSV DNA are also used to effectively diagnose HSV infection.

CMV is also a member of the herpesviridae family. Infection with CMV is common, with as much as 80% of those in the lower socioeconomic groups and about half of those in the upper and middle socioeconomic groups having the CMV antibody. Transmission can be vertical, through breast milk, sexual transmission, or nosocomially. Infected cells develop large intranuclear inclusions giving a characteristic "owl's eye" appearance. Congenital infection is characterized by neonatal jaundice, thrombocytopenia, pneumonia, hepatosplenomegaly, intracerebral calcifications, microcephaly, hearing loss, and chorioretinitis. CMV can also cause a mononucleosis syndrome in healthy individuals. In patients who are immunosuppressed, CMV is a cause of hepatitis, gastroenteritis, and interstitial pneumonitis (Table 3.3.3).

EBV is similar to other members of the herpesvirus family. EBV causes latent infection of B cells and pre-B cells, possibly contributing to its pathogenesis in malignant disorders. Transmission is through infected oral secretions. EBV classically causes infectious mononucleosis, which is characterized by a prodrome of fatigue and malaise, followed by lymphadenopathy and tonsillitis and pharyngitis, and is sometimes associated with hepatosplenomegaly. Complications of EBV include aplastic anemia, hemolytic anemia, pancytopenia, encephalitis, aseptic meningitis, splenic rupture, and pneumonia (Table 3.3.3). EBV infection is associated with the development of Burkitt lymphoma, Hodgkin disease, and nasopharyngeal carcinoma.

VZV is the etiologic agent for chickenpox and shingles. VZV is also similar to other members of the herpesvirus family. Transmission is by contact with infected airborne droplets. The primary disease is manifested by chickenpox, which is an extremely contagious infection with a pruritic vesicular rash and fever. VZV establishes latency in sensory ganglia during the primary infection. Complications of the primary infection can include superinfection of the skin, encephalitis, and aseptic meningitis. Severe complications occur more frequently in patients who are immunosuppressed, and can include varicella pneumonia, glomerulonephritis, and purpura fulminans. Zoster occurs primarily in adults in the presence of impaired cell-mediated immunity. The primary manifestation of zoster is a vesicular skin rash confined to one or several dermatomal regions (see Fig. 3.3.6).

HHV 6 and 7 are important pathogens in immunocompromised patients, particularly with human immunodeficiency virus (HIV) infection. HHV-6 has been known to cause the disease roseola (exanthema subitum) and aseptic meningitis and febrile seizures in children. In immunosuppressed children, HHV-6 has been described as a cause of fulminant hepatitis. HHV-7 has been described as causing a febrile illness in children similar to roseola.

Poxviruses are brick-shaped large viruses and include variola virus and molluscum contagiosum virus. Smallpox, caused by variola virus, is a disease that has regained interest because of its potential as a biologic warfare agent (Table 3.3.3). Transmission occurs through contact with infected respiratory secretions and skin lesions. The classic manifestations of smallpox include a prodrome of fever and myalgias, followed by characteristic cutaneous lesions on the face and extremities (see Fig. 3.3.7). The eruptions become vesicular and commonly umbilicated.

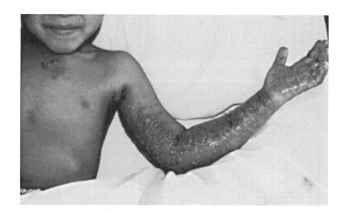

Figure 3.3.6 Herpes zoster in an otherwise healthy child. Note the dermatomal distribution of this unusually severe form, which required skin grafts to restore full range of motion. (From Gorbach SL, Bartlett JG, Blacklow NR. *Infectious diseases.* 3rd ed. Philadelphia, PA: Lippincott Williams & Wilkins; 2003:1199.)

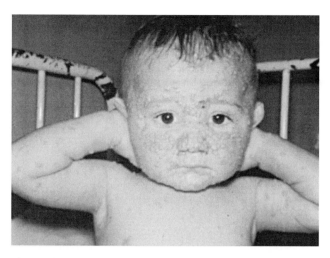

Figure 3.3.7 Appearance of rash of smallpox on day 6 and 7. All of the lesions are in the same stage of development. (From Gorbach SL, Bartlett JG, Blacklow NR. *Infectious diseases.* 3rd ed. Philadelphia, PA: Lippincott Williams & Wilkins; 2003:1208.)

A hemorrhagic form of smallpox also existed that was almost uniformly fatal. With the development of a smallpox vaccine, the disease has since been eradicated.

Parvovirus B19 is a naked DNA virus with an icosahedral shape. Parvovirus B19 is the cause of erythema infectiosum, an acute febrile illness with a characteristic exanthem (see Fig. 3.3.8). Other significant manifestations include hydrops fetalis, aplastic crisis in patients with an underlying hemolytic disease, hepatitis, myocarditis, aseptic meningitis, and encephalitis (Table 3.3.3).

RNA Viruses

Hepatitis A virus (HAV) is a naked RNA virus in the Picornaviridae family. Replication occurs in the liver, and transmission is fecal–oral. Clinical manifestations include an asymptomatic infection, or an acute hepatitis with abdominal pain, nausea, anorexia, and vomiting. Infection with HAV is similar to other forms of viral hepatitis. Complications include a relapsing course in up to 10% of patients, a fulminant hepatitis associated with encephalopathy and sepsis.

Hepatitis E virus (HEV) is a cause of outbreaks of viral hepatitis. Transmission occurs through oral ingestion without any seasonal variation. Clinical manifestations include a gastroenteritis and hepatitis similar to other forms of viral hepatitis (Table 3.3.3). In pregnant women, Hepatitis E is associated with a high risk of fetal and maternal mortality and the development of acute liver failure.

Hepatitis C virus (HCV) is a single-stranded RNA virus thought to infect up to 3% of the world's population. Transmission is perinatal, intrafamilial, sexual, and transfusion-associated. Severe hepatitis is uncommon in adults with HCV infection. Coinfection of HCV and HIV

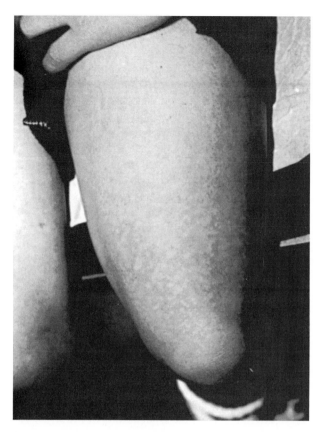

Figure 3.3.8 A lacy or reticular pattern of erythema, as evident on the thigh, is characteristic of erythema infectiosum. (From Gorbach SL, Bartlett JG, Blacklow NR. *Infectious diseases.* 3rd ed. Philadelphia, PA: Lippincott Williams & Wilkins; 2003:1220.)

should be considered. The long-term clinical course in children is less severe than infection in adults, with lower incidence of progression to cirrhosis.

Influenza is a single-stranded RNA virus classified as an orthomyxovirus. The three major types are A, B, and C, with types A and B being the main pathogens in humans. Influenza causes worldwide disease with seasonal variation. Transmission is through inhalation of infected airborne droplets by coughing and sneezing. Manifestations of influenza infection include a febrile illness with cough, coryza, anorexia, nausea, vomiting, and abdominal pain. Complications include febrile seizures, croup, secondary bacterial pneumonia, myositis, and encephalopathy (Table 3.3.3). Reye syndrome has been associated with influenza virus and the use of salicylates, and is characterized by cerebral edema and fatty degeneration of the liver. Primary prevention with vaccination is recommended for children who are at high-risk for chronic lung disease, heart disease and immunosuppression, and for those on chronic salicylate therapy.

Respiratory syncytial virus (RSV) remains one of the most clinically significant causes of disease in infants and children. RSV is a single-stranded, nonsegmented RNA virus in the family Paramyxoviridae. Peak activity of RSV occurs between November and May. RSV is the most common cause of bronchiolitis and pneumonia in infants and young children. Transmission in humans is through infected respiratory droplets or secretions. Pathologically, RSV causes a peribronchiolar mononuclear infiltration with epithelial necrosis of the small airways, leading to plugging, atelectasis, and hyperinflation. Infection can range from a mild upper respiratory illness to severe lower respiratory tract disease (Table 3.3.3). Among those presenting for medical attention, bronchiolitis and pneumonia are common manifestations. Progressive respiratory compromise requiring mechanical ventilation may occur. Nosocomial spread of RSV through environmental contamination is an increasing problem associated with significant morbidity among patients with chronic illnesses and those receiving immunosuppressive therapy. Infection control procedures are important means of limiting nosocomial spread of RSV. Primary prevention is achieved with the use of an RSV monoclonal antibody (palivizumab) in high-risk infants and young children during the RSV season to reduce the risk of significant disease.

Rotaviruses are one of the primary causes of gastroenteritis in children. Rotavirus is a member of the family Reoviridae and contains three outer shells with icosahedral symmetry. Transmission is fecal–oral. Once infection has occurred, rotavirus causes denuding of intestinal villi. The exact mechanism of inducing diarrhea in humans is incompletely understood, and it may be multifactorial. Manifestations include watery diarrhea, vomiting, and dehydration, which may require hospitalization (Table 3.3.3). Other less common manifestations that have been associated with rotavirus include meningitis, encephalitis, and pneumonia, although a direct causality cannot be determined. In 1998, a vaccine was licensed for use in the United States; however, it was removed from use after 15 cases of intussusception were noted following vaccination.

HIV is an RNA retrovirus in the Lentivirinae family that is trophic for CD4$^+$ cells. The virus has two RNA strands that are encased within a core that is surrounded by membrane receptor molecules. Three gene sequences known as *gag*, *env*, and *pol* code for the molecules that provide security to the RNA strands. The *gag* gene codes for the core proteins including the p24 antigen. The *env* gene codes for the envelope proteins, which serve to bind cells to the virus. The *pol* gene encodes for the reverse transcriptase, which assists the virus in creating viral DNA for inclusion in the cell's genome. HIV is discussed in greater detail elsewhere in this book (see Chapter 21).

FUNGI

Fungi represent significant morbidity and mortality in patients who are immunocompromised and critically ill. The classification of fungi depends largely on their mode of reproduction, either sexually or asexually, and on their growth pattern (yeast or mold). Yeasts are unicellular and reproduce by asexual budding; molds are multicellular and form as long filaments (hyphae). In some fungi, the hyphae can form walls (septate hyphae), whereas in others they do not (nonseptate hyphae). Several important fungi such as histoplasma and candida are dimorphic; that is, they form different structures at different temperatures. At body temperature, they exist as yeasts and at ambient temperature as molds. Most clinically significant fungi are obligate aerobes, whereas some are facultative anaerobes.

Among the clinically significant fungi, the *Candida* sp. play an increasing role in nosocomial infections. *Candida* does not have a capsule, and is dimorphic. A combination of infecting dose and host factors play a role in the development of candidiasis. The extent of *Candida* infection can vary from a localized skin infection to severe systemic disease. Risk factors for hospitalized patients for nosocomial fungal bloodstream infections include indwelling bladder catheters, multiple antibiotics, and the presence of a central line. Clinically, *Candida* sp. cause urinary tract infections, peritonitis following abdominal surgery or peritoneal dialysis, and pneumonia. Fungal endocarditis can commonly be associated with sterile blood cultures. Disseminated disease most likely affects patients with acquired immunodeficiency syndrome, postorgan-transplantation patients, patients with cancer, patients with central lines, and patients undergoing hyperalimentation. The brain, liver, spleen, kidney, and lungs are the most commonly affected sites of disseminated disease.

Aspergillus is also a significant pathogen in patients with compromised immunity. Reproduction is primarily through the formation of asexual spores, and the response against *Aspergillus* is mainly through phagocytosis. Invasive disease is seen more commonly in patients with neutropenia and can manifest as pneumonia, pulmonary infarction, osteomyelitis, endocarditis, and aspergillomas of the urinary tract and CNS.

Cryptococcus neoformans is found in the soil associated with avian feces and is the cause of cryptococcosis. Replication occurs through budding, and infection is by inhalation and hematogenous dissemination. Infection can occur in immunocompetent individuals, but the most severe disease is found in patients with impaired cell-mediated immunity. Clinical manifestations include meningitis (most common) and disseminated disease.

Histoplasmosis, caused by *Histoplasma capsulatum*, is the most common systemic fungal pathogen worldwide. Like *Cryptococcus*, infection is usually by inhalation of aerosolized spores located in avian feces. Clinical manifestations include pneumonitis, often presenting with wheezing, and disseminated disease presenting as failure to thrive, fever, and hepatosplenomegaly. In patients who are immunocompromised, disseminated disease can occur, with worsening hypoxia, progressive pulmonary infiltrates, leukopenia, and disseminated intravascular coagulation. A sepsislike syndrome and meningitis can also be seen with Histoplasmosis.

Pneumocystis Carinii (Now Classified Under Fungi)

Pneumocystis carinii, also known as *Pneumocystis jiroveci*, plays an interesting role, both clinically and in terms of taxonomy. Most recently classified as a fungus, it was originally identified as a parasite. Although *P. carinii* are more similar to fungi than parasites, classic antifungal drugs do not have any effect on *P. carinii*. Transmission of *P. carinii* to humans is not well understood. More than 90% of adults possess antibodies to *P. carinii*, indicating a high prevalence of asymptomatic infection. Increased recognition of *Pneumocystis* pneumonia has occurred with the acquired immunodeficiency syndrome (AIDS) epidemic, although the disease has been reported with other forms of immunodeficiency, including severe combined immunodeficiency, congenital hypogammaglobulinemia, and DiGeorge syndrome.

Clinical disease is characterized histologically by an initial stage of trophozoites and cysts attaching to alveolar walls. Alveolar cells then desquamate, leading to an extensive alveolitis. In children who are immunocompromised, clinical manifestations include tachypnea, cough, and fever, with an increased alveolar–arterial oxygen (A–a) gradient. The clinical course is variable, and depends on the immune status of the host. Radiographically, diffuse, bilateral infiltrates are common, but any pattern of disease can be seen.

The diagnosis includes use of the methenamine silver nitrate staining method of Gomori on aspirates and secretions to demonstrate cyst forms. The most reliable means for confirming *Pneumocystis carinii* pneumonia (PCP) is through the use of invasive tests such as needle aspiration and open lung biopsy. Bronchoscopy with bronchopulmonary lavage is useful as a diagnostic procedure.

PROTOZOAL AND HELMINTHIC INFECTIONS

Human parasites include the Protozoa (flagellates, amoebae, ciliates, microsporidia, coccidian, sporozoans), Platyhelminthes (cestodes, trematodes), Nematodes (roundworms), Acanthocephala, and Arthropoda. Summarizing each of these divisions in terms of the pathophysiology and reproductive cycles is difficult, as variations exist within each group.

Among the clinically significant Protozoa are the *Plasmodium* sp., *Naegleria* sp., and *Toxoplasma* sp. Malaria remains a significant health problem worldwide, with up to 2.7 million deaths per year. About half of these deaths occur in children under 5 years of age. The most prevalent

regions include Oceania, the Indian subcontinent, Africa, Southeast Asia, the Middle East, South America, and Central America. An increasing number of cases are being reported in the United States due to increasing travel to high-risk regions.

Plasmodium sp., including *Plasmodium falciparum*, *Plasmodium malariae*, and *Plasmodium vivax*, are transmitted to humans in the infective sporozoite stage through the bite of the female anopheline mosquito. The organisms asexually reproduce in the liver of the host and proliferate. At 1 to 2 weeks, these schizonts release merozoites that infect red blood cells. In this erythrocytic phase, both asexual and sexual replication occurs. In the asexual phase, red blood cells are eventually lysed, releasing merozoites; in the sexual phase, the parasites will differentiate into gametocytes, which, when ingested by a mosquito, will complete the life cycle and be able to infect another host.

Classic manifestations of malaria include fever, chills, myalgias, and gastrointestinal symptoms. Thrombocytopenia, leukopenia, and anemia can also be seen. Cerebral malaria is a severe complication of *P. falciparum* and is characterized by depressed mental status, seizures, and signs of increased intracranial pressure. Other complications include severe anemia, pulmonary edema (usually a late manifestation), and renal failure, which may require dialysis. The first-line therapy for severe, complicated malaria and for those unable to tolerate oral therapy is intravenous quinidine gluconate. Because of the increased likelihood of arrhythmias with this therapy, cardiac monitoring such as in an ICU setting is required.

Naegleria are free-living amoebae that cause fulminant meningoencephalitis. Usually the organism is acquired through swimming in untreated, warm water. The disease is characterized by a nonspecific prodrome, followed by rapidly progressing meningitis and death. Because the clinical presentation is similar to other forms of bacterial meningitis, patient history and a high index of suspicion are critical to make the diagnosis.

Toxoplasmosis is caused by *Toxoplasma gondii*, an obligate intracellular parasite. The host of *Toxoplasma* is the cat family and transmission to humans is through cat feces and undercooked meat. Infection with *Toxoplasma* is usually asymptomatic, but patients may present with fatigue and lymphadenopathy. However, in patients who are immunocompromised, manifestations can include pneumonitis, myocarditis, and encephalitis. Congenital infection occurs as a result of a primary maternal infection. The risk of maternal transmission increases over the duration of the pregnancy, with the highest risk in the third trimester. Clinical manifestations of congenital toxoplasmosis include hepatosplenomegaly, seizures, cerebral calcifications, fever, and CSF mononuclear pleocytosis. Uncommonly, pneumonitis and myocarditis may be seen.

Schistosomiasis is one of the significant helminthic infections. Five species of *Schistosoma* cause human disease: *Schistosoma mansoni*, *Schistosoma japonicum*, *Schistosoma haematobium, Schistosoma intercalatum,* and *Schistosoma mekongi.* These organisms are unique in their ability to live within the human vascular system. The intermediate host is the freshwater snail, and infections occur by contact with infected water. Once in the human bloodstream, the parasites migrate to the lungs, go across to the systemic circulation, and eventually end up in the portal system. They then travel to species-specific organs where they produce eggs. IgE and IgG antibodies to egg antigens are produced, with the immune complex deposition causing the clinical manifestations of rash, fever, and myalgias. Pneumonitis, usually self-resolving, may occur. Significant complications include hepatosplenic disease, seen with *S. japonicum* and *S. mansoni,* which is characterized by portal hypertension and hepatosplenomegaly. Progression of the parasites to the pulmonary vasculature can lead to cor pulmonale; migration to cerebral vessels can lead to seizures or cranial nerve defects.

CONCLUSION

Infectious diseases are an important component of practice in the PICU. Intensivists need to have a working knowledge of the different microbial agents and the diseases that they can cause in different patient populations.

THE CLINICIAN AND THE CLINICAL MICROBIOLOGY LABORATORY

Joseph M. Campos

Infections in pediatric critical care patients usually place patients at serious risk of morbidity and mortality. Clinical suspicion of infection is first aroused when patients exhibit one or more of the following signs and symptoms: fever, apnea, lethargy, irritability, anorexia, vomiting, jaundice, hepatomegaly, and diarrhea. When it is not possible to localize the site of infection from a history and physical examination, one of the next steps is to launch a laboratory test workup—initially to confirm the suspicion of infection and then to identify the specific cause. Some of the initial laboratory results received may provide only nonspecific evidence of infection (e.g., complete blood cell count and differential, sedimentation rate, quantitative C-reactive protein, and measurement of cytokine levels). Microbiology tests that confirm the existence of infection, identify the etiologic agent, and determine the antimicrobial susceptibility of the etiologic agent is the subject of the remainder of this chapter.

SPECIMEN SELECTION, COLLECTION, AND PROCESSING

The success that the microbiology laboratory will have in identifying the etiology of infection depends on selecting, collecting, and transporting suitable specimens to the laboratory. The site(s) of specimen collection must be chosen with care to afford the greatest likelihood of detecting microbial pathogens, their toxins, or the antibodies generated by the host. Specimen collection must be performed in a manner that minimizes contamination with endogenous host microflora. Delivery of specimens to the laboratory must be undertaken under conditions that maintain the viability of infectious agents and preserve the integrity of their components and extracellular products. Transport conditions that inhibit the growth of contaminating microflora must be chosen or the duration of transit must be brief enough to limit the growth of microorganisms. Table 3.3.4 shows guidelines for collection and transport of microbiology specimens from pediatric critical care patients.

Blood

The importance of employing aseptic technique during the collection of blood culture specimens cannot be overstated. The venipuncture site, as well as the rubber stoppers on the collection tubes or blood culture bottles, should be disinfected with a rapidly acting agent such as chlorhexidine, tincture of iodine, or povidone-iodine before introduction of a sterile needle. One bacterial or fungal contaminant introduced into a blood culture bottle can jeopardize the correct interpretation of a blood culture result. Moreover, contaminated blood cultures lead to unnecessary use of financial and personnel resources. Blood culture contamination rates should be <2% in children hospitalized in an ICU.

Current recommendations call for the collection of 0.5 to 10 mL of blood from children per blood culture bottle, depending on the age and size of the child. Less than optimal quantities of blood compromises the sensitivity of culture. Collection of paired specimens from two separate venipuncture sites or from and indwelling line plus a venipuncture site is recommended to help interpret the clinical significance of positive results. A lessening incidence of anaerobic bacteremia and a growing incidence of fungemia have led to the discontinuation of routine anaerobic blood cultures and an allocation of more blood to aerobic or fungal blood cultures. Anaerobic blood cultures should be reserved for clinical situations in which anaerobic bacteremia is a likely possibility (e.g., patients with neutropenia and those with problems in which seeding of microorganisms from the respiratory, gastrointestinal, and urogenital tracts is possible). The general consensus is that no more than three blood cultures per 24-hour period are necessary to recognize uncomplicated bacteremia.

TABLE 3.3.4
GUIDELINES FOR COLLECTION OF MICROBIOLOGY SPECIMENS FROM PEDIATRIC CRITICAL CARE PATIENTS

Specimen	Container	Other Considerations
Anaerobic culture		
Pus, aspirate	Anaerobic transport device, B30	Deliver to the laboratory immediately
Rayon/Dacron swab	Anaerobic transport device	Deliver to the laboratory immediately. Preparation of smears from a swab specimen requires a separate swab
Blood for culture		
Bacteria (aerobic)	Aerobic blood culture bottle	0.5–10 mL of blood
Bacteria (anaerobic)	Anaerobic blood culture bottle	0.5–10 mL of blood (should only be ordered in situations in which anaerobic bacteremia is likely)
Fungi	Fungal blood culture bottle or lysis direct plating tube	0.5–10 mL of blood (most yeasts will also grow well in an aerobic blood culture bottle collected for bacteria)
Mycobacteria	Heparinized tube or lysis direct plating tube	0.5–10 mL of blood
Body fluid for culture		
CSF	Sterile, leak-proof tube	Deliver to the laboratory immediately. 2 mL for each culture type (bacterial, fungal, mycobacterial, viral) is optimal
Synovial, peritoneal, pleural, etc.	Sterile, leak-proof tube	Deliver to the laboratory immediately. 2 mL for each culture type (bacterial, fungal, mycobacterial, viral) is optimal
Body fluid for antigen detection	Sterile, leak-proof tube	0.5 mL is required
Catheter tip (intravenous)	Sterile, leak-proof tube	Disinfect skin surrounding insertion site, remove catheter, clip off tip aseptically into sterile tube
Respiratory tract		
Throat (R/O *Corynebacterium diphtheriae*)	Rayon/Dacron swab	Notify the laboratory to R/O *C. diphtheriae*
Nasopharynx (R/O *Bordetella pertussis*)	Calcium alginate mini-tip swab (in lab-specified container for nucleic acid detection, in charcoal transport medium for culture, smear on two microscope slides for antigen detection)	Notify the laboratory if *B. pertussis* is suspected. PCR is more sensitive than culture, which is more sensitive than antigen detection
Nasopharynx (R/O *Chlamydia trachomatis*)	Calcium alginate mini-tip swab (smear on microscope slide for antigen detection, in lab-specified container for nucleic acid detection, in viral transport medium for culture)	Check with laboratory to determine whether nucleic acid detection test has been validated for diagnostic use
Endotracheal aspirate	Sterile, leak-proof container	Deliver to the laboratory immediately
Sputum for bacterial pathogens	Sterile, leak-proof container	Collect at least 2 mL from a deep cough and deliver to the laboratory immediately
Sputum for fungal and mycobacterial pathogens	Sterile, leak-proof container	Collect at least 5 mL from a deep cough and deliver to the laboratory immediately
Serum		
Infectious disease serology	Red top tube	Collect at least 2 mL of blood
Stool		
Bacteria	Leak-proof container; rayon/Dacron swab	Deliver to the laboratory immediately. Notify laboratory if enterohemorrhagic *Escherichia coli* or *Vibrio* spp. is suspected
Clostridium difficile toxin	Leak-proof container	25 g of stool required. Deliver to the laboratory on wet ice immediately
Clostridium botulinum toxin	Leak-proof container	25 g of stool required. Deliver to the laboratory on wet ice immediately
Tissue	Pea-sized piece of tissue bathed in sterile, nonbacteriostatic normal saline in a sterile, leak-proof container	Deliver to the laboratory immediately
Urine		
Clean catch or catheterized	Sterile, leak-proof container	Deliver to the laboratory on wet ice immediately. Bagged urine specimens strongly discouraged
Suprapubic aspiration	Sterile, leak-proof container; anaerobic transport device of anaerobic culture desired	Deliver to the laboratory on wet ice immediately
Fungal/mycobacterial culture	Sterile, leak-proof container	10 mL of urine required. Deliver to the laboratory on wet ice immediately
Wound/abscess/pus	Sterile, leak-proof container; capped needleless syringe, rayon/Dacron swab; anaerobic transport device for anaerobic culture	Preparation of smears from a swab specimen requires a separate swab

CSF, cerebrospinal fluid; PCR, polymerase chain reaction.

Body Fluids

CSF, synovial fluid, pleural fluid, peritoneal fluid, pericardial fluid, and fluids from other closed cavity body sites should be collected in sterile, leak-proof containers and delivered promptly to the laboratory. The same aseptic technique described in the preceding text for collection of blood samples also applies to collection of body fluids.

Urine

Only catheterized or suprapubically aspirated urine specimens should be collected from critical care patients. "Bagged" specimens are strongly discouraged because of the high potential for contamination and should be used only as a last resort. Catheterized specimens collected from female and uncircumcised male patients should be preceded by disinfection of the periurethral area. Despite proper disinfection, catheterized specimens inevitably are contaminated with small numbers of microorganisms, and care must be taken to prevent excessive growth of contaminants during transport to the laboratory. Maintenance of specimens at 4°C during transport or transport of specimens in commercially available boric acid preservative tubes are effective. Inoculation of agar dipslide culture devices immediately after specimen collection is also helpful in eliminating problems associated with contaminant overgrowth. Suprapubically aspirated urine essentially is a closed cavity body fluid and should be handled in the manner described in the preceding text for other body fluids.

Stool

Some enteric pathogens are harmed by changes that occur in stool maintained at room temperature after defecation. Continuing anaerobic metabolism (fermentation) results in the accumulation of acidic waste products that can kill microorganisms and damage the structural integrity of parasitic elements. pH-stabilized stool transport medium (e.g., buffered glycerolized saline) should be used if specimens cannot be tested immediately. Unfortunately, *Campylobacter* spp. do not survive well in buffered glycerolized saline, and, for detection of this pathogen, Cary-Blair stool transport medium is recommended. Stool for ova and parasite examination should be brought to the laboratory promptly after collection or placed in a formalin-based or polyvinyl alcohol–based (PVA) preservative. Stool for toxin studies (e.g., *C. difficile*, *C. botulinum*, or *E. coli* toxins) should be brought to the laboratory immediately or refrigerated to prevent loss of heat-labile activity.

Respiratory Tract Specimens

Diagnosis of lower respiratory tract infections often depends on examination of sputum, endotracheal, or gastric aspirates. Such specimens are inevitably contaminated with upper respiratory tract microorganisms, which can interfere with clinicians attempting to determine the etiology of infection. Another difficulty is that, all too often, the specimen labeled as sputum is nothing more than saliva. If a patient is unable and cannot be induced to expectorate genuine sputum from the lower respiratory tract, collection of a more invasive specimen should be considered. Aspiration of respiratory tract secretions during bronchoscopy using a suction apparatus that is protected from contamination with upper respiratory tract flora (bronchoalveolar lavage) is a frequently chosen option. Percutaneous needle aspiration of an abscess or empyema cavity and open lung biopsy are other alternatives to be considered. Collection of gastric aspirates is often relied on as an alternative to sputum for diagnosis of pulmonary tuberculosis in children. All lower respiratory tract specimens should be transported promptly to the laboratory or refrigerated until transport is possible.

Tissue

Tissue biopsies are strongly recommended for establishing the etiology of infection. A pea-sized piece of tissue delivered to the laboratory in a timely manner can be homogenized in sterile broth and used to prepare smears and inoculate cultures for aerobic/anaerobic bacteria, mycobacteria, viruses, and fungi. The primary concerns are drying of the specimen during transport and, when anaerobic infection is suspected, extended exposure of the specimen to atmospheric oxygen. Placement of tissue in a small quantity of sterile, nonbacteriostatic saline prevents drying, and delivery of tissue to the laboratory in an anaerobic transport device can allay these concerns.

Swab Specimens

Swab specimens should be considered a last resort because growth yields are always lower than those achieved by culturing the corresponding aspirate, exudate, pus, body fluid, or tissue homogenate. In addition, most microbiology laboratories require that separate swabs be submitted when multiple cultures from the same specimen site are requested. The convenience and simplicity of the use of swabs have convinced many practitioners to rely on them routinely for collection of specimens, often to the detriment of culture results.

When swabs are used for specimen collection, sterile rayon, Dacron, cotton, and calcium alginate swabs are commercially available. Because cotton is a plant fiber that contains vegetable oils that may be toxic to some microorganisms, swabs comprised of synthetic fibers are universally preferred. For the same reason, swabs with plastic shafts are superior to swabs with wooden shafts. A liquid or semisolid transport medium is often present in the swab container and is intended to maintain the viability of microorganisms during transport.

Specimens for Anaerobic Culture

Oxygen is a metabolic poison for obligate anaerobes, resulting in the intracellular accumulation of toxic metabolites. Detecting these microorganisms by culture is contingent on their survival during specimen collection, transport, inoculation, and incubation. Anaerobic specimen transport devices that include chemical processes to eliminate oxygen from specimens and from the atmosphere within the specimen container are commercially available. Microbiology laboratories should not accept specimens for anaerobic culture unless steps have been taken to ensure the survival of anaerobes.

DETECTION, IDENTIFICATION, AND ANTIMICROBIAL SUSCEPTIBILITY DETERMINATION

Microscopy

Conventional light microscopy is a central element in the early diagnosis of infectious diseases. Visualization of microorganisms and evidence of inflammation in specimens can strongly influence clinician decision making during the initial stages of patient management. The remainder of this section deals with the microscopic analyses of import to the critical care physician.

Gram Stain

The Gram stain, first described more than a century ago, remains an effective means for detecting most bacteria and many fungi in clinical specimens. Gram-positive microorganisms appear purple under the microscope, whereas gram-negative bacteria are pinkish red. Knowledge of the Gram reaction is a major help to clinicians in selecting initial antimicrobial therapy because antimicrobial agents frequently have predictable activity against gram-positive and gram-negative bacteria.

Gram stain reports should be unambiguous, concise, and informative. They should note the quantity of microorganisms seen and the presence of inflammatory cells and epithelial cells. Further characterization of inflammatory cells as mononuclear and polymorphonuclear is feasible but attempting to provide an accurate description of inflammatory cell types is not. Such information should be derived from examination of Wright- or Giemsa-stained smears.

Detection of more than one microorganism per 960x to 1,000x oil immersion field indicates the presence of at least 100,000 colony forming units per mL (cfu per mL) in an uncentrifuged specimen. This relationship is particularly helpful when examining Gram-stained smears of urine. Many laboratories routinely stain sputa to assess whether specimens contain material from the lower respiratory tract or consist primarily of saliva. Inflammatory cells should greatly outnumber epithelial cells in sputa collected from patients with lower respiratory tract infections.

Acid-fast Stain

Mycobacterium sp., *Nocardia* sp., *Legionella micdadei*, and the oocysts of *Cryptosporidium*, *Cyclospora*, and *Isospora* are detectable in acid-fast–stained smears. Several staining procedures are in current use, but all are based on the same principle—retention of tightly bound dyes in cell or oocyst walls after exposure to strong aqueous decolorization agents. Depending on the dye component of the primary stain, smears are examined with a conventional light microscope or ultraviolet light–equipped microscope. Non–acid-fast material is stained with a differently colored or fluorescence-quenching counterstain that facilitates recognition of acid-fast microorganisms.

Calcofluor White Stain

Certain dyes, such as calcofluor white M2R or Tinopal CBS-X, are added to laundry detergents to enhance the "whiteness" of clothing. The appearance of enhanced "whiteness" is attributable to the fluorescence emitted by bound dyes exposed to the ultraviolet light in sunlight and artificial light. The same dyes also bind efficiently to the polysaccharides found in fungal cell walls. Specimen smears can be stained with one of these dyes and then examined microscopically with ultraviolet illumination. Stained fungi emit a bluish white fluorescence that is easily recognized against an unstained background.

India Ink Preparation

The India ink preparation is a negative-staining technique for rapid, presumptive identification of *C. neoformans* in body fluid specimens. In a positive specimen, the microscopic carbon particles in India ink are unable to penetrate the thick polysaccharide capsule of *C. neoformans*, resulting in the formation of a distinctive halo around the organism. Because of the clinical ramification of a positive result, it is recommended that encapsulated budding yeast cells be noted in the wet mount before concluding that a test is positive.

Similar to all microscopic wet mount procedures, India ink preparations are likely to be reported as negative if fewer than 10,000 microorganisms per mL of specimen are present. A much more sensitive, and almost as rapid, test is the latex particle agglutination (PA) assay for cryptococcal antigen.

Giemsa or Wright Stain

Microscopic examination of Giemsa- or Wright-stained blood smears is the procedure of choice for recognizing patients with blood-borne parasitic infections, including malaria, babesiosis, trypanosomiasis, and filariasis. Both thick and thin smears should be prepared from fresh (preferred) or ethylene diamine tetra-acetic acid (EDTA)-anticoagulated blood. The thick smear is left unfixed and the thin smear is fixed with methanol before staining. The staining process lyses almost all of the blood cells in the thick smear, leaving intracellular parasites adherent to the microscope slide. Thick smears should be stained only with Giemsa reagents because Wright-stain reagents contain an alcohol fixative that will prevent blood cell lysis. Staining of thin smears leaves the blood cell morphologies intact, which may be required for correct identification of blood parasites.

Antigen Detection

A very large number of immunoassays for direct detection of microbial antigens in patient specimens have been developed during the last 30 years. The primary advantage of these assays is the speed with which results are available, when compared to routine culture. The disadvantages of antigen detection include a lower sensitivity and/or specificity than culture, greater expense than culture, and an inability to determine the antimicrobial susceptibility of microorganisms whose susceptibility is not predictable.

Immunofluorescence

Immunofluorescent antigen detection assays can be configured in two ways. Direct immunofluorescence is a technique in which antibody conjugated with a fluorescent dye reacts directly with microbial antigens present in specimen smears. Indirect immunofluorescence begins with an unconjugated antibody reacting with antigens present in specimen smears, followed by reaction with an antibody conjugate directed against the first antibody.

Numerous immunofluorescent antigen detection assays are used by the current microbiology laboratories. The more useful assays for patients in critical care units include those that detect antigens of *C. trachomatis*, *Legionella* spp., *Bordetella pertussis*, *P. carinii*, HSV, VZV, RSV, influenza virus, parainfluenza virus, and adenovirus.

The major advantages of these assays are the rapidity of test results (30 to 60 minutes) and the ability to visually assess the quality of antigen-negative specimens.

Particle Agglutination

Another widely used method for rapid detection of bacterial and fungal antigens is PA. In this procedure, microscopic particles (e.g., latex, charcoal, erythrocytes, *and S. aureus* cells) are coated with antibodies directed against the microbial antigens of interest. In the presence of soluble antigen, the particles agglutinate to form visible clumps. Specimens that are amenable to PA testing include urine, nonviscous body fluids, and liquid specimen extracts (e.g., nitrous acid extracts of pharyngeal swabs for group streptococcal antigen detection). Testing of viscous specimens is not possible because of nonspecific agglutination of particle suspensions.

Commercial products are available for assays that detect groups A and B *Streptococcus*, *H. influenzae* Type b, *S. pneumoniae*, *N. meningitidis*, *E. coli* K1, and *C. neoformans* antigens, among others. Standard assays call for use of two different suspensions of microscopic particles. Particles in one suspension (test suspension) are coated with antibodies directed against the antigen being sought, and particles in the other (control suspension) are coated with nonspecific antibodies of the same class used to prepare the test suspension. A positive result is indicated by agglutination of particles only in the test suspension.

The advantages of PA assays are the rapidity of their results (usually <10 minutes), better sensitivity than the immunofluorescence methods, and relatively low cost.

Enzyme Immunoassay

Enzyme immunoassay (EIA) was introduced in the 1970s as a more convenient and equally sensitive replacement for radioimmunoassay. EIAs have been configured to detect either microbial antigens or antibodies and are available in both rapid (time to test results <30 minutes) and conventional (time to test results 1 to 4 hours) assay formats. Since then, rapid EIAs have been largely replaced by simpler, more rapid methods. Conventional antigen detection EIAs are still widely used and are currently available for detection of HBV surface and e antigens, HIV-1 p24 antigen, and the capsid/envelope antigens of RSV, influenza A and B viruses, rotavirus, HSV, and VZV. In addition, EIAs for detection of microbial toxins (e.g., *C. difficile* toxins A and B and *E. coli* Shigalike toxins I and II) are also available.

There are several advantages that EIAs hold over other assay methods. They generally are an order of magnitude, or greater, more sensitive than PA assays. Most users agree that manual detection of a colored endpoint is more accurate and requires less training than detection of a PA or immunofluorescence endpoint. Finally, EIAs lend themselves well to being read with laboratory equipment (e.g., spectrophotometer), which aids in differentiating weakly positive and negative results. The cost of reagents, however, is generally higher than those for PA and immunofluorescence.

Immunochromatography

One of the more recent antigen detection assay formats to become commercially available is known as immunochromatography. The principle of this method involves reaction of microbial antigens with antibodies conjugated to colored particles. The immune complexes that form then flow (chromatograph) through a membrane reaction region coated with capture antibodies to the same microbial antigens. A positive signal is indicated by retention of the colored particles in the reaction region of the test device. The chromatography continues until the advancing "front" encounters a second set of capture antibodies directed against nonmicrobial antigenic components of the migrating particles. The completion of the assay is indicated by the appearance of a colored signal in the control region of the test device. Assays for detection of a wide variety of microbial antigens and antibodies are available in this test format, including assays for Group A streptococcal antigen, influenza A and B antigens, RSV antigens, rotavirus antigens, and *C. difficile* toxins A and B.

The primary advantage of the immunochromatography method is the simplicity and the rapidity of the assays. These assays are so easy to perform that the U.S. Food and Drug Administration (FDA) has assigned many of them to the "waived" category of test device, lending them suitable for use at the point of care. Assay times are less than 20 minutes and are frequently less than 10 minutes. The sensitivity of the results and the cost of reagents are comparable to that for PA or immunofluorescence assays.

Molecular Methods

The development of molecular diagnostic tests for the diagnosis of infectious diseases ranks as one of the most important advances ever that has occurred in clinical microbiology laboratories. These methods use microorganism-specific nucleic acid probes to detect the presence of homologous nucleic acid sequences in clinical specimens. Probe targets may be DNA or RNA and may be detected in specimens directly or after they have been amplified in number to make their detection easier. At this time, assays licensed by the FDA are commercially available for detection of *C. trachomatis*, *N. gonorrhoeae*, *M. tuberculosis*, groups A and B *Streptococcus*, HIV-1, and hepatitis B and C viruses, with many more on the horizon. Detection of nucleic acid sequences for virtually all infectious agents has already been described in the peer-reviewed scientific literature. Once the performance of such methods (known as home-brew assays) has been carefully validated by a laboratory, they can be used for patient testing.

Several target-amplification assays and one signal-amplification assay are commercially available for quantifying the number of viral nucleic acid targets present in clinical specimens. These so-called viral load assays are used initially for assessing the severity of infection and then for monitoring the success of antiviral therapy over time. "Viral load" assays for HIV-1, hepatitis B, hepatitis C, Epstein-Barr, CMV, and BK viruses, among others, are available in FDA-licensed or home-brew formats.

The main advantages of molecular diagnostic assays are the rapidity of test results compared to culture and the increased sensitivity these assays have over microscopy, antigen detection, and, oftentimes, culture. Results are available in 1 to 4 hours, compared to the several days that may be required for culture. The major disadvantages of these assays are their higher reagent costs and the ease with which specimen-to-specimen contamination with probe targets can occur.

Culture

For most infectious diseases, culture remains the mainstay for definitive diagnosis. Liquid and/or solid growth media are available for growth of most bacteria and fungi. Well-characterized eukaryotic cell lines are available for growth of many viruses and chlamydiae. Some difficult-to-culture agents are still being inoculated to chicken eggs or live animals to confirm the presence of microorganisms in clinical specimens.

There are three categories of growth media in common use by clinical microbiology laboratories: nonselective, selective, and differential. Nonselective media (e.g., 5% sheep blood agar, chocolate agar) support the growth of a wide variety of microorganisms at relatively rapid growth rates. Selective media (e.g., *Campylobacter* blood agar) contain additives that are intended to inhibit the growth of all but a select group of microorganisms. Differential media (e.g., MacConkey agar) display characteristics of growing microorganisms that aid in their presumptive identification. It is not unusual for growth media to belong to more than one of these categories (e.g., MacConkey agar, in addition to being a differential medium, is also a selective medium).

A large number of cell culture lines are available to laboratories for propagating agents that are obligately intracellular pathogens (e.g., viruses and chlamydiae). Many cell culture lines in current use originated from human tissue, some from tissues of other mammals, and others from tissues of lower animals. No cell culture line supports the growth of all agents; therefore, clinicians must inform the laboratory about the agents that are being sought in order to obtain optimal results.

Bacterial Culture

Growth of bacteria on culture media depends on selecting appropriate environmental conditions. The composition of the culture media, the content of the incubation atmosphere, the temperature of incubation, and the length of culture incubation are critical elements.

There is a wide choice of growth media to select from when inoculating bacterial cultures. Most laboratories base their media selections on the type of specimen or the site of specimen collection. The pathogens most likely to cause infection at the site from which specimens are obtained dictate the assortment of culture media to be inoculated. Therefore, it is essential that clinicians inform the laboratory of the source of specimens or whether unusual pathogens are suspected so that appropriate media are inoculated.

The standard incubation temperature for bacterial cultures is 35°C to 37°C. Other incubation temperatures are used when circumstances warrant. The incubation atmosphere for aerobic cultures on blood-containing or chocolatized blood-containing agar media should be enriched with 5% to 10% CO_2. Elevated CO_2 levels stimulate the growth of many bacteria, and a few important pathogens actually require the presence of added CO_2.

The duration of culture incubation varies with the pathogens being sought. Agar media cultures for most bacteria are routinely held for 48 to 72 hours. When slow-growing or fastidious pathogens are suspected, the laboratory should be prepared to extend the culture incubation time to as long as 8 weeks, as in the case of *M. tuberculosis*.

Once growth has occurred, bacteria can be categorized quickly on the basis of their growth characteristics and the results of a few quick tests. Knowledge of the organism's oxygen and carbon dioxide requirements, its colonial and Gram-stain morphology, and its catalase and oxidase test reactions greatly narrows the list of possible identifications. With this knowledge at hand, specific testing can be performed to obtain the definitive identification of the organism.

Bacterial Oxygen Requirements

All bacteria can be assigned to one of five categories of oxygen requirement: obligate aerobes, microaerophilic aerobes, facultative anaerobes, aerotolerant anaerobes, and obligate anaerobes. Obligate aerobes generate energy exclusively from oxygen-dependent metabolism (aerobic respiration). Microaerophilic aerobes likewise exhibit a requirement for oxygen but at a level considerably lower than the toxic level present in an ambient atmosphere. Facultative anaerobes derive energy by either oxygen-dependent or oxygen-independent fermentative metabolism. Because considerably more energy can be produced per mole of substrate during aerobic respiration, this group of bacteria, given a choice, always prefers oxygen-dependent metabolism. Aerotolerant anaerobes rely exclusively on fermentation as a source of energy, yet they can tolerate ambient levels of oxygen. Obligate anaerobes also obtain their energy from fermentation, but their growth is inhibited or they are actually killed by the presence of oxygen in the atmosphere.

Bacterial Gram-Stain Morphology

The Gram-stain morphology of a microorganism consists of its Gram reaction (gram-positive or -negative) and its structural shape (e.g., spherical or rodlike). Information about the arrangement of microorganisms, as viewed under a microscope (e.g., pairs, chains, clusters) may be helpful, but it can sometimes be misleading.

Colony Morphology

The physical appearance of well-isolated colonies growing on agar media and the condition of the media immediately surrounding the colonies can be extremely helpful during microorganism identification. The size, shape, opacity, and even the odor of colonies are features that aid in the identification of isolates. Observation of partial or complete hemolysis of erythrocytes in growth media near the edge of bacterial colonies is useful in obtaining a preliminary identification of isolates.

Bacterial Catalase and Oxidase Reactions

Bacteria that engage in aerobic respiration, for the most part, produce an enzymatic hemeprotein known as catalase that is at least partially responsible for eliminating intracellular hydrogen peroxide, a toxic by-product of oxygen-dependent metabolism. Because oxygen is not used during metabolism, aerotolerant and obligate anaerobes are usually catalase negative. The results of the catalase test, which requires no more than 30 seconds to perform in the laboratory, can be used to differentiate staphylococci from streptococci.

Another enzyme manufactured by some aerobic bacteria is cytochrome oxidase, which catalyzes the reduction of molecular oxygen to water during oxidative metabolism. The results of the oxidase test in the laboratory, which likewise requires no more than 30 seconds to perform, are useful in distinguishing members of the *Neisseria/Moraxella* genera, most *Pseudomonas* sp., and genera within the *Vibrionaceae* family from other gram-negative bacteria.

Anaerobic Bacterial Culture

Properly collected specimens from appropriate body sites that are transported to the laboratory under suitable conditions can be inoculated to nonselective and selective culture media for recovery of anaerobes. After inoculation, culture media should be placed in an anaerobic environment without undue delay. Anaerobic cultures should be incubated at $35°C$ to $37°C$. Because anaerobes grow at a slower rate than obligate aerobes and facultative anaerobes, culture plates should be incubated for at least 5 days. A companion set of aerobically incubated growth media should be inoculated from the same specimens to allow comparison of culture results. Facultative and oxygen tolerant anaerobes will grow on both sets of media—obligate anaerobes will grow only on the media incubated in an oxygen-free atmosphere.

Mycobacterial Culture

Mycobacteria are obligate aerobes that differ from most other microorganisms in that the composition of their cell walls makes them acid-fast. They also, for the most part, exhibit very slow rates of growth. In contrast to a small group of "rapidly growing" species, which form visible colonies on solid media in less than 7 days, pathogenic species yield positive cultures after 3 to 8 weeks of incubation. More and more laboratories are also inoculating specimens to bottles containing selective broth media to reduce the time to detection of positive cultures to 2 to 4 weeks. Incubating cultures are monitored for growth on a regular basis. Depending on the culture system used, the evidence of growth may be a release of $^{14}CO_2$ into the bottle atmosphere, fluorescence of the medium when illuminated by ultraviolet light, or detection of growth with a continuously monitoring blood culture instrument adapted for use with mycobacterial cultures. Liquid media cultures should be incubated for at least 4 weeks and solid media cultures for at least 8 weeks before negative results are reported.

The slow growth rate of these microorganisms places the laboratory at a definite disadvantage when trying to recover mycobacteria from contaminated specimens such as sputum. Such specimens are pretreated to eradicate nonmycobacteria that otherwise would interfere with the laboratory's ability to detect mycobacterial growth. Because the number of mycobacteria present in specimens collected from infected patients is often very low, concentration of specimens by centrifugation is a standard practice. Viscous specimens such as sputum must be chemically digested if centrifugation is to have any benefit.

Years ago, mycobacteria were classified as "typical" or "atypical." Typical mycobacteria referred to *M. tuberculosis* and *M. bovis*. The atypical mycobacteria included members of all other species except *M. leprae*. Today, the preferred term for the "atypical" group is nontuberculous mycobacteria, or MOTT (an acronym for mycobacteria other than *tuberculosis*).

Fungal Culture

The medically important fungi are a diverse group of microorganisms that cause a wide spectrum of infections. They can be classified into three groups: yeasts, molds, and dimorphic fungi. The latter group grows in the laboratory either as a yeast or a mold, depending on the incubation conditions. Fungi are sometimes grouped by the types of infections they cause. Dermatophyte fungi infect the hair, nails, and superficial layers of the skin. The fungi that cause phaeohyphomycosis, chromomycosis, and mycetoma infect the subcutaneous layers of the skin. Finally, fungi that cause disseminated infections affecting multiple organs and body sites are termed the *deep fungi.*

Most of the clinically significant fungal isolates recovered by laboratories are yeasts. Most yeast grow equally well on fungal and bacterial culture media. Likewise, some clinically significant molds, especially those that cause opportunistic infections in immunocompromised patients, grow readily and fairly rapidly on bacterial culture media.

One reason that laboratories offer fungal cultures is to enable detection of slow-growing fungi in specimens harboring large numbers of rapidly growing bacteria. Overgrowth of bacteria on nonselective media can easily inhibit or hide the growth of fungi. Selective culture media can be made inhibitory to bacteria by maintaining a low pH (e.g., Sabouraud dextrose agar) or by including antibacterial agents in the media (e.g., gentamicin and chloramphenicol). Another important reason for performing fungal cultures is the incubation conditions. Several clinically important fungi either grow poorly or do not grow at all at the standard incubator temperature of 35°C to 37°C. Therefore, fungal cultures are routinely incubated at 25°C to 30°C to allow the growth of dermatophytes and other fungi unable to tolerate higher temperatures.

Generally speaking, fungal cultures should be inoculated to a medium lacking antimicrobial agents (e.g., Sabouraud dextrose agar) and a medium containing blood, antibacterial agents, and the antifungal agent cycloheximide (e.g., brain heart infusion agar with sheep blood, chloramphenicol, gentamicin, and cycloheximide). Cycloheximide is an antifungal agent that prevents the growth of many of saprophytic fungi that occasionally contaminate nonselective media. The occasions in which specialized media are needed (e.g., cultures to rule out *Malassezia furfur*) should be communicated to the mycology laboratory. One should also keep in mind that a few important fungal pathogens (e.g., *C. neoformans*) do not grow on cycloheximide-containing media. Therefore, it is advisable to inoculate at least one cycloheximide-free medium for all fungal cultures.

Viral and Chlamydial Culture

Viruses are the smallest known infectious agents, ranging in diameter from 25 to 300 nm. Their physical structure consists of a nucleic acid polymer surrounded by a proteinaceous coat (capsid), which, in turn, may be surrounded by a host cell membrane–derived envelope. The nucleic acid polymer may be DNA or RNA, either single-stranded or double-stranded. Most human viruses are icosahedral or spherical in shape, but brick-shaped, bullet-shaped, and filamentous morphologies are known.

Cell lines for propagation of viruses are grown as monolayers on coverslips, in test tubes, in wells of microtiter trays, or in flat-sided bottles. If a particular virus is suspected, inoculation of one or more cell lines known to support the growth of the virus is necessary. If an unknown virus is suspected, cell lines that can support the growth of a variety of viruses should be inoculated.

The growth and detection of many viruses can be accelerated by the use of the shell vial technique. Specimens are inoculated by high-speed centrifugation onto a cell culture monolayer growing on the surface of a small coverslip housed in small shell vials. These cultures are examined after 24 to 72 hours of incubation for the presence of early viral antigens, usually by direct immunofluorescence.

Chlamydiae structurally resemble gram-negative bacteria but are unable to propagate in an extracellular environment. They lack the ability to generate energy and depend on the host cell as a source for adenosine triphosphate (ATP). The infectious stage is the elementary body, a small (0.25 to 0.35 μm in diameter) particle that preferentially adheres to and is taken up by mucosal columnar epithelial cells. A phagocytosed elementary body reorganizes into a metabolically active reticulate body that undergoes several cycles of division to form multiple elementary bodies. The elementary bodies then leave the host cell and infect neighboring cells or susceptible cells in a new host.

Specimens for *C. trachomatis* culture should be placed in the *Chlamydia* transport medium (e.g., 2-sucrose phosphate broth) immediately after collection. After arrival in the laboratory, specimens are inoculated to cycloheximide-treated McCoy cells by centrifuging specimens onto the cells. After 48 to 72 hours of incubation at 35°C, cell cultures are examined for the presence of inclusion bodies by staining with Giemsa, iodine, or immunofluorescence reagents.

Antimicrobial Susceptibility Testing

Antimicrobial resistance in bacteria and fungi is a growing problem of global proportions. One of the most important functions of the microbiology laboratory is production of antimicrobial susceptibility data for clinically significant microorganisms grown in cultures. These results aid clinicians in replacing empirically selected broad-spectrum antimicrobial agents with narrow-spectrum specific antimicrobial therapy.

There are two features of antimicrobial susceptibility testing that clinicians should consider as they review reports:

1. Standardized testing methods exist for a limited list of microorganisms. The reproducibility of results for microorganisms not on the list cannot be assured.
2. Test results are obtained in a controlled laboratory environment, which is much less complex than the site of a human infection. Therefore, test results can only predict the clinical efficacy of antimicrobial therapy, an assumption that clearly does not always hold.

Agar Diffusion. In this method, a microorganism suspension is inoculated to the surface of an agar plate with a swab. Filter paper disks impregnated with antimicrobial agents are applied to the agar surface. The antimicrobial agents diffuse into the agar in a radial manner, and, depending on the effectiveness of the antimicrobial agent, a zone of growth inhibition surrounds each disk. The diameters of the inhibitory zones are measured and compared to a reference chart that interprets the zone diameter for each agent as indicating a susceptible (S), intermediately susceptible (I), or resistant (R) result.

A variant of the disk diffusion method that is growing in popularity is the E-test method. This approach uses a calibrated, narrow, rectangular plastic strip that is impregnated with an antimicrobial agent concentration gradient. The test is performed in the same manner as the agar disk diffusion method except that an elliptical zone of growth inhibition forms. The intersection of the zone with the calibrated strip indicates the minimum inhibitory concentration (MIC) of the antimicrobial agent.

Broth Dilution. The broth dilution method is the reference method for antimicrobial susceptibility testing. Test results are obtained from a series of test tubes, wells of a microtiter tray, or tiny chambers of a clear plastic card, each of which contains antimicrobial agents of known varying concentrations. A microorganism suspension is inoculated into each tube, well, or chamber and incubated. The MIC is determined by visual or instrument-assisted examination of the test cultures for evidence of growth. The MIC is the lowest antimicrobial agent concentration that inhibits visible growth of the microorganism.

The broth dilution method can also be used to determine the minimum bactericidal concentration (MBC) of antimicrobial agents. The MBC is the lowest antimicrobial agent concentration that kills at least 99.9% of the original organism inoculum. Tubes or wells displaying no visible growth after incubation during an MIC determination are subcultured to determine the viable count of the survivors. If the viable count ratio of the survivors to the original inoculum is ≤0.001, killing has occurred; if the ratio is >0.001, killing has not occurred.

Agar Dilution. The agar dilution method is another means of determining antimicrobial agent MICs. This method is well suited for testing large groups of isolates simultaneously versus identical ranges of antimicrobial agent concentrations. In this method, agar test media containing antimicrobial agents at different concentrations are inoculated with small volume spots of test organism suspensions. After incubation, the MIC is the lowest antimicrobial concentration that inhibits visible growth on the agar surface.

β-Lactamase Test. The β-lactam antimicrobial agents include the penicillin, cephalosporin, cephamycin, azobactam, and carbapenem classes of antimicrobial agents. The most common mechanism of resistance to these agents is bacterial enzymatic hydrolysis of the β-lactam ring.

The β-lactamase test is a rapid means of determining whether an isolate produces a particular type of β-lactamase that is effective against certain penicillins. However, it should be remembered that many β-lactamases cannot be detected by the standard β-lactamase test and that bacteria may become resistant to β-lactam agents by mechanisms unrelated to β-lactamase production. Therefore, a positive result indicates resistance to certain penicillins, but a negative result does not guarantee susceptibility.

The test in general use today is known as the chromogenic cephalosporin test and uses a substrate that changes color when the β-lactam ring is broken. The test is performed by applying a heavy suspension of the microorganism to a piece of filter paper or to the surface of a filter paper disk that contains the β-lactam substrate. The test is incubated for as long as 30 minutes at room temperature and examined for a color change. Most positive test results are evident in less than 1 minute.

Special Tests

Clinical situations occasionally warrant requests for special tests involving antimicrobial agents. The laboratory's ability to accommodate such requests varies with the difficulty of the test procedure and the staffing level/sophistication of the laboratory. Generally, laboratories that are unable to perform special tests will forward isolates or specimens to reference laboratories for testing.

Anaerobic Susceptibility Testing. In most instances, the testing of anaerobic gram-negative bacilli for β-lactamase production is all that is required to guide antimicrobial management of anaerobic infections. However, in regions of the world with high endemic rates of resistance to agents used for treating anaerobic infections or if individual patients fail seemingly appropriate antimicrobial therapy, there may be a need to perform a more comprehensive testing.

The current standardized method for anaerobic susceptibility testing is the agar dilution method. Broth dilution and E test methods may also be performed, although there are no standardized procedures available.

Mycobacterial Susceptibility Testing. Most hospital laboratories do not recover sufficient numbers of clinically significant mycobacteria to warrant maintenance of the materials and expertise necessary for mycobacterial susceptibility testing. Testing, for the most part, is performed by reference laboratories and by laboratories located in large urban hospitals.

The reference susceptibility test method is the agar proportion method, which entails the elution of antimicrobial agents from filter paper disks immersed in agar. Mycobacterial suspensions with known cell densities are inoculated to media containing antimycobacterial agents at clinically relevant concentrations. After sufficient incubation for visible growth to be apparent, the number of colonies growing on antimicrobial agent–containing agar is determined. If the count is less than 1% of the number observed on the antimicrobial agent–free control agar, then the isolate is considered susceptible. Colony numbers greater than 1% of the control indicate resistance.

A more rapid method than the agar proportion method involves the use of radiometry. Isolates are inoculated to antimicrobial agent–containing broth media supplemented with ^{14}C-labeled growth substrates. The quantitative release of $^{14}CO_2$ during growth is compared radiometrically to that occurring in a control antimycobacterial agent–free broth. The advantage of the radiometric method is that results can be obtained in a shorter time frame.

Fungal Susceptibility Testing. A standardized broth dilution method is available for testing *Candida* spp. and *C. neoformans*. It is performed in much the same way as the broth dilution test for rapidly growing aerobic bacteria, except that a special growth medium is used and that the incubation period is extended. A similar method has been standardized for testing the filamentous fungi that cause invasive infections. Laboratories should embark on fungal susceptibility testing only if there is sufficient demand

for testing to ensure the maintenance of competency for performing these tests.

Antimicrobial Agent Synergy Testing. When more than one antimicrobial agent is administered to a patient, the effect of the combination on microorganisms may be additive, antagonistic, or synergistic. An additive effect is noted when the combined antimicrobial activity approximates the sum of the activities exhibited by the agents individually. An antagonistic effect results when the activity of the combination is markedly less than the sum of the individual activities. A synergistic effect is observed when the activity of the combination is markedly greater than the sum of the individual activities. Under most circumstances, clinicians prescribing antimicrobial agents in combination rely on their own past experience or the experience of others documented in the medical literature to guide their decision making. On rare occasions, however, it may be desirable to test a patient's isolate versus a pair of antimicrobial agents to determine whether the combination is synergistic. Such testing is difficult, time-consuming, and expensive, and should be performed only when the results are clinically necessary.

The checkerboard titration method of synergy testing is usually performed in microtiter trays. MICs of two antimicrobial agents are determined individually and in combination by testing the isolate versus stepwise concentrations of the agents alone and then testing the isolate versus the stepwise concentration combinations of the agents together. Synergy is observed when the MIC of one or both of the agents is reduced by at least fourfold in the presence of a subinhibitory concentration of the other agent.

The kill curve method of synergy testing is performed in broth culture. Serial viable counts of the test microorganism following exposure to each antimicrobial agent alone are compared to serial viable counts of the test microorganism following exposure to the antimicrobial agents in combination. The kill curve is constructed by plotting the number of surviving bacteria in each culture versus time. Antimicrobial agent synergy is defined as observing at least 10-fold fewer survivors in the culture containing the agents in combination than in either of the cultures containing the agents individually.

Serology

The antigen detection, nucleic acid detection, and culture methods discussed earlier provide direct, etiologically specific evidence of infection. This kind of evidence is preferable to antibody detection, in almost every circumstance, because the latter offers only indirect evidence of infection. However, situations exist in which antigen detection, nucleic acid detection, and culture methods are either unavailable or may generate results that are insensitive, nonspecific, or ambiguous. Antibody detection can be diagnostically important at times like this or when it is necessary to document previous infection or prior immunization with a specific infectious agent.

IgM antibodies generally appear 1 to 2 weeks after onset of infection and typically persist for 2 to 3 months. The presence of microorganism-specific IgM in sera suggests current or very recent infection. Diagnosis of congenital infections in newborns is facilitated by finding microorganism-specific IgM in cord blood samples because IgM molecules are too large to cross the fetal placenta. Serum IgG, on the other hand, freely crosses the fetal placenta. The presence of microorganism-specific IgG in cord bloods may be due to passively acquired maternal antibodies.

Serum IgG antibody titers begin rising 2 to 3 weeks after infection and may remain detectable for life. The existence of microorganism-specific IgG in individual specimens may be unrelated to a patient's current health problem because of the lengthy period over which IgG may be produced following infection. Much more useful from a clinical standpoint are antibody assays conducted on sera collected 2 to 4 weeks apart during the acute and convalescent phases of infection. Such specimens can be tested simultaneously using the same lots of reagents. Demonstration of a fourfold (or greater) rise or fall in titer of microorganism-specific IgG is considered serologic evidence of recent infection. A twofold rise or fall in titer is not clinically significant and may reflect specimen-to-specimen variation in test performance.

Rheumatoid factor (IgM antibodies directed against the heavy chain of IgG immunoglobulins) may interfere with assays for IgM-specific antibodies. This is especially so in newborns who frequently manufacture IgM antibodies directed against "foreign" maternal IgG. The microorganism-specific, transplacentally acquired, maternal IgG in uninfected infants can react with assay antigen(s). Rheumatoid factor in the same specimen can bind to these maternal IgG–antigen immune complexes, leading to the erroneous conclusion that microorganism-specific IgM has been detected—in other words, a false-positive IgM result is produced.

False-positive IgM results can be circumvented by separating IgM and IgG immunoglobulin fractions before performing the assay. Ion exchange chromatography using inexpensive, disposable minicolumns; sucrose gradient ultracentrifugation; affinity chromatography using protein A–coated Sepharose beads; or pretreatment of sera with precipitating antihuman-IgG antisera have all been used to achieve this goal.

Methods for Detection of Antibodies

Laboratories currently use a wide spectrum of assay methods for detecting antibodies.

Particle Agglutination/Agglutination Inhibition

PA assays are popular because of the simplicity and rapidity of these procedures. Most commercially available PA assays involve the use of antigen-coated latex particles, charcoal particles, bentonite particles, or erythrocytes. Specimens are mixed with antigen-coated particles on a glass or cardboard slide, placed on a mechanical rotator for 2 to 10 minutes, and examined for macroscopic PA. The PA assays for antibodies are similar in principle to the PA assays for microbial antigens described earlier, with the exception that particles are coated with antigens instead of antibodies.

Immunofluorescence

Immunofluorescence assays for detecting antibodies require a microscope equipped to provide ultraviolet illumination. Assays are based on the indirect fluorescent antibody (IFA) method, in contrast to the direct fluorescent antibody (DFA) procedure described earlier for antigen detection. IFAs differ from DFAs in that the antibody–fluorescent dye conjugate is directed against human IgG or IgM instead of infectious agent antigens. IFAs for detection of antibodies are performed by applying patient sera to smears containing infectious agents or host cells expressing infectious agent antigens. After incubation and careful rinsing, smears are flooded with antihuman IgG or IgM antibody conjugates. A second incubation-rinse cycle follows, and then smears are examined microscopically or with instrumentation for ultraviolet light–induced fluorescence.

Enzyme Immunoassay

EIA for antibody detection have grown rapidly in popularity since their introduction because EIAs lend themselves well to automation and instrumentation. EIAs for antibodies are indirect assays that include use of an antihuman IgG or IgM antibody conjugates. The relationship between direct and indirect EIAs is analogous to that between direct and IFA assays described earlier.

Indirect EIAs are 2- to 24-hour procedures. The assay is performed by incubating specimens with microorganism antigens attached to a solid phase (e.g., a plastic bead, paddle, or the walls of a microtiter tray or tube). The solid phase is thoroughly rinsed and bathed in a solution of the enzyme–anti-IgG/IgM conjugate. The incubation-rinse cycle is repeated, followed by addition of the enzyme substrate. The enzyme–antibody conjugate catalyzes conversion of the colorless substrate to a colored end product. The assay is read manually by the eye or with a spectrophotometer. The intensity of color development correlates with the amount of antibody present in the specimen.

THE ANTIMICROBIAL AGENTS

Sumati Nambiar and John N. van den Anker

The pediatric intensivist has available a number of antimicrobial agents in different classes to assist in treating diseases caused by microbial agents. This section provides insight into the different drugs available to treat infectious diseases in the PICU, and their spectrum of activity, mechanism of action, dosage, and adverse events (see Table 3.3.5).

ANTIBIOTICS

The Penicillins

Penicillins are derived from the mold *Penicillium*. All penicillins contain the 6-aminopenicillanic acid nucleus composed of a β-lactam ring and a five-member thiazolidine ring. The penicillins are categorized into four major groups, as shown in Table 3.3.6.

Natural Penicillins
Mechanism of Action
Penicillin interferes with bacterial cell wall synthesis by reacting with one or more penicillin-binding proteins (PBPs). PBPs are bacterial enzymes involved in cell wall synthesis (Table 3.3.5).

Spectrum of Activity
Penicillins have activity against gram-positive cocci and bacilli; gram-negative bacteria such as *N. gonorrhoeae*, *H. influenzae*, and *N. meningitidis*; anaerobic bacteria; and *Spirochetes* (Table 3.3.5). Penicillin resistance is mediated mainly through production of β-lactamase. Alteration of PBPs accounts for penicillin resistance among pneumococci, some strains of *H. influenzae*, and some *Neisseria* spp.

Principles of Dosing
The dosing of antibiotics is based on a balance between maximal efficacy and minimal toxicity, as well as on induction of resistance. Most of the time, dosing has to be based on surrogate markers to determine the relationships between dosing regimens, susceptibility of microorganisms, and efficacy. The three surrogate markers, or pharmacodynamic indices, predominantly used are area under the serum concentration time curve to minimum inhibitory concentration ratio (AUC/MIC), peak concentration to MIC ratio (Cmax/MIC), and the time the concentration remains above the MIC (T > MIC). In this way, the concentration–effect relationships for antibacterial agents against microorganisms can be adequately described and, when combined with pharmacokinetic knowledge, used to rationalize dosing.

In general, antibacterial agents can be divided in two groups (lactam agents and other agents). The efficacy of all β-lactam agents (penicillins, penicillinase-resistant penicillins, the extended-spectrum penicillin derivatives, cephalosporins, carbapenems, and the monobactams) depends on the time the free, non–protein-bound concentration remains above the MIC of the microorganism. The efficacy of virtually all other antibacterial agents is related

to the AUC/MIC ratio and the Cmax/MIC ratio. This has important consequences for the design of dosing regimens. It means that, for β-lactam agents, the frequency of dosing is an important factor in determining outcome. Indeed, maintaining the concentration above the MIC during the whole dosing interval has become the standard of care. This is in contrast to the aminoglycosides and fluoroquinolones, the total daily dose of which—as reflected by the AUC or peak concentration—is the most important determinant of efficacy. These latter antibiotics should therefore be given once daily.

Clinical Uses
Penicillin is effective in the treatment of infections caused by *S. pyogenes*, group B streptococci, meningococci, susceptible *S. pneumoniae*, enterococci, and gonococci. Infections caused by anaerobic mouth flora are generally susceptible to penicillins (Table 3.3.5).

Adverse Reactions
Allergic reactions are the major adverse effects associated with penicillins. Severe and occasionally fatal anaphylaxis can occur. This relates to the ability of penicillins to combine with proteins to produce hapten–protein complexes, which induce immune responses, leading to allergic reactions (Table 3.3.5). Anaphylactic reactions are estimated to occur in 0.01% to 0.05% of persons receiving penicillins. In patients with a history of life-threatening reaction to penicillin, it may be prudent to avoid other β-lactam agents. However, if no other options are available, a trial of desensitization may be attempted. Protocols have been developed for desensitization using both oral and parenteral routes. Desensitization should be performed only under close supervision. During desensitization, if mild reactions such as pruritus, fleeting urticaria, or rhinitis develop, the same dose is repeated until the patient tolerates it without systemic symptoms. However, if more serious reactions develop, the dose is withheld and, if desensitization is continued, a reduced dose should be used. Hematologic toxicity including Coombs-positive hemolytic anemia, leukopenia, and thrombocytopenia can occur with penicillin use. Sodium overload and hypokalemia can occur with massive doses of penicillin.

Aminopenicillins
Aminopenicillins have a free amino group at the α position on the β-lactam ring of the penicillin nucleus, which increases their ability to penetrate the outer membranes of gram-negative organisms.

Spectrum of Activity
Compared to penicillin G, ampicillin has increased *in vitro* efficacy against most strains of enterococci and *L. monocytogenes*, as well as against some gram-negative pathogens, such as non–β-lactamase-producing strains of *H. influenzae* and *N. gonorrhoeae* (Table 3.3.5).

TABLE 3.3.5
COMMON CHARACTERISTICS ASSOCIATED WITH DIFFERENT CLASSES OF ANTIMICROBIAL AGENTS

Class	Spectrum of Activity	Mechanism of Action/Resistance	Principles of Dosing	Dosing Guidelines (mg/kg/d)	Adverse Drug Events
Antibacterial agents					
Penicillins			Time > MIC		Hypersensitivity reactions, anaphylaxis, Coombs-positive hemolytic anemia, leukopenia, and thrombocytopenia
Natural penicillins Crystalline penicillin	Staphylococci, streptococci, *Neisseria gonorrhoeae, Haemophilus influenzae, Neisseria meningitidis,* anaerobes, *Spirochetes*	Inhibit cell-wall synthesis	Time > MIC	Mild-moderate infections 25–50,000 U in four doses IV Severe infections 250,000–400,000 U in four–six doses IV	
Aminopenicillins Ampicillin	More active against enterococci and *Listeria monocytogenes,* non–β-lactamase-producing strains of *H. influenzae,* and *N. gonorrhoeae*	Inhibit cell-wall synthesis	Time > MIC	100–150 mg in four doses IV Meningitis: 200–400 mg in four doses IV	
Extended-spectrum penicillins		Inhibit cell-wall synthesis	Time > MIC		Hypokalemia, platelet dysfunction, prolonged bleeding time
Ticarcillin ± clavulanate Piperacillin ± tazobactam			Time > MIC Time > MIC	200–300 mg in four doses IV 240 mg in four–six doses IV	
Penicillinase-resistant penicillins		Inhibit cell-wall synthesis	Time > MIC		Elevated liver enzymes
Oxacillin Nafcillin			Time > MIC Time > MIC	150–200 mg in four doses IV 100–150 mg in four doses IV	
Cephalosporins	No activity against MRSA, *Enterococcus, L. monocytogenes, Legionella, Stenotrophomonas maltophilia*	Inhibit cell-wall synthesis	Time > MIC Time > MIC		β-Lactam class allergic reactions. Patients with IgE-mediated anaphylaxis to penicillins can have cross sensitivity
First generation	MSSA, Streptococci, some gram-negative bacteria		Time > MIC		
Cefazolin			Time > MIC	50–150 mg in three–four doses	
Second generation	Better activity against *H. influenzae, M. catarrhalis, N. meningitidis, N. gonorrhoeae*		Time > MIC		
Cefuroxime			Time > MIC	100–150 mg in three doses	

Drug	Spectrum/Activity	Mechanism	PK/PD parameter	Dose	Notes/Adverse effects
Cefoxitin	Enterobacteriaceae, B. fragilis, staphylococci		Time > MIC	80–160 mg in four–six doses	
Third Generation	β-lactamase + Enterobacteriaceae, penicillin-resistant S. pneumoniae, S. pyogenes, S. aureus		Time > MIC		
Cefotaxime			Time > MIC	150–200 mg in three–four doses	
Ceftriaxone			Time > MIC	80–100 mg in one–two doses	
Ceftazidime	Pseudomonas aeruginosa, poor activity against S. aureus		Time > MIC	125–150 mg in three doses	
Fourth Generation					
Cefepime	Resistant to several β-lactamases		Time > MIC	150 mg in three doses	
Carbapenems	Streptococci, MSSA, Enterobacteriaceae, P. aeruginosa, and anaerobes. Enterococcus faecium is resistant	Inhibit cell-wall synthesis	Time > MIC		β-Lactam class allergic reactions. Patients with IgE-mediated anaphylaxis to penicillins or cephalosporins can have cross sensitivity to carbapenems
Imipenem	Has better gram-positive activity than meropenem or ertapenem. Some activity against Enterococcus faecalis		Time > MIC	40–60 mg in three doses IV	Imipenem can cause seizures, especially with high doses and in patients with renal failure
Meropenem	More active against Pseudomonas, B. cepacia		Time > MIC	60–120 mg in three doses	
Ertapenem	Less active against Pseudomonas, Acinetobacter		Time > MIC	Adults: 1 g q24h	
Monobactams					
Aztreonam	Gram-negative bacteria only		Time > MIC	120 mg in four doses	Skin rashes, nausea and diarrhea
Aminoglycosides		Inhibit protein synthesis			Nephrotoxicity, ototoxicity
Gentamicin	Enterobacteriaceae, P. aeruginosa		Cmax/MIC; AUC/MIC	3–7.5 mg in three doses	
Tobramycin	Additional activity against S. aureus. Most active against P. aeruginosa		Cmax/MIC; AUC/MIC	3–7.5 mg in three doses	

(continued)

TABLE 3.3.5 (continued)

Class	Spectrum of Activity	Mechanism of Action/Resistance	Principles of Dosing	Dosing Guidelines (mg/kg/d)	Adverse Drug Events
Amikacin	Most active against resistant gram-negative organisms, e.g., Enterobacteriaceae		Cmax/MIC; AUC/MIC	15–22.5 mg in three doses	
Lincosamides Clindamycin	Staphylococci streptococci, anaerobes, Plasmodium, Babesia, Toxoplasma	Inhibit protein synthesis	AUC/MIC	25–40 mg in three–four doses	Diarrhea, C. difficile colitis, rash
Sulfonamides Trimethoprim-sulfamethoxazole	Gram-positive and negative bacteria, Pneumocystis carinii	Inhibit folic acid synthesis	Not known	8–12 mg trimethoprim in two doses PCP: 20 mg of trimethoprim in four doses IV	Hypersensitivity reactions including Stevens-Johnson syndrome
Macrolides Erythromycin	Staphylococci, streptococci, Bacillus, Corynebacterium, Legionella, Bordetella, Campylobacter	Inhibit protein synthesis	AUC/MIC	PO: 30–50 mg in two–four doses IV: 15–50 mg in four doses	Gastric irritation, cholestatic jaundice
Clarithromycin	In addition to above, Mycobacteria, H. influenzae, Ureaplasma, Helicobacter pylori		AUC/MIC	15 mg in two doses PO	Nausea, rash, diarrhea, elevation in transaminases
Azithromycin	Similar to clarithromycin, better activity against H. influenzae		Cmax/MIC; AUC/MIC	5–12 mg once daily PO	Less gastrointestinal symptoms than erythromycin, elevation in transaminases
Fluoroquinolones		Inhibit DNA synthesis	Cmax/MIC; AUC/MIC		
Ciprofloxacin	Enterobacteriaceae and P. aeruginosa, less activity against staphylococci and streptococci		Cmax/MIC; AUC/MIC	30 mg in two doses	Rash, tremors, seizures, increase in liver enzymes, evidence of arthropathy in puppies
Levofloxacin	P. aeruginosa, Enterobacteriaceae staphylococci, streptococci, Chlamydia, Mycoplasma, Legionella and Mycobacteria		Cmax/MIC; AUC/MIC	500 mg once a day (adult dose)	Same as ciprofloxacin
Tetracyclines Doxycycline	Gram-positive and gram-negative bacteria, Chlamydia, Rickettsia, Mycoplasma	Inhibit protein synthesis	AUC/MIC	2–4 mg in one–two doses (daily adult dose 100–200 mg)	Staining of teeth, hepatotoxicity, tissue injury if extravasation occurs

Drug	Spectrum	Mechanism of action	PK/PD	Dose	Adverse effects
Glycopeptides Vancomycin	Gram-positive cocci only, active against MRSA	Inhibit cell-wall synthesis	AUC/MIC	40–60 mg in four doses, in meningitis 60-mg dose should be used	Red-man syndrome, nephrotoxicity, ototoxicity
Oxazolidinones Linezolid	Gram-positive cocci only, includes MSSA, MRSA, VRE and Streptococci	Bind to the 50S ribosomal subunit and inhibits protein synthesis	AUC/MIC	30 mg/kg in three doses, ≥12 y: 600 mg/dose q12h, IV/PO	Thrombocytopenia, myelosuppression, neuropathy
Streptogramins Quinupristin/dalfopristin	Gram-positive cocci only, including MSSA, MRSA, VREF and Streptococci. No activity against E. faecalis	Bind to ribosomes and disrupts protein synthesis	AUC/MIC	7.5 mg/kg q8–12h	Infusion site reactions, myalgia, arthralgia, hyperbilirubinemia, drug interactions
Chloramphenicol	Gram-positive and gram-negative bacteria, Chlamydia, Rickettsia, Mycoplasma, anaerobes	Inhibit protein synthesis	AUC/MIC	50–100 mg/kg/d in four divided doses	Idiosyncratic or dose-dependent bone marrow suppression; maintain peak between 15–25 mg/L, trough <12 mg/L
Metronidazole	Anaerobes, G. lamblia, E. histolytica, T. vaginalis; poor activity: anaerobic cocci, Actinomyces, Propionibacterium	Disrupting DNA synthesis	AUC/MIC	15–35 mg/kg/d in three doses	Neurotoxicity, metallic after taste
Rifampin	Mycobacteria, S aureus, N. meningitidis, H. influenzae, and Legionella	Inhibit RNA synthesis	Not known	20 mg/kg/d in two doses	Orange discoloration of secretions, hepatotoxicity, drug interactions, rapid development of resistance if used as monotherapy
Antimalarials Quinidine gluconate	All Plasmodium	May act on the digestive vesicles of intraerythrocytic parasites		10 mg/kg loading dose, maximum 600 mg over 1–2 h, followed by continuous infusion of 0.02 mg/kg/min till PO	Hypotension, prolonged QTc syndrome, hypoglycemia, tinnitus, headache
Antiviral agents Acyclovir	Herpes simplex, varicella-zoster	Inhibit synthesis of viral DNA by competitively inhibiting DNA polymerases	AUC/IC$_{90}$	IV acyclovir HSV encephalitis/varicella: 30 mg/kg/d in three divided doses Neonatal HSV: 60 mg/kg/d in three divided doses	Neurotoxicity, nephrotoxicity, obstructive uropathy, skin rash
Ganciclovir	Cytomegalovirus, Herpes simplex, varicella-zoster, Herpes B	Inhibit synthesis of viral DNA by competitively inhibiting DNA polymerases	AUC/IC$_{90}$	10 mg/kg/d IV in two divided doses	Myelosuppression, CNS side effects such as headache, confusion, psychosis and seizures

(continued)

TABLE 3.3.5 (*continued*)

Class	Spectrum of Activity	Mechanism of Action/Resistance	Principles of Dosing	Dosing Guidelines (mg/kg/d)	Adverse Drug Events
Valganciclovir Foscarnet	Same as ganciclovir Cytomegalovirus, Herpes simplex, varicella-zoster, including ganciclovir-resistant CMV and acyclovir-resistant HSV	Same as ganciclovir Direct inhibition of DNA polymerase	AUC/IC$_{90}$ Not known	900 mg twice a day PO CMV retinitis: 180 mg/kg/d in three divided doses for 3 wk, then 90–120 mg/kg once a day Acyclovir-resistant HSV: 80–120 mg/kg/d in two–three divided doses	Nephrotoxicity, metabolic abnormalities such as hypocalcemia, hypomagnesemia, hypophosphatemia, and hypokalemia, CNS effects such as seizures, tremors, hallucinations
Cidofovir	Herpes simplex including acyclovir or foscarnet-resistant strains, CMV including ganciclovir or foscarnet resistant strains, EBV, HHV-6, HHV-8, papillomaviruses, polyoma viruses, poxviruses, and adenoviruses	Inhibits synthesis of viral DNA by competitively inhibiting DNA polymerases	Not known	Induction: 5 mg/kg IV weekly for 2 wk Maintenance: 5 mg/kg every 2 wk; should be coadministered with probenecid	Nephrotoxicity, neutropenia
Lamivudine	Hepatitis B virus, HIV	Inhibits hepatitis B DNA polymerase	AUC/IC$_{90}$	3 mg/kg/d, PO maximum 100 mg/d	Elevation of transaminases
Adefovir	Hepatitis B, pox and herpesviruses	Inhibits synthesis of viral DNA by competitively inhibiting DNA polymerases	AUC/IC$_{90}$	10 mg/d PO	Headache, diarrhea, abdominal discomfort, and asthenia Higher doses can cause nephrotoxicity
Amantadine	Influenza A virus	Blocks the viral M2 protein ion channel, thereby interfering with viral uncoating	Not known	5 mg/kg/d in two divided doses	Central nervous system side effects
Rimantadine	Influenza A virus	Blocks the viral M2 protein ion channel, thereby interfering with viral uncoating	Not known	5 mg/kg/d in two divided doses	Central nervous system side effects
Ribavirin	Myxoviruses, paramyxoviruses, flavivirus, adenovirus	Alters cellular nucleotide pools, inhibits viral RNA synthesis	Not known	6 g in 300 mL delivered over 18 h by small particle generator	Anemia with oral/IV use, aerosol can cause plugging of ventilator circuits, transient wheezing

Agent	Organisms	Mechanism of action	PK/PD parameter	Dose	Adverse effects
Oseltamivir	Influenza A and B virus	Inhibits viral neuraminidase protein	AUC/IC_{90}	≤15 kg 30 mg b.i.d. PO >15–23 kg 45 mg b.i.d. PO >23–40 kg 60 mg b.i.d. PO >40 kg: 75 mg b.i.d. PO	Nausea and vomiting
Zanamivir	Influenza A and B virus	Inhibit viral neuraminidase protein	AUC/IC_{90}	≥7 y: two inhalations of 5 mg each	Bronchospasm
Antifungal agents					
Polyene Antifungals Amphotericin B Amphotericin B lipid complex Amphotericin B colloidal dispersion Liposomal amphotericin	*Aspergillus, Candida* spp., *Cryptococcus,* dimorphic fungi	Bind to ergosterol in fungal cell membrane, alters cell permeability and causes cell death	Cmax/MIC: large doses are most effective; achievement of optimal peak concentrations is important; postantifungal effect present	Amphotericin B: 0.25–0.5 mg/kg initially, increase as tolerated to 0.5–1.5 mg/kg IV ABLC: 5 mg/kg IV ABCD: 3–6 mg/kg IV Liposomal amphotericin: 3–5 mg/kg IV	Fever, chills, hypotension, headache, cardiac arrhythmias; nephrotoxicity less with lipid formulations
Azoles		Inhibit cell membrane sterols			
Triazoles Itraconazole	*Aspergillus, Candida* spp., *Cryptococcus,* dimorphic fungi		AUC/MIC	5–10 mg/kg/d, as single or two divided doses	Rash, hypokalemia, thrombocytopenia, leukopenia
Fluconazole	*Candida* spp., *Cryptococcus,* dimorphic fungi		AUC/MIC	3–6 mg/kg/d, IV single dose; PO 6 mg/kg on day 1, 3 mg/kg/d thereafter	Hepatotoxicity, drug interactions
Voriconazole	*Aspergillus, Candida* spp., *Scedosporium*		AUC/MIC	6 mg/kg q12h on day 1 followed by 4 mg/kg q12h Maintenance dose: Wt ≥40 kg, 200 mg q12h, <40 kg 100 mg q12h	Visual disturbance, rash, increased liver function tests
Flucytosine	*Candida* spp., *Cryptococcus*	Fluorine analog of cytosine, inhibits RNA and DNA synthesis	Time >MIC: for efficacy plasma concentrations >40 mg/L; to prevent toxicity concentrations <90 mg/L	50150 mg/kg/d in four divided doses	Bone marrow suppression, renal dysfunction, rash, neuropathy, hepatotoxicity
Echinocandins Caspofungin	*Aspergillus, Candida* spp., dimorphic fungi	Inhibit synthesis of β-1,3 D-glucan, an integral component of the fungal cell wall	Cmax/MIC; postantifungal effect present	70 mg loading dose, then 50 mg once daily IV	Symptoms of histamine release, hepatotoxicity especially if coadministered with cyclosporin

MIC, minimum inhibitory concentration; MRSA, methicillin-resistant Staphylococcus aureus; MSSA, methicillin-susceptible Staphylococcus aureus; AUC/MIC, area under the serum concentration time curve to minimum inhibitory concentration ratio; Cmax/MIC, peak concentration to MIC ratio; AUC/IC_{90}, area under the serum concentration time curve/inhibitory concentration 90th percentile.

TABLE 3.3.6

TYPES OF PENICILLINS

Natural Penicillins	Aminopenicillins	Penicillinase-Resistant Penicillins	Extended-Spectrum Penicillins
Penicillin G	Amoxicillin	Cloxacillin	Carbenicillin
Penicillin V	Ampicillin	Dicloxacillin	Ticarcillin
Penicillin G procaine		Oxacillin	Piperacillin
Benzathine penicillin G		Nafcillin	Mezlocillin
		Methicillin	Azlocillin

Clinical Uses

Parenteral ampicillin is widely used in neonates with sepsis because of its activity against *L. monocytogenes*. Amoxicillin is used in combination with clarithromycin and a proton pump inhibitor for the treatment of *Helicobacter pylori* infections. Amoxicillin is the drug of choice for acute otitis media, sinusitis, and other respiratory tract infections. Amoxicillin is also used for the treatment of certain clinical manifestations of Lyme disease such as erythema migrans, isolated facial palsy, and arthritis.

Adverse Events

The incidence of hypersensitivity reactions with aminopenicillins is similar to that of natural penicillins. There is a slightly higher incidence of maculopapular rash associated with ampicillin use in patients with intercurrent viral illnesses, especially due to EBV.

Antistaphylococcal Penicillins

These semisynthetic penicillin derivatives are resistant to staphylococcal penicillinases.

They are active against isolates of *S. aureus* resistant to other penicillins and have less but adequate activity against streptococci. Enterococci, gram-negative cocci, *L. monocytogenes*, and anaerobes are resistant to these penicillins (Table 3.3.5). Resistance to semisynthetic penicillins among staphylococci is related to the presence of the *mecA* gene, which results in the synthesis of a unique PBP, PBP2a, that has low affinity for methicillin and other β-lactam antibiotics.

Adverse Events

Interstitial nephritis manifesting clinically as fever, rash, eosinophilia, proteinuria, eosinophiluria, and hematuria is more commonly reported with methicillin use. Elevated levels of transaminases and cholestasis, usually without jaundice, have been reported with oxacillin use. Liver enzyme levels usually return to normal after discontinuation of therapy.

Extended-Spectrum Penicillins

Spectrum of Activity

The extended-spectrum penicillins have a broader spectrum of activity than other penicillins. Ticarcillin is active against *Pseudomonas* and some β-lactamase–producing Enterobacteriaceae but is less active than ampicillin against streptococci and relatively inactive against enterococci. Piperacillin is similar to ampicillin in activity against gram-positive species. It also has good activity against anaerobic cocci and bacilli, members of the Enterobacteriaceae family, and *P. aeruginosa*. The extended-spectrum penicillins are susceptible to hydrolysis by β-lactamases of both gram-positive and gram-negative bacteria. The extended-spectrum penicillins are generally used as fixed combination preparations with β-lactamase inhibitors. The β-lactamase inhibitors are compounds that inhibit many β-lactamases and additionally have weak antibacterial activity. Clavulanic acid is the most efficient inhibitor of staphylococcal β-lactamase. There are no significant differences in activity between the inhibitors with respect to anaerobes; therefore, they should be considered comparable with respect to extending anaerobic coverage to their partner antibiotic in treating mixed infections.

Clinical Uses

Extended-spectrum penicillins are generally used in combination with aminoglycosides for gram-negative infections such as hospital-acquired pneumonia, intra-abdominal infections, and certain complicated skin infections such as burns and trauma.

Adverse Events

The occurrence of hypersensitivity reactions in extended-spectrum penicillins is similar to that of natural penicillins. Hypokalemia, neutropenia, platelet dysfunction, and prolonged bleeding times have been observed with the use of extended-spectrum penicillins. They can inhibit platelet aggregation by binding to the adenosine diphosphate (ADP) receptor on platelets.

Cephalosporins

Cephalosporins are semisynthetic derivatives of a 7-aminocephalosporanic acid nucleus. Like penicillins, cephalosporins possess a β-lactam ring. The cephamycins are similar to cephalosporins but have a methoxy group at position 7 of the β-lactam ring. The cephamycins are discussed along with the second-generation cephalosporins.

Mechanism of Action

Cephalosporins interfere with the synthesis of peptidoglycan in the bacterial cell wall (Table 3.3.5). They bind to and inactivate PBPs. Three mechanisms of resistance to cephalosporins that have been described include inactivation by bacterial β-lactamases, alteration of PBPs, and alteration of bacterial permeability to cephalosporins.

Classification

Cephalosporins are classified into generations on the basis of their spectrum of microbiologic activity (Table 3.3.5). This classification reflects increasing stability of the higher generations to various bacterial β-lactamases. None of the cephalosporins are effective against organisms such as methicillin-resistant *S. aureus* (MRSA), *Enterococcus*, *L. monocytogenes*, *L. pneumophila*, *S. maltophilia*, *C. difficile*, and *C. jejuni*.

The first-generation cephalosporins have good activity against gram-positive cocci and relatively modest activity against many gram-negative bacteria. The second-generation cephalosporins are more active against gram-negative bacteria and have variable activity against gram-positive cocci. They have improved activity against *H. influenzae*, *M. catarrhalis*, *N. meningitidis*, and *N. gonorrhoeae*. The cephamycins have inferior activity against staphylococci but are active against some Enterobacteriaceae and *B. fragilis*. Third-generation cephalosporins are more active against the Enterobacteriaceae, including the β-lactamase–producing strains. They are also active against *S. pneumoniae* (including those with relative penicillin resistance); *S. pyogenes*; and, with the exception of ceftazidime, have clinically useful activity against *S. aureus*. They have excellent activity against *H. influenzae*, *M. catarrhalis*, *N. meningitidis*, and *N. gonorrhoeae*. Ceftazidime and cefoperazone have good antipseudomonal activity.

Fourth-generation cephalosporins have a greater spectrum of activity compared to the third-generation agents. They are stable against the chromosomally mediated AmpC β-lactamases. They are active against Enterobacteriaceae, *P. aeruginosa*, *H. influenzae*, and *Neisseria* sp. They are also effective against gram-positive cocci including methicillin-susceptible *S. aureus* (MSSA), *S. pneumoniae*, and other streptococci.

Clinical Uses

First-Generation Agents

Members of this class are widely used in the treatment of skin and soft-tissue infections. Cefazolin is used commonly for preoperative prophylaxis for surgical procedures involving foreign-body implantation and clean and clean–contaminated procedures in which there is a high risk of infection.

Second-Generation Agents

Oral second-generation agents are commonly used for the treatment of respiratory infections including community-acquired pneumonia, sinusitis, and otitis media.

Cephamycins such as cefoxitin and cefotetan are used in the treatment of intra-abdominal infections, pelvic inflammatory disease, infected decubitus ulcers, and mixed aerobic–anaerobic soft-tissue infections in which gram-negative bacteria and anaerobes are likely to be involved.

Third-Generation Agents

Cefotaxime and ceftriaxone have similar antibacterial activity. Because of its protein binding, ceftriaxone can be used once daily for most infections except meningitis, which should be treated with a 12-hourly regimen. Ceftriaxone and cefotaxime are effective in the treatment of bacterial meningitis caused by *S. pneumoniae*, *H. influenzae*, and *N. meningitidis*. Vancomycin is given in addition to cefotaxime or ceftriaxone for the empiric therapy for meningitis in children to cover for pneumococci with penicillin resistance. Third-generation cephalosporins are also useful in the treatment of nosocomial infections caused by susceptible gram-negative bacilli, including pneumonia, wound infections, and complicated urinary tract infections. Because of its antipseudomonal activity, the use of ceftazidime should be restricted to the treatment of infections caused by *P. aeruginosa*. Ceftazidime has been used in combination with aminoglycosides in the treatment of febrile neutropenia. As a single agent, ceftazidime is often used for the treatment of acute exacerbation of chronic pulmonary disease in patients with cystic fibrosis.

Fourth-Generation Agents

The use of fourth-generation cephalosporins should be limited to the empiric treatment of nosocomial infections in which there is a high likelihood of AmpC β-lactamase-producing organisms. Cefepime is indicated for the treatment of nosocomial infections when extended-spectrum β-lactamase (ESBL) or chromosomally induced β-lactamase resistance is present.

Adverse Reactions

Hypersensitivity reactions are the most common adverse events seen with cephalosporins. History of prior immediate hypersensitivity reaction to β-lactams should preclude the use of cephalosporins. Cephalosporins are generally safe in patients with history of prior non—IgE-mediated nonsevere reactions. Some delayed hypersensitivity reactions are compound-specific and not class-specific. Hence, some patients who develop hypersensitivity reactions to second-generation cephalosporins can tolerate a third-generation agent.

Granulocytopenia, anemia, and immune-mediated thrombocytopenia have been associated with cephalosporin use. Interstitial nephritis and acute tubular necrosis can occur rarely in association with cephalosporin use. Biliary pseudolithiasis can occur with ceftriaxone use. Several cephalosporins have been implicated in triggering seizures, particularly in patients with renal impairment, when the dosage was not reduced. Ceftriaxone has been associated with fatal immune-mediated hemolytic anemia in patients with underlying HIV infection, sickle cell disease, and leukemia.

Carbapenems

Carbapenems are derivatives of thienamycin, a compound produced by the soil organism *Streptomyces cattleya*. These compounds contain a β-lactam ring fused to a five-member ring similar to that of penicillin. Carbapenems bind to PBPs and therefore inhibit cell wall synthesis (Table 3.3.5). Imipenem is metabolized by the dehydropeptidase I (DHP-I) found in renal brush border and hence is coadministered with cilastatin, a DHP-I inhibitor. Meropenem and ertapenem are stable to DHP-I.

Spectrum of Activity
Carbapenems have a broader spectrum of activity than other β-lactams and are fairly similar in their antibacterial activities. All have good activity against hemolytic streptococci, penicillin-susceptible *S. pneumoniae*, and MSSA (Table 3.3.5). They are active against most species of Enterobacteriaceae and *P. aeruginosa*. *E. faecium* is resistant to the carbapenems. Anaerobic organisms including *B. fragilis*, *Clostridium* sp., and *Fusobacterium* sp. are also susceptible. The carbapenems possess stability against a wide variety of β-lactamases.

Imipenem is bacteriostatic against penicillin-susceptible strains of *E. faecalis*. Meropenem and ertapenem are less active against gram-positive organisms and more active against gram-negative aerobes than imipenem. Meropenem has greater activity against *B. cepacia* than imipenem. Ertapenem has less activity against *Pseudomonas* and *Acinetobacter*. Meropenem is the most active carbapenem against *Pseudomonas*. *Nocardia* spp. is inhibited by imipenem and meropenem.

Clinical Uses
The carbapenems should be reserved for the treatment of serious polymicrobial infections or aerobic gram-negative bacteria infections that are resistant to other β-lactam agents. Carbapenems are often used for the treatment of nosocomial pneumonia, intra-abdominal infections, soft-tissue infections, and pulmonary exacerbation in patients with cystic fibrosis and febrile neutropenia. Meropenem is approved for the treatment of bacterial meningitis in children 3 months of age and older. Ertapenem has a long half-life and hence is administered once a day. It is not approved for use in children.

Adverse Reactions
The carbapenems are generally well tolerated. β-Lactam class allergic reactions are the most common drug-related clinical adverse events reported. Patients with IgE-mediated anaphylaxis to penicillins or cephalosporins can have cross sensitivity to carbapenems. Imipenem can cause seizures, especially with high doses and in patients with renal failure.

Monobactams

Aztreonam
Aztreonam is a monocyclic β-lactam compound originally isolated from *Chromobacterium violaceum*. It differs from other β-lactams structurally in its unique monocyclic β-lactam nucleus. Aztreonam is the only currently available synthetic monobactam antibiotic.

Mechanism of Action
Aztreonam inhibits bacterial cell wall synthesis. It has a high affinity for penicillin-binding protein 3 (PBP3) present in gram-negative bacteria.

Spectrum of Activity
Aztreonam exhibits *in vitro* activity against gram-negative pathogens, including members of the Enterobacteriaceae family and *P. aeruginosa*. It is less active than ceftazidime or imipenem against most strains of *P. aeruginosa*. Aztreonam has no significant antibacterial activity against gram-positive organisms or anaerobes. Aztreonam resistance may be mediated by β-lactamases or by alterations in outer membrane porin proteins.

Clinical Uses
Patients with IgE-mediated anaphylactic reaction to penicillins or cephalosporins appear not to react to aztreonam. Aztreonam can be used to treat a variety of infections such as those of the urinary tract, respiratory tract, skin and skin structure, and intra-abdominal infections. Because its spectrum of activity is limited to gram-negative organisms, aztreonam should not be used as a single agent for empiric therapy in seriously ill patients if gram-positive or anaerobic infections are a possibility (Table 3.3.5).

Adverse Reactions
Aztreonam is relatively well tolerated. Adverse reactions reported include skin rashes, nausea, and diarrhea.

Aminoglycosides
Aminoglycosides are natural or semisynthetic derivatives of *Streptomyces* or *Micromonospora* sp. Gentamicin, amikacin, and tobramycin are the commonly used aminoglycosides.

Mechanism of Action

Aminoglycosides inhibit protein synthesis by binding to the 30S subunit of ribosomes.

Spectrum of Activity

The activity of aminoglycosides is primarily against gram-negative organisms including Enterobacteriaceae, *Pseudomonas*, and *Acinetobacter* (Table 3.3.5). It has limited activity against MSSA. Tobramycin has the greatest antipseudomonal activity. Amikacin is the most active against organisms that are resistant to other aminoglycosides. Streptomycin and gentamicin are active against *Brucella* and *Francisella*. Amikacin has activity against certain nontuberculous mycobacterial species. Streptomycin and kanamycin have antituberculous activity.

Clinical Uses

Aminoglycosides are commonly used for the treatment of gram-negative bacillary infections. Because of its synergistic activity against group B streptococci and *Enterococcus*, gentamicin is used in combination with penicillins for the treatment of infections caused by these organisms. Aerosolized tobramycin is used in patients with cystic fibrosis.

Amikacin is more effective than other aminoglycosides against many nosocomial Enterobacteriaceae. In addition to treatment of tuberculosis, streptomycin is effective in the treatment of tularemia, plague, and brucellosis.

Adverse Reactions

All aminoglycosides have ototoxic and nephrotoxic potential (Table 3.3.5). Ototoxicity is characterized by both hearing loss and vestibular dysfunction. Amikacin and kanamycin are more likely to cause cochlear damage, and streptomycin and gentamicin are more likely to cause vestibular dysfunction. Aminoglycoside-induced nephrotoxicity is usually a reversible nonoliguric renal failure. Aminoglycosides can cause neuromuscular blockade when coadministered with anesthetic agents or neuromuscular relaxants.

Lincosamides

Clindamycin and lincomycin are lincosamides. Lincomycin has no advantages over clindamycin and is not generally used.

Mechanism of Action

Clindamycin acts by binding to the 50S ribosomal subunit and inhibiting protein synthesis.

Spectrum of Activity

Clindamycin is active against most gram-positive cocci including staphylococci, *S. pneumoniae*, and other streptococci (Table 3.3.5). It has no activity against enterococci. It is also active against anaerobes including *Actinomyces*, *Bacteroides*, and *Peptococcus*. Clindamycin is effective against certain protozoans such as *Plasmodium*, *Babesia*, and *Toxoplasma*.

Clinical Uses

Clindamycin is useful in the treatment of intra-abdominal, gynecologic, and osteoarticular infections. Clindamycin has good penetration of most tissues, especially the bone. However, it does not attain adequate levels in the CSF even in the presence of meningeal inflammation. Clindamycin is an acceptable alternative in patients with IgE-mediated anaphylaxis. Clindamycin has activity against some community-acquired MRSA strains. It is also effective in the treatment of toxoplasmosis, *P. falciparum* malaria, and in the treatment of babesiosis in combination with quinine.

Adverse Reactions

The main adverse event associated with clindamycin use has been the development of *C. difficile*—associated diarrhea and pseudomembranous colitis (Table 3.3.5). Other adverse reactions include elevation of hepatic enzyme levels, skin rash, and eosinophilia.

Macrolides

Erythromycin

Mechanism of Action

Erythromycin is a naturally occurring macrolide that acts by binding to the 50S ribosomal subunit and inhibiting protein synthesis.

Spectrum of Activity

Erythromycin is active against staphylococci, streptococci, *Legionella*, *Bordetella*, *Chlamydia*, *Mycoplasma*, and *Ureaplasma*.

Clinical Uses

Erythromycin is the drug of choice for the treatment of pertussis, diphtheria, *C. trachomatis* pneumonia, or conjunctivitis.

Adverse Reactions

The most common adverse effect of erythromycins is gastrointestinal discomfort (Table 3.3.5). They can also cause reversible cholestatic jaundice. Prolonged QT interval, ventricular tachycardia, and local irritation can occur with intravenous administration.

Macrolides are potent inhibitors of CYP3A4 and, hence, care should be exercised if coadministered with other drugs metabolized through this system.

Clarithromycin and Azithromycin

Clarithromycin and azithromycin are semisynthetic derivatives of erythromycin. They have better oral bioavailability, fewer gastrointestinal side effects, and a broader spectrum of activity.

Spectrum of Activity

Clarithromycin has greater activity than erythromycin against most streptococci including *S. pyogenes*, *S. pneumoniae*, and MSSA (Table 3.3.5). Azithromycin is less active than erythromycin against these organisms. Azithromycin is more active than both erythromycin and clarithromycin against gram-negative bacteria, especially *H. influenzae* and *M. catarrhalis*. Clarithromycin is more active than azithromycin against *M. avium* complex. Both have good activity against *Mycoplasma*, *Chlamydia*, and *Legionella*.

Clinical Uses

Both clarithromycin and azithromycin are effective in the treatment of several respiratory tract infections including pharyngitis, sinusitis, and community-acquired pneumonia.

Although both have *in vitro* activity against *B. pertussis*, limited clinical data are available for this use. Erythromycin is still considered the drug of choice. Clarithromycin and azithromycin are used for the treatment of *M. avium* infections. Clarithromycin is also used for the prophylaxis of *M. avium* infections and for the treatment of other nontuberculous mycobacterial infections. A single 1-g dose of azithromycin is effective in the treatment of chlamydial infections. Clarithromycin is useful in the treatment of *H. pylori* peptic ulcer disease in combination with other agents.

Adverse Reactions

Gastrointestinal adverse reactions are less than that seen with erythromycin. Elevation of levels of transaminases and reversible cholestatic hepatitis has been reported during therapy.

Sulfonamides

The sulfonamides are synthetic analogs of *p*-amino benzene sulfonamide. They are generally used in a 5:1 combination with trimethoprim. Trimethoprim is a 2,4 diamino pyrimidine.

Mechanism of Action

Sulfonamides act sequentially by inhibiting enzymes of the folic acid pathway, thereby inhibiting DNA synthesis. They inhibit incorporation of *p*-aminobenzoic acid (PABA) into tetrahydropteroic acid, and trimethoprim interferes with conversion of dihydrofolate to tetrahydrofolate.

Spectrum of Activity

The spectrum of activity for sulfonamides includes some strains of staphylococci, streptococci, *Nocardia*, certain Enterobacteriaceae, and *P. carinii*.

Clinical Uses

In an ICU, the main use for sulfonamides is for the treatment of *P. carinii* pneumonia. They are also useful therapy for brucellosis, nocardiosis, and some cases of gram-negative bacteremias.

Adverse Effects

The most frequent adverse effects of sulfonamides are skin reactions, including the potential to cause Stevens-Johnson syndrome. The frequency of adverse events is higher in patients with AIDS.

Tetracyclines

Tetracyclines are semisynthetic agents that contain the four-member tetracycline nucleus.

Mechanism of Action

Tetracyclines act by inhibiting protein synthesis by binding to the 30S and 50S ribosomal subunits (Table 3.3.5). They are available as oral and intravenous formulations. Doxycycline is the preferred formulation for intravenous use.

Spectrum of Activity

Tetracyclines have a broad spectrum of activity, including some gram-negative and gram-positive bacteria, *Rickettsia*, *Chlamydia*, and *Mycoplasma* sp. (Table 3.3.5). Doxycycline is also active against *Plasmodium* spp. Resistance to tetracyclines is usually due to efflux pumps or by ribosomal protection.

Adverse Reactions

Tetracyclines can inhibit bone growth in neonates and cause staining and deformation of nonerupted teeth. Other adverse effects include hepatotoxicity, nephrotoxicity, pseudotumor cerebri, and photosensitivity reactions (Table 3.3.5). Intravenous administration can cause pain, phlebitis, and tissue damage if extravasation occurs. Absorption of tetracyclines is reduced if coadministered with food or antacids.

Clinical Uses

Tetracyclines are effective in the treatment of a variety of infections, including those due to *Rickettsia*, *Chlamydia*, and *Mycoplasma*; early Lyme disease; and brucellosis. In certain clinical conditions, such as Rocky Mountain spotted fever, ehrlichiosis, cholera, and anthrax, the use of doxycycline is justified in children younger than 8 years. Doxycycline is recommended for the treatment of inhalational and cutaneous anthrax and for postexposure prophylaxis against inhalational anthrax. It is also recommended for the treatment and postexposure prophylaxis against plague and tularemia.

Chloramphenicol

Chloramphenicol is a synthetic antibacterial agent that is still used in many parts of the developing world. In the United States, it is used primarily as an alternative in patients with infections due to resistant organisms.

Mechanism of Action
Chloramphenicol inhibits protein synthesis by binding to the 50S subunit of 70S ribosomes.

Spectrum of Activity
Chloramphenicol is active against streptococci; gram-negative bacteria including *Salmonella*, *Shigella*, and Enterobacteriaceae; and anaerobes including *B. fragilis*, *Clostridium*, and *Fusobacterium*. It is also active against *Rickettsia*, *Chlamydia*, and *Mycoplasma* (Table 3.3.5).

Clinical Uses
Chloramphenicol is used clinically in the treatment of rickettsial infections such as Rocky Mountain spotted fever, typhus, and Q fever. It is also effective in the treatment of typhoid fever in areas of the world where the bacterium is still susceptible and where alternate therapies are not available. It has also been used for the treatment of bacterial meningitis due to *S. pneumoniae*, *H. influenzae*, and *N. meningitidis* in penicillin-allergic patients. Chloramphenicol has activity against vancomycin-resistant *E. faecium*. Chloramphenicol is an alternative for the treatment and postexposure prophylaxis against plague and for the treatment of tularemia.

Adverse Reactions
The main adverse reaction associated with chloramphenicol is bone marrow suppression, which can be caused by two different mechanisms (Table 3.3.5). One is a dose-dependent, reversible suppression, which usually occurs after 1 week of therapy, and the other is an irreversible idiosyncratic aplastic anemia. Idiosyncratic anemia occurs in approximately 1 in 25,000 to 40,000 patients. In neonates, gray baby syndrome characterized by abdominal distension, vomiting, cyanosis, circulatory collapse, and death can occur. This syndrome results from the limited ability of the neonate to conjugate chloramphenicol. Serum levels of chloramphenicol should be monitored; peak levels should be 10 to 20 μg per mL in patients with nonmeningeal infections and 15 to 25 μg per mL in patients with meningeal infections. Trough levels should be less than 12 μg per mL.

Rifamycins

The rifamycin class of antibacterial agents includes rifampin, rifabutin, rifapentine, and rifaximin.

Mechanism of Action
Rifampins suppress RNA synthesis by inhibiting transcription of DNA-dependent RNA polymerase.

Spectrum of Activity
Rifampin is active against mycobacteria, and other organisms including *S. aureus*, *N. meningitidis*, *H. influenzae*, and *Legionella*. Rifabutin is highly active against *M. avium* complex. Compared to rifampin, rifapentine has slightly less activity against staphylococci. Resistance to rifampin results from mutations in the *rpo*B gene encoding the β subunit of RNA polymerase.

Clinical Uses
In addition to its role in the treatment of mycobacterial infections, rifampin is used for the prophylaxis of contacts of patients with infection due to *H. influenzae* Type b or *N. meningitidis*. In combination with other agents, rifampin is used for the treatment of serious infections by *S. aureus*, such as endocarditis, osteomyelitis, and orthopedic implant infections. In children with infected ventriculoperitoneal shunts or vascular grafts, due to *S. aureus* or coagulase-negative staphylococci, addition of rifampin may result in better bacteriologic cure. Rifabutin is generally used for the treatment of *M. avium* infections in patients with HIV. In patients receiving protease inhibitors, rifabutin should generally be avoided. Rifapentine is approved for the treatment of tuberculosis. Resistance develops rapidly if rifampin is used alone for treatment. Cross-resistance can occur between rifampin and other rifamycins.

Adverse Reactions
Rifampin can cause hepatotoxicity, orange coloration of urine, and other biologic secretions (Table 3.3.5). Sensitization to rifampin, characterized by flulike illness, shocklike syndrome, acute hemolytic anemia, or thrombocytopenia, is more common with intermittent therapy. Rifabutin can cause leukopenia, anemia, and thrombocytopenia. Rifapentine has an adverse event profile similar to that of rifampin. Rifamycins are potent inducers of CYP3A4. This can result in increased metabolism and hence reduction in serum levels of the coadministered drug(s) being metabolized by this system. Rifabutin is the least potent inducer of this enzyme system.

Metronidazole

Metronidazole is a synthetic 5-nitroimidazole agent that has antibacterial and antiprotozoal properties.

Mechanism of Action
The 5-nitro group of metronidazole is reduced intracellularly to unstable intermediate compounds that cause disruption of DNA synthesis.

Spectrum of Activity
Metronidazole is active against anaerobes, including *B. fragilis*, *Clostridium*, and *Prevotella*. It has variable activity against gram-positive cocci, such as *Peptococcus*, and gram-positive

bacilli, such as *Actinomyces* and some *Propionibacterium* spp. Resistance to metronidazole has been reported in some isolates of *B. fragilis* and other anaerobes, and among *H. pylori*, *Trichomonas*, and *Giardia*.

Clinical Uses

Metronidazole has very good tissue penetration and is therefore effective in the treatment of brain abscess and intra-abdominal infections. Because anaerobic infections are generally polymicrobial, metronidazole is not used as monotherapy. It is also used for the therapy for *C. difficile*–associated diarrhea, *H. pylori* peptic ulcer disease, trichomoniasis, intestinal and hepatic amebiasis, and giardiasis (Table 3.3.5).

Adverse Effects

Metronidazole is associated with neurotoxicity, including peripheral neuropathy, headache, seizures, and encephalopathy, and is usually seen in patients who receive prolonged therapy or high doses. It commonly causes a metallic taste after oral and intravenous administration.

Oxazolidinones

Linezolid
Mechanism of Action
Linezolid is the only approved member of this class of synthetic compounds. It acts by binding to the 50S ribosomal subunit and inhibiting protein synthesis. It is available as an oral and intravenous formulation.

Spectrum of Activity
Linezolid is active against gram-positive organisms including staphylococci, streptococci, and enterococci. Linezolid is effective against MRSA and VRE. Resistance to linezolid has been described among isolates of *S. aureus* and VRE.

Clinical Uses
Linezolid is currently approved for the treatment of skin and soft-tissue infections, infections caused by vancomycin-resistant *E. faecium* (VREF), and community-acquired and hospital-acquired pneumonia.

Adverse Reactions
Adverse events associated with linezolid use include thrombocytopenia, myelosuppression, peripheral and optic neuropathy, and lactic acidosis. Linezolid is a weak monoamine oxidase inhibitor. No cases of serotonin syndrome were reported during clinical trials.

Streptogramins

Quinupristin-Dalfopristin
Mechanism of Action
Quinupristin-dalfopristin is a 30:70 water-soluble combination of two streptogramin antibiotics and is available

only as an intravenous formulation. It acts by binding to ribosomes and disrupting protein synthesis.

Spectrum of Activity
Quinupristin-dalfopristin is active against staphylococci including methicillin-resistant strains; streptococci; and *E. faecium*, including vancomycin-resistant strains (Table 3.3.5). *E. faecalis* is intrinsically resistant to quinupristin-dalfopristin.

Clinical Uses
Quinupristin-dalfopristin is currently approved for the treatment of VREF infections and skin and skin structure infections caused by MSSA or *S. pyogenes*. The drug has not been approved for use in children. The recommended dosing for adults is 7.5 mg per kg every 8 hours for VREF infections and every 12 hours for skin and soft-tissue infections. This dose has been reported to be safe in children.

Adverse Reactions
Infusion site reactions such as pain, inflammation, edema, and thrombophlebitis can occur in patients receiving quinupristin-dalfopristin through a peripheral vein (Table 3.3.5). The drug is incompatible with normal saline and has to be administered in 5% dextrose. It can also cause arthralgia and myalgia, usually with no elevation in creatine phosphokinase (CPK) values. It is a potent inhibitor of CYP3A4 and hence should be used with caution in patients taking drugs metabolized through this system.

Lipopeptides

Daptomycin
Daptomycin is a cyclic lipopeptide antibacterial agent derived from the fermentation of *Streptomyces roseosporus*.

Mechanism of Action
Daptomycin binds to bacterial membranes and causes a rapid depolarization of membrane potential. The loss of membrane potential leads to inhibition of protein, DNA, and RNA synthesis, resulting in bacterial cell death.

Spectrum of Activity
In vitro, daptomycin is bactericidal against staphylococci (methicillin susceptible and resistant), streptococci, and enterococci (vancomycin susceptible and resistant).

Clinical Uses
Daptomycin is currently approved for use in adults at a dosage of 4 mg per kg every 24 hours for the treatment of complicated skin infections.

Adverse Reactions
Elevations in CPK levels can occur during daptomycin therapy. Patients should be monitored for the development

of muscle pain or weakness. Also, CPK levels should be monitored weekly, and daptomycin should be discontinued in patients with unexplained signs and symptoms of myopathy in conjunction with CPK elevation >1,000 U per L (approximately 5 × upper limit of normal [ULN]), or in patients without reported symptoms who have marked elevations in CPK levels (>10 × ULN). On the basis of animal data, there is a possibility of developing neuropathy in patients receiving daptomycin.

Quinolones

Quinolones are synthetic antibacterial agents. Nalidixic acid is a nonfluorinated quinolone, whereas most clinically useful quinolones are fluorinated. The fluoroquinolones have a broader spectrum of activity compared to the nonfluorinated quinolones.

Mechanism of Action
The quinolones act by inhibiting DNA gyrase and topoisomerase IV, thereby inhibiting DNA replication.

Spectrum of Activity
Quinolones have good activity against most gram-negative bacteria, including Enterobacteriaceae and *P. aeruginosa*, and are less active against staphylococci and streptococci. Levofloxacin has an expanded spectrum that includes most gram-positive and gram-negative organisms, *Chlamydia*, *Mycoplasma*, and *Legionella*. Ciprofloxacin is the most active quinolone against *P. aeruginosa*. Fluoroquinolone resistance is probably related to mutations in the DNA gyrase or alteration in outer membrane protein.

Clinical Uses
Quinolones are being increasingly used in pediatric patients. Most experience with use in children has been in patients with cystic fibrosis. Their main role in pediatric patients is in the treatment of bronchopulmonary infections in patients with cystic fibrosis, complicated urinary tract infections, chronic suppurative otitis media, multidrug-resistant gram-negative infections, resistant salmonella or shigella infections, and resistant mycobacterial infections. Ciprofloxacin is recommended for the treatment of inhalational and cutaneous anthrax and also for the postexposure prophylaxis of inhalational anthrax in children. It is also recommended for the treatment and postexposure prophylaxis against plague. It is an alternative drug for the treatment of tularemia in children.

Adverse Reactions
Quinolones are generally well tolerated. Gastrointestinal symptoms such as anorexia, nausea, and vomiting are commonly seen. Neurologic effects such as headache, tremors, confusion, and insomnia have been reported. Quinolones can cause prolongation of the QT interval and should be avoided or used with caution in patients taking antiarrhythmics. Elevation in levels of liver enzymes, creatinine, and blood urea nitrogen (BUN), and hematologic abnormalities such as eosinophilia, leukopenia, and thrombocytopenia can also occur with quinolone therapy. Quinolones inhibit cytochrome P-450 activity and hence can interfere with the metabolism of certain drugs. Absorption of quinolones is significantly reduced if administered concomitantly with magnesium and aluminum salts.

Fluoroquinolone antibiotics are not recommended for use in patients younger than 18 years because of concerns of cartilage and joint toxicity initially observed in juvenile animal studies. The mechanism of quinolone-induced joint toxicity is not clear. Weight-bearing joints such as the hips, knees, and shoulders seem particularly prone. Fluoroquinolones have been used in children with difficult-to-treat infections for whom the benefit of quinolone therapy may outweigh the risks. Review of safety data of ciprofloxacin-treated children showed that the rates of arthralgia and quinolone-induced cartilage toxicity were low.

ANTIVIRALS

Antiviral agents are used for the treatment and prevention of viral disease. The virus needs to multiply actively for the drug to exert its antiviral activity. Hence, they have no effect on latent viruses. Antiviral agents can interfere with virus entry, viral genome replication, or viral assembly or release. Resistance to antivirals is seen more often in patients with high viral load, infections with viruses that have high intrinsic mutation rates, and with selective drug pressure, as seen in patients who have received prolonged or multiple courses of therapy.

Nucleoside Analogs

Acyclovir and Valacyclovir
Acyclovir is an analog of 2'-deoxyguanosine. Valacyclovir is the L-valyl ester of acyclovir that is rapidly converted in the body to acyclovir. It is available only as an oral formulation, and its bioavailability is three to five times that of acyclovir.

Mechanism of Action
In the body, acyclovir is converted to acyclovir triphosphate, which inhibits synthesis of viral DNA by competing with 2'-deoxyguanosine triphosphate as a substrate for viral DNA. Incorporation of acyclovir into viral DNA stops DNA synthesis, and this is an irreversible process. Acyclovir triphosphate is far less toxic to human cellular DNA polymerase compared to viral DNA polymerase. Oral bioavailability of acyclovir is only 15% to 25%.

Spectrum of Activity
Acyclovir is effective for the treatment of infections caused by HSV types 1 and 2 and VZV (Table 3.3.5). Its activity

against HSV is 10-fold higher than that against VZV. EBV is only moderately susceptible *in vitro*, and its activity against CMV is limited. The antiviral spectrum of valacyclovir is similar to that of acyclovir.

Clinical Uses

Acyclovir is effective for the treatment of HSV infections including genital herpes, herpes labialis, HSV encephalitis, neonatal HSV infections, and VZV infections including primary varicella, and herpes zoster in immunocompetent and immunocompromised patients. The dose of acyclovir and valacyclovir should be reduced in patients with impaired renal function.

Adverse Reactions

Precipitation of acyclovir crystals in renal tubules can occur if the maximum solubility of free acyclovir is exceeded or if the drug is administered by bolus injection. Renal failure, in some cases resulting in death, has been observed with acyclovir therapy. Concomitant use of other nephrotoxic drugs, preexisting renal disease, and dehydration make further renal impairment with acyclovir more likely.

Thrombotic thrombocytopenic purpura/hemolytic uremic syndrome (TTP/HUS) has been reported in immunocompromised patients receiving acyclovir therapy. Patients receiving acyclovir can develop encephalopathic changes characterized by lethargy, obtundation, tremors, confusion, hallucinations, seizures, or coma.

Ganciclovir and Valganciclovir

Ganciclovir is a nucleoside analog of guanosine. Valganciclovir is the L-valyl ester of ganciclovir and is rapidly converted to ganciclovir after oral administration.

Mechanism of Action

In vivo, ganciclovir is converted to ganciclovir triphosphate, which in turn inhibits viral DNA polymerase. The half-life of ganciclovir triphosphate in CMV-infected cells is 16.5 hours compared to 2.5 hours with acyclovir. The higher intracellular concentrations of ganciclovir triphosphate and its prolonged intracellular half-life make it far superior to acyclovir in inhibiting the replication of CMV. The oral bioavailability of ganciclovir is 6% to 9%.

Spectrum of Activity

Ganciclovir has been shown to be active against CMV and HSV in human clinical studies.

Clinical Uses

Ganciclovir is currently approved for the treatment and chronic suppression of CMV retinitis in immunocompromised patients and in the prevention of CMV disease in transplant recipients. Valganciclovir is indicated for the treatment of CMV retinitis in patients with AIDS. It is also indicated for the prevention of CMV disease in kidney, heart, and kidney–pancreas transplantation patients at high risk (donor CMV seropositive/recipient CMV seronegative [D+/R−]).

Ganciclovir has been shown to be effective in the treatment of CMV pneumonia and gastrointestinal tract infections in patients with AIDS and in solid-organ transplant recipients. In bone marrow transplant recipients, better outcomes are reported when CMV pneumonia is treated in combination with intravenous immunoglobulin or CMV immunoglobulin. Intravenous ganciclovir prophylaxis has also been used in bone-marrow and solid-organ transplant recipients. Intravenous ganciclovir is recommended for initial treatment of herpes B virus infections, particularly with CNS involvement. The dose of ganciclovir and valganciclovir should be reduced in patients with impaired renal function.

Adverse Reactions

Myelosuppression is the major dose-limiting toxicity of ganciclovir. Granulocytopenia and thrombocytopenia occur in approximately 25% of patients receiving ganciclovir. Other adverse events include CNS side effects such as headache, confusion, psychosis, and seizures.

Penciclovir

Penciclovir is structurally similar to ganciclovir. Its metabolism and mechanism of action is similar to that of acyclovir. Its oral bioavailability is poor, and it is currently approved only as a topical formulation for the treatment of herpes labialis.

Famciclovir

Famciclovir is the diacetyl-6-deoxy analog of penciclovir. It is well absorbed after oral administration and rapidly metabolized to penciclovir, which is effective against genital herpes and herpes zoster infections.

Cidofovir

Cidofovir is an acyclic phosphonate nucleoside analog. Because it contains a phosphonate group, viral specific enzymes are not required for initial phosphorylation.

Mechanism of Action

Cidofovir is converted to its active diphosphate form, which inhibits viral DNA synthesis by competitive inhibition of DNA polymerase. The active form of the drug has a much higher affinity for viral DNA polymerase compared to cellular polymerase.

Spectrum of Activity

Cidofovir has inhibitory activity against human herpesviruses, including CMV, EBV, HHV-6, and HHV-8, and other DNA viruses including papillomaviruses, polyoma viruses, poxviruses, and adenoviruses (Table 3.3.5). Because it is phosphorylated by cellular enzymes and not by viral enzymes, cidofovir is active against acyclovir- and foscarnet-resistant HSV isolates and ganciclovir- and foscarnet-resistant CMV isolates.

Clinical Uses

Intravenous cidofovir is approved for the treatment of CMV retinitis in patients with AIDS. It has been used to treat acyclovir- or foscarnet-resistant mucocutaneous HSV infections, invasive adenoviral infections in transplant recipients, and refractory BK virus–associated nephropathy in renal transplantation patients. The dose of penciclovir, famciclovir, and cidofovir should be reduced in patients with impaired renal function.

Adverse Reactions

Nephrotoxicity is the major side effect of intravenous cidofovir. Cidofovir causes proximal renal tubular dysfunction including proteinuria, glycosuria, azotemia, metabolic acidosis, and, less commonly, Fanconi syndrome. To reduce the potential for nephrotoxicity, cidofovir is coadministered with probenecid preceded by intravenous hydration. Neutropenia develops in about one fourth of patients.

Ribavirin

Mechanism of Action

Ribavirin is a synthetic guanosine analog. It is converted by intracellular enzymes to its 5'-phosphate derivatives.

Mechanism of Action

The active metabolites of ribavirin interfere with the capping and elongation of messenger RNA.

Spectrum of Activity

In vitro ribavirin has activity against a variety of RNA and DNA viruses including myxoviruses, paramyxoviruses, arenaviruses, bunyaviruses, herpesviruses, and adenoviruses. It does not inhibit severe acute respiratory syndrome SARS coronavirus *in vitro*.

Clinical Uses

Ribavirin is available as oral, intravenous, and aerosolized formulations. Ribavirin aerosol is approved for the treatment of RSV bronchiolitis in hospitalized children. Oral ribavirin is approved for the treatment of chronic hepatitis C infection in combination with interferons.

Clinical efficacy has been demonstrated in infections due to Lassa fever, hemorrhagic fever with renal syndrome, and certain other hemorrhagic fevers.

Aerosolized ribavirin in combination with intravenous immunoglobulin appears to have some benefit in bone marrow transplant recipients with RSV pneumonia. Ribavirin has not been very effective in the treatment of infections due to other respiratory infections such as parainfluenza and influenza. Ribavirin should not be used in patients with chronic kidney disease because of the high risk of severe anemia.

Adverse Reactions

Systemic ribavirin causes dose-dependent anemia due to hemolysis and at higher dosages because of bone marrow suppression. Other reported adverse effects include elevation of serum bilirubin, pruritus, myalgia, rash, and cough. Aerosolized ribavirin may cause conjunctival irritation, bronchospasm, and rash. Health care workers can be exposed to ribavirin while working with infants receiving aerosolized ribavirin. Because ribavirin has been shown to be teratogenic in animal species, it is contraindicated in pregnant women or in women likely to become pregnant during exposure to the drug. When ribavirin is used in conjunction with mechanical ventilation, care should be taken to prevent plugging of valves and tubing.

Other Nucleoside Analogs

Lamivudine

Lamivudine is a cytidine analog that is metabolized intracellularly to lamivudine triphosphate, which inhibits hepatitis B DNA polymerase in addition to HIV reverse transcriptase. It is effective as monotherapy for the treatment of chronic hepatitis B. At doses used to treat chronic hepatitis B, it is generally well tolerated. Lamivudine-resistant strains are usually susceptible to adefovir. The dose of lamivudine should be reduced in patients with impaired renal function.

Adefovir

Adefovir dipivoxil is a diester prodrug of adefovir. It is an adenosine analog that has *in vitro* activity against a range of DNA and RNA viruses including hepatitis B, HIV, and pox and herpesviruses. Intracellularly, it is converted to adefovir diphosphate. Adefovir dipivoxil is approved for treatment of chronic hepatitis B. Main adverse events reported are headache, diarrhea, abdominal discomfort, and asthenia (Table 3.3.5). At higher doses it can cause nephrotoxicity. The dose of adefovir should be reduced in patients with impaired renal function.

Inorganic Pyrophosphate Analogs

Foscarnet

Foscarnet is an inorganic pyrophosphate analog with good activity against human herpesviruses.

Mechanism of Action

Unlike nucleosides, foscarnet sodium does not require phosphorylation by thymidine kinase or other kinases. It directly inhibits viral DNA polymerase by blocking the pyrophosphate binding site. It is available only as an intravenous formulation.

Spectrum of Activity

Foscarnet inhibits replication of herpesviruses *in vitro*, including CMV and HSV-1 and HSV-2. It is inhibitory for most ganciclovir-resistant CMV and acyclovir-resistant HSV and VZV (Table 3.3.5). Resistance to foscarnet is caused by point mutations in DNA polymerase of HSV and CMV. Foscarnet-selected CMV mutations generally do not cause cross-resistance to ganciclovir or cidofovir, but simultaneous resistance to all three drugs has been reported.

Clinical Uses

Foscarnet is approved for the treatment of CMV retinitis in patients with AIDS, ganciclovir-resistant CMV infections, and acyclovir-resistant HSV or VZV infections. The dose of foscarnet should be reduced in patients with impaired renal function.

Adverse Reactions

Nephrotoxicity is the major dose-limiting side effect. Risk factors for nephrotoxicity include high doses, rapid infusion, dehydration, and concurrent use of other nephrotoxic agents. Azotemia, proteinuria, acute tubular necrosis, crystalluria, and renal tubular acidosis have been described with foscarnet administration. Foscarnet can cause metabolic abnormalities such as hypocalcemia, hypomagnesemia, hypophosphatemia, and hypokalemia. Intravenous foscarnet should be administered at a fixed rate using an infusion pump to minimize the possibility of acute metabolic abnormalities. Other side effects include headache, tremors, rash, diarrhea, abnormal liver function test results, and painful genital ulcerations.

Tricyclic Amines

Amantadine and Rimantadine

Amantadine and rimantadine are symmetric tricyclic amines. Their activity is limited to influenza A viruses.

Mechanism of Action

Both drugs inhibit the replication of influenza A viruses by blocking the viral M2 protein ion channel, thereby interfering with viral uncoating. They have no effect on influenza B virus. Both drugs have good oral bioavailability.

Clinical Uses

Amantadine and rimantadine are used for the treatment and prevention of influenza A infections. For the treatment of influenza A, the drugs should be started within 48 hours of onset of symptoms. Both drugs are approximately 70% to 90% protective against clinical illness caused by influenza A. The dose of amantadine should be reduced in patients with impaired renal insufficiency, but the dose of rimantadine should be reduced only in patients with a creatinine clearance of 10 mL per minute or less.

Adverse Reactions

Amantadine causes anxiety, insomnia, confusion, and other CNS side effects in approximately 10% to 30% of healthy subjects. Severe neurotoxic reactions such as tremors, hallucinations, or seizures may be seen in patients receiving high doses. Cardiac arrhythmias and death can occur with elevated serum amantadine levels. The risk of CNS side effects is lower with rimantadine.

Neuraminidase Inhibitors

Zanamivir and Oseltamivir

Zanamivir and oseltamivir are related drugs that interfere with the function of the influenza neuraminidase enzyme and are effective against influenza A and B viruses. Zanamivir is inhaled through the mouth, whereas oseltamivir is given orally.

Mechanism of Action

Zanamivir and oseltamivir act by inhibition of the neuraminidase enzyme, with subsequent interference with deaggregation and release of viral progeny. Neuraminidase enzyme permits the virus to penetrate the surface of cells and is also necessary for the optimal release of virus from infected cells.

Clinical Uses

Both drugs are approved for the treatment of influenza A or B infections in persons who have been symptomatic for less than 48 hours. The efficacy of zanamivir has been demonstrated in preventing naturally occurring influenza illness. Administration of oseltamivir for 6 weeks during the peak of influenza season has been shown to reduce the risk of contracting influenza.

Zanamivir is approved for adults and children 7 years of age or older, and oseltamivir is approved for children 1 year of age and older. Reductions in the dose are recommended in patients with a creatinine clearance of less than 30 mL per minute, but precise guidelines for use in patients with renal insufficiency are not yet available.

Adverse Reactions

The most common adverse effects of oseltamivir are nausea and vomiting. Zanamivir has been associated with bronchospasm in some individuals and is generally not recommended for use in patients with underlying airway disease.

ANTIFUNGALS

Antifungal agents are available for topical and systemic use. This section discusses most systemic antifungals, with the exception of those used to treat dermatophytic infections. Some of the newer antifungals have been discussed, although pediatric data is limited.

Polyene Antifungals

Amphotericin B–based formulations

Amphotericin B (AmB) is a polyene macrolide antifungal. It is available as a colloidal suspension with the detergent sodium deoxycholate and as lipid-based formulations.

Mechanism of Action

AmB acts by binding to ergosterol in the fungal cell membrane, thereby altering cell permeability and causing cell death (Table 3.3.5).

Spectrum of Activity

AmB is effective against most *Candida* sp. Some species, especially *C. lusitaniae*, can have reduced susceptibility. *Scedosporium apiospermum* and *Fusarium* sp. are often resistant (Table 3.3.5).

Principles of Dosing

Clearance of AmB from plasma is slow, with a β-half-life of 24 to 48 hours and a terminal half-life of 15 days and longer. Dose adjustment is not necessary in patients with unrelated renal or hepatic dysfunction. Hemodialysis does not affect plasma concentrations of AmB. Infants and children seem to clear the drug from plasma more rapidly than adults. AmB displays concentration-dependent fungicidal activity (Cmax/MIC) and exhibits a postantifungal effect of up to 12-hour duration. There is no need to monitor AmB concentrations.

Clinical Uses

AmB deoxycholate is indicated for the treatment of candidiasis. *C. albicans* usually responds to 0.5 to 1 mg/kg/day; higher doses may be needed for nonalbicans species. Infections with invasive aspergillosis or mucormycosis are treated with 1.5 mg/kg/day. AmB is also effective in the treatment of infections due to *C. neoformans*, *H. capsulatum*, *Sporothrix schenckii*, and *Zygomycetes*. Local instillation of AmB has been used in certain infections such as candida cystitis or coccidioidal meningitis.

Adverse Reactions

Infusion-related adverse effects include fever, chills, nausea, vomiting, diarrhea, and headache. These reactions are usually more common after the first few infusions. Less commonly reported adverse events include hypotension, cardiac arrhythmias, neurotoxicity manifesting as hyperthermia, confusion, psychotic behavior, and convulsions.

Pretreatment with acetaminophen, with or without diphenhydramine, and/or hydrocortisone often reduces febrile reactions. In children refractory to conventional premedication regimen, meperidine and ibuprofen have shown to be effective. Slowing the infusion rate may also be beneficial. The most significant toxicities of AmB are nephrotoxicity and myelosuppression (Table 3.3.5). It has a vasoconstrictive effect on the afferent renal arterioles, resulting in reduced renal blood flow. Hypokalemia, hypomagnesemia, and renal tubular acidosis can occur during AmB therapy.

Lipid Formulations

Three lipid-based formulations are available in the United States; one is a liposomal formulation and the other two are aggregates of lipids and AmB. AmB lipid complex (ABLC) is a phospholipid ribbon structure consisting of almost equimolar concentrations of AmB and lipid. AmB colloidal dispersion (ABCD) consists of disclike colloidal particles of cholesterol sulfate and AmB. Liposomal AmB consists of AmB incorporated into the lipid bilayer of a liposome.

The lipid formulations offer certain advantages over conventional AmB, including increased daily dose of the parent drug, high tissue concentrations in the primary reticuloendothelial organs (lungs, liver, and spleen), decrease in infusion-associated side effects (especially liposomal AmB), and reduction in nephrotoxicity. Lipid formulations of AmB do not achieve adequate levels in the kidney and hence may have reduced effectiveness in infections of the kidney or bladder. Superiority in clinical efficacy has however not been definitively established. Moreover, these formulations are considerably more expensive than conventional AmB. Most experts recommend restricting use of the lipid formulations to patients with renal dysfunction, to those intolerant of or unresponsive to AmB deoxycholate, or as initial therapy for critically ill patients with *Aspergillus* infections that require high-dose AmB.

Azoles

Azoles are composed of two classes, the imidazoles and triazoles, on the basis of the presence of two or three nitrogen atoms in the azole ring.

Mechanism of Action

Azole antifungal agents inhibit fungal cytochrome P-450–dependent 14α-sterol demethylase, resulting in depletion of ergosterol, the major sterol in fungal cell membranes.

Triazoles

Fluconazole and Itraconazole

Spectrum of Activity. Fluconazole (FLC) and itraconazole (ITC) are both triazoles with activity against dermatophytes, *Candida*, *C. neoformans*, and dimorphic fungi. *C. krusei* and *C. glabrata* are intrinsically more resistant to azoles. Development of FLC resistance has been documented in *Candida* spp. ITC has activity against *Aspergillus* sp. Both are available as oral and intravenous formulations.

Principles of Dosing. FLC exhibits linear plasma pharmacokinetics, independent of route and formulation, which supports once-daily dosing. Steady state is reached in 4 to 7 days with once-daily dosing, but this might be reached more rapidly by doubling the dose on the first day of treatment. Dose adjustments are needed if there is renal impairment but not with hepatic impairment. FLC is dialyzable. For optimal efficacy, the area under the concentration-time curve is the most predictive pharmacodynamic parameter.

The drug exerts a concentration-dependent postantifungal effect of 1 to 4 hours.

With ITC, steady state is reached in 7 to 14 days with once-daily dosing, but this might be reached more rapidly by doubling the dose over the first 2 to 3 days. Dosing adjustments are indicated with hepatic impairment. More importantly, intravenous ITC is contraindicated with a creatinine clearance <30 mL per minute because of the impaired elimination of hydroxypropyl-β-cyclodextrin, which is used as a solubilizer. There are no data to support the optimal way for predicting efficacy.

Clinical Uses. FLC is effective in the treatment of oropharyngeal and esophageal candidiasis and of candidemia in immunocompetent hosts and in preventing relapse of cryptococcal meningitis in patients with AIDS. AmB remains the treatment of choice in patients with neutropenia and with hepatosplenic or disseminated candidiasis. FLC is not indicated for treatment of aspergillosis. ITC is approved for the treatment of blastomycosis, histoplasmosis, and aspergillosis.

Adverse Reactions. The most common adverse events with triazoles are nausea, vomiting, diarrhea, elevation in transaminases, and skin rash. The triazoles can cause significant drug interactions mainly by altering hepatic metabolism through the cytochrome P-450 system. ITC needs an acidic environment for absorption; hence, antacids and H_2-receptor antagonists can decrease its bioavailability.

Voriconazole

Voriconazole (VCZ) is a triazole antifungal agent. The intravenous formulation contains the solubilizing agent sulfobutyl ether cyclodextrin sodium (SBECD), which can accumulate in patients with moderate to severe renal impairment.

Spectrum of Activity. VCZ has *in vitro* activity against isolates of *Aspergillus* spp.; *Candida* spp. including *C. albicans*, *C. parapsilosis*, *C. krusei*, and *C. glabrata*; *S. apiospermum*; and *Fusarium* spp. VCZ also has activity against isolates of *C. neoformans*, *Trichosporon* spp., and variety of molds such as *Blastomyces dermatitidis*, *Coccidioides immitis*, and *H. capsulatum*.

Principles of Dosing. VCZ exerts nonlinear pharmacokinetics and has a plasma half-life of 6 hours, with elimination primarily occurring by oxidative hepatic metabolism. The major isoenzyme involved in VCZ metabolism is CYP2C19, but CYP2C9 and CYP3A4 also play a role. There is a large interindividual variability in disposition, partly explained by the polymorphically expressed CYP2C19. In patients with mild to moderate hepatic impairment,

dosing adjustment is indicated. For the oral formulation, no changes are needed if there is renal impairment, but intravenous VCZ is contraindicated with a creatinine clearance <50 mL per minute because of the impaired elimination of its intravenous carrier. For optimal efficacy, the area under the concentration-time curve is the most predictive pharmacodynamic parameter.

Clinical Uses. The recommended dosage of VCZ for the treatment of adults is 6 mg per kg intravenously every 12 hours for two doses, followed by 4 mg per kg every 12 hours. Oral maintenance dosages are 200 mg every 12 hours for patients weighing >40 kg and 100 mg for patients weighing ≤40 kg. It is approved for the treatment of acute invasive aspergillosis, candidemia in non-neutropenic hosts, disseminated candidiasis, esophageal candidiasis, and serious fungal infections caused by *Scedosporium apiospermum* and *Fusarium* spp. Limited data is available on use of VCZ in pediatric patients using the same dosing regimen as in adults.

Adverse Reactions. Drugs cleared through the CYP450 system may interact with VCZ. Coadministration of VCZ with rifampin, rifabutin, efavirenz, ritonavir, carbamazepine, long-acting barbiturates, sirolimus, cisapride, quinidine, or ergot alkaloids is contraindicated. The most common adverse events with VCZ include visual disturbances such as transient altered perception of light, photopsia, chromatopsia, or photophobia. Visual adverse events tend to occur early in therapy and disappear on stopping therapy. Hepatic enzyme abnormalities, mainly elevated transaminases and, less commonly, elevation in alkaline phosphatases and bilirubin, occur during VCZ therapy. Monitoring of hepatic enzymes during therapy is recommended. Skin reactions including photosensitivity reactions can also occur.

Other Azoles

Ketoconazole

Ketoconazole is an imidazole that has activity against yeast, such as *Candida* spp. and *Cryptococcus*, and dimorphic fungi, including *Histoplasma*, *Coccidioides*, and *Blastomyces*. Ketoconazole can cause elevation in hepatic enzymes and, rarely, fatal hepatic necrosis. It also has the potential for drug interactions with several drugs. With the availability of newer antifungals, ketoconazole is not used very frequently. Posaconazole, a derivative of ITC, and ravuconazole, a derivative of FLC, have a spectrum of activity including yeasts and molds. Both drugs are not yet approved for use.

Echinocandin lipopeptides

Caspofungin is the only FDA-approved echinocandin. Others such as micafungin and anidulafungin are under development. They have poor bioavailability and hence need to be administered intravenously.

Mechanism of Action

Echinocandins noncompetitively inhibit synthesis of β-1,3 D-glucan, which is an integral component of the fungal cell wall, but it is not present in mammalian cells.

Caspofungin

Spectrum of Activity

Caspofungin has *in vitro* activity against *Candida* spp., *Aspergillus* spp., and some dimorphic molds such as *H. capsulatum*, *C. immitis*, and *B. dermatides* (Table 3.3.5). Certain yeasts such as *C. neoformans* and *Trichosporon* are resistant to caspofungin. Activity against molds such as *Fusarium* spp., *Scedosporium* spp., and *Zygomycetes* is also limited.

Principles of Dosing

Caspofungin has a β-half-life of between 10 and 15 hours that allows for once-daily dosing. They are metabolized by the liver and slowly excreted into urine and feces. It exerts concentration-dependent fungicidal activity and prolonged postantifungal effects of up to 12-hour duration.

Clinical Uses

Caspofungin is indicated for empiric therapy for presumed fungal infections in patients with febrile neutropenia, treatment of candidemia, esophageal candidiasis, and treatment of invasive aspergillosis in patients who are refractory to or intolerant of other therapies. A 70-mg loading dose should be administered on day 1, followed by 50 mg daily thereafter for all indications. Patients with esophageal candidiasis were studied with a 50-mg daily dose.

Adverse Reactions

Caspofungin is relatively well tolerated. Possible histamine-mediated symptoms including rash, facial swelling, pruritus, sensation of warmth, or bronchospasm can occur (Table 3.3.5). Anaphylaxis can occur during administration of caspofungin. Abnormal liver function test results have been reported with caspofungin therapy, more so in patients receiving concomitant cyclosporin.

Flucytosine

Mechanism of Action and Spectrum of Activity

Flucytosine is a fluorine analog of cytosine that inhibits RNA and DNA synthesis. Because of rapid development of resistance, it is not useful as a single antifungal agent. Its spectrum of activity is limited to *Candida* spp., *C. neoformans*, and some molds.

Principles of Dosing

Flucytosine displays concentration-dependent antifungal activity. Peak plasma concentrations 2 hours postdosing between 40 and 60 mg per L correlate with antifungal efficacy. Monitoring of plasma concentrations is essential to avoid toxicity (goal: <90 mg per L) and optimize efficacy (goal: >40 mg per L).

Clinical Uses

Flucytosine is given in combination with amphotericin B in patients with certain *Candida* infections such as meningitis, endocarditis, and hepatosplenic disease, and in patients with cryptococcal meningitis.

Adverse Effects

Adverse effects include nausea, vomiting, diarrhea, rash, and headache. Significant adverse events are hepatotoxicity, bone marrow suppression, and enterocolitis (Table 3.3.5). Myelosuppression is dose-related. Hepatic function, renal function, and leukocyte and platelet counts should be monitored during therapy.

ACKNOWLEDGMENTS

Supported in part by grant KO-8 HS14009-01, Agency for Healthcare Research and Quality, Rockville, MD.

Supported in part by grant 1 U10HD045993-02, National Institute of Child Health and Development, Bethesda, MD.

RECOMMENDED READINGS

1. American Academy of Pediatrics. Antimicrobial agents and related therapy. In: Pickering LK, ed. *Red book: 2003 report of the committee on infectious diseases.* 26th ed. Elk Grove Village, IL: American Academy of Pediatrics; 2003:693–771.
2. Balfour HH Jr. Antiviral drugs. *N Engl J Med.* 1999;340(16): 1255–1268.
3. Boucher HW, Groll AH, Chiou CC, et al. Newer systemic antifungal agents: Pharmacokinetics, safety and efficacy. *Drugs.* 2004;64(18):1997–2020.
4. Bowlware KL, Stull T. Antibacterial agents in pediatrics. *Infect Dis Clin North Am.* 2004;18(3):513–531.
5. Couch RB. Prevention and treatment of influenza. *N Engl J Med.* 2000;343(24):1778–1787.
6. Crumpacker CS. Ganciclovir. *N Engl J Med.* 1996;335(10): 721–729.
7. Denning DW. Echinocandin antifungal drugs. *Lancet.* 2003; 362(9390):1142–1151.
8. Dennis DT, Inglesby TV, Henderson DA, et al. Consensus statement: Tularemia as a biological weapon: Medical and public health management. *JAMA.* 2001;285(21):2763–2773.
9. Feigin R, Cherry JD, Demmler GJ, eds. *Texbook of pediatric infectious diseases.* 5th ed. Philadelphia, PA: WB Saunders; 2004:2110–2133.
10. Gorbach SL, Bartlett JG, Blacklow NR. *Infectious diseases.* 3rd ed. Philadelphia, PA: Lippincott Williams & Wilkins; 2003.
11. Mausner JS, Bahn AK. *Epidemiology—an introductory text.* 2nd ed. Philadelphia, PA: WB Saunders; 1985.

12. Grady R. Safety profile of quinolone antibiotics in the pediatric population. *Pediatr Infect Dis J.* 2003;22:1128–1132.

13. Hoog M, van den Anker JN. Aminoglycosides and glycopeptides. In: Yaffe SJ, Aranda JV, eds. *Neonatal and pediatric pharmacology therapeutic principles in practice.* 3rd ed. Philadelphia, PA: Lippincott Williams & Wilkins; 2005:377–401.

14. Inglesby TV, Dennis DT, Henderson DA, et al. Plague as a biological weapon: Medical and public health management. *JAMA.* 2000;283(17):2281–2290.

15. Inglesby TV, O'Toole T, Henderson DA, et al. Anthrax as a biological weapon, 2002: updated recommendations for management. *JAMA.* 2002;287(17):2236–2252.

16. Levison ME. Pharmacodynamics of antimicrobial drugs. *Infect Dis Clin North Am.* 2004;18(3):451–465.

17. Loeffler AM, Drew RH, Perfect JR, et al. Safety and efficacy of quinupristin/dalfopristin for treatment of invasive gram-positive infections in pediatric patients. *Pediatr Infect Dis J.* 2002; 21:950–956.

18. Nambiar S, Rodriguez WJ. Penicillins, Beta-lactamase inhibitors, cephalosporins and other Beta-lactams. In: Yaffe SJ, Aranda JV, eds. *Neonatal and pediatric pharmacology therapeutic principles in practice.* 3rd ed. Philadelphia, PA: Lippincott Williams & Wilkins; 2005:361–376.

19. Pickering LK, ed. *Red book: 2003 report of the committee of infectious diseases.* 26th ed. Elk Grove Village, IL: American Academy of Pediatrics; 2003:561–573.

20. Riegelman RK. *Studying a study and testing a test.* 4th ed. Philadelphia, PA: Lippincott Williams & Wilkins; 2000.

21. Rothman KJ, Greenland S. *Modern epidemiology.* 2nd ed. Philadelphia, PA: Lippincott Williams & Wilkins; 1998.

22. Wassertheil-Smoller Sylvia. *Biostatistics and epidemiology a primer for health and biomedical professionals.* 3rd ed. New York: Springer Publishing; 2004.

23. Weiss ME, Adkinson NF Jr. β-Lactam Allergy. In: Mandell GL, Douglas RG, Bennett JE, eds. *Principles and practice of infectious diseases.* 6th ed. Philadelphia, PA: Elsevier 2005:318–326.

Hematology and Oncology

Edward C. Wong   Naomi L. C. Luban

OXYGEN TRANSPORT

Oxygen transport is a critically important physiologic process that results from the intricate modulation of hemoglobin synthesis, formation of red blood cells (RBCs) containing oxygen-laden hemoglobin molecules, and the off-loading of oxygen. This physiologic process is intricately involved at both DNA transcriptional and hemodynamic levels. In this chapter, we describe these physiologic processes and the key pathologic events that alter this transport process.

Hemoglobin Synthesis

Globin Synthesis

Hemoglobin is a tetrameric molecule consisting of two α-globin chains and two non–α-globin chains containing four heme moieties (see Fig. 4.1). The key to the formation of hemoglobin is the synthesis of globin chains, which is dependent on the transcription of precursor messenger RNA (mRNA) from genomic DNA. Transcription is followed by processing of the mRNA molecule to mature cytoplasmic mRNA and translation of the mature mRNA to produce globin molecules.[1,2]

The organization of the globin genes in humans is divided into two major groups (see Fig. 4.2). The β-globin-like (or non–α-globin) cluster genes are located on chromosome 11 and consist of the genes for β, γ, δ, and ε. The other major group of genes (collectively called the *α-globin gene cluster*) are located on chromosome 16 and include the genes for α- and ζ-globin. There are a variety of specific, highly conserved DNA sequences within a short distance upstream and downstream from each gene called *cis-acting elements* (promoter, enhancer, silencers,

etc.), which are binding sites for a number of trans-acting factors, the nuclear protein products of remote genes. Often, cis-acting elements may occur within the introns of the gene. It should be noted that although there are similarities, each gene has its own unique set of regulatory sequences and trans-activating factors, which are critical for globin protein expression.

A major control point for the expression of the β-globin genes is the locus control region (LCR), which is approximately 5- to 25-kb upstream from the β-globin gene cluster (see Fig. 4.3). This site contains important binding sites for trans-acting factors and consists of at least five separate DNAse hypersensitivity (HS) domains, HS-1 to HS-5, each containing several bindings sites for a variety of trans-activating factors. The LCR has several important functions that distinguish it. One important function is the transcription of all globin genes on chromosome 11. Deletion of the LCR markedly reduces or silences all β-globin genes. This occurs in several different types of thalassemia. Interestingly, the LCR continues to function when its location is experimentally varied. Importantly, significant erythroid expression of novel gene function requires the LCR. High-level expression of human β-globin genes also requires LCR. Similarly, a distant (40 kb) upstream regulatory complex on chromosome 16, called *HS-40*, serves a similar function for the α-globin gene cluster. Deletion of HS-40 largely silences α gene expression; it is also required for similar expression of trans genes.

Despite this similarity in these locus control "like" regions and the likelihood that both the α- and β-globin genes arose out of a duplication of a common ancestral globin gene, they lie in very different genomic contexts (Fig. 4.3). The β-globin gene cluster is adenine and thymidine rich, with no CpG islands, whereas the α-globin

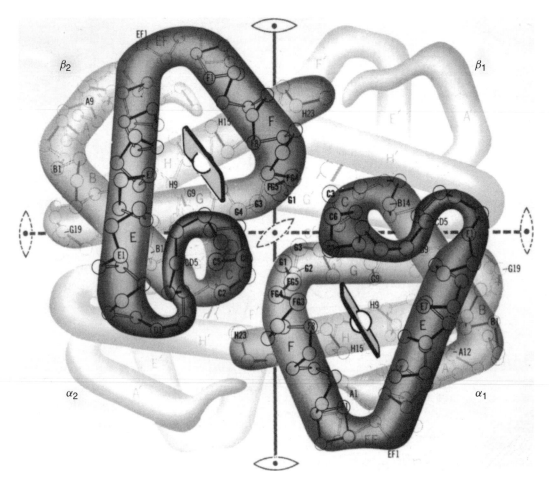

Figure 4.1 Tetramer formation of hemoglobin demonstrating the close proximity of FG corner of the α_1 chain with the C helix of the β_2 chain. This increases the oxygen affinity of the β_2 chain and demonstrates the phenomenon of cooperativity of the hemoglobin molecule. (From Dickerson RE, Geis I. eds. *Hemoglobin: Structure, function, evolution, and pathology.* Menlo Park, CA: Benjamin/Cummings; 1983:36. Rights owned by Howard Hughes Medical Institute. Not to be reproduced without permission.)

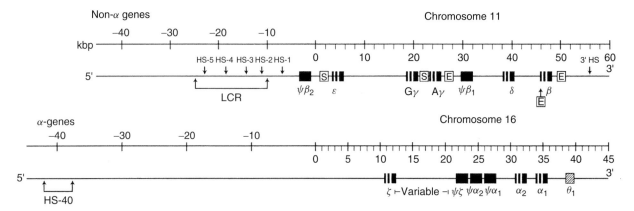

Figure 4.2 Map of the location of the α- and β-globin and related genes with corresponding pseudogenes and upstream and downstream cis-acting elements involved in transcriptional regulation on chromosomes 11 and 16. The θ_1 gene on chromosome 16 is transcribed but not translated. Filled areas indicate exons. Enhancer and silencer sequences are indicated by *E* and *S*, respectively. Promoter regions are located 5' to each gene but are not shown. (From Woodson RD. Hemoglobin synthesis, structure, and oxygen transport. In: Simon TL, Dzik WN, Snyder EL, et al., eds. *Rossi's principles of transfusion medicine*, 3rd ed. Philadelphia, PA: Lippincott Williams & Wilkins; 2002:26.)

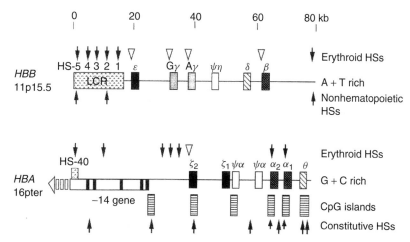

Figure 4.3 Chromatin structure differences between the α- and β-globin gene locus region. The β-globin gene locus control region (LCR) and related HS-40 region for the α-globin gene on chromosomes 16 and 11, respectively. The globin genes and distal control regions are shown in boxes. In both gene clusters, both nonhematopoietic and erythroid DNAse hypersensitivity (HS) sites are indicated with *arrows*. HS sites that occur at specific developmental stages are shown as open triangles. CpG islands (*boxes with horizontal lines*) are indicated. Both the LCR and HS-40 region are critical for α- and β-globin gene expression. Hb B, β-globin gene; Hb A, α-globin gene; HBA, hemoglobin A; HBB, hemoglobin B. (From Hardison R. Organization, evolution, and regulation of the globin genes. In: Steinberg MH, Forget BG, Higgs DR, et al., eds. *Disorders of hemoglobin: Genetics, pathophysiology, and clinical management.* Cambridge, MA: Cambridge University Press; 2001:103.)

gene cluster contains many CpG islands. Because of this difference in cytosine and guanine content, the α-globin gene cluster is not methylated in any cell type, whereas the β-globin gene cluster is subject to tissue-specific DNA methylation. Therefore, the α-globin gene, in contrast to the β-globin gene, has many features of constitutively expressed "housekeeping genes." These striking differences in the number and location of these CpG islands and degree of DNA methylation reflect differences in replication of the gene clusters. The α-globin gene clusters are replicated early in S phase from multiple points of origin within a large C + G rich region within the cluster in both nonerythroid and erythroid cells, whereas the β-globin gene cluster is replicated only in S phase in erythroid cells from a single point of origin close to the promoter of β-globin gene.[3]

There are families of trans-acting factors that bind to the regulatory domains. The most notable include GATA-1, friend of GATA (FOG), and erythroid Kruppel-like factor (EKLF) trans-activating factors. These trans-acting factors have little or no expression or function in nonhematopoietic tissues but are specific regulators of hematopoietic cell function. Each is indispensable for globin expression. There are other important trans-acting factors including activator protein-1 (AP-1)/nuclear factor-erythroid 2 (NF-E2) and related family proteins, basic Kruppel-like factor (BKLF), possibly others essentially restricted to hematopoietic tissue, and other ubiquitous factors that probably modulate

globin transcription control. None of these, however, are essential for globin gene expression.

The complex system of regulatory domains and various binding factors results in exquisite temporal control of tissue-specific gene expression. Intense investigation is under way to understand how these domains and trans-acting factors interact to activate and modulate gene transcription. Several DNA-based topology related models have been proposed to explain how the remote and nearby sequences interact to initiate (or derepress) transcription; however, none of these models can explain experimental observations. At the present time, it is felt that the interactions largely represent an ever-changing three-dimensional construct that can influence transcription in multiple ways. It is likely that similarly complex control systems regulate transcription of other erythroid enzymes.

After initiation, globin transcription by RNA polymerase results in a completely complementary RNA molecule, called *precursor mRNA*, which typically extends 41 to 57 bases downstream (in the 3' direction) beyond the protein-encoded portion. This precursor mRNA typically ends with a tail of 100 or more adenylic acid residues, the poly (A) tail. This precursor mRNA undergoes several processing steps including a process called *capping*, in which the 5' end is fitted with two or three specific nucleotides, which undergo specific linking and methylation. This capping process and the presence of at least three well-conserved base sequences downstream from the cap and upstream from the 5' end of the gene are important in later protein synthesis. When capping occurs, the poly (A) tail is reduced to 50 to 70 residues.

Within the structural portion of the gene and its initial complementary RNA transcript are noncoding intervening sequences or introns that are recognized and excised by spliceosomes. This results in mature mRNA, which codes for functionally or structurally important domains of the protein product. After formation, mature globin mRNA is transported to the cytoplasm, where it attaches to several ribosomal subunits. With the appropriate translation initiation factors, this mRNA serves as the template for synthesis of the globin molecule. Translation starts at a unique start codon at the 5' end of the mRNA and amino acids, in turn, are added by a specific transfer RNA in a 5' to 3" direction until a stop codon is reached, resulting in the release of a complete protein chain. Many additional globin chains are derived from this mRNA template. Because of its unusual stability compared to other mRNAs, the globin mRNA allows hemoglobin production to continue in reticulocytes for several days after loss of the nucleus.

Disorders of nearly every step in transcription and subsequent translation have been observed with respect to globin production.[4] Several hundred hemoglobin mutants can be identified on the basis of base sequence abnormalities (single-base substitutions, deletions, insertions, missense mutations, frame shifts, crossovers) within the globin exons. A similar paradigm exists with respect to the thalassemia syndromes, which, with rare exceptions, results in the reduced or absent production of selected globin chain. There are a tremendous number (in the hundreds) of known single-base substitutions, missense mutations, frame shifts, and deletions that affect flanking regulatory domains (such as LCR and HS-40), the various introns and exons or even entire clusters of genes, the poly (A) signal sequence, the cap site, mRNA processing and translation. These same abnormalities extend even to critical trans-acting factors that can result in reduction or absent production of globin chains.

Heme Synthesis

The structure of the heme consists of a porphyrin or tetrapyrrole ring with a central iron atom surrounded by four nitrogen atoms. The ability to reversibly bind oxygen or electrons is a central function of many critically important molecules including hemoglobin, myoglobin, cytochromes, peroxidases, and catalase. Because the heme moiety absorbs light strongly, the color of the heme changes with the degree of oxygenation and oxidation and accounts for the characteristic red color of hemoglobin in an oxygenated state.

The heme synthesis (see Fig. 4.4) begins with the formation of 5-aminolevulinic acid (ALA) from succinyl-coenzyme A and glycine by ALA synthase. This reaction occurs on the inner mitochondrial membrane and requires pyridoxal-5'-phosphate as a cofactor. This requirement for pyridoxal-5'-phosphate explains the response to large doses of pyridoxine observed occasionally in patients with mutant ALA synthase enzymes, which results in a hereditary X-linked form of sideroblastic anemia. Porphobilinogen forms two molecules of ALA, which combine in the cytoplasm through ALA dehydratase. In turn, four molecules of porphobilinogen then form one molecule of uroporphyrinogen III. This results from the action of porphobilinogen deaminase producing primarily hydroxymethylbilane. Hydroxymethylbilane is subsequently converted to uroporphyrinogen III by uroporphyrinogen III cosynthase. Uroporphyrinogen III is converted to coproporphyrinogen III by uroporphyrinogen decarboxylase. This process converts the four acetates to methyl residues. In the mitochondria, coproporphyrinogen III is converted to protoporphyrin IX through oxidative decarboxylation of propionate groups to vinyl residues by coproporphyrinogen III oxidase and oxidation by protoporphyrin oxidase of the four ethylene bridges between the pyrrole groups. Lastly, ferrochelatase inserts iron into the porphyrin ring.[5]

There are a variety of deficiencies and abnormalities of these enzymes that underscore several disorders (see Table 4.1). Most of the inherited forms of porphyria, including the most common X-linked version of hereditary sideroblastic anemia and certain other hematologic disorders, are explained by enzymatic deficiencies. Chronic exposure to lead is the most common acquired cause of inhibition of several heme synthesis enzymes, most notably ALA dehydratase, coporphyrinogen oxidase, and ferrochelatase. The liver is the principal site of overproduction of porphyrin in most of these disorders with the exception of congenital erythropoietic protoporphyria and protoporphyria, in which the bone marrow is the principle source of the elevated porphyrin molecules.

All of the genes involved in heme synthesis have been cloned and mapped to their chromosomal loci with many mutations now identified. Although the liver and other tissues synthesize heme, there is a separate set of control mechanisms that operate in erythroid cells to generate the extremely high rate of heme synthesis. Linked to the high rate of heme synthesis is the temporal appearance of the pathway of normoblast maturation that is tightly linked to iron availability and globin synthesis. In red blood cell precursors, expression of ALA synthase (ALAS2), unlike its counterpart in other tissues (ALAS1) is the result of gene transcription on the X chromosome. Erythropoietin (EPO) triggers this transcription through the EPO receptor. This process is dependent on transcription factors such as GATA-1, TATA-binding protein (TBP), and very possibly EKLF. In contrast, constitutive expression of a similar ALA synthase gene (ALAS1) in nonerythroid tissues is regulated by different regulatory sequences on chromosome 3. Interestingly, the expression of several other heme synthetic enzymes is regulated in conjunction with ALAS2 synthesis, as inhibition of ALAS2 production by antisense mRNAs techniques results in decreased production of these enzymes including globin synthesis. Both

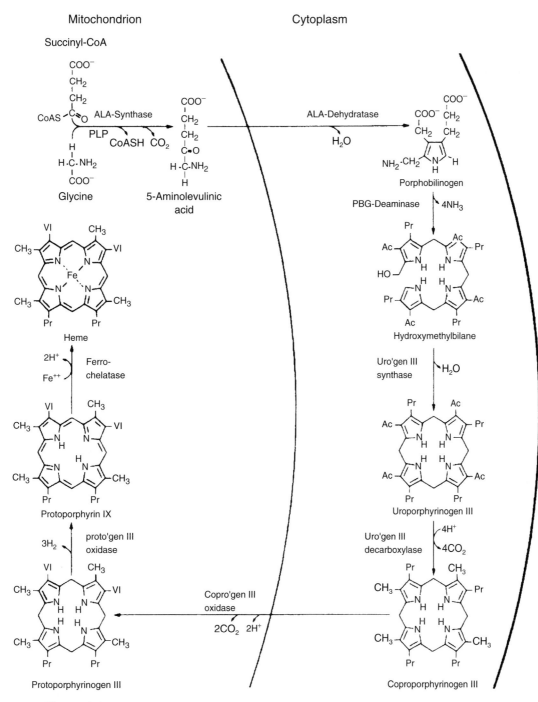

Figure 4.4 Synthesis of heme. Synthesis of heme starts with the formation of 5-aminolevulinic acid (ALA) from glycine and succinyl-CoA through the action of ALA synthase in the mitochondria. In the cytosol the action of ALA dehydratase results in the formation of porphobilinogen, which subsequently undergoes deamination by porphobilinogen (PBG) deaminase, removal of H_2O by uroporphyrinogen III synthase and further decarboxylation by uroporphyrinogen III decarboxylase to eventually form coproporphyrinogen III. In the mitochondria, coproporphyrinogen III oxidase and protoporphyrinogen oxidase further oxidizes coproporphyrinogen III to protoporphyrin IX which, in turn, has Fe^{2+} added by ferrochelatase. See text for details. (From Bottomley SS, Muller-Eberhard U. Pathophysiology of heme synthesis. *Semin Hematol.* 1988;25:284.)

TABLE 4.1

CLINICAL DISORDERS ASSOCIATED WITH DEFICIENCY OR DYSFUNCTION OF HEME SYNTHESIS ENZYMES

Enzyme Deficiency or Dysfunction	Disorder
ALAS2	X-linked hereditary sideroblastic anemia
ALA dehydratase	ALA dehydratase deficiency porphyria[a]
Porphobilinogen deaminase	Acute intermittent porphyria
Uroporphyrinogen III synthase	Porphyria cutanea tarda[b], hepatoerythropoietic porphyria
Uroporphyrinogen decarboxylase	Coproporphyria, harderoporphyria[a]
Coproporphyrinogen oxidase	Variegate porphyria
Ferrochelatase	Erythropoietic protoporphyria[a]

ALAS2, aminolevulinic acid synthase 2.
[a]Acquired deficiency caused by lead exposure.
[b]Associated with hepatitis C-induced liver disease and hereditary hemochromatosis.

erythroid and ubiquitous (nonerythroid) versions of ALA dehydratase, are derived from the same gene, have identical exons, but undergo alternative splicing secondarily as a result of either erythroid or ubiquitous promoters. Similarly, the erythroid and ubiquitous (nonerythroid) isoforms of the third enzyme, porphobilinogen deaminase, also undergo alternative splicing secondarily to different promoters. Both ALA dehydratase and porphobilinogen deaminase erythroid genes possess putatively GATA-1 and NF-E2 domains, indicative of an erythroid tissue-specific control of transcription. Finally, erythroid-specific control elements are also present in the last three genes, coproporphyrinogen III oxidase, protoporphyrin oxidase, and ferrochelatase involved in heme synthesis.

Another major difference between control of heme synthesis in erythroid cells and nonerythroid cells is the tight regulation related to iron availability and globin synthesis. Translation of ALAS2 appears to be controlled by an iron-responsive element in the mRNA, which binds iron regulator proteins such as iron regulatory protein-1 (IRP-1), which regulates mRNA translation of other proteins involved in iron metabolism such as ferritin and transferrin receptors.[6] Therefore, it is likely that upregulation of ALAS2 production is influenced by increased ferritin, which results in decreased IRP binding to ALAS2 mRNA, resulting in stabilization of the ALAS2 message, and subsequently increased translation. This tightly couples heme synthesis to cellular iron availability. Porphobilinogen deaminase is another potential control point in which there is a several-fold increase in basal activity with acceleration of

erythropoiesis. This enzyme is also inhibited by elevated heme levels. Remarkably, heme synthesis is tightly coupled to globin synthesis with heme synthesis directly inducing globin synthesis. This process is terminated or occurs at a reduced rate when globin synthesis is blocked or reduced. Likewise, globin synthesis does not occur if ALAS2 is nonfunctional. The final result is a multitiered control system that allows hemoglobin to be produced at a high rate avoiding both free heme and globin accumulation (see Fig. 4.5).

Tetramer Assembly

In the cytoplasm, the binding of the heme ring to globin occurs during globin transcription or just after globin transcription as the globin molecule establishes its secondary and tertiary structure. There is spontaneous formation of α(non-α) dimers from α and non-α chains in the cytoplasm of the maturing normoblast and reticulocyte.[7] After the first few months of life in the healthy neonate nearly all of the dimers consist of α and β chains. The formation of heterodimers is related to the difference in electrostatic charge at physiologic pH between positively charged α-globin chains and the negatively charged non-α-globin chains and by the high number of contact points between the α- and non-α-globin proteins. This charge-dependent relationship explains why in variant hemoglobins, the ratio of hemoglobin A to hemoglobin X is not normally 1:1. For example, in the common β-chain variants such as S, C, and E, the β chains are less negatively charged than normal α chains. This results in the production of less variant hemoglobin as compared to normal hemoglobin A. This phenomenon is accentuated when α-chain availability is limited such as in α thalassemia.

Within the erythrocyte and its precursors, the formation of tetramers from dimers also occurs spontaneously, largely as a result of high intracellular dimer concentration. Within the red blood cell, hemoglobin levels can reach as high as 5 mmol per L, which is close to maximal solubility and strongly favors the formation of tetramers. When two or more types of dimers are produced in a cell (e.g., $\alpha\beta^A$ and $\alpha\beta^S$), for example, when sickle cell trait is present, the resulting tetramers are commonly represented as combinations of like dimers ($\alpha_2\beta_2^A$ and $\alpha_2\beta_2^S$). However, mixtures of dimers can result in hybrid ($\alpha_2\beta^A\beta^S$), as well as nonhybrid tetramers, within the erythrocyte. Excess globin chains are for the most part removed by cellular proteases except when thalassemia is present. Under conditions in which hemoglobin concentrations are much lower, for example, in intravascular hemolysis, dimer formation is favored. From a diagnostic perspective, evaluation for the presence of hemoglobin variants using standard hemoglobin electrophoresis usually involves analysis of dimers as under most conditions employed in hemoglobin electrophoresis, tetramers will dissociate into dimers.

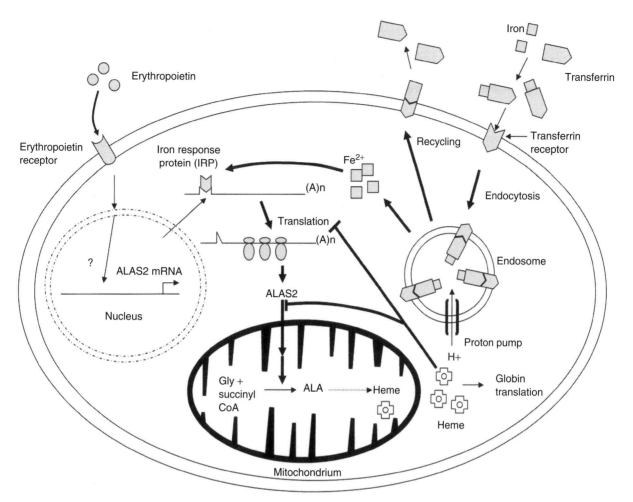

Figure 4.5 Overall positive and negative control of heme synthesis. Erythropoietin enhances transcription and expression of ALAS2 in erythroid precursors. Once ALAS2 transverses the mitochondrial membrane, heme synthesis is initiated from succinylcoenzyme A and glycine. Availability of iron regulates translation of ALAS2 by iron regulatory protein, which binds to an iron-responsive cis-acting element in ALASA2 mRNA and stabilizes ALAS2 mRNA. Heme stimulates globin synthesis while inhibiting ALAS2 translation and translocation to the mitochondrium. ALAS2, erythrocyte isoform of ALA synthase; Gly, glycine; succinyl-CoA, succinylcoenzyme A.

Various Hemoglobins in Humans

By 6 months of age, the principal hemoglobin species produced in the child is Hb A, which has the structural formula, $\alpha_2\beta_2^A$. In contrast, Hb F ($\alpha_2\gamma_2$) and Hb A_2 ($\alpha_2\delta_2$) are present in small amounts, typically at <2% and approximately 2% to 3%, respectively. During intrauterine life, there is an orderly succession of embryonic and fetal hemoglobins (see Fig. 4.6).

The more important physiologic hemoglobin during gestation and in the first few months of extrauterine life is Hb F. Hb F is the principal hemoglobin after the first few weeks of gestation and during late pregnancy and, in the early months of life is replaced by Hb A. A major characteristic of Hb F is that it binds oxygen with a higher affinity than does Hb A (i.e., the partial pressure of oxygen at which hemoglobin 50% saturated with oxygen [P_{50}] of Hb F is lower) and is therefore better suited for oxygen transport during intrauterine life. The reason for this switch from Hb F to Hb A is not well understood and is under intense investigation. Of interest is the observation that the 5′ to 3′ order of genes in the β-globin gene cluster is identical to the appearance of the respective hemoglobins during fetal development. In mice studies, experimentally varying the position of the globin genes results in an identical change in the order of appearance of hemoglobins in the embryo.[8,9]

Post-translationally, hemoglobin undergoes nonenzymatic glycosylation during the life of the red cell, resulting in Hb A_{1c}, which is produced by N-terminal attachment of glucose to the β-globin chain by a ketoamine linkage. Given the 120-day erythrocyte life span, the level of Hb A_{1c} provides a useful overall measure of diabetic control. Hb A_{1c} has poor oxygen affinity, but because it is a very small percentage of the overall hemoglobin content of the red cell, oxygen delivery is not significantly altered.

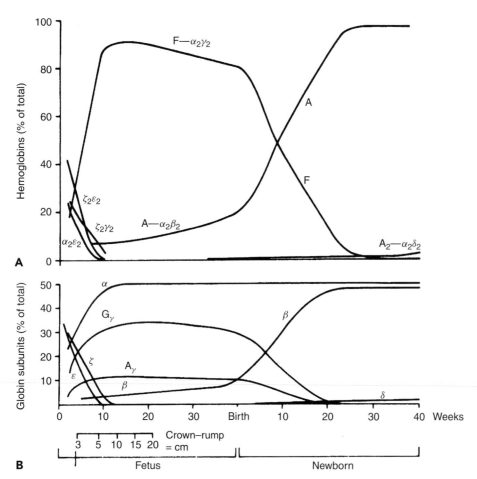

Figure 4.6 Time course of intrauterine and postnatal hemoglobin formation. **A:** It illustrates the formation of embryonic hemoglobins, Gower 1 and 2 ($\zeta_2\varepsilon_2$ and $\alpha_2\varepsilon_2$) and Portland ($\zeta_2\gamma_2$), hemoglobin F ($\alpha_2\gamma_2$ [$\alpha_2^G\gamma_2$ and $\alpha_2^A\gamma_2$]), and hemoglobin A ($\alpha_2\beta_2$) and A$_2$ ($\alpha_2\delta_2$) from conception through birth and 40 weeks postnatally. **B:** It illustrates the percentages of the embryonic and adult globin chains during the same period. (From Bunn HF, Forget BG. *Hemoglobin: Molecular, genetic and clinical aspects*. Philadelphia, PA: WB Saunders; 1986:68.)

Hemoglobin Function

There are major aspects of hemoglobin function that relate directly to its role as an oxygen transporter and hence oxygen delivery. These include (i) its co-operative and reversible binding to oxygen, (ii) pH, (iii) carbon dioxide, (iv) chloride, (v) 2,3-bisphosphoglycerate (2,3-BPG), (vi) temperature, and (vii) nitric oxide.

Oxygen–Hemoglobin Binding

Because of the presence of four heme moieties, a molecule of hemoglobin can bind maximally four molecules of oxygen. This allows a maximum binding of 1.39 mL oxygen per g of hemoglobin. Given that there are only small amounts of methemoglobin and carboxyhemoglobin normally present, and allowing for a small amount of dissolved oxygen, this translates to approximately 20 mL oxygen per dL in normal arterial blood when the hemoglobin concentration is 15 g per dL.

Oxygen equilibrium curves (OEC) for myoglobin and hemoglobin under physiologic conditions are seen in Figure 4.7. Comparing the curves for myoglobin and hemoglobin is instructive. Although the curve for myoglobin is a hyperbola, the hemoglobin curve is sigmoidal. This sigmoidicity results from cooperativity related to

heme–heme interaction, which results from the alteration of the oxygen affinity of one subunit of the hemoglobin tetramer, when another subunit binds oxygen. Because myoglobin contains only one heme moiety, it does not demonstrate heme–heme interaction and therefore no cooperativity. Additionally, the presence of two different types of globin chains is a prerequisite for cooperativity and therefore, a tetramer such as Hb Bart ($\beta4$), which is composed of four identical β-globin chains, does not demonstrate cooperativity. This degree of cooperativity can be determined when data are replotted as the log of the fractional hemoglobin–oxygen saturation versus log PO_2. This analysis gives a slope of 1.0 for myoglobin (no cooperativity) and a slope of 2.8 for hemoglobin (moderate cooperativity), with maximal cooperativity resulting in a slope of 4 (see Fig. 4.8).

Oxygenation of the hemoglobin starts in one of the α-heme subunits, which has high oxygen affinity under physiologic conditions. Binding of the first oxygen results in an increased oxygen affinity of the other subunits. This subsequent oxygenation of the second subunit occurs at a lower PO_2 than would be required if cooperativity were not present. By the time the last subunit is oxygenated, the last heme group binds oxygen approximately 300 times more

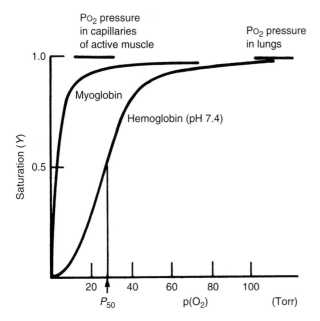

Figure 4.7 Comparison of oxygen dissociation curves of myoglobin and hemoglobin. Myoglobin oxygenation saturation as function of Po₂ demonstrates a hyperbola at relatively low Po₂, while the curve for hemoglobin demonstrates sigmoidicity across a greater range of Po₂ indicating cooperatively. Myoglobin can more effectively release oxygen at Po₂ ranges that are seen in actively metabolizing tissue such as muscle. (From Woodson RD. Hemoglobin synthesis, structure, and oxygen transport. In: Simon TL, Dzik WN, Snyder EL, et al., eds. *Rossi's principles of transfusion medicine*, 3rd ed. Philadelphia, PA: Lippincott Williams & Wilkins; 2002:32.)

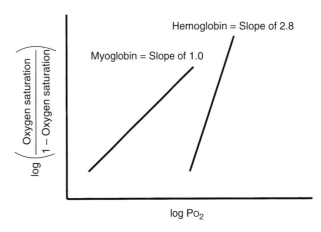

Figure 4.8 Comparison of simplified Hill plots of myoglobin and hemoglobin comparing log of the oxygen fractional saturation versus log Po₂. Myoglobin demonstrates a slope of 1.0 (no cooperativity), while hemoglobin demonstrates a slope of 2.8 (cooperativity).

tightly than does the first subunit. Conversely, release of the first molecule of oxygen from hemoglobin facilitates release of subsequent molecules because oxygen affinity of the remaining oxygenated subunits decreases. As a result of cooperativity, most molecules tend toward being fully oxygenated or fully deoxygenated, with few intermediates present.

The phenomenon of cooperativity has great biologic importance because it results in nearly full saturation of hemoglobin at Po₂ values ordinarily present in the pulmonary alveoli. Likewise, the markedly steep slope with relatively small decreases in tissue Po₂ permits large fractions of bound oxygen to be released as blood flows through tissue. For example, 25% of oxygen is released when Po₂ falls from arterial levels to 40 mm Hg. In contrast, approximately 50% of oxygen is released when Po₂ decreases from 40 to 20 mm Hg of bound oxygen. This allows a large diffusion gradient for oxygen diffusion from the interior of the red blood cell to relatively hypoxic cells distant from the microvasculature.

The effect of a shift of the OEC to the right (P_{50} of 36 mm Hg) or left (P_{50} of 16 mm Hg) is seen in Figure 4.9. When the curve is shifted to the right, more oxygen is released for any given decrease in pressure. For example, at a Po₂

of 27 mm Hg (see nonshifted OEC), whole blood releases 54% of its bound oxygen, whereas the right-shifted curve releases 72%. By contrast, the curve to the left, typically of stored blood releases only 22% of oxygen for the same decrease in Po₂. Physiologically, as blood passes through the microvasculature, the OEC shifts to the right allowing for greater release of oxygen for the same Po₂.

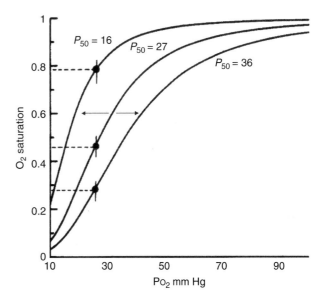

Figure 4.9 Comparison of left-shifted ($P_{50} = 16$), nonshifted ($P_{50} = 27$), and right-shifted ($P_{50} = 36$) hemoglobin oxygen equilibrium curves (OECs) illustrating the ability of left-shifted or right-shifted hemoglobins to off-load oxygen. A left-shifted OEC compared to right-shifted OEC has clearly a greater ability to off-load oxygen under conditions seen in metabolically active tissues. (Modified from Schultz RM, Liebman MN. Proteins II: Structure-function relationship of protein families. In: Devlin TM, ed. *Textbook of biochemistry*, 3rd ed. New York: Wiley-Liss; 1992:126.)

In contrast, a left-shifted OEC is able to deliver more oxygen when alveolar P_{O_2} is markedly reduced, as at very high altitudes or in the developing fetus. Under these conditions, assuming the leftward shift in the OEC depicted in Figure 4.9, approximately 40% more oxygen is released in the microvasculature when P_{O_2} is decreased from an arterial value of 35 to 15 mm Hg with the left-shifted curve than with the right-shifted curve. This explains why a leftward-shifted OEC is necessarily seen in nearly all fetuses compared to the maternal (adult) curve and why a left-lying OEC is necessary for the survival of animals and humans living in high-altitude areas.

The OEC has been discussed so far under equilibrium conditions; under pathologic conditions, the OEC undergoes continued alteration to maintain critical oxygen transport needs. It should be noted that because hemoglobin combines with four molecules of oxygen, there are a number of intermediate compounds that have their own reversible reactions for oxygen release. Factors that modify the OEC do so by altering the ratios between the on-and-off rate constants, which are themselves under the influence of a variety of physiologic influences.

Molecular Basis of Oxygen–Hemoglobin Cooperativity

Key research into the molecular basis of hemoglobin function has resulted in a detailed mechanistic explanation of the co-operative effect of how oxygenation of one heme group contributes to the alteration of oxygen affinity of distant heme groups associated with different globin chains in hemoglobin. Hemoglobin is a globular, tetrameric molecule with a molecular weight of 64,500 Da. Its diameter ranges from 50 to 65 Å. Each globin chain exists for the most part as an α helix folded at several inflection points (Fig. 4.1). Between the E and F helices in an interior crevice of the folded globin chain, heme is surrounded by mostly uncharged amino acid residues. This nonpolar environment partially protects the central heme iron from oxidation. In contrast, the external polar amino acids of hemoglobin are hydrophilic and allow hemoglobin to maintain its solubility. The central iron atom is surrounded by four tetrapyrrole rings, which provide four of six possible coordination positions. A fifth position is provided by a covalent linkage to the nitrogen of a particular histidine called the *proximal histidine* (residues 87 and 92 in α and β chains, respectively). Because the outermost electrons of iron are located in a higher orbital when hemoglobin is in a deoxygenated state, the effective atomic diameter of iron is such that the iron molecule cannot quite fit in the plane of the ring between the tetrapyrrole nitrogens and is therefore slightly outside the plane of the ring. This displacement depends on the globin molecule (0.22 and 0.19 Å in α and β_1 subunits, respectively). As seen in Figure 4.10, this "out of plane" position of the iron molecules displaces the proximal histidines and bends or "tents" the heme ring resulting in subunit strain.[10] In the process of oxygenation,

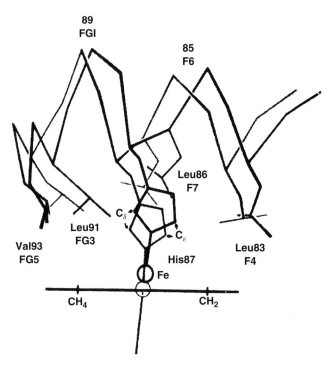

Figure 4.10 Conformational changes in the globin chain resulting from oxygenation of the heme iron atom. Heavy lines depict deoxygenated state. (From Baldwin J, Chothia C. Hemoglobin: The structural changes related to ligand binding and its allosteric mechanism. *J Mol Biol.* 1979;129:192, Figure 6A.)

the oxygen molecule binds to the iron on the side of the heme ring opposite from the proximal histidine, and forms a hydrogen bond with the imidazole nitrogen of the distal histidine (residue 58 in α chains and 63 in β chains). This results in an effective decrease of the iron diameter because the outer iron electrons drop into a lower orbital. As a consequence, the iron molecule is no longer displaced from the plane of the ring and allows the proximal histidine to move closer to the ring, reducing overall ring strain, resulting in further shifts in other parts of the subunit. These shifts involve particularly the FG helical corner, which has a series of contacts with the C corner of the β chain (β_2) of the opposite dimer. During oxygenation, a number of the 14 salt bridges in deoxyhemoglobin between subunits and within β subunits loosen or break and after two to three subunits are oxygenated, the entire tetramer converts from a taut, constrained (lower oxygen affinity) state (T) to a relaxed (higher oxygen affinity) state (R).

This attainment of a relaxed hemoglobin state markedly decreases oxygen affinity. This transition is accompanied by a rotation of the two $\alpha\beta$ dimers away from one another by 12 to 15 degrees and a lateral movement of one with respect to the other of 0.8 Å. These intramolecular movements of the molecule were detected with x-ray crystallography by Dr. Max Perutz, who formulated a comprehensive model of oxygen cooperativity of hemoglobin. This model, with a few minor adjustments, has remained remarkably correct since the original description.[11]

TABLE 4.2

SUMMARY OF THE EFFECTS OF VARIOUS LIGANDS, METHEMOGLOBIN FORMATION, AND TEMPERATURE ON THE OXYGEN–HEMOGLOBIN AFFINITY

Increased Oxygen Affinity	Decreased Oxygen Affinity
Oxygen binding	Oxygen release
Carbon monoxide	2,3-bisphosphoglycerate
pH <6	pH >6
Methemoglobin	Chloride ion
Decreased temperature	Increased temperature
	Nitric oxide?

Linked Functions of Hemoglobin

Oxygenation and deoxygenation of hemoglobin are not isolated events: There are changes in the binding affinity of hemoglobin for its other ligands such as hydrogen ions, carbon dioxide, chloride ions, 2,3-BPG (2,3-BPG, formally known as 2,3-diphosphoglycerate [2,3-DPG]), and nitric oxide, which alters oxygen affinity. Likewise, when oxygen saturation is held constant, a change in the amount of any other bound ligand evokes changes in the affinity of hemoglobin for the other ligands. The effects of these ligands and methemoglobin formation and temperature on oxygen affinity are summarized in Table 4.2.

Bohr Effect

From a physiologic perspective, an increase in hydrogen ions shifts the OEC to the right, and a decrease shifts it to the left. This is termed the *Bohr effect* (also called *alkaline Bohr effect* by chemists) and is used to describe the relationship between hydrogen ions and oxygen affinity. Often the Bohr effect is described as a change in oxygen affinity with a change in carbon dioxide concentration. However, the carbon dioxide effect has been shown to comprise both a pH and a small non-pH-independent carbon dioxide–specific effect on blood oxygen affinity. Physiologists often use the term *carbon dioxide Bohr effect* to denote the change in oxygen affinity caused by a change in P_{CO_2} related to pH and carbon dioxide–specific effects together and the term *hydrogen ion* Bohr effect to denote the specific change in P_{50} caused by a change in the pH at constant P_{O_2} (pH effect *per se*). Because of the high concentration of hemoglobin present in blood, hemoglobin serves as a very important buffer of hydrogen ions. Although not physiologically relevant, there is another phenomenon at low (subphysiologic) pH (<6.0) called the *acid Bohr effect* in which an increased pH or decrease in hydrogen ion concentration has the opposite effect on oxygen affinity.

There is a molecular basis for the Bohr (alkaline) effect. When hydrogen ions are added to hemoglobin, amino acid residues (such as the imidazole ring of histidine), which have pK values close physiologic pH, are titrated. Therefore, when protonation occurs, hydrogen bond formation is favored at the C termini, resulting in a strengthened T structure. Protonation also increases the charge density of anionic groups lining the central cavity, increasing mutual repulsion and shifts the molecule toward the T structure. This portion of the (alkaline) Bohr effect requires the presence of chloride, whereas that associated with hydrogen bonds is chloride independent. Under physiologic conditions, the following equation can describe the relationship between oxygen affinity and pH in whole blood: $\Delta \log P_{50}/\Delta pH = -0.40$. Overall, decreasing pH by 0.10 will increase the P_{50} of whole blood 2.5 to 3.0 mm Hg. It should be noted that a corollary to the (alkaline) Bohr effect is that oxygenation will release hydrogen ions from hemoglobin and conversely that deoxygenation will cause uptake of hydrogen ions.

Carbon Dioxide Effect

In addition to its effect on pH, carbon dioxide can affect hemoglobin–oxygen affinity by the following reaction:

$$Hb\text{-}O_2\text{-}NH_2 + CO_2 \leftrightarrow Hb\text{-}NH\text{-}CO_2^- + H^+ + O_2$$

This carbamylation occurs primarily at the N-terminal amino groups of the β-globin chains under physiologic conditions. Similarly, there is a reciprocal relationship between carbon dioxide and oxygen binding to hemoglobin. Although carbon dioxide decreases the affinity of the molecule for oxygen, oxygen uptake will, in turn, decrease the ability of carbon dioxide to bind to hemoglobin.

Hemoglobin also participates directly, to a limited extent, in carbon dioxide transport. At relatively high oxygen saturation (approximately 50%) with other factors constant, a 40-mm Hg increase in P_{CO_2} will increase whole-blood P_{50} by approximately 0.8 mm Hg. Although this is not clinically important, at both low oxygen saturations and low 2,3-BPG concentration, this can be of some significance.

Chloride Effect

Chloride also has a reciprocal relationship with oxygen to hemoglobin in a similar manner as pH and carbon dioxide. Chloride interacts with positively charged sites on the hemoglobin molecule and alters oxygen affinity by the following reaction:

$$Hb\text{-}NH_3^+Cl^- + O_2 \leftrightarrow HbO_2\text{-}NH_2 + H^+ + Cl^-$$

Importantly, the chloride ion accounts for approximately one half of the (alkaline) Bohr effect. The binding of chloride neutralizes positively charged residues within the central cavity. This is thought to increase the P_{50} by decreasing mutual repulsion within the central cavity allowing it to decrease in size, shifting the equilibrium toward the more constrained T structure. When the chloride ion concentration decreases from 0.15 to 0.02 M in a 2,3-BPG–free hemoglobin solution, the P_{50} decreases from 16 to 10 mm Hg, resulting in decrease of the Bohr effect by approximately 50%.

2,3-Bisphosphoglycerate Effect

2,3-BPG is a highly charged molecule with approximately 3.5 negative charges at pH 7.2. This molecule is approximately at the same molar concentration as hemoglobin and binds to specific molecular groups—β terminal amino valines, β143 histidine, and β82 lysine—of deoxyhemoglobin. This helps to internally constrain the tetramer, reducing its oxygen affinity by the following reaction:

$$Hb\text{–}BPG + O_2 \leftrightarrow HbO_2 + BPG$$

A decrease in the intracellular concentration of 2,3-BPG from normal (approximately 5 mmol per L) to 0 decreases the P_{50} from approximately 27 to 16 mm Hg. Although there is limited effect of 2,3-BPG concentration beyond a 2,3-BPG to hemoglobin ratio of greater than 1.0, on P_{50}, because 2,3-BPG is an acidic molecule, it lowers red cell pH and thereby increases the P_{50} through the Bohr effect. Interestingly, unlike the situation for Hb A, 2,3-BPG does not interact significantly with Hb F. This mainly is a result of replacement of the β143 histidine, a principal site of 2,3-BPG interaction, with serine. This partially accounts for the increased oxygen affinity of fetal and neonatal cells relative to that of adult cells. Again, like pH, CO_2, and chloride, 2,3-BPG exhibits a reciprocal relationship between oxygen and itself on hemoglobin binding.

Nitric Oxide Effect

Nitric oxide interacts with the iron in deoxygenated hemoglobin to generate Hb–Fe^{2+}–NO and with the iron in oxyhemoglobin to yield methemoglobin (Fe^{3+}–Hb) with the production of nitrate:

$$Hb\text{–}Fe^{2+} + NO \leftrightarrow Hb\text{–}Fe^{2+}\text{–}NO$$
$$Hb\text{–}O_2\text{–}Fe^{2+} + NO \leftrightarrow Hb\text{–}Fe^{3+} + NO_3^{-}$$

Methemoglobin has several functions. One of these is its well-known ability to increase the oxygen affinity of unaffected subunits. A second function is to act as the scavenging system for the elimination of nitric oxide. A third involves its binding to the β cysteine 93 thiol group producing the adduct S-nitrosyl-Hb (SNO–Hb). This thiol group is invariant across mammals and birds. It has been postulated that SNO–Hb is produced in the lungs when hemoglobin is in the "R" or relaxed, oxygenated state. When hemoglobin loses oxygen in the microcirculation, hemoglobin transitions from the "R" or relaxed to the "T" or taut configuration, allowing release of nitric oxide from the Cys93 site. Subsequently, this nitric oxide may modulate small vessel tone and therefore blood flow. This third function has been difficult to reconcile with the role of hemoglobin being a major nitric oxide scavenger. This paradox has been addressed by several investigators who

suggested that nitric oxide scavenging does not occur *in vivo*. Furthermore, some studies have suggested that the nitric oxide liberated as SNO is prevented from rebinding by Fe^{2+} and that facilitated diffusion through erythrocyte glutathione across the red blood cell to the endothelium occurs for SNO.[12–14] Controversy in the physiologic relevance of SNO–Hb has come from studies of nitric oxide inhalation in normal volunteers where measurement of S-nitrosation of hemoglobin β-chain cysteine 93 demonstrated only a fraction of the level of nitrosyl (heme) hemoglobin and without a detectable arterial–venous gradient.[15] Furthermore, examination of forearm blood flow under periods of rest (with and without inhibition of nitric oxide) followed by exercise revealed no significant arterial–venous gradient of SNO–Hb and only small amounts of low-molecular-weight SNO and S-nitroso-albumin.[16] Another study has found that SNO–Hb is unstable in the reductive environment of the erythrocyte and that β cysteine 93 is maintained in a reduced state.[17] Furthermore, under cycling conditions of oxygenation and deoxygenation, nitric oxide did not demonstrate reversible intermolecular transfer from heme to β cysteine 93. The use of ^{15}N-labeled nitrite in this study demonstrated that previous results demonstrating this transfer may have been caused by the presence of exogenous nitrite.[18] Indeed, it has been shown that nitric oxide can be produced in the red cell under hypoxic conditions by a deoxyhemoglobin-mediated nitrite reduction reaction, a potentially new mechanism of nitric oxide delivery to hypoxic endothelium.[19] Recently, Han et al.[20] have observed that hypoxic conditions that allow the formation of HbFe(II)NO increase nitric oxide consumption explaining the hypoxic pulmonary vasoconstriction and the rebound seen upon termination of nitric oxide inhalation therapy. They postulate under hypoxic conditions and exposure to nitric oxide, where the nitric oxide/heme ratio is low, nitric oxide is bound primarily to the α heme moiety and results in a markedly shifted "T" state of hemoglobin, which causes displacement of ankyrin from the erythrocyte skeletal membrane. This displacement of ankyrin from the cytoskeleton allows nitric oxide entry, which is normally blocked by ankyrin binding to the band 3 protein. Evidence for a modulatory role of nitric oxide uptake by the RBC cytoskeleton has come from cytoskeletal altering experiments where the band 3 binding is altered using chemical cross-linkers.[21] Therefore, to date, the physiologic role of SNO–Hb as a key mediator of nitric oxide transport and function is controversial; that the role of hemoglobin as a scavenger of nitric oxide is still held by several investigators as a potentially important mechanism of nitric oxide loss. This is especially evident in the postulated role of plasma hemoglobin and superoxide in hemolytic anemia-associated pulmonary hypertension found in sickle cell disease.[22,23] It should be noted that experimental studies are difficult to perform because of the minute amounts of SNO–Hb present, the presence of other pathways of nitric oxide synthesis and metabolism, the fact that Fe^{3+} produced by nitric oxide also influences oxygen affinity and methodologic issues.[24] Future studies are necessary to clarify the influence of nitrite reduction and nitric oxide on normal hemoglobin function and will be pertinent to the development of blood substitutes.

Temperature Effect

The influence of temperature on the OEC is seen in the following equation with other factors being constant and in the physiologic range: $\Delta \log P_{50} / \Delta T = 0.023$. Overall, increasing body temperature by $5°C$ increases P_{50} approximately 7 mm Hg. Therefore, under conditions of extreme muscular exercise or increased in body temperature, there is a significant rightward shift of the OEC.

Interactions between Different Effectors of the Oxygen Equilibrium Curves

Many of the previously mentioned factors are not mutually exclusive. For example, the degree of the Bohr effect is influenced not only by pH and P_{CO_2} but also by 2,3-BPG and other anion concentrations and temperature. Several of these interactions are discussed in the subsequent text.

Effects of Carbon Monoxide and Hemoglobin Oxidation

These two effects are listed together because they have similar effects on the hemoglobin–oxygen affinity. The binding of carbon monoxide to heme iron forms carboxyhemoglobin, whereas the oxidation of Fe^{2+} to Fe^{3+} forms methemoglobin. Both of these effects render normal oxygen-binding sites unavailable for oxygen binding, shifting the OEC of the remaining unaltered subunits to the left. These effects are largely related to the stabilization of the T structure. This decreased total oxygen binding and increased affinity for bound oxygen explains the clinical severity of carbon monoxide poisoning and to a lesser extent, methemoglobinemia.[25]

Hemoglobin Variants

Variant hemoglobins possess amino acid substitutions or deletions, which in the large majority, produce no alteration of function. However, clinical consequences are likely if the mutation results in disruption of a structural portion of hemoglobin where intramolecular movements may alter the relationship between T and R states and result in altered position or shape of the OEC. Similarly, mutations at sites where hydrogen ions, 2,3-BPG, or other ligands attach may also cause functional consequences, such as a reduced Bohr or 2,3-BPG effect. Several other mutations have been noted to result in significant methemoglobin formation, enhanced denaturation of the hemoglobin molecule, and sickling. Many of these mutations also result in shortened red cell survival. However, despite many detailed functional studies and detailed three-dimensional x-ray crystallographic map of hemoglobin, our understanding of hemoglobin structure and function is not yet complete.[25]

Pathophysiologic Consideration of Shifts in the Oxygen Equilibrium Curves

Under conditions in which hydrogen ion, carbon dioxide, and temperature (i.e., overall metabolism) are increased, hemoglobin plays several critical roles. First, the high hemoglobin concentration in blood provides a powerful buffer for excess hydrogen ions. Therefore, the generation of large amounts of lactic acid, as in muscular exercise or other active metabolic processes, results in relatively little change in red blood cell and plasma pH. Second, because of the linked functions between oxygen and hydrogen ions (and other physiologic conditions such as increased P_{CO_2} and temperature), more oxygen is released locally when tissues are metabolically active or hyperthermic as, for example, during exercise. Conversely as blood enters the lung with decreased temperature, decreased P_{CO_2}, and increased pH, oxygen affinity is increased allowing efficient oxygen loading in the pulmonary capillaries.

The intracellular level of 2,3-BPG markedly affects the position of the OEC *in vivo*. In anemia and heart disease, for example, intracellular levels are increased. This causes a rightward shift of the OEC, thereby improving oxygen release under conditions in which oxygen transport is decreased.

Because there are mutant hemoglobins that have intrinsic rightward or leftward shifts of the OEC, erythrocytosis or anemia can result. This is largely a result of a renal EPO response that compensates for changes in the OEC. For example, patients with sickle cell disease have rightward shifts in the OEC. This explains why these patients appear to tolerate severe anemia relatively well.

Another important interaction is the effect that pH has on 2,3-BPG modulation of oxygen affinity. Initially, a very rapid change in oxygen affinity occurs when pH changes. This is followed by a slower effect through intracellular 2,3-BPG that shifts the OEC in the opposite direction. For example, when pH decreases the OEC is immediately shifted to the right. After several hours, the increase in intracellular pH decreases 2,3-BPG concentration and restores the OEC to approximately its starting position. Similar physiologic changes occur but in a converse manner when alkalosis is present. Sudden increases in pH may render the OEC inappropriately left-shifted for several hours until synthesis of 2,3-BPG occurs. Other physiologic changes such as vasoconstriction secondary to alkalosis may also result in inappropriate decrease in oxygen transport.

Stored Blood. Blood for transfusion is collected in anticoagulant/preservative solutions designed to ensure adequate *in vivo* survival and restoration of red cell mass. Stored blood does, however, undergo a series of metabolic phenomena known as the *storage lesion*. During refrigerated storage, there is a leftward shift of the OEC of stored blood, resulting in a P_{50} of 16 mm Hg versus normal P_{50} of 27 mm Hg. This is largely because of the marked decrease of intracellular 2,3-BPG in the red blood cells. Although, the rate of decrease in 2,3-BPG level depends on variables such as the final room temperature, rate of cooling of the whole blood unit to room temperature, time that the whole blood is held before component preparation, use of additive solution, the temperature during refrigeration, and pH of the red cell unit, all currently licensed additive systems and storage conditions yield blood units with low levels of 2,3-BPG after 7 to 10 days. This is seen in Figures 4.11 and 4.12.[26,27] When such blood is transfused, several hours are required for the return of 2,3-BPG levels and P_{50} to normal as seen in Figure 4.13.[28] With small volume transfusions (<15 mL per kg) there is little clinical consequence; neonates transfused with blood using different additives regenerate 2,3-BPG.[29-31] However, with massive transfusion of blood older than 7 to 10 days old, most RBCs will be stored red cells, which have a marked increased in oxygen affinity and may result in decreased ability to release oxygen. Although this can be compensated partially by the presence of acidosis (through the Bohr effect), which results in increased oxygen affinity at the tissue level, the overall *in vivo* blood oxygen affinity would still be greater than even with 2,3-BPG–replete RBCs at any given pH. At the present time, it is unclear whether the use of 2,3-BPG depleted RBCs harms patients who may already have massive blood loss and underlying disease, which may be affected by decreased oxygen transport. A relatively healthy patient likely has a sufficient physiologic reserve to deal with the limitation imposed by the leftward OEC shift. However, when the blood flow response is limited as a result of existing coronary or cerebral vascular disease, an increase in oxygen affinity will decrease oxygen consumption and greatly impair the function of the heart and brain. Although there is no definitive proof that seriously ill patients require blood with normal 2,3-BPG levels, a reasonable argument can be made that these patients should avoid massive transfusion with blood of high oxygen affinity (low or absent 2,3-BPG). To date, there has been only one prospective, randomized, double-blind study of red cell transfusion in anemic, nonbleeding, euvolemic, adult intensive care patients comparing fresh (≤5 days) versus older blood (≥20 days) leukoreduced red blood cells. In this study, the authors found that there were no clinically significant differences in gastric tonometry or global indices of tissue oxygenation 5 hours after transfusion, and concluded that fresh blood is not routinely needed in critically ill patients.[32] However, this study was limited in several aspects; it included a heterogeneous patient population, small study number, and the lack of transfusion criteria. Clearly, further studies are needed to evaluate the appropriate red cell products to use in critically ill pediatric patients.

Novel Therapies. Recently, a number of clinical trials have been performed that involve the modification of the OEC. One involves the drug, RSR13 (2-[4-[[(3,5-di-

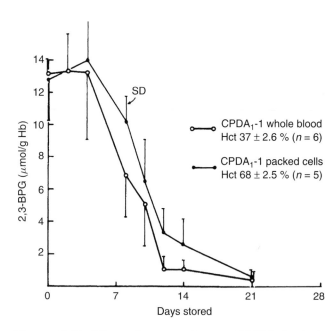

Figure 4.11 Effect of storage time on 2,3-BPG levels in whole blood and packed red blood cell (RBC) in citrate-phosphate-dextrose supplemented with 0.26 mmol per L adenine. CPDA-1, citrate-phosphate-dextrose-adenine; 2,3-BPG, 2,3-bisphosphoglycerate. (From Valeri CR, Valeri DA, Gray A, et al. Viability and function of red blood cell concentrates stored at 4°C for 35 days in CPDA-1, CPDA-2, or CPDA-3. *Transfusion.* 1982;22:212.)

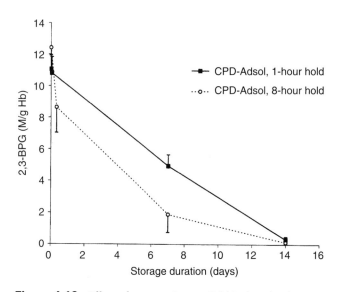

Figure 4.12 Effect of storage time on 2,3-bisphosphoglycerate (2,3-BPG) levels in packed cells collected in citrate-phosphate-dextrose (CPD) and stored in adenine-glucose-mannitol (Adsol) solution. (From Woodson RD. Hemoglobin synthesis, structure, and oxygen transport. In: Simon TL, Dzik WN, Snyder EL, et al., eds. *Rossi's principles of transfusion medicine*, 3rd ed. Philadelphia, PA: Lippincott Williams & Wilkins; 2002:39, with permission. Figure derived from Moroff G, Holme S, Keegan T, et al. Storage of ADSOL-preserved red cells at 2.5 and 5.5 degrees C: Comparable retention of in vitro properties. *Vox Sang.* 1990;59:136–139.)

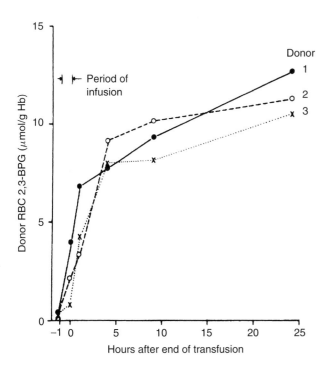

Figure 4.13 *In vivo* recovery of 2,3-bisphosphoglycerate (2,3-BPG) levels of transfused autologous red cells within 25 hours after transfusion in three patients. Autologous red cells were radiolabeled with ^{51}Cr and recovered by differential agglutination and assayed for 2,3-BPG levels. (From Beutler E, Wood L. The *in vivo* regeneration of red cell 2,3-diphosphoglyceric acid (DPG) after transfusion of stored blood. *J Lab Clin Med.* 1969;74:302, with permission.)

methylanilino)carbonyl]methyl]phenoxyl]-2-methylpropionic acid). This drug can cross the red cell membrane and interact with hemoglobin, causing a rightward shift of the OEC. Several animal models of ischemia have shown that this drug improves oxygen delivery.[33,34] Currently, human trials are in process in ischemia and as an adjunct to radiation therapy for malignant tumors. Another approach is the use of inosital hexaphosphate, which, like RSR13, produces a rightward shift of the OEC of human hemoglobin. Use of either compound with stored autologous or allogeneic blood could permit retention of a rightward OEC shift and eliminate the potential oxygen transport problems described in the preceding text. Still other approaches include the use of hemoglobin-based substitutes, reviewed in Reference 35.[35]

Oxygen Delivery

One of the most critical physiologic processes in the human body is oxygen transport. This system involves oxygen diffusion from the lungs coupled to intravascular red blood cell transport and release of heme-bound oxygen to metabolically active tissues. The amount of oxygen transported and delivered to tissues can be described by the following equation:

Oxygen delivery (Do_2)
$$= \text{Cardiac output (CO)}$$
$$\times \text{Arterial oxygen content (Ca}o_2)$$

Normally, 1 g of hemoglobin when fully saturated will bind 1.39 mL of oxygen. A small, but negligible amount of oxygen is dissolved in plasma which can be calculated by multiplying the partial pressure of oxygen by the solubility coefficient of oxygen ($k = 0.0001$ mL per mm Hg). Under most conditions this is so negligible that the arterial oxygen content can be estimated from the following equation:

$\text{Ca}o_2$ (mL per L)
$$= \%o_2 \text{ saturation} \times 1.39 \text{ (mL per g)} \times \text{[Hb]}$$

Therefore, oxygen delivery (Do_2) can be estimated after substituting for $\text{Ca}o_2$ using the following equation:

$$Do_2 = \text{CO} \times \%o_2 \text{ saturation} \times 1.39 \text{ (mL per g)} \times \text{[Hb]}$$

Where [Hb] is hemoglobin concentration in grams per deciliter. Therefore, decreased oxygen delivery can result from low hemoglobin concentration, decreased cardiac output, or poor hemoglobin saturation. In the typical resting state, the amount of oxygen delivered to tissues is twofold to fourfold in excess of oxygen consumption. In the resting state, oxygen consumption is relatively independent of the amount of oxygen delivered. However, once oxygen delivery begins to equal oxygen consumption (the critical level of oxygen delivery), the amount of oxygen consumed will be dependent on oxygen delivery (see Fig. 4.14). From a clinical perspective, a number of factors such as basal metabolic rate, specific organ or tissue involved, underlying disease, age, and genetic predisposition can alter this dependence and alter the critical level of oxygen delivery.

Adaptive Mechanisms to Anemia

It is important to realize that the regulation of oxygen transport is under the influence of several interactive control mechanisms, which can be altered under a variety of physiologic conditions. These control mechanisms range from alterations at the molecular level resulting in increased erythrocyte production to changes in cardiovascular hemodynamics and microcirculatory response.

Although there are many intracellular and extracellular factors, one of the key regulators of erythrocyte production is the interaction of EPO and the EPO receptor.[36] EPO is a 30.4-kDa glycoprotein that is produced primarily by the kidneys with a small amount produced by the liver. When there is a decrease in erythrocytes, such as with hemorrhage or hemolysis, oxygen delivery decreases and tissue hypoxia results. In response to tissue hypoxia, the kidneys and the liver respond with increased EPO production. The molecular mechanism involves post-translational induction of a transcription factor, hypoxia inducible factor-1 (HIF-1), a dimer composed of HIF-1α and HIF-1β, to an enhancer region that is 3′

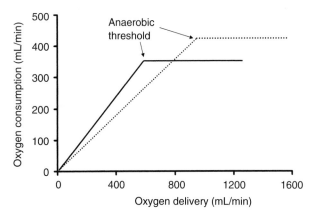

Figure 4.14 Demonstration of the biphasic relationship between oxygen consumption and oxygen delivery. The *solid line* represents the dependence of oxygen consumption on oxygen delivery. At low levels of oxygen delivery, oxygen consumption demonstrates a linear dependence on oxygen delivery. However, at some level of oxygen delivery, maximal oxygen consumption is surpassed (anaerobic threshold). However, increased oxygen consumption can occur in the presence of sepsis and acute respiratory distress syndrome (*dotted line*) elevating the anaerobic threshold.

to the *EPO* gene polyadenylation signal. Both HIF-1β and HIF-1α are constitutively expressed; however, under normal conditions, HIF-1α is undetectable because it is rapidly degraded through a ubiquitin-proteasome pathway. However, under hypoxic conditions, this degradation pathway becomes inactivated and intracellular HIF-1α increases, resulting in dimer formation with HIF-1β, which in turn binds to the 3′ enhancer region of EPO described in the preceding text. This enhancer region with the HIF-1 and other transcriptional factors, hepatocyte nuclear factor-4 (HNF-4) and p300, interact with the upstream promoter region of EPO to initiate mRNA production, which eventually results in EPO production and increased circulating EPO levels. Cells that produce EPO do so in an all-or-none fashion, allowing for rapid increases in EPO levels when tissue hypoxia occurs. Recruitment of renal cortical interstitial cells adjacent to the proximal tubules is largely responsible for the rapid increase in EPO level. This recruitment of cells actively producing EPO increases in an exponential fashion with linear decreases in hematocrit. This results in exponential increases in EPO in a similar fashion. The only patients with anemia who do not respond in this fashion to tissue hypoxia associated with anemia are those patients with renal disease who do not have the same number of functioning renal cortical cells as other patients.

EPO has several potential effects on erythroid progenitor cells. These include stimulation of proliferation, induction of termination differentiation, and promotion of cell survival. However, as the CFU-E (colony forming unit-erythroid) progenitor is always in the S phase of the cell cycle, it has been difficult to discern an effect of EPO on this progenitor, which has the highest number of EPO

receptors. Furthermore, EPO has only been able to effect partial differentiation, an effect only seen in cell lines. It is likely that EPO has an effect on cell survival likely through an inhibition of programmed cell death (apoptosis). This is thought to occur through EPO induction of Bcl-X_L, which binds and inhibits the action of Bax, a proapoptotic protein.[37] Depending on the stage of erythroid differentiation, there is a tremendous variation in the level of EPO needed for cell survival. This does not appear to be dependent on either the affinity of the EPO receptors or the number of EPO receptors. Furthermore, in different clinical scenarios there is a great deal of variation of the EPO level needed to maintain erythroid progenitor survival. For example, patients with chronic renal failure need very low levels of EPO to maintain survival of erythroid progenitor cells, whereas conditions involving acute blood loss or hemolysis require very high levels of EPO for continued cell survival.

Figure 4.15 demonstrates a possible model for different responses to EPO in different physiologic and pathologic states.[36] This model takes into account suppression of programmed cell death by EPO and the heterogeneity of the EPO dependence. In this model, there is an EPO-dependent stage and an EPO-independent stage. These stages correspond to the CFU-E through the reticulocyte stages. Under normal conditions (see Fig. 4.15A), with an average survival of 40% in the EPO-dependent stages, most cells undergo apoptosis with only a few cells surviving, allowing for a daily adult production of approximately 200 billion RBCs per day. Given that the life span of circulating erythrocytes in neonates ranges from 13 to 35 days, whereas in adults the erythrocyte life span is approximately 120 days, erythropoiesis is especially active in the neonatal population which is seen in higher reticulocyte reference ranges. In contrast, in conditions involving acute blood loss or hemolysis (see Fig. 4.15B), EPO levels are markedly increased. This results in a greater number of erythroid progenitor cells surviving to the EPO-independent stage, which results in several-fold higher rate of erythrocyte production. In conditions involving decreased production of EPO (see Fig. 4.15C), such as in chronic renal failure, the survival rate markedly decreases to levels much less than normal. This, in turn, results in the survival of a much smaller fraction of erythrocyte progenitors reaching the EPO-independent stage and erythrocyte production is much decreased. This is largely the rationale for the use of EPO in patients with chronic renal failure. Finally, under conditions in which erythropoiesis is ineffective (see Fig. 4.15D), such as seen in megaloblastic anemias and thalassemia, EPO levels are elevated, but there is an increased rate of apoptosis with progressive cell maturation of erythroid precursors. This pathologic apoptotic process extends to the EPO-independent stages, resulting in decreased erythrocyte production.

Erythropoiesis requires a sufficient supply of nutrients to produce the large number of erythrocytes needed for oxygen transport. The large DNA synthesis component

Figure 4.15 Proposed model of erythropoiesis incorporating suppression of programmed cell death (apoptosis) and heterogeneity in erythropoietin (EPO) dependence of erythroid progenitor cells. The period of EPO dependence starts at the colony forming unit-erythroid (CFU-E) stage and ends at the basophilic erythroblast stage. The time post-EPO dependence (EPO-independent period) includes the polychromatic erythroblast to the reticulocyte stage. The values in the figure indicate the fraction of surviving cells. **A:** Normal erythropoiesis. **B:** Acute hemolysis or blood loss associated with elevated EPO levels. **C:** Chronic renal failure associated with decreased EPO production. **D:** Ineffective erythropoiesis associated with high EPO levels, but increased apoptosis throughout both EPO-dependent and independent periods. See text for details. (From Koury MJ. Red blood cell production and kinetics. In: Simon TL, Dzik WH, Snyder EL, et al., eds. *Rossi's principles of transfusion medicine*, 3rd ed. Philadelphia, PA: Lippincott Williams & Wilkins; 2002:21.)

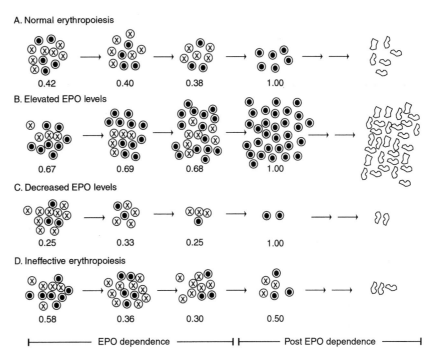

of erythropoiesis requires that adequate levels of both folate and vitamin B_{12} be available, whereas the need for hemoglobin production requires that iron be readily available. When any of these nutrients are not available erythrocyte production markedly decreases and anemia results. As a result of decreased oxygen transport (because of the decreased number of erythrocytes), there is a marked increase in EPO levels, which increases the survival of the pool of the erythroid progenitor cells and only partially compensates for decreased erythrocyte production.

Folate is a necessary cofactor for many enzymes involved in erythroid progenitor cells. When vitamin B_{12} is deficient, folate is trapped in the methyltetrahydrofolate form and is not available as the methylenetetrahydrofolate form, which is necessary for thymidine synthesis or the formyltetrahydrofolate form, which is necessary for purine synthesis.[38] Vitamin B_{12} deficiency is similar to folate deficiency in that folate is not available for DNA synthesis. This results in accumulation of erythroid progenitor cells in the S phase of the cell cycle, which is rapidly followed by apoptosis.[39,40] Cells that are most susceptible to this apoptosis include EPO-dependent cells and cells beginning to produce hemoglobin. Because of the high EPO levels, the erythroid progenitor cells consist of a large proportion of CFU-E cells in the presence of reticulocytopenia. Given the elevated apoptotic rates and therefore very high cell turnover rates, increased serum lactate dehydrogenase, serum bilirubin, and iron turnover is seen.

The mechanisms by which iron deficiency results in decreased erythropoiesis are several. These include decreased erythrocyte life span, ineffective erythropoiesis,

and impaired maturation of late-stage erythroblasts. Experimental ferrokinetic studies suggest that although EPO levels and CFU-E cells are increased, iron deficiency in a degree of ineffective erythropoiesis exists, but not to the extent seen in vitamin B_{12} or folate deficiency or thalassemia.[41] The ineffective erythropoiesis and decreased maturation rate of late-stage erythroblasts may be related to the observation that iron uptake is greatest before the beginning of hemoglobin synthesis, during EPO dependence, occurring during the highest rate of cell proliferation.[42] The decreased red cell survival of iron deficient cells is related to the increased rigidity of the plasma membrane of these cells, which results in increased hemolysis and removal by the reticuloendothelial system.[43]

There are a number of dyserythropoietic disorders such as myelodysplastic syndrome, aplastic anemia, Fanconi anemia, and myeloid leukemias, which are associated with a reduction of erythroid progenitor cells. In contrast, acute lymphoblastic leukemia results in inhibition of erythroid progenitor maturation and increased apoptosis. This leads to the reticulocytopenia and anemia seen in these patients. Polycythemia vera, by contrast, is associated with increased numbers of erythroid progenitor cells, which are very sensitive to EPO and insulinlike growth factor.[44,45] Therefore, these cells survive longer and many circulating erythrocytes are observed.

There are many diseases that affect erythropoiesis by virtue of their displacement of hematopoietic cells in the bone marrow. These include myelofibrosis, metastatic tumors, and lymphoid neoplasms. The most common cause of secondary inhibition of erythropoiesis, however, is anemia of chronic disease, also known as *anemia of inflammation*. Like iron deficiency, several mechanisms are thought to contribute to the impairment of erythropoiesis. These include: increased sequestration of iron by macrophages, cytokine-mediated inhibition of both EPO production by the kidneys (resulting in increased apoptosis) and erythroid progenitor cell growth, and decreased life span of circulating erythrocytes. Recently, a link between hepcidin and anemia of chronic disease has been elucidated.[46] Animal and human studies have demonstrated that mediators of inflammation such as lipopolysaccharide and interleukin-6 (IL-6) can upregulate hepcidin expression by hepatocytes.[47–49] Several transgenic mouse models, furthermore, have demonstrated that hepcidin is a predominant negative regulator of iron absorption in the intestine and iron release from macrophages.[50] Recently, Weinstein et al.[51] reported on several patients who had large hepatic adenomas that overexpressed hepcidin mRNA and had severe iron-refractory microcytic anemia. Resection of their tumors led to full reversal of their hematologic abnormalities. This is an area of intense investigation as the molecular mechanisms by which hepcidin alters iron metabolism is not fully understood. In the future, this may lead to hepcidin antagonists, which may be useful in the treating anemia of chronic disease, a condition often resistant to EPO and iron therapy. Until these new therapies become a reality, resolution of the underlying disease is necessary to treat this cause of anemia.

Other physiologic adaptations to anemia include physiologic alterations of the OEC.[52] As mentioned previously, increased pH or temperature, as well as decreased intracellular 2,3-BPG concentration, all result in a rightward shift of the oxyhemoglobin dissociation curve, whereas opposite changes result in a leftward shift. Anemia increases 2,3-BPG synthesis in RBCs, causing a rightward shift in the OEC, and results in the release of more oxygen at a given P_{O_2} despite decreased oxygen content of the blood because of anemia. There is also a small influence related to the Bohr effect; however, this is of little clinical significance as it necessitates a relatively large change in pH to cause a significant change in the P_{50}; this is despite the ability of the Bohr effect to initiate a rapid rightward shift of the OEC, which enhances off-loading of oxygen from hemoglobin. It is important to realize that assessing the degree of hemoglobin–oxygen saturation can be problematic as arterial specimens are processed at standard temperature and pH, which does not reflect microcirculatory conditions (such as pH, temperature, and other disease processes), that would affect the OEC.

Hemodynamic adaptations to the development of anemia have come from studies of normovolemic hemodilution in relatively healthy patients in whom there has been documentation of increased cardiac output secondary to increased heart rate and stroke volume, increased sympathetic activity, increased myocardial contractility, decreased systemic vascular resistance, and a redistribution of cardiac output from toward the heart and the brain away from the splanchnic circulation. The most important factor affecting response, however, is the patient's left ventricular preload. When intravascular volume is high or stable after anemia (such as normovolemic hemodilution), increases in cardiac output have been reported when the hemoglobin ranges from 7 to 12 g per dL. This increase has been postulated to be a result of two mechanisms: (i) reduced blood viscosity and (ii) increased sympathetic stimulation. Reduced blood viscosity will enhance cardiac output by decreasing both preload and afterload while sympathetic stimulation increases heart rate and contractility.[53] In the case of blood loss, however, both hypovolemia and anemia can result in tissue hypoxia through decreased cardiac output and decreased oxygen carrying capacity. To compensate for these changes and to protect vital organs, the body will attempt compensatory changes in myocardial contractility and heart rate, increase vascular tone through increased sympathetic activity and divert blood flow from the skeletal, cutaneous, and splanchnic circulation toward the cerebral and coronary circulation. In contrast to hypervolemic or normovolemic anemia, however, blood viscosity does not appear to play a predominant role in affecting cardiac output.

There are several important interactions between blood flow, viscosity, and cardiac output. Intravascularly, blood flow alters whole blood viscosity, and blood viscosity modulates cardiac output. Based on the Poiseuille-Hagan law, blood flow is directly proportional to the fourth power of the radius and pressure. It is inversely proportional to the length of the vessel and to blood viscosity.[53] Where flow is slowest (such as at the postcapillary venules) viscosity is the highest, while in the aorta (where flow is fastest) viscosity is the lowest. With anemia, viscosity at the postcapillary venules decreases resulting in increased venous return and left ventricular preload. This is the most important contribution to increased cardiac output provided that cardiac function is normal during normovolemic hemodilution. As mentioned previously, decreased left ventricular afterload can contribute to increased cardiac output during anemia.[54]

The inverse relationship between hemoglobin level and cardiac output has led many investigators to study the optimal hemoglobin level that optimizes oxygen transport. On the basis of a canine model,[55] it was found that optimal oxygen delivery occurred at hematocrits between 40% and 60%, whereas others suggest optimal hematocrits between 40% and 45% (hemoglobin concentration 13 to 15 g per dL).[56] A widely quoted study[57] found that peak oxygen transport occurs at hematocrit of 30% (hemoglobin concentration of 10 g per dL). A major problem with these studies is their reliance on global measures of oxygen delivery, which largely ignore blood flow difference between different organs and ignores the effect of pathologic processes on the adaptive responses to anemia. For example, in critically ill patients, these hemodynamic adaptations are unlikely to be fully functional and decreased hemoglobin levels, which would be easily tolerated by relatively normal individuals, may be suboptimal.

There are several putative microvascular responses to anemia including (i) recruitment and activation of previously closed capillaries, (ii) capillary flow enhancement, and (iii) increased oxygen extraction from existing capillaries. These responses are affected by the degree of anemia, the specific tissue in question and the underlying disease. A decreased whole blood viscosity is an advantage in the capillary system. This is because the hematocrit in the capillaries is highest compared to other parts of the vascular tree. When anemia occurs there is a disproportionate decrease in whole blood viscosity, which results in improved capillary blood flow to tissues. However, with severe anemia, the benefit of improved capillary flow may be offset by decreased transit time (and oxygen diffusion time) in the capillaries, resulting in overall decreased oxygen delivery.[58,59] In contrast, in the presence of a severely elevated hematocrit, microcirculatory stasis may occur resulting in decreased blood flow and decreased oxygen delivery.

From a transfusion standpoint, transfusion of older, stored, RBCs (>7 to 10 days old) has a theoretical risk of delivering less oxygen to tissues because of markedly decreased 2,3-BPG level, which results in a leftward shift of the OEC. In addition, these red cells are less deformable with theoretical potential for impeding flow in the microcirculation.[60,61] These two phenomena, part of the red cell storage lesion, however, are reversible in the 24 to 48 hours post-transfusion.[62] Of interest is the contraindication of the transfusion of sickle trait blood to neonates and to patients with sickle cell disease. This is based on studies demonstrating that leukoreduction of sickle cell trait blood is affected by the degree of oxygenation of the RBCs before filtration[63] and reports of sickling of sickle trait blood in patients with hypoxia.[64] The goal of transfusion is to reduce intravascular sickling by diluting or replacing the patient's sickled cells with nonsickled (Hb A) blood from a normal donor. Use of sickle trait blood defeats this purpose. Furthermore, sepsis has been postulated to affect red blood cell deformability. Under inappropriate microcirculatory adaptive responses, red cell transfusion, especially of older blood, is theorized to adversely affect microcirculatory flow and oxygen delivery at the tissue level.[65] However, a study by Friedlander et al.[66] suggests that transfused RBCs improve overall red blood cell deformability by dilution of autologous RBCs, which, under conditions of sepsis, are more rigid then transfused RBCs.

There are a number of diseases that can potentially limit the adaptive mechanisms. Diseases that affect the heart, and specifically the left ventricle, are especially prone to the effects of anemia because 60% to 75% of the oxygen delivered by the coronary circulation is consumed by the myocardium. Because of the high myocardial oxygen extraction, oxygen delivery to the myocardium can only increase by an increasing coronary blood flow, which itself is dependent primarily on the duration of diastoli. Diseases that result in tachycardia will decrease the duration of diastole and if there is significant coronary stenosis, oxygen delivery to the myocardium may be inadequate resulting in myocardial dysfunction. Animal studies have shown that hemoglobin levels as low as 7 g per dL are well tolerated if the coronary circulation is normal.[67] However, if there is moderate to high-grade coronary stenosis, animal models have shown that myocardial dysfunction and ischemia will occur earlier compared to controls with normal hemoglobin levels.[68] Human studies have been inconclusive; however, several recent adult studies have demonstrated that moderate anemia is poorly tolerated in perioperative and critically ill patients with cardiovascular disease.[69,70]

Studies from patients undergoing normovolemic hemodilution have shown that cerebral blood flow increases by 50% to 500% secondary to increased cardiac output, which is diverted from other less critical areas of the body.[71,72] At the present time, there is little evidence that moderate levels of anemia worsen already present cerebrovascular disease. Although patients with high intracranial pressures after traumatic brain injury may have a theoretical risk from increased blood flow in the presence of normovolemic or hypervolemic hemodilution, there may actually be a benefit in patients who develop subarachnoid hemorrhage.[73] This may be related to improved oxygen delivery through decreased blood viscosity and reduction in vasospasm. However, because of the redistribution toward the cerebrovascular and coronary arteries, there is the continued danger that less vital organs may be affected, for example, the kidneys and gastrointestinal tract.[74] In addition, in critically ill patients, the increased metabolic demands, possible impairment of cardiac function, and microcirculatory changes may affect oxygen delivery to other organs.[75,76]

TRANSFUSION PHYSIOLOGY

Risks of Anemia

Much of what we know about the risks of anemia comes not only from careful studies of normovolemic hemodilution in both adults and children but also from studies involving Jehovah's Witness patients. Early studies in cardiopulmonary bypass in children, for example, delineated relatively safe degrees of hemodilution to a hematocrit of 20% when performed under hypothermic conditions and hypotensive anesthesia.[77]

However, only recently has a series of studies permitted an understanding of detailed cardiovascular and metabolic responses.[78] In these studies healthy adult volunteers were compared to healthy adult patients undergoing acute, severe normovolemic hemodilution to 5 g per dL with 5% albumin replacement. Systemic vascular resistance decreased with increased heart rate, stroke volume, and cardiac index with no decrease in blood pressure. Remarkably, there was no evidence of inadequate oxygenation with small significant changes in oxygen consumption and no change in plasma lactate levels. No clinically significant ST changes on Holter monitoring occurred. In a comparison of patients who were well hydrated and warmed prior to the start of normovolemic hemodilution (well perfused) versus patients who were not deliberately well perfused, there was no difference in subcutaneous wound oxygen tension at a hemoglobin of 5 g per dL. Increases in subcutaneous perfusion and flow indices appeared to compensate for the decreased oxygen content of the blood at the lower hemoglobin concentration and suggest that severe isovolemic hemodilution to 5 g per dL would not impair wound healing. However, hemodilution less than 7 g per dL was associated with decreased self-scored energy levels, reversible with autologous RBC transfusion and reversible impairment of cognitive function with increased reaction time and degradation of immediate and delayed memory at hemoglobin concentrations of 6 g per dL or below. Many of these physiologic changes could be reasonably extrapolated to children, particularly adolescents; however, in very small infants with complex congenital heart defects, compensatory mechanisms are unlikely to be operating normally and it is important to examine pediatric studies in detail.

Other physiologic studies of hemodilution in pediatric surgery patients comes from studies by Fontana et al.[79] which found that extreme hemodilution could be performed under hypothermic conditions, hypotensive anesthesia, and 100% FIO_2 ventilation. In this study eight children underwent spinal fusion with extreme acute normovolemic hemodilution (ANH) to a mean hemoglobin ($\pm SD$) of 3.0 $\pm$ 0.8 g per dL. The mean ($\pm SD$) mixed venous oxygen saturation decreased from 90.8% $\pm$ 5.4% to 72.3% $\pm$ 7.8%, whereas the mean ($\pm SD$) oxygen extraction ratio increased from 17.3% $\pm$ 6.2% to 44.4% $\pm$ 5.9%. Mean ($\pm SD$) oxygen delivery decreased from 532.1 $\pm$ 138.1 mL/minute/m^2 to 260.2 $\pm$ 57.1 mL/minute/m^2 while global oxygen consumption did not decrease and plasma lactate did not appreciably increase. To compensate for the changes, central venous pressure increased and peripheral resistance decreased during hemodilution. Cardiac index increased, heart rate remained essentially constant and left ventricular stroke work index did not decrease significantly. Patients underwent hyperoxic ventilation at a fraction of inspired oxygen (FIO_2) of 1.0. There were no clinically adverse outcomes. This study suggested that more severe ANH (<15% hematocrit) may be clinically acceptable for young, healthy patients if hyperoxic anesthesia is employed.

Criticism of these studies, which examined the physiologic effects of extreme hemodilution, include the lack of studies of specific organ function that may be affected by decreased oxygen delivery at these lower hematocrits. Although nonspecific measurements such as mixed venous oxygen saturation, plasma lactate, and physiologic monitoring are useful, such measurements may not adequately reflect the effect of decreased oxygen delivery to individual organs with different oxygenation thresholds. Although animal studies can be used to ascertain specific organ safety (as was initially used to ascertain safety in the early clinical assessment of hemodilution), these are no substitute for actual organ-specific oxygen delivery measurement in children; however, it is unlikely that given the vulnerability of children as research subjects such studies will be forthcoming.

Another criticism of these studies is the confounding effect of techniques to lower global oxygen use or to maintain greater oxygenation on the hemodynamic and oxygenation safety of the study patients. The use of moderate to deep hypothermia (30°C to 32°C) not only increases the amount of dissolved oxygen, but together with general anesthesia also decreases tissue oxygen demands. Hypotensive anesthesia also decreases oxygen demands on the cardiovascular system. Hyperoxic ventilation used by Fontana et al.[79] offered a margin of safety for very severe hemodilution or any intraoperative hemorrhage that increases surgical risk. This technique is currently under evaluation and currently is used in patients who have religious reasons for avoiding transfusion (i.e., Jehovah's Witnesses). Therefore, the safety of hemodilution in children must take into account anesthetic techniques, which either improve tissue oxygenation or minimize global oxygen consumption. Because intraoperative hemorrhage can dramatically increase surgical risk, hemodilution in children can only be recommended to a level of 20% based on studies of Jehovah's Witness children undergoing cardiopulmonary bypass with bloodless prime and moderate to deep hypothermia.[77]

Transfusion Thresholds

Transfusion guidelines in neonatal and pediatric practice are difficult to establish. Practices and policies vary and are often based on small studies with limited statistical power. Furthermore, many patients requiring transfusion support often need highly specialized products, in small volumes, intensely during critical illness. The fact that neonatal and pediatric patients also survive their disease per event and have a normal life expectancy drives the need to select the safest products. Two recent reviews detail guidelines for transfusion threshold in pediatric patients.[80,81] Table 4.3 details data-driven consensus guidelines from the United States.

The observation that infants may be asymptomatic with low hemoglobin concentrations, whereas others are symptomatic with similar or higher hemoglobin concentrations supports the concept that hemoglobin alone is an inadequate measure of the need to transfuse. Compensatory

TABLE 4.3

CONSENSUS DRIVEN GUIDELINES FOR THE TRANSFUSION OF PACKED RBCS TO PEDIATRIC PATIENTS GREATER OR LESS THAN 4 MONTHS OF AGE

Patients <4 mo of Age:

1. Hct <20% with low reticulocyte count and symptoms of anemia[a]
2. Hct <30% with an infant:
   a. On <35% hood O_2
   b. On O_2 by nasal canula
   c. On continuous positive airway pressure and/or intermittent mandatory ventilation with mechanical ventilation with mean airway pressure <6 cm H_2O
   d. With significant apnea or bradycardia[b]
   e. With significant tachycardia or tachypnea[c]
   f. With low weight gain[d]
3. Hct <35% with an infant:
   a. On >35% hood O_2
   b. On continuous positive airway pressure/intermittent mandatory ventilation with mean airway pressure $\geq$6–8 cm H_2O
4. Hct <45% with an infant:
   a. On ECMO
   b. With congenital cyanotic heart disease

Patients >4 mo of Age:

1. Emergency surgical procedure in patient with significant preoperative anemia
2. Preoperative anemia when other corrective therapy is not available
3. Intraoperative blood loss $\geq$15% total blood volume
4. Hct <24%:
   a. In perioperative period, with signs and symptoms of anemia
   b. While on chemotherapy/radiotherapy
   c. Chronic congenital or acquired symptomatic anemia
5. Acute blood loss with hypovolemia not responsive to other therapy
6. Hct <40% with:
   a. Severe pulmonary disease
   b. ECMO
7. Sickle cell disease:
   a. Cerebrovascular accident
   b. Acute chest syndrome
   c. Splenic sequestration
   d. Recurrent priapism
   e. Preoperatively when general anesthesia is planned to reach Hb 10 g/dL
8. Chronic transfusion programs for disorders of RBC production (such as β thalassemia major and Diamond-Blackfan syndrome unresponsive to therapy)

[a]Tachycardia, tachypnea, poor feeding.
[b]More than six episodes in 12 h or two episodes in 24 h requiring bag and mask ventilation while receiving therapeutic doses of methylxanthines.
[c]Heart rate >180 beats/min for 24 h, respiratory rate >80 breaths/min for 24 h.
[d]Gain of <10 g/d observed over 4 d while receiving $\geq$100 kcal/kg/d.
ECMO, extracorporeal-membrane oxygenation; Hct, hematocrit.

responses in the infant to decreased tissue oxygen concentration include increases in heart rate, cardiac output, and cerebral blood flow and therefore are similar to the adult and older child. Cerebral fractional oxygen extraction (FOE) increases to maintain low cerebral oxygen delivery, likely because of low cerebral blood flow. Another adaptive mechanism is the progressive shift to anaerobic respiration, which results in an increase in lactic acid. Several authors have studied FOE and lactic acid as surrogates for transfusion; post-transfusion decrease in lactic acid, for example, might reflect improved oxygen delivery. However, there are technical and biological variables that affect both FOE

and lactic acid measurement which include fasting, cold, increased activity, hemolysis, and venous occlusion, especially when the specimen is obtained from a peripheral vein. In a well-conceived study that attempted to avoid these variables, capillary whole blood lactic acid was analyzed pretransfusion and 48 hours post-transfusion in 18 premature infants. Lactic acid measurements did not correlate with either respiratory rate or bradycardiac episodes when regression analysis was performed.[82] The high coefficient of variation of 19.8% of repeated measures of lactic acid likely contributed to the poor correlation. Some have suggested that an elevated lactic acid results from the catecholamine surge associated with sepsis or injury. In this circumstance, post-transfusion lactate might well fall, but as a result of a fall in catecholamine response rather than from improvement in anaerobic metabolism.

Utilizing a different approach, Wardle et al. support the use of near infrared spectroscopy (NIRS) measurement of FOE as a guide to transfusion.[83,84] Preliminary data suggests that a normal FOE might obviate the need to transfuse RBCs. In a pilot study, 37 infants were randomized to one of two groups: transfusion decision was based on peripheral FOE or conventional protocol based on hemoglobin. The NIRS group (56 transfusions) was determined by an FOE of 0.47 while the conventional group received 84 transfusions. Of the 56 transfusions given in the NIRS group, 33 (59%) were given because of clinical concerns. Other measurements like paired pre- and post-transfusion measurements of oxygen consumption (Vo_2), mixed venous oxygen saturation (MVo_2) and hemoglobin–oxygen dissociation curve alone or in combination would theoretically demonstrate post-transfusion improvement in oxygen delivery, but are impractical.

Mock et al.[85] correlated hematocrit to RBC volume in 26 premature infants of birth weight less than 1,300 g, studied on 43 occasions using a nonradioactive biotinylated RBC-labeling flow cytometric method. Their goal was to develop an accurate RBC volume measurement and establish the relationship between circulating red cell volume and hematocrit and to assess whether poor correlations between hematocrit and RBC volume were due to artifact or unique preterm physiology. They hypothesized that if RBC volume and hematocrit were correlated, then hematocrit could be used as a decisive test for transfusion need. Despite good correlation between the two assays ($r = 0.907$), the circulatory RBC volume ranges for premature infants at a given hematocrit were so broad as to make the RBC volume measurement of questionable clinical significance, and raised issues about the use of either hematocrit alone or a specific RBC volume measurement.

Establishing a physiologic basis for transfusion triggers in the pediatric intensive care unit (PICU) setting is as problematic as in the neonatal intensive care unit (NICU). To date, three prospective epidemiologic surveys[86–88] and one retrospective survey[89] have addressed the characteristics of children transfused in the PICU setting. None were randomized or controlled. Marked variability in practice patterns was shown and there was little consistency among the three studies to guide the practitioner. Two prospective observational studies of hospitalized anemic children in Africa suggest that a hemoglobin more than 5 g per dL decreased mortality in chronically anemic children. No guidance was provided for acute anemia exacerbating chronic anemia.[90,91] Generalization from adult data[92] may be inappropriate because of the differences in diagnoses, physiologic variability over time in children, better health status of children and differences in cardiovascular physiology. An international multicenter noninferiority trial (transfusion requirements in pediatric intensive care units [TRIPICU]) will study a restrictive (threshold Hb 7 per dL) versus liberal (threshold 9.5 g per dL) transfusion strategy to study the proportion of children who develop or progress to multisystem organ failure syndrome.[93] This study may well provide valuable guidance on transfusion criteria for the critically ill child.

Considerations on dose and administration for bleeding patients include (i) consideration of the degree and rate of blood loss, (ii) hemodynamic assessment, and (iii) comorbid conditions. Considerations for surgical patients include maintaining adequate Do_2 well beyond the anaerobic threshold while minimizing allogeneic exposure. However, it should be mentioned that current methods of monitoring effective circulatory blood volume and utilization of oxygen at the tissue level have limitations. In high-risk patients, it may be necessary to measure right and left ventricular filling pressure by means of central venous pressure and pulmonary artery catheters to better ascertain cardiac function. Continuous monitoring of cardiac output is also possible with pulmonary arterial catheters or esophageal Doppler techniques. However, there is little data on whether invasive monitoring and different treatment strategies cause more good than harm. Most experienced anesthesiologists and critical care physicians have developed an approach to management of blood loss and hemodynamic instability. Considerations are different for the patients with chronic anemia where compensation may have developed. There is usually increased blood flow as a result of decreased viscosity, greater release of oxygen caused by higher levels of 2,3-BPG and increased cardiac output.

Guidelines by the American Society of Anesthesiologists are by far the most rigorously developed and methodologically sound.[94] The College of American Pathologists and the UK Blood Transfusion Task Force have updated red cell transfusion guidelines.[95,96] Because there have been no randomized clinical trials in pediatric patients, clinical practice has largely been extrapolated from adult studies and/or expert opinion.

Coagulation

There has been a tremendous evolutionary pressure in the development of the coagulation system to maintain blood in a fluid state under normal physiologic conditions but allow rapid reaction to vascular injury while preventing blood loss by rapid sealing of the intravascular defect. Unfortunately, this mechanism may result in thrombosis if the initial stimulus is unregulated, either because of dysregulated inhibitory pathways or if the ability of the natural anticoagulant mechanisms are overwhelmed by the initial stimulus. (For a detailed in-depth review, see Reference 97.)

The key to the maintenance of blood fluidity is the vascular endothelium, which inhibits blood coagulation and platelet aggregation while promoting fibrinolysis. It also

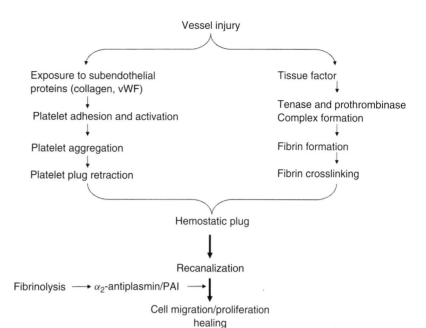

Figure 4.16 Summary of the effects of vessel injury on the formation of the hemostatic plug with subsequent healing. See text for details. Not shown are the inhibitory factors that modulate and limit this process. PAI, plasminogen activator inhibitor; vWF, von Willebrand factor.

acts to separate blood cells and plasma factors from highly reactive elements (such as collagen, laminin, vitronectin, von Willebrand factor [vWF], and tissue factor [TF]) in the subendothelial and deeper layers of the vessel wall. Many of these elements are responsible for platelet adhesion and aggregation and initiation of blood coagulation. During vessel injury, blood is exposed to these reactive elements stimulating primary platelet plug formation and activating blood coagulation. Exposure to subendothelial collagen consequently results in the exposure and assembly of platelet glycoproteins IIb and IIIa, which, in turn, bind circulating fibrinogen and vWF, which, in turn, promote platelet recruitment and aggregation. This results in α granule secretion, which is mediated by several intracellular platelet biochemical reactions such as thromboxane A_2 synthesis, targeted protein phosphorylation, and intracellular calcium translocations. Various coagulation factors such as factor V, secreted by platelets or derived from plasma, when present on the platelet surface initiate the assemblage of various enzyme–cofactor complexes resulting in accelerated factor X and prothrombin activation. Thrombin is produced, which, in turn, catalyzes its own production by further activation of factor V and VIII and stimulating further platelet activation and secretion (see Fig. 4.16).

Modulation of these processes occurs by a variety of compounds including antithrombotic lipids such as prostacyclin, or prostaglandin I_2 (PGI_2), proteins (such as thrombomodulin), inorganic compounds such as nitric oxide, and polysaccharides (heparin), by surface binding enzymes such as adenosine diphosphatase (ADPase) (CD39), and by several plasma protease inhibitors, including antithrombin-III (AT-III), C1-inhibitor (C1-INH), α_1-antitrypsin, and α_2-macroglobulin. Thrombin acts on fibrinogen, which forms fibrin monomers that undergo

spontaneous polymerization to form the fibrin clot. Factor XIIIa, which is activated by thrombin, improves the resistance of the clot to fibrinolysis.

Plasminogen, a major zymogen that plays a critical role in fibrinolysis, is converted to plasmin by plasminogen activators produced by endothelial cells. This process is modulated by several plasminogen activator inhibitors. These include α_2-antiplasmin, plasminogen activator inhibitor (PAI-1) and thrombin-activatable fibrinolysis inhibitor (TAFI). The presence of α_2-antiplasmin in solution prevents plasmin from acting on fibrinogen. PAI-1, itself, prevents early lysis of the clot by neutralizing tissue plasminogen activator (tPA), whereas TAFI, a carboxypeptidase B proenzyme, decreases fibrinolytic degradation of fibrin strands. Therefore, with more thrombin generation, more fibrin is formed and is further protected from fibrinolysis by TAFI. Wound healing occurs when the clot is dissolved and there is deposition of collagen and formation of fibrous tissue.

Endothelium

The endothelium plays a key role in the maintenance of blood fluidity because of its critical roles in the production of inhibitors of blood coagulation and platelet aggregation, modulation of vascular tone and permeability, and provision of a protective role as a barrier separating hemostatic blood components from reactive subendothelial sites and structures such as the basement membrane and extracellular matrix, which contain adhesive proteins, collagen, fibronectin, laminin, vitronectin, and vWF. One of the principle mechanisms by which the endothelium inhibits coagulation is the synthesis and secretion of thrombomodulin and heparan sulfate. Endothelial synthesis and secretion of tPA, urokinase plasminogen activator (uPA), and plasminogen activator inhibitors also regulate the action of plasmin, whereas platelet aggregation is inhibited by endothelial PGI$_2$ and nitric oxide. Other actions of the endothelium include the regulation of vessel wall tone by endothelin synthesis, which induces vasoconstriction and PGI$_2$ and nitric oxide, which produces vasodilation.

Abnormal extravascular bleeding can occur if there are structural abnormalities of the vessel wall or extracellular supporting structures which lead to inappropriate vasoconstrictive responses, or if there is abnormal physiologic fibrinolysis, which is not controlled by plasminogen activator inhibitor. Immune complex and virally mediated endothelial damage can also result in bleeding. Breakdown of endothelial wall integrity secondary to vasculitic disorders or release of proteolytic enzymes in inflammatory states may also contribute to petechial hemorrhage. Despite the presence of large, biologically active platelets seen in idiopathic thrombocytopenic purpura, fenestration, and attenuation of the vascular endothelium may also contribute to the petechia seen in this disorder.[98]

Stimulation of endothelial cells by enzymes such as thrombin, hypoxia; fluid shear stress; oxidants; cytokines such as IL-1, tumor necrosis factor and γ-interferon; synthetic hormones such as desmopressin acetate; and endotoxin results in the loss of endothelial thrombogenic protection. TF and PAI-1 synthesis is induced, whereas thrombomodulin is reduced by cytokines and endotoxin. Desmopressin acetate induces the release of vWF into the blood and therefore high-molecular-weight vWF multimers are lost from the endothelial surface, which could assist in platelet adhesion to the injured vessel wall. By contrast, endothelial cells contain many receptors that are involved in adhesion. These include integrins such as the very late antigen (VLA) type (that bind to fibronectin, collagen, and laminin), the vitronectin receptor, and intercellular adhesion molecules such as intercellular adhesion molecule-1 (ICAM-1) and ICAM-2, and vascular cell adhesion molecule-1 (VCAM-1), which act as counter receptors for leukocyte integrins. The stimulated endothelial cells also synthesize chemokines such as monocyte chemoattractant protein, IL-8, and regulated upon activation, normal T-cell expressed and secreted (RANTES). Furthermore, the rolling interaction of platelets and leukocytes on the endothelial cell (which occurs before adhesion to the endothelium) is mediated by E selectin and P selectin, which is stored in Weibel-Palade bodies in endothelial cells.

Endothelium in different parts of the vascular tree differs in structure and function.[99] For example, the expression of thrombomodulin, vWF, and the family of selectin molecules is quite variable. Thromboxane A$_2$ is synthesized primarily by the pulmonary arterial endothelium. *In vivo*, there is differential expression of various mediators in response to *Escherichia coli* sepsis, traumatic shock, and blood flow as well as different signaling molecules such as thrombin, IL-1α, and platelet-derived growth factor.

Endothelial proliferation becomes especially prominent at sites of hemodynamic stress or injury. Maintenance of endothelial junctional apposition involves both intracellular contractile proteins and extracellular molecules such as cadherin and platelet–endothelial cell adhesion molecule. Any stimulus and signal that can influence expression or interaction of these molecules can clearly affect the ability of the endothelium to maintain vascular integrity. Furthermore, passage of macromolecules across the endothelium occurs through intercellular junctions, by endocytosis, and through transendothelial pores. Therefore, increased fenestration and attenuation of endothelium will increase vessel permeability. This occurs through vasodilation, with thrombocytopenia, and by high doses of heparin. In the case of thrombocytopenia, petechiae develop because of extravasation of erythrocytes principally through postcapillary venular interendothelial channels. The loss of endothelial barrier function associated with thrombocytopenia, which results in petechial formation may be related either to the loss of delivery of platelet-derived serotonin and norepinephrine to the microvasculature or failure of primary platelet plug formation.

Another feature of endothelial cells is its highly negatively charged surface. This feature is important in limiting hemostasis and preventing extravasation of platelets. This negatively charged surface combined with endothelial antithrombotic properties (PGI$_2$ synthesis and release, which inhibits platelet aggregation, presence of surface-bound molecules such as thrombomodulin and heparan sulfate) limit the spread of fibrin formation and are important in limiting the intravascular extension of the hemostatic reaction. Heparan sulfate activates AT in a similar manner as heparin and catalyzes the inhibition of thrombin and factor Xa. Adenosine diphosphate (ADP), which also activates platelet aggregation is affected by the presence of endogenous cell–associated ADPase (CD39), which cleaves ADP to adenosine monophosphate (AMP).

The mechanism by which thrombomodulin limits the spread of fibrin formation from a site of vessel injury includes binding thrombin, which reduces thrombin's ability to cleave fibrinogen and activate platelets, and prevention of activation of factor V and VIII. Because thrombomodulin enhances the ability of thrombin to activate protein C through the endothelial cell protein C receptor, there is inactivation of already formed factors Va and VIIIa by protein C. Protein C also is involved in enhancing fibrinolysis, most likely through inhibition of plasminogen activators. AT along with heparan sulfate inactivates thrombin binding to thrombomodulin. Proteins that inhibit protein C activity include protein C inhibitor (PAI-3) and α_1-proteinase inhibitor, whereas protein S, is a cofactor for protein C activity. Protein S levels and activity are, in turn, controlled by C4b, which binds protein S inhibiting its activity. The enhancement of fibrinolysis by protein C also may be dependent on protein S. Therefore the action of thrombomodulin limits hemostasis by activating inhibitory proteins

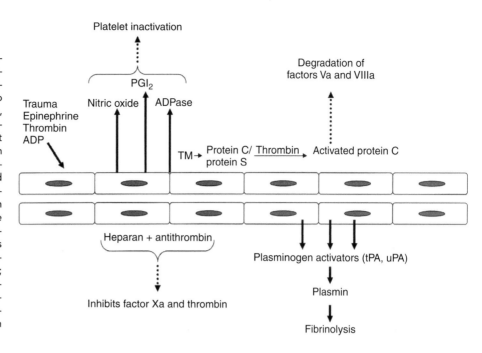

Figure 4.17 Depiction of the antithrombotic properties of endothelium. Under a variety of external stimuli, endothelial cells are induced to form nitric oxide, PGI_2, and ADPase, which inactivate platelets. The presence of thrombomodulin is important in the activation of protein C, which degrades factors Va and VIIIa. Plasminogen activators are also released which result in the formation of plasmin, which is critically important in the fibrinolytic process. The presence of heparan on the surface of the endothelium with antithrombin inhibits the action of factor Xa and thrombin. ADP, adenosine diphosphate; PGI_2, prostacyclin; ADPase, adenosine diphosphatase; TM, thrombomodulin; tPA, tissue plasminogen activator; uPA, urokinase plasminogen activator.

(most notably protein C) in the coagulation cascade and by enhancing fibrinolysis (see Fig. 4.17).

Stimuli such as epinephrine, thrombin, and trauma stimulate PGI_2 synthesis by endothelial cells. Other agonists including histamine, bradykinin, and acetylcholine are important in the stimulation of endothelial cell guanylate cyclase which catalyzes the formation of intracellular cyclic guanosine 3′,5′-monophosphate (cGMP), which stimulates nitric oxide synthesis. Therefore, when endothelial cells are exposed to appropriate stimuli, both vasodilation and platelet inhibition are modulated. Stimulated endothelial cells produce endothelins, a group of proteins, which are involved in counter-regulatory actions including vasoconstriction. Endothelial cells are also involved in the production of plasminogen activators, which promote fibrinolysis and which can aggravate bleeding in susceptible patients. From a clinical perspective, synthetic and natural fibrinolytic inhibitors have been shown to inhibit this bleeding tendency. Natural inhibitors to plasminogen activators such as PAI-1 are expressed with different time courses depending on stimuli. The rare congenital deficiency of PAI-1 results in a bleeding tendency that implies that uninhibited fibrinolysis disrupts hemostasis.

Endothelial cells can also be stimulated to induce a procoagulant response that results in synthesis and release of PAI-1, release of vWF, exposure to TF, and decreased cell surface-associated thrombomodulin. The marked decrease in postoperative and post-traumatic fibrinolytic activity is associated with increased circulating PAI-1 levels mediated by cytokines elaborated as a response to tissue damage. In these clinical scenarios, when thrombin is bound to thrombomodulin, there is more efficient activation of TAFI. Although these responses protect the newly formed clot

from dissolution, it is likely that these same processes contribute to the well-known postoperative risk of venous thrombosis.

The complex interaction between many of these mediators and countermediators from the endothelium, including arterial and venous vasomotor regulation, influences clot formation, and eventual wound healing. Although these processes act in concert to maintain normal hemostasis, on occasion the response is excessive and leads to intravascular thrombosis. Mediators of the hemostatic response including plasminogen, AT, kininogen, platelet factor 4, and collagen, are also important in other physiologic processes such as angiogenesis.

Platelets

Platelets are critical to hemostasis (see Fig. 4.18). Normally functioning platelets will adhere and spread on the exposed subendothelium of an injured blood vessel with secretion of platelet constituents, which stimulate hemostasis and wound healing, and the formation of large platelet aggregates. The platelet surface then becomes an important site for clotting factor binding and acceleration of coagulation, which, in turn, results in the formation of a fibrin mesh that strengthens a fragile platelet plug. The clot retracts into a smaller volume, an intrinsic platelet process.

Platelets adhere only to exposed endothelium. vWF, fibronectin, and fibrinogen are present at these exposed sites providing the base for adhesion through the platelet glycoprotein Ib/IX/V complex (vWF) and integrin receptors. These adhesive proteins are thought to participate in the formation of a bridge from platelets to subendothelial connective tissue. Two primary platelet diseases,

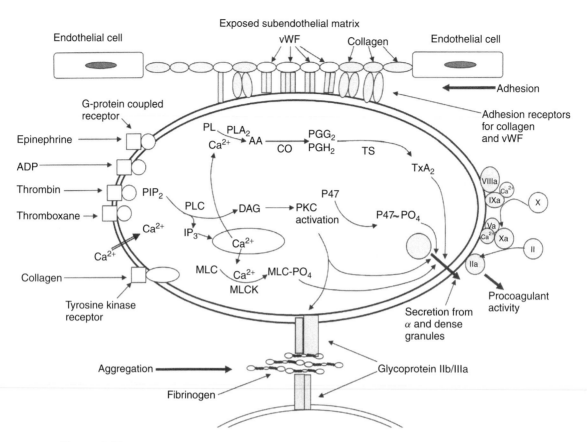

Figure 4.18 Summary of platelet function. The exposure of the subendothelial matrix to platelets initiates adhesion through platelet receptors for collagen and von Willebrand factor (vWF). Platelet aggregation is mediated by glycoprotein IIb/IIIa through fibrinogen. A variety of agonists, such as ADP, thrombin, thromboxane, epinephrine, and collagen and others, activate platelets through a number of intracellular signaling mechanisms related to the specific receptor many of which are G-protein–coupled receptors. The result of these intracellular signals results in the secretion of α granule and dense granule contents, which leads to further platelet activation, and platelet plug formation. The surface of platelets acts a procoagulant surface for the formation of tenase (VIIIa, IXa, Ca^{2+}) and prothrombinase (Va, Xa, Ca^{2+}) complexes that act in concert to produce thrombin. ADP, adenosine disphosphate; PIP_2, phosphatidyl inositol bisphosphate; PLC, phospholipase C; IP_3, inositol trisphosphate; MLC, myosin light chain; MLC-PO_4, phosphorylated myosin light chain; MLCK, myosin light chain kinase; DAG, diacylglycerol; PKC, protein kinase C, PL, phospholipids; AA, arachidonic acid; PLA_2, phospholipase A_2; CO, cyclooxygenase; PGG_2, prostaglandin G_2; PGH_2, prostaglandin H_2; TS, thromboxane synthetase; TxA_2, thromboxane A_2.

Bernard-Soulier disease (BSD) and von Willebrand disease (vWD) illustrate the importance of these adhesion molecules and receptors. In BSD, patients lack glycoprotein Ib/IX, whereas in vWD, vWF may be markedly decreased secondarily to quantitative or qualitative defects. At high shear rates (i.e., >800 per second), such as is found in arteries in the microvasculature, plasma vWF is required for normal adhesion of platelets to subendothelium. At low shear rates, adhesion of platelets to subendothelium is normal in patients with these disorders, suggesting that other proteins can at least partially substitute for the adhesive properties of vWF. In addition to vWF-dependent adhesion, other adhesive processes include interactions of collagen with the platelet glycoprotein Ia-IIa and platelet glycoprotein VI (CD36), which results in the activation of

intracellular signaling pathways. Abnormalities in either of these platelet receptors for collagen can result in bleeding defects.

After adhering to the exposed subendothelium, platelets undergo shape change (spreading) and form an initial basal layer of adherent activated platelets. This layer acts as a nidus for additional platelets adherence and activation resulting in a mass of aggregated platelets, the platelet plug. Critical to platelet aggregation is a conformation change in glycoprotein IIb/IIIa, which results in increased ability to bind fibrinogen, as well as vWF, fibronectin, and vitronectin. The divalent structure of fibrinogen likely allows bridging from platelet to platelet, thereby allowing aggregation. Other platelet integrins function as receptors for adhesive plasma proteins. The vitronectin receptor, for example, is a platelet integrin, which is present on the surface of both blood cells and endothelial cells. It should be noted that vWF and collagen are the major molecules that interact with resting platelets. This is in contrast to fibrinogen, which binds with high affinity to the glycoprotein Ib/IIIa (also an integrin) on only activated platelets. Demonstration of the importance of both glycoprotein IIb/IIIa and fibrinogen come from the bleeding tendency seen in patients with Glanzmann thrombasthenia, a congenital disorder in which the glycoprotein IIb/IIIa complex is deficient or absent, and in congenital afibrinogenemia.[100,101] Although there are numerous agonists of platelet aggregation, those having the greatest physiologic relevance include thrombin, ADP, collagen, arachidonic acid, and epinephrine. Platelet aggregation assays can detect abnormalities in platelet granule content (storage defect) and defects in platelet receptors for these agonists and whether the intracellular signaling of platelets is intact. Many of these agonists, except for epinephrine, induce platelet shape change.

There are specific receptors for these agonists. Many of these receptors are G-protein–coupled receptors that result in hydrolysis of guanosine triphosphate. Several of these receptors are coupled to ion-permeable channels in the platelet membrane, modulating transmembrane calcium ion flux. Other receptors are linked to protein tyrosine kinases (TK) that result in phosphorylation of sites on the receptor protein. Many of these intracellular signaling events are coupled to microtubule formation, which results in loss of the platelet discoid shape, central movement of platelet storage granules, and pseudopod formation. Stimulatory agonists activate phospholipase C, which breaks down phosphatidylinositol bisphosphate (PIP_2) to inositol trisphosphate (IP_3) and diacylglycerol. IP_3 is a key intracellular mediator as it reacts with receptors on dense tubular system, which is analogous to the sarcoplasmic reticulum of muscle, leading to release and increase of intracellular calcium. Rare familial abnormalities in a G-protein–coupled receptors and phospholipase C have been associated with mild bleeding tendencies.[102,103]

Many intracellular processes involved in platelet activation are calcium-dependent, including myosin light chain phosphorylation and release of arachidonic acid from membrane phospholipids by phospholipase A_2. Phospholipase A_2 acts on phosphatidylcholine located on the inner surface of membrane lipid bilayer to release arachidonic acid. Arachidonic acid is converted to PG endoperoxides (PGG_2 and then PGH_2) by cyclooxygenase and peroxidase and then to thromboxane A_2 by thromboxane synthase. Thromboxane A_2 is an unstable, potent platelet agonist with a half-life of less than a minute. Thromboxane A_2 is converted nonenzymatically to thromboxane B_2 and other more stable PGs such as PGD_2, which may modulate platelet activity. Aspirin alkylates the reactive serine in cyclooxygenase, irreversibly inactivating the enzyme and therefore exposure to aspirin irreversibly inactivates

platelets. Another intracellular signaling pathway includes a calcium-dependent neutral cysteine protease (calpain), which may participate in changes in the cytoskeletal protein remodeling, intracellular receptor protein cleavage and thrombin-induced activation of platelets.[104]

Diacylglycerol that results from the action of phospholipase C activates protein kinase C. Protein kinase C phosphorylates a number of proteins including pleckstrin, a 47-kDa protein whose phosphorylation reflects the degree of activation of the protein kinase C. Counter-regulatory proteins to protein kinases are phosphatases that provide negative feedback and decrease intracellular levels of ionized calcium by IP_3. It is believed that diacylglycerol is responsible for "calcium-independent" reactions that occur during platelet activation. Diacylglycerol may also act in concert with elevated intracellular calcium levels to activate protein kinase C and further secretion of platelet granules.

Platelets contain several classes of granules including α granules (containing fibrinogen, vWF, factor V, high-molecular-weight kininogen [HMWK], fibronectin, α_1-antitrypsin, β-thromboglobulin, platelet factor 4, and platelet-derived growth factor), dense bodies (containing serotonin, adenosine triphosphate [ATP], ADP, pyrophosphate, and calcium), and lysosomes. With platelet activation, changes occur in the cytoskeletal contractile apparatus associated with actin polymerization and myosin phosphorylation, with central migration of these granules. In the presence of elevated intracellular calcium levels, there is fusion of the granules with the intracellular canaliculi, leading to extracellular secretion of the granule contents.

With the release of ADP from dense granules, several receptors become activated. These include $P2X_1$, $P2Y_1$, and P2TAC. Although the $P2X_1$ receptor is an ADP-operated calcium channel, there is no functional abnormality when this receptor is defective. By contrast, the $P2Y_1$ receptor mediates shape change by activating phospholipase C, while P2TAC decreases stimulated adenylate cyclase activity and reduces platelet adenosine 3′,5′-cyclic monophosphate (cAMP) levels.[105] Both $P2Y_1$ and P2TAC are required for aggregation. Epinephrine, in contrast, binds to the α_2-adrenergic receptor, whereas thromboxane A_2 and PGH_2 bind to their own receptors. Together, all of these interactions result in elaboration of additional fibrinogen-binding sites through G-protein–coupled signaling.

During platelet activation, specific plasma clotting factors, such as activated factor V (Va), become bound to platelet receptors. These newly acquired receptors, together with anionic phospholipids allow the platelets to be an important binding site for prothrombin to thrombin conversion by factor Xa. A similar system for the binding of factor IXa and conversion of factor X to Xa also exists.

Intracellular cAMP along with other intracellular mediators modulate many aspects of platelet activation. Intracellular platelet adenylate cyclase maintains intracellular levels of cAMP by converting ATP to cAMP. PG D_2 in

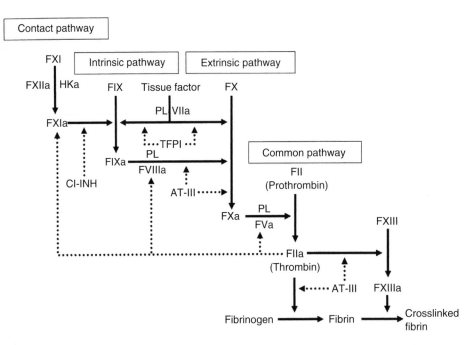

Figure 4.19 Summary of the clotting cascade. Tissue factor is considered the central initiating factor. Upon exposure to blood, tissue factor complexes with activator factor VIIa (FVIIa) and phospholipid (PL) to convert factor IX to IXa and factor X to Xa. A "contact" pathway involving activated high-molecular-weight kininogen (HKa) with activated factor XII converts factor XI to XIa which also contributes to the formation of the activated factor IX (FIXa) which contributes to the "intrinsic" pathway of coagulation. The "extrinsic pathway" involves tissue factor, which is expressed on a number of cells including damaged endothelium. The complex of factor Xa, factor Va, and phospholipids result in the formation of thrombin (FIIa). Thrombin together with activated factor XIII (FXIIIa) result in cross-linked fibrin. *Dashed arrows* indicate inhibitory feedback actions (from thrombin) or specific inhibitor actions. TFPI, tissue factor pathway inhibitor; AT-III, antithrombin-III; CI-INH, CI-inhibitor.

platelets and PGI_2 (prostacyclin) in endothelial cells modulate cAMP levels. Breakdown of cAMP occurs through action of cyclic nucleotide phosphodiesterases that cleave cAMP to AMP. cGMP inhibits PDE3A, the major cAMP phosphodiesterase in platelets. Therefore, mediators that increase cGMP will also inhibit platelet activation by decreasing cAMP levels. Another mechanism by which cAMP inhibits platelet action is through stimulation of a protein kinase that phosphorylates an ATP-dependent calcium-pump that removes calcium from the cytosol. Depending on its intracellular concentration, cAMP can inhibit platelet aggregation, secretion, and shape change, as well as platelet adhesion, and is therefore a key counter-regulatory molecule in platelet activation and aggregation.

Other counter-regulatory mechanisms of platelet activation include an ADPase on the endothelial cell surface as well as thrombomodulin, which inhibits thrombin. Furthermore, the production of nitric oxide by endothelial cells with agonists, such as ATP, inhibits platelet function by raising platelet cGMP levels. There is some evidence that platelets can form nitric oxide from L-arginine resulting in a rise in cGMP concentration, which down-regulates cAMP levels to inhibit platelet activity.

Coagulation Pathways

Traditionally, coagulation has been divided into intrinsic and extrinsic pathways because of *in vitro* laboratory testing. This artificial division should be abandoned because TF/factor VIIa complex activates factor IX as well as factor X and therefore there is cross talk between these pathways. The traditional pathways will be discussed with special emphasis on these newer concepts (see Fig. 4.19).

Extrinsic Coagulation Pathways

Blood coagulation is initiated by the extrinsic system, which involves both blood and vascular components. TF, an intrinsic membrane protein composed of a single polypeptide chain, is critical in this pathway.[106] TF is expressed constitutively on most cells (other than hepatocytes) that do not normally contact the blood. However, after vascular injury, the blood is exposed to TF that is constituently expressed. Alternatively, TF biosynthesis can be induced by cytokines such as tumor necrosis factor and IL-1 as a result of endotoxin effects on monocytes and endothelial cells. TF ultimately functions as a factor VII cofactor in the extrinsic pathway and as a factor V cofactor in the "final common pathway." A key regulator of this pathway is tissue factor pathway inhibitor (TFPI), a protein that in association with factor Xa inhibits the TF/factor VII complex. TFPI is a protein produced by endothelial cells and consists of three kunitz domains. The first domain binds to and inhibits factor VIIa-TF and the second, factor Xa. Therefore, the direct activation of factor Xa is rapidly down-regulated. Ligation of factor Xa is required for TFPI to inhibit TF-factor VIIa. In the presence of TFPI, the major pathway for the propagation of coagulation becomes the intrinsic pathway, which is activated by factor IXa.

Factor VII, a vitamin-K–dependent protein, is the major coagulation factor involved in the initiation of the intrinsic pathway. It is synthesized as a prozymogen and converted to a serine proteinase by proteolytic cleavage. Common to vitamin-K–dependent proteins are unique γ-glutamyl carboxyl acid (Gla) residues at the N-terminal end of the molecule that require vitamin K for proper synthesis by hepatocytes. This post-translational modification is necessary for the binding of calcium to two carboxyl groups of a Gla residue. These moieties are a necessary bridge for coagulant protein binding to the phospholipid surface. Other plasma proteins that require Gla residue post-translational modification include factors II, IX, and X and protein C and S and are therefore dependent on adequate intake of vitamin K.

The TF/FVIIa complex and factor Xa activate factor IX and factor X. FVIIa represents approximately 1% of total factor VII and is largely the result of autoactivation of factor VII. The TF/factor VIIa complex, when formed, is present primarily on activated monocytes or endothelial cells although it is felt more recently that the platelet surface may be the major site of the complex for maintenance of normal hemostasis. The complex's principal substrates include factors IX and X. When either are cleaved by the TF/factor VIIa complex, membrane bound serine proteases result. Factor VIII acts as a cofactor for factor IX in the conversion of factor X to factor Xa (intrinsic pathway) while factor V acts as the cofactor to factor Xa for conversion of prothrombin to thrombin (common pathway).

Factor VIII exists in plasma largely in a noncovalent complex with vWF, which allows a tremendous increase in its plasma half-life. In the absence of factor VIII (hemophilia A) or IX (hemophilia B), a hemorrhagic state is induced. The factor IXa-VIIIa complex is the most important activator of factor X. Clinically, hemophilia A and B are similar and likely result from the absence of proper "tenase" complex necessary for factor X activation. Clinical severity is dependent on the concentration of either factor VIII or IX. Extreme deficiencies (<1%) result in spontaneous joint hemorrhage (hemarthroses), whereas mild symptoms may occur at levels between 5% and 30% except in serious trauma or surgery. In these cases, activity greater than 30% is necessary for normal hemostasis.

Normal individuals are unlikely to develop the hemorrhagic condition seen in hemophilia A or B because of the presence of high levels of either factor as compared to carriers. Although the TF/VIIa complex can directly convert factor X to Xa, congenital deficiencies in factor VII or X produce a similar hemorrhagic condition, which can only be distinguished by specific coagulation factor assay. To date, there has been no description of a TF deficiency state.

Intrinsic Coagulation Pathways

The intrinsic pathway depends on the TF/factor VIIa complex independent activation of factor IX by a dimeric serine protease, factor XIa. In this pathway, the activation of factor IX requires only ionized calcium (hence "intrinsic") in contrast to the requirement for TF found on cellular membranes (hence "extrinsic" pathway). Although deficiencies in the contact system proteins such as factor XII, HMWK and prekallikrein result in the *in vitro* prolongation of the activated partial thromboplastin time (aPTT), only a deficiency of factor XI is associated with a hemorrhagic tendency. The importance of the contact system becomes manifest during interaction of blood with a foreign surface, for example, in cardiopulmonary bypass. The zymogen factor XII (Hagemen factor) binds to negatively charged surfaces such as kaolin, dextran sulfate, and sulfatides and while bound to this surface (through its heavy chain) initiates autoactivation. The light chain of factor XII contains a serine protease that converts prekallikrein and factor XI to kallikrein and factor XIa, respectively. Kallikrein cleaves the HMWK to produce bradykinin and a kinin-free kininogen (HKa). This activated kininogen has a 10-fold greater ability to bind to the surface than prekallikrein, allowing it to associate more with the urokinase receptor on the endothelial cell, leading to enhanced fibrinolysis and inhibition of angiogenesis. Currently it is felt that these proteins participate instead in the initiation of the inflammatory response, complement activation, fibrinolysis, angiogenesis, and kinin formation.

There are a number of negative feedback mechanisms. One such mechanism occurs through factor XIa cleavage of the light chain of HMWK, which destroys its cofactor activity and allows factor XIa to dissociate from the activating surface. Similarly, although thrombin activates factors V and VIII, activation of protein C leads to the destruction of factor Va and VIIIa. Although deficiency of proteins involved in the contact system pathway results in minimal generation of thrombin and a prolonged *in vitro* aPTT, there either appears to be no effect *in vivo* or at least unrelated or opposite effect. HMWK, for example, has antithrombotic activity after endothelial injury, which may predispose to thrombosis in deficiency. Factor XII deficiency has been implicated as a risk factor in venous and possibly arterial thrombosis. Even factor XI deficiency results only in a mild disorder of hemostasis in half the affected individuals. Therefore, blood coagulation *in vivo* is likely initiated by factor IX or X through TF/VIIa mechanisms.

Coagulation Common Pathway

The initiation of the common pathway begins with the formation of factor Xa from either the extrinsic or intrinsic pathway. Its critical role is to convert prothrombin to thrombin. Prothrombin has distinct functional domains devoted to calcium binding to phospholipids. The mature prothrombin molecule contains a Gla domain, which can bind Ca^{2+} along with phospholipid, other domains that can interact with factor V, an activation peptide region, and a portion containing the catalytic center, a precursor serine proteinase domain. After cleavage by factor Xa, the N-terminal Gla portion of prothrombin (fragment 1.2) is removed and the resultant two-chain thrombin molecule detaches from the phospholipid surface. Fragment 1.2 is often used as a marker of thrombin generation. The prothrombinase complex (consisting of factor Xa, factor V, phospholipids, and calcium) provides a more than 300,000-fold increased rate for prothrombin activation than that achieved by factor Xa and prothrombin alone. The source of factor V that participates in the prothrombinase complex on the platelet membrane is likely supplied by platelet α granules or fusion with the platelet plasma membrane. This factor V serves as a receptor for factor Xa binding to the activated platelet. Because of this involvement of the platelet, the bleeding manifestation of factor V deficiency sometimes resemble that seen in qualitative platelet disorders. There are alternative pathways for prothrombin activation by factor Xa independent of factor V that have been described in malignant cells, hypoxic endothelial cells, and macrophages. Of notable importance is that a mutation in the 3′ untranslated regions, G20120 → A results in elevated prothrombin levels and is implicated as a common cause of hypercoagulability. (See Chapter 25 for a review of prothrombotic conditions in infants and children.)

The cellular location of coagulation complexes is important. Activated monocytes localize the extrinsic system because they not only express TF after they are activated but also have receptors for factor X and the integrin MAC-1 (CD11b/CD18), the latter of which is important in leukocyte adhesion. Factor Xa, once formed, binds to a receptor on monocytes called *effector proteinase receptor 1* or to factor Va, which binds to cells. Furthermore, platelets bind factor IX and XIa and as mentioned previously, platelets secrete factor Va, which serves as a locus for binding factor Xa, thrombin, itself will bind to protease-activated receptors 1 and 4 on platelets. Recently, the clinical efficacy of NovoSeven (recombinant activated factor VII) has been explained in large part by the central role of the platelet as a localizing surface to maintain effective hemostasis.[107]

Inhibition of Coagulation

There are several plasma proteolytic inhibitors, which limit and control the extent and speed of both coagulation and fibrinolysis. For example, the major inhibitor of the contact system is C1-INH, which accounts for approximately 95% of the plasma inhibitory capacity for factor XIIa and more than 50% for kallikrein. However, hereditary deficiency of C1-INH results in angioedema rather than bleeding. In similar fashion although α_1-antitrypsin is the major inhibitor of factor XIa, its more critical role is inhibiting neutrophil elastase, resulting in emphysema because of the lack of inhibition of the effects of elastase in the lung.

In contrast, congenital AT-III deficiency is associated with a strikingly increased risk of venous thromboembolism. AT-III is a member of the serpin gene family and has broad activity against serine proteinases in the coagulation cascade. AT-III is primarily an inhibitor of thrombin but also has activity of against factor Xa (common pathway), IXa, XIIa (and its fragments), plasma kallikrein–HMWK (extrinsic pathway), and factor VIIa-TF (intrinsic pathway). However, even a 40% to 50% decrease in AT-III levels predisposes to thrombosis. This is despite the fact that enough circulating AT-III is present to neutralize three times the total amount of thrombin that could form in the blood. AT-III inactivates thrombin by forming a covalent arginine linkage to the catalytic-site serine of thrombin. This inactivates thrombin irreversibly. This inhibition is enhanced by heparin, a highly negatively charged sulfated polysaccharide, which is closely related to heparan sulfate found on the endothelial cells. Heparin binds to a basic group in AT-III, increasing its rate of thrombin inactivation. However, once thrombin binds fibrin, it becomes resistant to AT-III and even more so to the AT-III/heparin complex. Another regulatory protein, heparin cofactor II, is a serine protease inhibitor that selectively inactivates thrombin (not factor Xa) in the presence of heparin or dermatan sulfate.

The α_2-macroglobulin is another major inhibitor of many procoagulant and fibrinolytic proteins. Although many enzymes become trapped in the cage structure of this inhibitor, the complex may be actually protective against other inhibitors. Severe α_2-macroglobulin deficiency has not been associated with a clinical disorder. Another plasma protein, α_2-antiplasmin, prevents systemic plasmin fibrinogenolysis in response to life-threatening stimuli. This limits the fibrinolytic response to thrombi in the affected region and allows hemostatic plugs to remain intact until healing is complete. In α_2-antiplasmin deficiency, the hemostatic plugs dissolve before healing has occurred and a hemorrhage state results. Still other proteins such as PAI-1 and protein C inhibitor are important in the regulation of procoagulant activity. For example, congenital deficiency of PAI-1 results in a hemorrhagic tendency. By contrast, protein C inhibitor, a serine protease inhibitor, inactivates protein C, preventing its inactivation of factor Va and VIIIa and therefore functions as a potential procoagulant molecule (see Table 4.4).

TABLE 4.4

PROTEASE INHIBITORS OF THE CONTACT AND PATHWAY AND FIBRINOLYTIC SYSTEM

Inhibitor	Molecular Weight (Da)	Plasma Concentration (μg/mL)	Major Target Enzyme(s)
α_1 Protease inhibitor	55,000	2,500	Factor XIa, elastase
α_2-Macroglobulin	725,000	2,500	Kallikrein, plasmin, thrombin
Antithrombin-III	62,000	900	Factor Xa, thrombin
Cl-inhibitor	105,000	240	Factor XIIa, kallikrein
α_2-Antiplasmin	67,000	70	Plasmin
Heparin cofactor II	65,000	40	Thrombin
Plasminogen activator inhibitor-1	50,000	10	tPA, urokinase
Protein C inhibitor	53,000	5	Protein C, kallikrein
Tissue factor pathway inhibitor	43,000	0.1	Factor VIIa and factor Xa through tissue factor inhibition

Fibrin Formation

Thrombin has a critical role in fibrin formation by its action on multiple substrates, including factors XIII, V, and VIII; platelet membrane glycoprotein V; protein S, protein C, and fibrinogen. In so doing, thrombin affects the rate and extent of the hemostatic plug formation, influencing its form, and rate of formation. Thrombin can both promote formation and dissolution of the hemostatic plug. Thrombin, for example, in association with factors V and VIII causes an increase in the tenase and prothrombinase complexes, resulting in a rapid increase of thrombin activity and fibrin strand formation. Conversely, the important role of thrombin in limiting coagulation is seen in its ability to activate protein C which, in turn, hydrolyzes activated factor V. Because of a mutation in factor V_{Leiden}, the codon at position 506 is changed from an arginine to glutamine. This makes this site resistant to activated protein C (aPC) and is the basis for one of the most common genetic causes of venous thrombosis. Thrombin is also important in fostering platelet aggregation. However, this is dependent on the relative activity of both the intrinsic or extrinsic clotting systems during coagulation. For example, if there is marked thrombin generation because of the exposure of TF by activated endothelial cells, tumor cells, or macrophages (extrinsic pathway), then the generation of thrombin will more likely contribute to platelet activation and recruitment (see Fig. 4.20).

The formation of fibrin is considered to be the second phase in hemostasis, the first phase being the formation of the platelet plug. Fibrinogen is a large glycoprotein of 340 kDa and is found in high concentration in

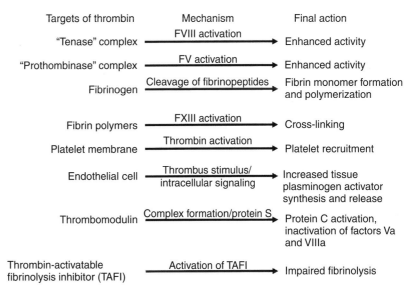

Figure 4.20 Functions of thrombin. Thrombin contributes to the formation of the tenase and prothrombinase complexes through factor VIII and V activation. Fibrin polymerization is initiated by the cleavage of fibrinopeptides and which is enhanced by cross-linking by factor XIII, which is activated by thrombin. Thrombin is not only a potent platelet agonist but also increases the release and synthesis of tissue plasminogen activator and together with thrombomodulin, endothelial cell receptor protein and protein S, activate protein C which serves to help limit the thrombotic process.

both plasma and platelet α granules. Fibrinogen is a dimer composed of two identical heterotrimers. This heterotrimer is composed of Aα, Bβ, and γ polypeptides linked by coiled-coil segments. The central domain, which consists of N-terminals of each chain bound in a disulfide knot, is the binding site for thrombin. Thrombin binds to this central domain and cleaves off fibrinopeptides A and B, producing fibrin monomer. Fibrin polymer formation occurs by spontaneous partial overlapping of fibrin monomer molecules. Fibrin strands or broad sheets of fibrin are formed when the protofibrils interact laterally. Resistance to plasmin degradation and chemical dissolution by 6 M urea is related to cross-linking of these fibrin strands by thrombin-activated factor XIII. Both cross-linking by factor XIIIa and the degree of lateral strand association contributing to the tensile strength of the clot. In the early stages of fibrin formation, the protofibrils are cross-linked initially between γ chains of fibrin molecules. These covalent cross-links occur between lysine and glutamine residues in the γ chain region of individual fibrin molecules creating "end to end" links. After the formation of these γ chain covalent links, slower cross-linking between α chain occurs. Because there are multiple lysine and glutamine acceptor and receptor residues in the α chains, multiple cross-links can occur creating an intricate cross-linked meshwork. Once mature, the fibrin fiber contains approximately 100 cross-linked protofibrils. Factor XIIIa also contributes to continued fibrin clot integrity by attachment of α_2-antiplasmin to fibrin, which may protect the clot against further fibrinolysis (see Fig. 4.21).

This fibrin network binds and surrounds the platelet plug and assists in the attachment of the platelet plug to the vessel wall. This occurs through interactions to platelet glycoproteins and adhesion proteins such as thrombospondin,

fibronectin, and platelet fibrinogen (from platelet α granules). These proteins serve as molecular bridges between plasma proteins and intracellular platelet cytoskeletal proteins, between platelet and the vessel wall, and between fibrin strands and the subendothelium. For instance, fibronectin is cross-linked by factor XIIIa to fibrin. Because fibronectin possesses a separate binding site for collagen, this could result in bridging fibrin to the vessel wall. vWF binds either platelet glycoprotein Ib or IIb/IIIa and is associated with the subendothelium. Platelet glycoprotein IIb/IIIa undergoes a conformational change on platelet activation to expose a fibrinogen-binding site. This links changes in intracellular actin formation and therefore clot retraction and vessel-wall constriction to platelet activation, aggregation, and primary platelet plug formation.

Because the end product of the coagulation cascade is fibrin, there is tremendous potential for either hemorrhagic or thrombotic disease resulting from alterations of fibrinogen structure, concentration, or interaction with either thrombin or factor XIII. If there is poor fibrin polymerization or inadequate cross-linking, a hemorrhagic condition may result. A dysfunctional or absent factor XIII, can contribute to both a hemorrhage condition and inadequate wound healing. The most common acquired disorders of fibrinogen include syndromes associated with disseminated intravascular coagulation (DIC), which reflect excessive or inappropriate coagulation or proteolytic degradation of plasma fibrinogen. Rarer disorders include dysfunctional fibrinogen molecules resulting in dysfibrinogenemia. All of these disorders can result in a variety of hemorrhage and thrombotic manifestations depending on the underlying pathologic process.

There are several mechanisms for controlling the extent and duration of local hemostasis including vascular

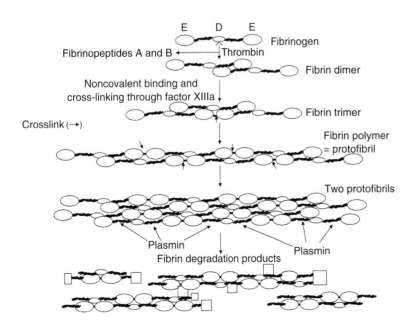

Figure 4.21 Formation of cross-linked fibrin. Cleavage of fibrinopeptides A and B from the central E domain of fibrinogen, results in the formation of soluble fibrin monomers that interact noncovalently to form fibrin dimers. Cross-linking of these dimers through the γ chains of contingent terminal D domains occurs through the action of activated factor XIIIa (FXIIIa). Eventually, a protofibril consisting of two fibrin strands is formed. These protofibrils interact laterally to form long fibrin stands or broad fibrin sheets. Continued cross-linking by FXIIIa provides increased tensile strength and resistance to plasmin degradation. The action of plasmin results in the formation of cross-linked and un-cross-linked fibrin degradation products.

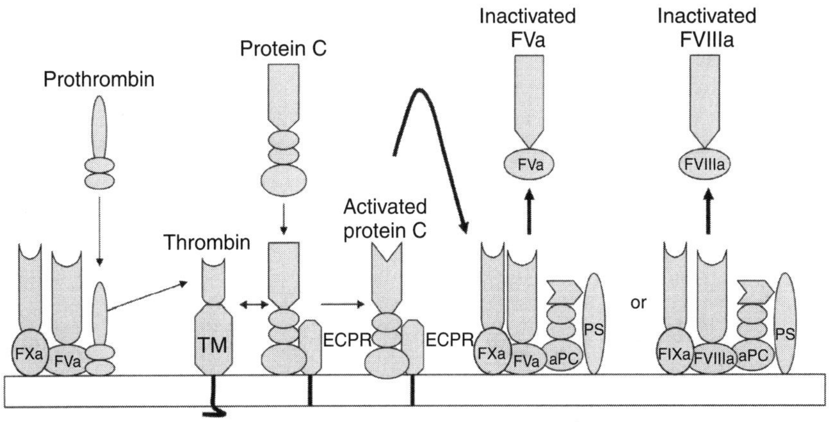

Figure 4.22 Model of the protein C anticoagulant system. Prothrombin complexes with activated factor V (FVa) and X (FXa) to form thrombin. Thrombin complexes with thrombomodulin (TM) and together with endothelial cell protein receptor with bound protein C, activates protein C (aPC). Released activated protein C binds to free protein S (PS) and together inactivates factor Va (FVa) and VI-IIa (FVIIIa). ECPR, endothelial cell protein C receptor.

flow, hemodilution, proteolytic feedback by thrombin, inhibition by plasma proteins and endothelial cell-localized protein C activation, and fibrinolysis. Probably the initial limiting mechanism is vascular flow, which can detach small platelet clumps that are loosely attached to the platelet plug or the vessel wall. Second, thrombin present in the hemostatic plug, which contributes to the factor V and VIII activation, may later initiate inactivation of these same factors in the presence of thrombomodulin, an endothelial cell membrane protein. Third, there is diffusion of soluble activated coagulant proteins such as factor Xa or thrombin, which bind inhibitory plasma proteins. As previously mentioned, AT-III is a major inhibitor, which complexes with thrombin, other serine proteases involved in coagulation, and plasmin. Although thrombin can be readily inactivated by AT-III in plasma, AT-III cannot inactivate thrombin while it is bound to fibrin. Even heparin, which accelerates AT-III inactivation of thrombin in solution, cannot completely inactivate thrombin bound to fibrin. Cleavage of fibrinopeptides from fibrinogen is still possible by fibrin-bound thrombin. Fourth, thrombin that diffuses into the endothelial cell surface can bind to thrombomodulin. The thrombin/thrombomodulin complex is a receptor for protein C. The interaction of the complex with protein C (protein S is a cofactor) results in release of activated form of protein C, which is released from the endothelium and inactivates nearby factor VIIIa and factor Va, limiting the action of thrombin itself. Additionally, an endothelial cell protein C receptor has been identified and characterized and shown to be expressed on the endothelial cell surface. In the presence of an endothelial cell protein C receptor, the activation of protein C is enhanced (see Fig. 4.22). Patients with congenital antigenic or functional deficiencies of protein C, protein S, and AT-III have been described who have lifelong tendency for thromboembolic disease.

FIBRINOLYTIC SYSTEM

Another mechanism for limiting clot formation is fibrinolysis. Fibrinolysis is the ultimate mechanism that counteracts the clot formation process. The dissolution or solubility of the fibrin clot at the correct time is necessary for wound healing and is required for angiogenesis as well as vessel recanalization after clot formation. Endothelial cells release tPA after stimulation by thrombin, which binds tightly to fibrin; fibrin serves as cofactor enabling efficient activation of plasminogen to plasmin to tPA. Plasminogen also binds to fibrin. Fibrin localizes both the activator and zymogen. Plasmin cleaves fibrinogen or fibrin, or both, to produce degradation products, which inhibit fibrin polymerization and thrombin action, thereby serving as natural anticoagulants, especially in DIC. Plasmin exerts a positive feedback by cleavage of an N-terminal peptide from the native glu-plasminogen, converting it to lys-plasminogen, which undergoes a large conformational change rendering it much more susceptible to activation. Therefore, fibrinolysis resembles the cascade mechanism of coagulation because of the paradigm of zymogen to enzyme conversion and feedback potential and inhibition. Timing of fibrinolysis is important as initially, during hemostatic plug formation, there is the need for fibrin formation. In response to the need for a hemostatic plug, platelets, and endothelial cells release plasminogen activator inhibitors. However, after clot formation, endothelial cells produce tPA, which allows conversion of plasminogen to the serine protease, plasmin for clot lysis or limitation of clot formation.

Another plasminogen activator, which is synthesized and released by endothelial cells, is uPA. In contrast to the release of tPA by thrombin and subsequent binding to fibrin, prourokinase is expressed on the surface by binding to the urokinase plasminogen activator receptor (uPAR), which then undergoes autoactivation. One mechanism that may account for the enhanced fibrinolysis that occurs with activation of the contact system is as follows. HMWK, after being cleaved, produces bradykinin and HKa. Bradykinin enhances release of tPA, which undergoes conversion to a two-chain form by plasmin and sequentially binds to fibrin. Meanwhile HKa binds endothelial uPAR closely to prourokinase. HMWK circulates in complex with

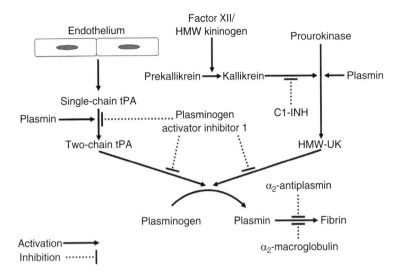

Figure 4.23 Model of fibrinolytic system. Plasmin formation forms a positive feedback loop in the formation of additional plasmin from plasminogen. Endothelial cells secrete tissue plasminogen activator (tPA) as a single chain, which is converted to a two-chain form by the action of plasmin. This two-chain form converts plasminogen to plasmin. Prourokinase is also converted by plasmin and kallikrein to high-molecular-weight urokinase (HMW-UK), which also contributes to plasmin formation. A number of major inhibitors (plasminogen activator inhibitor-1, C1-INH], α_2-antiplasmin, and α_2-macroglobulin) and their sites of action are depicted. The factor XII/high-molecular-weight kininogen (HMWK) pathway may come into play during the contact pathway activation. Activation is indicated by the *arrows*, while inhibition is indicated by *dashed lines with bar.*

prekallikrein, which is converted to kallikrein by an endothelial cell membrane cysteine protease. Kallikrein (as well as plasmin) is known to activate prourokinase to urokinase. The process by which endothelial perturbation contributes to the initiation of the uPA pathway is supported by a study demonstrating that peptides that inhibit the HK-prekallikrein (or kallikrein) interaction prevent the formation of plasmin on the endothelial cell surface (see Fig. 4.23).

In much the same manner that thrombin leads to accelerated factor Xa formation and consequently more thrombin generation, plasmin, in very simplistic fashion, also exerts positive feedback by cleaving an activation peptide from plasminogen rendering it more susceptible to surface binding and subsequent activation by plasminogen activator. Interestingly, plasmin is made more reactive by binding to fibrin through lysine binding sites within its kringle structures. Lipoprotein A, a protein with multiple kringle structures and rich in histidine can modulate this fibrin–plasminogen interaction by inhibiting plasminogen binding to fibrin through its occupation of plasminogen binding sites.

The small amount of plasma plasminogen that binds fibrin during clot formation influences subsequent fibrinolysis. The presence of α_2-antiplasmin bound to fibrin by factor XIIIa, creates an ongoing balancing act between procoagulant and profibrinolytic mediators. The ratio of profibrinolytic plasminogen and plasminogen activator molecules to antifibrinolytic α_2-antiplasmin molecules is important to the extent and timing of clot dissolution; the location of these molecules on the fibrin strand is also important. Congenital deficiencies of α_2-antiplasmin and PAI-1, another inhibitor of plasminogen activator, can result in a hemorrhagic disorder.

An important connection between the coagulation and fibrinolytic pathways is thrombin/thrombomodulin-mediated activation of protein C and TAFI. Protein C

activation leads to inactivation of factor Va and VIIIa and limits further clotting. TAFI activation, by contrast, enhances stability of fibrin by cleaving the C-terminal lysine residues from fibrin, preventing plasminogen, plasmin or tPA from binding to fibrin and secondarily inhibiting fibrinolysis. Under clinical scenarios of deficient procoagulant proteins such as factor VIII or IX (such as in hemophilia A and B), thrombin generation and fibrin formation are deficient but because of low TAFI formation, fibrinolysis occurs unimpeded. This combination of decreased fibrin formation and unbridled fibrinolysis likely contributes to the bleeding diathesis seen in hemophilia. By contrast, patients with protein C deficiency have a thrombotic tendency because of decreased inhibition of factors Va and VIIIa. The tendency for thrombosis may be the result of continuously high production of thrombin, which leads to excessive TAFI formation, which, in turn, leads to further thrombus formation because of the resistance to fibrinolytic mechanisms by TAFI.

Once plasmin forms on the hemostatic plug, fibrin degradation is initiated. However, the dissolution of the clot will occur only if there is a proper balance between factors which favor the hemostatic plug, such as procoagulant pathways and platelet aggregation, versus factors that do not favor the hemostatic plugs, such as coagulation inhibitors, profibrinolytic, and antifibrinolytic reactions. Furthermore, cellular mechanisms for both coagulation and lysis (in leukocytes, platelets, and endothelial cells) must be factored in before the dissolution of the clot can occur. Elastase, a neutral serine proteinase, released from the primary granules of neutrophils, likely contributes to the local fibrinolytic potential.

During hemostatic plug dissolution, plasmin releases fibrin degradation products into the circulation, some of which represent unique cross-linked derivatives such as D-dimer that can be distinguished from fibrinogen degradation products. The circulating degradation products

TABLE 4.5

COMPARISON OF THE PLASMA CONCENTRATIONS OF COMPONENTS OF THE FIBRINOLYTIC SYSTEM OF HEALTHY FULL-TERM INFANTS AND HEALTHY PREMATURE INFANTS (30 TO 36 WEEKS GESTATION) IN THE FIRST 6 MONTHS OF LIFE VERSUS ADULT LEVELS

| | Healthy Full-term Infants | | | | | | | | | |
| | Day 1 | | Day 30 | | Day 90 | | Day 180 | | Adult | |
	M	B	M	B	M	B	M	B	M	B
Plasminogen (U/mL)	1.95	(1.25–2.65)	1.98	(1.26–2.70)	2.48	(1.74–3.22)	3.01	(2.21–3.81)	3.36	(2.48–4.24)
tPA (ng/mL)	9.6	(5.0–18.9)	4.1	(1.0–6.0)[a]	2.1	(1.0–5.0)[a]	2.8	(1.0–6.0)[a]	4.9	(1.4–8.4)
α_2AP (U/mL)	0.85	(0.55–1.15)	1.00	(0.76–1.24)[a]	1.08	(0.76–1.40)[a]	1.11	(0.83–1.39)[a]	1.02	(0.68–1.36)
PAI-1 (U/mL)	6.4	(2.0–15.1)	3.4	(0.0–8.8)[a]	7.2	(1.0–15.3)	8.1	(6.0–13.0)	3.6	(0.0–11.0)

| | Healthy Premature Infants (30 to 36 wk Gestation) | | | | | | | | | |
| | Day 1 | | Day 30 | | Day 90 | | Day 180 | | Adult | |
	M	B	M	B	M	B	M	B	M	B
Plasminogen (U/mL)	1.70	(1.12–2.48)[b]	1.81	(1.09–2.53)	2.38	(1.58–3.18)	2.75	(1.91–3.59)[b]	3.36	(2.48–4.24)
tPA (ng/mL)	8.48	(3.00–16.70)	4.13	(2.00–7.79)[a]	3.31	(2.00–5.07)[a]	3.48	(2.00–5.85)[a]	4.96	(1.46–8.46)
α_2AP (U/mL)	0.78	(0.40–1.16)	0.89	(0.55–1.23)[b]	1.06	(0.64–1.48)[a]	1.15	(0.77–1.53)[a]	1.02	(0.68–1.36)
PAI-1 (U/mL)	5.4	(0.0–12.2)[a,b]	4.3	(0.0–10.9)[a]	4.8	(1.0–11.8)[a,b]	4.9	(1.0–10.2)[a,b]	3.6	(0.0–11.0)

[a]Values that are indistinguishable from those of the adult.
[b]Values that are different from those of the full-term infant.
All values are given as mean (M) followed by the lower and upper boundary encompassing 95% of the population (B) tPA, tissue plasminogen activator; α_2AP, α_2-antiplasmin; PAI-1, plasminogen activator inhibitor-1.
Modified from Tables 2 and 3 in reference 108 and Tables 3 and 4 in reference 109.

serve as a diagnostic marker of thrombin or factor XIIIa activity as well as plasmin activity, reflecting prior clot formation and ongoing fibrinolysis. The clot surface as well as circulating fibrin derivatives may possess a small but significant amount of active thrombin that could serve to propagate the coagulant process elsewhere in the circulation. Active plasmin molecules also may be released into the circulation during fibrinolysis, but just as free thrombin is neutralized by AT-III, plasmin is extremely susceptible in solution to inhibition by α_2-antiplasmin. This reaction clearly serves to limit fibrinolysis to the clot, just as AT-III serves to prevent disseminated coagulation by released thrombin.

When hemostatic plug formation is defective (e.g., in hemophilia), naturally occurring fibrinolysis may aggravate bleeding; and therefore, the use of epsilon aminocaproic acid (Amicar) aids in hemostasis in these patients. This mechanism may be seen in the bleeding that occurs with factor XIII deficiency, α_2-antiplasmin deficiency and after dextran infusion. In the case of factor XIII deficiency, the lack of cross-linking leads to decreased resistance to plasmin action and failure to cross-link inhibitors to the fibrin clot. This ultimately leads to increased fibrinolysis and increased bleeding tendency.

It must always be remembered that the procoagulant and fibrinolytic system of infants and children are constantly evolving. Table 4.5 shows age-specific reference ranges for components of the fibrinolytic system in both healthy premature and full-term infants in the first 6 months of life compared to adults.[108,109] As Figure 4.24 shows, there are tremendous changes in coagulation factor levels, especially in the first 6 months and the few years of life, which continue through preadolescence.[110] Therefore, evaluation of prothrombotic and fibrinolytic potential must always consider the age-dependent concentrations of these interactive procoagulant and anticoagulant systems.

In summary, there are a tremendous number of processes involving endothelial cells, platelets, and plasma factors, which are involved in the delicate balance between coagulation, the formation of the hemostatic plug, and clot dissolution. Normally, in response to bleeding there is a rapid, efficient, and targeted hemostatic response that avoids a disseminated and prolonged thrombogenic response to the site of injury. However, perturbations in any portion of this intricate process can produce an imbalance in hemostasis resulting in a hemorrhagic or thrombotic disorder. Although our therapeutic interventions are targeted toward the perceived hemostatic imbalance that occurs in pathologic diseases, caution must be made in our ability to make therapeutic interventions, as our knowledge of hemostasis remains limited. This is especially so in a

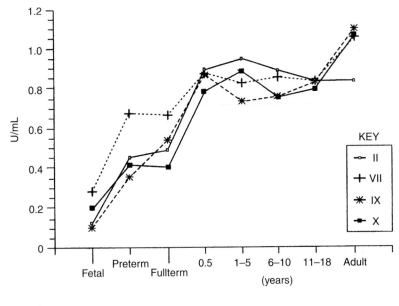

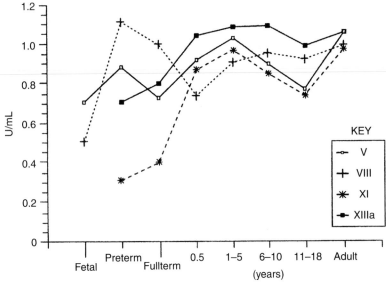

Figure 4.24 Coagulation levels as a function of age. Selected coagulation factors are depicted. (From Andrew M. Developmental hemostasis: Relevance to thromboembolic complications in pediatric patients. *Thromb Haemost* 1995;74 (1 Suppl):416, with permission.)

dynamically changing coagulation system of neonates and children.

REFERENCES

1. Dickerson RE, Geis I. *Hemoglobin: Structure, function, evolution, and pathology.* Menlo Park, CA: Benjamin Cummings; 1983.
2. Woodson RD. Hemoglobin synthesis, structure, and oxygen transport. In: Simon TL, Dzik WN, Snyder EL, et al., eds. *Rossi's principles of transfusion medicine.* 3rd ed. Philadelphia, PA: Lippincott Williams & Wilkins; 2002:25–42.
3. Hardison R. Organization, evolution, and regulation of the globin genes. In: Steinberg MH, Forget BG, Higgs DR, et al., eds. *Disorders of hemoglobin: Genetics, pathophysiology, and clinical management.* Cambridge, MA: Cambridge University Press; 2001.
4. Orkin SH, Nathan DG. The thalassemias. In: Nathan DG, Orkin SH, Ginsburg D, et al., eds. *Nathan and Oski's hematology of infancy and childhood.* 6th ed. Philadelphia, PA: WB Saunders; 2003:842–919.
5. Bottomley SS, Muller-Eberhard U. Pathophysiology of heme synthesis. *Semin Hematol.* 1988;25:282–302.
6. Sadlon TJ, Dell 'Oso T, Surinya KH, et al., Regulation of erythroid 5-aminolevulinate synthase expression during erythropoiesis. *Int J Biochem Cell Biol.* 1999;31:1153–1167.
7. Bunn HF, Forget BG. *Hemoglobin: Molecular, genetic and clinical aspects.* Philadelphia, PA: WB Saunders; 1986.
8. Li Q, Peterson KR, Stamatoyannopoulos G. Developmental control of epsilon- and gamma-globin genes. *Ann N Y Acad Sci.* 1998;850:10–17.
9. Dillon N, Trimborn T, Strouboulis J, et al., The effect of distance on long-range chromatin interactions. *Mol Cell.* 1997;1:131–139.
10. Baldwin J, Chothia C. Haemoglobin: The structural changes related to ligand binding and its allosteric mechanism. *J Mol Biol.* 1979;129:175–220.
11. Perutz MF, Wilkinson AJ, Paoli M, et al., The stereochemical mechanism of the cooperative effects in hemoglobin revisited. *Annu Rev Biophys Biomol Struct.* 1998;27:1–34.
12. Gow AJ, Stamler JS. Reactions between nitric oxide and haemoglobin under physiological conditions. *Nature.* 1998;391:169–173.

13. Gow AJ, Luchsinger BP, Pawloski JR, et al., The oxyhemoglobin reaction of nitric oxide. *Proc Natl Acad Sci U S A.* 1999;96:9027–9032.

14. Singel DJ, Stamler JS. Chemical physiology of blood flow regulation by red blood cells: The role of nitric oxide and s-nitrosohemoglobin. *Ann Rev Biochem.* 2005;67:99–145.

15. Gladwin MT, Ognibene FP, Pannell LK, et al., Relative role of heme nitrosylation and β-cysteine 93 nitrosation in the transport and metabolism of nitric oxide by hemoglobin in the human circulation. *Proc Natl Acad Sci U S A.* 2000;97:9943–9948.

16. Gladwin MT, Shelhamer JH, Schechter AN, et al., Role of circulating nitrite and s-nitrohemoglobin in the regulation of regional blood flow in humans. *Proc Natl Acad Sci U S A.* 2000;97:11482–11487.

17. Gladwin MT, Wang X, Reiter DC, et al., S-nitrosohemoglobin is unstable in the reductive erythrocyte environment and lacks O_2/NO-linked allosteric function. *J Biol Chem.* 2002;277:27818–27828.

18. Xu X, Cho M, Spencer N, et al., Measurements of nitric oxide on the heme iron and β-93 thiol of human hemoglobin during cycles of oxygenation and deoxygenation. *Proc Natl Acad Sci U S A.* 2003;100:11303–11308.

19. Nagababu E, Ramasamy S, Abernethy DR, et al., Active nitric oxide produced in the red cell under hypoxic conditions by deoxyhemoglobin-mediated nitrite reduction. *J Biol Chem.* 2003;278:26349–26356.

20. Han TH, Qamirani E, Nelson AG, et al., Regulation of nitric oxide consumption by hypoxic red blood cells. *Proc Natl Acad Sci U S A.* 2003;100:12504–12509.

21. Huang K-T, Han TH, Hyduke DR, et al., Modulation of nitric oxide bioavailability by erythrocytes. *Proc Natl Acad Sci U S A.* 2001;98:11771–11776.

22. Jison ML, Gladwin MT. Hemolytic anemia-associated pulmonary hypertension of sickle cell disease and the nitric oxide/arginine pathway. *Am J Respir Crit Care Med.* 2003;168:3–4.

23. Morris CR, Morris SM, Hagar W, et al., Arginine therapy: A new treatment for pulmonary hypertension in sickle cell disease? *Am J Respir Crit Care Med.* 2003;168:63–39.

24. Stamler JS. S-nitrosothiols in the blood: Roles, amounts, and methods of analysis. *Circ Res.* 2004;94:414–417.

25. Nagel RL. Hemoglobins: Normal and abnormal. In: Nathan DG, Orkin SH, Ginsburg D, et al., eds. *Nathan and Oski's hematology of infancy and childhood.* 6th ed. Philadelphia, PA: WB Saunders; 2003:745–789.

26. Valeri CR, Valeri DA, Gray A, et al., Viability and function of red blood cell concentrates stored at 4 degrees C for 35 days in CPDA-1, CPDA-2, or CPDA-3. *Transfusion.* 1982;22:210–216.

27. Moroff G, Holme S, Keegan T, et al., Storage of ADSOL-preserved red cells at 2.5 and 5.5 degrees C: Comparable retention of in vitro properties. *Vox Sang.* 1990;59:136–139.

28. Beutler E, Wood L. The in vivo regeneration of red cell 2,3-diphosphoglyceric acid (DPG) after transfusion of stored blood. *J Lab Clin Med.* 1969;74:300–304.

29. Rock G, Poon A, Haddad S, et al., Nutricel as an additive solution for neonatal transfusion. *Transfus Sci.* 1999;20:29–36.

30. Strauss RG, Burmeister LF, Johnson K, et al., Feasibility and safety of AS-3 red blood cells for neonatal transfusions. *J Pediatr.* 2000;136:215–219.

31. Strauss RG, Burmeister LF, Johnson K, et al., AS-1 red cells for neonatal transfusions: A randomized trial assessing donor exposure and safety. *Transfusion.* 1996;36:873–878.

32. Walsh TS, McArdle F, McLellan SA, et al., Does the storage time of transfused red blood cells influence regional or global indexes of tissue oxygenation in anemic critically ill patients? *Crit Care Med.* 2004;32:364–371.

33. Watson JC, Doppenberg EMR, Bullock MR, et al., Effects of the allosteric modification of hemoglobin on brain oxygen and infarct size in a feline model of stroke. *Stroke.* 1997;28:1624–1630.

34. Miyake M, Grinberg OY, Hou H, et al., The effect of RSR13, a synthetic allosteric modifier of hemoglobin, on brain tissue PO_2 (measured by EPR oximetry) following severe hemorrhagic shock in rats. *Adv Exp Med Biol.* 2003;530:319–329.

35. Buechler PW, Alayash AI. Toxicities of hemoglobin solutions: In search of in-vitro and in-vivo model systems. *Transfusion.* 2004;44:1516–1530.

36. Koury MJ. Red blood cell production and kinetics. In: Simon TL, Dzik WH, Snyder EL, et al., eds. *Rossi's principles of transfusion medicine.* Philadelphia, PA: Lippincott, Williams & Wilkins; 2002:14–24.

37. Gregoli PA, Bondurant MC. The roles of bcl-xL and apopain in the control of erythropoiesis by erythropoietin. *Blood.* 1997;90:630–640.

38. Herbert V, Zalusky R. Interrelations of vitamin B_{12} and folic acid metabolism: Folic acid clearance studies. *J Clin Invest.* 1962;41:1263–1276.

39. Koury MJ, Price JO, Hicks GG. Apoptosis in megaloblastic anemia occurs during DNA synthesis by a p53-independent, nucleoside-reversible mechanism. *Blood.* 2000;96:3249–3255.

40. Koury MJ, Horne DW, Brown ZA, et al., Apoptosis of late stage erythroblasts in megaloblastic anemia: Association with DNA damage and macrocyte production. *Blood.* 1997;89:4617–4623.

41. Finch CA, Deubelbeiss K, Cook JD, et al., Ferrokinetics in man. *Medicine (Baltimore).* 1970;49:17–53.

42. Sawyer ST, Krantz SB. Transferrin receptor number, synthesis and endocytosis during erythropoietin-induced maturation of Friend virus-infected erythroid cells. *J Biol Chem.* 1986;261:9187–9195.

43. Anderson C, Aronson I, Jacobs P. Erythropoiesis: Erythrocyte deformability is reduced and fragility increased by iron deficiency. *Hematology.* 2000;4:457–460.

44. Eaves CJ, Eaves AC. Erythropoietin (Ep) dose-response curves for three classes of erythroid progenitors in normal human marrow and in patients with polycythemia vera. *Blood.* 1978;52:1196–1210.

45. Correa PN, Eskinazi D, Axelrod AA. Circulating erythroid progenitors in polycythemia vera are hypersensitive to insulin-like growth factor-1 in vitro: Studies in an improved serum-free medium. *Blood.* 1994;83:99–112.

46. Roy CN, Weinstein DA, Andrews NC. 2002 E. Mead Johnson Award for research in pediatrics lecture: The molecular biology of the anemia of chronic disease: A hypothesis. *Pediatr Res.* 2003;53:507–512.

47. Lee P, Peng H, Gelbart T, et al., The IL-6- and lipopolysaccharide-induced transcription of hepcidin in HFE-, transferrin receptor 2-, and β2-microglobulin-deficient hepatocytes. *Proc Natl Acad Sci U S A.* 2004;101:9263–9265.

48. Nemeth E, Valore EV, Territo M, et al., Hepcidin, a putative mediator of anemia of inflammation, is a type II acute-phase protein. *Blood.* 2003;101:2461–2463.

49. Nicolas G, Chauvet C, Viatte L, et al., The gene encoding the iron regulatory peptide hepcidin is regulated by anemia, hypoxia, and inflammation. *J Clin Invest.* 2002;110:1037–1044.

50. Ganz T. Hepcidin, a key regulator of iron metabolism and mediator of anemia of inflammation. *Blood.* 2003;102:783–788.

51. Weinstein DA, Roy CN, Fleming MD, et al., Inappropriate expression of hepcidin is associated with iron refractory anemia: Implications for the anemia of chronic disease. *Blood.* 2002;100:3776–3781.

52. Carson JL, Hébert P. Anemia and red blood cell transfusion. In: Simon TL, Dzik WH, Snyder EL, et al., eds. *Rossi's principles of transfusion medicine.* 3rd ed. Philadelphia, PA: Lippincott Williams & Wilkins; 2002:149–164.

53. Spahn Dr, Leone BJ, Reves JG, et al., Cardiovascular and coronary physiology of acute isovolemic hemodilution: A review of nonoxygen-carrying and oxygen-carrying solutions. *Anesth Analg.* 1994;78:1000–1021.

54. Murray JF, Escobar E, Rapaport E. Effects of blood viscosity on hemodynamic responses in acute normovolemic anemia. *Am J Physiol.* 1969;216:638–642.

55. Richardson TQ, Guyton AC. Effects of polycythemia and anemia on cardiac output and other circulatory factors. *Am J Physiol.* 1959;197:1167–1170.

56. Fan FC, Chen RYZ, Schuessler GB, et al., Effects of hematocrit variations on regional hemodynamics and oxygen transport in the dog. *Am J Physiol.* 1980;238:H545–H552.

57. Messmer K, Lewis DH, Sunder-Plassmann L, et al., Acute normovolemic hemodilution. *Eur Surg Res.* 1972;4:55–70.

58. Mirhashemi S, Ertefai S, Messmer K. Medol analysis of the enhancement of tissue oxygenation by hemodilution due to increased microvascular flow velocity. *Microvasc Res.* 1987;34:290–301.

59. Gutierrez G. The rate of oxygen release and its effect on capillary O_2 tension: A mathematical analysis. *Respir Physiol*. 1986;63: 79–96.

60. LaCelle PL. Alteration of deformability of the erythrocyte membrane in stored blood. *Transfusion*. 1969;9:238–245.

61. Simchon S, Jan KM, Chien S. Influence of reduced red cell deformability on regional blood flow. *Am J Physiol*. 1987;253: H898–H903.

62. Valeri CR, Hirsch NM. Restoration in vivo of erythrocyte adenosine triphosphate, 2,3-diphosphoglycerate, potassium ion, and sodium ion concentrations following the transfusion of acid-citrate-dextrose-stored human red blood cells. *J Lab Clin Med*. 1969;673:722–733.

63. Stroncek DF, Byrne KM, Noguchi CT, et al., Increasing hemoglobin oxygen saturation levels in sickle trait donor whole blood prevents hemoglobin S polymerization and allows effective white blood cell reduction by filtration. *Transfusion*. 2004;44:1293–1299.

64. Novak RW, Brown RE. Multiple renal and splenic infarctions in a neonate following transfusion with sickle trait blood. *Clin Pediatr (Philadelphia)*. 1982;21:239–241.

65. Hurd TC, Dasmahaptra KS, Rush BF, et al., Red blood cell deformability in human and experimental sepsis. *Arch Surg*. 1988;123:217–220.

66. Friedlander MH, Simon R, Machiedo GW. The relationship of packed cell transfusion to red blood cell deformability in systemic inflammatory response syndrome patients. *Shock*. 1998;9:84–88.

67. Habler OP, Kleen MS, Podtschaske AH, et al., The effect of acute normovolemic hemodilution (ANH) on myocardial contractility in anesthetized dogs. *Anesth Analg*. 1996;83:451–458.

68. Spahn DR, Smith LR, Venonee CD, et al., Acute isovolemic hemodilution and blood transfusion effects on regional function and metabolism in myocardium with compromised coronary blood flow. *J Thorac Cardiovasc Surg*. 1993;105:694–704.

69. Carson JL, Duff A, Poses RM, et al., Effect of anaemia and cardiovascular disease on surgical mortality and morbidity. *Lancet*. 1996;348:1055–1060.

70. Lam HTC, Schweitzer SO, Petz L, et al., Effectiveness of a prospective physician self-audit transfusion-monitoring system. *Transfusion*. 1997;37:577–584.

71. Korosue K, Heros RC. Mechanism of cerebral blood flow augmentation by hemodilution in rabbits. *Stroke*. 1992;23: 1487–1493.

72. Tu YK, Liu HM. Effects of isovolemic hemodilution on hemodynamics, cerebral perfusion, and cerebral vascular reactivity. *Stroke*. 1996;27:441–445.

73. Awad IA, Carter LP, Spetzler RF, et al., Clinical vasospasm after subarachnoid hemorrhage: Response to hypervolemic hemodilution and arterial hypertension. *Stroke*. 1987;18:365–372.

74. Nelson DP, Samsel RW, Wood LD, et al., Pathological supply dependence of systemic and intestinal O_2 uptake during endotoxemia. *J Appl Physiol*. 1988;64:2410–2419.

75. Gutierrez G, Lund N, Bryan-Brown CW. Cellular oxygen utilization during multiple organ failure. *Crit Care Clin*. 1989;5: 271–287.

76. Parillo JE, Parker MM, Natanson C, et al., Septic shock in humans: Advances in the understanding of pathogenesis, cardiovascular dysfunction, and therapy. *Ann Intern Med*. 1990;113: 227–242.

77. Stein JI, Gombotz H, Rigler B, et al., Open heart surgery in children of Jehovah's Witnesses: Extreme hemodilution on cardiopulmonary bypass. *Pediatr Cardiol*. 1991;12:170–174.

78. Wong EC. Acute normovolemic hemodilution: A critical evaluation of its safety and utility in pediatric patients. *Transfu Altern Transfu Med*. 2004;6:10–21.

79. Fontana JL, Welborn L, Mongan PD, et al., Oxygen consumption and cardiovascular function in children during profound intraoperative nomovolemic hemodilution. *Anesth Analg*. 1995;80:219–225.

80. Roseff SD, Luban NL, Manno CS. Guidelines for assessing appropriateness of pediatric transfusion. *Transfusion*. 2002; 42:1398–1413.

81. Gibson BE, Todd A, Roberts I, et al., British Committee for Standards in Haematology Transfusion Task Force: Writing group. Transfusion guidelines for neonates and older children. *Br J Haematol*. 2004;124:433–453.

82. Frey B, Losa M. The value of capillary whole blood lactate for blood transfusion requirements in anemia of prematurity. *Intensive Care Med*. 2001;27:222–227.

83. Wardle SP, Weindling M. Peripheral fractional oxygen extraction and other measures of tissue oxygenation to guide blood transfusions in preterm infants. *Semin Perinat*. 2001;25:60–64.

84. Wardle SP, Garr R, Yoxall CW, et al., A pilot randomised controlled trial of peripheral fractional oxygen extraction to guide blood transfusions in preterm infants. *Arch Dis Child Neonatal Ed*. 2002;86:F22–F27.

85. Mock DM, Bell EF, Lankford GL. Hematocrit correlates well with circulating red blood cell volume in very low birth weight infants. *Pediatr Res*. 2001;50:525–531.

86. Laverdiere C, Gauvin F, Hebert PC, et al., Survey on transfusion practices of pediatric intensivists. *Pediatr Crit Care Med*. 2002;3:335–340.

87. Armano R, Gauvin F, Toledano B, et al., Determinants of red blood cell transfusions in a pediatric critical care unit: A prospective descriptive epidemiological study. *Pedatr Crit Care Med*. 2003;4:A186.

88. Nahum E, Ben-Ari J, Schonfeld T. Blood transfusion policy among European pediatric intensive care physicians. *J Intensive Care Med*. 2004;19:38–43.

89. Goodman AM, Pollack MM, Patel KM, et al., Pediatric red blood cell transfusions increase resource use. *J Pediatr*. 2003;142:123–127.

90. Lackritz EM, Campbell CC, Ruebush TK, et al., Effect of blood transfusion on survival among children in a Kenyan hospital. *Lancet*. 1992;340:524–528.

91. English M, Ahmed M, Ngando C, et al., Blood transfusion for severe anaemia in children in a Kenyan hospital. *Lancet*. 2002; 359:494–495.

92. Hebert PC, Wells G, Blajchman MA, et al., Transfusion Requirements in Critical Care Investigators, Canadian Critical Care Trials Group. A multicenter, randomized, controlled clinical trial of transfusion requirements in critical care. *N Engl J Med*. 1999;340:409–417.

93. Desmet L, Lacroix J. Transfusion in pediatrics. *Crit Care Clin*. 2004;20:299–311.

94. Practice guidelines for blood component therapy: A report by the American Society of Anesthesiologists Task Force on Blood Component Therapy. *Anesthesiology*. 1996;84:732–747.

95. Simon TL, Alverson DC, Aubuchon J, et al., Practice parameter for the use of red blood cell transfusions: Developed by the Red Blood Cell Administration Practice Guideline Development. *Arch Pathol Lab Med*. 1998;122:130–138.

96. Murphy MF, Wallington TB, Kelsey P, et al., British Committee for Standards in Haematology, Blood Transfusion Task Force Guidelines for the clinical use of red cell transfusions. *Br J Haematol*. 2001;113:24–31.

97. Colman RW, Hirsh J, Marder VJ, et al., eds. *Hemostasis and thrombosis*, 4th ed. Philadelphia, PA: Lippincott Williams & Wilkins; 2001.

98. Kitchens CS. The anatomic basis of purpura. *Prog Hemost Thromb*. 1982;5:211–244.

99. Rosenberg RD, Aird WC. Vascular-bed-specific hemostasis and hypercoagulable states. *N Engl J Med*. 1999;340:1555–1564.

100. Nurden AT, Caen JP. The different glycoprotein abnormalities in thrombasthenic and Bernard-Soulier platelets. *Semin Hematol*. 1979;16:24–250.

101. al-Mondhiry H, Ehmann WC. Congenital afibrinogenemia. *Am J Hematol*. 1994;46:343–347.

102. Gabbeta J, Yang X, Kowalska MA, et al., Platelet signal transduction defect with G-alpha subunit dysfunction and diminished G-alpha-q in a patient with abnormal platelet responses. *Proc Natl Acad Sci U S A*. 1997;94:8750–8755.

103. Lee SB, Rao AK, Lee KH, et al., Decreased expression of phospholipase C-beta 2 isozyme in human platelets with impaired function. *Blood*. 1996;88:1684–1691.

104. Serrano K, Devine DV. Vinculin is proteolyzed by calpain during platelet aggregation: 95 kDa cleavage fragment associates with the platelet cytoskeleton. *Cell Motil Cytoskeleton*. 2004; 58:242–252. Aug;

105. Murugappan S, Shankar H, Kunapuli SP. Platelet receptors for adenine nucleotides and thromboxane A2. *Semin Thromb Hemost.* 2004;30:411–418.

106. Price GC, Thompson SA, Kam PC. Tissue factor and tissue factor pathway inhibitor. *Anaesthesia.* 2004;59:483–492.

107. Abshire TC. Dose optimization of recombinant factor VIIa for control of mild to moderate bleeds in inhibitor patients: Improved efficacy with higher dosing. *Semin Hematol.* 2004;41(1 Suppl 1):3–7.

108. Andrew M, Paes B, Milner R, et al., The development of the human coagulation system in the full term infant. *Blood.* 1987;70:165–172.

109. Andrew M, Paes B, Milner R, et al., Development of the coagulation system in the healthy premature infant. *Blood.* 1988; 72:1651–1657.

110. Andrew M. Developmental hemostasis: Relevance to thromboembolic complications in pediatric patients. *Thromb Haemost.* 1995;74(1 Suppl):415–424.

Cardiac Physiology and Pathophysiology

John T. Berger III   *Richard A. Jonas*

Acute severe myocardial dysfunction remains a significant cause of mortality and morbidity in children requiring intensive care. The heart is one of the most common organs to fail in critical illness, and this failure can arise from many disease processes including sepsis, congenital heart disease, trauma, and even predominantly respiratory illnesses such as respiratory synctial virus (RSV) infection.[1,2] A basic understanding of cardiac anatomy and function is essential for the intensivist to diagnose and manage cardiovascular abnormalities. Chapter 5.1 describes cardiac function from several different levels including the myocyte, and the intact heart and its interaction with the respiratory system. Additional sections focus on unique cardiac pathophysiologies encountered in the intensive care unit.

Cardiomyocyte Function

5.1

Steven M. Schwartz

The clinical management of children with heart disease is essentially the practice of applied cardiovascular physiology. Underlying the clinically apparent physiology, however, are cellular and molecular processes that are subject to developmental regulation and that dictate the cardiovascular response to disease. Complex and highly integrated pathways of signal transduction and protein synthesis change the molecular composition of the myocardium throughout the fetal and newborn periods, and when the mature heart is exposed to chronic stressors. Structural elements, contractile proteins, ion channels, and even nonmyocyte cardiac cells are vital components in the process of myocardial maturation and in the response to critical illness. Understanding these processes helps develop new therapeutic targets and advance our understanding of conventional drugs such as angiotensin converting enzyme (ACE) inhibitors and β-adrenergic agonists. It is therefore becoming progressively important for the clinician to understand the mechanisms that underlie cardiac function and dysfunction.

The molecular and cellular pathways that form the basis of cardiac maturation and function have been studied in a number of species and at various stages of development. Although there is general consensus regarding many important principles, the precise contribution of developmental physiology to human pediatric heart disease remains an active field of study. It is unclear exactly when the human heart assumes characteristics of the mature, adult heart. This is particularly relevant to clinical medicine in that we often rely on the outcome of studies in adults to guide our management decisions in children. It is therefore essential that the pediatric intensive care physician understands the basic cellular processes that contribute to myocardial function and the way in which these may change during postnatal development. The purpose of this section is to review the key elements involved in generating cardiac contraction and relaxation and the key systems involved in regulating these processes. Particular emphasis has been placed on the differences between the neonatal and mature hearts.

CELLULAR AND MOLECULAR BASIS OF CARDIAC CONTRACTILITY

Myocardial contraction is initiated by a large increase in available intracellular calcium, which, in turn, leads to movement of the contractile elements of the sarcomere. A sharp decrease in calcium availability then brings about diastolic relaxation.

Contractile Elements

The primary contractile elements of the sarcomere (see Fig. 5.1.1) are the thin filament, comprised primarily of monomers of α-actin arranged into two long, intertwined strands that are anchored at the Z disks, and the thick filament, consisting of myosin molecules joined together at the tail with the globular heads protruding from this central axis. In most mammalian species including humans, both actin and myosin exist in several isoforms, the expression of which is regulated in both tissue-specific and developmentally specific manners. Actin isoforms include both cardiac and skeletal α-actin. In the fetal and neonatal human ventricle, most of the actin is cardiac α-actin, but, as the heart matures, a progressively greater proportion of skeletal α-actin is incorporated into the sarcomere.[3] The regulation of myosin is more complex than that of actin. The myosin molecule is constructed of two heavy and four light chains. The heavy chains form the rod of the molecule that comprises the thick filament. The cardiac myosin heavy chain exists as either the α- or the β-myosin heavy chain. There are three isoforms of myosin. The V1 isoform contains two α chains, the V2 isoform contains one α and one β chain, and the V3 isoform contains two β chains. The V3 isoform is the predominant myosin isoform present in the human ventricle during development and throughout

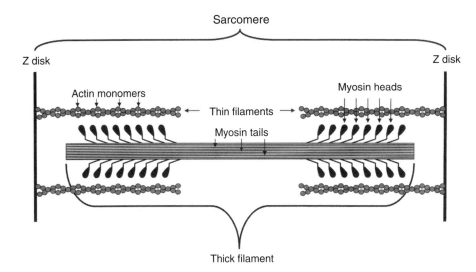

Figure 5.1.1 Organization of the sarcomere. The sarcomere is composed of thin filaments made up of two intertwined strands of repeating actin monomers, and thick filaments made up of the tails of myosin molecules. The heads of the myosin molecules protrude from the thick filament and are poised to attach to the actin strands. The actin strands are anchored at the z disks that form the lateral edges of the sarcomere.

maturation.[4] In rodents, the V3 isoform predominates in the fetal heart but the adult ventricle is virtually all V1, a fact that may limit the applicability of some rodent models of heart failure. The myosin head is composed of the light chains and generates the movement of the actin filament along the length of the thick filament. The myosin head binds to actin and undergoes a conformational change driven by the hydrolysis of adenosine triphosphate (ATP) (see Fig. 5.1.2). The cycle of attachment of the myosin head to actin and hydrolysis of ATP with pivoting of the myosin head causes movement of the actin filament and shortening of the sarcomere.

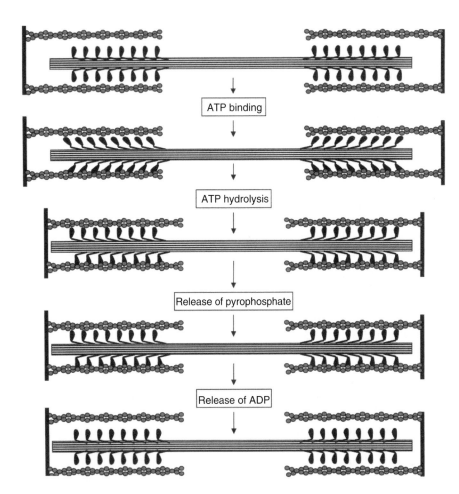

Figure 5.1.2 Adenosine triphosphate (ATP) binding and hydrolysis drive the shortening of the sarcomere. Contraction of the sarcomere occurs when myosin binds to ATP. The myosin head undergoes a conformational change and binds to actin. Hydrolysis of ATP drives pivoting of the myosin head, causing shortening of the sarcomere. Pyrophosphate (Pi) and adenosine diphosphate (ADP) are then released by myosin, allowing release of actin from myosin. The cycle repeats throughout systole.

One particularly interesting aspect of the way in which the mature heart responds to pressure overload is that there is, at least in many species, a re-expression of the fetal genetic program. Rodent models of cardiac hypertrophy show the isoforms of actin and myosin present in the fetal heart, β-myosin heavy chain and α-skeletal actin, re-emerge during the development of cardiac hypertrophy.[5] The β-myosin heavy chain has a slower velocity of shortening but better energetics and calcium response than does α-myosin, which may confer some advantage in the overloaded or hypertrophied heart. Although there is some evidence that hypertrophied human ventricles have a relative increase in β-myosin compared to α-myosin, the β-myosin predominance of the human ventricle makes the importance of isoform switching in human hypertrophy unclear.

Troponin and Tropomyosin

Troponin and tropomyosin regulate the binding of myosin to actin (see Fig. 5.1.3). Tropomyosin winds around the thin filament in the groove between the two strands of actin monomers. Tropomyosin strengthens the actin filament and increases myosin binding. The troponin complex consists of three elements: troponin I (TnI), troponin C (TnC) and troponin T (TnT). The troponin complex makes the binding of actin and myosin a calcium-dependent process. TnI inhibits the interaction of actin and myosin. There are two isoforms of TnI: cardiac and skeletal muscle isoforms. The neonatal heart contains mostly the skeletal isoform, but the cardiac isoform predominates as the heart matures.[6] TnI is affected by numerous stimuli, including β-adrenergic–receptor activation and ischemia-reperfusion injury,[7,8] and the appearance of cardiac TnI in serum is a highly specific marker of myocardial injury. TnC binds calcium and initiates a conformational shift that releases the inhibition of actin–myosin binding caused by TnI. TnT attaches the troponin complex to tropomyosin.

Anchoring Proteins

The contractile apparatus within the cardiomyocyte must be able to communicate with the extracellular matrix. This communication can translate external biomechanical stress, such as pressure overload, to the cytoplasm and can also signal intracellular events to neighboring cells. Some of the most important proteins responsible for this function are the integrins, a family of heterodimeric transmembrane receptors composed of α and β subunits. Because of the large number of different subunits and splice variants, there are numerous potential α/β heterodimers, but only a subset of these has been detected in the heart. Seven of the (at least) 18 α subunits and the β_1 isoform have been reliably detected in the myocardial tissue, although there is some suggestion that the β_3 and β_5 isoforms may also be present. Like many other structural elements, there is developmental regulation of integrin expression, and isoform expression may change in response to a variety of stimuli.[9] In addition to structural-anchoring proteins, it is important to realize that other signaling molecules may also be anchored to either the cell membrane or other membranous structures within the cell. Ion channels and protein kinases may be anchored in place so as to effectively compartmentalize their effects. For example, protein kinase A (PKA), a major signaling molecule in adrenergic-receptor signaling, can have numerous effects, depending on the target molecules. The specific substrates for PKA depend largely on their proximity to the activated receptor and PKA, a relationship maintained by A-kinase anchoring proteins (AKAP). Other proteins can be regulated in a

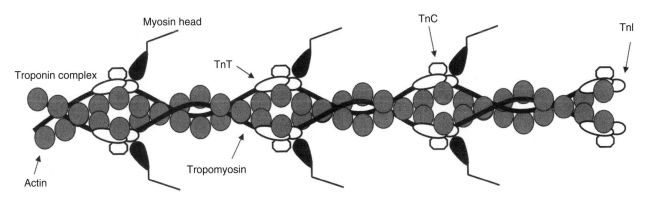

Figure 5.1.3 Tropomyosin and the troponin complex. Troponin and tropomyosin regulate the binding of myosin to actin. Tropomyosin winds around the thin filament in the groove between the two strands of actin monomers to strengthen the actin filament and increase myosin binding. The troponin complex consists of three elements: troponin I (TnI), troponin C (TnC), and troponin T (TnT). TnI inhibits the interaction of actin and myosin. TnC binds calcium and initiates a conformational shift that releases inhibition of actin–myosin binding caused by TnI. TnT binds the troponin complex to tropomyosin.

similar fashion, and therefore, compartmentalization is an essential principle to understand the means by which cardiac function can be manipulated by various agents and/or diseases.

Calcium Cycling

The binding and release of actin and myosin, and therefore, cardiac contraction and relaxation, are mediated by cyclic fluctuations in cytoplasmic calcium concentration. The cardiomyocyte is highly specialized to allow rapid release and resequestration of calcium. The degree to which these calcium fluxes are dependent on intracellular versus extracellular sources of calcium is subject to maturational forces and may explain some differences between neonatal and adult heart responses to various stimuli.

Calcium influx into the cardiomyocyte is initiated during phase 2 of the action potential with the slow inward calcium current generated by the L-type calcium channels (see Fig. 5.1.4). These channels consist of multiple subunits, with the α_{1c} subunit forming the core of the channel. The other subunits modify the function of the α-subunit and potentially allow modification of channel activity in response to stimuli such as β-adrenergic–receptor activation. The channel is voltage-gated, which means, when a certain level of depolarization is achieved, the channel opens and calcium flows into the cell. In the neonatal heart, the increase in cytosolic calcium from the L-type calcium channels contributes directly and significantly to the calcium that binds to TnC and causes cardiac contraction (excitation–contraction coupling).[10,11] The increase in intracellular calcium caused by the slow inward calcium current activates the ryanodine receptor (RyR) and causes further calcium release from the sarcoplasmic reticulum (SR). In the adult heart, the calcium released from the SR accounts for the overwhelming majority of

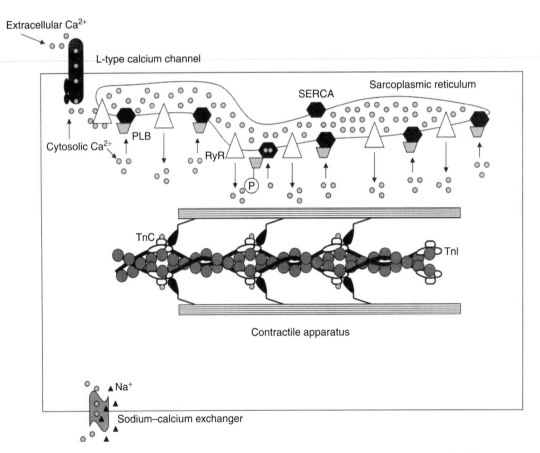

Figure 5.1.4 Myocardial calcium cycling. Extracellular calcium enters the cell through voltage-gated (L-type) calcium channels on the cell membrane. The influx of extracellular calcium initiates massive calcium release from the sarcoplasmic reticulum through the ryanodine receptor (RyR). Cytosolic calcium binds to Troponin C (TnC), causing a conformational change in troponin I (TnI) and allowing myosin to bind to actin and to initiate sarcomere shortening. In diastole, calcium is resequestered in the sarcoplasmic reticulum by the sarcoplasmic reticulum calcium ATPase (SERCA). SERCA itself is gated by phospholamban (PLB), which, in its dephosphorylated state, inhibits reuptake of calcium by SERCA. A small amount of calcium is pumped out of the cell by sodium–calcium exchanger on the cell surface.

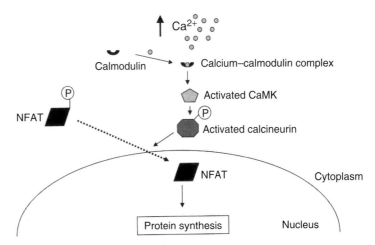

Figure 5.1.5 Calcium-mediated hypertrophic signaling. Persistently elevated intracellular calcium levels lead to binding of calcium to calmodulin and activation of calcium/calmodulin-dependent protein kinase (CaMK). Activated CaMK phosphorylates calcineurin, which then dephosphorylates nuclear factor of activated T cells (NFAT). In its dephosphorylated state, NFAT can translocate from the cytoplasm to the nucleus and initiate protein synthesis.

calcium that is bound by TnC, minimizing the direct effect of the L-type channels on contractility.

The switch from systolic contraction to diastolic relaxation is initiated by resequestration of the calcium from the cytosol back into the SR and/or the extracellular space. Most of the calcium removal is by the sarcoplasmic reticulum calcium ATPase (SERCA). This pump is present on the membrane of the SR and actively transports calcium back into the SR. The pump is regulated by the multimeric protein phospholamban (PLB), which in the dephosphorylated state inhibits reuptake of calcium by SERCA. PLB can be phosphorylated by any of the three protein kinases including PKA (also known as *cyclic adenosine monophosphate* (cAMP)-*dependent protein kinase*). A much smaller amount of calcium is removed from the cell by the sodium–calcium exchanger, which may have increased importance in the neonatal heart trans-sarcolemmal calcium fluxes because of the relative immaturity of the SR system.[12–14]

Although the predominant effects of calcium fluxes in the cardiomyocyte are initiation of contraction and relaxation, calcium also plays a vital role in intracellular signaling. Intracellular calcium levels are sensed by calmodulin (see Fig. 5.1.5). Binding of calcium to calmodulin activates calcium/calmodulin-dependent protein kinase (CaMK) that subsequently activates an important downstream effector, calcineurin. Activated calcineurin dephosphorylates nuclear factor of activated T cells (NFAT), a DNA transcription factor, that is then able to translocate from the cytoplasm to the nucleus and initiate protein synthesis, which provides a mechanism whereby information about cardiac function can directly lead to structural changes in the myocyte.

NONMYOCYTES

In addition to contractile cells, the myocardium contains fibroblasts, vascular cells including endothelium, and noncellular elements such as collagen. These cells and proteins participate both actively and passively in determining systolic and diastolic properties of the myocardium and in signaling cascades that result in functional and structural responses to various stressors.

In the healthy heart, collagen exists as a fine latticework surrounding myocytes and blood vessels. Collagen fibers and the cytoskeleton of the cellular components of the myocardium impart a passive elastic quality to the myocardium as a whole, which has important implications for diastolic function. As the ventricle begins to fill in early diastole, active relaxation caused by calcium sequestration is the primary determinant of myocardial compliance. At high filling volumes, as can occur in volume overload lesions and myocardial dysfunction, a greater portion of the axial stress is borne by collagenous elements of the myocardium. Many of the signals that inform cardiomyocytes of increased load may be channeled through the extracellular matrix by connections between this matrix and the myocyte. There is evidence of signaling between myocytes, fibroblasts, and endothelial cells, both through biomechanical transduction and through paracrine release of such potent growth stimuli as angiotensin II.[15] The end result is that increases in loading stimulate not only cardiomyocyte hypertrophy but also fibroblast proliferation and collagen production. This is important from a clinical standpoint because cardiac disease is associated with significant fibrosis and loss of myocytes, which limits the response to therapies primarily targeted to improve myocyte function such as dopamine, dobutamine, or milrinone.

ADRENERGIC RECEPTORS AND INTRACELLULAR SIGNALING

Although there are many receptor systems on the cardiomyocyte membrane that enable the heart to respond to a variety of stimuli, the β-adrenergic system remains the one most commonly manipulated by intensive care physicians. Both β_1- and β_2-adrenergic receptors couple to

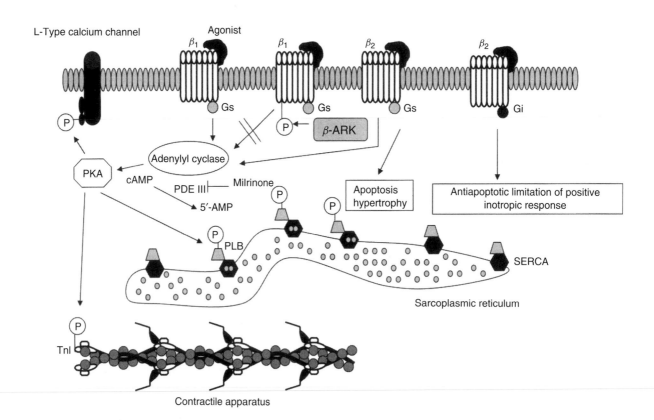

Figure 5.1.6 β-Adrenergic signaling. β₁-Adrenergic and β₂-adrenergic receptors couple to stimulatory G proteins (Gs). Agonist binding activates adenylyl cyclase, which increases cyclic adenosine monophosphate (cAMP) and activates protein kinase A (PKA). PKA phosphorylates L-type calcium channels, phospholamban (PLB), and troponin I (TnI) among other proteins. cAMP is degraded to 5'-AMP by phosphodiesterase III (PDE III), which is inhibited by milrinone. Activation of Gs also promotes apoptosis and hypertrophy, whereas activation of the inhibitory G protein, Gi, by β₂ receptors has antiapoptotic effects and may limit the positive inotropic response to β-adrenergic agonists. Increased levels of the β-adrenergic receptor kinase (β-ARK) phosphorylate the receptors and render them less responsive to agonist. SERCA, sarcoplasmic reticulum calcium ATPase; PKA, protein kinase A.

adenylyl cyclase by means of the stimulatory G protein (Gs) (see Fig. 5.1.6). This enzyme forms cAMP, which activates PKA. PKA phosphorylates TnI, PLB, and L-type calcium channels. Consequently, the L-type calcium channels increase calcium transport, the troponin complex becomes more calcium responsive, and calcium is resequestered into the SR more rapidly. Myocardial cAMP is degraded by phosphodiesterase III (PDE III). This enzyme can be inhibited by specific PDE inhibitors such as milrinone and inamrinone. This provides a receptor-independent mechanism to bring about the same salutary effects as β-adrenergic agonists, even in the presence of decreased β-adrenergic–receptor responsiveness or downregulation, which can occur in many situations, including after cardiopulmonary bypass.[16] PDE inhibitors may also enhance calcium flux through the reverse activity of the sodium–calcium exchanger and improve ventricular function by a mechanism unrelated to increases in cAMP. As noted previously, increased influx of extracellular calcium may be particularly significant in neonates.

Acutely then, the predominant effect of adrenergic stimulation of the myocardium is to increase inotropy and chronotropy. Diastolic function is also enhanced. Chronic exposure to adrenergic agonists results in more complex and comprehensive effects on the cardiomyocyte. Overexpression of β₁ receptors in mice is associated with increased contractility, both at baseline and in response to adrenergic stimulation over the first 15 weeks of life.[17] Longer exposure and higher levels of β₁ expression, however, have resulted in depression of contractile function and myocyte hypertrophy, fibrosis, and apoptosis.[17] Similar deleterious effects have occurred in mice overexpressing a Gs protein,[18] suggesting that this is a potential mechanism for the adverse consequences of prolonged β-adrenergic stimulation.

β₂-Adrenergic receptors appear to couple to inhibitory G proteins (Gi) in addition to Gs.[19] Gi is thought to oppose the effects of Gs to some degree, including limiting the acute positive inotropic response to adrenergic stimulation and offering some protection from apoptosis. Transgenic mice with cardiac-specific overexpression of β₂-adrenergic receptors show increased contractility, similar to that observed early in β_1 overexpression, but without the long-term decompensation.[20] At very high levels of overexpression, though, these mice develop dilated cardiomyopathy,[21] perhaps because of relative amounts of Gs and Gi signaling. The complex nature of adrenergic signaling in which there is a short-term positive effect coupled with long-term adverse effects is a pattern followed by many other myocardial signaling cascades, including those involved in calcium handling and the renin–angiotensin system.

Another intriguing aspect of β-adrenergic signaling is polymorphic variation. Polymorphisms are normal variants in genetic sequences in the population that do not, by definition, cause disease but may alter the course of a specific disease by conferring variable responsiveness to therapeutic drugs or modifying the natural progression of the disease. Although polymorphisms that affect cardiovascular disease have not been studied to any great extent in the pediatric population, they are obviously present. Polymorphic variants of both β_1- and β_2-adrenergic receptors have been identified in the adult population and although they are not associated with altered exercise performance or increased risk of cardiomyopathy in healthy subjects, it appears increasingly clear that they are important modifying factors for individuals with either asthma or cardiomyopathy. β_1-Adrenergic–receptor polymorphisms have been identified at two loci that are likely to be important in either receptor downregulation or G protein–coupling. Patients with heart failure who have one of these polymorphisms have decreased exercise tolerance, and this polymorphism has also been associated with an increased risk of systemic hypertension. There are three potentially important polymorphisms that have been identified in the β_2 receptor, also associated with either receptor downregulation or coupling to G proteins. One of these, a threonine/isoleucine (Thr/Ile) polymorphism at position 164 shows significantly reduced adenylyl cyclase activity in the Ile164, both at baseline and in response to epinephrine, than the Thr164 when expressed in recombinant cells.[22] Population studies have shown that 95% of the adult population is homozygous, Thr, and 5% heterozygous, Thr/Ile. Transgenic mice that express the Ile form of the receptor in the myocardium show decreased receptor coupling to adenylyl cyclase and decreased physiologic responsiveness to the β-adrenergic agonist, isoproterenol.[23] Studies in humans, likewise, suggest that this particular polymorphism is an important modifier of cardiovascular disease. Heterozygous heart failure patients have decreased exercise tolerance,[24] and 1-year survival for adults with heart failure, who are homozygous for Thr164, is 76% compared to 42% for heterozygous individuals.[20] Even healthy subjects heterozygous at the 164 locus show a blunted cardiovascular response to intravenous terbutaline. These findings clearly imply that the β_2-adrenergic–receptor polymorphism at position 164 can have a major effect on the outcome in individuals with cardiovascular disease and that variable response of the receptor to β-adrenergic agonists may be a key underlying mechanism.

SUMMARY

The cardiovascular system is very dynamic in its response to both physiologic and developmental stimuli. Structural, contractile, and regulatory proteins all undergo changes in form and function. Furthermore, the effects of genetics and other modifying factors may also be subject to maturational forces. Treatment of critically ill patients with cardiovascular disease must therefore take into consideration the differences between the neonatal and more mature heart, in terms of intrinsic function and response to disease. Although direct knowledge of human developmental cardiac physiology remains limited, it is clear that infants are not "little adults," and future studies must focus on the features unique to the immature heart.

REFERENCES

1. Proulx F, Gauthier M, Nadeau D, et al. Timing and predictors of death in pediatric patients with multiple organ system failure. *Crit Care Med*. 1994;22:1025–1031.
2. Kim KK, Frankel LR. The need for inotropic support in a subgroup of infants with severe life-threatening respiratory syncytial viral infection. *J Invest Med*. 1997;45:469–473.
3. Boheler KR, Carrier L, de la Bastie D, et al. Skeletal actin mRNA increases in the human heart during ontogenic development and is the major isoform of control and failing adult hearts. *J Clin Invest*. 1991;88:323–330.
4. Bouvagnet P, Neveu S, Montoya M. Development changes in the human cardiac isomyosin distribution: An immunohistochemical study using monoclonal antibodies. *Circ Res*. 1987;61: 329–336.
5. Izumo S, Nadal-Ginard B, Mahdavi V, et al. Protooncogene induction and reprogramming of cardiac gene expression produced by pressure overload. *Proc Natl Acad Sci U S A*. 1988;85: 339–343.
6. Sasse S, Brand NJ, Kyprianou P, et al. Troponin I gene expression during human cardiac development and in end-stage heart failure. *Circ Res*. 1993;72:932–938.
7. Schwartz SM, Duffy JY, Pearl JM, et al. Glucocorticoids preserve calpastatin and troponin I during cardiopulmonary bypass in immature pigs. *Pediatr Res*. 2003;54:91–97.
8. McDonough JL, Arrell DK, Van Eyk JE. Troponin I degradation and covalent complex formation accompanies myocardial ischemia/reperfusion injury. *Circ Res*. 1999;84:9–20.
9. Ross RS, Borg TK. Integrins and the myocardium. *Circ Res*. 2001; 88:1112–1119.
10. Osaka T, Joyner RW. Developmental changes in calcium currents of rabbit ventricular cells. *Circ Res*. 1991;68:788–796.
11. Katsube Y, Yokoshiki H, Nguyen L, et al. L-type Ca2+ currents in ventricular myocytes from neonatal and adult rats. *Can J Physiol Pharmacol*. 1998;76:873–881.
12. Hanson GL, Schilling WP, Michael LH. Sodium-potassium pump and sodium-calcium exchange in adult and neonatal canine cardiac sarcolemma. *Am J Physiol*. 1993;264:H320–H326.
13. Boucek RJ, Shelton M Jr., Artman M, et al. Comparative effects of verapamil, nifedipine, and diltiazem on contractile function in the isolated immature and adult rabbit heart. *Pediatr Res*. 1984;18:948–952.
14. Klitzner TS, Friedman WF. A diminished role for the sarcoplasmic reticulum in newborn myocardial contraction: Effects of ryanodine. *Pediatr Res*. 1989;26:98–101.

15. Sadoshima J, Xu Y, Slayter HS. Autocrine release of angiotensin II mediates stretch-induced hypertrophy of cardiac myocytes in vitro. *Cell.* 1993;75:977–984.

16. Schwinn DA, Leone BJ, Spahn DR, et al. Desensitization of myocardial beta-adrenergic receptors during cardiopulmonary bypass. Evidence for early uncoupling and late downregulation. *Circulation.* 1991;84:2559–2567.

17. Engelhardt S, Hein L, Wiesmann F. Progressive hypertrophy and heart failure in beta1-adrenergic receptor transgenic mice. *Proc Natl Acad Sci U S A.* 1999;96:7059–7064.

18. Iwase M, Uechi M, Vatner DE, et al. Cardiomyopathy induced by cardiac Gs alpha overexpression. *Am J Physiol.* 1997; 272:H585–H589.

19. Xiao RP, Avdonin P, Zhou YY, et al. Coupling of beta2-adrenoceptor to Gi proteins and its physiological relevance in murine cardiac myocytes. *Circ Res.* 1999;84:43–52.

20. Bittner HB, Chen EP, Milano CA, et al. Functional analysis of myocardial performance in murine hearts overexpressing the human beta 2-adrenergic receptor. *J Mol Cell Cardiol.* 1997;29:961–967.

21. Liggett SB, Tepe NM, Lorenz JN, et al. Early and delayed consequences of beta(2)-adrenergic receptor overexpression in mouse hearts: Critical role for expression level. *Circulation.* 2000; 101:1707–1714.

22. Liggett SB, Wagoner LE, Craft LL, et al. The Ile164 beta2-adrenergic receptor polymorphism adversely affects the outcome of congestive heart failure. *J Clin Invest.* 1998;102: 1534–1539.

23. Turki J, Lorenz JN, Green SA, et al. Myocardial signaling defects and impaired cardiac function of a human beta 2-adrenergic receptor polymorphism expressed in transgenic mice. *Proc Natl Acad Sci U S A.* 1996;93:10483–10488.

24. Wagoner LE, Craft LL, Singh B, et al. Polymorphisms of the beta(2)-adrenergic receptor determine exercise capacity in patients with heart failure. *Circ Res.* 2000;86:834–840.

Cardiac Performance

John T. Berger III

WHAT IS CARDIAC FUNCTION?

The purpose of the cardiovascular system is to deliver adequate oxygen and metabolic substrates to meet the body's demands. Cardiovascular function can be measured at several levels: intrinsic cardiac muscle function (i.e., contractility), pump performance, and adequacy of oxygen delivery. A single measure of these performance categories may not provide sufficient information for other categories. For example, measures of cardiac output provide limited information about adequacy of cardiac output or myocardial contractility. Patients with severe dilated cardiomyopathy have preserved cardiac output and are without signs of cardiogenic shock such as acidosis or oliguria but have severely depressed contractility and poor pump performance. Patients with septic shock may have increased cardiac output, but the output may still be insufficient to meet metabolic demands representing inadequate cardiovascular function.

When considering cardiac function and cardiac output in the past, there is a tendency to focus primarily on left systolic ventricular function. Ultimately, cardiac output is related to the interaction of the left and right ventricle, as well as the arterial and venous circulations. Although adult patients present primarily with left ventricular (LV) dysfunction due to ischemic disease, children frequently have predominantly right ventricular (RV) dysfunction because of pulmonary hypertension or congenital heart disease. Furthermore, patients may have preserved systolic or contractile function and still have diminished cardiac output related to diastolic dysfunction. For instance, a subgroup of patients after tetralogy of Fallot repair have diastolic RV dysfunction despite preserved systolic dysfunction. Compared to patients without diastolic dysfunction, they have evidence of low cardiac output (acidosis, oliguria) and longer lengths of intensive care unit (ICU) stay.[1] Studies in adults with congestive heart failure (CHF) have shown that a substantial proportion have preserved systolic function. When faced with a patient with inadequate cardiac output,

the astute clinician considers the function of the left and right ventricles, as well as systolic and diastolic variables.

DETERMINANTS OF CARDIAC PERFORMANCE

Cardiac pump function is determined by several interdependent factors including preload, afterload, contractility, diastolic filling, and heart rate. The first four variables determine stroke volume, the volume of blood ejected from the ventricle. Cardiac output is the product of stroke volume and heart rate. Although pump function of the heart is a major determinant of cardiac output, interactions of the heart with the vasculature and nervous system are equally crucial. Although it is useful to consider each variable independently, as described in the subsequent text, this represents a simplification of the fundamental function of myocardium. Even at the level of the sarcomere these factors are interrelated. Changes in preload, heart rate, and afterload each alter cytosolic calcium or its interaction with contractile elements and hence alter intrinsic myocardial contraction. Furthermore, diseases usually act on more than one determinant of cardiac function such as dilated cardiomyopathy, in which contractility and diastolic function are altered. Therapies employed in the ICU also alter multiple factors. The commonly used drug, milrinone, increases contractility but also decreases afterload, which may be the more important effect in decompensated CHF.

Preload

Isolated cardiac muscle strips have been used to understand the effects of load on muscle contraction (see Fig. 5.2.1). A muscle strip is tied to a lever and the other end to a force transducer. Weights are attached to the lever to stretch the muscle before contraction (preload). Other weights can be added to the lever after the initial length is set (afterload). The muscle is then stimulated to contract. Instruments

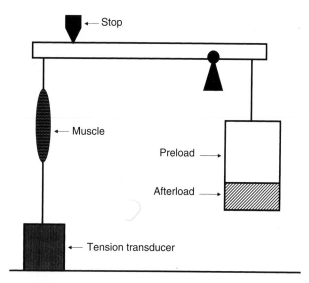

Figure 5.2.1 Starling experiment. A muscle strip is attached to a pressure transducer. A weight is attached to the lever to stretch the muscle and establish its resting tension, preload. A stop is applied and additional weight, afterload, is attached, which because of the stop is only sensed when the muscle is contracting.

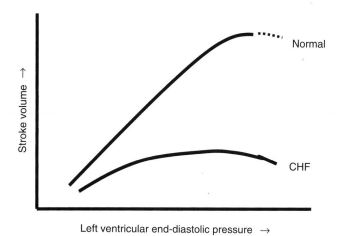

Figure 5.2.2 Idealized Frank-Starling relationship. With increasing left ventricular end-diastolic pressure, there is an increase in stroke volume or cardiac output. The position of each curve is determined by the contractility of the heart. Depressed contractility shifts the curve downward. CHF, congestive heart failure.

can measure multiple variables including muscle length, sarcomere length, and calcium entry.

Preload is the load on a muscle before contraction has started. In isolated cardiac muscle strips, the length to which a muscle is stretched before activation independently determines the active force (tension) developed with muscle stimulation. The amount of active tension developed during stimulation can be measured at various lengths and plotted to produce an active length–tension curve. The active length–tension curve in cardiac muscle has a steep ascending limb and a very small descending limb. The descending limb represents decreased active tension if a myocardial cell is overstretched.

In skeletal muscle, the length–tension relationship relates to the overlapping of actin and myosin filaments and the formation of more cross-bridges. In cardiac muscle, the molecular basis of the length–tension relationship is more complex as myocardium normally functions within a very narrow length range. The increase in force development is caused by an increase in calcium sensitivity of the myofilaments with increasing length.[2,3] In other words, for the same cytosolic calcium concentration, tension steeply increases as the length of the myofiber is increased. The mechanism of length dependence of calcium sensitivity is not certain and is certainly multifactorial. Factors, including changes in calcium binding to troponin C, reduced lateral separation of thick and thin filaments, and the stretch of titin, an intrasarcomeric filament, have all been suggested.[4]

Preload in Intact Heart

Simple translation of the length–tension relationship of isolated muscle to the heart is not straightforward because

of the three-dimensional structure of the heart and the organization and alignment of myocytes. The heart as a pump generates pressure rather than tension and ejects a volume rather than a reduction in length. Preload is more accurately described therefore as the ventricular wall stress at end diastole. In 1895, Otto Frank correlated the length–tension observations made with muscle strips to volume–pressure changes that occur in the intact heart.[5] He observed that if the heart is not allowed to eject, increased preload results in increased pressure generation. In 1918, E. H. Starling proposed that a larger preload results in a larger stroke volume if the heart is permitted to eject and afterload is held constant. These combined observations, the Frank-Starling law or relationship, state that if preload is increased stroke volume and capability for pressure generation are increased (see Fig. 5.2.2).

In clinical practice, different variables have been used to substitute muscle fiber length and tension development when describing the Frank-Starling relationship. When trying to understand preload–performance relationships, it is important to know the assumptions made when using surrogate variables. In the ICU, preload is often estimated by end-diastolic pressure because of the ease of measurement. There are limitations to using end-diastolic pressure as a surrogate for end-diastolic volume. First, the diastolic pressure–volume relationship or compliance in the ventricle is curvilinear (see Fig. 5.2.3). At low levels of end-diastolic pressure and volume, large increases in ventricular volume produce only small changes in ventricular pressure. When end-diastolic volume (EDV) is high, small changes in volume produce proportionally larger increases in ventricular pressure. Second, alterations in intrinsic diastolic properties, such as those seen with myocardial edema or in pericardial tamponade, will change diastolic pressure without reflecting a change in diastolic

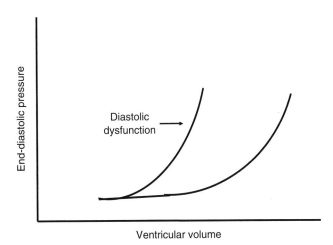

Figure 5.2.3 Ventricular compliance curve. In the normally compliant ventricle as ventricular volume increases, end-diastolic pressure increases only a small amount. However, at very large ventricular volumes, pressure rises rapidly with very small increases in ventricular volume, indicating decreased compliance. Disease processes like myocardial fibrosis, hypertrophy, or edema cause intrinsic diastolic dysfunction represented by a shift of the compliance curve to the left.

volume. A rising end-diastolic pressure in these conditions reflects increased myocardial stiffness and not increased preload. Under certain conditions of decreased diastolic function and high end-diastolic pressure, further increases in end-diastolic pressure may result in lower preload by inhibiting venous return (see section on venous–cardiac coupling).

Afterload

In the isolated muscle strip, afterload is the load that resists contraction after stimulation (Fig. 5.2.1). A stimulated muscle fiber contracts isometrically until it develops enough force to overcome the mass opposing shortening. Once the mass is overcome, shortening begins. The tension that develops before the shortening is afterload. If preload is held constant, an increased afterload will decrease the rate and extent of fiber shortening.

Afterload in the Intact Heart

An understanding of afterload is particularly important in patients with cardiac disease because afterload is a major determinant of not only cardiac output but also myocardial oxygen consumption. In the intact ventricle, afterload is the force opposing ventricular contraction and ejection of blood. Major components of afterload include arterial vessel elastance, vascular resistance, and ventricular wall stress. Systole is a dynamic process. Variables such as ventricular size, and wall thickness are constantly changing and therefore instantaneous afterload is also changing during systole. Two important representations of afterload *in vivo* are systolic wall stress and arterial impedance.

In the intact ventricle, wall stress or load per cross-sectional area during ventricular ejection is analogous to tension of the isolated muscle strip as a representation of afterload. The relationship between pressure and stress is influenced by the size and shape of the ventricle. This relationship is approximated by the law of Laplace, which, as applied to a thick-walled sphere, states that the wall stress (T) is equal to the pressure (p) within the sphere times the radius (r) divided by two times the wall thickness (h):

$$T = p \times r/2h$$

Laplace law, although an oversimplification due to the complex geometry and dynamic changes of the LV, highlights important cardiac physiology. A dilated ventricle with a larger radius has a higher systolic wall stress. The greater the pressure developed within the ventricle for a given radius, the greater the wall stress. Additionally, the pressure in Laplace law is the transmural pressure (LV intracavitary pressure—pericardial pressure). Consequently, when intrathoracic pressure becomes very negative, as during labored breathing, transmural pressure and afterload increase on the LV. This partially explains the benefit of positive end-expiratory pressure (PEEP) in patients with left ventricular dysfunction. Finally, the increased wall thickness that occurs with ventricular hypertrophy decreases wall stress.

Another method to describe afterload is to consider the vascular opposition to ventricular ejection. Traditionally, vascular resistance has been used as the measure of afterload because of its ease of calculation in the ICU. Resistance is the opposition to flow in a continuous or steady state system and ignores the pulsatile nature of blood flow. Resistance equals the pressure difference across the vascular bed (mean arterial pressure—central venous pressure [CVP] for the systemic circulation) divided by the mean flow or cardiac output:

$$R = P/Q = 8\,\mu L/\pi r^4$$

where R is vascular resistance, P is mean pressure, Q is mean flow, μ is blood viscosity, L is length of vascular system, and r is vessel radius. Vascular resistance reflects the contribution of the distal vasculature to afterload and is a function of the diameter, length, and number of small arterioles. In humans, the greatest influence on resistance is the radius of the arteriolar bed. In children who have compliant great vessels, vascular resistance is the most important component but not the only component of afterload.

Because blood flow is pulsatile, there are dynamic forces that oppose cardiac ejection in addition to static forces. Arterial input impedance, defined as the opposition to flow in a pulsatile system, is a better measure of afterload. Arterial input impedance is determined by density and viscosity of blood, aortic wall compliance, vessel diameter, pulsatility of the flow, and the reflected pressure waves generated at branch points. Clinically, the arterial input impedance is determined by dividing the aortic pressure by the aortic flow at that instant. Although it is possible to measure arterial impedance, these measurements are time-consuming and technically demanding, which has limited its utility for routine patient monitoring.

The differences between impedance and resistance as estimates of afterload are illustrated when aortic compliance is altered. Afterload increases when aortic compliance decreases. In an experimental model, when the aorta is replaced with a stiff tube graft, the measured aortic impedance increases, whereas cardiac output and systolic blood pressure are unchanged compared to control animals. The pulse pressure was wider in the grafted animals and consequently mean arterial pressure was lower and resistance was unchanged. As a response to the increased afterload, the ventricles in the experimental animals hypertrophied.[6] Resistance calculations, while allowing simultaneous assessment of pressure and flow, are oversimplifications of true afterload.

Contractility

Contractility is the load-independent ability of cardiac muscle to generate force. Contractility is difficult to understand, and physicians confuse contractility with global systolic function. Cardiac contractility is independent of fiber length and load imposed on the contracting muscle. At the molecular level increased contractility can be explained by the enhanced interaction of calcium and the contractile proteins, producing greater extent and velocity of fiber shortening. Factors that increase contractility include exercise, adrenergic stimulation, and vasoactive agents (catecholamines, phosphodiesterase inhibitors). Contractility, like afterload, is an important determinant of myocardial oxygen consumption.

Changes in contractility can be demonstrated in isolated muscle strips when calcium or catecholamines are added. Graphically, the length–tension curve (Frank-Starling curve) shifts upward and to the left. Many indices have attempted to describe contractility in the critically ill patient that by definition must be independent of loading conditions and heart. Unfortunately, there is no gold standard that completely isolates myocardial function from the loading conditions and heart rate. Furthermore, at the molecular level, contractility, heart rate, and load are interrelated and are therefore not independent variables.

Diastolic Function and Dysfunction

Abnormal diastolic function is now recognized as a major component of myocardial dysfunction that presents in the ICU. Critically ill patients may have markedly reduced cardiac output solely because of diastolic dysfunction such as postoperative tetralogy of Fallot patients.[1]

Diastole has four phases: isovolumic relaxation, early rapid filling, diastasis or slow filling, and late filling due to atrial systole. Isovolumic relaxation is an energy-dependent process whereby the intraventricular pressure rapidly falls

without an increase of ventricular volume. Most of the LV filling occurs in the early rapid filling phase in normal functioning hearts after the atrioventricular valves open. Diastasis is the period between early rapid filling and atrial systole, when there is usually very little ventricular filling. Atrial systole or the late filling phase typically provides 15% of the ventricular filling at end diastole. Atrial systole provides a larger relative contribution to ventricular filling in patients with diastolic or combined diastolic/systolic dysfunction. Loss of atrioventricular synchrony, as seen with arrhythmias, is therefore associated with more profound reduction in cardiac output in patients with abnormal myocardial function than in those without.

Diastolic mechanics can be described as two distinct components, active relaxation and passive stiffness, of the myocardium. These determinants are interdependent, similar to the interdependence of ventricular load and contractility. Relaxation is an energy-dependent process involving the disassociation of calcium from myofilaments, its removal from the cytosol, and the uncoupling of actin–myosin cross-bridges. Relaxation occurs rapidly, although it is not yet complete when the atrioventricular valve opens. Like systolic variables of ventricular function, relaxation rates are influenced by heart rate, loading conditions, myocardial health, and any other factor that alters calcium-myofilament interaction. In patients with normal myocardium, a greater afterload increases the rate of relaxation, whereas in patients with CHF, the relaxation rate is reduced with increased afterload.[7] The assessment of relaxation is difficult. Relaxation occurs over a very short period (milliseconds). The rate of relaxation can be evaluated using measures such as the time constant of relaxation (τ) or $-dP/dt$. Unfortunately, as highlighted in the preceding text, alterations in the relaxation rate may or may not reflect intrinsic changes in diastolic function.

Once the actin–myosin cross-bridges are uncoupled, ventricular mechanical properties are determined by passive viscoelastic factors such as myocardial mass (hypertrophy), extracellular matrix, noncontractile myocyte proteins, coronary vasculature, and ventricular geometry. These passive factors determine the end-diastolic pressure–volume relationship, which is inherently nonlinear (Fig. 5.2.3). A change in the passive component of diastole is represented by a change in this relationship. A leftward and upward shift of the pressure–volume relationship occurs in patients with severe ventricular hypertrophy. These patients have a smaller EDV and higher end-diastolic pressure. Instantaneous chamber stiffness ($\Delta P/\Delta V$), the reciprocal of compliance, and instantaneous compliance are often used to describe the intrinsic diastolic properties of myocardium. Instantaneous stiffness and compliance are load dependent and do not uniquely describe diastolic properties. Specifically, as ventricle volume nears total capacity, pressure rises more rapidly (greater slope of the stiffness curve). A severely hypervolemic patient may have a normal diastolic function but a high end-diastolic pressure because of an overstretched ventricle. Alternatively, the patient may have identical end-diastolic pressure but small ventricular volume, indicating abnormal diastolic function. In addition, pericardial constraint, atrial function, and adrenergic tone can alter measurements of diastolic properties.

Diastolic dysfunction may be considered present when there is an alteration in active or passive properties. The slowing of relaxation delays the onset of filling and therefore decreases the rate of filling at a fixed heart rate. This may change the shape of the instantaneous pressure–volume relationship in early diastole and result in increased atrial pressure to achieve normal filling. Conversely, the ventricular compliance may be altered by myocardial edema or hypertrophy, which will in turn affect the rate of relaxation. Understanding diastolic function explains the limitation of preload augmentation. If a patient's ventricle is operating on the steep portion of the end-diastolic pressure–volume relationship, volume loads result in markedly elevated end-diastolic pressure, which then limits venous return and possibly impairs coronary perfusion.

Heart Rate and Cardiac Synchronization

The heart rate is an important determinant of cardiac output, especially in the neonate's heart where other mechanisms of increasing cardiac output are limited. When stroke volume is held constant, cardiac output is a linear function of heart rate. Heart rate, however, influences other factors of cardiac performance including preload, myocardial blood flow, and contractility. An increased heart rate increases the force of ventricular contraction. This increase in inotropy can be demonstrated in isolated muscle strips when preload, afterload, and extracellular calcium concentration are held constant. This phenomenon is called the *force–frequency relationship*. The increased inotropy is due to increased cytosolic calcium because of decreased time for calcium sequestration in diastole. Excessive heart rates, however, can interfere with myocardial blood supply and ventricular preload. As outlined in the subsequent text, most of the blood flow to the LV occurs in diastole. Consequently, excessive tachycardia may cause subendocardial ischemia and ventricular dysfunction.

The LV ejects blood in a corkscrew motion requiring synchronized activation of myofibers for optimal cardiac performance. There is growing realization that not only the heart but also the sequence of electrical activation can have a profound impact on cardiac function. Patients with dilated cardiomyopathy have significant intraventricular and/or interventricular dyssynchrony. Cardiac resynchronization therapy improves LV systolic function by synchronizing the activation of the interventricular septum and left ventricular free wall using a multilead pacemaker. This therapy improves patient's symptoms, exercise tolerance, and survival.[8]

PRESSURE–VOLUME LOOPS

Because the determinants of cardiac function are interrelated, a useful way to understand cardiac function is to construct a pressure–volume loop of a complete cardiac cycle. The diagram demonstrates the four phases of the cardiac cycle (see Fig. 5.2.4). Point A is end diastole and represents the preload on the ventricle. Isovolumic contraction is demonstrated by the increase in pressure from point A to B. The ejection phase begins at point B with the opening of the aortic valve. Point C heralds the end of the ejection phase as the aortic valve closes and isovolumic relaxation begins. When LV pressure drops below the left atrial pressure, ventricular filling begins (Point D). The line from D to A represents ventricular filling. The difference between line AB and CD represents stroke volume.

Two curves or relationships constrain each pressure–volume loop. First, the end-systolic pressure–volume curve is generated by holding preload and contractility constant as seen in Figure 5.2.4. The end-systolic pressure–volume relationship is a load-independent measure of contractility. This relationship is relatively linear, and increases in steepness indicate increased contractility.[9] The end-systolic point of any individual cardiac cycle on this curve is determined by the afterload and inotropic state. Increases in afterload result in decreased stroke volume if the contractile state of the myocardium does not change (see Fig. 5.2.5).

Second, the end-diastolic pressure–volume point is determined by the preload and intrinsic diastolic properties of the heart. The end-diastolic pressure–volume curve

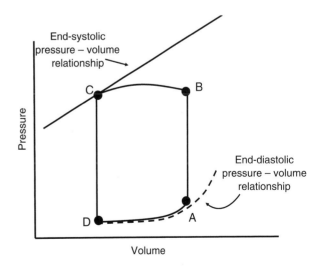

Figure 5.2.4 Pressure–volume loop. *A,* end diastole, *A* to *B,* isovolumic contraction, *B* to *C,* ejection phase; *C,* end systole; *C* to *D,* isovolumic relaxation; *D* to *A,* ventricular filling. The *solid line* represents the end-systolic pressure–volume relationship and represents a load-independent measure of contractility. The *dashed line* represents the end-diastolic pressure–volume relationship.

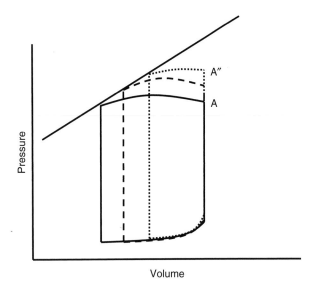

Figure 5.2.5 Effects of isolated increases in afterload. Increases in afterload (point *A* to *A″*) result in decreased stroke volume unless other compensatory changes occur.

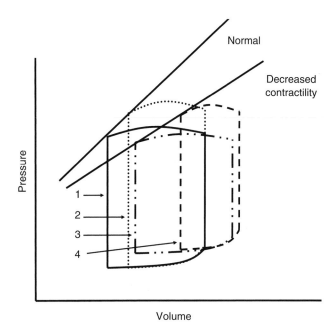

Figure 5.2.6 Effects of changes in contractility on ventricular performance. Loop 1 (*solid line*) represents normal function. Loop 3 (*dot-dash line*) represents a cardiac cycle from a patient with dilated cardiomyopathy with depressed contractility. Note the higher diastolic pressures for any given volume indicating diastolic dysfunction. Also, the curve is shifted to the right (i.e., higher preload) in order to maintain stroke volume. Loops 2 (*dotted line*) and 4 (*dashed line*) represent the response to increased afterload for the normal and impaired heart, respectively. Note the greater reduction in stroke volume in the failing heart for similar increases in afterload.

reflects the intrinsic diastolic properties of the heart. Any increased preload moves the end-diastolic point along the curve and generally results in an increased stroke volume until ventricular compliance decreases. When ventricular volume becomes very large, end-diastolic compliance falls, end-diastolic pressure rises, and further increases in stroke volume cease. This is represented by the curvilinear portion of the end-diastolic pressure–volume relationship. This translates to the plateau on the Frank-Starling curve. Alterations in the intrinsic diastolic properties of the heart are represented by changes in the end-diastolic pressure–volume curve. Patients who have restrictive cardiomyopathy and diastolic dysfunction have a shift of the end-diastolic pressure–volume relationship upward and rightward, indicating a higher ventricular pressure is required to achieve same ventricular filling.

Pressure–volume loops are useful for describing the interrelationship between loading conditions and contractility in the intact heart (see Fig. 5.2.6). Loop 1 represents a normal contraction. Loop 3 is from a patient with impaired contractility as might be seen in dilated cardiomyopathy. A much larger EDV is required to maintain an adequate stroke volume. Additionally, the diastolic limb of the curve is shifted upwards, indicating decreased diastolic function. When exposed to an acute increase in afterload, the failing myocardium has much greater reduction in stroke volume as compared to the normal heart (curves 4 vs. 2).

INTEGRATED CARDIAC AND VASCULAR FUNCTION

Under most conditions, the heart is able to pump all of the venous return that it receives and cardiac output equals the summation of the venous return of the various organs. Consequently, regulation of the vasculature by autoregulatory mechanisms and cardiovascular reflexes determines cardiac output. Venous return to the heart is determined by the difference between the mean systemic pressure and the right atrial pressure (see Fig. 5.2.7). Venous return diminishes when right atrial pressure increases without parallel increase in mean systemic pressure as occurs with the institution of positive pressure ventilation. Venous return is maximum at a right atrial pressure of zero. Venous return does not increase when the right atrial pressure drops below zero because of inflow limitation. The veins at the entrance in the thorax are exposed to atmospheric pressure, and as the intraluminal pressure falls below zero, the vessels collapse and flow decreases. Flow increases only when the intraluminal pressure rises above zero.

Pressure differences determine venous return and hence cardiac output. Mean systemic pressure is the mean pressure throughout the arterial and venous circulation when the heart is at a standstill. The pressure is determined by the capacitance and the relative filling of the entire circulation. Mean systemic pressure can be increased by increased intravascular volume or by peripheral vasoconstriction and is represented by a shift of the venous return to the right (dotted line in Fig. 5.2.7). A fluid bolus increases mean

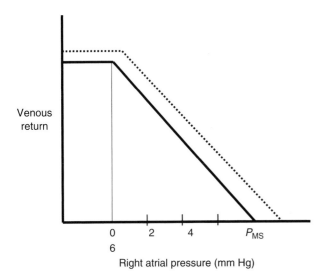

Figure 5.2.7 Normal venous return curve. Venous return increases as the pressure gradient between right atrial pressure and mean systemic pressure increases. Venous return is maximum when right atrial pressure is 0 mm Hg. Volume expansion increases P_{MS} and hence venous return for any given right atrial pressure (*dotted line*). *Solid line*, normal curve; *dotted line*, volume expansion; P_{MS}, mean systemic pressure.

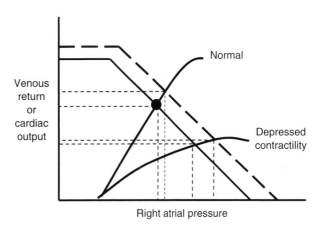

Figure 5.2.8 Venous return and cardiac output coupling. Over time, cardiac output and venous return are equal, as represented by the intersection of the Frank-Starling curve and venous return curve (*dot*). In a patient with depressed cardiac contractility (*lower curve*), the intersection shifts downward and to the right indicating a lower cardiac output and venous return at a higher atrial pressure compared to normal.

systemic pressure. Venous return, and hence preload, only increases if the gradient between mean systemic pressure and the right atrium increases. If a fluid bolus increases the mean systemic and right atrial pressures by the same amount as when the ventricle is on the steep portion of the compliance curve, venous return is constant and cardiac output does not increase. These concepts highlight the dangers of considering atrial pressure to be the same as preload. If the heart becomes less compliant or if contractility decreases, the same EDV will be maintained at a higher atrial pressure and venous return will decrease.

Venous return and cardiac output are coupled (i.e., equal over any given time) because blood flows in a circle in the intact circulation. This interplay is shown in Figure 5.2.8. The intersection of the venous return curve and the Frank-Starling curve represents the steady state of the circulation at any given time. The intersection is a function of the complex and interrelated forces affecting cardiac and vascular function. Using this curve, it is now apparent that patients with normal contractility are preload responsive. A fluid challenge shifts the venous return curve rightward, and in a patient with normal contractility, cardiac output increases a large amount while right atrial pressure does not. In the patient with impaired contractility, the Frank-Starling curve shifts to the right along the same venous return curve. The intercept point is at a much higher atrial pressure and lower cardiac output/venous return. In this patient with poor contractility, a fluid bolus results in only a small increase in cardiac output and a large increase in mean systemic and right atrial pressures. The increase in mean systemic pressure results in fluid retention and edema.

The heart is also coupled to the arterial system, although forces are opposite of venous coupling. An increase in arterial pressure decreases cardiac output, but in the circulation, increased arterial pressure increases arterial flow. In patients with normal cardiovascular function, cardiac output is insensitive to changes in blood pressure and afterload because of the contractile reserve of myocardium. In other words, large changes in blood pressure do not result in decreases in cardiac output. In patients with impaired myocardial function, small increases in afterload may compromise cardiac output.

MYOCARDIAL OXYGEN CONSUMPTION AND SUPPLY

The myocardium extracts 60% to 75% of the oxygen from blood compared to an average extraction of approximately 30% for the rest of the body. The low oxygen tension of coronary venous blood requires that any increased myocardial oxygen demand must be met with increased flow rather than increased extraction. The primary mechanisms controlling myocardial flow are autoregulation and local metabolic signals such as adenosine, CO_2, and acidosis. In addition, myocardial contraction during systole abolishes and can even reverse capillary blood flow in the LV. The coronary perfusion pressure (aortic pressure minus left ventricular pressure) is essentially zero during systole, and LV blood flow occurs predominantly during diastole. In conditions in which diastolic blood pressure is low, such as patent ductus arteriosus (PDA) or central shunt, systolic blood flow to the systemic ventricle becomes a much larger percentage of total flow.

Myocardial oxygen consumption is linked to myocardial work. Myocardial oxygen consumption can be broken

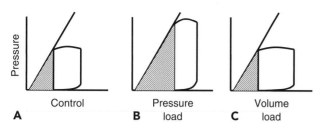

Figure 5.2.9 Myocardial work depicted by pressure–volume loops. The area within the pressure–volume loop represents external work. Internal work is represented by the shaded area. Figure (**A**) represents the control case. Figures (**B**) and (**C**) demonstrate the changes in work associated with a pressure or volume load. Note the large increase in internal work with a pressure load.

down into three major components: basal metabolism, external work, and internal work. Basal metabolism is the smallest component and varies with changes in heart rate but not contractility. Another component is utilized for excitation–contraction coupling and it varies with the contractile state of the heart. The largest component of myocardial oxygen consumption is used for mechanical work of the heart, internal and external. External work is the work of the heart as it ejects blood against a pressure. Using a pressure–volume loop, external work is the area within the pressure–volume loop (see Fig. 5.2.9). Internal work is the energy used to generate force that occurs independent of muscle shortening and is often referred to as "pressure-work." The amount of energy varies with the afterload and contractility. In the pressure-loaded heart, myocardial oxygen consumption increases as internal work increases to maintain the high wall stress at end systole.[10] Conversely, a volume-loaded heart increases myocardial consumption to a much less extent as internal work is unchanged (Fig. 5.2.9C).

MEASUREMENT OF CARDIAC FUNCTION

Questions to Answer about Cardiac Function

The accurate assessment of cardiac function in the ICU is essential as high prevalence of cardiac dysfunction during critical illness and as treatments for cardiac dysfunction have narrow therapeutic windows. Modern ICUs have many noninvasive and invasive systems to assess cardiac function. Clinicians routinely analyze multiple variables such as heart rate, blood pressure, and pulse oximetry from most patients in order to formulate hemodynamic diagnoses and therapies. Regardless of monitoring technique, cardiac function should be assessed at three levels:

A. What is the cardiac output?
B. Is the cardiac output adequate to meet the patient's metabolic demand?

C. Why is the cardiac output depressed or inadequate? Is the inadequacy a result of depressed systolic or diastolic function, excessive demand, adverse cardiopulmonary interactions, or a combination?

Diagnostic confusion occurs when a clinician relies on single variables to assess cardiac function or uses the wrong test to answer a question. For example, measurement of cardiac output by thermodilution provides limited assessment of myocardial contractility or the adequacy of cardiac output. Conversely, the determination of depressed contractility as seen in patients with dilated cardiomyopathy does not mean that cardiac output is decreased. The clinician should address all three questions in critically ill patients.

Efficacy of Invasive Monitoring

As a patient's severity of illness increases, there is a tendency to place more invasive monitoring devices on the assumption that more detailed physiologic information about the patient will improve clinical outcome. Whether this assumption is "true" has been difficult to prove, and recent studies have suggested that the general use of advanced monitoring techniques such as pulmonary artery catheterization are associated with higher patient mortality in the ICU.[11] Ideal monitors allow clinicians to detect derangements that would otherwise escape detection and prompt changes in therapy, which improves survival and or quality of life. In reality, few monitoring techniques can claim benefit at this level.

Rationale for Advanced Monitoring

The rationale for advanced monitoring is based on two lines of evidence, physiology and empiric data. Although clinical and laboratory examination is crucial, the derived information has limitations and can be misleading because of the many confounding conditions (e.g., hypothermia, diuretics, other organ dysfunctions) present in the critically ill patient. The need for appropriate monitoring is underscored by the observation that clinicians cannot reliably predict cardiac output from the clinical information in children.[12] Failure to detect poor hemodynamic function is associated with worse outcome. In children with septic shock, persistently low cardiac output is associated with a higher mortality.[13] Consequently, accurate and repeated assessments of cardiac function are important, especially as severity of illness increases. A recent randomized trial has shown improvement in mortality by the use of invasive monitoring.[14] A total of 263 adults with severe sepsis or septic shock were randomized to goal-directed therapy guided by continuous mixed venous saturation measurement versus standard resuscitation. Patients in the intervention group had an almost 30% decrease in mortality. This study is one of the very few studies to demonstrate a clear benefit of invasive monitoring.

Rationale Against Advanced Monitoring

Recent clinical studies have suggested that the general use of pulmonary artery catheters in adults does not improve survival and may cause actual harm and higher mortality.[11,15] The causes of increased mortality are not completely clear in these studies, but it could include inappropriate patient selection,[16] inaccurate data collection, inappropriate therapeutic goals (e.g., use of vasoactive agents to achieve "supranormal" cardiac output), or complications of right heart catheterization (see Table 5.2.1). Most important, physicians may be misinterpreting the derived information. Despite the use of pulmonary artery catheters for at least two decades, many ICU physicians lack knowledge of this modality.[17] Monitors are useful only if the clinician can correctly interpret and act on the information derived.

Accurate hemodynamic monitoring requires that the clinician has sufficient understanding of the underlying physiology, methodologies, and limitations of the monitoring techniques. Each technique described in the subsequent text has limitations such as invasiveness, low signal-to-noise ratios, or the inability to provide continuous information. The use of a single tool or monitor as the sole guide to therapy is prone to a high chance of error. More important, clinicians do not use single tests but rather integrate historical, clinical, laboratory, and monitored data to determine management. Whether to use a specific monitor depends on the hemodynamic questions, as well as on the risks and benefits of a technique.

What is Cardiac Output?

Accurate detection and treatment of low cardiac output states are essential in the critical care unit because low cardiac output is associated with higher mortality in some populations.[13] Mean arterial blood pressure is often used as a surrogate for cardiac output and as a therapeutic goal. Blood pressure, however, is a function of vascular resistance and cardiac output. A low blood pressure may be related to low systemic resistance, requiring a vasopressor or low cardiac output or both. Measurement of flow or cardiac output may be crucial in select populations. Cardiac output measurements represent the interplay of systolic (heart rate, preload, afterload, contractility) and diastolic function. Measurement does not delineate which elements, such as contractility or loading conditions, are normal or abnormal in an individual patient. Consequently, identification of a low flow state by measuring cardiac output warrants additional investigation to determine the underlying cause of depressed flow. Additionally, cardiac output measurements must be interpreted in the context of a patient's disease and course. For example, a fall in the cardiac output is common on the first postoperative night after cardiac surgery. This decrease does not require the same interventions nor does it imply the same prognosis as in a patient with septic shock.[18]

Common indications to measure cardiac output include congenital or acquired heart disease, multisystem organ failure, shock states, complex cardiopulmonary interactions, and clinical research. Over the last several years, there has been a trend toward less invasive and continuous monitoring rather than intermittent methods. In general, noninvasive methods are easier to use but are less accurate. However the loss in accuracy is probably acceptable, given the ability to follow continuous trends in the ICU.

Methods to measure cardiac output include dilution techniques, the Fick principle, and Doppler ultrasound.

Indicator Dilution Techniques

Indicator dilution techniques derived from principles developed by Stewart and Hamilton represent the commonest method for measuring cardiac output. Briefly, blood flow can be calculated after the central venous injection of an indicator by measuring the change in the indicator concentration over time at a point downstream from the injection. The calculation is valid as long as several conditions are met, including complete mixing of the indicator and blood, no loss of the indicator between injection and measurement (i.e., no anatomical shunt), and no valve regurgitation. Available indicators include dyes (e.g., Indocyanine green), temperature, and lithium chloride. Intermittent measurements of the cardiac output are made by injecting in a central systemic vein and measuring the indicator either in the pulmonary artery or from an arterial line.

Pulmonary Artery Thermodilution

The most common indicator technique is thermodilution using a thermistor catheter placed in the pulmonary artery. Additionally, this technique is the clinical reference against which new technologies are compared. A specific volume of saline at a specific temperature is injected rapidly through the proximal port of the catheter into the right atrium. The

---

TABLE 5.2.1

COMPLICATIONS OF PULMONARY ARTERY CATHETERIZATION

Arrhythmias—PVCs, ventricular tachycardia, bradycardia, and RBBB
Pneumothorax
Bleeding
Pulmonary infarction
Emboli
Pulmonary artery rupture
Balloon rupture
Catheter knotting
Infection
Valve damage
Therapeutic misadventure due to inaccurate measurements or interpretation

PVC, pulmonary ventricular contraction; RBBB, right bundle branch block.

change in temperature of blood passing the thermistor is used to calculate the cardiac output:

$$\text{Cardiac output} = [(V_i \times S_i \times C_i)(T_b - T_i)60]/(S_b \times C_b) \\ \times \int_0^\infty T_{b(t)}dt$$

where V_i is the injectate volume, S_i and S_b are the specific gravities of the injectate and blood; C_i and C_b are the specific hearts of injectate and blood; T_i and T_b are the respective temperatures; and $T_{b(t)}dt$ is the area under the temperature curve.

Meticulous attention to detail is required to minimize the numerous sources of error. Falsely elevated cardiac output will occur with slow injection rates and small volumes. Falsely depressed cardiac output will occur with solution cooler or injection volumes larger than values used for computations. Additionally, changes in ventilation can produce changes in tricuspid valve regurgitation and alter measured cardiac output. Consequently, three to five injections are generally averaged for each determination of cardiac output.

The use of invasive pulmonary artery catheters to measure cardiac output and pulmonary catheter wedge pressure is not without risk, danger, or controversy (Table 5.2.1). Furthermore, the use of pulmonary artery catheters in adults has been associated with increased mortality risk.[11,15] A more recent study has suggested that pulmonary artery catheterization may be appropriate in more selected populations. A retrospective analysis of 7,310 adult patients showed that pulmonary artery catheterization improved survival in patients with high severity of illness while increasing mortality in patients with low severity of illness.[16]

In summary, pulmonary artery thermodilution technique provides reliable cardiac output determinations if performed correctly. It has a proven clinical record and provides additional pressure and mixed venous saturation data. The disadvantages of this technique include difficulty of access in small-sized patients, less accuracy at low flow states, significant mortality and morbidity risk, and the ability to only obtain intermittent information.

Transpulmonary Thermodilution

Transpulmonary thermodilution is another thermodilution technique that measures temperature change in a large systemic artery rather than the pulmonary artery. The technique has been validated in children and infants as small as 2.5 kg.[19] The advantages of transpulmonary over pulmonary artery thermodilution include avoidance of right heart catheterization, better reproducibility, and less measurement variability with mechanical ventilation. The presence of intracardiac shunts or valvular regurgitation limits the utility of this technique, which is similar to pulmonary artery thermodilution. An additional limitation is the potential for limb ischemia caused by femoral artery cannulation.

Lithium Dilution

Lithium dilution is another indicator technique that has been validated in adults and children.[20] The indicator sensor is attached to a pre-existing peripheral line and comprises a lithium sensitive electrode. After systemic venous injection of isotonic lithium, arterial blood is pumped past the electrode, which converts a change in voltage to a change in lithium concentration using the Nernst equation. The principle advantage of this technique is the utilization of pre-existing monitoring lines (i.e., neither femoral artery nor pulmonary artery cannulation is required). The lithium may be injected peripherally. The disadvantages of this method are the need for blood sampling with each measurement and the need to avoid administration of medications containing an electric charge (e.g., muscle relaxants, lithium). As in all indicator dilution methods, abnormal intracardiac shunts could result in erroneous measurements.

Fick Principle

Another major methodology for measuring cardiac output is based on the Fick principle. The Fick principle for flow measurement relates cardiac output to oxygen consumption and the arteriovenous oxygen content difference. The calculation requires measurement of the patient's oxygen consumption and oxygen content of arterial and mixed venous blood:

$$CO = V_{O_2}/(Ca_{O_2} - Cv_{O_2})$$

where CO = cardiac output, V_{O_2} = systemic oxygen consumption, and Ca_{O_2} and Cv_{O_2} = oxygen content of arterial and mixed venous blood, respectively.

Oxygen content of blood is the sum of oxygen in blood bound to hemoglobin and the amount in plasma. The binding capacity of oxygen for hemoglobin is 1.36 mL/g/dL. Consequently, the content of oxygen is [1.36 mL/g $\times$ Hb (g/dL) $\times$ O_2 saturation $+$ 0.003 (mL/mm/dL) Pa_{O_2}] $\times$ 10 dL/L. In patients in whom the Pa_{O_2} is less than 100 mm Hg, the contribution of dissolved oxygen can be ignored and the equation simplified:

$$CO = V_{O_2}/[(\text{Ao Sat} - \text{Pa Sat}) \times 13.6 \times \text{Hb}]$$

where Ao Sat and Pa Sat are the aortic and pulmonary artery saturations respectively.

The ability to use this technique in the ICU has become possible with the development of portable metabolic carts to measure systemic oxygen consumption. Oxygen consumption is determined by measuring the carbon dioxide and oxygen concentrations in inspired and expired gases. Determinations of cardiac output have correlated well with thermodilution cardiac outputs when cardiac output was low but not elevated.[21] The sources of error in this method center primarily on the measurement of V_{O_2}. The reliability of V_{O_2} measurements is decreased by metabolic instability, high inspired oxygen fractions, and respiratory circuit leaks. V_{O_2} from metabolic carts represent lung and systemic oxygen consumption, which may overestimate cardiac output in conditions of acute lung injury, in which lung V_{O_2} is increased.[22] Additionally, this method still requires pulmonary artery catheterization to obtain mixed venous oxygenation samples.

The Fick principle is the underlying basis for continuously or intermittently monitoring mixed venous oxygen content or saturation. If one assumes that systemic oxygen consumption is stable and that arterial saturation is not different from baseline state, then changes in mixed venous oxygen saturation indicate changes in cardiac output. The use of continuous monitors in superior vena cava (SVC) has been shown to improve mortality in diverse populations such as adults with severe sepsis[14] and infants after repair of hypoplastic left heart syndrome.[23] The technique avoids pulmonary artery catheterization and allows flow calculations in patients with intracardiac shunts. The major limitation is lack of recognition when oxygen consumption changes, such as occurs with agitation or fever. Additionally, if measuring SVC saturation, factors that alter cerebral blood flow such as acidosis may lead to changes not associated with changes in cardiac output.

Noninvasive Fick Using Carbon Dioxide

The Fick principle can be applied to any gas diffusing through the lungs, including carbon dioxide. Cardiac output can be measured less invasively (i.e., without the need for pulmonary artery catheterization) by estimating mixed venous CO_2 from expired CO_2 using a partial rebreathing technique. A recent pediatric study in patients undergoing cardiac catheterization showed reasonable agreement (bias, -0.18 L/minute/m^2; precision, ± 1.49 L per minute) between thermodilution cardiac output measurements and a commercially available monitor.[24] Current technology requires ventilating patients with at least 200 mL, which limits the technique to patients >8 kg. Additionally, data in critically ill children with lung disease and/or hemodynamic instability is lacking.

Doppler Echocardiography

Flow in a vessel is equal to the product of flow velocity in a vessel and its cross-sectional area. Echocardiography can measure cardiac output by combining the Doppler-derived aortic velocity–time integral (VTI) with a determination of cross-sectional area by two-dimensional (2D) echocardiography. Echocardiography probes can be placed in the suprasternal notch or in the esophagus to measure ascending or descending aortic blood flow. Both sites calculate cardiac output without coronary blood flow because measurement is made after takeoff of the coronary arteries. Therefore, cardiac output measure by this method will be less than output measured by indicator dilution technique. The principle advantage of this technique is its noninvasiveness and the fact that it avoids the need for central venous catheters. There are several potential sources of inaccuracy with this technique, including incorrect measurement of aortic diameter and incorrect angle of Doppler interrogation. Consequently, the technique is rarely used in the ICU because of the need for a skilled technician and concerns of interuser and intrauser variability. A reliable way to apply a continuous probe has not been adequately refined.

Is Cardiac Output Adequate to Meet the Patient's Metabolic Demand?

Integration of the cardiac output measurement into the assessment of the patient is essential before making therapeutic decisions. Is the cardiac output appropriate in the context of a patient's disease and history? Does the cardiac output supply enough oxygen to meet metabolic demands? Global indicators of adequate oxygen supply include serum lactate levels and acid–base balance. Regional indicators include clinical examination of capillary refill, urine output, and level of consciousness. Regional monitors such as gastric tonometry and near infrared spectrometry are also gaining popularity.

Why is Cardiac Output Depressed?

Once the realization that cardiac output is insufficient for metabolic demands, it is imperative to seek out the reason. Cardiac output is the end result of several interrelated variables: heart rate, preload, afterload, contractility, diastolic function, and cardiac synchronization. Quantification of these individual components poses two major challenges including imprecise methods for measurement and their interrelatedness.

Preload Assessment Using Central Venous Pressure and Pulmonary Artery Occlusion Pressure

The most commonly used measures of preload are CVP (right side of the heart) and pulmonary artery occlusion pressure (PAOP) (left side of the heart). CVP is the pressure in the large veins before the right atrium and can be measured in the SVC or right atrium. Monitoring of CVP from a femoral approach correlates well with right atrial pressure and is a reasonable alternative in pediatric patients without significant abdominal pathology.[25] The advantage of CVP monitoring includes ease (frequently patients require central access for medications) and the ability to continuously collect data.

Left ventricular preload may be monitored using PAOP or direct measurements of left atrial pressure. The use of CVP as a marker of left ventricular filling is discouraged given the frequent discordance of CVP and PAOP. PAOP reflects left atrial pressure when there is a continuous column of blood between the catheter and the atrium. Consequently, the catheter tip must reside in West zone 3, where pulmonary alveolar pressure does not exceed pulmonary venous pressure. The placement of the catheter in West zone 1 will result in erroneous measurements and is easily recognizable by respiratory variation in the occlusion pressure waveform.

TABLE 5.2.2

CAUSES OF ELEVATED CENTRAL VENOUS PRESSURE

Hypervolemia
Right ventricular dysfunction
Pulmonary artery hypertension
Pulmonary stenosis
Tricuspid stenosis
Tricuspid regurgitation
Catheter tip malposition in RV
Elevated intrathoracic pressure

RV, right ventricle.

Over the last two decades, studies in healthy and critically ill patients show that CVP and PAOP fail to correlate with end-diastolic ventricular volume or stroke volume.[26] Additionally, neither CVP nor PAOP is a reliable indicator of a patient's cardiac response to volume loading. Many factors limit the use of pressure as a monitor of ventricular preload. Patients with atrioventricular valve disease (regurgitation or stenosis), pulmonary hypertension, or undergoing mechanical ventilation can have simultaneously elevated CVP and inadequate ventricular volume (see Table 5.2.2). Most important, if a patient has decreased ventricular compliance or diastolic dysfunction small changes in ventricular volume will result in large changes in pressure. Even if single pressure measurements do not correlate well with EDV, CVP monitoring can be useful in trending changes in volume status over time or in response to therapy if myocardial compliance remains constant. Unfortunately, many patients in the ICU have simultaneous changes in myocardial compliance and volume status, which make interpretation of CVP changes more challenging.

Limitations in the use of CVP and PAOP in identifying preload abnormalities have led to the development of other tools. Analysis of arterial pulse pressure variation is one such technique that has been clinically validated to be a reliable preload indicator in adults.[27] Patients with a baseline pulse pressure variation greater than 15% always increased cardiac output in response to fluid administration. The correlation between pulse pressure variation and cardiac output augmentation had a close linear correlation.

Afterload Assessment

Clinical measures of afterload include arterial impedance, peripheral vascular resistance systolic wall stress, and mean blood pressure. The most accurate measures of afterload, systolic wall stress and arterial impedance are unfortunately difficult to measure and trend in the ICU. An understanding of the changes in afterload are particularly important in patients with cardiac disease as afterload is a major determinant of not only cardiac output but also myocardial oxygen consumption.

Arterial input impedance, the opposition to flow in a pulsatile system, can be determined using fast Fourier analysis of high-fidelity measurements of aortic pressure and flow signals.[28] This technique has provided valuable insight into the pathophysiology of several disease states such as septic shock and pulmonary hypertension. These measurements are time-consuming and technically demanding, which has limited its utility for routine patient monitoring.

The most common clinical measure of afterload is calculated as systemic vascular resistance (SVR). Peripheral SVR is calculated as the pressure difference across the circulation (Mean arterial pressure—CVP for systemic circulation) divided by mean aortic flow or cardiac output. Using resistance calculations to represent afterload has several pitfalls. Resistance calculations fail to include the contributions of aortic elastance and wave reflections from the distal vasculature and may provide misleading information in the ICU. A study showed discordant changes in SVR measurements and end-systolic wall stress as measured by echocardiogram. In this animal study, norepinephrine increased SVR by 21% but decreased wall stress by 9%.[29] Finally, vascular resistance is not independently measured but calculated resulting in another source of error. Nevertheless, trends in SVR are useful in properly selected patients and generally mirror ventricular afterload.

Mean arterial pressure is used sometimes as an estimate of afterload. This is of little use. Mean arterial pressure is the product of cardiac output and resistance. Consequently, if there is comparable but opposite changes in resistance and flow, then the blood pressure will remain the same and significant changes in afterload will be missed. A recent study of critically ill children confirmed that blood pressure was a poor predictor of myocardial function assessed by wall stress analysis and Doppler cardiac output.[30]

Echocardiography can be used to estimate end-systolic meridional wall stress from the M-mode image:[31]

$$\text{Wall stress} = 1.35P * D/4H * (1 + H/D)$$

where P = mean arterial pressure, D = LV internal diameter, and H = posterior wall thickness.

End-systolic wall stress is used as a measure because the effects of preload are eliminated. The use of echocardiographic wall stress analysis is time intensive and repeated measures in the ICU are not practical. Additionally, calculation of meridional wall stress tends to underestimate afterload in patients with thick ventricular walls and overstated in thin-walled ventricles.[32]

Contractility Assessment

The development of a practical bedside measure of contractility has been elusive. In isolated muscle strips, loading conditions can be controlled and the effect of an intervention on force and velocity of muscle shortening can be used to measure the contractile state of the muscle. Such determinations in individual patients is difficult in whom loading conditions are interrelated and not easily controlled. Many drugs that affect contractility also affect vascular tone and alter myocardial loading. Many indices have been proposed but there is no absolute measure of contractility and no gold standard for comparison. The indices studied can be divided into isovolumic (pre-ejection) phase, ejection phase, or measures derived from pressure–volume relationships.

Isovolumic Indexes

Historically, the maximum first derivative of left ventricular pressure (dP/dt_{max}) has been used as the index of contractility.[33] Normally, dP/dt_{max} occurs before aortic valve opening and therefore is relatively independent of afterload. However, in patients with severe LV dysfunction or arterial vasodilation, as seen in severe sepsis, aortic valve opening is delayed and afterload conditions can affect dP/dt_{max}, which is very sensitive to changes in preload. dP/dt_{max} has wide variation between individuals and is therefore not useful for assessing initial contractility. This measurement depends on highly accurate measurements of dP/dt, which is usually beyond the capabilities of pressure measurement systems in the ICU.

Recently, tissue Doppler imaging has been used to measure myocardial acceleration during isovolumic contraction.[34] Isovolumic contraction describes the rate of change of contractile force and is a surrogate of dP/dt_{max}. Tissue Doppler imaging by analyzing movement of myocardium rather than blood allows functional assessments independent of ventricular geometry. By varying loading conditions as well as contractile state, the investigators were able to show that isovolumic contraction was unaffected by preload or afterload and was highly sensitive to changes in contractility.[33] This promising technique may prove useful as automated tissue Doppler imaging becomes more readily available.

Ejection Phase Indices

Frequently, the extent of ventricular ejection is substituted for a measure of ventricular contractility. Common measures include ejection fraction, fractional shortening, and velocity of shortening. Ejection fraction can be measured by echocardiogram, angiogram, or other radiologic techniques, whereas the other measures are derived from echocardiograms (see subsequent text). All of these measurements are influenced by load and contractility and, therefore, reflect systolic performance rather than contractility.

Pressure–Volume Relationships

The slope of the end-systolic pressure–volume relationship varies as a function of contractility (Fig. 5.2.6) and is not affected by changes in loading conditions.[35] There are practical limitations of using the end-systolic pressure–volume relationship as a clinical measure. First, defining the relationship requires measurement of pressure–volume loops over a range of loading conditions. Such alterations are not clinically practical and may induce reflexively mediated changes in heart rate and contractility. Second, the slope of the relationship varies with the subject's size, and a normal range has not been established. Despite these limitations, pressure–volume loops are powerful tools for understanding the interrelated function of the ventricle.

ECHOCARDIOGRAPHY

Echocardiography supplies a vast amount of structural and functional information in children with congenital and acquired heart disease and is a powerful diagnostic tool in the ICU. The accuracy of echocardiography is dependent on the skill of the user, but portable echo machines have allowed critical care physicians to measure basic cardiac parameters.[36] Echocardiography utilizes several basic modes including M-mode, 2D, Doppler (blood and tissue), and color Doppler, which in the hands of a trained clinician provides vast amounts of information, including indices of systolic and diastolic function, regional myocardial abnormalities, valve regurgitation or stenosis, pericardial disease, and cardiac structure. Diagnostic limitations of echocardiography are caused by inadequate acoustic windows, artifacts, and, most important, misinterpretation. In the postoperative patient with limited suboptimal windows, transesophageal echocardiogram should be considered in cases of complicated or protracted recovery.

A complete description of echocardiography is beyond this text, but basic techniques relevant in the ICU have been discussed.

M-mode echocardiography is a unidimensional view with high temporal and axial resolution and is used primarily for assessing left ventricular size and function (see Fig. 5.2.10). In 2D imaging, a rapidly moving ultrasound beam generates multiple M-mode lines, which construct a cross-sectional image of the heart from various views. The Doppler principle states that the change in frequency of an ultrasonic beam after it strikes a moving object is proportional to the velocity of the object, either blood or more recently tissue. Doppler ultrasound can be used to calculate cardiac output, pressure gradients across stenotic regions, as well as provide qualitative information about shunts, and valve regurgitation. Flow is calculated by measuring the Doppler flow signal or VTI through a structure with a known diameter. Using either the transthoracic or transesophageal approach, cardiac output can be calculated by measuring the VTI just above the aortic valve and 2D measurement of the LV outflow tract dimension. This technique has led to the development of continuous esophageal probes to measure cardiac output. The disadvantages of this technique include need for user expertise in assuring the correct windows and signal angles. Additionally, small changes in aortic diameter occur during the cardiac cycle, and care must be taken to correctly measure it during early systole.

Doppler measurements may also be used to calculate pressure gradients not easily assessable by invasive pressure

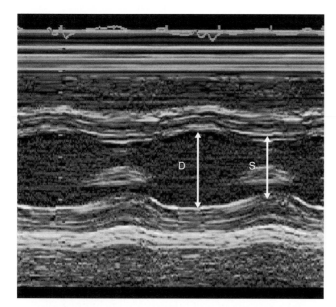

Figure 5.2.10 M-mode echocardiogram of the left ventricle from a parasternal short axis. Two cardiac cycles are depicted. The *arrows* represent the left ventricular internal cavity dimension in diastole (*D*) and systole (*S*) (see color Figure 5.2.10.)

measurements such as RV pressure or pressure gradients across cardiac valves (see Fig. 5.2.11). The pressure decrease across a stenotic area is measured using the Bernoulli equation. For fluid flowing through a rigid tube, the flow is equal to the velocity of the fluid times the cross-sectional area. If there is narrowing, the fluid must accelerate to maintain the constant volume flow over time. The acceleration of fluid is achieved by a drop in pressure across the obstruction. The Bernoulli equation may be simplified if velocity proximal to an obstruction and viscous friction are negligible: Consequently, a pressure drop (ΔP) equals a constant times the postobstruction velocity (V_2) squared. The following describes the relationship between pressure and velocity acceleration:

$$\Delta P = 4(V_2)^2$$

Underestimation of the pressure gradient is possible if the angle of interrogation is too large or overestimated if the preobstruction velocity is not negligible. By measuring the velocity of a tricuspid valve regurgitant jet, one can estimate the RV pressures. By measuring the velocity across the aortic valve, one can determine the extent of aortic stenosis.

Common Measures of Cardiac Function Obtained by Echocardiography

Two common measures of systolic myocardial performance are the shortening fraction (M-mode) and ejection fraction (2D) of the LV. Both ejection fraction and shortening fraction are influenced by loading conditions (preload and afterload) and heart rate and therefore do not reflect contractility. Once systolic dysfunction is identified, further

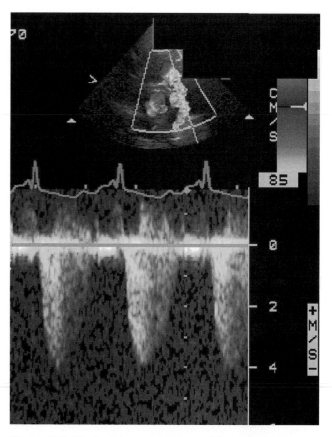

Figure 5.2.11 Doppler measurement of flow across a stenotic pulmonary valve. The velocity measures 4 m per second, which represents a pressure gradient of 64 mm Hg across the valve. $\Delta P = 4 \times (4)^2$ (see color Figure 5.2.11.)

investigation into the underlying cause(s) is required. The shortening fraction is from a parasternal short axis views as follows:

$$SF = (LVIDd - LVIDs)/LVIDd \times 100$$

where LVIDd = LV internal diameter in diastole, LVIDs = LV internal diameter in systole, and SF = fractional shortening (Fig. 5.2.10). The fractional shortening has normal range of 30% to 45%. Because M-mode echocardiography uses a single dimension, it cannot be used in the presence of wall motion abnormalities or ventricles with abnormal shapes.

The 2D ejection fraction of the LV is typically calculated using the modified Simpson rule, although other methods exist. The volume of the ventricle at end systole and end diastole is calculated by dividing the ventricle into stacked slices and summating the volume of each slice. It is most accurate when two orthogonal planes are used.

%EF = 100 × (end-diastolic volume
    −end-systolic volume)/end-diastolic volume.

The geometric assumptions are used in calculating ejection fraction and, consequently, the technique cannot be applied to the irregularly shaped RV or patients with only one ventricle.

Another measure of cardiac systolic function is the mean velocity of circumferential fiber shortening normalized for end-diastolic dimension (VcFc) and is calculated from the M-mode image:

$$VcFc = LVIDd - LVIDs/LVIDd/LV \text{ ejection time} \times (RR \text{ interval})^{1/2}$$

This measure of systolic function corrects for heart rate and preload and is a closer measure of contractility than ejection fraction. To obtain a true reflection of contractility, VcFc can be plotted against wall stress. The wall stress–VcFc relationship reflects contractility independent of loading conditions, but it is cumbersome and is not routinely used.[37]

REFERENCES

1. Cullen S, Shore D, Redington A. Characterization of right ventricular diastolic performance after complete repair of tetralogy of Fallot. Restrictive physiology predicts slow postoperative recovery. *Circulation.* 1995;91:1782–1789.
2. Kentish JC, Wrzosek A. Changes in force and cytosolic Ca^{2+} concentration after length changes in isolated rat ventricular trabeculae. *J of Physiology.* 1998;506:431–444.
3. Moss RL, Razumova M, Fitzsimons DP. Myosin crossbridge activation of cardiac thin filaments. Implications for myocardial function in health and disease. *Circ Res.* 2004;94:1290–1300.
4. Fukuda N, Sasaki D, Ishiwata S, et al. Length dependence of tension generation in rat skinned cardiac muscle. Role of Titin in the Frank-Starling Mechanism of the heart. *Circulation.* 2001;104:1639–1645.
5. Dreyer Wj, Mayer DC, Neish SR. Cardiac contractility and pump function. In: Garson A, Bricker JT, Fisher DJ, eds. *The science and practice of pediatric cardiology.* 2nd ed. Baltimore: Williams and Wilkens; 1998:213.
6. Morita S, Asou T, Yasui H, et al. Inelastic vascular prothesis for proximal aorta increases pulsatile arterial load and causes left ventricular hypertrophy in dogs. *J Thorac Cardiovasc Surg.* 2002;124:768–774.
7. Eichhorn EJ, Willard JE, Alvarez L. Are contraction and relaxation coupled in patients with and without congestive heart failure? *Circulation.* 1985;85:2132–2139.
8. McAlister FA, Ezekowitz Wiebe N. Systematic review: Cardiac resynchronization patients with symptomatic heart failure. *Ann Intern Med.* 2004;141:381–390.
9. Suga H, Sagawa K. Instantaneous pressure-volume relationships and their ratio in the excised, supported canine left ventricle. *Circ Res.* 1974;35:117–126.
10. Suga H, Hisano R, Hirata S, et al. Mechanism of higher oxygen consumption rate: Pressure loaded vs. volume loaded heart. *Am J Physiol.* 1982;242:H942–H948.
11. Connors AF, Speroff T, Dawson NV, et al. The effectiveness of right heart catheterization in the initial care of critically ill patients. Support Investigators. *JAMA.* 1996;276:889–897.
12. Tibby SM, Hatherill Marsh MJ, Murdoch IA. Clinician's abilities to estimate cardiac index in ventilated children and infants. *Arch Dis Child.* 1997;77:516–518.
13. Ceneviva G, Paschall JA, Maffei F, et al. Hemodynamic support in fluid-refractory pediatric septic shock. *Pediatrics.* 1998;102:e19.
14. Rivers E, Nguyen B, Havstad S, et al. Early goal-directed therapy in the treatment of severe sepsis and septic shock. *N Engl J Med.* 2001;345:1368–1377.
15. Sandham JK, Hull RD, Brant RF, et al. A randomized controlled trial of the use of pulmonary artery catheters in high risk surgical patients. *N Engl J Med.* 2003;348:5–14.
16. Chittock DR, Dhingra VK, Ronco JJ. Severity of illness and risk of death associated with pulmonary artery catheter use. *Crit Care Med.* 2004;32:911–915.
17. Gnaegi A, Feihl F, Perret C. Intensive care physician's insufficient knowledge of right-heart catheterization at the bedside: Time to act? *Crit Care Med.* 1997;25:213–220.
18. Wernovsky G, Wypij D, Jonas RA, et al. Postoperative course and hemodynamic profile after the arterial switch operation in neonates and infants: Comparison of low-flow cardiopulmonary bypass versus circulatory arrest. *Circulation.* 1995;92:2226–2235.
19. Tibby SM, Hatherill M, Marsh MJ, et al. Clinical validation of cardiac output measurements using femoral artery thermodilution with direct Fick in ventilated children and infants. *Intensive Care Med.* 1997;23:987–991.
20. Jonas MM, Tanser SJ. Lithium dilution measurement of cardiac output and arterial pulse waveform analysis: An indicator dilution calibrated beat by beat system for continuous estimation of cardiac output. *Curr Opin Crit Care.* 2002;8:257–261.
21. Wippermann CF, Huth RG, Schmidt FX, et al. Continuous measurement of cardiac output by Fick principle in infants and children: Comparison with thermodilution method. *Intensive Care Med.* 1996;22:467–471.
22. Tibby SM, Murdoch IA. Measurement of cardiac output and tissue perfusion. *Curr Opin Pediatr.* 2002;14:3030–3306.
23. Tweddell JS, Hoffman GM, Mussatto KA, et al. Improved survival of patients undergoing palliation of hypoplastic left heart syndrome: Lessons learned from 115 consecutive patients. *Circulation.* 2002;106(suppl I):I-82–I-89.
24. Levy RJ, Chiavacci RM, Nicolson SC, et al. An evaluation of non-invasive cardiac output measurement using partial carbon dioxide rebreathing in children. *Anesth Analg.* 2004;99:1642–1647.
25. Chait HI, Kuhn MA, Baum VC. Inferior vena cava pressure reliably predicts right atrial pressure in pediatric cardiac surgical pressures. *Crit Care Med.* 1994;22:219–224.
26. Kumar A, Anel R, Bunnell E, et al. Pulmonary artery occlusion pressure and central venous pressure fail to predict ventricular filling volume, cardiac performance or the response to volume infusion in normal subjects. *Crit Care Med.* 2004;32:691–699.
27. Michard F, Boussat S, Chemla D, et al. Relation between Respiratory Changes in Arterial Pulse Pressure and Fluid Responsiveness in Septic Patients with Acute Circulatory Failure. *Am J Respir Crit Care Med.* 2000;162:134–138.
28. Milnor WR. Arterial impedance as ventricular afterload. *Circ Res.* 1975;36:565.
29. Lang RM, Borow KM, Neumann A, et al. Systemic vascular resistance: An unreliable index of left ventricular afterload. *Circulation.* 1986;74:1114–1123.
30. Courand JA, Marshall J, Chang Y, et al. Clinical applications of wall stress analysis in the pediatric intensive care unit. *Crit Care Med.* 2001;29:526–533.
31. Snider AR, Serwer GA, Ritter SB. *Echocardiography in pediatric heart disease.* 2nd ed. St. Louis, MO: Mosby; 1997:200.
32. Gentles TL, Colan SD. Wall stress misrepresents afterload in children and young adults with abnormal left ventricular geometry. *J Appl Physiol.* 2002;92:1053–1057.
33. Little WC. The left ventricular dP/dtmax—end-diastolic volume relation in closed chest dogs. *Circ Res.* 1985;56:808–815.
34. Vogel M, Schmidt MR, Kristiansen SB, et al. Validation of myocardial acceleration during isovolumic contraction as a novel noninvasive index of right ventricular contractility: Comparison with ventricular pressure-volume relations in an animal model. *Circulation.* 2002;105:1693–1699.
35. Suga H, Sagawa K, Shoukas AA. Load independence of the instantaneous pressure-volume ratio of the canine left ventricle and effects of epinephrine and heart rate on the ratio. *Circ Res.* 1973;32:314.
36. Spurney CF, Sable CA, Berger JT, et al. Use of a hand-carried ultrasound device by critical care physicians for the diagnosis of pericardial effusions, decreased cardiac function left ventricular enlargement in pediatric patients. *J Am Soc Echocardiogr.* 2005;18:313–310.
37. Colan Sd, Borow Km, Neumann A. Left ventricular end-systolic wall stress-velocity of fiber shortening relation: A load independent index of myocardial contractility. *J Am Coll Cardiol.* 1984;4:715–724.

Electrophysiology

John T. Berger III   *Jeffrey P. Moak*

The recognition and treatment of abnormal heart rhythms is essential for the treatment of critically ill children. Children admitted to intensive care units (ICUs) frequently experience arrhythmias, with one study showing that 29% of children admitted to large cardiac ICUs had an arrhythmia.[1] Children can experience arrhythmias in an otherwise normal heart or as a consequence of cardiac and noncardiac disease (see Table 5.3.1). Children who present with a significant arrhythmia should always undergo an investigation for an underlying disease and/or structural heart defect.

The pumping function of the heart is controlled by highly coordinated electrical impulses. These impulses are intrinsic to the heart but are modulated by the autonomic nervous system. Arrhythmias have important hemodynamic consequences that can lead to transient hypotension (syncope), shock, cardiac failure, and cardiac arrest. Tachyarrhythmias can decrease cardiac output by several different mechanisms: (i) decreased ventricular filling due to a shorter diastolic time; (ii) loss of atrioventricular (AV) synchrony (loss of the atrial "kick"); (iii) decreased coronary artery blood flow resulting in myocardial ischemia; or (iv) unfavorable length–tension relationship (Frank-Starling relationship) due to decreased preload. Bradyarrhythmias lead to decreased cardiac output when the heart is unable to compensatorily increase stroke volume, as seen in neonates and younger children. Consequently, it is very important to consider the interdependence of heart rate, preload, afterload, and contractility in the ensuing discussions.

Cardiac impulse initiation and conduction involves complex interactions between single cellular electrical events, intercellular electrical communication, and cardiac tissue structure. The aims of the following section are (i) to describe the anatomy of the conduction system within the heart, (ii) to describe the electrophysiology underlying normal myocardial depolarization and the regional variations, (iii) to describe the electrophysiologic

TABLE 5.3.1
SECONDARY SUBSTRATES FOR ARRHYTHMIA

Metabolic abnormalities	Hypoxemia
	Ischemia
	Acidemia
Electrolyte disturbances	Hypo- or hyperkalemia
	Hypo- or hypercalcemia
	Hypomagnesemia
Drug or toxin exposure	Antiarrhythmic agents
	Digoxin
	Sympathomimetic agents (e.g., cocaine)
	Drugs that prolong QT interval (see www.qtdrugs.org)
Myocardial abnormalities	Myocardial infarction
	Congenital heart disease (unrepaired or repaired)
	Cardiomyopathy
	Myocarditis
	Accessory atrioventricular pathways (WPW)
Channelopathies	Long QT syndromes
	Brugada syndrome
	Catecholaminergic ventricular tachycardia
Trauma	Surgical
	Commotio cordis

WPW, Wolff-Parkinson-White syndrome.

mechanisms of arrhythmias, and (iv) to highlight some of the molecular mechanisms of arrhythmias.

CARDIAC CONDUCTION SYSTEM

The normal cardiac rhythm is initiated in the sinoatrial (SA) node, located in the high right atrium at the junction of the right atrial appendage and the superior vena cava. A wave of depolarization spreads from the SA node throughout both atria, producing the P wave on the surface electrocardiogram. Both the parasympathetic and sympathetic nervous systems can affect the sinus rate, with the parasympathetic limb predominating. The SA node is the dominant pacemaker owing to its rapid rate of spontaneous depolarization and overdrive suppression of secondary pacemakers.

Preferential intranodal pathways functionally connect the SA node to the AV node, which rests at the base of the right atrium in the muscular AV septum. The AV node is complex, with three general divisions: a transitional zone, compact AV node, and a penetrating bundle. The penetrating bundle of His arises from the compact AV node as it penetrates the fibrous junction between the atrium and ventricles. Impulse conduction through the AV node is slow, causing a delay between atrial and ventricular activation. The delay allows time for optimal separation of atrial from ventricular contraction to contribute to diastolic filling of the ventricles. Within the ventricular septum, the His bundle divides into right and left bundle branches. The proximal portions of the bundle branches are insulated from the surrounding myocardium by fibrous tissue. The branches subdivide into a network of small Purkinje fibers that leads to coordinated depolarization of the ventricle. Impulse conduction over the Purkinje fibers is rapid.

ACTION POTENTIAL

Each heartbeat is initiated by a pulse of electrical activity, an action potential that begins in specialized pacemaker cells in the sinus node and spreads throughout the heart. The action potential is made possible by the electrochemical gradient that exists across the surface membrane of the cardiac myocyte. The shape and duration of the cardiac action potentials reflect the movement of ions (primarily Na^+, K^+, Ca^{2+}, and Cl^-) across the membrane through dozens of different ion channels and ion exchange pumps. Ion channels are transmembrane proteins that allow rapid movement of specific ions down electrochemical gradients. The macroscopic current produced by ion channels during each phase of the action potential is the product of the number of functional channels in the cell membrane, the probability that a channel is open, and the single channel conductance for an ion.

Opening and closing of ion channels occur through a process known as *gating* whereby changes in voltage, intracellular or extracellular ligands, or time lead to conformational changes of the channel pore allowing ion movement. Voltage gating is predominant in the cardiac tissue. Ion channels can be in an open, closed, or inactive state. For example, normal Na^+ channels associated with phase 0 depolarization close and do not reopen despite continuation of the depolarizing stimulus that has initiated the open state. The ionic gradients across the cell membrane are maintained by energy-consuming pumps such as the Na^+/K^+ ATPase pump. In general, Na^+ and Ca^{2+} channels favor membrane depolarization, whereas K^+ channels predominantly aid in repolarization of myocardial cells.

Mutated forms of ion channels associated with channelopathies may act aberrantly. In the case of the cardiac Na^+ channel, repolarization of the cell membrane to -55 mV is required before the channel will reopen. Mutations in the genes encoding for sarcolemma, as well as sacroplasmic ion channels, have been demonstrated in a variety of arrhythmias such as long QT syndrome (LQTS), Brugada syndrome, catecholamine-sensitive polymorphic ventricular tachycardia, and idiopathic ventricular fibrillation. There are five phases (0–4) to the cardiac action potential (see Fig. 5.3.1). The following discussion relates primarily to the action potential of the ventricle, as opposed to conduction tissue or atrial myocytes. Ventricular myocytes maintain a steady diastolic membrane potential of -85 mV because of the membrane's permeability to K^+ but not Na^+ or Ca^{2+}. Phase 0 represents myocyte depolarization and typically lasts <1 ms. When the myocyte is depolarized to a critical threshold, the threshold potential, a fast voltage-dependent Na^+ channel opens and Na^+ enters the cell. A stimulus of sufficient strength to reach threshold potential elicits a maximal response. Phase 1 is a period of rapid repolarization and results from inactivation of inward Na^+ current and a transient outward K^+ current with the opening of several potassium channels.

The plateau phase, phase 2, which lasts hundreds of milliseconds in the ventricle, is the result of a balance of inward and outward currents. Contributors to this phase include rapid and slow component of the delayed rectifier potassium currents (I_{Kr}, I_{Ks}), L-type calcium channel, and the Na^+/Ca^{2+} exchanger. As outward potassium currents increase and inward calcium current decrease, the action potential progresses to phase 3, rapid repolarization. Another inward rectifier K^+ current (I_{K1}) makes an increasingly important contribution to net membrane current as the resting potential is approached. During phase

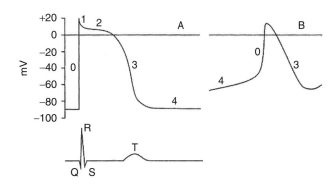

Figure 5.3.1 The 5 phases of the cardiac action potential. (From Topol E, ed. *Textbook of cardiovascular medicine*. 2nd ed. Philadelphia, PA: Lippincott Williams & Wilkins; 2002 from the CD-rom only chapter Mechanisms of Cardiac Arrhythmias.)

TABLE 5.3.2		
FACTORS THAT ALTER SPONTANEOUS AUTOMATICITY		
	Increase	**Decrease**
Autonomic nervous system	↑Sympathetic tone	↓Sympathetic tone
	↑Catecholamines	↓Catecholamines
	↓Parasympathetic tone	↑Parasympathetic tone
Metabolism	↑CO_2 or acidity	↓CO_2 or acidity
	↑Temperature	↓Temperature
	↓Oxygen	↑Oxygen
Electrolytes	↓K^+	↑K^+
	↑Ca^{2+}	↓Ca^{2+}

4, the heart is in diastole, and nonpacemaker cells maintain a resting membrane potential at −85 to −90 mV because of I_{K1}, which is inactivated as membrane potential as depolarization occurs and the cycle repeats.

Pacemaker cells in the SA and AV nodes and His-Purkinje system have different electrophysiologic properties as compared to the ventricular myocardium. Pacemaker cells display automaticity and undergo slow spontaneous depolarization during phase 4 and will spontaneously reach threshold potential to begin phase 0. Ventricular myocytes require an external stimulus to reach threshold potential. Three ionic currents can contribute to this spontaneous depolarization: deactivation of I_{Ks}, activation of an inward Na^+ current, and a hyperpolarization current (I_f) carried by Na^+ and K^+ ions. Pacemaker cells differ in terms of conduction velocity, shape, and duration of action potential as compared to ventricular myocytes. Finally, pacemaker cells differ in different tissues. For example, the SA and AV nodes have a paucity of I_{K1} channels. This difference in channel distribution partially explains the persistence of SA node function in hyperkalemia. Many factors may alter normal automaticity by changing the rate of diastolic depolarization, altering resting membrane potential, or altering the threshold potential and/or cycle length (see Table 5.3.2).

ELECTROPHYSIOLOGIC MECHANISMS OF ARRHYTHMIAS

A cardiac arrhythmia is an abnormality of initiation, timing, or sequence of cardiac depolarization, which can result in either tachycardia or bradycardia. Mechanisms of arrhythmias may be viewed from an electrophysiologic perspective or a molecular perspective. Mechanisms of tachyarrhythmias include abnormal automaticity, triggered activity, and re-entry (see Table 5.3.3). Mechanisms of bradycardia include abnormal impulse formation or impulse conduction. Understanding electrophysiologic mechanisms aids in diagnosis and is useful in predicting response to treatment. For example, arrhythmias caused by enhanced automaticity such as junctional ectopic tachycardia (JET) and atrial

TABLE 5.3.3	
ARRHYTHMIA MECHANISMS	
Conduction block	■ Sinus node exit block
	■ AV node block
	■ Bundle branch block
Re-entry	■ Atrial fibrillation/flutter
	■ Sinus node re-entrant tachycardia
	■ AV node re-entry tachycardia
	■ Permanent junctional re-entry tachycardia
	■ AV reciprocating tachycardia (accessory pathway tachycardia, WPW)
	■ Ventricular tachycardia
	■ Brugada syndrome
Enhanced automaticity	■ Atrial ectopic tachycardia
	■ Junctional ectopic tachycardia
	■ Accelerated junctional tachycardia
	■ Accelerated idioventricular tachycardia
	■ Ventricular tachycardia
Triggered activity	■ Digitalis toxicity
	■ *Torsade de pointes*
	■ Ventricular tachycardia

AV, atrioventricular; WPW, Wolff-Parkinson-White syndrome.

ectopic tachycardia (AET) will not respond to treatments such as cardioversion or adenosine.

Abnormal Automaticity

Automaticity is the ability of cardiac cells to initiate spontaneous action potentials. Under normal circumstances, the sinus node has the fastest spontaneous firing and is the predominant pacemaker. The AV node, His bundle, and Purkinje fibers fire at progressively slower rates and are usually suppressed by the activity of the sinus node. A lower subsidiary pacemaker may take over if a faster pacemaker fails to produce an escape rhythm.

Abnormal automaticity or spontaneous impulse generation can develop when pathologic conditions depolarize myocardial cells. For instance, an injury current can develop between a depolarized ischemic cell and normal cells, leading to repetitive activity in the normal cells. Cellular depolarization can result from medications, ischemia, metabolic disturbances, or local trauma.

Triggered Activity

Triggered activity refers to abnormal impulse generation from after-depolarizations from a preceding action potential. These after-depolarizations can occur early or late and represent oscillations of membrane potential. (see Fig. 5.3.2) When after-depolarizations are large enough to reach threshold potential, the resultant action potential is called *triggered*. Early after-depolarizations (EADs) are related to increased Ca^{2+} or Na^+ currents (calcium–sodium exchanger current) that maintain the plateau phase of the action potential. EADs are important in the genesis of *torsades de pointes*. EADs are facilitated by increased repolarization times, as seen with slow heart rates, congenital or acquired LQTS, hypokalemia, hypomagnesemia, hypocalcemia, and medications such as erythromycin, procainamide, or sotalol.

Delayed after-depolarizations (DADs) arise from the repolarized membrane (phase 4). DADs occur in states of increased intracellular Ca^{2+}. Two mechanisms have been proposed for DADs. Excessive intracellular Ca^{2+} can lead to further calcium release from sacroplasmic reticulum, activating a nonspecific cation inward current. The other mechanism is an inward current generated by the Na^+/Ca^{2+} exchanger. Classic examples of arrhythmias associated with DADs are arrhythmias secondary to digitalis toxicity. Digitalis inhibits Na^+/K^+ pump, resulting in increased Na^+

concentration, which in turn results in increased calcium through the Na^+/Ca^{2+} exchanger.

Re-entry

Re-entry is the most common mechanism for arrhythmia formation and occurs in the setting of abnormal impulse conduction. The abnormalities in impulse conduction can result from anomalous anatomic pathway (i.e., an accessory pathway as is seen in Wolff-Parkinson-White syndrome) or from poor impulse propagation. Poor pulse propagation may result from pathology, drugs, or hormonal modulation of the conduction system. Fibrotic changes in the heart associated with hypertrophy or injury can lead to areas of slow conduction and provide micro pathways, as well as macro pathways, for re-entry.

Three conditions are typically required for re-entry to occur (see Fig. 5.3.3): the presence of two electrical pathways, unidirectional block in one pathway, and slow conduction permitting recovery of excitability in the previously blocked area. AV reciprocating tachycardia is an example of re-entrant tachycardia. During sinus rhythm, the action potential activates the ventricle through the AV node and the accessory pathway. Supraventricular tachycardia (SVT) can be initiated when a premature atrial impulse blocks antegrade in the accessory pathway and conducts through the AV node (because of differences in refractory periods of the AP and AV node). The impulse then can return to the atria retrograde by the AP, resulting in a

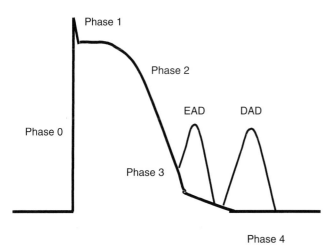

Figure 5.3.2 Early and delayed after-depolarizations. If an after-depolarization is large enough to reach threshold potential, arrhythmia may be triggered. EAD, early after-depolarization; DAD, delayed after-depolarization.

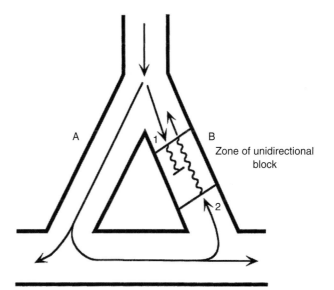

Figure 5.3.3 Three conditions are typically required for re-entry to occur: the presence of two electrical pathways, unidirectional block in one pathway, and slow conduction permitting recovery of excitability in the previously blocked area. (From Topol E, ed. *Textbook of cardiovascular medicine.* 2nd ed. Philadelphia, PA: Lippincott Williams & Wilkins; 2002 from the CD-rom only chapter Mechanisms of Cardiac Arrhythmias.)

re-entrant circuit. Re-entrant tachycardias may be converted by inducing a transient block within a limb of the circuit, such as the use of adenosine to block the AV node.

Mechanisms of Bradyarrhythmias

Bradyarrhythmias arise from conduction block. The block may be physiologic, as occurs when a premature atrial impulse fails to conduct through an AV node, when still refractory. Conduction block may also occur from ischemia, direct trauma, infarction, or fibrosis. Right bundle branch block is frequently seen in patients after surgeries associated with right ventriculotomy (60% to 100% incidence after surgical repair of patients with tetralogy of Fallot).[2]

PATHOLOGIC SUBSTRATES OF ARRHYTHMIAS

Arrhythmias arise from abnormal electrophysiologic substrates that occur at the macroscopic, cellular, molecular, and/or ionic levels. These alterations may acutely or permanently change the electrical properties of the heart. On the macroscopic level, hypertrophy, accessory pathways, or surgical scars in cardiac tissue can change conduction or refractory periods that facilitate arrhythmias. Cellular alterations such as ischemia or hyperkalemia alter ion currents and produce arrhythmias. Finally, gene mutations can produce changes in ion channels that lead to arrhythmia and/or sudden cardiac death. The following examples of substrates for arrhythmias are presented to help integrate the genetic, molecular, electrical, and pathologic components to arrhythmias.

Channelopathies

Inherited abnormalities of ionic channel function can render children susceptible to arrhythmias. Familial LQTS such as Romano-Ward syndrome can arise from one of several different gene mutations, and seven forms of inherited LQTS have been described (LQTS 1 to 7).[3] In LQTS 2, approximately 100 mutations have been identified in gene coding for a channel of the delayed K^+ rectifying current (I_{Kr}). These mutations produce a loss of function in the channel and prolong the plateau phase of the action potential. Interestingly, different mutations can interfere by several different cellular mechanisms. Channel function is reduced either by reducing the number of functioning channels in the cell membrane because of abnormal protein trafficking, changing the probability that a channel is open, or by changing ion conductance of an individual channel.[3]

Other arrhythmia syndromes such as Brugada syndrome, idiopathic ventricular fibrillation, sudden infant death syndrome, and sick sinus syndrome have been linked to gene mutations that alter cardiac ion channels function.

Ischemia

Acute myocardial ischemia can produce multiple different electrophysiologic effects. Myocardial ischemia is associated with a rise in extracellular K^+, intracellular Ca^{2+} and fall in intracellular pH and adenosine triphosphate (ATP). These changes result in a partial depolarization of the resting membrane potential, slowing of conduction, and prolonged refractoriness. Abnormal automaticity, triggered activity, and re-entry can all result from these perturbations.

Electrolyte Disturbances

Patients in the ICU frequently have alterations in potassium, calcium, or magnesium, often a result of diuretic use and are at increased risk of arrhythmias. For instance, hypokalemia has several electrophysiologic effects. Hypokalemia hyperpolarizes the resting membrane potential and consequently slows conduction. In addition, hypokalemia delays repolarization by prolonging the action potential duration.[4] This may lead to after-depolarizations and triggered activity, which could ultimately manifest clinically as ventricular arrhythmias. Hypocalcemia also prolongs the QT interval and may result in EADs and triggered arrhythmias such as *torsade de pointes*.

Congenital Heart Disease

Children with congenital heart disease are susceptible to arrhythmias before and after surgery. The substrates for development of arrhythmias include surgical scarring, myocyte hypertrophy from pressure and volume overload, and dilation.

REFERENCES

1. Hoffman TM, Wernovsky G, Wieand TS, et al. The incidence of arrhythmias in a pediatric cardiac intensive care unit. *Pediatr Cardiol*. 2002;23:598–604.
2. Kongrad E. Prognosis for patients with congenital heart defects and postoperative intraventricular conduction defects. *Circulation*. 1978;57:867–880.
3. Deslisle BP, Anson BD, Rajamani S, et al. Biology of cardiac arrhythmias: Ion channel protein trafficking. *Circ Res*. 2004;94:1418–1428.
4. Ramaswamy K, Hamdan MH. Ischemia, metabolic disturbances and arrhythmogenesis: Mechanisms and management. *Crit Care Med*. 2000;28:N151–N157.

Cardiopulmonary Interactions

John T. Berger III

The cardiorespiratory system functions as a single unit to provide adequate oxygen delivery. The complex interactions between the cardiac and respiratory system are influenced by a complex interaction of many factors, including cardiac anatomy, myocardial function, circulating blood volume, blood flow distribution, autonomic nervous system function, intrathoracic pressure (ITP), and lung volume. The interactions found in healthy individuals are often exaggerated in patients with pulmonary and/or cardiac disease.

An understanding of cardiopulmonary interactions is central in the management of critically ill children, especially those with heart disease. A single respiratory intervention may affect cardiac function in many different ways and net effects are sometimes difficult to predict. For instance, patients with left ventricular (LV) failure usually benefit from positive pressure ventilation, whereas patients with predominantly right ventricular (RV) failure do not. Ventilation not only affects steady state hemodynamics but also produces beat-to-beat effects and the effect of these dynamic changes range from minimal alterations, when cardiopulmonary function is normal or nearly normal, to profound, when there is cardiopulmonary dysfunction.

Ventilation affects cardiovascular function by several mechanisms. Inspiration increases lung volume and causes diaphragmatic descent, altering the relationship between intrathoracic and extrathoracic structures. Inspiration requires changes in ITP, positive or negative, which effects cardiac function independent of changes in lung volume. Ventilation also alters acid–base balance, oxygen tensions, and neurohormonal activity, which can affect cardiac function. The following section will focus on the effect of spontaneous and positive pressure ventilation on cardiac function. These interactions are first discussed as separate processes although they usually coexist in the clinical setting. Second, cardiopulmonary interactions in specific patient populations will be reviewed to emphasize how these principles enable rationale optimization of therapies.

EFFECTS OF CHANGES IN INTRATHORACIC PRESSURE ON CARDIAC FUNCTION

Effects on Venous Return and Right Ventricular Preload

Venous return to the right atrium is determined by the pressure gradient between mean systemic venous pressure (P_{MS}) and right atrial pressure (P_{RA}). P_{RA} represents the back pressure to venous return. Because the right atrium is an intrathoracic structure, respiratory-induced changes in ITP directly affect P_{RA} and therefore the pressure gradient for venous return. During a spontaneous inspiration P_{RA} falls, intra-abdominal pressure increases as the diaphragm descends, and the peripheral venous pressure remains constant. The increased gradient between the extra- and intrathoracic cavities produces increased venous return. When P_{RA} drops to zero relative to the atmosphere, venous return is maximized (see Fig. 5.2.7). Venous return does not increase when the P_{RA} drops below zero due to inflow limitation. The veins at the entrance in the thorax are exposed to atmospheric pressure and, as ITP and the transmitted intraluminal pressure fall below zero, the vessels collapse and flow decreases. Flow increases only when the intraluminal pressure rises above zero.

Positive pressure mechanical ventilation inhibits venous return to the right atrium. When ITP becomes positive, venous flow into the right atrium decelerates and right ventricular filling falls. The impairment in cardiac output is most commonly seen in patients with hypovolemia where P_{MS} is already low. Conversely, in patients with hypervolemia the fall in venous return is less because there is a greater systemic to atrial pressure gradient because of a relatively high P_{MS}. The application of positive end-expiratory pressure (PEEP) causes an increase in intrathoracic volume and pressure and causes the diaphragm to descend, which pressurizes the abdominal cavity. Consequently, both P_{MS} and P_{RA} rise, and the pressure gradient for venous return may be relatively unchanged.[1] This was demonstrated in a study of adults after coronary artery bypass surgery. As mean airway pressure was progressively increased from 0 to 20 cm H_2O, venous return was maintained because intra-abdominal pressure increased in parallel with P_{RA} and cardiac output was unchanged.[2] Clearly, there are certain clinical situations where positive pressure ventilation will decrease cardiac output by decreasing venous return. These situations typically occur in patients with low circulating blood volume (dehydration, septic shock). Cardiac output in these patients can by restored by volume loading or increasing vasomotor tone.

Effects on Left Ventricular Preload

Changes in systemic venous return that occur during spontaneous ventilation directly and indirectly change LV preload. The RV volume increases during spontaneous inspiration causing a leftward shift of the intraventricular septum, which decreases LV compliance and consequently decreases LV filling.[3] Additionally, the increase in RV volume causes the pericardial pressure to rise, which further compromises LV compliance and impedes pulmonary venous return.[4] The decrease in LV compliance and preload because of ventricular interdependence is a major mechanism of pulsus paradoxus in patients with pericardial effusion and tamponade.

During mechanical ventilation, positive pressure ventilation reduces LV preload by decreasing venous return,

intraventricular dependence, direct compression, or combinations of these basic etiologies. When cardiac contractility is normal, a sustained increase in ITP reduces RV filling by reducing the pressure gradient for venous return. This has two opposite effects on LV preload. First, the ventricles share a common wall, the intraventricular septum, and the filling of one ventricle effects the other (i.e., intraventricular dependence). The reduction in RV volume during inspiration leads to an increase in LV compliance and hence LV end-diastolic volume. Second, because the RV and LV are in series, any reduction in venous return and RV output must eventually decrease the LV preload.[5] Third, as the lung volume increases, the lungs may physically constrain the heart and interfere with ventricular filling by compressing the ventricles. A recent study in normal dogs demonstrated that positive pressure ventilation reduced LV preload more by LV compression from the lungs than reductions in venous return.[6] However, when LV contractility was reduced, the same study showed less change in LV end-diastolic volume as a result of the reduced effect of external lung pressure.

When respiratory disease or excessive PEEP leads to afterload-induced RV dysfunction (e.g., increased pulmonary vascular resistance [PVR]) and increased RV end-diastolic volume, intraventricular interdependence becomes more important. As PEEP was increased from 0 to 30 cm H_2O in patients with acute respiratory distress syndrome (ARDS), RV afterload increased, RV end-diastolic volume increased, the intraventricular septum shifted leftward, LV diastolic dimensions were reduced, and cardiac output decreased. Volume administration did not restore cardiac output.[7]

Effects of Ventilation on Left Ventricle Afterload

LV afterload can be defined as LV systolic wall stress, which is a function of the transmural LV pressure and the radius of the LV. The transmural pressure of the LV, or pressure

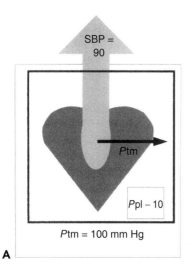

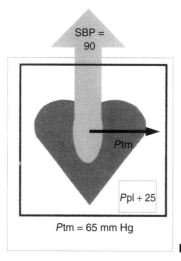

A

B

Figure 5.4.1 Effects of ventilation on left ventricular (LV) afterload. **A:** During a spontaneous inspiration, pleural pressure falls to −10 mm Hg producing an LV transmural pressure of 100 mm Hg during systole. **B:** During a positive pressure inspiration, pleural pressure increases to 25 mm Hg resulting in a reduced LV transmural pressure of 65 mm Hg. The positive intrathoracic pressure (ITP) has reduced LV afterload if cardiac output remains constant. Ptm, transmural pressure; SBP, Extra-thoracic systolic blood pressure; Ppl, pleural pressure.

across the LV wall, is intravascular systolic pressure minus the pleural pressure. A decrease in ITP with a constant systemic arterial pressure will result in increased LV wall tension and increased afterload (see Fig. 5.4.1). Conversely, an increased transthoracic pressure reduces the transmural pressure gradient and lowers LV afterload.

The effects of negative ITP on LV afterload are negligible in patients with normal myocardial and respiratory function because the pressure changes induced by ITP changes are small compared to intravascular pressures and the effects of ventilation on right ventricular preload predominate. However, when inspiratory pleural pressure is very negative (e.g., upper airway obstruction), LV afterload is greatly increased, even precipitating pulmonary edema.[8]

CARDIOVASCULAR EFFECTS OF CHANGES IN LUNG VOLUME

Ventilation Effects on Right Ventricle Afterload

PVR is the main determinant of RV afterload and is directly affected by changes in lung volume. Changes in lung volume affect PVR by two mechanisms: (i) passive compression of pulmonary blood vessels and (ii) hypoxic pulmonary vasoconstriction.

PVR is lowest at functional residual capacity (FRC) and PVR increases when lung volume rises or falls below FRC (see Fig. 5.4.2). The pulmonary vasculature can be divided into intra-alveolar and extra-alveolar blood vessels; total

PVR depends on the tone of each compartment. When the lung volume falls below FRC, two events occur that can independently raise PVR. First, extra-alveolar blood vessels become more tortuous and tend to collapse. Second and more significantly, terminal airways close at low lung volumes producing alveolar collapse and hypoxia, resulting in hypoxic pulmonary vasoconstriction.[9,10] As lung volumes increase to FRC, extra-alveolar vessels straighten, alveolar hypoxia decreases, and PVR falls. When the lung inflates above FRC, intra-alveolar blood vessels are compressed and PVR rises. Therefore, PVR rises at either extreme of lung volume.

Mechanical ventilation can increase or decrease PVR. It can reduce hypoxic pulmonary vasoconstriction by enriching alveolar oxygen tension, re-expanding collapsed alveoli, or reversing respiratory acidosis. Conversely, in patients with hyperinflated lungs, right ventricular dysfunction, or pulmonary hypertension, it can increase PVR by further increasing lung volumes, increasing PVR, and increasing RV afterload. Small changes in lung volume in some patients produce acute cor pulmonale.

Lung Volume Affects Autonomic Tone

The lungs are extensively supplied with nerve fibers and receptors. Lung inflation induces changes in autonomic output that alters instantaneous and steady state cardiac function. The most commonly described response is heart rate acceleration during inspiration with normal tidal volumes caused by a withdrawal in vagal tone. If the lungs are hyperinflated, however, heart rate decreases because of vagal overstimulation and reflex arteriolar dilation.[11]

RESPIRATORY EFFECTS OF CARDIAC DYSFUNCTION

The preceding discussion has focused primarily on the effects of ventilation on circulation; however, the effects of circulation on ventilation (also see Chapter 6.7). Abnormal cardiac function alters respiratory function by impairing gas exchange. For example, acute severe reductions in pulmonary blood flow caused by pulmonary hypertension increase airways resistance and decrease lung compliance as well as increasing RV afterload.[12] Patients with increased pulmonary blood flow such as those with a large ventricular septal defect (VSD) have increased airways resistance in both large and small airways. The increased airways resistance in small airways is a result of interstitial edema and vascular compression.[13]

Spontaneous respiration normally requires a small fraction of total systemic oxygen delivery to meet the demands of respiratory muscles. The respiratory muscles have an abundant arterial supply such that blood flow is not a limiting factor for ventilatory function. In patients with lung

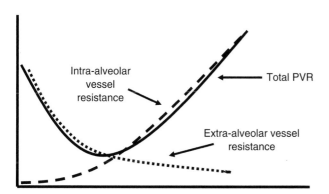

Figure 5.4.2 Relation between lung volume and pulmonary vascular resistance (PVR). Total PVR is the sum of resistance of the intra-alveolar and extra-alveolar blood vessels. Intra-alveolar vessels are compressed and resistance rises as lung volume increases from residual volume to total lung capacity (*dashed line*). When lung volume falls below functional residual capacity (FRC), extra-alveolar vessels become tortuous and collapse increasing their resistance (*dotted line*). Additionally, at low lung volumes, alveolar hypoxia causes hypoxic pulmonary vasoconstriction. The combined effect of lung volume on total pulmonary vascular resistance produces an asymmetric U-shaped curve (*solid line*) with minimal PVR at FRC.

disease, the metabolic demand of respiratory muscles can rise to 25% to 30% of total oxygen delivery because of the increased work of breathing.[14] If cardiac output is limited, respiratory muscle function is reduced as a result of limited oxygen delivery. Respiratory muscle failure caused by the inability to increase cardiac output is an important cause of failure to wean from mechanical ventilation even in patients without primary cardiac disease.[15] For example, adult patients who successfully extubated increase their cardiac output and oxygen transport, whereas those who failed weaning did not.

CARDIOPULMONARY INTERACTIONS IN SELECTED INTENSIVE CARE UNIT POPULATIONS

From the preceding discussion, it can be seen that ventilation has profound effects on cardiovascular function, and those effects vary depending on the dominant physiologic conditions. Patients with increased work of breathing, hypervolemia, or impaired left (systemic) ventricular dysfunction benefit from positive pressure ventilation because of its ability to decrease oxygen demand and enhance LV systolic function. Conversely, patients with hypovolemia, hyperinflation, or RV dysfunction, have profound cardiovascular instability with mechanical ventilation.

Initiation of Mechanical Ventilation in Patients with Hypovolemia

A common example of heart-lung interaction in the pediatric ICU is intubation and initiation of mechanical ventilation. In patients with sepsis, trauma, or dehydration, the initiation of mechanical ventilation may result in cardiovascular collapse. The predominant effect of initiating positive pressure breathing is the reduction in systemic venous return. The onset of positive pressure ventilation in this population exaggerates physiologic hypovolemia and will be especially evident in patients who are vasodilated secondary to sepsis. For example, application of PEEP in adults with P_{RA} <10 mm Hg was associated with a decreased cardiac output while patients whose P_{RA} was >10 mm Hg had fewer alterations in cardiac output.[16] Providing volume to counter the reduction in preload, or minimizing the ITP, or both, may be important in minimizing the cardiac effects of initiating mechanical ventilation.

Left Ventricular Failure

LV failure is characterized by increased intrathoracic blood volume caused by reduced LV compliance and high systemic afterload. The failing myocardium is very sensitive to alterations in afterload but not preload as it is usually operating on the flat portion of the Frank-Starling curve. Additionally, patients even with optimally treated congestive heart failure (CHF) have increased lung water, decreased lung compliance, increased work of breathing, and increased systemic oxygen demand because of increased oxygen needs from increased work of breathing. In these patients, spontaneous breathing with decreased lung compliance also results in greater inspiratory effort, resulting in greater negative pleural pressure further raising LV afterload. Positive pressure ventilation in these patients improves cardiac function in several ways including decreasing LV afterload, decreasing LV preload, and reducing oxygen delivery requirement of the inspiratory muscle.[17] Additional physiologic benefits include the restoration of lung volumes and improved RV afterload in patients with atelectasis and pulmonary edema. Several studies have confirmed that cardiac output is unchanged or improved in patients with CHF during mechanical ventilation. Even chronic nocturnal continuous positive airway pressure (CPAP) improves LV contractile function, decreases catecholamine levels, and may improve long-term survival.[18] Noninvasive positive pressure ventilation has become popular in patients with acute decompensation of ventricular dysfunction as a method of improving cardiac performance. In contrast, weaning mechanical ventilation can unmask cardiac dysfunction in otherwise stable patients with compromised cardiac function and may require vasoactive drugs. Rasanen et al. showed that decreasing levels of ventilation in patients with myocardial ischemia worsened the ischemia and could be minimized by preventing negative swings in intrapleural pressure.[19]

Acute Lung Injury and Mechanical Ventilation

The RV normally pumps into a low-resistance, high-compliance circuit. ARDS, by injuring the microvasculature, increases RV afterload. The institution of mechanical ventilation may further impair RV function and can result in acute RV failure for the reasons described previously. Older studies detected cor pulmonale in 61% of adults with ARDS ventilated with relatively large tidal volumes.[20] A more recent study of adults ventilated with a lung protective strategy (plateau pressure <30 cm H_2O) showed a reduced incidence of cor pulmonale.[21] This reduction may be related to changes in ventilation strategy in which ITP and tidal volume are reduced.

Patients with Passive Pulmonary Blood Flow

Patients who have had bidirectional Glenn or Fontan procedures present unique cardiopulmonary interaction physiology. The central feature of this physiology is the absence of a ventricle to pump blood through the pulmonary circulation. Mean systemic venous pressure (P_{MS}) in not only the driving pressure for blood returning into the thorax but also for pulmonary arterial flow. Consequently, the amount of blood flow is exquisitely sensitive to ITP and phasically varies with the respiratory cycle. Pulmonary blood flow is enhanced with inspiration but is reduced or reversed when ITP is positive.[22] Clinical studies have shown that steady state cardiac output is augmented by 42% when ventilating patients with Fontan circulation with negative pressure as compared to positive pressure.[23]

Additional complexity occurs in patients with bidirectional Glenn circulation in which the superior vena cava is connected directly to the pulmonary artery. In this population, pulmonary blood flow is almost exclusively derived from cerebral blood return with only a minor contribution from the upper extremities. Consequently, cerebral blood flow autoregulatory mechanisms influence pulmonary blood flow more significantly as compared to patients with normal two-ventricle circulation. Hypoxia and acidemia vasodilates the cerebral circulation, whereas pulmonary vessels constrict.

The success of the bidirectional Glenn procedure relies on an unobstructed, low-resistance pulmonary vascular bed. Postoperative hypoxemia in these patients has often been attributed to elevated PVR as a consequence of cardiopulmonary bypass. Unfortunately, hyperventilation and conventional treatments aimed at lowering PVR are ineffective. Recent studies have shown that the cerebral autoregulatory controls predominate over pulmonary autoregulation whereby hypercarbic acidosis increases cerebral and pulmonary blood flow, oxygen saturation, and cerebral oxygen delivery.[24,25] Cerebral oxygen delivery was not increased by hyperoxia despite higher oxygen content of arterial blood.[25] A strategy of permissive hypercapnia may improve oxygenation in these patients despite the increase in PVR.

REFERENCES

1. Pinsky MR. Recent advances in the clinical application of heart-lung interactions. *Curr Opin Crit Care.* 2002;8:26–31.
2. Van den Berg PCM, Jansen JRC, Pinsky MR. Effect of positive pressure on venous return in volume-loaded cardiac surgical patients. *J Appl Physiol.* 2002;92:1223–1231.
3. Brinker JA, Weiss I, Lappe DL, et al. Leftward septal displacement during right ventricular loading in man. *Circulation.* 1980;61:626–633.
4. Shekerdemian L, Bohn D. Cardiovascular effects of mechanical ventilation. *Arch Dis Child.* 1999;80:475–480.
5. Scharf SM, Brown R, Souanders N, et al. Hemodynamic effects of positive pressure ventilation. *J Appl Physiol.* 1980;49:124–131.
6. Denault AY, Goscsan J, Pinsky MR. Dynamic effects of positive pressure ventilation on canine left ventricular pressure-volume relations. *J Appl Physiol.* 2001;91:298–308.
7. Jardin F, Farcot J-C, Boisante L, et al. Influence of positive end-expiratory pressure on left ventricular performance. *N Engl J Med.* 1981;304:387–392.
8. Stalcup SA, Mellins RB. Mechanical forces producing pulmonary edema in acute asthma. *N engl J Med.* 1977;297:592–596.
9. Madden JA, Dawson CA, Harder DR. Hypoxic induced activation in small isolated pulmonary arteries from the cat. *J Appl Physiol.* 1985;59:1110–1115.
10. Chang AC, Zucker H, Hickey PR. Pulmonary vascular resistance in infants after cardiac surgery: Role of carbon dioxide and hydrogen ion. *Crit Care Med.* 1995;23:568–574.
11. Shepherd JT. The lungs as receptor sites for cardiovascular regulation. *Circulation.* 1981;63:1–10.
12. Schulze-Neick I, Penny DJ, Derrick GP, et al. Pulmonary vascular-bronchial interactions: Acute reductions in pulmonary blood flow alters lung mechanics. *Heart.* 2000;84:284–289.
13. Bancalari E, Jess MJ, Gelban H, et al. Lung mechanics in congenital heart disease with increased and decreased pulmonary blood flow. *J Pediatr.* 1977;90:192–195.
14. Stock MC, Davis DW, Manning JW, et al. Lung mechanics and oxygen consumption during spontaneous ventilation and severe heart failure. *Chest.* 1992;102(1):279–283.
15. Jubran A, Mathru M, Dries D, et al. Continuous recordings of mixed venous oxygen saturation during weaning from mechanical ventilation and the ramifications thereof. *Am J Respir Crit Care Med.* 1998;158:1763–1769.
16. Jellinek H, Krafft P, Fitzgerald RD, et al. Right atrial pressure predicts hemodynamic response to apneic positive airway pressure. *Crit Care Med.* 2000;28:672–678.
17. Naughton MT, Rahman A, Hara K, et al. Effect of continuous positive airway pressure on intrathoracic and left ventricular transmural pressures in patients with congestive heart failure. *Circulation.* 1995;91:1725–1731.
18. Yan AT, Bradley TD, Liu PP. The role of continuous positive airway pressure in the treatment of congestive heart failure. *Chest.* 2001;120:1675–1685.
19. Rasanen J, Nikki P, Heikkila J. Acute myocardial infarction complicated by respiratory failure: The effects of mechanical ventilation. *Chest.* 1984;85:21–28.
20. Jardin F, Gueret P, Dubourg O, et al. Two-dimensional echocardiographic evaluation of right ventricular size and contractility in acute respiratory failure. *Crit Care Med.* 1985;13:952–956.
21. Vieillard-Baron A, Schmitt JM, Augarde R, et al. Acute cor pulmonale in acute respiratory distress syndrome submitted to protective ventilation: Incidence, clinical implications and prognosis. *Crit Care Med.* 2001;29:1551–1555.
22. Redington AN, Penny D, Shinebourne EA. Pulmonary blood flow after total cavopulmonary shunt. *Br Heart J.* 1991;65:213–217.
23. Shekerdemian LS, Bush A, Shore DF, et al. Cardiopulmonary Interactions after Fontan Operations. Augmentation of cardiac output using negative pressure ventilation. *Circulation.* 1997;96:3934–3942.
24. Fogel MA, Durning S, Wernovsky G, et al. Brain versus Lung: Hierarchy of feedback loops in single ventricle patients with superior cavopulmonary connection. *Circulation.* 2004;110(suppl II):II–147–II–152.
25. Hoskote A, Li J, Hickey C, et al. The effects of carbon dioxide on oxygenation and systemic, cerebral and pulmonary vascular hemodynamics after the bi-directional superior cavopulmonary anastomosis. *J Am Coll Cardiol.* 2004;44:1501–1509.

Pathophysiology of Chronic Myocardial Dysfunction

5.5

J. Carter Ralphe

Heart failure is a syndrome of cardiac dysfunction that results in circulatory congestion and neuroendocrine responses. It results from primary myocardial dysfunction, volume overload, or pressure overload of the heart. Heart failure may manifest as diastolic and/or systolic dysfunction. The primary problem is the inability of the myocardium to generate force for given loading conditions. The increase in intravascular volume produced by activation of the rennin–angiotensin–aldosterone (RAA) system should increase cardiac output by the Frank-Starling mechanism. However, the failing myocardium is less responsive to myocardial stretch and the cardiac output does not increase[1] (see Figure 5.2.2). Additionally, as volume is increased, ventricular compliance is eventually exceeded and chamber pressure rises sharply with even small increases in ventricular volume. This results in increased atrial and venous pressures and in development of circulatory congestion (systemic or pulmonary edema). In contrast to decreased sensitivity of preload augmentation, the failing myocardium is extremely sensitive to increased afterload whereby increased afterload significantly decreases cardiac output (see Fig. 5.5.1). The activation of the maladaptive neurohormonal systems promotes progressive myocardial injury. Chronic remodeling including cardiomyocyte hypertrophy, fibroblast hyperplasia, and altered gene expression affects both the composition of the contractile proteins and the energetic function of the heart cell and results in the downward spiral exhibited in untreated chronic heart failure.

The earliest response to diminished cardiac output is the retention of salt and water by the kidneys under the

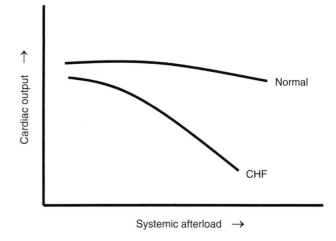

Figure 5.5.1 Reduced afterload reserve of failing myocardium. The failing ventricle is very sensitive to increases in afterload. As afterload increases, cardiac output falls because the myocardium is unable to compensate. CHF, congestive heart failure.

influence of the RAA system. An associated increase in adrenergic activity also contributes to the early neurohormonal activation that acutely increases cardiac filling volume and contractility. These two neurohormonal systems interact with each other in such a way that activation of one system leads to the activation of the other. For example, rennin release from the kidney is an adrenergic-receptor–mediated response, and angiotensin II facilitates presynaptic norepinephrine release. These initial mechanisms that compensate for decreased cardiac output rapidly become deleterious when the dysfunction persists, leading to progressive cardiac remodeling.

Pediatric heart failure often differs from that seen in adults in its presentation, its underlying etiology, and aspects of its pathophysiology. This latter difference is based on important differences between the immature and mature myocardium.[2] The immature heart compared to that of the adult has a higher collagen content, rendering it less compliant and therefore requiring higher filling pressures to ensure adequate cardiac output. The developing and immature heart expresses different isoforms of cardiac actin, myosin subunits, and troponin than the adult heart. Additionally, the immature heart uses glucose rather than fatty acids for adenosine triphosphate (ATP) production. Of perhaps greatest importance is that the immature heart has a relatively undeveloped sarcoplasmic reticulum calcium exchanger, which renders the movement of intracellular calcium less efficient. Rapid, substantial changes in intracellular calcium are an absolute requirement for systolic contraction and diastolic relaxation. Increase in intracellular calcium concentration is the primary mechanism for increasing contractile force and is the predominant effect of the long-standing medication for heart failure, digoxin. Because of decreased compliance and a relatively diminished capacity to increase contractile force (inotropy), the young pediatric heart is much more reliant on the rate to maintain output. These differences not only impact the manifestation of heart failure in young patients but also imply that the response of the pediatric patient to pharmacologic intervention may be quite different than the response of the adult patient. Application of treatments shown to be effective in adults to children must be approached cautiously and the outcomes monitored carefully.

Chronic heart failure in children is commonly due to either cardiomyopathy (postinfectious, genetic, metabolic, or unknown) or congenital heart disease. As many as 20% of the children born with a congenital heart defect will continue to have chronic failure despite appropriate surgical intervention. Defects often result in either pressure overload (e.g., valvar stenosis, coarctation of the aorta) or volume overload due to intracardiac shunts (e.g., ventricular or atrial septal defects). Occasionally, heart failure is related to underlying rhythm abnormalities (supraventricular tachycardia, atrial flutter, or ventricular tachycardia) or is secondary to genetic defects such as Duchenne muscular dystrophy or Marfan syndrome. These patients often present with varying degrees of decompensated failure. Understanding the basic mechanisms of heart failure and how the body attempts to compensate for this dysfunction, however ill-fated, is important for the successful management of children with this defect.

NEUROHORMONAL ACTIVATION

Neurohormonal activation is the complex response of the body to augment cardiac output by increasing heart rate,

TABLE 5.5.1

NEUROHORMONAL FACTORS ALTERED IN PATIENTS WITH CONGESTIVE HEART FAILURE

Norepinephrine	Vasoactive intestinal peptide
Epinephrine	Arginine vasopressin
Renin	Substance P
Angiotensin II	Growth hormone
Aldosterone	Atrial natriuretic peptide
Endothelin	B-type natriuretic peptide
Adrenomedullin	Nitric oxide
Tumor necrosis factor-α	Prostacyclin
Cortisol	Bradykinin
Neurokinin A	

contractility, preload, and myocardial contractile elements. The response involves many inter-related systems including the RAA axis, the sympathetic nervous system, endothelin, vasopressin, and cytokines. There is also coactivation of counter-regulatory systems such as natriuretic peptides and prostaglandins (see Table 5.5.1). These mechanisms are helpful when responding to acute stress, but when left unchecked, they exert a wide array of negative effects on the heart and the vasculature that result in worsening failure and progressive symptoms (see Table 5.5.2).

The Renin–Angiotensin–Aldosterone Axis

In the classic paradigm of heart failure, the kidneys respond to decreased oxygen delivery by increasing the secretion of renin, angiotensin II, and catecholamines, which effectively increase the reabsorption of sodium and water by the proximal renal tubules. Increased rennin and angiotensin II levels stimulate release of aldosterone from the adrenal glands, resulting in still further sodium and water reabsorption by the distal tubules. Initially, the expanded blood volume is beneficial, increasing stroke volumes on the basis of the Frank-Starling mechanism. Eventually, chamber dilation due to volume overload decreases the mechanical

TABLE 5.5.2

SIGNS OF CONGESTIVE HEART FAILURE

Increased Sympathetic Activity	Salt and Water Retention
Irritability	Cardiomegaly
Anorexia	Hepatomegaly
Sweating	Jugular venous distension
Tachycardia	Extremity edema
Oliguria	Pulmonary edema and tachypnea
Cool extremities	

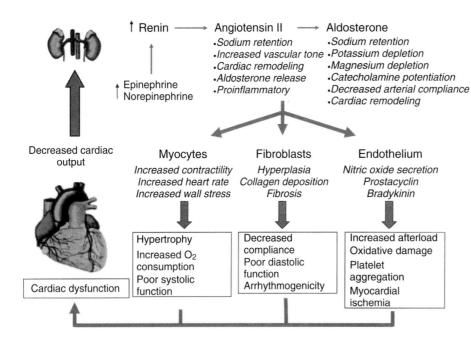

Figure 5.5.2 Renin–angiotensin–aldosterone (RAA) system activation. Decreased cardiac output leads to increased renin and angiotensin II activity. Chronic RAA activity leads to ventricular remodeling and worsening myocardial function.

efficiency of the ventricle, reducing systolic function, and increases wall stress and myocardial oxygen consumption.

Angiotensin II has a number of biologic effects in addition to promoting aldosterone release and sodium retention (Fig. 5.5.2). Angiotensin II causes constriction of vascular smooth muscle, a potential positive influence early in failure because a reapportionment of cardiac output to vital organs including the brain and heart is necessary. Ultimately, the vasoconstriction becomes deleterious by increasing aortic impedance and placing additional load on the failing myocardium. Long-term, angiotensin II acts as a myocardial growth hormone, stimulating both myocyte hypertrophy and fibroblast hyperplasia.[3] The hypertrophic response, as well as the increased fibroblasts (with increased collagen deposition), renders the ventricular wall thickened and poorly compliant. Consequently, expansion of blood volume produces increased end-diastolic ventricular pressures rather than augmented cardiac output. Central and/or pulmonary venous pressure increases and fluid begins to back up into the capillary beds and leak into the soft tissues.

The importance of blocking the RAA system to prevent progressive cardiac dysfunction is highlighted by the beneficial effects of angiotensin-converting enzyme (ACE) inhibitors, which have shown efficacy in improving long-term survival and form a cornerstone in the medical management of adult heart failure. An immediate beneficial effect of the ACE inhibitor class is the achievement of afterload reduction, thereby decreasing the workload of the heart and allowing for an improvement in systolic function. Long-term use of ACE inhibitor is believed to slow the adverse ventricular remodeling that occurs in heart failure, although definitive trials in children have not been done. More recently, subtypes of the angiotensin receptor (AR) have been identified with unique distribution

in the myocardium and vasculature, each having somewhat unique downstream effects. Selective blockade of AR1 and AR2 is now achievable, opening the possibility of tailoring treatment to the individual.

Aldosterone inhibition is another target in the treatment of heart failure that has shown great benefit. Aldosterone, in addition to its effects in the kidney, exerts many of the same influences in the heart as angiotensin. Aldosterone causes vascular and myocardial remodeling, fibroblast proliferation, and increased collagen secretion. In addition to the hemodynamic effects due to the resultant stiff and poorly compliant ventricle, the cardiac fibrosis secondary to neurohormonal activation is also associated with increased arrhythmias and sudden death.[4] Although increased by renin activation, some aldosterone is produced independent of the renin–angiotensin system. The aldosterone receptor inhibitor, spironolactone, added to a regimen of ACE inhibitor, β-blocker, and loop diuretic reduces overall mortality, mortality from sudden cardiac death, and hospitalizations in adults with congestive heart failure (CHF).[5]

Adrenergic Activation

Myocardial dysfunction results in an early and sustained increase in catecholamine release. Although initially improving cardiac output through increases in contractility and heart rate, and direct renin release by the renal juxtaglomerular cells, sustained adrenergic stimulation rapidly becomes detrimental by the direct toxicity and stimulation of RAA system (Table 5.5.2). Plasma norepinephrine levels are a powerful predictor of mortality in adults with CHF.[6] Excessive norepinephrine is directly toxic to the cardiomyocyte.[7] Sympathetic activation of the heart alters contractile and metabolic proteins and leads to myocyte hypertrophy.

As the myocardium hypertrophies and undergoes fibrotic changes, the decreased compliance, elevated end-diastolic pressures, and increased wall stress all combine to decrease coronary perfusion and coronary reserve. With increased oxygen consumption and decreased delivery, myocardial performance is further compromised.

The shift from treating CHF with adrenergic agonists to blocking sympathetic stimulation emphasizes the importance of sympathetic activation in the progression of chronic myocardial failure. Several studies have shown increased mortality in patients treated with inotropes like dobutamine.[8] Instead, β-blocker therapy has been shown in multiple large adult trials to be beneficial in the treatment of heart failure. In children, the use of β-blockers has been slow to become accepted for other than a few indications including arrhythmias and aortic root dilatation. This reluctance may be due in part to the concern that the immature heart is more rate-dependent for maintaining cardiac output than its mature counterpart and that β-blockers decrease heart rate. Several small trials have nonetheless demonstrated that β-blockers both reduce the clinical symptoms of heart failure and decrease neurohormonal activation.[9,10] These agents effectively decrease activity of the RAA axis, decrease cardiac afterload by lowering vascular resistance, decrease myocardial oxygen demand while simultaneously improving coronary blood flow, and reduce myocardial arrhythmogenicity. Further, β-blockade reverses adverse ventricular remodeling.

The Natriuretic Peptides

Atrial natriuretic peptide (ANP) and brain natriuretic peptide (BNP) are made and released from the atrial and ventricular myocardium, respectively. They are continuously produced and secreted, but their secretion is increased by stretching of the wall, as occurs commonly in CHF.[11] The natriuretic peptides counter the hormonal systems that exacerbate heart failure, and therefore represent a unique defense against the seemingly relentless downward spiral of heart failure. Both peptides inhibit several hormonal systems including the RAA system, endothelins (which are potent vasoconstrictors), cytokines, and vasopressin. They decrease cardiac preload without inducing a compensatory oxygen-consuming tachycardia by modulating the sympathetic and parasympathetic nervous systems. They act directly on the kidneys to increase glomerular filtration, resulting in natriuresis and diuresis. A synthetic recombinant BNP, nesiritide, is now available for use in humans. Early trials in adults demonstrate that nesiritide provides global improvement in status, decreases both right atrial pressure and systemic vascular resistance, and improves cardiac output.

The fact that BNP has a basal secretion rate and that its levels are increased with ventricular stretch makes it a marker for heart failure and treatment response. BNP can serve a prognostic function in acute coronary syndrome and myocardial infarction. Preliminary studies in adults with CHF indicate that BNP levels might be useful in monitoring responsiveness to drug therapy.[11,12]

MOLECULAR PATHOPHYSIOLOGY AND THE FUTURE OF HEART FAILURE

The future of chronic heart failure management lies in the translation of the explosive growth in understanding the molecular mechanisms of heart failure into specifically targeted therapies. Areas of intense research interest include defining the role of oxidative stress and hypoxia in myocardial dysfunction. The generation of reactive oxygen species within myocytes causes oxidative damage to cellular macromolecules and is associated with failure. Hypoxic tissue injury increases the generation of reactive oxygen species and decreases the efficiency of the cellular mechanisms to neutralize the reactive oxygen species. Heart failure has been shown to result in the increased generation of reactive oxygen species, thereby providing the setting for a cycle of ongoing tissue damage and worsening myocardial function.[13] Newer antioxidant therapies including allopurinol, the xanthine oxidase inhibitor traditionally used to treat hyperuricemia, and carvedilol, a β-blocker that has antioxidant function in addition to blocking β-receptors, show promise as adjuncts to traditional heart failure medications.

An additional area of renewed interest is the role of intracellular calcium handling during heart failure. Perturbations in calcium release from sarcoplasmic reticulum by the ryanodine receptor, as well as its reuptake by the sarcoplasmic reticulum calcium ATPase (SERCA), play a key role in the development and worsening of failure. Recent advances have shown that calcium cycling abnormalities precede the observed depression of mechanical function.[14] This may have a potential for the development of diagnostic tools and treatment modalities that may allow earlier detection and reversal of heart failure. Additional areas of interest include transcriptional reprogramming, mitochondrial energy metabolism, and programmed cell death (apoptosis).

Much of the research involves adults, not children. Before any innovations can be applied to the pediatric population, careful trials will need to assess pediatric efficacy and untoward pediatric-specific side effects. The interest in developing treatments aimed at modifying calcium handling is a good example of a treatment for use in adults that may be expected to have very different effects in children. The application of high-throughput technologies such as genomics and proteomics, as well as increasingly sophisticated bioinformatics platforms, should greatly accelerate the pace of both discovery and development of suitable treatment options for heart failure. The unique physiology of the immature heart will require careful study of all new agents before widespread adoption to the pediatric patient with myocardial failure. Meanwhile, the available approach of using digoxin, diuretics, ACE inhibitors, and possibly β-blockers with added antioxidant capabilities provide the clinician with powerful tools to modify the often relentless course of chronic heart failure.

REFERENCES

1. Schwinger RH, Bohm M, Koch A, et al. The failing human heart is unable to use the Frank-Starling mechanism. *Circ Res.* 1994;74:959–969.
2. Schwartz SM, Duffy JY, Pearl JM, et al. Cellular and molecular aspects of myocardial dysfunction. *Crit Care Med.* 2001; 29:S214–S219.
3. Buchhorn R, Hammersen A, Bartmus D, et al. The pathogenesis of heart failure in infants with congenital heart disease. *Cardiol Young.* 2001;11:498–504.
4. Khan NU, Movahed A. The role of aldosterone and aldosterone-receptor antagonists in heart failure. *Rev Cardiovasc Med.* 2004; 5:71–81.
5. Deswal A, Yao D. Aldosterone receptor blockers in the treatment of heart failure. *Curr Treat Options Cardiovasc Med.* 2004;6:327–334.
6. Cohn Jn, Levine TB, Olivari MT, et al. Plasma norepinephrine as a guide to prognosis in patients with chronic congestive heart failure. *NEJM.* 1984;311:819–823.
7. Mann DL, Kent R, Parsons B, et al. Adrenergic effects on the biology of the adult mammalian cardiocyte. *Circulation.* 1992; 85:790–804.
8. Felker GM, O'Connor CM. Inotropic therapy for heart failure: An evidence based report. *Am Heart J.* 2001;142:393–401.
9. Buchhorn R, Hulpke-Wette M, Hilgers R, et al. Propranolol treatment of congestive heart failure in infants with congenital heart disease: The CHF-PRO-INFANT Trial. Congestive heart failure in infants treated with propranolol. *Int J Cardiol.* 2001;79: 167–173.
10. Giardini A, Formigari R, Bronzetti G, et al. Modulation of neurohormonal activity after treatment of children in heart failure with carvedilol. *Cardiol Young.* 2003;13:333–336.
11. Suttner SW, Boldt J. Natriuretic peptide system: Physiology and clinical utility: *Curr Opin Crit Care.* 2004;10:336–341.
12. Abassi Z, Karram T, Ellaham S, et al. Implications of the natriuretic peptide system in the pathogenesis of heart failure: Diagnostic and therapeutic importance. *Pharmacol Ther.* 2004;102:223–241.
13. Giordano FJ. Oxygen, oxidative stress, hypoxia, and heart failure. *J Clin Invest.* 2005;115:500–508.
14. Yano M, Ikeda Y, Matsuzaki M. Altered intracellular calcium handling in heart failure. *J Clin Invest.* 2005;115:556–564.

Cardiopulmonary Resuscitation

Vinay Nadkarni   Robert A. Berg

Approximately 450,000 North Americans die from cardiac arrest each year, nearly 90% in prehospital settings. The incidence of unexpected childhood cardiopulmonary arrest is approximately 16,000 American children per year.[1] Only 30% of out-of-hospital pediatric cardiac arrest patients receive bystander cardiopulmonary resuscitation (CPR).[1] Therefore, it is not surprising that the outcome following cardiac arrest in children has been reported to be very poor. Animal studies and human data both suggest that well-performed CPR for children can be quite effective. Prompt early action by laypersons in the prehospital setting or by a provider in the in-patient setting is generally more effective than late heroic efforts by intensive care life-support providers. The quality of CPR provided in and out of hospital settings is often poor, with numerous interruptions of chest compressions and overventilation.

EPIDEMIOLOGY OF CARDIAC ARREST IN CHILDREN

Pediatric cardiac arrests most frequently result from global asphyxia secondary to respiratory failure rather than from a sudden arrhythmic cardiac event. Sudden infant death syndrome (SIDS) is the leading cause of out-of-hospital pediatric cardiac arrest, followed by trauma, airway obstruction, and submersion.[2] Rare causes include congenital cardiac disease, poisoning, and central nervous system disease. Approximately 2% to 4% of the children admitted to a pediatric intensive care unit (ICU) have a cardiac arrest. Primary cardiac disease is present in patients having a cardiac arrest in an ICU as compared to out-of-hospital cardiac arrest.

The outcome of CPR vary depending on the location of the cardiac arrest, presenting echocardiogram (ECG) rhythm, duration of cardiac arrest, availability and quality of resuscitation, and the patient's preexisting medical condition. Initial return of spontaneous circulation (ROSC) occurs in 5% to 64% of pediatric patients. The outcome of CPR in children out of hospital settings remains dismal with reported 5% to 10% survival to hospital discharge. Survival is poor among patients with trauma and better in patients with a respiratory or submersion etiology. Survival is also improved in witnessed cardiac arrest and with pulseless electrical activity or ventricular fibrillation (VF) as the presenting arrest rhythm. In-hospital CPR has better survival outcomes, although results vary depending on patient location, diagnosis, and severity of illness. Survival to hospital discharge after cardiac arrest in a pediatric intensive care unit (PICU) is 15% to 27%.[3] Improved rates of survival to hospital discharge (44%) have been reported in pediatric cardiac ICU environment, where mechanical cardiopulmonary support is available.[4] Many survivors (10% to 83%) have significant neurologic disability.

THE FOUR PHASES OF CARDIAC ARREST AND CARDIOPULMONARY RESUSCITATION

There are at least four phases of cardiac arrest: (i) prearrest, (ii) no flow (untreated cardiac arrest), (iii) low flow (CPR), and (iv) postresuscitation. Interventions to improve outcome of pediatric cardiac arrest should optimize therapies targeted to the phase of resuscitation, as suggested in Table 5.6.1. The prearrest phase provides the opportunity to have the largest impact on patient survival by preventing cardiopulmonary arrest. Interventions during the prearrest phase focus on prevention, with special attention to early recognition and treatment of respiratory

TABLE 5.6.1
PHASES OF CARDIAC ARREST AND RESUSCITATION

Phase	Interventions
Prearrest phase (protect)	■ Optimize community education regarding child safety ■ Optimize patient monitoring ■ Prioritize interventions to avoid progression of respiratory failure and/or shock to cardiac arrest
Arrest (no flow) phase (preserve)	■ Minimize interval to BLS and ACLS/organized response ■ Preserve cardiac and cerebral substrate ■ Minimize interval to defibrillation, when indicated
Low-flow (CPR) phase (resuscitate)	■ Push hard, push fast, minimize interruptions in compressions ■ Titrate CPR to optimize myocardial blood flow (coronary perfusion pressures and exhaled CO_2) ■ Consider adjuncts to improve vital organ perfusion during CPR ■ Match oxygen delivery to oxygen demand ■ Consider extracorporeal CPR if standard CPR/ALS is not promptly successful
Postresuscitation phase (immediate) (hours to days)	■ Optimize cardiac output and cerebral perfusion ■ Treat arrhythmias, if indicated ■ Avoid hyperglycemia, hyperthermia, hyperventilation ■ Consider mild resuscitative systemic hypothermia (for 24–48 h following resuscitation)
Postresuscitation phase rehabilitation (regenerate)	■ Early intervention with occupational and physical therapy ■ Bioengineering and technology interface ■ Possible future role for stem cell transplant

BLS, basic life support; ACLS, advanced cardiovascular life support; CPR, cardiopulmonary resuscitation; ALS, advanced life support.

failure and shock in children. Specifically, the mobilization of medical emergency response teams to address rapid restoration of oxygenation, ventilation, and monitoring may improve outcome. Interventions during the no-flow phase of untreated cardiac arrest focus on early recognition of cardiac arrest and initiation of basic and advanced life support. When there is insufficient oxygen delivery to the brain or heart, CPR should be started. The goal of effective CPR is to optimize coronary perfusion pressure and blood flow to critical organs during the low-flow phase. Basic life support with continuous effective chest compressions (e.g., push hard, push fast, allow full chest recoil, minimize interruptions, and do not overventilate) is the emphasis in this phase. Improved rates of ROSC and long-term survival are associated with close monitoring of cardiac output using exhaled carbon dioxide and pulse pressure. Optimal CPR is frequently not provided, even in highly monitored in-patient environments.

The postresuscitation stage is a high-risk period for continuing brain injury, ventricular arrhythmias, and other reperfusion injuries. Injured cells can hibernate, die, or partially or fully recover function. Interventions such as systemic hypothermia during the immediate postresuscitation phase strive to minimize reperfusion injury and support cellular recovery. Overventilation is frequent and can have adverse effects during and following CPR.[5] The postarrest phase may have the most potential for innovative advances in the understanding of cell injury and death, inflammation, apoptosis, and hibernation, ultimately leading to novel interventions (see Chapter 7). Thoughtful attention to management of temperature, glucose, blood pressure, coagulation, ventilation, and carbon dioxide may be particularly important in this phase. The rehabilitation stage concentrates on salvage of injured cells, recruitment of hibernating cells, and re-engineering of reflex and voluntary communications of these cell and organ systems to improve functional outcome.

The specific phase of resuscitation should dictate the timing, intensity, duration, and focus of interventions. Emerging data suggest that interventions that can improve short-term outcome during one phase may be deleterious during another. For instance, intense vasoconstriction during the low-flow phase of cardiac arrest may improve coronary perfusion pressure and probability of ROSC.[6] The same intense vasoconstriction during the postresuscitation phase may increase left ventricular afterload and worsen myocardial strain and dysfunction.[6] Current understanding of the physiology of cardiac arrest and recovery only enables the crude titration of blood pressure, global oxygen delivery and consumption, body temperature, inflammation, coagulation, and other physiologic parameters in an attempt to optimize outcome. Future strategies will likely take advantage of emerging discoveries and knowledge of cellular inflammation, thrombosis, reperfusion, mediator cascades, cellular markers of injury and recovery, and transplantation technology.

INTERVENTIONS DURING THE LOW-FLOW PHASE: CARDIOPULMONARY RESUSCITATION

Airway and Breathing

The most common precipitating event for cardiac arrests in children is respiratory insufficiency. Therefore, providing adequate ventilation and oxygenation must remain the first priority. Effective ventilation does not necessarily require an endotracheal tube. A randomized, controlled study comparing outcomes of children with out-of-hospital respiratory arrest who received bag-mask ventilation compared to bag-mask ventilation followed by tracheal intubation did not demonstrate that prehospital placement of a tracheal tube improves outcome.[7] Effective bag-mask ventilation skills remain the cornerstone of providing effective emergency ventilation. Emergency airway techniques such as transtracheal jet ventilation and emergency cricothyroidotomy are rarely, if ever, required during CPR.

Provision of adequate oxygen delivery to meet the metabolic demand and removal of carbon dioxide are the goal of initial assisted breathing. During CPR, cardiac output and pulmonary blood flow are approximately 10% to 25% of that during normal sinus rhythm. Consequently, much less ventilation is necessary for adequate gas exchange from the blood traversing the pulmonary circulation during CPR. There is evidence that overventilation during CPR can be harmful by interfering with blood circulation.

Circulation

Blood is circulated during CPR by at least two different mechanisms: (i) the cardiac pump (direct compression of the heart between the sternum and the spine) and (ii) the thoracic pump (increases intrathoracic pressure, generating a gradient for blood to flow from the pulmonary vasculature, through the heart, and into the peripheral circulation). Underlying the cardiac pump mechanism, ventricular compression causes the atrioventricular valves to close and blood to be ejected into the aorta. During the relaxation phase, ventricular pressure falls and the atrioventricular valves open. This sequence of events occurs during open chest CPR. The cardiac pump mechanism also predominates in young children because of the relatively compliant thoracic wall. In children, from infancy through adolescence, the heart is immediately posterior to the lower third of the sternum, suggesting that focusing compressions in this area may optimize the cardiac pump in pediatric CPR. In older patients, several observations are inconsistent with the cardiac pump hypothesis. For example, echocardiographic studies of CPR show that the atrioventricular valves remain open during blood ejection. This supports the thoracic pump hypothesis and suggests that the heart is a passive conduit during CPR.

Variables Affecting the Effectiveness of Chest Compressions

Ratio of Compressions to Ventilation

Ideal compression–ventilation ratios for pediatric patients are unknown. Current compression–ventilation ratios and tidal volumes recommended during CPR are based on rational conjecture, tradition, and educational retention theory. Recent physiologic estimates suggest that the amount of ventilation provided should match, but not exceed, perfusion and should be titrated to the phase of resuscitation (no flow, low flow, high flow). The benefits of positive pressure ventilation (increased arterial content of oxygen) must be balanced against the adverse consequence of decreased circulation. Coronary perfusion pressure is higher after 15 uninterrupted compressions than after 5 and falls during ventilation.[8] In adult cardiac arrest, increasing the number of chest compressions to as many as 50 between ventilations or eliminating ventilation during bystander CPR may result in better hemodynamics and increased rates of ROSC. In animal models of sudden VF cardiac arrest, acceptable Pao_2 and $Paco_2$ persist with sudden cardiac arrest for 4 to 8 minutes in the absence of any rescue breathing.

Why is rescue breathing not necessary for such long periods in VF, yet quite important in asphyxia? Immediately after an acute VF cardiac arrest, aortic oxygen and carbon dioxide concentrations do not vary from the prearrest state. Therefore, when chest compressions are initiated, the blood flowing from the aorta to the coronary circulation has adequate oxygen content at an acceptable pH. Myocardial oxygen delivery is limited more by blood flow than by oxygen content. Adequate oxygenation and ventilation can continue without rescue breathing because of chest compression–induced gas exchange and spontaneous gasping ventilation during CPR.

Foregoing ventilation in the pediatric patient is not prudent because respiratory arrest and asphyxia generally precede pediatric cardiac arrest. During asphyxia, blood continues to flow to tissues, and arterial and venous oxygen saturation decrease while carbon dioxide and lactate levels increase for many minutes. In addition, continued pulmonary blood flow before the cardiac arrest depletes the pulmonary oxygen reservoir. Therefore, asphyxial arrests result in significant arterial hypoxemia and acidemia before resuscitation. Children with asphyxial cardiac arrests typically have a significantly higher $Paco_2$ and lower Pao_2 at the onset of cardiac arrest and following tracheal intubation than adults.[9]

Maximizing systemic oxygen delivery during single-rescuer CPR requires a trade-off between time spent doing chest compressions and time spent doing mouth-to-mouth ventilations. Theoretically, neither compression-only nor ventilation-only CPR can sustain systemic oxygen delivery. Some intermediate value of the compression-to-ventilation ratio is needed. The best intermediate value depends upon many factors including the compression rate, the tidal volume, the blood flow generated by compressions, and the time that compressions are interrupted to perform ventilations. A chest compression-to-ventilation ratio of 15:2 delivered the same minute ventilation as CPR with a chest compression-to-ventilation ratio of 5:1 in a mannequin model of pediatric CPR, but the number of chest compressions delivered was 48% higher with the 15:2 ratio.[10]

Duty Cycle

Duty cycle is the ratio of time of compression phase to the entire compression–relaxation cycle. In a model of human adult cardiac arrest, cardiac output and coronary blood flow are optimized when chest compressions last for 30% of the total cycle time. As the duration of CPR increases, the optimal duty cycle may increase to 50%. In a juvenile swine model, a relaxation period of 250 to 300 millisecond (a duty cycle of 40% to 50% if 120 compressions are delivered per minute) correlates with improved cerebral perfusion pressure when compared to shorter duty cycles of 30%.

Circumferential versus Focal Sternal Compressions

In adults and animal models of cardiac arrest, circumferential (vest) CPR improves CPR hemodynamics dramatically. In smaller infants, it is often possible to encircle the chest with both hands and depress the sternum with the thumbs, while compressing the thorax circumferentially. In an infant model of CPR, this "two-thumb" method of compression resulted in higher systolic and diastolic blood pressures and a higher pulse pressure than the traditional two-finger compression of the sternum.

Open Chest Cardiopulmonary Resuscitation

Excellent standard closed chest CPR generates a cerebral blood flow that is approximately 50% of the normal value. By contrast, open chest CPR can generate a cerebral blood flow that approaches the normal value. Although open chest massage improves coronary perfusion pressure and increases the chance of successful defibrillation in animals and humans, performing a thoracotomy to allow open chest CPR is impractical in many situations. A retrospective review of 27 cases of CPR following pediatric blunt trauma (15 with open chest CPR and 12 with closed chest CPR) demonstrated that open chest CPR increased hospital cost without altering rates of ROSC or survival to discharge.[11] However, survival in both groups was 0%, indicating that the population may have been too severely injured or too late in the process to benefit from this aggressive therapy. Earlier institution of open chest CPR may warrant reconsideration in select special resuscitation circumstances.

MONITORING EFFECTIVENESS OF CARDIOPULMONARY RESUSCITATION

Adequate myocardial perfusion pressure (MPP) is necessary for ROSC in CPR. MPP is the difference between aortic relaxation pressure and right atrial relaxation pressure. Without an arterial line, monitoring of the aortic relaxation or "diastolic" pressure is difficult.

The generation of exhaled carbon dioxide depends upon pulmonary blood flow. Therefore, circulation generated by chest compressions can be assessed to an extent by measuring end-tidal carbon dioxide. Chest compressions can be titrated to exhaled carbon dioxide as an index of pulmonary perfusion and cardiac output. In adults with cardiac arrest, an end-tidal carbon dioxide of >10 mm Hg is associated with ROSC and with hospital survival. In an animal model, end-tidal carbon dioxide during CPR correlates with coronary perfusion pressure and with ROSC.

In pediatric animal models of asphyxial cardiac arrest, end-tidal carbon dioxide is high at the initiation of CPR (likely representing exhalation of carbon dioxide that accumulates in the tissues and venous system while the animals are apneic but not pulseless) and then falls to levels similar to those seen during adult CPR.[12] Although end-tidal carbon dioxide monitoring is useful during pediatric CPR, pediatric-specific data is limited.

MECHANICAL DEVICES TO IMPROVE CARDIOPULMONARY RESUSCITATION HEMODYNAMICS

The goal of mechanical adjuncts to CPR is to increase cardiac output by increasing the action of the cardiac, thoracic, or abdominal pump or to provide artificial circulation to vital tissue beds. Potentially beneficial mechanical devices under development include pneumatic vests and bands, active compression–decompression and interposed abdominal compression CPR techniques, and inspiratory impedance threshold valves to increase venous return and cardiac output. None of these adjuncts to CPR has yet been adequately evaluated specifically in children.

Extracorporeal Membrane Oxygenation–Cardiopulmonary Resuscitation

The use of venoarterial extracorporeal membrane oxygenation (ECMO) to establish circulation and provide controlled reperfusion following cardiac arrest has been reported, but prospective, controlled studies are lacking. Nevertheless, these series of studies have reported extraordinary results with the use of an ECMO as a rescue therapy for pediatric cardiac arrests, especially from potentially reversible acute postoperative myocardial dysfunction or arrhythmias.[13] In one study, 11 children who had cardiac arrest in the PICU after cardiac surgery were placed on ECMO during CPR after 20 to 110 minutes of CPR. Prolonged CPR was continued until ECMO cannulae, circuits, and personnel were available. Six of these 11 children were long-term survivors without apparent neurologic sequelae. More recently, two centers have reported eight additional pediatric cardiac patients provided with mechanical cardiopulmonary support within 20 minutes of the initiation of CPR; all eight patients survived to hospital discharge. CPR and ECMO are not curative treatments. They are simply cardiopulmonary supportive measures that may allow tissue perfusion and viability until recovery from the precipitating disease process. Potential advantages of

ECMO include its ability to maintain tight control of physiologic parameters following resuscitation. For example, blood flow rates, oxygenation, ventilation, and body temperature can be manipulated precisely through the ECMO circuit.

MEDICATION USE DURING CARDIAC ARREST

Vasopressors

During CPR, epinephrine's α-adrenergic effect on vascular tone is most important. The α-adrenergic action increases systemic vascular resistance, increasing diastolic blood pressure, which in turn increases coronary perfusion pressure and blood flow and the likelihood of ROSC. Epinephrine also increases cerebral blood flow during CPR because peripheral vasoconstriction directs a greater proportion of flow to the cerebral circulation. The β-adrenergic effect increases myocardial contractility and heart rate and relaxes smooth muscles in the skeletal muscle vascular bed and bronchi, although this effect is of less importance. Epinephrine also increases the vigor and intensity of VF, increasing the likelihood of successful defibrillation.

High-dose epinephrine (0.05 to 0.2 mg per kg) improves myocardial and cerebral blood flow during CPR more than the standard-dose epinephrine (0.01 to 0.02 mg per kg) and may increase the incidence of initial ROSC. Administration of high-dose epinephrine, however, can worsen a patient's postresuscitation hemodynamic condition, with increased myocardial oxygen demand, hypertension, and myocardial necrosis. Retrospective studies indicate that the use of high-dose epinephrine in adults or children does not improve survival and may be associated with a worse neurologic outcome. A randomized, controlled trial of rescue high-dose epinephrine versus standard-dose epinephrine following failed initial standard-dose epinephrine in pediatric in-hospital cardiac arrest demonstrated a worse 24-hour survival in the high-dose epinephrine group (1/27 vs. 6/23, p <0.05).[14] High-dose epinephrine cannot be recommended routinely for initial therapy or rescue therapy.

Wide variability in catecholamine pharmacokinetics and pharmacodynamics dictate individual titration of therapy in non–cardiac arrest situations. Therefore, it is likely that a life-saving dose during CPR for one patient may be life threatening to another. Perhaps, high-dose epinephrine should be considered as an alternative to standard-dose epinephrine in special circumstances of refractory pediatric cardiac arrest (e.g., patient on high-dose epinephrine infusion before cardiac arrest) and/or when continuous direct arterial blood-pressure monitoring allows titration of the epinephrine dosage to diastolic (relaxation phase) arterial pressure during CPR. Nevertheless, high-dose epinephrine has not been demonstrated to improve outcome and should be used with caution.

Vasopressin is a long-acting endogenous hormone that acts at specific receptors to mediate systemic vasoconstriction (V_1 receptor) and reabsorption of water in the renal tubule (V_2 receptor). In experimental models of cardiac arrest, vasopressin increases blood flow to the heart and brain and improves long-term survival compared to epinephrine. Vasopressin may decrease splanchnic blood flow during and following CPR. In a small trial in adults, vasopressin had comparable efficacy to epinephrine. In a pediatric porcine model of prolonged VF, the use of vasopressin and epinephrine in combination resulted in higher left ventricular blood flow than either pressors alone, and both vasopressin alone and vasopressin plus epinephrine resulted in superior cerebral blood flow than epinephrine alone.[15] By contrast, in a pediatric porcine model of *asphyxial* cardiac arrest, ROSC was more likely in piglets treated with epinephrine than in those treated with vasopressin. A case series of four children who received vasopressin during six prolonged cardiac arrest events suggests that the use of bolus vasopressin may result in ROSC when standard medications have failed.[16] Vasopressin has also been reported to be useful in low cardiac output states associated with sepsis syndrome and organ recovery in children. Although vasopressin will not likely replace epinephrine as a first-line agent in pediatric cardiac arrest, there is preliminary data to suggest that its use in conjunction with epinephrine in pediatric cardiac arrest deserves further investigation.

Calcium

The indications for calcium administration during CPR are limited to a few specific indications, although its use is reported to be high. In the absence of hypocalcemia, the administration of calcium does not improve outcome in cardiac arrest and may worsen reperfusion injury. Calcium administration is indicated for hypocalcemia, hyperkalemia, hypermagnesemia, and calcium channel blocker overdose.

Buffer Solutions

Cardiac arrest results in lactic acidosis from inadequate organ blood flow and poor oxygenation. Acidosis depresses myocardial function and responsiveness to catecholamines, reduces systemic vascular resistance, and inhibits defibrillation. Nevertheless, the routine use of sodium bicarbonate for a child who has a cardiac arrest is not recommended. Clinical trials involving critically ill adults with severe metabolic acidosis did not demonstrate a beneficial effect of sodium bicarbonate. However, the presence of acidosis may depress the action of catecholamines, and so the use of sodium bicarbonate may be considered in an acidemic child who is refractory to catecholamine administration. The administration of sodium bicarbonate is also indicated in the patient with a tricyclic antidepressant overdose, hyperkalemia, hypermagnesemia, or sodium channel blocker poisoning.

The buffering action of bicarbonate occurs when a hydrogen cation and a bicarbonate anion combine to form carbon dioxide and water. If carbon dioxide is not effectively cleared through ventilation, its buildup will counterbalance the buffering effect of bicarbonate. Other side effects of using sodium bicarbonate include hypernatremia, hyperosmolarity, and metabolic alkalosis. Excessive alkalosis decreases calcium and potassium concentration and shifts the oxyhemoglobin dissociation curve to the left.

VENTRICULAR FIBRILLATION IN CHILDREN

VF has been an underappreciated pediatric problem. Two important studies demonstrated VF as the initial rhythm in 19% to 24% of out-of-hospital pediatric cardiac arrest patients.[17,18] Most previous investigations had indicated an incidence of VF in the range of 6% to 10% but had included substantial numbers of babies with SIDS. In special circumstances, such as tricyclic antidepressant overdose, cardiomyopathy, postcardiac surgery, and prolonged QT syndromes, VF and pulseless ventricular tachycardia (VT) are more likely presenting rhythms. VF can also occur secondary to asphyxia. It is well documented among near-drowning patients. In careful prospective studies of VF among asphyxiated piglets, the incidence was between 28% and 33% at some time during the cardiac arrest. This is supported by data from the American Heart Association (AHA) National Registry of CPR, which suggests that a shockable rhythm is the *initial* rhythm seen in 7% of all in-hospital pediatric cardiac arrest events requiring chest compressions and in 15% of all pulseless cardiac arrest events.[3] Further, up to 25% of pulseless cardiac arrest patients exhibit a shockable rhythm at some point during their cardiac arrest management.

The treatment of choice for short-duration VF is prompt defibrillation. The high-voltage countershock terminates VF by simultaneously depolarizing and causing a sustained contraction of myocardium. This allows spontaneous cardiac contractions to begin. The success of defibrillation decreases with increased duration of VF. The recommended defibrillation dose is 2 J per kg, but the data supporting this recommendation is minimal. Gutgesell et al. retrospectively evaluated the efficacy of their strategy to defibrillate with 2 J per kg.[19] Shocks within 10 J of 2 J per kg resulted in successful defibrillation in 91% of the defibrillation attempts.

Antiarrhythmic Medications: Lidocaine and Amiodarone

Administration of antiarrhythmic medications should not delay administration of countershock in a patient with VF. However, after unsuccessful attempts at electrical defibrillation, medications to increase the effectiveness of defibrillation should be considered. In both pediatric and adult patients, the current first-line medication in VF is epinephrine. If epinephrine with or without vasopressin and a subsequent repeat attempt to defibrillate are unsuccessful, lidocaine or amiodarone should be considered.

Lidocaine has been recommended traditionally for shock-resistant VF in adults and children. However, the only antiarrhythmic agent that has been prospectively determined to improve survival to hospital admission in the setting of shock-resistant VF when compared to placebo is amiodarone. In a study of shock-resistant out-of-hospital VF, patients receiving amiodarone had a higher rate of survival to hospital admission than patients receiving lidocaine. Both studies did not include children. There are no published comparisons of antiarrhythmic medications for pediatric refractory VF.

POSTRESUSCITATION INTERVENTIONS

Postresuscitation myocardial function and hypoxic–ischemic encephalopathy, with associated multiple organ failure, is common following cardiac arrest in children. Key neurologic support measures are given in detail in Chapter 7. Goal-directed therapy targets for temperature, blood pressure, ventilation, and blood glucose have been associated with improved outcomes following resuscitation.

LIMITATIONS TO UNDERSTANDING PEDIATRIC CARDIAC ARREST AND CARDIOPULMONARY RESUSCITATION

Our knowledge of the epidemiology and appropriate treatment of pediatric cardiac arrest has been limited, in part, because we have lumped diverse diseases and pathophysiologies. Pediatric studies tend to include all pediatric cardiac arrests, including those secondary to sudden respiratory failure (e.g., drowning, foreign body aspiration), progressive respiratory failure from infections and/or neuromuscular diseases, trauma, SIDS, septic shock, hypovolemic shock, anaphylaxis, primary cardiomyopathy, primary arrhythmia (e.g., VF or VT), and drug intoxications. Some pediatric studies have reported lumped respiratory arrests with cardiac arrests, and many have included both prehospital and in-hospital cardiac arrests in their data. Moreover, many of the cardiac arrest patients in these studies had been dead for a prolonged period (e.g., SIDS), and, therefore, data such as initial cardiac rhythm of asystole and lack of response to therapy are not helpful in terms of understanding the etiology, pathophysiology, or appropriate therapy. Quality of CPR is generally poor and not easily accounted for in prior studies of cardiac arrest. Finally, most pediatric cardiac arrest studies have suffered from inadequate and nonuniform data collection. In response to this issue, international resuscitation experts have established

Utstein-style international consensus guidelines for uniform reporting of cardiac arrest data.[20]

CONCLUSION

Pediatric cardiac arrests most frequently result from global asphyxia secondary to respiratory failure (hypoxia and ischemia) rather than from a sudden arrhythmic cardiac event. Outcomes following pediatric cardiac arrest and CPR are often poor but appear to be improving. The evolving understanding of pathophysiologic events before, during, and after pediatric cardiac arrest contribute to these improvements. Matching the timing, sequence, intensity, and duration of therapeutic interventions to prevent cardiac arrest, and protect, preserve, and promote restoration of intact neurologic survival is of the highest priority. By strategically focusing therapies to four specific phases and pathophysiology of cardiac arrest and resuscitation and improving the quality of a few critical interventions, there is great promise that critical care interventions will lead the way to more successful cardiopulmonary and cerebral resuscitation in children.

REFERENCES

1. Young KD, Seidel JS. Pediatric cardiopulmonary resuscitation: A collective review. *Ann Emerg Med.* 1999;33(2):195–205.
2. American Heart Association in collaboration with International Liaison Committee on Resuscitation. Guidelines 2000 for cardiopulmonary resuscitation and emergency cardiovascular care: International Consensus on Science, Part 6: Advanced cardiovascular life support: 7B: understanding the algorithm approach to ACLS. *Circulation.* 2000;102(suppl I)(8):I140–I141.
3. Reis AG, Nadkarni V, Perondo MB, et al. A prospective investigation into the epidemiology of in-hospital pediatric cardiopulmonary resuscitation using the international Utstein reporting style. *Pediatrics.* 2002;109(2):200–209.
4. Parra DA, Totapally BR, Zalui E, et al. Outcome of cardiopulmonary resuscitation in a pediatric cardiac intensive care unit. *Crit Care Med.* 2000;28(9):3296–3300.
5. Aufderheide TP, Lurie KG. Death by hyperventilation: A common and life-threatening problem during cardiopulmonary resuscitation. *Crit Care Med.* 2004;32(9 Suppl):S345–S351.
6. Yakaitis RW, Otto CW, Blitt CD. Relative importance of alpha and beta adrenergic receptors during resuscitation. *Crit Care Med.* 1979;7(7):293–296.
7. Gausche M, Lewis RJ, Stratton SJ, et al. Effect of out-of-hospital pediatric endotracheal intubation on survival and neurological outcome: A controlled clinical trial. *JAMA.* 2000;283(6):783–790.
8. Paradis NA, Martin GB, Rivers EP, et al. Coronary perfusion pressure and the return of spontaneous circulation in human cardiopulmonary resuscitation. *JAMA.* 1990;263(8):1106–1113.
9. Berg RA, Henry C, Otto CW, et al. Initial end-tidal CO_2 is markedly elevated during cardiopulmonary resuscitation after asphyxial cardiac arrest. *Pediatr Emerg Care.* 1996;12(4):245–248.
10. Kinney SB, Tibballs J. An analysis of the efficacy of bag-valve-mask ventilation and chest compression during different compression-ventilation ratios in manikin-simulated paediatric resuscitation. *Resuscitation.* 2000;43(2):115–120.
11. Sheikh A, Brogan T. Outcome and cost of open- and closed-chest cardiopulmonary resuscitation in pediatric cardiac arrests. *Pediatrics.* 1994;93(3):392–398.
12. Bhende MS, Thompson AE. Evaluation of an end-tidal CO2 detector during pediatric cardiopulmonary resuscitation. *Pediatrics.* 1995;95(3):395–399.
13. Morris MC, Wernovsky G, Nadkarni VM. Survival outcomes after extracorporeal cardiopulmonary resuscitation instituted during active chest compressions following refractory in-hospital pediatric cardiac arrest. *Pediatr Crit Care Med.* 2004;5(5):440–446.
14. Perondi MB, Reis AG, Paiva EF, et al. A comparison of high-dose and standard-dose epinephrine in children with cardiac arrest. *N Engl J Med.* 2004;350(17):1722–1730.
15. Voelckel WG, Lurie KG, McKnite S, et al. Comparison of epinephrine and vasopressin in a pediatric porcine model of asphyxial cardiac arrest. *Crit Care Med.* 2000;28)12):3777–3783.
16. Mann K, Berg RA, Nadkarni V. Beneficial effects of vasopressin in prolonged pediatric cardiac arrest: A case series. *Resuscitation.* 2002;52(2):149–156.
17. Hickey RW, Cohen DM, Strausbaugh S, et al. Pediatric patients requiring CPR in the prehospital setting. *Ann Emerg Med.* 1995;25(4):495–501.
18. Mogayzel C, Quan L, Graves JR, et al. Out-of-hospital ventricular fibrillation in children and adolescents: Causes and outcomes. *Ann Emerg Med.* 1995;25(4):484–491.
19. Gutgesell HP, Tacker WA, Geddes LA, et al. Energy dose for ventricular defibrillation of children. *Pediatrics.* 1976;58(6):898–901.
20. Idris AH, Becker LB, Ornato JP, et al. Utstein-style guidelines for uniform reporting of laboratory CPR research. A statement for healthcare professionals from a Task Force of the American Heart Association, the American College of Emergency Physicians, the American College of Cardiology, the European Resuscitation Council, the Heart and Stroke Foundation of Canada, the Institute of Critical Care Medicine, the Safar Center for Resuscitation Research, and the Society for Academic Emergency Medicine. *Resuscitation.* 1996;33(1):69–84.

Pulmonology

Heidi J. Dalton   *Mark J. Heulitt*

"... and God breathed into his nostrils the breath of life, and the man became a living being" Genesis 2:7

This chapter's focus is to expose the reader to the important principles of respiratory physiology and to serve as a primer to other chapters that utilize these principles. First, the important components of the respiratory tree outside the lungs are described; then, the lung development, function, response to injury, and interactions with other organs are considered in more detail.

Airway Structures and Functions

Heidi J. Dalton

EXTRATHORACIC

Nose

The primary responsibility of the upper respiratory tract is to condition inspired air to protect the delicate distal lung units. The nose, sinuses, pharynx, and larynx work together to provide decontamination, warming, and humidification of inspired air.

The nose is a network of epithelial cells lying over a capillary plexus supported by bony plates called *turbinates*. The function of the vascular and epithelial structures is controlled by humoral and neural mediators. The tissue of the nose is constantly bathed by thin, watery secretions that function to trap foreign material and add humidity to inspired air. When breathing normally, the inspired air is heated rapidly to body temperature and the humidity is increased to 90%. An intricate system of baffles in the nose accomplishes these functions and also accounts for a higher resistance to airflow than when breathing through the mouth. During exercise, mouth breathing may predominate over nasal breathing to allow for higher airflow. As inspired dry, cold air bypasses the nose and enters the lower airways directly through the mouth, bronchial tree irritation may result in bronchospasm. Mechanically ventilated patients and those with a tracheostomy require artificially humidified air to prevent drying or irritation of the bronchial tree that accompanies bypassing the humidification function of the nose.

Sinuses

The sinuses communicate with the nasal passages by narrow openings that can become occluded when inflammation occurs. The cilia within the sinuses propel secretions toward this opening into the nasal cavity. The purpose of the sinuses is unknown, although they may insulate the cranial vault and increase the resonance of the voice. If sinusitis occurs, secretions, referred to as *postnasal drip*, may drain into the pharynx and become aspirated into the respiratory tract, especially during sleep, causing chronic bronchial irritation.

Pharynx

The pharynx is divided into the nasopharynx, which consists of the adenoids, tonsils and eustachian tubes, and the oropharynx, which acts as the entry to the larynx and esophagus. The epiglottis is an important oropharyngeal structure situated at the base of the tongue to protect the laryngeal opening during swallowing and to prevent the aspiration of oral material into the trachea. Infants have an elongated epiglottis, which is positioned high in the pharynx and almost meets the soft palate, creating a direct pathway from the nose to the lungs for air entry. Infants are obligate nose breathers. If either partial or complete occlusion of the nasopharynx occurs, dramatic increases in the work of breathing and respiratory failure can result. Infants with difficulty in feeding, retractions, or obstructive apnea can benefit from an investigation of the nasal airway. The epiglottis is longer and floppier in infants and young children than in adults. Therefore, a straight laryngoscope blade, which allows direct lifting of the epiglottis, may facilitate intubation, whereas in older children and adults, a curved laryngoscope blade that fits above the epiglottis to lift the soft tissues of the neck and expose the vocal cords and trachea may be preferred.

Vocal Cords

The vocal cords sit below the epiglottis at the entry to the trachea. The vocal cords are important for phonation and are a defense mechanism to prevent aspiration of foreign material into the trachea and lungs. For material that bypasses this important mechanism, coughing is the backup method to clear secretions collecting in the larger airways. When the vocal cords close and the respiratory and abdominal muscles contract, high pressure is generated in the lower airways. When the vocal cords open suddenly, a rush of air from the lower airways expels foreign material from the lungs. Injury or paralysis to one or both vocal cords may change voice tone or cause hoarseness. Bilateral vocal cord paralysis causes symptoms of inspiratory stridor, hoarseness, dyspnea, and anxiety.

INTRATHORACIC

Trachea

The trachea extends from the base of the neck to the level of the second anterior rib, where it branches into the right and left main bronchi. The bifurcation point is called *the carina*. The left bronchus projects off the trachea at an angle of 50 to 100 degrees, which is a much sharper angle than the right bronchus. The right bronchus is also larger than the left. These two characteristics may explain why aspirated material more frequently enters the right rather than the left side of the major airways. Upon entering the thorax, the right bronchus branches almost immediately into the upper lobe and intermediate bronchi. There are three main lobar bronchi on the right and two on the left. These continue to branch into the segmental bronchi, ten on the right and nine on the left.

The tracheal walls are held open anteriorly by horseshoe-shaped cartilaginous rings while fibrous bands form the posterior aspect. The airway grows both in length and diameter with age. Until the age of 5 years, the airway's anterior portion grows faster than the distal segments, resulting in a relative narrowing of the distal portion of the airway. Because resistance to airflow is inversely proportional to the fourth power of the radius during laminar flow and to the fifth power of the radius during turbulent flow, this distal narrowing explains the susceptibility of young infants with lower airway infections and inflammation to respiratory failure.

Cartilaginous support reaches the level of the segmental bronchi by the 12th gestational week. From birth to 2 months of age, the cartilage increases in depth, and during childhood, it increases in area. The weaker cartilage in infants and young children predisposes them to dynamic airway collapse in circumstances of high expiratory flow and increased airway resistance, as occurs with crying, bronchiolitis, and asthma.

Mucous glands in the major bronchi are innervated by both the sympathetic and parasympathetic nervous systems, which connect to the brain through the vagus nerve. Receptors within the bronchi initiate the cough reflex, and cause mucous secretion and bronchoconstriction. Substance P and neurokinins appear to mediate these reactions within the airway. Irritation within one area of the bronchi can affect the entire airway.

RECOMMENDED READINGS

1. Staub NC, Albertine KH. The structure of the lungs relative to their principal function. In: Murray JF, Nadel JA, eds. *Textbook of respiratory medicine*. Philadelphia, PA: WB Saunders; 1988:12–16.
2. Garrity ER Jr, Shart JT. Respiratory muscles: Function and dysfunction. *AACP Pulm Crit Care Update*. 19862:Lesson 10.
3. Carden DL, Matthay MA, George RB. Functional anatomy of the respiratory system. In: George RB, Light RW, Matthay MA, et al., eds. *Chest medicine: Essentials of pulmonary and critical care medicine*. Vol. 1. Philadelphia, PA: Lippincott Williams & Wilkins; 2000:1–10.

Embryologic and Postnatal Airway and Lung Development

Angela T. Wratney   *Ronald C. Sanders Jr*   *Heidi J. Dalton*

EMBRYOLOGIC DEVELOPMENT

Prenatal lung development is divided into four stages on the basis of the histologic characteristics (see Fig. 6.2.1). Sequential branching of airway and vascular structures through these stages constructs a template upon which the adult lung develops and functions.

Lung development begins with the formation of a laryngotracheal groove within the endodermal epithelium of the embryonic anterior pharynx at 5 weeks of gestation. This groove or outpouching becomes the tracheal rudiment that gives rise to two primary bronchial buds, which are the future lung anlage (primordium) (see Fig. 6.2.2). These bronchial buds grow and undergo a series of branching events into the surrounding mesenchyme. The surrounding mesenchyme influences the proliferation, migration, and differentiation of these branches. The proximal mesenchyme stimulates the development of the trachea and upper bronchi, whereas more peripheral mesenchyme stimulates the growth of bronchioles and terminal bronchioles. Distally, the mesenchyme facilitates the creation of alveoli. Mesenchymal–epithelial interactions are critical to the development of the lung primordium. These interactions depend upon an interplay of local growth factors and inhibitors. The mesenchymal branching occurs through 23 generations and is completed by 40 weeks gestation.

Pseudoglandular Stage (5 to 16 Weeks)

This stage is characterized by the glandular appearance of the tissue sections. Progressive airway branching and vascular differentiation characterize the pseudoglandular stage.

Vascular system changes that occur during gestation result in the aortic outflow tract becoming connected to the fourth aortic arch while the pulmonary outflow tract becomes connected to the sixth aortic arch. The connection, which remains between the pulmonary tract and the descending aorta, is called *the ductus arteriosus*. Differentiation within the vascular system creates two sources of blood supply for the lung, the bronchial, and pulmonary circulations. The bronchial circulation supplies the conducting airways, connective tissue, and pleura from the trachea to the terminal bronchioles. The bronchial arteries supply only a small fraction of the total pulmonary blood flow and do not participate in gas exchange. By 16 weeks gestation, the development of the bronchial circulation is complete.

The pulmonary arterial circulation eventually forms the capillary network necessary for gas exchange. These arteries course along the branching airways, infiltrating toward the center of the lobules and dividing extensively in the periphery of the fetal lung. Pulmonary veins and lymphatics develop along a separate pathway, coursing between the branching airways within the connective tissue septa, which demarcate each pulmonary segment.

Canalicular Stage (16 to 25 Weeks)

Pulmonary development in the canalicular stage integrates the developing capillary network with peripherally developing respiratory units. Vascularization occurs by

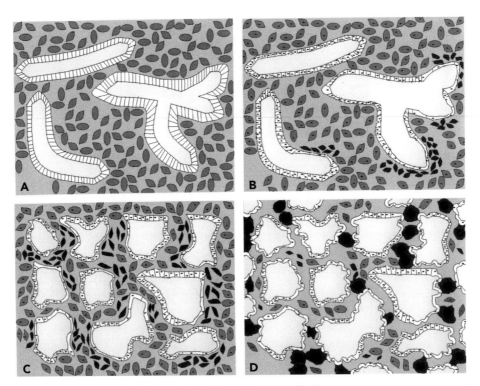

Figure 6.2.1 The prenatal phase of lung development is divided into four stages on the basis of the histologic characteristics. **A:** The first stage is the pseudoglandular stage, which occurs from 5 to 16 weeks and is characterized by its glandular appearance. The primordial lung begins differentiating into cells that are destined to be airway and respiratory cells. **B:** The canalicular stage takes place from 16 to 25 weeks, and it exhibits further differentiation of bronchi, bronchioles, and alveoli. The hallmark of the canalicular stage is the development of the pulmonary capillary system facilitated by the close interaction of primitive angioblasts (vasculogenesis) with the distal pulmonary epithelium. (Note: The other postulated mechanism of pulmonary vascular development, angiogenesis, is not shown here.) **C:** The terminal-sac stage continues after the canalicular stage and is recognized by the appearance of saccules, which will continue to divide by means of ridges or secondary crests. Alveoli are seen as early as 32 weeks and will continue to expand their surface area greatly. **D:** The alveolar stage begins at birth, with additional alveolar development and growth occurring along with vascular network enhancement.

two different mechanisms, angiogenesis and vasculogenesis. Angiogenesis is the creation of blood vessels by the branching and spreading of preexisting vasculature. Vasculogenesis is the construction of vessels from individual angioblasts. The pulmonary vasculature is thought to arise by means of vasculogenesis or a combination of angiogenesis and vasculogenesis. Lung vessels exist initially as capillarylike structures in 70% of the lung during the pseudoglandular stage. These structures account for approximately 90% of the pulmonary vessels in the terminal-sac stage. More importantly, the branching bronchial epithelium exhibits staining for vascular endothelial growth factor (VEGF) that is most intense at the distal airways. VEGF assists with the proliferation of pulmonary capillaries noted in the terminal areas of the lung. Once formed, this dense pulmonary capillary network organizes more tightly around the distal airways. The capillary network expands as the parenchymal interstitial thickness decreases, eventually forming a single capillary tightly adjacent to

the alveolar epithelium. During this stage of development, the total surface area of the air–blood barrier increases exponentially.

In synchrony with the development of the pulmonary circulation, the conducting airways dichotomously branch to form approximately 17 generations of bronchi at the level of the terminal bronchioles. Distal growth, beyond the terminal bronchioles, forms the future gas exchange portions of the lung known as the *terminal respiratory unit* (TRU).

The TRU is composed of respiratory bronchioles, alveolar ducts, and alveolar sacs (see Fig. 6.2.3). The alveolar ducts are small canals completely lined with alveolar sacs. As development progresses, the alveolar epithelium flattens into individual cells (alveolar type I cells) that function alongside cuboidal cells (alveolar type II cells). Alveolar type I cells appear by 20 to 24 weeks gestation. At a gestational age of 24 weeks, both alveolar type I and type II cells are present. The formation of groups of two to

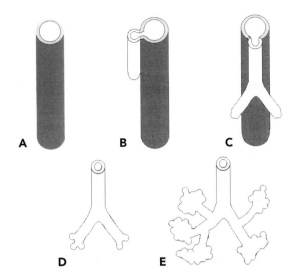

Figure 6.2.2 The lung anlage (primordium) arises from the **(A)** embryonic pharynx as a **(B)** laryngotracheal groove on the anterior surface. Shortly thereafter, the **(C)** two bronchial buds are formed. From the bronchial buds, a series of asymmetric branching and expansion events **(D,E)** occur into the surrounding mesenchyme that give rise to a right trilobed lung and a left bilobed lung.

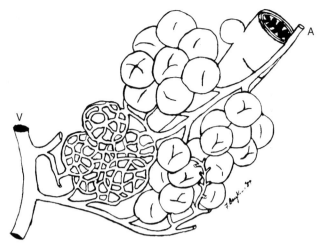

Figure 6.2.3 A terminal respiratory unit (TRU), which is the basic gas exchange unit of the lungs. The pulmonary artery branch (A) enters the center of the TRU along with the terminal bronchiole. It anastomoses with the pulmonary venule in the alveolar walls, forming a dense capillary network for gas exchange. Venous drainage is to the periphery of the TRU, where the venous branches (V) lie. They coalesce to form the major pulmonary veins, which carry oxygenated blood. (From George RB, Light RW, Matthay MA, et al. *Chest medicine: Essentials of pulmonary and critical care medicine.* 4th ed. Philadelphia, PA: Lippincott Williams & Wilkins; 2000:21.)

four respiratory bronchioles, each communicating with six to seven generations of alveolar ducts, is critical to the development of the expansive cross-sectional surface area needed for efficient gas exchange within the lung.

Saccular Stage (25 Weeks to Term)

Transformation of the immature saccular lung with limited gas exchange capacity to a mature lung with a large internal surface area requires thinning of the alveolar walls, growth of the dense capillary network, and extensive subdivision of gas exchange units into alveoli. Alveolar ducts branch, elongate, and dilate until mature alveoli form in the 30-week fetus. Alveoli are common by 36 weeks of gestation (see Fig. 6.2.4). The alveolar epithelium accounts for approximately 25% of the total cells in the lung and is composed almost exclusively of type I and type II cells. Flat type I cells cover 95% of the alveolar surface area, with thinned processes fused along the capillary basement membrane. These type I epithelial cells, originally characterized as *la petite alvéolaire cellule*, are flat, with little cytoplasm, few organelles, and numerous pinocytic vesicles. Type II epithelial cells, initially known as *la grande alvéolaire cellule*, are cuboidal and possess microvilli on their apical surface. Although type II cells outnumber type I cells by a ratio of 2:1, type I cells cover 93% of the air–lung interface. Type I cells serve to facilitate gas exchange and water transport through a specialized structure known as *aquaporins*. Type II cells contain cytoplasmic lamellar bodies and are responsible for the production of pulmonary surfactant. In addition, type II cells are the progenitor cells of the alveolar epithelium capable of replicating to

replace both type I and type II cells that are lost following lung injury.

By the end of gestation, the walls of the mature alveolar sacs appear as if they are composed almost completely of capillaries. The alveolar capillaries are a single, nonfenestrated, endothelial cell layer without a muscular media and connected by tight junctions. These capillaries thin to form an almost continuous sheet of blood in the alveolar wall with a diameter just sufficient to allow for the passage of a red blood cell (10 μm). This architecture maximizes the gas exchange potential. Branches from the pulmonary arteries feed into this capillary mesh at intervals. Unlike capillaries in the systemic circulation, most pulmonary capillaries are surrounded by air and not supportive tissue. Although this improves the surface area for gas exchange, it also poses an increased risk for rupture at high intravascular pressures.

Following oxygenation, blood flows from the pulmonary capillaries to the pulmonary veins at the level of the terminal bronchioles. These smaller veins merge and form the four pulmonary veins that empty into the left atrium. Some blood from the bronchial system also empties into the pulmonary veins. The bronchial arteries branch off the systemic circulation to supply the tissues of the lung. Because bronchial blood flow does not participate in gas exchange, venous return from the bronchial vessels is deoxygenated. This bronchial flow mixed with the pulmonary venous return accounts for a large part of the shunt fraction noted within normal lungs.

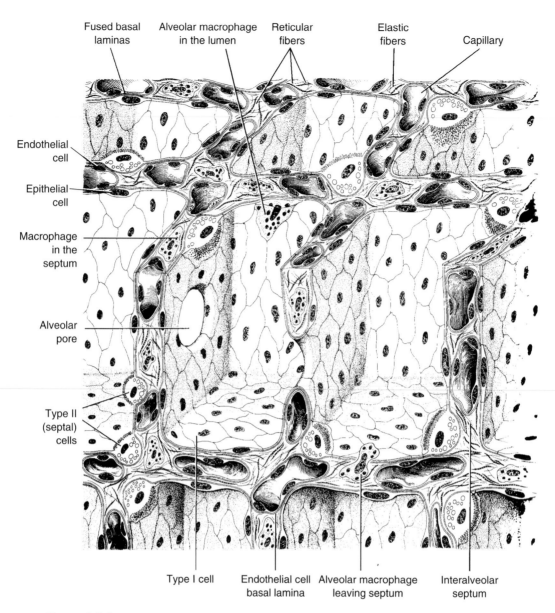

Figure 6.2.4 Three-dimensional schematic diagram of pulmonary alveoli. Observe the capillaries, connective tissue, and macrophages. These cells can also be seen in the alveolar lumens or passing into them. Alveolar pores are numerous. Type I cells are flat and attenuated. Type II cells are identified by their abundant apical microvilli. The alveoli are lined by a continuous epithelial layer. (From Junqueira LC, Carneiro J, Long JA. *Basic histology.* 5th ed. Los Altos, CA: Lange Medical Publications; 1986:390.)

The pulmonary arterial system is extremely compliant, estimated at 7 mL per mm Hg, and can accommodate large changes in stroke volume from the right heart. This arrangement between alveoli and capillaries also regulates fluid and solute exchange within the lung parenchyma. The alveolar epithelium forms a barrier that limits water and solute movement into the alveolar space. Protein adhesion within the tight junctions of the alveolar epithelium controls the movement of fluid both into and out of the alveolus. The epithelium may also assist in the reabsorption of fluid within the alveolus. The thin endothelium of the pulmonary capillary has cell–cell junctions, which accounts for most fluid and solutes across the vascular endothelium. These junctions consist of occludins and cadherins. The pulmonary endothelial cells can express adhesion molecules, which can contribute to increased fluid leak after a lung insult. The adhesive proteins produced may interact with other receptors to mediate leukocyte activity and tissue migration following lung injury (see Fig. 6.2.5). Some fluid may also leak from junctions between the alveolar walls and the arterioles and venules.

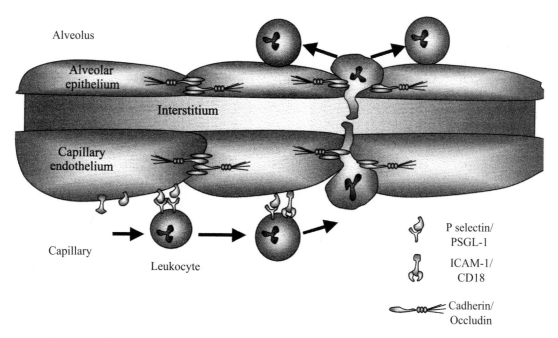

Figure 6.2.5 The interaction of the adhesion glycoprotein, P selectin, on the alveolar endothelium with P selectin glycoprotein ligand-1 (PSGL-1) on white blood cells mediates leukocyte rolling along the vascular wall. The interaction of endothelial intercellular adhesion molecule-1 (ICAM-1) with the leukocyte adhesive determinant, CD 18, contributes to firm leukocyte adhesion and extravascular migration. These events contribute to leukocyte movement in the lung and alter the barrier properties of the alveolar–capillary membrane. (From George RB, Light RW, Matthay MA, et al. *Chest medicine: Essentials of pulmonary and critical care medicine.* 4th ed. Philadelphia, PA: Lippincott Williams & Wilkins; 2000:15.)

POSTNATAL LUNG DEVELOPMENT AND FUNCTION

At birth, pulmonary development remains incomplete. The immature neonatal lung will continue to develop for several years. The adult lung contains 23 to 25 bronchial branches, 60,000 TRUs, 500,000 alveolar ducts, and 300 to 500 million alveoli. At birth, the neonatal lung has approximately 17 to 20 bronchi and approximately 50 million formed alveoli. In early childhood, the lung will undergo bronchiolar branching, continued alveolar formation and maturation, and a corresponding increase in lung volume and size. Although the neonatal lung retains remarkable growth potential, its long-term potential can be adversely affected by insults caused within this vulnerable period.

As the lung matures, three collateral anatomic channels develop, which allow ventilation to an obstructed airway (see Fig. 6.2.6). These paths consist of passages between alveolar sacs that can distribute gas between one another and are called *pores of Kohn*. These openings are noted in the 1st or 2nd year of life and appear as holes in the alveolus. Epithelial-lined canals known as *Lambert channels* allow communication between a bronchiole and its adjacent alveolus. These channels develop after 6 to 8 years of age. Interbronchiolar connections, although not present in normal lungs, may also be present in diseased lungs,

particularly those affecting the small airways. These three types of collateral ventilation can increase physiologic dead space and ventilation–perfusion mismatch by allowing airflow into lung segments that are distal to the obstructed airways; however, they help prevent these distal segments from becoming atelectatic.

Alveoli participate in efficient gas exchange only after birth. The fetal lungs are filled with fluid that contains surfactant, mucus, and a small amount of protein, which maintains airway patency and indirectly influences the size

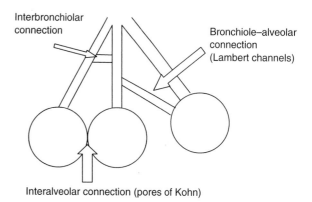

Figure 6.2.6 Alternative ventilatory channels.

and growth of the lung. Most of the lung fluid is rapidly resorbed into the blood and lymph capillaries during labor in an epinephrine-mediated process that results in cessation of fluid production and augmentation of fluid removal. At birth, lung inflation stimulates the active uptake of sodium across the type II epithelial cells, leading to the clearance of residual alveolar fluid.

Changes in postnatal lung function also influence the ductus arteriosus. In the fetus, approximately 8% of the cardiac output flows through the ductus arteriosus to perfuse the pulmonary circulation, whereas 68% of cardiac flow is directed to the descending aorta. As oxygen tension increases in the pulmonary circulation after birth and local prostaglandin E (PGE) activity falls, ductal closure begins. By 10 days of age, complete ductal closure occurs. Failure of the ductus to close can result in severe hypoxia and poor systemic oxygenation.

Other Aspects of Lung Development and Function

The interstitium is bound by the epithelial and endothelial basement membranes. It contains approximately 37% of all cells in the pulmonary parenchyma and is composed predominantly of mesenchymal cells, lymphocytes, inflammatory cells, pericytes, and stroma. Neutrophils are rarely found in the interstitium. In addition, several connective tissue macromolecules exist here and include collagens type I and III, elastin, fibronectin, and proteoglycans. Type IV collagen, laminin, and fibronectin are macromolecules that are typically found in the basement membranes.

RECOMMENDED READINGS

1. Warburton D, Schwarz M, Tefft D, et al. The molecular basis of lung morphogenesis. *Mech Dev.* 2000;92(1):55–81.
2. Merkus PJ, Ten Have-Opbroek AA, Quanjer PH. Human lung growth: A review. *Pediatr Pulmonol.* 1996;21(6):383–397.
3. Shannon JM, Hyatt BA. Epithelial-mesenchymal interactions in the developing lung. *Annu Rev Physiol.* 2004;66:625–645.
4. Warburton D, Zhao J, Berberich MA, et al. Molecular embryology of the lung: Then, now, and in the future. *Am J Physiol.* 1999;276(5 Pt 1):L697–L704.
5. Sadler T. Chapter 13: Respiratory system. *Langman's medical embryology.* 5th ed. Baltimore, MD: Williams & Wilkins; 1985:215–223.
6. Maeda S, Suzuki S, Suzuki T, et al. Analysis of intrapulmonary vessels and epithelial-endothelial interactions in the human developing lung. *Lab Invest.* 2002;82(3):293–301.
7. Cutz E. Cytomorphology and differentiation of airway epithelium in developing human lung. In: McDowell EM, ed. *Lung carcinomas.* Edinburgh: Churchill Livingstone; 1987:1–41.
8. Crapo JD, Barry BE, Gehr P, et al. Cell number and cell characteristics of the normal human lung. *Am Rev Respir Dis.* 1982;126(2):332–337.
9. Berthiaume Y, Hans GF, Matthay MA. Lung edema clearance: 20 years of progress. Invited review: Alveolar edema fluid clearance in the injured lung. *J Appl Physiol.* 2002;93:2007–2213.
10. West JB. *Respiratory physiology.* 5th ed. Coryell Patricia A, ed. Philadelphia, PA: Williams & Wilkins; 1995.
11. Meyrick B, Reid L. The alveolar wall. *Br J Dis Chest.* 1970; 64(3):121–140.
12. Morrell NW, Roberts CM, Biggs T, et al. Collateral ventilation and gas exchange during airway occlusion in the normal human lung. *Am Rev Respir Dis.* 1993;147:535–539.
13. Terry RB, Traystman RJ, Newball HH, et al. Collateral ventilation in man. *N Engl J Med.* 1978;298:10.
14. Jobe AH. The respiratory system. In: Faranoff AA, Martin RJ, eds. *Neonatal-perinatal medicine: Diseases of the fetus and infant,* 7th ed. Philadelphia, PA: Mosby; 2002:973–991.
15. American Thoracic Society Documents. Mechanisms and limits of induced postnatal lung growth. *Am J Resp Crit Care Med.* 2004;170:319–343.
16. Inselman LS, Mellins RB. Medical progress: Growth and development of the lung. *J Pediatr.* 1981;98:1–15.
17. Lines A, Hooper SB, Harding R. Lung liquid production rates and volumes do not decrease before labor in healthy fetal sheep. *J Appl Physiol.* 1997;82:927.
18. Hummler E, Barker P, Gatzy J. Early death due to defective neonatal lung liquid clearance in α-ENaC-deficient mice. *Nat Genet.* 1996;12:325.
19. NIH Consensus. Development panel on the effect of corticosteroids for fetal maturation on perinatal outcomes. *JAMA.* 1995; 273:413.

Defense Mechanisms of the Pulmonary Tree

K. Alex Daneshmand   *Ronald C. Sanders Jr*   *Heidi J. Dalton*

The lung has several defense mechanisms to protect it from injury caused by inspired particles and infectious and non-infectious agents. Large inspired particles (>10 μm) are trapped by the upper respiratory passages. Smaller particles (2 to 10 μm) are trapped in the bronchial tree. Extremely small particles (0.5 to 3 μm) become deposited within the terminal respiratory unit, and particles <0.2 μm are generally exhaled. Particle size is the property used by modern nebulizers to deposit medication particles deep into the respiratory tract.

Inhaled particles may be removed by three systems within the lung: the mucociliary elevator, the phagocytes, and lymphohematogenous drainage system. The mucociliary elevator is a highly efficient system that moves particles from the terminal bronchioles to the large airways, where they can be expectorated. The cells in the main bronchi are ciliated epithelial cells, goblet cells, and mucous cells. Smaller bronchi and bronchioles contain goblet cells, which secrete mucous. At the level of the smallest bronchioles, the epithelium is lined by a material, which contains surfactant and is produced by Clara cells and type II alveolar cells (see Fig. 6.3.1)

The mucous produced contains a viscous layer that acts to trap deposited particles. It is also elastic and allows the movement of the cilia to propel it proximally. Cilia within the liquid portion of the mucous beat rhythmically to help move the mucous toward the larynx. Appropriate composition and amount of mucous are needed to provide optimal mucociliary action. Abnormalities in cilia motion can be influenced by congenital, toxic, or infectious conditions. Interestingly, it is the beating of the cilia during embryologic development that pushes the heart to the left. In patients with congenital immobile cilia syndrome,

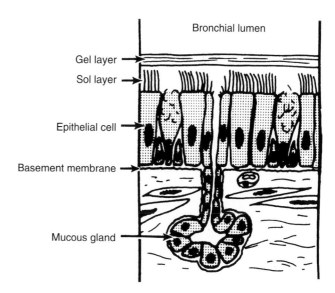

Figure 6.3.1 The mucociliary elevator. The gel layer of mucus is propelled toward the trachea by the movement of the cilia on the surface of the cells. (From George RB, Light RW, Matthay MA, et al. *Chest medicine: Essentials of pulmonary and critical care medicine.* 4th ed. Philadelphia, PA: Lippincott Williams & Wilkins; 2000:21.)

the triad of situs inversus, bronchiectasis, and sinusitis constitutes Kartagener syndrome.

Alveolar macrophages are the primary inflammatory cells of the lung capable of phagocytosis, cytokine production, destruction, and lung tissue remodeling. These cells can phagocytose bacteria, inert particles, surfactant, and other extracellular components of the alveoli recognized as foreign, thereby playing a role in the metabolic turnover of the lung. Macrophages can also release cytokines, which can recruit other inflammatory cells to the lung.

Chemotactic factors for neutrophils, such as leukotriene B_4 or interleukin-8, are released by macrophages. In addition to these functions, macrophages regulate parenchymal cells by releasing proteases, which can degrade the extracellular matrix of the lung and are important in the repair and remodeling of lung tissue following injury.

The lymphatic system is important for fluid clearance and protection of the pulmonary system. Two lymphatic systems exist within the human lung: a superficial network that exists in the pleura and a deep network that courses along with the pulmonary arteries, veins, and bronchi. Anastomoses exist between the two systems in the pleura and near the lung hilum. The lymphatic walls are lined with endothelium and have less elastic tissue than either pulmonary arteries or pulmonary veins. They also contain valves near and within the visceral pleura. A network of lymphatics drain the lungs and course through the visceral pleura toward the hila. The pleural space is drained by lymphatics in the parietal pleura. Parietal pleural lymphatics drain the pleural space through small openings called *stomata* (2 to 6 μm in diameter), which drain into lymph vessels called *lacuna*. Both stomata and lacuna are found predominantly in the mediastinal and intercostal pleura in the lower portion of the thorax. All lymph eventually drains into central veins. A large amount of parietal pleural lymph fluid drains into the parasternal lymph nodes located in the second and third interspaces. The biopsy of these nodes may be helpful in distinguishing the etiology of a pleural effusion. High hydrostatic pressure in the pulmonary circulation leads to an increase in pleural fluid formation, whereas elevated pressure in the systemic circulation will decrease the rate of pleural fluid absorption.

RECOMMENDED READINGS

1. Weinacker A. Chapter 11: Pleural disease. In: Ali J, Summer WR, Levitzky MG, eds. *Pulmonary pathophysiology.* New York: McGraw-Hill; 1999:239–267.
2. Broaddus VC, Winer-Kronish JP, Berthiaume Y, et al. Removal of pleural liquid and protein by lymphatics in awake sheep. *J Appl Physiol.* 1988;64:384–390.

Movement of Fluids and Solutes and Blood Flow within the Lung

Angela T. Wratney   *Heidi J. Dalton*

An abnormality in fluid movement within the lung results in pulmonary edema. Two types of pulmonary edema exist: high-pressure edema, usually resulting from cardiogenic causes, and permeability edema, resulting from increases in the leakage of fluid from microvessels or alveoli within the lung. Understanding these fluid fluxes helps to identify the etiology and treatment of the edema.

HIGH-PRESSURE EDEMA

Under normal conditions, fluid from the lung moves toward the interstitial space, where it is removed by the lymphatics. The quantity of fluid leaving the vascular space can be determined by the Starling equation. The Starling equation defines the movement of fluid across a semipermeable membrane and is abbreviated as:

$$\dot{Q} = K[(P_c - P_i) - \sigma(\pi_c - \pi_i)]$$

where $\dot{Q}$ represents the transvascular flow of fluid, K is the permeability coefficient of the membrane (determined by the ease of fluid passage and the surface area available for fluid flux), and σ is the reflection coefficient (see Table 6.4.1), which is a measure of the restriction to movement of plasma protein across the capillary membrane. If σ is 0, there is no restriction to protein movement whereas a σ of 1 indicates that the restriction is absolute. The σ within the lung is estimated to be 0.65.

P_c represents the hydrostatic pressure within the vascular lumen, whereas P_i is the hydrostatic pressure in the interstitial space surrounding the microvessels. π_c represents the plasma protein osmotic pressure within the circulation, whereas π_i is the osmotic pressure of the proteins within the perivascular interstitial space. Normally, the permeability of the pulmonary capillaries allows some fluid to leave the vessel but restricts protein movement. Therefore, most of the fluid filtration ($\dot{Q}$) in the lung depends on the difference between hydrostatic and protein osmotic pressures.

Hydrostatic pressure in the interstitium (P_i) approximates alveolar pressure and is assumed to be 0, but the exact pressure is affected by the lung's elastic recoil and alveolar surface tension. The hydrostatic pressure of the pulmonary capillary (P_c) depends on gravity and the depth of the vessel within the lung. Therefore, hydrostatic pressure is influenced by whether the vessel is in lung zone 1, 2, or 3 (see subsequent text). It is also related to the height of the vessel from the heart and commonly measures 4 to 17 mm Hg, with an average of 9 mm Hg. The best estimation of P_c can be obtained by the following equation:

$$P_c = WP + \gamma(PAP - WP)$$

where PAP is the pulmonary artery pressure, WP is the wedge pressure, and γ is the ratio of postcapillary (venous) resistance to the total pulmonary vascular resistance (PVR). Under normal conditions, WP is a good estimate of P_c. Therefore, the major component of hydrostatic force responsible for fluid filtration in the lung is from the pulmonary capillaries. The normal hydrostatic pressure in the capillaries averages approximately 9 mm Hg $(P_c - P_i) = (9 - 0)$.

The microvasculature's colloid oncotic pressure is estimated at 25 mm Hg, whereas that of the interstitium

TABLE 6.4.1
STARLING EQUATION

$$\dot{Q} = K[(Pmv - Ppmv) - (\pi mv - \pi pmv)]$$

Transvascular fluid flow = permeability fluid flux × [hydrostatic pressure − protein osmotic pressure] Then, substituting estimated values for the variables under normal conditions:

$$\dot{Q} = K[(10 - 0) - (25 - 19)]$$
$$\dot{Q} = K[10 - 6] = K \times 4$$

1. Net calculated transvascular fluid flow ($\dot{Q}$) is positive from the capillary lumen into the perimicrovascular interstitial space
2. Note that the protein osmotic pressure gradient normally opposes fluid filtration out of the vessels. If the gradient were abolished, i.e., if protein osmotic pressure were assumed to be equal on both sides of the capillary, then the calculated transvascular fluid flow would more than double
3. Also, if permeability (K) increases, there are two apparent effects: (a) transvascular fluid flux increases, even at normal hydrostatic pressures, and (b) the protein osmotic pressure difference across the capillary membrane decreases as proteins leak into the interstitium, further increasing transvascular fluid flux

From George RB, Light RW, Matthay MA, et al. *Chest medicine: Essentials of pulmonary and critical care medicine.* 4th ed. Philadelphia, PA: Lippincott Williams & Wilkins; 2000:577.

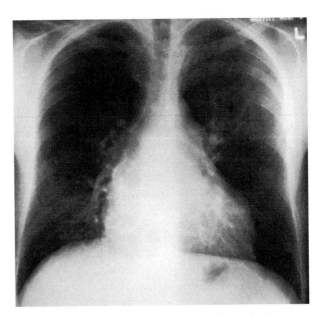

Figure 6.4.1 A posteroanterior chest radiograph of a patient with interstitial pulmonary edema secondary to left ventricular heart failure. Pulmonary capillary wedge pressure is measured at 20 mm Hg. Prominent vascular markings are present in the left upper lobe. Prominent Kerley B lines are visible in the left lower lobe, indicating fluid-filled interlobular septae. (From George RB, Light RW, Matthay MA, et al. *Chest medicine: Essentials of pulmonary and critical care medicine.* 4th ed. Philadelphia, PA: Lippincott Williams & Wilkins; 2000:579.)

(π_i) is at 15 to 19 mm Hg, thereby creating an oncotic gradient across the membrane from the vasculature to the interstitium of the lung. Because the capillary hydrostatic pressure is greater than that of the interstitium, fluid moves from the microvasculature into the interstitium surrounding the alveoli and continues to flow into the extra-alveolar interstitium because of the negative pressure in this space relative to the alveolar area. The loose connective tissue, which predominates in the extra-alveolar space, can act as a sponge to drain the fluid away from the alveolar wall. In adults, the fluid flux into the interstitium is approximately 10 to 20 mL per hour. It is estimated that the interstitial space of the lung can absorb approximately 500 mL of edema fluid. This interstitial fluid flows to the lymphatic system and then to the venous system, which drains into the superior vena cava.

When the hydrostatic pressure in the microvasculature increases, the rate of fluid flux into the interstitium increases. Left heart failure is a common cause of increased hydrostatic pressure in the microvasculature. As left ventricular end-diastolic pressures rise, a concomitant rise in left atrial pressure is transmitted to the microvasculature and fluid flux into the interstitium increases. Mild elevations in left atrial pressure of 14 to 20 mm Hg results in an increase in pulmonary edema that is confined to the interstitium. This may be visualized on the chest radiograph as Kerley B lines, which outline the interlobular septae within the lung

and are not seen under normal conditions (see Fig. 6.4.1). Symptoms of mild dyspnea may be present at this time. At higher levels of left atrial pressure (25 to 30 mm Hg), the ability of the interstitium to absorb fluid and the ability of the lymphatics to drain collected fluid is exceeded. Clinically, high-pressure cardiogenic edema is the most common form of pulmonary edema. Reduction of elevated left atrial pressure may restore the flux of fluid to normal. This can be accomplished by reducing systemic venous return; sitting the patient upright; and administering medications such as morphine, nitroglycerin, or nitroprusside that will decrease systemic venous return and left ventricular preload. Diuretics may reduce extracellular volume and reduce systemic venous tone. Improving cardiac function may also lower atrial filling pressures.

In addition to the ability of lung lymph flow to help remove edema fluid, other mechanisms of defense exist. When fluid and solute flow into the interstitium increases, the protein concentration within the interstitium is diluted. This results in an increased oncotic force, which favors protein reabsorption back into the vasculature to restore the normal gradient. Patients with low plasma protein are more likely to develop pulmonary edema at lower levels of left atrial pressure. When the lymphatics exceed their ability to remove fluid, edema fluid can break through the tight walls of the alveolar epithelium and cause flooding in the alveolar air spaces. Hypoxemia begins to occur at this stage.

PERMEABILITY EDEMA

The second form of pulmonary edema results from an increase in permeability of the capillary membrane, usually because of an acute lung injury. Both fluid and protein flow into the interstitial space and therefore the protein content of the edema fluid will be much higher than that noted with cardiogenic pulmonary edema. Infection, cytokines, sepsis, toxins and gastric aspiration are a few of the initiating events that can result in permeability edema. Although the best treatment of permeability edema would be to give a medication that would restore normal permeability to the vasculature, no such therapy exists. Treatment of the underlying condition remains the best alternative at the current time.

DISTRIBUTION OF BLOOD FLOW WITHIN THE LUNG

The distribution of blood flow within the lung depends on gravity, pulmonary vascular pressures, and resistance. Perfusion to the lung is inversely related to the height of the pulmonary artery above or below the heart (see Fig. 6.4.2). Decreased pulmonary artery perfusion occurs to lung segments above the heart and is increased for lung segments below the heart. Perfusion is also influenced by the collapsibility of pulmonary capillaries. The interdependencies of alveolar, pulmonary artery, and pulmonary venous pressures that influence lung perfusion are described as the zones of West. Zone 1 refers to areas where alveolar pressure is greater than pulmonary artery and pulmonary venous pressure. This zone corresponds to the apex of the lung in the upright patient. These segments are ventilated but poorly perfused and thereby increase dead space ventilation. In the middle of the lung, called *zone 2*, pulmonary artery pressure is greater than alveolar pressure and pulmonary venous pressure. Blood flow in this zone depends on the difference between pulmonary arterial and alveolar pressures. At the base of the lung, zone 3 conditions, in which alveolar pressure is lower than both pulmonary arterial and venous pressure, occur. Flow is determined by the difference between pulmonary artery and venous pressures. In this zone, perivascular pressure is increased and lung expansion is reduced, resulting in uneven ventilation and perfusion.

RECOMMENDED READINGS

1. Krapo JD, Barry BE, Gehr P, et al. Cell number and cell characteristics of the normal human lung. *Am Rev Respir Dis.* 1982;126(2):332–337.

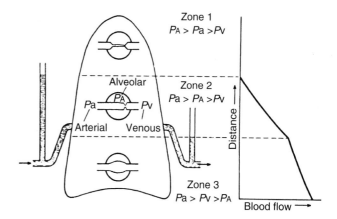

Figure 6.4.2 The zones of West illustrating regional changes in blood flow on the basis of hydrostatic pressure differences affecting the capillaries. Pa, pulmonary artery pressure; PA, alveolar pressure; Pv, pulmonary venous pressure. (From George RB, Light RW, Matthay MA, et al. *Chest medicine: Essentials of pulmonary and critical care medicine.* 4th ed. Philadelphia, PA: Lippincott Williams & Wilkins; 2000:16; adapted from West JB, Dollery CT, Naimark A. Distribution of blood flow in isolated lungs: Relation to vascular and alveolar pressure. *J Appl Physiol.* 1964;19:713.)

2. Berthiaume Y, Hans GF, Matthay MA. Lung edema clearance: 20 years of progress. Invited review: Alveolar edema fluid clearance in the injured lung. *J Appl Physiol.* 2002;93:2007–2213.
3. West JB. *Respiratory physiology.* 5th ed. Coryell Patricia A, ed. Philadelphia, PA: Williams & Wilkins; 1995.
4. Meyrick B, Reid L. The alveolar wall. *Br J Dis Chest.* 1970;64(3):121–140.
5. Morrell NW, Roberts CM, Biggs T, et al. Collateral ventilation and gas exchange during airway occlusion in the normal human lung. *Am Rev Respir Dis.* 1993;147:535–539.
6. Terry RB, Traystman RJ, Newball HH, et al. Collateral ventilation in man. *N Engl J Med.* 1978;298:10.
7. Lines A, Hooper SB, Harding R, et al. Lung liquid production rates and volumes do not decrease before labor in healthy fetal sheep. *J Appl Physiol.* 1997;82:927.
8. Gluecker T, Patrizio C, Schnyder P, et al. Clinical and radiologic features of pulmonary edema. *Radiographics.* 1999;19:1507–1531.
9. Gattinoni L, Bombino M, Pelosi P, et al. Lung structure and function in different stages of severe adult respiratory distress syndrome. *J Am Med Assoc.* 1994;271:1772–1779.
10. Prewitt RM, McCarthy J, Wood LDH. Treatment of acute low pressure pulmonary edema in dogs: Relative effects of hydrostatic and oncotic pressure, nitroprusside, and positive end-expiratory pressure. *J Clin Invest.* 1981;67:409–441.
11. Ware LB, Matthay MA. Medical progress: The acute respiratory distress syndrome. *N Engl J Med.* 2000;342:1334–1349.
12. Walther FJ, Siassi B, Ramadan NA, et al. Cardiac output in newborn infants with transient myocardial dysfunction. *J Pediatr.* 1985;107:781.
13. Staub NC. Pulmonary edema. *Physiol Rev.* 1974;54:678.
14. Chollet-Martin S, Jourdain B, Gilbert C, et al. Interactions between neutrophils and cytokines in blood and alveolar spaces during ARDS. *Am J Respir Crit Care Med.* 1996;153:594–601.
15. Fein A, Grossman RF, Jones JG, et al. The value of edema fluid protein measurement in patients with pulmonary edema. *Am J Med.* 1979;67:32.

Alveolar Function

Douglas F. Willson

ROLE OF SURFACTANT

Pulmonary surfactant serves two primary functions in the lung: (i) it is a "surface-acting agent" that lowers surface tension at the aqueous–air interface of the alveolar surface and (ii) the surfactant, specifically its component hydrophilic surfactant proteins (SP)-A and SP-D (known as *collectins*), is an important component of the innate immune response in the lung. Its function as a surface tension–lowering agent is of primary clinical interest and is the focus of this chapter.

Surface tension refers to the potential energy that exists at the interface between two substances or phases of matter because of unbalanced intermolecular forces at the interface. The surface tension at the air–water interface is approximately 70 dynes per cm and is a function of the strong cohesive forces between water molecules (van der Waals forces) relative to those between gas molecules, which are negligible because of the large distances between molecules. In a three-dimensional construct such as a bubble, these unopposed attractive forces result in a net inward force tending to make the bubble collapse (see Fig. 6.5.1). Mathematically, surface tension can be expressed by the Laplace law, which states that the pressure (P) within an elastic sphere is directly proportional to the tension (T) of the wall and inversely proportional to the radius (r) of the curvature:

$$P = 2 \times \frac{T}{r}$$

Applying this principle to the alveolus, P is the pressure inside the alveoli, T represents the surface tension at the interface, and r is the alveolar radius. The presence of surfactant in the liquid lining the alveoli allows the surface tension to change as the surface area of the alveolus changes.

Surfactants are molecules that have an energetic preference for interfaces because of their amphipathic nature (i.e., having both polar and nonpolar moieties in their

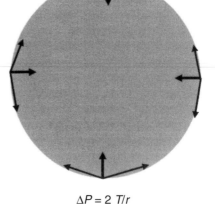

$$\Delta P = 2\ T/r$$

where ΔP = pressure to keep "bubble" inflated
   T = surface tension
   r = radius of sphere

Figure 6.5.1   Surface tension in a bubble. Intermolecular attraction between molecules of the liquid result in a net inward vector, the magnitude of which is determined by the radius of curvature of the bubble and the surface tension at the liquid–gas interface.

structure). The phospholipids in the pulmonary surfactant have polar phosphate "heads" and nonpolar lipid "tails" that orient with the polar phosphate head to the aqueous alveolar hypophase and the nonpolar lipid moieties to the gas phase. In doing so, their internal bond energy is substituted for the surface tension at the interface, and surface tension at the interface is decreased.

Pulmonary surfactant lowers surface tension in a dynamic rather than static manner (see Fig. 6.5.2). As the alveolar "bubble" size decreases during exhalation, the surfactant film is compressed and surface tension approaches zero. As the "bubble" radius increases with inspiration, the surfactant film is expanded and surface tension proportionately increases, compensating for the effects of the

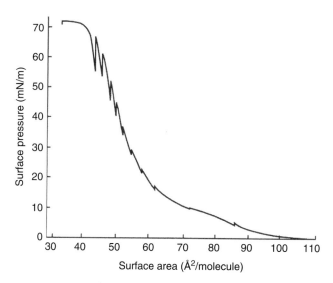

Figure 6.5.2 Dynamic surface pressure relaxation in a dynamically compressed dipalmitoylphosphatidylcholine (DPPC) surface film. Compressed DPPC films at the air–water interface achieve dynamic surface pressures in excess of equilibrium values. When compression is halted at a fixed area, dynamic surface pressures relax toward equilibrium over a timescale that varies with the extent of the film compression.

TABLE 6.5.1	
SURFACTANT COMPOSITION[a]	
Lipid	90%–95%
Phospholipid	78%
Saturated phosphatidylcholine	45%
Unsaturated phosphatidylcholine	20%
Phosphatidylglycerol	8%
Other phospholipids	5%
Neutral lipids	10%
Other lipids	2%
Protein[b]	5%–10%
Loosely associated, mainly serum	0%–5%
Apoproteins (SP-A, SP-B, SP-C)	5%–10%

SP, surfactant protein.
[a]Values are the approximate percentage masses of individual components in the surfactant isolated from alveolar washings by sedimentation and density gradient centrifugation. This material contains many different surfactant structures including lamellar body contents, tubular myelin, and variably sized vesicles. The composition of each structure may differ from the average composition presented.
[b]The protein content varies as a function of the purification procedure used. Serum proteins are the major loosely associated protein group, but several lung-specific proteins that have no known role in surfactant function have also been identified in surfactant preparations. From Rooney SA. The surfactant system and lung phospholipid biochemistry. *Am Rev Respir Dis*. 1985;131:439–460.

increasing radius (remember the Laplace law, $\Delta P = 2T/r$). This dynamic variation in surface tension is responsible for the ability of alveoli of different sizes to coexist in the lung. If surfactants were not present, the Laplace law would mandate a need for greater pressure to keep an alveolus open as its radius decreases with declining lung volume. This would promote atelectasis at low lung volumes, result in small alveoli emptying into larger ones, and require high pressures to reopen alveoli that have collapsed. In surfactant-lined alveoli, as the radius decreases, the surface area over which the surfactant is distributed also decreases. In surfactant-deficient states, some alveoli collapse while some patent alveoli overexpand, generating ineffective gas exchange within a nonhomogeneously inflated lung. The consequences of surfactant deficiency are seen commonly in the diffuse atelectasis in preterm infants with infant respiratory distress syndrome.

SURFACTANT COMPOSITION AND PHARMACEUTICAL SURFACTANTS

Natural surfactant is a complex mixture of phospholipids, neutral lipids, and protein (see Table 6.5.1). Phospholipids constitute the major component (80% by weight), with the other two components being neutral lipids and proteins. Each of the components and their balance are important in adsorption, film formation, and film behavior at the alveolar surface.

Four surfactant proteins have been identified, SP-A, B, C, and D. SP-A and SP-D are large, hydrophilic proteins in the collectin family that are integral in the innate immune system. SP-B and SP-C are small, hydrophobic proteins present in approximately equal amounts (1% to 2%) and are vital in adsorption (spreading) and film formation. SP-B and SP-C can be extracted with the phospholipids in commercial surfactants, whereas the hydrophilic proteins SP-A and SP-D are lost during the extraction process. The presence of SP-B and SP-C is probably the primary reason for the greater efficacy of "natural" relative to synthetic surfactants. An excellent review of the structure of the alveoli and the role of surfactant is offered by Gatto et al.

Although surfactant seems to be produced by type II cells in the lung, its synthesis can be affected by glucocorticoids, estrogens, and androgens. Secretion of surfactant from type II cells can be stimulated by β-adrenergic and cholinergic agonists and by factors such as hyperinflation within the lung parenchyma. Surfactant has a quick turnover rate and is catabolized by Type II epithelial cells and alveolar macrophages.

Maternal corticosteroid treatment significantly improves fetal lung development by maturation of type II cells and enhancement of the gas exchange surface area. Maternal steroid treatment is considered a standard of care for the delivery of preterm infants between 24 to 34 weeks gestational age.

RECOMMENDED READINGS

1. Notter RH. *Lung surfactants. Basic science and clinical applications.* New York: Marcel Dekker; 2000:16.

2. Tabak SA, Notter RH, Ultman JS, et al. Relaxation effects in the surface pressure behavior of dipalmitoyl lecithin. *J Colloid Interf Sci.* 1977;60:117–1255.

3. Rooney SA. The surfactant system and lung phospholipid biochemistry. *Am Rev Respir Dis.* 1985;131:439–460.

4. Bernhard W, Mottaghian J, Gebert A, et al. Commercial versus native surfactants: Surface activity, molecular components, and the effect of calcium. *Am J Respir Crit Care Med.* 2000;162:1524–1533.

5. Egan EA, Notter RH, Kwong MS, et al. Natural and artificial lung surfactant replacement therapy in premature lambs. *J Appl Physiol.* 1983;55:875–883.

6. Horbar JD, Wright LL, Soll RF, et al. A multicenter randomized trial comparing two surfactants for the treatment of neonatal respiratory distress syndrome. National Institute of Child Health and Human Development Neonatal Research Network. *J Pediatr.* 1993;123:757–766.

7. Gatto LA, Fluck RR, Nieman GF. Alveolar mechanics in the acutely injured lung: Role of alveolar instability in the pathogenesis of ventilator induced lung injury. *Respir Care.* 2004;49(9):1045–1055.

8. Hummler E, Barker P, Gatzy J, et al. Early death due to defective neonatal lung liquid clearance in α-ENaC-deficient mice. *Nat Genet.* 1996;12:325.

9. Bunton TE, Plopper CG. Triamcinolone-induced structural alterations in the development of the lung of the fetal rhesus macaque. *Am J Obstet Gynecol.* 1984;148:203.

10. Ikegami M, Polk D, Tabor B, et al. Corticosteroid and thyrotropin releasing hormone effects on preterm sheep lung function. *J Appl Physiol.* 1991;70:2268.

11. NIH Consensus Development panel on the effect of corticosteroids for fetal maturation on perinatal outcomes. *JAMA.* 1995;273:413.

Pulmonary Gas Exchange

Angela T. Wratney   Ira M. Cheifetz

Pulmonary gas exchange requires the efficient movement of gas from the atmosphere to the alveoli, across the air–capillary interface, and into the capillary red blood cell (RBC). Because of the expansiveness of this network and the small diameter of the capillaries, pulmonary capillary blood flow traverses the alveoli as a thin sheet of RBCs, which promotes efficient gas exchange. Gas exchange is so efficient that although each RBC spends an average of 0.8 seconds in the capillary, alveolar gas exchange is usually complete within 0.25 seconds.

ALVEOLAR VENTILATION

The conducting airways extend from the nose to the terminal bronchioles and function as a conduit for gas to be warmed as it flows to the respiratory lung units. A portion of each tidal breath remains in the conducting airways, estimated at approximately 25% of the breath, while the remainder passes to the alveolar–capillary membrane, where gas exchange occurs. The conducting airways do not participate in gas exchange of oxygen and carbon dioxide with blood and, therefore, comprise the anatomic dead space. This is expressed as follows:

$$V_T = V_D + V_A$$

where V_T is the total volume of the tidal breath, V_D is the volume of dead space ventilation, and V_A is the volume of alveolar ventilation. Alveolar ventilation (VA) is the product of the volume of the tidal breath that reaches the alveoli ($V_A = V_T - V_D$) and the respiratory rate per minute (f).

$$VA = V_A \times f$$

Universal Gas Law

The universal gas law relates the pressure (P), temperature (T), and volume (V) of an ideal gas where n = number of moles of gas and R = the proportionality gas constant.

$$n \times R = P \times V/T$$

As long as T, n, and R are constant, the equation becomes:

$$P_1 \times V_1/T_1 = P_2 \times V_2/T_2$$

Therefore, in any volume of gas, the total gas pressure is equal to the sum of the individual pressures if each molecular species were present alone in the volume of gas. Room air at 37°C and sea level is composed of 0% carbon dioxide, 79% nitrogen, and a percent of fractional inspired oxygen (FiO_2) of 21% generating a barometric pressure (P_B) of 760 mm Hg. As air is inspired through the conducting airways, it is warmed and saturated with water vapor. At 37°C, the pressure contribution to inspired air is P_{BH_2O} is 47 mm Hg.

Alveolar Gas Equation

The alveolar gas equation determines the alveolar partial pressure of oxygen (P_{AO_2}) and is used clinically to relate the alveolar–arterial oxygen tension gradient (A-a gradient; $P_{AO_2} - P_{aO_2}$):

$$P_{AO_2} = P_{IO_2} - \frac{P_{aCO_2}}{R} \quad \text{where } P_{IO_2} = F_{IO_2} \times (P_B - P_{H_2O})$$

The normal partial pressure of alveolar carbon dioxide (P_{aCO_2}) in the prealveolar capillary is 40 mm Hg, and the respiratory quotient (R) is normally 0.8. The inspired oxygen tension (P_{IO_2}) in the alveolus is a product of the fraction of oxygen in the tidal gas and the barometric pressures of the gases present. For example, the alveolar oxygen tension of inspired room air ($F_{IO_2} = 0.21$) versus F_{IO_2} of 1.0 at sea level and $37°C$ can be calculated as follows:

at room temperature: $P_{AO_2} = 0.21 \times (760$ mm Hg

$$- 47 \text{ mm Hg}) - 40/0.8$$
$$= 0.21 \times (713) - 50$$
$$= 150 - 50$$
$$= 100 \text{ mm Hg}$$

at 100% F_{IO_2}: $P_{AO_2} = 1.0 \times (760$ mm Hg

$$- 47 \text{ mm Hg}) - 40/0.8$$
$$= 663 \text{ mm Hg}$$

At higher altitudes, the concentration (%) of oxygen remains the same, but the partial pressure decreases. The total P_B of inspired air at higher altitudes also decreases. P_{AO_2} is lower, creating a lower driving pressure across the capillary membrane and a decrease in Pa_{O_2}.

The A-a gradient is used clinically to detect oxygenation defects. A physiologic gradient exists in which the arterial oxygen tension is 5 to 15 mm Hg less than the alveolar oxygen tension because of the venous bronchial bloodflow and thesbian (cardiac) venous admixture, which mix into the pulmonary vein outflow. An abnormally large A-a gradient is caused by many conditions or pathophysiologic states, including hypoventilation, airway obstruction, diffusion abnormalities, ventilation–perfusion mismatch, and hemoglobinopathies, which disturb alveolar gas exchange or oxygen binding in the capillary.

ALVEOLAR–CAPILLARY INTERFACE

Oxygen uptake and transport into the capillary is controlled in two phases: (i) uptake by diffusion through the alveolar–capillary interface and (ii) transport within the pulmonary capillaries whether bound by hemoglobin or dissolved within the plasma.

Diffusion of Gas

Oxygen and carbon dioxide move between air and blood by simple diffusion from areas of high to low partial pressure. The Fick law of diffusion states that the rate of gas transfer through a sheet of tissue is proportional to the tissue area and the difference in gas partial pressure between the two sides is inversely proportional to the tissue thickness.

Fick law: $V_{O_2} = D \times A(P_{AO_2} - Pa_{O_2})/L^2$

where V_{O_2} = oxygen consumption; D = the diffusion coefficient which integrates the properties of the molecular size and solubility of the gas; A = the effective available alveolar surface area; and L = the distance for diffusion (see Fig. 6.6.1). The characteristics of the alveolar–capillary membrane make it suitable for efficient gas exchange.

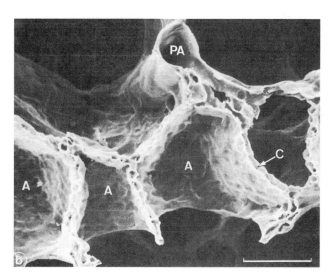

Figure 6.6.1 Blood flow in pulmonary capillaries (C) surrounds the alveoli (A) in a dense vascular network. PA, pulmonary arteriole; marker = 50 μg. (From Weibel ER. Design and morphology of the pulmonary gas exchanger. In: Crystal RG, West JB, Weibel WR, et al., eds. *The lung: Scientific foundations.* Philadelphia, PA: Lippincott-Raven; 1997:1147–1159.)

Recall that the surface area of the blood–gas barrier is extremely large (70 to 80 m^2) and that the membrane is extremely thin (0.3 μm—essentially the diameter of a single RBC). Therefore, the rate of diffusion is rapid; diffusion limitations are extremely rare.

The partial pressure of oxygen is typically the net driving force ($P_{AO_2} - Pa_{O_2}$) for oxygen uptake. As blood passes the alveoli, the partial pressure of oxygen in the capillary (P_{O_2}) rises so that, under typical resting conditions, it equilibrates to that of the alveoli (P_{AO_2}) approximately one third of the way along the capillary. The RBC typically passes two to three alveoli during its course through the lungs. Each RBC remains in the capillary bed for <1 second, and oxygen diffusion and hemoglobin binding occur in milliseconds. This brief time is sufficient for the complete exchange of oxygen and carbon dioxide between the alveoli and the capillary blood.

Abnormal gases present in inspired air can be particularly dangerous both because of their physical gas properties and the pathologic effects they exert at the tissue level. Carbon monoxide is an odorless gas present in toxic amounts in automobile exhaust or formed from combustion during a fire. Carbon monoxide diffuses extremely rapidly across the capillary interface and binds tightly to the hemoglobin molecule. Carbon monoxide occupies the hemoglobin–oxygen–binding sites, thereby reducing capillary oxygen content and impairing oxygen transport to the tissue beds. Signs of tissue hypoxia will exist despite a normal hemoglobin level and normal Pa_{O_2}. Administration of high oxygen mixtures will help eliminate carbon monoxide and improve tissue oxygenation.

Oxygen Transport

Oxygen transport in the capillary blood occurs predominantly by binding with hemoglobin within the capillary RBC and secondarily by dissolving within the plasma. The total blood oxygen content, a combination of the oxygen bound to hemoglobin and the dissolved component, is calculated by:

$$\text{Oxygen content (vol\%)} = [O_2 \text{ sat (\%)} \times 1.39 \text{ mL } O_2 \text{ per L}$$
$$\times \text{ Hb (g per dL)}] + [0.003 \text{ mL}$$
$$\times \text{PaO}_2 \text{ (mm Hg)}]$$

Oxygen content is normally in the range of 20.8 mL oxygen per 100 mL blood.

Dissolved oxygen is normally a minor contribution to total blood oxygen content. However, at significantly higher partial pressures, such as in hyperbaric oxygen therapy, where the PaO_2 may exceed 2,000 mm Hg, the dissolved oxygen may contribute significantly to total oxygen content in the blood. The dissolved plasma component may also have a greater role in hemoglobinopathies, where hemoglobin may not be fully saturated with oxygen, or in severe anemia.

Oxygen is predominantly transported in the RBC bound to hemoglobin. Hemoglobin is composed of four polypeptide chains (globin), each containing a central iron–porphyrin ring (heme). The polypeptide protein chains may be a mixture of several types (e.g., α, β, or γ chains), each differing in their amino acid sequences. Normal adult hemoglobin (Hb A) is composed of two α and two β chains ($\alpha_2\beta_2$). Fetal hemoglobin (Hb F) is composed of two α and two γ chains ($\alpha_2\gamma_2$). Hemoglobin S (sickle) has valine instead of glutamic acid in the β chain. This single amino acid substitution causes deoxygenated hemoglobin to sickle.

Oxygen–Hemoglobin Dissociation Curve

The physiologic properties of oxygen–hemoglobin binding and dissociation underlie the principles of gas transport from the alveolus to the tissues. These properties are reflected by the oxyhemoglobin dissociation curve. The propensity for hemoglobin to bind oxygen is affected by the type of hemoglobin, the biochemical environment, and the redox state of the iron in the hemoglobin molecule (see Fig. 6.6.2).

Shape of the Oxyhemoglobin Curve

The sigmoid shape of the oxyhemoglobin curve results from a molecular interaction between the four heme groups. As each oxygen molecule binds to heme, the binding affinity of subsequent hemoglobin subunits for oxygen is increased, creating a nonlinear relationship for hemoglobin saturation. This is an important physiologic attribute for the pulmonary bed, where the increase in oxygen affinity ensures maximal saturation of hemoglobin. Hemoglobin remains fully saturated until capillary PO_2 is <70 mm

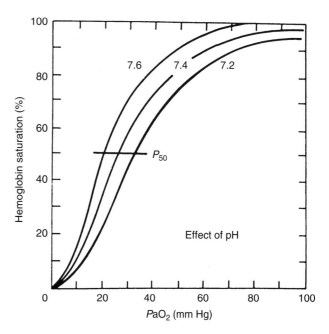

Figure 6.6.2 The oxyhemoglobin dissociation curve. The effects of shifts in pH on the affinity of hemoglobin for oxygen (the Bohr effect) are shown. Acidosis shifts the curve toward the right and therefore increases oxygen delivery at the tissue level. The affinity of hemoglobin for oxygen is expressed as the P_{50} (the PaO_2 at which the hemoglobin is 50% saturated). (From George RB, Light RW, Matthay MA, et al. *Chest medicine: Essentials of pulmonary and critical care medicine.* 4th ed. Philadelphia, PA: Lippincott Williams & Wilkins; 2000:54.)

Hg. At this inflection point, the steep downward slope of the sigmoidal curve indicates a partial pressure gradient favoring oxygen unloading from the systemic capillaries to the tissues. Maximal oxygen unloading occurs across a broad range of capillary oxygen tensions (20 to 60 mm Hg). This ability to unload oxygen at a range of oxygen tensions is essential because the tissue PO_2 varies throughout the body, ranging from being very low in the myocardium to being high in the kidneys. The steep portion of the curve allows optimal oxygen unloading in different tissue beds because small changes in PCO_2 result in significant oxygen release.

Left- or Rightward Shift of the Oxyhemoglobin Curve

Biochemical factors of the RBC may shift the oxyhemoglobin dissociation curve and alter the propensity for oxygen binding or unloading. The position of the curve depends upon the conditions of pH; temperature; PaCO_2; PaO_2; and presence of 2,3-diphosphoglycerate (2,3-DPG), which is an organic phosphate formed primarily in the RBC as a by-product of anaerobic metabolism that readily binds hemoglobin, reducing its affinity for oxygen and promoting the release of oxygen to the tissues (rightward shift). Other metabolic factors that shift the oxyhemoglobin curve to the right are increased temperature, increased PaCO_2, and decreased pH. These factors favor oxygen unloading to the tissue at a higher P_{CO_2}. A leftward shift in the oxyhemoglobin curve, favoring a greater affinity for oxygen binding, may occur with decreased temperature, decreased Pa_{CO_2}, increased pH, or decreased 2,3-DPG levels. These factors promote greater oxygen uptake and binding affinity at any P_{CO_2}. Passage of blood through the pulmonary circuit results in lowering of the Pa_{CO_2} levels as carbon dioxide is unloaded from the capillaries. This increases the affinity of hemoglobin for oxygen binding in the pulmonary circulation.

Of importance in transfusion medicine, the concentration of 2,3-DPG decreases in stored units of RBCs because of decreased metabolic activity. Recent research has investigated the physiologic alterations, if any, in tissue oxygen delivery that occur because of the relatively decreased capacity for these transfused RBCs to unload oxygen.

Altered Hemoglobin

Alterations in the redox state of iron or in the structure of the globin chains significantly affects the oxygen carrying capacity of the hemoglobin and change the sigmoidal shape of the curve. Normally, the heme iron is in the ferrous or reduced state (Fe^{2+}). Reducing enzymes present within the RBC maintains the iron in this functional state. Altered states of iron or the presence of abnormal hemoglobin disturb the physical interactions of hemoglobin molecules, resulting in an abnormal shape of the oxyhemoglobin curve. Methemoglobin is produced from exposure to nitrates or sulfates and converts iron to the ferric or oxidized state (Fe^{3+}). Carbon monoxide occupies oxygen-binding sites and disrupts heme group interactions. These forms of hemoglobin will not bind oxygen efficiently or transfer oxygen at a lower capillary PO_2, thereby significantly impairing systemic oxygen delivery.

Carbon Dioxide Transport

In addition to transporting oxygen from the pulmonary vasculature to the tissues, RBCs must also carry carbon dioxide produced in metabolically active tissues to the alveolar–capillary bed for removal. Carbon dioxide is transported in three forms: (i) dissolved in the blood (5%), (ii) as bicarbonate (HCO_3^-) ion (90%), and (iii) carried by deoxygenated hemoglobin or plasma proteins as carbamino-CO_2 (5%).

Carbon dioxide gas enters the RBC and reacts with water (through carbonic anhydrase) to form HCO_3^- and H^+ (see Fig. 6.6.3). These ions (HCO_3^- and H^+) serve essential functions in capillary gas transport. While HCO_3^- diffuses into the plasma, chloride enters the RBC to maintain electric neutrality; this movement constitutes the "chloride shift." When the blood reaches the pulmonary vascular bed, these processes are reversed. Chloride enters the plasma and

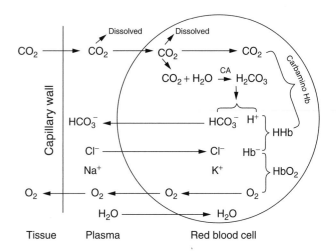

Figure 6.6.3 Carbon dioxide dissociation curve for a patient with a normal level of saturated hemoglobin. The curve shifts to the right in polycythemia and to the left in anemia. Oxygenation shifts the curve to the right and hypoxemia shifts it to the left (Haldane effect). (From George RB, Light RW, Matthay MA, et al. *Chest medicine: Essentials of pulmonary and critical care medicine.* 4th ed. Philadelphia, PA: Lippincott Williams & Wilkins; 2000:47.)

HCO_3^- enters the RBC, where it again forms carbon dioxide and water, thereby releasing carbon dioxide into the alveoli. The chloride shift involves the movement of bicarbonate to ultimately effect the release of carbon dioxide and water. Carbon dioxide diffuses down its partial pressure gradient into the capillary blood.

The H^+ formed during this process plays a significant role in effecting hemoglobin carbon dioxide binding and oxygen release (Haldane effect). Deoxygenated hemoglobin is a proton acceptor. Therefore, at the tissue level, carbon dioxide diffuses into the capillary RBC to produce HCO_3^- and H^+ ions. H^+ binds readily to hemoglobin, which promotes the release of bound oxygen to the tissues (shifts the oxyhemoglobin curve to the right) while enhancing carbon dioxide uptake. Deoxygenated hemoglobin has a greater affinity for binding carbon dioxide (forming carbamino-CO_2), thereby removing carbon dioxide from the systemic tissue beds. Oxygenated hemoglobin is relatively acidic (donates H^+), promoting carbon dioxide unloading in the lung.

The integration of the dense pulmonary capillary network within the specialized architecture of the alveolar air sacs (alveolar–capillary interface) creates an extensive surface area for gas exchange. Diffusion of oxygen and carbon dioxide across the alveolar–capillary membrane depends upon partial pressure gradients. The physiologic properties of hemoglobin and its response to the biochemical environment dictate the ability of the capillary RBCs to maximally unload oxygen to the tissues and return carbon dioxide to the alveoli.

RECOMMENDED READINGS

1. Collins VJ Transport of oxygen and carbon dioxide. In: *Physiologic and pharmacologic bases of anesthesia*. Philadelphia, PA: Williams & Wilkins; 1996:76–87.
2. Morisaki H, Sibbald WJ. Tissue oxygen delivery and the microcirculation. *Crit Care Clin*. 2004;20(2):213–223.
3. Hebert PC, Blajchman MA, Cook DJ, et al. Do transfusion requirements in critical care blood transfusions improve outcomes related to mechanical ventilation? *Chest*. 2001;119(6):1850–1857.
4. West JB. *Respiratory Physiology*. 5th ed. Baltimore: Williams & Wilkins; 1998:1–78.
5. Jobe AH. The respiratory system. In: Faranoff AA, Martin RJ, eds. *Neonatal-perinatal medicine: Diseases of the fetus and infant*. 7th ed. Philadelphia, PA: Mosby; 2002:973–991.
6. Crapo JD, Barry BE, Gehr P, et al. Cell number and cell characteristics of the normal human lung. *Am Rev Respir Dis*. 1982; 126:332–337.
7. Inselman LS, Mellins RB. Medical progress: Growth and development of the lung. *J Pediatr*. 1981;98:1–15.
8. American Thoracic Society Documents. Mechanisms and limits of induced postnatal lung growth. *Am J Respir Crit Care Med*. 2004;170:319–343.
9. Lines A, Hooper SB, Harding R, et al. Lung liquid production rates and volumes do not decrease before labor in healthy fetal sheep. *J Appl Physiol*. 1997;82:927.
10. Van Golde LM, Batenburg JJ, Robertson B, et al. The pulmonary surfactant system: Biochemical aspects and functional significance. *Physiol Rev*. 1988;68:374.

Respiratory System Physiology

Mark J. Heulitt   Paul Ouellet

The rapid gas exchange that occurs in the lungs is accomplished by a well-coordinated interaction of the lungs with the central nervous system, the diaphragm, chest wall musculature, and the circulatory system. The primary functions of the lungs are to supply oxygen and to remove carbon dioxide from the tissues of the body. To accomplish this, two inter-related processes must occur: ventilation, the movement of air between the environment and the alveoli, and gas exchange, the transfer of oxygen and carbon dioxide between the alveolar gas and the mixed venous blood entering the lungs.

Only approximately 10% of the lung is occupied by solid tissue, with the remainder being filled with air and blood. Supporting structures of the lung must be delicate enough to allow gas exchange, yet strong enough to maintain architectural integrity and sustain alveolar structure. Two inter-related systems exist to perform the functions of the lung: (i) airways for ventilation, divided into the conducting airways (dead-air space) and the gas exchange portions, and the (ii) circulatory system for perfusion. Both operate under low pressures.

RESPIRATORY MUSCLES

Movement of gas in and out of the lungs requires a balance of forces. Inspiration is active, whereas expiration is passive. When the inspiratory muscles contract, there are outward-acting forces. These forces are produced by changes in the pressure of the respiratory system (P_{RS}) and that of the muscles (P_{MUS}). During expiration, gas movement is caused by pressure changes in the lung (P_L) and in the chest wall (P_{CW}). The elastic recoil of the lung and chest wall generates these pressures $P_{RS} + P_{MUS} = P_L + P_{CW}$. The pressure of the respiratory system can be further divided into P_{ALV}

and P_{bs}, $P_{RS} = P_{ALV} - P_{bs}$, where P_{ALV} is alveolar pressure and P_{bs} is the pressure of the body surface. Both pressures are usually atmospheric. P_{MUS} is generated by inspiratory muscles including the diaphragm, external intercostals, and accessory muscles. The diaphragm is the principle muscle of respiration, whereas the intercostals function primarily to elevate the lower ribs. Accessory muscles, such as the sternocleidomastoid, do not normally participate in quiet breathing but serve an important role in situations in which inspiratory efforts are increased. Use of the sternocleidomastoid is depicted by the elevation of the upper part of the sternum noted in infants with respiratory distress. Abdominal muscles are needed to help with expiration. In adults, the diaphragm descends with inspiration and the lower ribs elevate, leading to lung expansion. In infants, however, the shape of the thorax and the compliant nature of the chest wall make breathing more difficult. In infants, the cross-section of the thorax is circular because of the placement of their ribs and the horizontal position of the diaphragm. When the diaphragm contracts, there is less efficient expansion of the lungs because the compliant chest wall allows the lower ribs to descend rather than elevate. This results in subcostal retractions and dissipates much of the force of diaphragmatic contraction into merely deforming the chest wall instead of improving inspiration. The increased workload on the diaphragm makes infants prone to muscle fatigue in situations of increased inspiratory effort. There are also fewer type I muscle fibers in the diaphragm of infants. These fibers are the slow-twitch, high-oxidative type, which are more resistant to fatigue. As children grow, changes in the orientation of the rib cage to a less horizontal position, an increase in the bulk of the muscles attached to the rib cage, and an increase in type I fibers all result in an increase in the maximum inspiratory pressures that can be generated and result in stiffening of the chest wall.

LUNG VOLUMES

As illustrated in Figure 6.7.1, lung volumes can be subdivided as a percentage of total lung capacity (TLC) and phases of respiration (inspiration, expiration, and rest). Total volume contained in the lung at the end of a maximal inspiration is subdivided into volumes and capacities. The volumes do not overlap and, when added together at a maximal inspiration, equal the TLC. The TLC is larger in patients who are taller, younger, and of the male gender. TLC is the sum of the vital capacity (VC) and the residual volume (RV). VC is the maximum volume of air that can be forcefully expelled from the lungs following a maximal inspiration. It is called a capacity because it is the sum of inspiratory reserve volume (IRV), tidal volume (TV), and expiratory reserve volume (ERV) $VC = IRV + TV + ERV = TLC - RV$. RV is the volume of air remaining in the lungs after a maximal expiration. It is normally approximately 25% of TLC. This is the only lung volume that cannot be measured with a spirometer.

Most lung diseases reduce VC. Importantly, ventilation is not affected under these conditions because even during maximal exercise, the entire VC is not used to breathe. VC can be reduced both by pulmonary and extrapulmonary factors. Pulmonary factors include an absolute reduction in distensible lung tissue (e.g., pneumonectomy, atelectasis), increase in stiffness of lungs (e.g., alveolar edema, respiratory distress syndrome, surfactant abnormalities, or infiltrative interstitial lung diseases), and increase in RV (e.g., emphysema, asthma, or lung cysts). Extrapulmonary factors that can reduce VC are limitations of thoracic expansion (thoracic deformities e.g., kyphoscoliosis), pleural fibrosis, limitations of diaphragmatic descent (e.g., ascites or increased abdominal pressure), and nerve or muscle dysfunction. Examples of nerve and muscle dysfunction include pain from surgery or rib fracture and primary neuromuscular disease (e.g., Guillain-Barré syndrome).

The resting lung volume is the functional residual capacity (FRC). It represents the quantity of air remaining in the lungs at the end of a spontaneous expiration. FRC in adults is defined as the static passive balance of forces between the lung and chest wall. Depending upon the position of the patient, FRC is approximately 50% of TLC in upright position and approximately 40% in supine position. The FRC of infants is reduced to approximately 10% of TLC because of the limited chest wall movement that occurs with expiration. The decreased elastic recoil of the lung coupled with the reduced inward recoil of the lung produces this low chest wall movement.

MODEL OF THE RESPIRATORY SYSTEM

The respiratory system can be represented by a collection of physical components interacting with one another and their environment. Although *in vivo* analysis demonstrates that the lungs do not function as a single compartment, analyzing the respiratory system in a linear model simplifies the presentation.

A single balloon on a pipe is the simplest model that represents a single-compartment model of breathing by inflation and deflation of the balloon. The model, demonstrated in Figure 6.7.2, has a single mechanical degree of freedom because its state is completely defined by its compartmental volume. By choosing the dimensions of the conduit, a resistance similar to a particular set of pulmonary airways can be assigned. By choosing the stiffness of the spring that helps inflate or deflate the balloon, the compartment can be assigned an elastance similar to an *in vivo* lung. This model has some deficiencies because the airway is more complex than a simple pipe and it now appears that the alveoli are not physically independent structures but are interconnected. However, to lay the groundwork for the understanding of respiratory mechanics, this simple model of a balloon on a pipe will suffice.

Referring to Figure 6.7.2, assume that the tension in the spring increases linearly as the spring is stretched past its relaxed length. This means that the elastic recoil pressure (P_{EL}) inside the compartment increases linearly with the volume (V) of the compartment; therefore, $P_{EL} = EV$. E is defined as the elastance of the compartment and is a

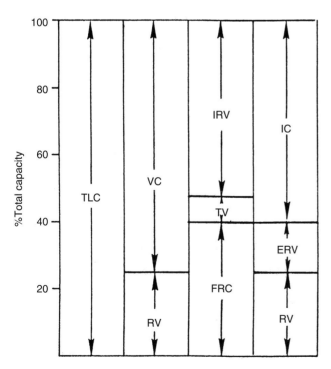

Figure 6.7.1 Subdivisions of lung volume. TLC, total lung capacity; VC, vital capacity; IRV, inspiratory reserve volume; TV, tidal volume; FRC, functional residual capacity; ERV, expiratory reserve volume; RV, residual volume; IC, inspiratory capacity. (From George RB, Light RW, Matthay MA, et al. *Chest medicine: Essentials of pulmonary and critical care medicine.* 4th ed. Philadelphia, PA: Lippincott Williams & Wilkins; 2000:27.)

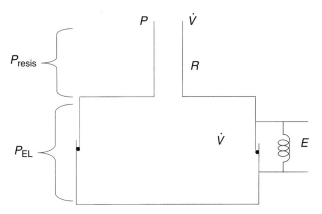

Figure 6.7.2 Single-compartment linear model. R, resistance; E, elastance; P, total pressure; $\dot{V}$, flow; P_{resis}, pressure necessary to overcome resistant elements; P_{EL}, pressure necessary to overcome elastic elements.

constant, secondary to the linear relationship between P_{EL} and V. Compliance is the inverse of elastance. Assuming that the pressure difference (ΔP) between the proximal and distal ends of the conduit increases linearly with flow ($\dot{V}$), $\Delta P = R\dot{V}$. R is defined as the resistance of the pipe and $\dot{V}$ is the derivative of V with respect to time (i.e., the flow through the conduit). The relation at any moment (t) between the pressure applied at the opening of the model [$P(t)$] and the volume in the model [$V(t)$] during emptying of this compartment can be described as a first-order model, in which total pressure across the model is the sum of P and ΔP, plus the resting pressure P_0:

$$P(t) = E \times V(t) + R \times \dot{V}(t) + P_0$$

where E = elastance of the balloon, R = resistance of the pipe, and $\dot{V}$ = flow through the opening. Using regression analysis, E and R can be calculated from $P(t)$, $V(t)$, and $V'(t)$.

What R and E represent depends on the type of pressure used for P in the equation of motion of the model. For example, the lung pressure is reflected by the transpulmonary pressure (P_{ao}[airway opening] $- P_{es}$[esophageal]); the chest wall pressure is reflected by the P_{es}; and, in mechanically ventilated patients, the respiratory system pressure is reflected by P_{ao}. The values of R and E, as applied to the respiratory system, reflect the resistance of the airways and the elastance of the respiratory system, whereas $V(t)$ is the volume increase from FRC when the mouth pressure is zero.

The important components of this linear model are the time constant (τ), compliance (C) or elastance (E), and resistance (R). The relation of these is given by the equations:

$$\tau = C \times R \text{ or } \tau = \frac{R}{E}$$

Each of these components is discussed separately. It is important to note that the respiratory system is not a linear system because compliance and resistance are not constants but are dependent on the volume, volume history, and flow.

ELASTIC PROPERTIES OF THE RESPIRATORY SYSTEM

The respiratory system is composed of a collection of elastic structures. The response to a force applied to the elastic structure of the respiratory system is to resist deformation by producing an opposing force, known as *elastic recoil*, to return the structure to its relaxed state. Because of the lung recoil pressure, the alveolar gas pressure is greater than the pressure on the pleural surface. In the respiratory system, this opposing force produces a pressure known as *the elastic recoil pressure* (P_{EL}). The force required to stretch an elastic structure depends on the volume at which the outward recoil of the chest wall balances the inward recoil. This point is known as the *elastic equilibrium volume* (EEV). The pressure of the elastic recoil or P_{EL} divided by the lung volume (V) gives a measure of the elastic properties of respiratory system and is called *elastance* (E):

$$E = \frac{P_{EL}}{V}$$

When lung volume is plotted on the ordinate (y-axis) and P_{EL} is plotted on the abscissa (x-axis), the slope of the static pressure–volume curve is equivalent to the reciprocal of elastance, called *compliance*.

For ventilation of the lungs to occur, forces must be produced to overcome the elastic, flow-resistive, and inertial properties of the lungs and the chest wall to create motion in the respiratory system. Normally, respiratory muscles produce these forces. Overcoming forces to move gas into the airway can be exemplified by moving a block of wood over a surface. The movement of the block is determined by the friction created between the block of wood and the surface and by the speed of the block's movement. The exact position of the block on the surface is irrelevant. In the lung, the pressure required to produce a flow of gas between the atmosphere and the alveoli must overcome the frictional resistance of the airways. This pressure is proportional to the rate at which volume is changing, or flow ($\dot{V}$), as follows:

$$P_{ao} - P_{ALV} = P_{fr}\alpha\dot{V}$$

where P_{ao} is pressure at the airway opening (usually atmospheric pressure). P_{ALV} is the alveolar pressure, and P_{fr} is the pressure required to overcome frictional resistance. The pressure required to produce a unit of flow is known as *flow resistance* (R).

$$R = P_{fr}/\dot{V}$$

If the respiratory system is modeled as a single compartment with a single constant elastance (E) and a single constant resistance (R), then the equation of motion describes the balance of forces acting on the system as follows:

$$P = EV + R\dot{V} + I\dot{V}$$

The inertance (I) is usually negligible and therefore ignored. Most of the pressure produced during tidal respiration is required to overcome the elastic forces, whereas a minimal is required to overcome the flow-resistant forces.

Traditionally, it was thought that little energy was dissipated by the tissues of the respiratory system and that most of the force developed during breathing was required to move gas through the airways. However, the lung parenchyma is a complex system consisting of alveolar walls composed of collagen, elastin, and proteoglycan macromolecules; an air–liquid interface of surfactant; and cells, which have the capacity to act in a contractile fashion, called *interstitial cells*. Airway smooth muscle exists in the terminal bronchioles and alveolar ducts. The interaction of all these components may well influence parenchymal mechanics in ways that have yet to be defined, contradicting previously held beliefs about energy consumption.

The energy expended while moving the tissue is called *the tissue viscance or resistance*. This is a non-Newtonian resistance. In other words, the viscosity depends upon the force applied. When measured during inspiration, the *tissue* resistance increases with increasing lung volume, whereas *airway* resistance falls. Tissue resistance contributes approximately 65% of respiratory system resistance at FRC in mechanically ventilated animals. It may increase by as much as 95% at higher lung volumes. The contribution of tissue resistance to respiratory system resistance in humans under the same circumstances is unknown.

Resistance is expressed as changes in pressure divided by changes in flow:

$$R = \frac{\Delta P}{\Delta \dot{V}}$$

The other part of elastic recoil depends upon the surface tension at the alveolar gas–liquid interface (surface forces). Surface tension is produced by the interface between air in the alveolus and the thin film of liquid that covers the alveolar surface. Surface tension in the alveolus is created by interacting water molecules that direct a force inward and could cause the alveoli to collapse. Remember the action described in Laplace equation where the pressure inside a bubble exceeds the pressure outside the bubble by twice the surface tension, divided by the radius. In other words, the smaller the bubble, the more the pressure inside it exceeds the pressure on the outside. Comparing two different alveoli with the same surface tension, the smaller the radius the greater the pressure created by a given surface tension. Air will flow from higher pressure (small alveoli) to lower pressure (larger alveoli) causing smaller alveoli to collapse more often. As discussed previously, the surface tension of the alveoli is affected by surfactants, which act to lower surface tension at the alveolar air–liquid interface and thereby decrease elastic recoil of the lungs.

COMPLIANCE AND ELASTANCE

Compliance is the degree to which a compartment will expand if the pressure in that compartment is changed. A balloon has a high compliance because a small pressure increase inside the balloon will greatly expand the balloon. A rigid tube has a low compliance because a small pressure increase inside the rigid tube will not result in a significant increase in the volume of the rigid tube. Two major forces contribute to lung compliance: tissue elastic forces and surface tension forces. The compliance (C) is determined by the change in elastic recoil pressure (ΔP) produced by a change in volume (ΔV).

$$C = \frac{\Delta V}{\Delta P}$$

The compliance of the lungs (C_L), chest wall (C_{CW}), and respiratory system (C_{RS}) can be determined by measuring the change in distending pressure and the associated change in volume. The distending pressure represents the pressure change across the structure.

$$C_L = \frac{\Delta V}{\Delta(P_{ao} - P_{PL})}$$
$$C_{CW} = \frac{\Delta V}{\Delta(P_{PL} - P_{bs})}$$
$$C_{RS} = \frac{\Delta V}{\Delta(P_{ao} - P_{bs})}$$

where P_{ao}, P_{PL}, and P_{bs} represent the pressure measured at the airway opening, the pleural pressure, and pressure at the body surface (atmospheric pressure), respectively. Lung volume and volume–pressure relationships (e.g., compliance) reflect parenchymal (air space) development, whereas airflow and pressure-flow relationships (resistance and conductance) predominantly reflect airway development. The lungs become stiffer (compliance decreases) at higher lung volumes. Both at the bedside and in the laboratory, pressure differences can be readily measured when the airways are open and when gas flow is either interrupted ("static" conditions) or kept so low ("quasistatic" conditions) that the pressure difference along the airways between the alveoli and the airway opening can be neglected. Therefore, lung recoil pressures can be evaluated directly from pressure differences noted between the airway opening and pleura (i.e., transpulmonary pressure).

Pulmonary compliance changes with growth and maturation, depending upon the number of expanded air spaces, the size and geometry of the air spaces, the characteristics of the surface-lining layer and the properties of the lung parenchyma. This is represented by changes in the shape of the volume–pressure curve. When these curves are corrected by expressing the volumes as a percentage of the maximal observed lung volume, they are more curved in infants than in older children (see Fig. 6.7.3). It is important to note that there may be boundaries for dynamic changes in alveolar size and shape during ventilation because of the tensile forces of the connective tissue and surface tension supporting the alveoli and alveolar ducts.

The change in shape of the volume–pressure curve represents the immature rather than the mature alveoli and hence the differences in the elastin–collagen ratio that exists

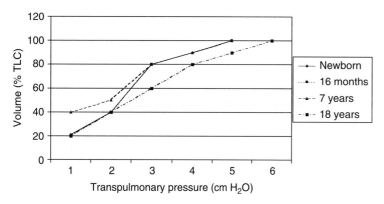

Figure 6.7.3 Deflation volume–pressure curves of the lung at different ages (obtained from studies on excised lungs). With increasing age up to young adulthood, the curves become straighter and, at a given lung volume, elastic recoil pressure is greater. The curve from elderly individuals resembles that of a 7-year-old's respiratory system. TLC, total lung capacity. (Adapted from Fagan DG. Post-mortem studies of the semistatic volume-pressure characteristics of infant's lungs. *Thorax.* 1976,31:534.)

with age. The lung volume at which airway closure occurs is higher in children younger than 7 years. Pressure–volume relationships are also more curvilinear in infants. Chest wall compliance is 50% greater in infants. Elastance is defined as the change in distending pressure divided by the associated change in volume. It is also the inverse of compliance. In stiff lungs, the elastance will be high while compliance will be low.

ELASTIC RECOIL OF THE RESPIRATORY SYSTEM

The example of forces involved in moving gas through the simple balloon on a pipe model can now be adapted to the respiratory system.

A series is created between the lungs and the chest wall by the forces within the pleural space. In the intact thorax, the inward recoil of the lungs is opposed by the outward recoil of the chest wall below its resting volume. Both the lungs and the chest wall recoil inward when this volume is exceeded.

By having a subject exhale in increments from TLC to RV, the pressure required to balance the elastic recoil of the lungs, chest wall, and respiratory system (elastic recoil pressure) may be determined. At each volume, the subject relaxes against a fixed obstruction with the glottis open, and the pressure difference across the lung, chest wall, and entire respiratory system is recorded. Pressure–volume curves are derived in this way for the respiratory system and its components. The static pressure–volume curves of the respiratory system, lung, and chest wall are different during inspiration and expiration. Therefore, lung volumes at a given transpulmonary pressure are higher during deflation than during inflation. This phenomenon is called *hysteresis*. Hysteresis is the failure of a system to follow identical paths of response on the application and withdrawal of a forcing agent, such as occurs during inspiration and expiration. The recoil pressures at the same lung volume are always less during deflation than inflation. Therefore, mechanical energy (work) expended during inflation is

greater than that recovered during deflation. This can be expressed mathematically as:

$$\int_{V_{min}}^{V_{max}} PdV > \int_{V_{max}}^{V_{min}} PdV$$

Hysteresis in the respiratory system depends on viscoelasticity, such as stress adaptation (i.e., a rate-dependent phenomenon) and on plasticity (i.e., a rate-independent phenomenon). In the lungs, hysteresis is due mainly to surface properties and alveolar recruitment–derecruitment. Surfactant is partly responsible for the hysteresis observed in the lung. More pressure must be exerted to open alveoli initially, but once open and inflated, the changes in surface tension produced by surfactant allow them to deflate more evenly. In comparison, the chest wall hysteresis is related to the action of both muscles and ligaments because both skeletal muscles and elastic fibers exhibit hysteresis. Hysteresis is negligible when volume changes are minimal, such as during quiet breathing. This is important because the area of the hysteresis loop represents energy lost from the system.

The resting volume of the respiratory system, the FRC, is the volume at which the elastic recoil of the lungs and the chest wall exactly balance each other. Above and below this equilibrium point, progressively increasing pressure is required to change the volume of the respiratory system. The total pressure required at each volume is the sum of the pressures required to overcome the elastic recoil of the lungs and chest wall.

FLOW RESISTANCE OF THE RESPIRATORY SYSTEM

The response of the lung to movement is governed by its response to the physical impedance of the respiratory system. The impedance can be categorized into (i) elastic resistance at the alveolar gas–liquid interface and (ii) tissue frictional resistance to gas flow. Under static conditions, pressure is required only to oppose the elastic recoil of the respiratory system. However, when the lungs and chest wall are in motion and movement of air into and out of the lungs occurs, pressure must also be provided to overcome the frictional or viscous forces. The ratio of this additional pressure (P) and the rate of airflow that it produces ($\dot{V}$) is defined as the resistance in the respiratory system.

$$R = \frac{P}{\dot{V}}$$

In other words, the flow ($\dot{V}$) measured at the mouth depends on the driving pressure (i.e., the pressure difference between alveoli [P_{ALV}] and mouth [P_{mo}]) and the airway resistance (R_{aw}):

$$\dot{V} = \frac{P_{mo} - P_{ALV}}{R_{aw}}$$

If the mouth pressure is 0 (i.e., atmospheric pressure), the driving pressure is the alveolar pressure.

Airways resistance (R_{aw}) is the sum of the peripheral airway resistance (peripheral intrathoracic airways <2 mm diameter; R_{awp}), the central airways resistance (large intrathoracic airways >2 mm diameter; R_{awc}), and the extrathoracic airways resistance (especially glottis; R_{ext}). In healthy individuals, R_{ext} accounts for 50% of the total R_{aw} and R_{awp} for approximately 15%. R_{awp} and R_{awc} are influenced by lung volume. Higher lung volumes give higher P_{EL} and therefore increase airway diameter. With increasing volumes during inspiration, the increased P_{EL} is counteracted by P_{PL}, resulting in increased radial distending force. This distending force is the transmural pressure and is the difference between pressure in (P_{in}) and pressure outside (P_{out}) the airway.

At 0 airflow, the pressure inside the airways (P_{in}) equals atmospheric pressure and transmural pressure (P_{tm}) equals the elastic recoil pressure (P_{EL}):

$$P_{in} = P_{mo}; P_{tm} = P_{EL}$$

The total respiratory resistance (R_{RS}) consists of the resistance of the airways (R_{aw}), the resistance of the lung (R_L), and the resistance of the chest wall (R_{CW}):

$$R_{RS} = R_{CW} + R_L + R_{aw}$$

In older children, R_{CW} and R_L represent only 10% to 20% of R_{RS}, but, in newborns, R_L could be higher.

Airway diameter of the intrathoracic airways approximates to a sigmoidal relationship with P_{tm}. This results in volume dependency of R_{aw}. At higher lung volumes R_{awp} decreases. The specific relation between R_{awp} (or its reciprocal conductance G_{aw} [$1/R_{aw}$]) and volume is mirrored by the specific R_{aw} (sR_{aw}) and specific G_{aw} (sG_{aw}):

$$sR_{aw} = \frac{R_{aw}}{V} \quad sG_{aw} = \frac{G_{aw}}{V}$$

The resistance of the airways (R_{aw}), lungs (airway and parenchyma) (R_L), chest wall (R_{CW}), and entire respiratory system (R_{RS}) can be calculated by measuring the rate of airflow and the associated trans-structural pressure by subtracting the amount required to overcome elastic recoil

from the total pressure:

$$R_{aw} = \frac{P_{ao} - P_{ALV}}{\dot{V}}$$
$$R_L = \frac{P_{ao} - P_{PL}}{\dot{V}}$$
$$R_{CW} = \frac{P_{PL} - P_{bs}}{\dot{V}}$$
$$R_{RS} = \frac{P_{ao} - P_{bs}}{\dot{V}}$$

where P_{ao}, P_{ALV}, P_{PL}, and P_{bs} represent the pressure at the airway opening, alveolar pressure, pleural pressure, and pressure at the body surface, respectively. The resistance of the lung parenchyma may be derived by subtracting airway resistance from total lung resistance.

The relationship between the flow rate and the airway pressure gradient is nonlinear because of the relative contribution of the various components of the respiratory system to the total pressure required to overcome the viscous forces. The viscous forces, and hence airway resistance, increases disproportionately as the flow rate increases. In contrast, the resistance of the chest wall and lung parenchyma remains constant over a wide range of flow rates. During quiet breathing by mouth, airway resistance accounts for >50% of the total respiratory system resistance. However, as flow rate increases, the contribution of the airways to total resistance progressively increases.

Changing patterns of airflow results in the nonlinear flow-resistance characteristic of the airways. Subsequently, as the flow rate to the airway increases, airflow becomes progressively more turbulent. Therefore, the more turbulent the flow, the greater the pressure required to overcome the viscous forces. Turbulence occurs at lower flow rates in the upper airway because of the tortuous geometry of the upper (extrathoracic) airway and because the glottic aperture is narrower than the lower (intrathoracic) airways. Therefore, the upper airway is responsible for most of the increase in airway resistance noted with an increase in flow rate. Studies have shown the resistance of the lower airways to be nearly constant up to flow rates of 2 L per second. For patients who are breathing quietly by mouth, the total airway resistance is divided almost equally between the upper and lower airways. As their effort increases (therefore flow rate increases), the ratio of upper to lower airway resistance progressively increases, as described in the preceding text.

Depending on whether laminar or turbulent flow predominates, resistance to airflow varies inversely with either the fourth or the fifth power of airway radius. Therefore, major changes in airway resistance occur by factors that affect airway diameter. During spontaneous lung inflation, airway diameter increases while airway resistance decreases. This is produced by two mechanisms. First, as lung volume increases, the increasing elastic recoil of the pulmonary parenchyma provides a tethering effect that results in dilation of the intrapulmonary airways. Second, extrapulmonary and large intrapulmonary airways are subject to

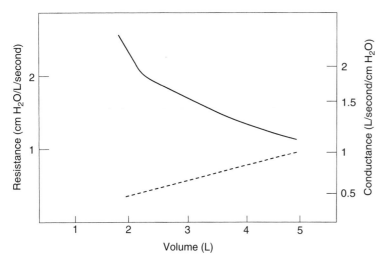

Figure 6.7.4 Relationship between lung volume and airway resistance (*solid line*) and conductance (*dashed line*). (Adapted from Briscoe WA, Dubois AB. The relation between airway resistance, airway conductance, and lung volume in subjects of different age and body size. *J Clin Invest.* 1958;37:1280.)

pleural pressure, which becomes increasingly negative during inspiration. This leads to an increasing pressure gradient across the airway wall, which favors expansion of the airway diameter. The change in airway resistance with lung volume is curvilinear and is illustrated in Figure 6.7.4. When the reciprocal of airway resistance, airway conductance (G_{aw}), is plotted against lung volume, this relation is nearly linear.

DYNAMIC CHANGE IN AIRWAY CALIBER DURING RESPIRATION

Airway caliber is partially dependent on the transmural pressure. The transmural pressure is the difference between interstitial pressure and atmospheric pressure. The external airway wall for the intrathoracic airways is subjected to the interstitial pressure in the lung, which is approximately equal to the pleural pressure. In contrast, the external walls of extrathoracic airways are subjected to atmospheric pressure. During inspiration, pleural pressure is negative

relative to atmospheric pressure. Alveolar pressure is approximately equal to pleural pressure, whereas pressure at the mouth is atmospheric. This pressure difference creates a gradient from the mouth to the alveoli. Extrathoracic airways tend to narrow during inspiration because the transmural pressure is positive. In contrast, the intrathoracic airway transmural pressure is negative, causing a tendency for these airways to dilate during inspiration. The degree of airway caliber change during inspiration depends on both the magnitude of the transmural pressure and the airway wall compliance. The point at which intrabronchial pressure becomes equal to the pleural pressure outside the bronchus is designated the equal pressure point (EPP) (see Fig. 6.7.5). At the end of inspiration, there is a relaxation of the inspiratory muscles, and therefore, the elastic recoil of the respiratory system produces a positive pleural and alveolar pressure. Because of the dynamic pressure changes described in the preceding text, there is a tendency for intrathoracic airways to narrow and for extrathoracic airways to dilate during expiration (see Fig. 6.7.6).

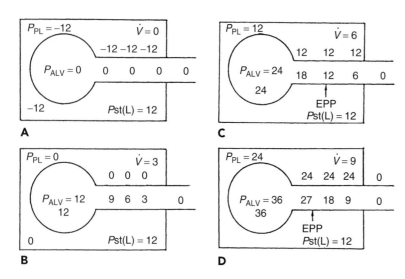

Figure 6.7.5 Equal pressure point (EPP) gas movement. **A:** The alveolar pressure is 0, so there is no flow. **B:** The increase in the alveolar pressure is equal to the static transpulmonary pressure of the lung Pst(L), so the pleural pressure is 0. Here, the EPP is at the airway opening. **C:** The alveolar pressure has increased, so the pleural pressure must be positive. The pressure drops from the alveolus to different points along the airway are greater because $\dot{V}$ is higher. Accordingly, the EPP moves closer to the alveolus. **D:** The P_{PL} has been increased even more, and the EPP has moved farther upstream because flow has increased. $\dot{V}$, rate of airflow; P_{PL}, pleural pressure; P_{ALV}, alveolar pressure. (From George RB, Light RW, Matthay MA, et al. *Chest medicine: Essentials of pulmonary and critical care medicine.* 4th ed. Philadelphia, PA: Lippincott Williams & Wilkins; 2000:35.)

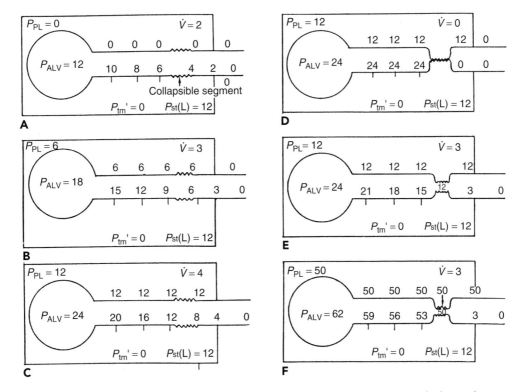

Figure 6.7.6   Effects of transmural pressure on airway caliber. In these diagrams, the lung volume is that giving a static transpulmonary pressure of the lung Pst(L) of 12, and it is assumed that P_{tm}' is zero. **A:** Pressures along the airways when P_{tm} still exceeds P_{tm}'. There is no collapse. **B:** Pressures along the airways when P_{tm} approaches P_{tm}'. Note that the flow rate increases from (**A**). **C:** Pressures along the airways when pleural pressures are further increased. Note that P_{tm} at the collapsible segment is now $8 - 12 = -4$, which is below $P_{tm}' = 0$, so this higher flow is impossible because the collapsible segment must collapse. **D:** Pressures along the airways when there is no flow. Now P_{tm} is $24 - 12 = 12$, so the airways must open. **E:** Pressure along the airways when the collapsible segment is partially collapsed such that $P_{tm} = P_{tm}'$. **F:** Pressures along the airways when the alveolar pressure is raised much higher. Note that the collapsible segment is more collapsed than in (**E**) and that the flows in (**B**), (**E**), and (**F**) are also identical. The airway pressures downstream from the collapsible segment in (**B**), (**E**), and (**F**) are also identical. $\dot{V}$, rate of airflow; P_{PL}, pleural pressure; P_{ALV}, alveolar pressure. (From George RB, Light RW, Matthay MA, et al. *Chest medicine: Essentials of pulmonary and critical care medicine.* 4th ed. Philadelphia, PA: Lippincott Williams & Wilkins; 2000:27.)

APPLIED FORCES

Ventilation of the lungs involves motion of the respiratory system, which is produced by the forces required to overcome the flow-resistive, inertial, and elastic properties of the lungs and chest wall. Under normal circumstances, these forces are produced by the respiratory muscles.

If ventilation is to occur, the opposing forces must be overcome by pressure applied to the respiratory system to create motion. At each instant, the applied pressure (P_{APP}) must equal the sum of the pressure required to balance the elastic recoil (P_{ER}) and the pressure lost to viscous forces (P_R).

$$P_{APP} = P_{ER} + P_R$$

Using the above equations this may be converted to:

$$P_{APP} = \frac{1}{C}V + R\dot{V}$$

This is known as *the equation of motion of the respiratory system.*

Figure 6.7.7 illustrates the pressure involved in respiration. Gradients must occur to allow for gas to flow into the lungs. Airway pressure gradient, which drives airflow into the lungs, is defined as:

$$P_M - P_{ALV}$$

P_M is the pressure at the mouth, which is normally atmospheric, and P_{ALV} is the alveolar pressure. Transpulmonary pressure (P_{TP}) is defined as:

$$P_{TP} = P_{ALV} - P_{PL}$$

P_{ALV} is the alveolar pressure and P_{PL} is the intrapleural pressure. The P_{TP} is equal to elastic recoil of the lungs when there is no airflow. The P_{TP} increases and decreases with lung volume. Trans–chest wall pressure (P_{TC}) is defined as:

$$P_{TC} = P_{PL} - P_{bs}$$

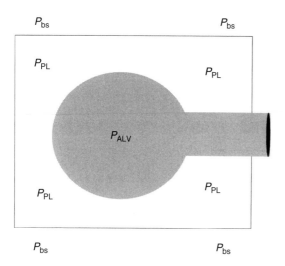

Figure 6.7.7 Pressure involved in respiration. Gradients must occur to allow for gas to flow into the lungs, P_{bs}, pressure of the body surface; P_{ALV}, alveolar pressure; P_{PL}, pleural pressure.

P_{PL} is the intrapleural pressure and P_{bs} is the pressure at the body surface. This pressure is usually the same as atmospheric pressure. P_{TC} is equal in magnitude to the elastic recoil of the chest when there is no airflow and, like P_{TP}, increases and decreases with lung volume.

The transmural pressure (P_{RS}) is defined as

$$P_{RS} = P_{ALV} - P_{bs}$$

P_{ALV} is the alveolar pressure and P_{bs} is the pressure at the body surface. P_{RS} represents the transmural pressure across the entire respiratory system including the lungs and the chest. The P_{RS} is equal to the net passive elastic recoil pressure of the whole respiratory system when the airflow is zero.

During inspiration, the respiratory muscles provide the applied force that expands the chest wall and the lungs and cause the alveolar and airway pressure to decrease. The net result of these actions is that the alveolar pressure becomes less than atmospheric pressure. This creates a pressure gradient from the mouth to the lungs, which results in airflow into the alveoli. Inflation of the lungs also results in the storage of potential energy within the elastic structures of the lung, which can be used to augment expiration. For gas flow to occur, there must be a balance of forces. Figure 6.7.8 illustrates these forces. Therefore, to inflate the lungs, there must be an increase in alveolar pressure, which is usually accomplished by the respiratory muscles during normal breathing or with positive pressure during mechanical ventilation. A decrease in body surface pressure, such as is provided with negative pressure ventilation (iron lung), will also result in lung inflation.

Expiration is usually passive under resting conditions (excluding disease states where the patient actively tries to empty their lungs); that is, the energy stored in the elastic recoil of the lungs and the chest wall produces the positive alveolar and airway pressures needed to overcome flow resistance and air is forced from the lungs. At times of increased ventilatory requirements, such as during exercise, contraction of the abdominal and internal intercostals muscles can aid in expiration.

INTERACTIONS BETWEEN THE LUNGS AND CHEST WALL

The lungs and the chest wall operate in series, and their compliance adds reciprocally to make total compliance.

$$\frac{1}{C_T} = \frac{1}{C_L} + \frac{1}{C_{CW}}$$

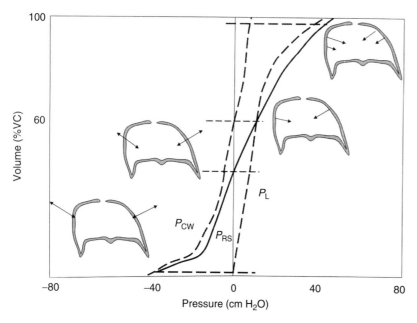

Figure 6.7.8 Pressure–volume relationship of the lung (P_L), chest wall (P_{CW}), and entire respiratory system (P_{RS}). *Large arrows* represent the elastic recoil of the lungs and the chest wall. VC, vital capacity. (Adapted from Agostoni E, Mead J. Statics of the respiratory system. In: Fenn WO, Rahn H. eds. *Handbook of physiology, respiration.* Washington, DC: AM Physiological Society; 1964;1:392.)

The chest wall is like a spring that may either be compressed or distended. Transthoracic pressure is negative at RV and FRC; that is, the chest wall is smaller than its unstressed volume and its tendency is to spring out. Normal tidal breathing is entirely in the negative pressure range for transthoracic pressure. When examining the compliance curve of the chest wall (lung volume vs. transthoracic pressure), pressure is 0 at approximately 65% of TLC. Therefore, the chest is at its unstressed volume and has no tendency to collapse or expand. Transthoracic pressure is positive at volumes above 65% TLC. The chest tends to collapse above its unstressed volume.

TIME CONSTANT OF EMPTYING

The time constant of the respiratory system (τ) is the time taken for the volume to be reduced by 63% when the respiratory system is allowed to empty passively and the volume–time profile is measured. The time constant characterizes the rate of variation of the function over a period. Short time constants imply a fast rate of change and long time constants imply a slow rate of change. If a single-compartment model of the respiratory system with a single, constant elastance and a single, constant resistance is used, then the following occurs:

$$\tau = \frac{R}{E}$$

In a single-compartment model, the volume–time profile can be represented by a single exponential decay.

In healthy adults, the time constant of the passive respiratory system is short, approximately 0.5 seconds. Such a short time constant allows the lungs to empty to the EEV at the end of each expiration. Therefore, FRC and EEV are equal. Because the respiratory system is relaxed at the end of expiration, inspiration can begin as soon as inspiratory muscle activity is initiated. The expiratory time constant is shorter in children, with values approximating 0.3 seconds in infants with normal lungs. Infants with hyaline membrane disease have stiffer than normal lungs and may have expiratory time constants as low as 0.1 seconds. Therefore, derecruitment of the lung in children, especially in those with stiff lungs, occurs rapidly and may explain the rapid fall in oxygen tension and the increase in atelectasis noted when these patients are removed from positive pressure ventilation. In the case of a patient with obstructive airway disease, such as asthma, resistance is increased, and the expiratory time constant is longer. Therefore, a longer time is required for the lungs to empty and return the respiratory system to EEV.

Patients with chronic airway obstruction frequently have carbon dioxide retention and an increased respiratory drive. This results in an increased respiratory rate with a shorter respiratory cycle and less time available for expiration. In this situation, the respiratory system frequently does not have the time to return to EEV before the next inspiration

starts. As a consequence, FRC occurs at a volume higher than EEV, causing the respiratory system not to be relaxed at the end of expiration. This lack of relaxation of the respiratory system at the end of expiration causes a positive recoil pressure. This pressure is called *intrinsic positive end-expiratory pressure* ($PEEP_i$). Before inspiratory flow can begin, the patient's inspiratory muscle must produce enough force to overcome the $PEEP_i$. This force represents a load that must be overcome by the inspiratory muscle before inspiratory flow can begin. This creates additional muscle work during inspiration. In patients with severe airway obstruction, this pressure can be as high as 15 to 20 cm H_2O.

ALVEOLAR VENTILATION

The volume of air entering the lungs each minute that actually participates in gas exchange is called *the alveolar ventilation* ($\dot{V}_A$). It is, therefore, the difference between the total volume of air entering the lungs each minute, the minute ventilation ($\dot{V}_E$) and the volume of air entering the lungs that does not participate in gas exchange, the dead space ($\dot{V}_D$).

$$\dot{V}_A = \dot{V}_E - \dot{V}_D$$

The type of total or physiologic dead space ($\dot{V}_D$) depends upon the location of the volume not participating in gas exchange, either in the anatomic airways or in the alveolus. The anatomic dead space is equal to the volume of airways proximal to the terminal respiratory units. Approximately 25% of each TV is lost in these conducting airways. The ultimate anatomic dead space volume depends on body size and equals approximately 1 mL per lb. This volume is divided almost equally between the upper and lower airways. The alveolar dead space is produced by all alveoli that are overventilated relative to their perfusion. Therefore, there is proportionally more gas than blood available for diffusion. The physiologic dead space is usually expressed as a fraction of the TV ($\dot{V}_D/\dot{V}_T$).

The alveolar ventilation is an important determinant of gas exchange because this, along with the rate at which tissue metabolism produces carbon dioxide ($\dot{V}_{CO_2}$) determines the P_{CO_2} of arterial blood.

$$P_{CO_2} \propto \frac{\dot{V}_{CO_2}}{\dot{V}_A}$$

When $\dot{V}_{CO_2}$ is constant, P_{CO_2} varies inversely with $\dot{V}_A$. It is evident that at given minute ventilation, the P_{CO_2} will vary directly with the amount of physiologic dead space. As dead space changes, the P_{CO_2} can be kept constant only by increasing $\dot{V}_A$ or decreasing $\dot{V}_E$ by an identical amount.

The measurement of dead space has evolved from the original description by Bohr in 1891, when dead space was considered simply as the gas lost in the conducting airways. $P_{E_{CO_2}}$ is the mixed expired carbon dioxide tension and Pa_{CO_2} is arterial blood carbon dioxide tension. Today, this has been modified so that physiologic dead space is measured by:

$$\frac{\dot{V}_D}{\dot{V}_T} = \frac{(Pa_{CO_2} - P\overline{E}_{CO_2})}{Pa_{CO_2}}$$

CONTROL OF RESPIRATION

Because the primary function of the respiratory system is gas exchange, there needs to be a precise regulation of blood–gas concentrations. Control of this system would require regulation of ventilatory requirements and feedback on system performance. Ventilatory requirements include functions such as cardiac output, carbon dioxide production, oxygen consumption, input from muscle afferents, and input from higher centers. The feedback system consists of the partial pressure of carbon dioxide and oxygen and the hydrogen ion concentration reaching the respiratory centers. The relation between ventilation (V) and alveolar carbon dioxide partial pressure (Pa_{CO_2}) can be described as:

$$V = S(Pa_{CO_2} - B)$$

where S is the slope of the line or sensitivity of the relationship and B is the intercept with Pa_{CO_2} axis. Hypoxia increases the sensitivity without altering the intercept. At very high levels of Pa_{O_2}, respiratory depression occurs.

The state of the respiratory system is important in the translation of the signals from the respiratory center for alveolar ventilation and gas exchange. Diseases of various components of the respiratory system are characteristically associated with increased mechanical loads. These loads may be elastic, resistive, inertial, or a combination thereof.

Asthma is an example of a disease that increases the resistance against which the patient must breathe. The patient's ability to keep the airway open is overwhelmed, resulting in airway narrowing. As a result of this airway narrowing, gas flow becomes turbulent, with increased energy dissipation in the airway. The primary ventilatory response to disorders with increased resistance is alterations in V_T and respiratory timing indices. A breathing pattern with a prolonged expiratory phase is optimal for lung emptying and for avoiding an increase in lung volume, with its resulting increase in elastic load. A shortened inspiratory phase may require high inspiratory flow, adding to the increased resistive load.

Increased elastic loading occurs when the respiratory system is stiffer than usual; this occurs with interstitial lung disease, severe cases of obesity, increased chest wall stiffness, or conditions of decreased muscle performance. The primary ventilatory response to these disorders is usually tachypnea, hypoxia, and a relatively normal or even low Pa_{CO_2}. Rapid shallow breathing, which minimizes the elastic load, may be seen.

PULMONARY FUNCTION TESTS

The use of pulmonary function testing can aid the clinician in both diagnostic and therapeutic decisions. To understand pulmonary function testing, certain physiologic and engineering principles must be elucidated. Because much of the discussion of pulmonary function testing in the pediatric intensive care unit (PICU) is in patients on positive pressure mechanical ventilation, this discussion focuses on these patients. As previously discussed, pulmonary function tests (PFTs) are based on the equation of motion that describes the pressure change at the airway opening during breathing. It is important to note that most bedside systems utilized in the PICU through the mechanical ventilator measure only pressure and flow, with volume being derived from an integration of flow.

Integration of Flow to Volume

Integration of flow ($\dot{V}$) measured at the airway opening to obtain volume can be performed utilizing a simple trapezoidal rule (see Figure 6.7.9). The trapezoidal rule joins adjacent sampled data points by straight lines and approximates the area under the curve by the area under all

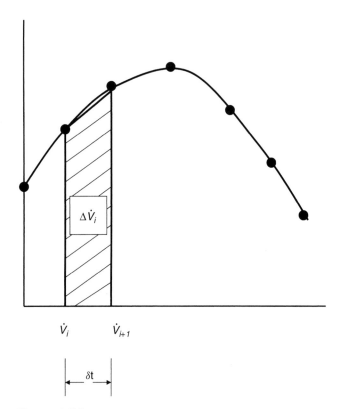

Figure 6.7.9 Integrating flow to volume. Volume (V) can be obtained by numerically integrating flow ($\dot{V}$) on a computer. The trapezoidal rule uses flow and time to obtain the volume of the integrated area under the flow curve.

the line segments. The formula for the trapezoidal rule is:

$$\dot{V} = V_0 + \sum_0^N \Delta \dot{V}_i$$

$$\text{where} \quad \Delta \dot{V}_i = \left(\frac{\dot{V}_i + \dot{V}_{i+1}}{2} \right) \delta t$$

δt is the time interval between data samples, and V_0 is the value of the volume at the start of the integration process.

Bedside Measurements

In Chapter 6.8, the clinical applications of bedside pulmonary function testing, as well as the interpretation of graphical interfaces, in patients on mechanical ventilation will be discussed. A common bedside measurement utilized in critically ill patients is the measurement of forced expiration for the detection of obstructive lung disease. The use of such measurements is derived from the observation that expiratory flow is independent over most of the expired VC as long as reasonable effort is made. Obtaining a reasonable effort is difficult in young children, and therefore, performance of PFT maneuvers is often not attempted. The physiologic mechanism for expiratory flow limitation is complex because of the high speed of air movement in the airways, the lower density, and the compliant nature of the airway.

RECOMMENDED READINGS

1. Hall JE. The promise of translational physiology. *Am J Physiol Lung Cell Mol Physiol.* 2002;283(2):L235–L236.
2. Fung YC. A model of the lung structure and its validation. *J Appl Physiol.* 1988;64(5):2132–2141.
3. Karlinsky JB, Snyder GL, Franzblaw C, et al. In vitro effects of elastase and collagenase on mechanical properties of hamster lungs. *Am Rev Respir Dis.* 1976;113:769–777.
4. Wright JR, Hawgood S. Pulmonary surfactant metabolism. *Clin Chest Med.* 1989;10(1):83.
5. Ludwig MS, Dreshaj I, Solway J, et al. Partitioning of the pulmonary resistance during constriction in the dog: Effects of volume history. *J Appl Physiol.* 1987;62(2):807–815.
6. Bangham AD. Lung surfactant: How it does and does not work. *Lung.* 1987;165:17–25.
7. Hills BA. What forces keep the air spaces of the lung dry? *Thorax.* 1982;37(10):713–717.
8. Hills BA. Water repellency induced by pulmonary surfactants. *J Physiol.* 1982;325:175–186.
9. Scapelli EM. The alveoli surface network: A new anatomy and its physiologic significance. *Anat Rec.* 1998;251(4):491–527.
10. Hills BA. An alternative view of the roles surfactant and the alveolar model. *J Appl Physiol.* 1999;87(5):1567–1583.
11. Scapelli EM, Hills BA. Opposing views on the alveolar surface, alveolar models, and the role of surfactant. *J Appl Physiol.* 2000;89(2):408–412.
12. Lachmann B. Open up the lung and keep the lung open. *Intens Care Med.* 1992;18(6):319–321.
13. Fagan DG. Post-mortem studies of the semistatic volume-pressure characteristics of infant's lungs. *Thorax.* 1976;31:534.
14. Mansell AL, Bryan C, Levison H. Airway closure in children. *J Appl Physiol.* 1988;319:1112.
15. Thorsteinsson A, Larsson A, Jonmarker C, et al. Pressure-volume relations of the respiratory system in healthy children. *Am J Respir Crit Care Med.* 1994;150:421.
16. Rahn H, Otis AB, Chadwick EL, et al. The pressure-volume diagram of the thorax and lung. *Am J Physiol.* 1946;146:161–178.
17. Murray JF, ed. *The Normal Lung.* Philadelphia, PA: WB Saunders; 1986.
18. Polgar G, String ST. The viscous resistance of the lung tissues in newborn infants. *J Pediatr (Rio J).* 1966;69:787.
19. Ferris BG, Mead J, Opie LH. Partitioning of respiratory flow resistance in man. *J Appl Physiol.* 1964;19:653–658.
20. Hogg JC, Williams J, Richardson JB, et al. Age as a factor in the distribution of lower airway conductance and in the pathologic anatomy of obstructive lung disease. *N Engl J Med.* 1970;282:1283.
21. Dubois AB. Resistance to breathing. In: Fenn WO, Rahn H, eds. *Handbook of physiology, respiration.* Vol. 1. Washington DC: AM Physiological Society; 1964:451–462.
22. Briscoe WA, Dubois AB. The relationship between airway resistance, airway conductance and lung volume in subjects of different age and body size. *J Clin Invest.* 1958;37:1279–1285.
23. Brody AW. Mechanical compliance and resistance of the lung-thorax calculated from the flow during passive expiration. *Am J Optom Physiol Opt.* 1954;178:189–196.
24. Kano S, Lanteri CJ, Pemberton PJ, et al. Fast versus slow ventilation for neonates. *Am Rev Respir Dis.* 1993;148:578–584.
25. West JB. *Ventilation/blood flow and gas exchange.* 3rd ed. London: Blackwell Scientific Publications; 1979.
26. West JB, Dollery CT. Distribution of blood flow and the pressure-flow relations of the whole lung. *J Appl Physiol.* 1964;19:713.
27. West JB, Dollery CT, Naimark A. Distribution of blood flow in isolated lung: Relation to vascular and alveolar pressure. *J Appl Physiol.* 1964;19:713.
28. Hughes JMB, Glazier JB, Maloney JE, et al. Effect of lung volume on the distribution of pulmonary blood flow in man. *Respir Physiol.* 1968;4:58.
29. Mellemgaard K. The alveolar-arterial oxygen difference: Its size and components in normal man. *Acta Physiol Scand.* 1966;67:10–20.
30. Radford EP. Ventilation standards for use in artificial respiration. *J Appl Physiol.* 1955;61:1560.
31. Roughton FJ. Average time spent by blood in human lung capillary and its relation to the rates of CD uptake and elimination in man. *Am J Physiol.* 1945;143:621.
32. Hogg JC. Varieties of airway narrowing in severe fatal asthma. *J Allergy Clin Immunol.* 1987;80(suppl, part 2):417–419.
33. Tay-Uyboco JS, Kwiatowski K, Cates DB, et al. Hypoxic airway constriction in infants of very low birth weight recovering from moderate to severe bronchopulmonary dysplasia. *J Pediatr.* 1989;115:456–459.
34. Hantos Z, Daroczy B, Klebniczki J, et al. Parameter estimation of transpulmonary mechanics by a nonlinear iterative model. *J Appl Physiol.* 1982;52(4):955–963.
35. Guttmann J, Eberhard L, Wolff G, et al. Maneuver free determination of compliance and resistance in ventilated ARDS patients. *Chest.* 1992;4:1235–1242.
36. Iotti GA, Braschi A, Brunner JX, et al. Respiratory mechanics by least squares fitting in mechanical ventilated patients, applications during paralysis and during pressure support ventilation. *Inten Care Med.* 1995;21(5):406–413.
37. Bates JHT. Assessment of mechanics. In: Marini JJ, Slutsky AS, eds. *Physiologic basis of ventilatory support.* New York: Marcel Dekker; 1998:231–259.
38. Heulitt M, Holt S, Thurman T. Reliability of measured tidal volume in mechanically ventilated young pigs with normal lungs. *Int Care Med.* 2005;31(9):1255–1261.
39. Sassoon CSH. Mechanical ventilator design and function: The trigger variable. *Respir Care.* 1992;37:1056–1069.
40. Heulitt MJ, Torres A, Anders M, et al. Comparison of total resistive work of breathing in two generations of ventilators in an animal model. *Pediatr Pulmonal.* 1996;22:58–66.
41. Otis A, Fenn W, Rahn H, et al. Mechanics of breathing in man. *J Appl Physiol.* 1950;2:592–607.
42. Beydon L, Chasse M, Harf A, et al. Inspiratory work of breathing during spontaneous ventilation using demand valves and continuous flow systems. *Am Rev Respir Dis.* 1988;138:300–304.
43. Banner M, Downs J, Kirby R, et al. Effects of expiratory resistance on inspiratory work of breathing. *Chest.* 1988;93(4):795–799.

44. Sanders R, Thurman T, Holt S, et al. Work of breathing associated with pressure support ventilation in two different ventilators: *Pediatr Pulmonal.* 2001;32:62–70

45. Nishimura M, Hess D, Kacmarek R. The response of flow-triggered infant ventilators. *Am J Respir Crit Care Med.* 1995;152 (6 Pt 1):1901–1909.

46. Carmack J, Torres A, Anders M, et al. Comparison of inspiratory work of breathing in young lambs during flow triggered and pressure triggered ventilation. *Respir Care.* 1995;40(1): 28–34.

47. Lanteri CJ, Sly PD. Changes in respiratory mechanics with age. *J Appl Physiol.* 1993;74(1):369–378.

48. Deoras KS, Wolfson MR, Bhutani VK, et al. Structural changes in the trachea of preterm lambs induced by ventilation. *Pediatr Res.* 1989;26:434–437.

49. Penn RB, Wolfson MR, Shaffer TH. Effect of ventilation on mechanical properties and pressure-flow relationships of immature airways. *Pediatr Res.* 1988;23:519–524.

50. Wolfson MR, Bhutani VK, Shaffer TH, et al. Mechanics and energetics of breathing helium in infants with bronchopulmonary dysplasia. *J Pediatr.* 1984;104:752–757.

51. Keens TG, Bryan AC, Levison H, et al. Developmental pattern of muscle fiber types in human respiratory muscles. *J Appl Physiol.* 1978;44:909–913.

52. Baumeister BL, el-Khatib M, Smith PG, et al. Evaluation of predictors of weaning from mechanical ventilation in pediatric patients. *Pediatr Pulmonal.* 1997;24(5):344–352.

53. Kondili E, Prinianakis G, Georgopoulos D. Patient-ventilator interaction. *Br J Anaesth.* 2003;91(1):106–119.

54. Nilsestuen JO, Hargett KD. Using ventilator graphics to identify patient-ventilator asynchrony. *Respir Care.* 2005;50(2):202–234.

55. Chao DC, Scheinhorn DJ, Stearn-Hassenpflug M. Patient-ventilator asynchrony in prolonged mechanical ventilation. *Chest.* 1997;112(6):1592–1599.

56. MacIntyre NR, Ho LI. Effects of initial flow rate and breath termination criteria on pressure support ventilation. *Chest.* 1991; 99(1):134–138.

57. Tokioka H, Tanaka T, Ishizu T, et al. The effect of breath termination criterion on breathing patterns and the work of breathing during pressure support ventilation. *Anesth Analg.* 2001;92(1): 161–165.

58. Heulitt MJ, Wankum P, Holt SJ, et al. Evaluation of the effects of an active exhalation valve and changing cycle off time during pressure support ventilation in a neonatal animal model. *Pediatr Res.* 2003;53:2711.

59. Katz JA, Ozanne GM, Zinn SE, et al. Time course and mechanisms of lung-volume increase with PEEP in acute pulmonary failure. *Anesthesiology.* 1981;54(1):9–16.

60. Matamis D, Lemaire F, Harf A, et al. Total respiratory pressure-volume curves in the adult respiratory distress syndrome. *Chest.* 1984;86(1):58–66.

61. Pelosi P, Cadringher P, Bottino N, et al. Sigh in acute respiratory distress syndrome. *Am J Respir Crit Care Med.* 1999;159(3): 872–880.

Mechanical Breathing

Mark J. Heulitt   Paul Ouellet   Richard T. Fiser

APPLIED PHYSIOLOGY

The same model describing the normal interaction between the airways and lungs can be applied to the interaction of the mechanical ventilator with the respiratory system. In simple terms, the lung–ventilator unit can be considered a tube with a balloon network at the end, with the tube representing the ventilator tubing, endotracheal tube and airways, and the balloon network of the alveoli. The movement of gas is determined by forces, displacements, and the rate of change of displacements of the components that are distensible.

In physiology, force is measured as pressure (pressure = force/area), displacement is measured as volume (volume = area × displacement), and the relevant rate of change is measured as flow (e.g., average flow = Δvolume/Δtime; instantaneous flow = dv/dt; the derivative of volume with respect to time). The pressure necessary to cause flow of gas into the airway and to increase the volume of gas in the lungs is the key component in positive pressure mechanical ventilation. The volume of gas (ΔV) to any lung unit (or the balloon in the simplified example), and the gas flow ($\dot{V}$) is related to the applied pressure (ΔP) by $\Delta P = \Delta V/C + \dot{V} \times R + k$ where R is the airway resistance and C is the lung compliance. This equation is known as the *equation of motion* for the respiratory system. The sum of the muscle pressures and the ventilator pressure is the applied pressure to the respiratory system. Muscle pressure is patient-generated but cannot be directly measured. Muscle pressure represents the pressure generated by the patient to expand the thoracic cage and lungs. In contrast, ventilator pressure is the trans-respiratory pressure generated by the ventilator during inspiration. Combinations of these pressures are generated when a patient is breathing on a positive pressure ventilator. For example, when respiratory muscles are at complete rest, the muscle pressure is 0; therefore, the ventilator must generate all the pressure necessary to deliver the tidal volume and inspiratory flow. The reverse is also true, and there are degrees of support depending upon the amount of force generated by the patient's respiratory muscles. The application of the equation of motion to the generation of gas flow is the next important step. Therefore, total pressure applied to the respiratory system (P_{RS}) of a ventilated patient is the sum of the pressure generated by the ventilator (measured at the airway) P_{AO} and the pressure developed by the respiratory muscles (P_{MUS}). Therefore,

$$P_{RS} = P_{AO} + P_{MUS} = \frac{V}{C} + \dot{V} \times R + k$$

where P_{RS} is the respiratory system pressure, P_{AO} is the airway pressure, P_{MUS} is the pressure developed by the respiratory muscles, $\dot{V}$ is flow, R being airway resistance, V/C being respiratory system compliance, and k is the constant that represents the alveolar end-expiratory pressure. P_{AO} and $\dot{V}$ can be measured by the pressure and flow transducers in the ventilator. Volume is derived mathematically from the integration of the flow waveform.

To generate a volume displacement, the total forces have to overcome elastic and resistive elements of the lung and airway/chest wall represented by V/C and $\dot{V} \times R$, respectively. V/C depends on both the volume insufflated in excess of resting volume and the respiratory system compliance. To generate gas flow, the total forces must overcome the resistive forces of the airway and the endotracheal tube against the driving pressure gradients. At any moment during inspiration, there must be a balance of forces opposing lung and chest wall expansion measured as the airway pressure (P_{AO}). The opposing pressures can be summarized as the sum of elastic recoil pressure ($P_{elastic}$), flow-resistive pressure ($P_{resistive}$), and inertance pressure ($P_{inertance}$) of the respiratory system, therefore:

$$P_{AO} = P_{elastic} + P_{resistive} + P_{inertance}$$

Inertial forces are usually negligible during conventional ventilation, which depends upon bulk convective flow, unlike in high-frequency ventilation, where volumes are at the level of dead space. Therefore, for conventional ventilation, the forces exemplified in the equation of motion can be expressed as:

$$P_{AO} = P_{elastic} + P_{resistive}$$

If the elastic forces are recognized as the product of elastance and volume ($P_{elastic} = E \times V$) and the resistive forces as the product of flow and resistance (Resistive $= \dot{V} \times R$), the formula can be rewritten as:

$$P_{AO} = (\text{Elastance} \times \text{Volume}) + (\text{Resistance} \times \text{Flow})$$

If compliance (the inverse of elastance) is substituted for elastance, the equation of motion, as described in the preceding text, becomes:

$$P_{AO} = \frac{\text{Volume}}{\text{Compliance}} + \text{Resistance} \times \text{Flow}$$

The quotient of volume displacement over compliance of the respiratory system represents the pressure necessary to overcome the elastic forces above the resting lung volume or functional residual capacity (FRC). The resting lung volume represents the quantity of air remaining in the lungs at the end of a spontaneous expiration. Pressure, flow, and volume are all measured relative to their baseline values. Therefore, the pressure necessary to cause inspiration is measured as the change in airway pressure above positive end-expiratory pressure (PEEP). For example, in a patient breathing spontaneously on continuous positive airway pressure (CPAP), the ventilator pressure is 0; the patient must utilize his respiratory muscles to generate all the work of breathing (WOB). The same can be applied to the volume during inspiration or the tidal volume, which is the change in volume above FRC. The pressure necessary to overcome the resistive forces of the respiratory system is the product of the maximum airway resistance (R_{MAX}) and inspiratory flow. Flow is measured relative to its end-expiratory value, which is usually 0, unless an intrinsic PEEP (PEEPi) is present.

FUNCTIONAL CHARACTERISTICS OF MECHANICAL VENTILATORS

For a discussion on mechanical ventilation, there must be differentiation between those variables that are directly controlled by clinicians and those that are indirectly controlled. For example, pressure, volume, and flow are directly controlled variables, as opposed to constants such as resistance and compliance, which are dependent upon the resistive and elastic properties of the respiratory system.

Each ventilator is a controller of pressure, flow, or volume in the equation of motion. The manner in which each variable is controlled, described as the mode of ventilation, determines how the ventilator delivers the mechanical breath. In the equation of motion, the form of any of the variables (pressure, volume, or flow) are expressed as

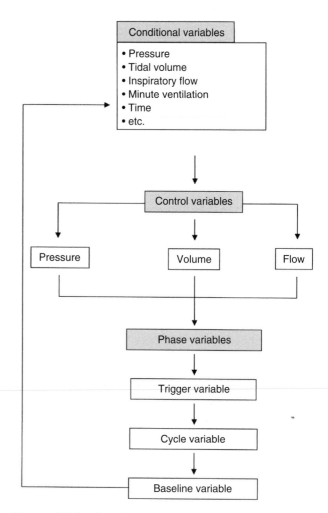

Figure 6.8.1 Flow chart to emphasize that each breath may have a different set of control and phase variables, depending on the mode of ventilation.

functions of time and can be predetermined. This serves as the theoretical basis for classifying ventilators as pressure, volume, or flow controllers (see Fig. 6.8.1). The necessary and sufficient criteria for determining the variable that is controlled are listed in Table 6.8.1. It is important to recognize that according to the equation of motion any ventilator can only directly control one variable at a time: pressure, volume, or flow. Therefore, a ventilator is simply a technology that controls the airway pressure waveform, the inspired volume waveform, or the inspiratory flow waveform. Therefore, pressure, volume, and flow are referred to in the context as control variables.

Most clinicians think of ventilators in terms of modes of ventilation. However, the mode of ventilation is a description of the way a mechanical breath is delivered. The determinants of how a mechanical breath is delivered are summarized not only in the control variables but also in the phase and conditional variables. Conditional variables are determinants of a response to a preset threshold. Control variables are the independent variables and include pressure, flow, or volume. In each phase, a particular

TABLE 6.8.1
VENTILATOR CONTROLLERS

Flow Controller Modes	Pressure Controller Modes	Volume Controller Modes
(Constant flow controller) Volume control, SIMV-VC	(Constant pressure controller) Pressure control, PRVC, SIMV-PC	(Variable flow controller) Volume control
Equation		
$Flow = \dfrac{Pressure}{Resistance}$	$Flow = \dfrac{Volume}{Compliance}$ $Pressure = Resistance \times Flow$	$Flow = Pressure \times Compliance$
Independent Variables		
Flow	Pressure	Volume
Dependent Variables		
Pressure	Volume Flow	Pressure
Limiting Variables		
Volume	Pressure	Volume
Trigger Variables		
Time Pressure Flow	Time Pressure Flow	Time Pressure Flow

SIMV-VC, synchronized intermittent mandatory ventilation–volume control; PRVC, pressure-regulated volume control; SIMV-PC, synchronized intermittent mandatory ventilation–pressure control.

variable is measured and is used to start, sustain, and end the phase. The phase variables include the trigger variable (determines the start of inspiration), limit variable (determines what sustains inspiration), and the cycle variable (determines the end of inspiration).

Control Variables

The control variables must overcome the elastic and resistive forces to allow gas delivery to the patient. The elastic components of the equation of motion related to pressure is:

$$Pressure = \frac{Volume}{Compliance}$$

If the clinician sets pressure as a function of time, volume varies directly with the compliance of the respiratory system. Pressure is the independent variable set by the clinician, and volume is the dependent variable determined by the level of pressure. As described in the preceding text, when the clinician presets the pressure pattern, the ventilator operates as a pressure controller. The volume becomes a function of compliance so that a decrease in compliance allows less volume to be delivered for the same pressure. During expiration, the elastic and resistive elements of the respiratory system are passive, and expiratory waveforms are not directly affected by the modes of ventilation or the controller.

For the resistive components of the equation of motion:

$$Pressure = Resistance \times Flow$$

As discussed in the preceding text on resistive elements, the clinician sets pressure as a function of time, allowing flow to vary with resistance. If resistance increases, flow is ultimately limited. Pressure is referred to as the independent variable and flow as the dependent variable. As previously discussed, expiration is passive and the expiratory profile is not directly affected by the mode of ventilation but rather by compliance and resistance. However, because the respiratory cycle is a set period, any change in the inspiratory time can influence expiratory time, and to a certain point, the expiratory profile.

When a ventilator operates as a constant pressure controller (e.g., in pressure control, pressure-regulated volume control [PRVC], and synchronized intermittent mandatory ventilation–pressure control [SIMV-PC]), pressure is an independent or controlled variable (see Table 6.8.1). The set pressure will be delivered and maintained constant throughout inspiration, independent of the resistive or elastic forces of the respiratory system. Although pressure is constant, the delivered tidal volume is a function of compliance and resistance, and the flow varies exponentially with time.

Figure 6.8.2 displays a waveform from a ventilator operating as a pressure controller. Under this condition, volume

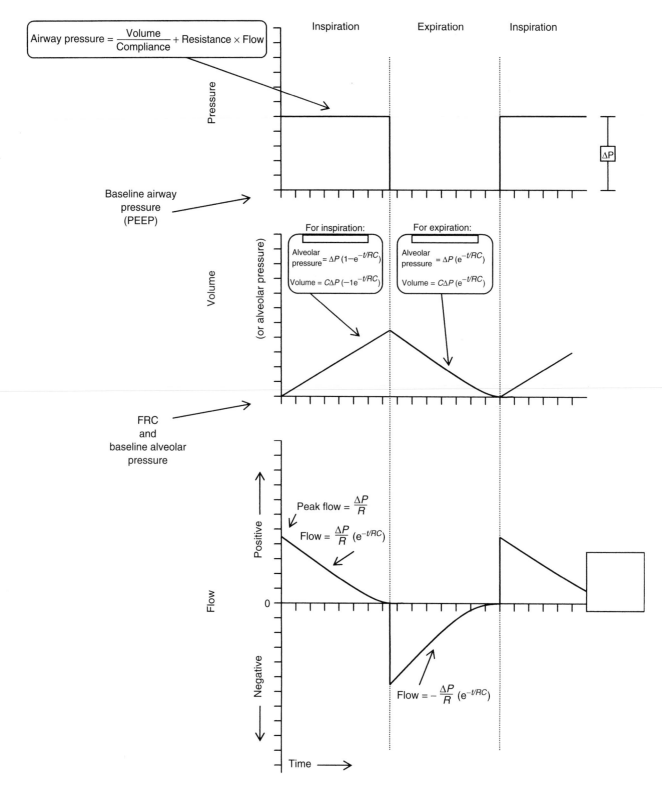

$$\text{Airway pressure} = \frac{\text{Volume}}{\text{Compliance}} + \text{Resistance} \times \text{Flow}$$

Inspiration   Expiration   Inspiration

Pressure

Baseline airway
pressure
(PEEP)

ΔP

Volume
(or alveolar pressure)

For inspiration:

Alveolar pressure $= \Delta P\,(1-e^{-t/RC})$

Volume $= C\Delta P\,(-1e^{-t/RC})$

For expiration:

Alveolar pressure $= \Delta P\,(e^{-t/RC})$

Volume $= C\Delta P\,(e^{-t/RC})$

FRC
and
baseline alveolar
pressure

Peak flow $= \dfrac{\Delta P}{R}$

Flow $= \dfrac{\Delta P}{R}\,(e^{-t/RC})$

Positive

0

Negative

Flow

Flow $= -\dfrac{\Delta P}{R}\,(e^{-t/RC})$

Time

Figure 6.8.2   Pressure–time, volume–time and flow–time waveforms from a ventilator operating as a pressure controller. Pressure is the independent variable (preset pattern); volume and flow are the dependent variables (function of compliance and resistance). ΔP, change in airway pressure; R, resistance; C, compliance; t, time; e, base of natural logarithm (approximately 2.72); PEEP, positive end-expiratory pressure; FRC, functional residual lung capacity.

and flow become the dependent variables, and their patterns will depend upon compliance and resistance. When a pressure pattern is preset (constant in a pressure control mode) flow–time and volume–time waveforms vary exponentially with time and are a function of compliance and resistance.

Flow and resistance are only associated with the resistive components of the equation of motion. The elastic component refers to volume and compliance. The resistive components of the equation of motion are:

$$Pressure = Resistance \times Flow$$

$$or\ Flow = \frac{Pressure}{Resistance}$$

Therefore, if the clinician sets flow as function of time, pressure varies with resistance. Flow is the independent variable, and pressure is the dependent variable. When a flow pattern is preset, the ventilator operates as a flow controller, the pressure is a function of resistance, and the inspiratory pressure-time waveform varies linearly with time. Volume increases linearly with time but does not have a direct relation to flow. Volume does have an indirect relationship to flow because volume is the integral of flow and flow is the derivative of volume.

Expiration is passive and the expiratory profile is not directly affected by mode of ventilation but rather by compliance and resistance, although the set inspiratory time can influence the expiratory time and to a certain point the expiratory profile.

When a ventilator operates as a constant flow controller (SIMV-VC), flow is the independent variable. Regardless of what the resistive or elastic forces of the respiratory system are, the set flow will be delivered and maintained constant throughout inspiration. Pressure and tidal volume will vary with time but are functions of compliance and resistance.

Figure 6.8.3 illustrates waveforms from a ventilator operating as a flow controller. Flow is the independent variable (controlled variable); pressure and volume are dependent variables. When a flow pattern is preset (constant in this case), pressure and volume are the dependent variables. With a preset flow pattern, pressure and volume vary linearly with time and are affected by compliance and resistance.

Modern ventilators operate as either a flow controller or a pressure controller. As a flow controller, the most common pattern is constant flow, also referred to as a square wave flow pattern. As a pressure controller, the only pressure pattern is a constant pressure, also referred to as square wave pressure pattern.

From the equation of motion, one can infer that with ventilator operating as a constant flow controller, the pressure and volume are linear functions of time. Different ventilators have the possibility of delivering different flow patterns.

Alternative flow patterns, beyond constant and exponentially decelerating flow, need to be controlled by a microprocessor that sequentially adjusts flow through an algorithm to produce the decelerating ramp, ascending ramp, and sinusoidal flow patterns. These flow patterns are used in various volume-cycled modes. The decelerating rate controlled by an algorithm produces a linear deceleration that does not reflect elastic and resistive elements of the respiratory system. A linear deceleration is often associated with flow-starvation asynchrony because flow is not a dependant variable in a volume-controlled mode. Not all ventilators can provide such flow patterns. The exponentially decreasing flow pattern is available with a pressure control mode.

Theoretically, it has been proposed that a decelerating flow favors better gas exchange and improves distribution of ventilation among lung units with heterogeneous time constants. However, neither animal nor clinical studies have documented this advantage.

Volume is associated with the elastic component of the equation. The resistive component refers to resistance and flow. The elastic components can be rearranged to indicate how volume is determined.

$$Volume = Pressure \times Compliance$$

If the clinician sets volume as a function of time, pressure then varies with compliance. Volume is an independent variable and pressure is a dependent variable. Expiration is passive, and the expiratory profile is not directly affected by the mode of ventilation but rather by compliance and resistance, although the set inspiratory time can influence the expiratory time and, to a certain point, the expiratory profile.

When a ventilator sets a volume pattern, it operates as a volume controller. However, to truly be a volume controller, the ventilator must measure volume directly to set the volume pattern. Most ventilators do not directly measure volume, rather, they calculate volume from flow over a period. Most ventilators use volume as a limiting variable; that is, inspiration stops when the preselected volume is reached. When inspiration stops at the preset volume, the ventilator is referred to as being volume-cycled, but it is actually a flow controller.

The relationship between the gas delivery and the resistive and elastic elements of the patient and ventilator system is important for understanding the delivery of a positive pressure breath to a patient.

Resistance in Mechanical Ventilation

To understand resistance during positive pressure mechanical ventilation, airflow, during both inspiration and expiration, as a measure of the flow-resistive elements of the respiratory system need to be considered. Resistance can be expressed as:

$$Airway\ resistance = \frac{\Delta Pressure}{Flow}$$

Airway resistance is affected by flow, tidal volume, and the dimensions of the gas delivery system, including the

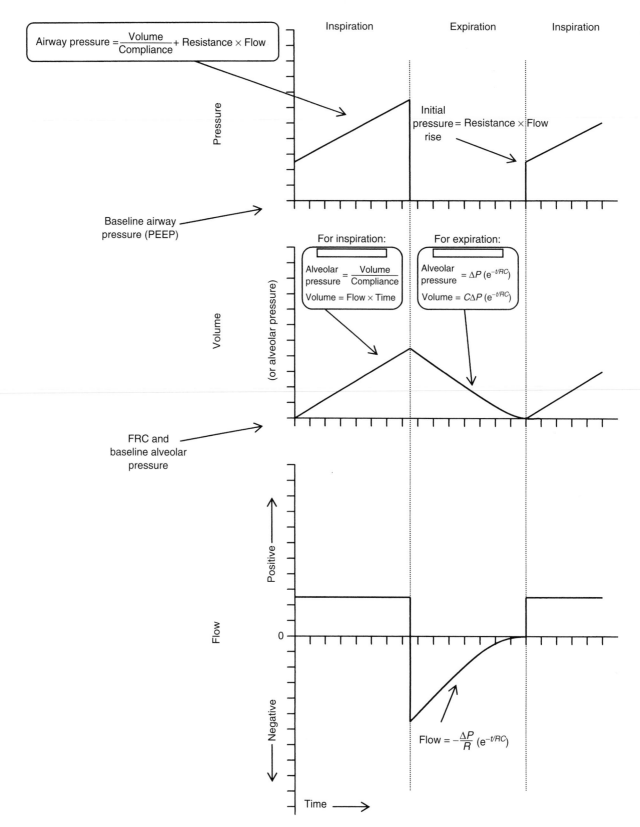

Figure 6.8.3 Pressure–time, volume–time, and flow–time waveforms from a ventilator operating as a flow controller. Flow is the independent variable (preset pattern); pressure and volume are the dependent variables (function of resistance and compliance). ΔP, change in airway pressure; R, resistance; C, compliance; t, time; e, base of natural logarithm (approximately 2.72); PEEP, positive end-expiratory pressure; FRC, functional residual lung capacity.

patient's endotracheal tube. In pediatric patients, resistance and gas flow are primarily caused by the endotracheal tube. When delivering a positive pressure breath with a set tidal volume and flow, the resistance created by the endotracheal tube is directly related to both the diameter and length of the tube. In examining resistance during positive pressure ventilation, the type of controller delivering the mechanical breath must be considered. For example if a mechanical breath operates as a pressure controller, (e.g., pressure control, pressure-regulated volume control, or SIMV-PC) the following relationship from the equation of motion occurs:

$$\text{Flow} = \frac{\text{Volume}}{\text{Compliance}}$$
$$\text{or Pressure} = \text{Resistance} \times \text{Flow}$$

The dependent variables are volume and flow and the independent variable is pressure. The resistive elements of both the respiratory system and breathing circuit are visualized in the flow–time and volume–time waveforms (see Figs. 6.8.4 and 6.8.5). Because pressure is the independent variable, it is held constant during inspiration, and a pressure–time waveform does not illustrate the effects of resistance. In contrast, because the rate of decay of flow is a function of resistance, a flow–time waveform illustrates resistance.

For ventilator modes that use a flow controller (e.g., volume control and SIMV-VC), Flow = Pressure/Resistance. The independent variable is flow and the dependent variable is pressure. When a ventilator operates in a constant flow mode, the resistive elements of the respiratory system and breathing circuit can be visualized and calculated with the pressure–time waveform, which begins with an exponential rise to a first step, followed by a linear rise to peak inspiratory pressure (PIP).

During the initial portion of inspiration, the first step is a function of flow and resistance, with the size of the step being directly related to the degree of resistance. The second

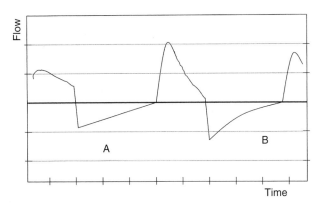

Figure 6.8.5 Flow–time waveform from a constant pressure mode of ventilation. Tracing A: increased resistance. There is a slow decay throughout inspiration, and inspiration stops before baseline is reached. With expiration, there is an abnormal linear decay to baseline. Tracing B: normal resistance. With inspiration and expiration, there is a normal exponential decay to baseline.

portion of the waveform is a linear increase to PIP, and is a function of flow being constant throughout inspiration and represents the elastic properties of the respiratory system.

As PIP is reached, a pause time or plateau is maintained while pressure inside the airways and the breathing circuit equilibrates at plateau pressure (P_{plateau}). Flow then stops while pressure equilibrates.

Figure 6.8.6 is a pressure–time waveform from a constant flow mode of ventilation and illustrates various elements related to resistive and elastic properties of the respiratory system.

Inspiratory resistance (R_I) is the difference between PIP and P_{plateau} over the flow values at PIP, as expressed by the following equation:

$$R_I = \frac{\text{PIP} - P_{\text{plateau}}}{\text{PIF}}$$

Expiratory resistance is the difference between P_{plateau} and total PEEP over flow value at the onset of exhalation, as

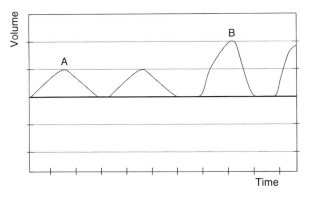

Figure 6.8.4 Volume–time waveform from a constant pressure mode of ventilation. Tracing A: increased resistance. With inspiration, there is an abnormal linear increase to tidal volume, normal exponential increase to tidal volume, and decreased inspired tidal volume compared with tracing B. With expiration, there is an abnormal linear decay to baseline. Tracing B: normal resistance. With inspiration, there is a normal exponential increase to tidal volume. With expiration, a normal exponential decay to baseline is seen.

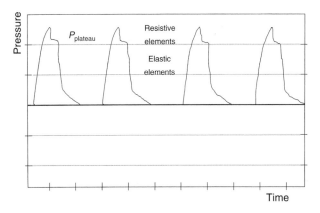

Figure 6.8.6 Pressure–time waveform from a constant flow mode illustrating resistive and elastic elements of the respiratory system.

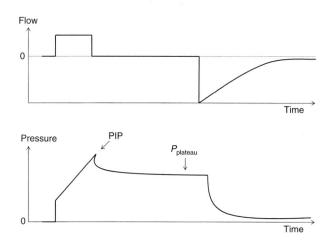

Figure 6.8.7 Flow–time and pressure–time waveforms (constant flow mode).

expected from the following equation:

$$R_E = \frac{P_{plateau} - PEEP_{TOT}}{Flow(onset)exhalation}$$

Figure 6.8.7 demonstrates flow–time and pressure–time waveforms from a constant flow mode of ventilation and illustrates various landmarks for resistance calculations.

PATIENTS WITH INCREASED AIRWAY RESISTANCE

Increased airway resistance in patients with obstructive lung disease is due to airway narrowing during exhalation. For example, in bronchial asthma, the patient has active bronchoconstriction of both large and peripheral airways, with peripheral airway narrowing secondary to airway inflammation; increased local blood flow; impaction of inspissated mucus; and increased airway microvascular leakage. Alveoli distal to these occluded airways continue to be ventilated because of collateral pathways from the better-preserved neighboring alveoli. As discussed previously, the act of breathing through narrowed airways imposes an additional load on the respiratory muscles that is exacerbated with increased airway resistance.

In patients with increased airway resistance, the resting volume at the end of exhalation is increased because of lower expiratory flows and short expiratory times. As a result, a positive recoil pressure (PEEPi) is created at the end of expiration, and a new resting state is established. This state of air trapping or dynamic hyperinflation is common in patients with obstructive lung disease such as asthma or bronchopulmonary dysplasia. Initially in these patients, hyperinflation tends to keep the airways open, reduces airway resistance, increases elastic recoil, and tends to improve expiratory flow. However, hyperinflation has several deleterious effects. The positive pressure within regions of hyperinflated lung increases the mean intrathoracic pressure and causes the inspiratory muscles

to operate at a volume higher than the resting volume. Respiratory muscle function becomes impaired because dynamic hyperinflation places the respiratory muscles at a considerable mechanical disadvantage. PEEPi imposes a substantial inspiratory threshold load as flow is limited because of a negative intrapleural pressure equal to the level of PEEPi that has to be generated before inspiratory flow can begin within the alveoli. This threshold load imposed by PEEPi may interfere with ventilator triggering by requiring the patient to overcome the imposed PEEPi before the trigger to begin inspiration is reached. Moreover, the ventilation–perfusion relationships can be impaired because the hyperinflated lung may compress adjacent areas of the normally inflated lung. PEEPi also decreases cardiac output by increasing intrathoracic pressure, thereby reducing venous return, and predisposes patients to barotraumas by causing dynamic hyperinflation. Therefore, a mainstay of therapy in patients with obstructive lung disease requiring mechanical ventilation would be to decrease dynamic hyperinflation.

ABNORMALITY OF GAS EXCHANGE

Several factors contribute to the development of gas exchange abnormalities in patients with obstructive lung disease. Airway obstruction creates regional hypoventilation and localized hypoxia from ventilation–perfusion mismatch. In addition, a concomitant interstitial process such as pneumonia may further exacerbate hypoxemia in these patients. Patients with acute asthma may initially compensate for hypoxemia by hyperventilation. However, hypoventilation develops in the presence of severe airway narrowing and dynamic hyperinflation when the respiratory muscles are unable to bear the excessive resistive and elastic loads. This may occur rapidly in infants and children because of anatomic instability of their chest wall, as well as underdeveloped diaphragmatic function. In patients with severe episodes of acute asthma, alveolar hypoventilation and hypercapnia may occur, thereby complicating gas exchange.

Patients with bronchopulmonary dysplasia also have acute hypoxic airway narrowing. Because the large airways are normally exposed to ambient concentrations of oxygen, the effect must occur in peripheral airways, where gas mixing in chronic lung disease (CLD) may be poor, leading to localized hypoxia, which may in turn lead to hypoxemia. The contribution of hypoxic airway narrowing to clinical disease is unknown but clearly represents a potential vicious cycle when present along with any underlying disorder of lung mechanics in CLD.

COMPLIANCE IN MECHANICAL VENTILATION

The elastic properties of the respiratory system are considered in this section. Compliance expresses the elastic components as a volume change divided by a pressure change, and can be expressed by the following general equation:

$$\text{Compliance} = \frac{\Delta \text{Volume}}{\Delta \text{Pressure}}$$

Total respiratory system compliance (C_{TS}) is related to lung compliance (C_{pulm}) and chest wall compliance (C_{CW}) by the following equation:

$$\frac{1}{C_{TS}} = \frac{1}{C_{pulm}} + \frac{1}{C_{CW}}$$

C_{TS} may be used to evaluate and modify various therapeutic interventions such as tidal volume and PEEP titration, paralysis, and patient positioning to identify interventions that may improve respiratory system compliance. However, in mechanical ventilation, the volume–pressure relation is most often monitored as total static compliance measured when there is no flow activity at the end of inspiration and expiration.

Chest Wall Compliance

Chest wall compliance (C_{CW}) can be calculated in patients by an esophageal balloon and an airway pneumotachograph. Chest wall compliance describes the changes in tidal volume (V_T) relative to the pleural pressure, reflected by the esophageal pressure (P_{eso}), and is expressed by the following equation:

$$C_{CW} = \frac{V_T}{P_{eso}}$$

To calculate chest wall compliance, the patient needs to be completely passive and not breathing spontaneously. Muscle relaxation and adequate sedation must be administered to spontaneously breathing patients. Chest wall compliance is an essential parameter for the calculation of total WOB using the Campbell diagram, as illustrated in Figure 6.8.8.

Chest wall compliance can usually be estimated at 4% of the vital capacity per cm H_2O in adults. Compliance in adults averages 100–200 mL per cm H_2O. In infants and children this value is markedly lower, averaging between 2.6–4.9 mL per cm H_2O.

Lung Compliance

Lung compliance (C_{pulm}) is not commonly calculated during mechanical ventilation for the same reason as chest wall compliance.

Lung compliance describes the change in tidal volume relative to the transpulmonary pressure ($P_{plateau} - P_{eso}$), where $P_{plateau}$ is the plateau pressure, also referred to as *alveolar pressure*, and P_{eso} is the esophageal pressure under the quasi-static condition.

Lung compliance is expressed by the following equation:

$$C_{pulm} = \frac{V_T}{P_{plateau} - P_{eso}}$$

Lung compliance can be obtained in passively or spontaneously breathing patients but is not commonly calculated

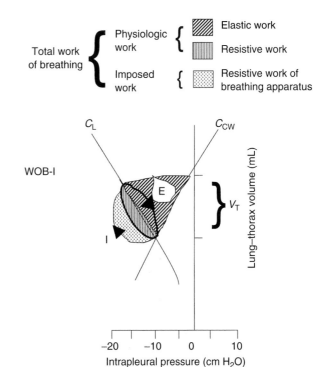

Figure 6.8.8 Campbell diagram, where WOB can be calculated using the area of the volume–pressure loop and lung compliance (C_L) and chest wall compliance (C_{CW}) curves. E, exhalation; I, inhalation; V_T tidal volume. (From Banner MJ, Kirby RR, Blanch PB. Differentiating total work of breathing into its component parts. Essential for appropriate interpretation. *Chest.* 1996;109(5):1141–1143.)

during mechanical breathing because of the complexity involved in the measurements.

TOTAL STATIC COMPLIANCE

Total static compliance of the respiratory system (Cst_{tot}) is frequently measured and monitored during mechanical ventilation.

Total static compliance is the pressure required to overcome the elastic forces of the respiratory system for a given tidal volume, and under a zero flow (static) condition. Static compliance therefore reflects the elastic properties of the respiratory system.

Specific measuring conditions must be met for a valid static compliance value: passive tidal volume (inspiration and expiration) and compressible volume correction for tubing; the plateau must have an end-inspiratory pause of at least 1 second, with a stable pressure of within 0.5 cm H_2O over two readings at least 10 millisecond apart.

Tidal static compliance describes the delivered tidal volume relative to the airway pressure under a static condition ($P_{plateau} - PEEP_{total}$), in which tidal volume must be corrected for compressible tubing volume. $P_{plateau}$ is the pressure during the pause time and $PEEP_{total}$ is the sum of the set PEEP and PEEPi; Cst_{tot} is expressed by the following

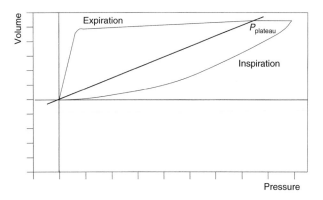

Figure 6.8.9 Volume–pressure loop from a constant flow mode of ventilation illustrating the static compliance slope.

equation:

$$Cst_{tot} = \frac{V_T}{P_{plateau} - PEEP_{total}}$$

Changes in static compliance represent changes in the lung elasticity. Therefore, any lung pathology that increases lung recoil or decreases lung volume will decrease static compliance. Normal values of static compliance in adults are 60 to 100 mL per cm H_2O or approximately 1 mL per cm H_2O/kg body weight.

The patient's static compliance will vary with tidal volume and PEEP because lung overdistension or collapse will affect static compliance. The titration of both tidal volume and PEEP can be accomplished by monitoring static compliance.

The volume–pressure loop from a constant flow mode of ventilation with pause time also allows the clinician to visualize the static compliance status. The slope of this loop (from the origin to $P_{plateau}$) is an estimate of static compliance. A flatter slope will be associated with decreased compliance. Figure 6.8.9 is a volume–pressure loop from a constant flow mode of ventilation with a pause time and illustrates the static compliance slope.

Compliance values are affected by the patient's size, state of relaxation, lung volume, and flow. The clinician should be cautious when interpreting actual values for compliance. Trended values rather than actual values are appropriate for monitoring the evolution of the elastic properties of the respiratory system throughout the period of ventilatory support.

DYNAMIC CHARACTERISTICS

Formerly known as the *effective dynamic compliance*, the dynamic characteristics (*DynChar*) have always been measured during mechanical ventilation.

We prefer to speak of dynamic characteristics rather than dynamic compliance because the relationship between volume and pressure during a dynamic event is subject to resistive forces in the system. In other words, during inspiration and expiration, gas flow constitutes a resistive element and volume/pressure is not truly compliance by definition because resistance is now a part of the relation. Flow and resistance therefore directly affect dynamic characteristics.

Endotracheal tube size is an important element in gas flow through the breathing circuit, affecting resistance and dynamic characteristics of the respiratory system. When delivering a set tidal volume at a set flow, smaller tubes will produce larger resistance to gas flow, thereby affecting dynamic characteristics. At normal flow of 50 to 80 L per minute, dynamic characteristic values are 10% to 20% lower than static compliance.

Total dynamic characteristics describe the components of total lung or parenchymal compliance plus the pressure required to overcome airway resistance to the delivery of a tidal volume. Dynamic characteristics reflect the resistive and elastic properties of the respiratory system.

Total dynamic characteristics are the tidal volume relative to the peak airway pressure under a dynamic condition and is expressed by the following relationship:

$$DynChar = \frac{V_T}{PIP - PEEP}$$

Dynamic characteristics are often displayed continuously breath by breath during mechanical ventilation. Normal values are 50 to 80 mL per cm H_2O in adults and 5 to 6 mL per cm H_2O in newborns. Trended values are clinically helpful in reflecting resistive and elastic properties of the respiratory system.

Figure 6.8.10 is a volume–pressure loop from a constant flow mode of ventilation. The slope of AC reflects the total dynamic characteristics of the respiratory system. The difference between static compliance and dynamic characteristics can be used as an indirect index of flow-resistive properties of the respiratory system. In mechanical ventilation, serial measurements of various components of the volume–pressure loop after changes in the relaxation state of the patient, tidal volume, and flow can provide useful information on the evolution of airways and parenchymal conditions of the patient. The volume–pressure loop should be monitored after any modifications in ventilatory strategies such as change in flow, tidal volume, respiratory rate, and patient relaxation state.

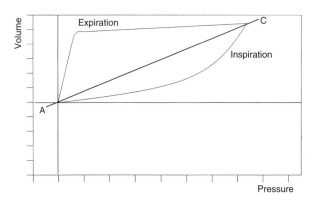

Figure 6.8.10 Volume–pressure loop from a constant flow mode of ventilation.

The equation of motion is as follows:

$$P_{RS} = P_{AO} = \frac{V}{C} + \dot{V} \times R + k$$

Therefore, the respective values of R_{RS} (resistance of the respiratory system), C_{RS} (compliance of the respiratory system), and k can be obtained by fitting the above equation to the sample values of P_{AO}, V, and $\dot{V}$ with a multiple linear regression analysis or linear squares fitting.

One of the most important methodologic limits of the single linear model is that it does not take into account the variation in R_{RS} and C_{RS} with lung volume, and it also neglects flow turbulence and inertial forces. R_{RS} can be underestimated during low-level pressure support ventilation (PSV) with high respiratory efforts.

TIME COURSE OF AIRWAY PRESSURE DURING CONSTANT FLOW INFLATION

The characteristics of inspiratory flow should be considered to understand the pressure–volume curve. During constant flow, volume control ventilation (VCV), the pressure–time curve has an almost vertical pressure increase related to the frictional forces generated by the gas flow. These frictional forces must be overcome to allow gas to move through the airways and the endotracheal tube. The curve shape then changes to a linear increase and follows a given slope to its maximum value (PIP), occurring at end inspiration. This course, which is normally linear, depends only on the respiratory system compliance. Under isovolumetric conditions, the curve loses its linearity and becomes either convex or concave, according to the increase or decrease in C_{RS}, as shown in Figure 6.8.11.

Similarly, during lung overdistension, the curve shape is concave and becomes linear and then convex as the preset V_T decreases, as shown in Figure 6.8.12.

VOLUME MEASUREMENT

The goals of modern mechanical ventilation in infants and children have focused on limiting tidal volume, thereby

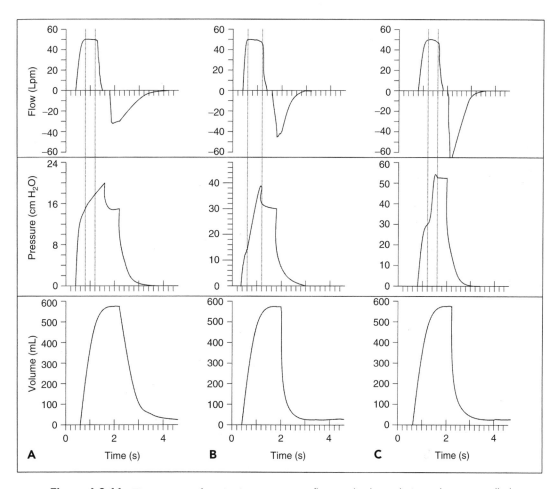

Figure 6.8.11 Time course of static airway pressure, flow, and volume during volume-controlled ventilation. From panel A to panel C, respiratory system compliance decreases. The constant flow phase is defined by the *dotted lines*, which show the elastic load on the pressure curve. As peak inspiratory pressure increases, the morphology of the curve changes, turning from concave to linear to convex.

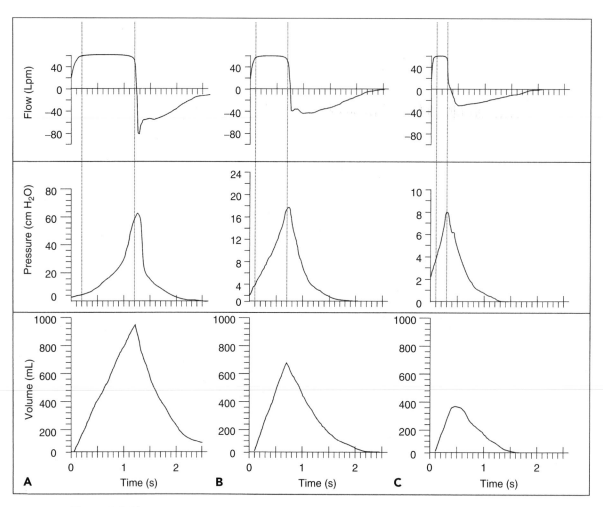

Figure 6.8.12 Time course of static airway pressure, flow, and volume during lung overdistension. From panel A to panel C, volume decreases and the shape of the airway pressure curve changes. Panel A shows the typical airway pressure curve aspect during lung overdistension.

preventing overdistension and volutrauma. Knowledge of both inspired and expired gas volumes is essential for using this lung-protective strategy. During the inflation phase of mechanical ventilation, pressure rises within the ventilator circuit, causing elongation and distension of the gas within the circuit. The volume stored in the circuit never reaches the patient, and therefore, the volume received is less than the set value. Compression volume can be calculated as the effective tidal volume, which is calculated as the ventilator-measured expired V_T − [circuit compensation × (peak inspiratory pressure [PI_{max}] − PEEP)].

However, the optimal site for monitoring volumes in infants and children is unclear. The inability to accurately measure tidal volumes at the expiratory valve of a conventional ventilator is caused by the difficulty in compensating for volume loss due to ventilator circuit compliance, the compliance of the humidifier, and factors such as changes in temperature, humidification, and secretions. Measuring tidal volumes at the proximal airway eliminates most circuit compliance and dead space factors.

A recommended site to obtain accurate volume measurements is at the proximal airway in infants and children. To measure volumes at the proximal airway, a pneumotachograph must be positioned at the patient's airway opening or endotracheal tube. Unfortunately, this technique has disadvantages, especially in infants and children. A pneumotachograph at the proximal opening is associated with increased dead space, particularly in infants with low tidal volumes. In addition, a pneumotachograph positioned at the proximal airway may be associated with impaired access to the endotracheal tube and airways, increased contamination of the pneumotachograph, and an increased risk of extubation because of the weight of the pneumotachograph.

We have stated that the effective tidal volume can be calculated as the ventilator-measured expired V_T − [circuit compensation × (peak inspiratory pressure [PI_{max}] − PEEP)]. However, this method fails to account for volume lost internally in the ventilator. Manufacturers have attempted to compensate for these volume losses by measuring compression volume loss in the system. The

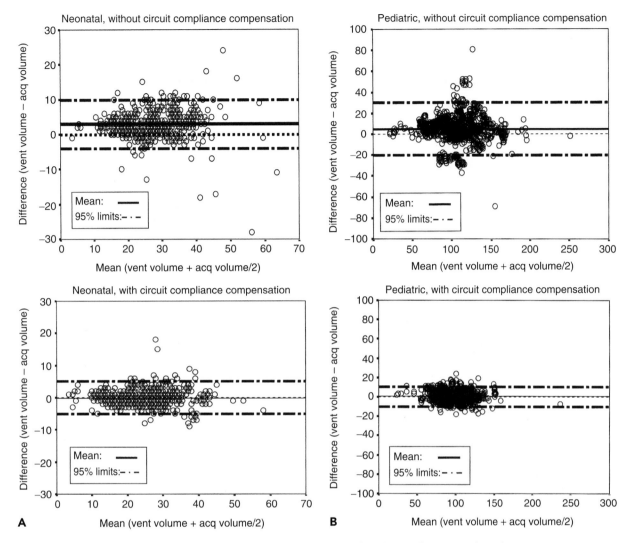

Figure 6.8.13 Bland-Altman plots in **(A)** neonatal animals and **(B)** pediatric animals, without **(top)** and with **(bottom)** circuit compliance compensation (difference plotted against the mean of the volumes obtained at the airway opening pneumotachograph [acq volume] and the ventilator [vent volume]).

compliance factor can be calculated as:

$$K_C = \frac{d_V}{(P_1 - P_0)} \,\text{mL per cm H}_2\text{O}$$

where K_C is the compliance factor, d_V is the total integrated volume, and P_0 and P_1 are start and target pressures. Recently published data demonstrates good agreement in volume measured at the ventilator with compensation as compared to the volume measured at the proximal airway (see Figures 6.8.13A and 6.8.13B). The use of circuit compliance compensation improved the agreement between the two volume methods for pediatric pigs; there was improvement in agreement between the two volume methods because of circuit compliance compensation (ccc: with circuit compliance compensation "on" was 0.97 and with circuit compliance compensation "off" was 0.88; $p = 0.027$). It is essential for the clinician to understand the

importance of the accuracy of the delivery of tidal volume to patients, especially in patients with small volumes such as infants.

PHASE VARIABLES

The control variable required for delivery of a breath by a mechanical ventilator and the interactions occurring with the delivery of that breath have been considered. Next, phase variables, which control the ventilator between the beginning of one breath and the initial phase of the next breath have to be discussed. Phase variables are important determinants of how a ventilator initiates, sustains, and ends inspiration and what it does between cycles. Because expiration is passive, it is not important for this discussion.

A specific variable is measured and used to initiate, sustain, and end each phase. The phase variables includes the trigger variable, which determines the initiation of inspiration; a limit variable, which determines what sustains inspiration; and a cycle variable, which determines the termination of inspiration.

The trigger variables and the physiologic principles of WOB are important to this understanding.

Patient Ventilatory Interactions—Trigger Variable

Patient ventilator system interactions can be initiated in two settings. The ventilator can deliver a controlled breath independent of the patient, or it can be co-ordinated with the patient's effort. Ventilators will measure one or more of the variables associated with the equation of motion (e.g., pressure, volume, flow, or time). Inspiration is initiated when one of these variables reaches a preset threshold. A patient triggered breath, sometimes known as *interactive ventilation*, provides patients with the ability to alter breathing patterns in response to their ventilatory demand. These systems require an interface between the ventilator and the patient that senses a signal from the patient to allow for rapid, measured responses from the ventilator to meet the patient's needs. In addition, the interface must pressurize the system to allow for the delivery of breath to the patient and to recognize the end of inspiration and thereby the termination of the breath. Ideally, if this interaction could be facilitated by direct interactions between the patient and ventilator, it could eliminate delays created by the temporary or relative unavailability of the caregiver at the patient's bedside.

Initial recognition of the signal from the patient to begin inspiration is commonly referred to as *triggering*, which can be subdivided into pretrigger and trigger phases. The pretrigger phase is the time from the onset of inspiration until triggering occurs. The trigger phase is the time from triggering until maximum flow occurs. The most common trigger variables are time and flow. In time triggering, the ventilator initiates a breath according to a set frequency independent of the patient's spontaneous efforts. In flow triggering, the ventilator senses the patient's inspiratory effort as a change in flow from the baseline and begins inspiration independent of the set frequency.

Ventilator features that affect the trigger phase include the response time of the ventilator and the presence of bias flow. Bias flow is a continuous delivery of fresh gas circulating through the inspiratory and expiratory limbs of the circuit. Theoretically, bias flow reduces WOB by making the flow available to satisfy the earliest demand of the patient during inspiration before the flow is initiated during the pretrigger phase. Phases of triggering can be quantified, as shown in Figure 6.8.14. Increased effort of the patient to trigger the ventilator and the delayed response of the ventilator to the patient's effort can be translated directly

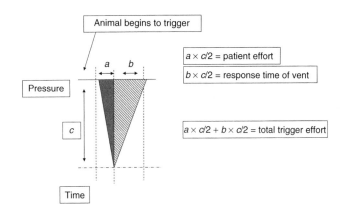

Figure 6.8.14 Demonstration of a single breath, with the triggering phase subdivided into the patient's effort and the ventilator response.

into increased WOB. Figure 6.8.15 illustrates a comparison between two ventilators in an animal model, where there is a marked difference between both response time and effort necessary to trigger the ventilator. In ventilator A, there is minimal effort for a rapid response to the animal's effort to trigger the ventilator. In contrast, there is a prolonged effort by the animal because of the delayed response of ventilator B. These differences translate into an increased WOB. Measured total WOB increased 20-fold between the two examples.

Current ventilator designs have improved patient ventilator interactions by improving both the signal sensed by the ventilator for triggering to occur and the response time of the ventilator. Today, all ventilators have the ability to utilize a flow signal as the trigger signal from the patient to the ventilator. Flow triggering has the advantage of allowing the patient to trigger the ventilator with less effort and faster response time.

Figure 6.8.16 demonstrates the differences between a flow-triggered and a pressure-triggered breath. In this example, of an animal model spontaneously breathing with PSV, it can be seen that the maximal deflection of pressure is greater in the pressure-triggered breath as compared to the flow-triggered breath. In this example, pressure-triggering sensitivity was set at -2 cm H_2O and flow-triggering sensitivity was set at 0.25 L per minute. Therefore, in pressure triggering, the patient must generate a pressure difference of at least 2 cm H_2O to trigger the ventilator. This process of creating somewhat seemingly small amounts of negative pressure is made increasingly more difficult in situations where the patients have smaller endotracheal tubes and in the presence of PEEPi.

Work of Breathing

Work is equal to the product of the force applied to an object and the distance the object travels; that is, work = force × distance, or $W = F \times D$.

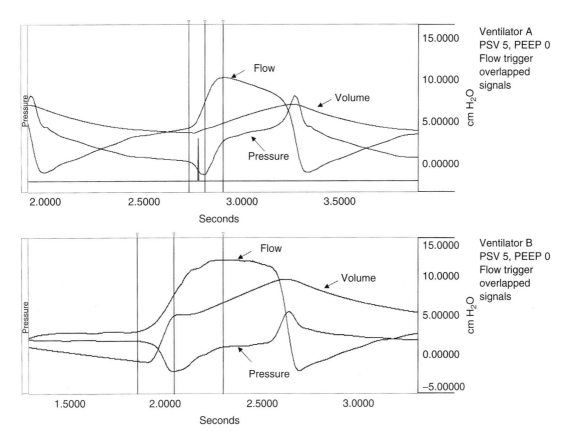

Figure 6.8.15 A comparison between two ventilators where there is a marked difference between both response time and effort necessary to trigger the ventilator. In ventilator A, there is minimal effort required and a rapid response to the animal's effort to trigger the ventilator. In contrast, in ventilator B, there is a prolonged effort by the animal because of the delayed response of the ventilator. These differences translate into an increased work of breathing (WOB). Measured total WOB increased 20-fold between the two examples. PEEP, positive end-expiratory pressure; PSV, pressure support ventilation. (From Sanders RC Jr, Thurman TL, Holt SJ, et al. Work of breathing associated with pressure support ventilation in two different ventilators. *Pediatr Pulmonol.* 2001;32(1):62–70.)

However, if we apply work into three dimensions that apply in the respiratory system, work becomes the pressure applied to yield a change in the volume of the system and can be expressed as:

$$W = P \times V$$
$$\text{or } W = \int_0^v P \times dv$$

where $\int_0^v P$ is the integral of the pressure across the respiratory system as a function of volume, and dv is the change in the volume of the respiratory system.

The concept of respiratory system work has been acknowledged since the seminal work of Otis et al. who identified the elastic forces of the chest wall and lungs, the viscous and turbulent resistance of air, and the nonelastic tissue impedance and inertia encountered while breathing. Basically, motion requires work. Work is performed when pressure changes the volume of the respiratory system and is the product of pressure and volume integrated over time with respect to volume. Work is performed by externally applied pressures from the ventilator through positive pressure, respiratory muscles, or both as the lungs expand and contract. To achieve normal ventilation, the body performs work, known as the WOB, to overcome the elastic and frictional resistance of the lungs and chest wall. Total WOB (WOB_T) is the sum of elastic work (WOB_E) and resistive work (WOB_R). Elastic WOB represents physiologic work that includes the work to expand the lungs and chest wall. Resistive WOB is considered a measure of imposed WOB and includes work caused by the breathing apparatus, such as the endotracheal tube, breathing circuit, and ventilator demand-flow system. Artificial airways and physiologic resistive work on the airways are responsible for a large part of the imposed resistive work, with the mechanical ventilator representing some of the remaining resistive work.

Clinicians have recognized the increased WOB in patients weaning from prolonged mechanical ventilation when the patient begins to breathe spontaneously and assumes work to breathe. Patient-related factors, equipment factors, and decision making affect weaning of patients

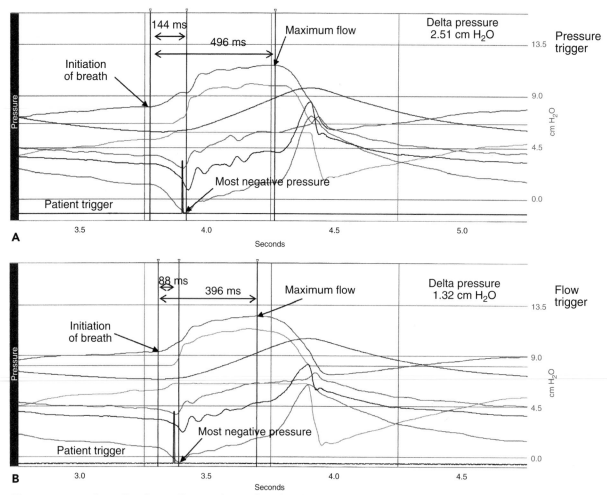

Figure 6.8.16 Illustration of two breaths, with ventilator set on **(A)** pressure triggering and **(B)** flow triggering. In a pressure-triggered breath, the response time and the effort necessary to trigger the ventilator (most negative pressure) are greater. (See color Figure 6.8.16A and B.)

from mechanical ventilation and, therefore, WOB. Equipment factors relate to the ability of the mechanical ventilator to meet patient demand. WOB varies with the device utilized. These equipment factors are important for patients with poor pulmonary reserve or high airway resistance, where the WOB associated with the equipment is increased. These equipment factors relate to the ability of the ventilator to meet the needs of the patient and are significantly more important in pediatric patients, where the equipment is often associated with an increased WOB.

Why are Children Different?

Infants and children are anatomically and physiologically different from adults. It is these differences that limit the direct application of adult studies to the care of young children on mechanical ventilation. These differences decrease with the child's growth. In a study of infants and children

intubated for elective surgery, the resistance of the respiratory system (R_{rs}) and airway resistance (R_{aw}) decreased as height increased. Comparing this relation with the reported power function of lung volume changes suggests that R_{rs} is actually lower, relative to the lung size in infants, than in older children; that is, increases in lung volumes are greater than decreases in resistance; therefore, specific resistance (resistance × volume) would increase with decreasing height. Therefore, it is speculated that the airways do not grow at the same rate as the increase in lung tissue, as reflected by increasing lung volumes. In infants, the lung volume may increase at a greater rate than the increase in airway diameter.

There are also detrimental effects of mechanical ventilation on the airways of infants. These include changes in the dimensions and mechanical properties of the airways. The extent of ventilation-induced deformation appears to be directly related to the compliance of the airway and inversely related to age. Anatomically, after mechanical ventilation, the airways are increased in tracheal diameter, with thinning of cartilage and muscle, disruption of the muscle–cartilage junction, and focal abrasions of the epithelium. In comparison to unexposed airways, airways exposed to mechanical ventilation are difficult to expand but easy to collapse and show a greater resistance to airflow. These findings result clinically in patients with increased dead space, flow limitation, increased airway resistance and WOB, and gas trapping.

Infants and young children also are at a mechanical disadvantage because of the high compliance and low elastic recoil of their chest walls. The child must perform more work, because of the distortion in the rib cage, to move the same tidal volume as a more mature patient. The chest wall's low elastic recoil places infants and young children at greater risk of lung collapse because most tidal breathing takes place in the range of the closing capacity of the lung. Also, infants have a reduced ability to generate muscle force because of the shape of their rib cage, location of the insertion of their diaphragm, reduced muscle mass, and oxidative capacity of muscle fibers.

Limit Variable

The limit variable sustains inspiration. Inspiration time is defined as the interval from the beginning of inspiratory flow to the beginning of expiratory flow. During inspiration, pressure, volume, and flow increase above their end-expiratory values. If one or more of these variables increase no higher than some preset value, this will be referred to as the *limit variable*. However, it is important to recognize that the limit variable determines the factors that sustain inspiration but differs from the cycle variable, which determines the end of inspiration. Therefore, a limit value does not terminate inspiration but increases to a preset value.

Cycle Variable

The cycle variable terminates inspiration once a preset value is obtained. The cycle variable is different for different modes of ventilation. In pressure support, the termination of the breath is traditionally triggered by the absolute level of flow or by a fixed percentage of peak inspiratory flow that is reached. Until recently, this gave the clinician little control over the cycling off of the ventilator because it relates to the patient's pathology. For example, for a patient with increased airway resistance and dynamic hyperinflation, it may be desirable to shorten the inspiratory time with a prolonged expiratory phase. By changing the cycle off variable, as illustrated in Figure 6.8.17, the patient's inspiratory phase can be shortened, allowing the patient a longer expiratory phase. The opposite is also true for patients with decreased pulmonary compliance, where the clinician might want to prolong the inspiratory phase with

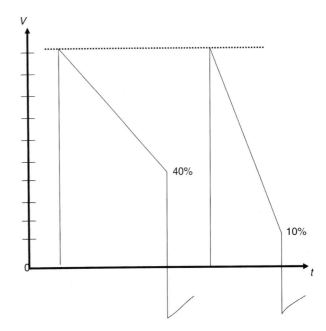

Figure 6.8.17 The figure illustrates two breaths with the cycle off set at 10% and 40%. When the cycle off is set at 40%, the inspiratory phase can be terminated earlier, thereby prolonging expiration. When the cycle off is set at 10%, the inspiratory phase is prolonged, thereby allowing the patient to spend more time in inspiration.

a shorter expiratory phase. The termination of the breath can be extended by delaying the beginning of expiration.

PATIENT–VENTILATOR ASYNCHRONY

Patient–ventilator asynchrony is the failure of two controllers to act in harmony. When a patient is on a mechanical ventilator, there are two controllers: the clinician-controlled mechanical pump of the ventilator and the patient's own respiratory muscle pump. The factors that affect patient–ventilator synchrony are listed in Table 6.8.2 and can be subdivided into equipment factors, patient factors, and decision-making factors. The evaluation of patient–ventilator synchrony can also be subdivided into four phases. These phases consist of issues of triggering, adequacy of flow delivery, adequate breath termination, and effects of PEEPi.

Trigger Asynchrony

Trigger asynchrony is defined as the presence of muscular effort with ventilator trigger. The incidence and occurrence of patient ventilator asynchrony is not well studied in pediatric patients. Clinical studies in adults have demonstrated trigger asynchrony in all of the common ventilator modes. Asynchrony occurs because of the failure of the patient's drive to breathe. This is found when additional support is provided by the base mode of the ventilator and when the

TABLE 6.8.2
VENTILATOR–PATIENT SYNCHRONY

Equipment Factors
Trigger variables
Sensitivity settings
Response time of the ventilator
Inspiratory flow characteristics
Mode of ventilation
Expiratory valve design
Design of PEEP valve and operation
External factors and equipment of the ventilator
Patient Factors
Sedation and pain control
Patient's inspiratory effort and drive
Patient's disease process
Intrinsic PEEP
Size of the airway
Presence of airway leak
Nutritional status
Patient homeostasis
Decision-Making Factors
Deleterious Effects
Patient fights the ventilator
Increased level of sedation
Higher work of breathing
Muscle damage
Ventilation–perfusion mismatch
Dynamic hyperinflation
Delayed or prolonged weaning
Prolonged intensive care or hospital stay
Higher costs

PEEP, positive end-expiratory pressure.

patient's drive to breathe decreases. Trigger asynchrony is also associated with the development of auto-PEEP.

Mechanically ventilated patients with obstructive lung disease who develop PEEPi have to generate a negative intrapleural pressure to match the value of PEEPi in addition to the ventilator sensitivity threshold level before triggering occurs and a ventilator breath is initiated. When inspiratory effort by the patient is less than the threshold value, the ventilator will not deliver a breath, causing effort with response from the ventilator. Therefore, dynamic hyperinflation (PEEPi) leads to frequent nontriggering of breaths in patients with obstructive lung disease. Such nontriggered breaths represent wasted breathing effort on the part of the patient and lead to patient–ventilator asynchrony. In assist-control modes, the ventilator must be set to respond to the patient's breathing effort in order to provide adequate support. In addition, application of external PEEP in mechanically ventilated patients with obstructive lung disease and PEEPi may reduce nontriggered breaths by narrowing the difference between mouth pressure and alveolar pressure at end-expiration. Application of external PEEP could reduce the elastic threshold load and WOB, particularly in patients with flow limitation during tidal expiration.

Flow Asynchrony

Flow asynchrony occurs whenever the patient and ventilator flows do not match. Flow from the ventilator can be a fixed flow pattern (such as in volume-controlled ventilation) or can vary (pressure control or pressure-regulated volume control). In volume control, flow is fixed so that a set level of flow is delivered with each breath. Because WOB is the sum of the work performed by the ventilator and the work performed by the patient, reduction in ventilator support or work will reduce the level of support. During ventilation with variable flow, the peak flow depends on the set target pressure, patient's effort, and respiratory system compliance and resistance. During pressure control, the clinician can set the target pressure and the rate of flow acceleration or rise time. The control flow of acceleration varies according to the manufacturer of the ventilator, but the principles remain the same. A slower rise time may limit the ability of the ventilator to meet the patient's inspiratory demand. Studies of flow asynchrony during pressure-controlled or PSV have implied that many patients require a rapid rise time to match increased ventilatory demand. MacIntyre et al., assessed whether adjustments in the initial flow or breath termination criteria affected patient–ventilator synchrony. The ventilator pattern response to PSV of 33 adult patients was studied under conditions with two parameters: seven different levels of delivered initial PSV flow, and, during PSV termination, at 50% and 25% of peak flow. They found that an optimal initial flow could be defined for a given PSV level, which resulted in the patient gaining a maximal pressure and volume from the ventilator. In addition, the initial PSV flows above and below this optimal flow were associated with faster breathing rates (or minute ventilation), shorter inspiratory times, smaller tidal volumes, and a tendency for airway pressure to not meet the preset value. In pediatric patients, increasing the rate of inspiratory flow, however, may have deleterious effects. Because pediatric patients have smaller endotracheal tubes, increased flow may lead to increased turbulence and, possibly, increased asynchrony.

Termination Asynchrony

Termination asynchrony occurs when neural inspiratory time and ventilator inspiratory time do not coincide. The ability of the ventilator mode to terminate a breath when the patient desires constitutes an important factor in reducing the incidence of dysynchrony. In conditions in which the patient experiences high airway resistance, such as bronchopulmonary dysplasia or chronic obstructive pulmonary disease, the inspiratory phase of a ventilator breath may be prolonged when selecting a mode that allows the patient to trigger spontaneous breaths. This situation can occur in PSV, resulting in early activation of expiratory muscles with premature termination of the ventilator breath.

Termination asynchrony can be caused by delayed termination or premature termination. The most common type of termination asynchrony is delayed termination. Generally, delayed termination results in dynamic hyperinflation, with resultant trigger delay and increased missed trigger attempts. Premature termination can also have deleterious effects with resultant asynchrony. In a study by Tokioka, premature termination led to substantially reduced V_T, increased respiratory rate, decreased inspiratory time, and increased WOB.

In later-generation ventilators, a solution to help alleviate termination asynchrony has been devised. This additional control allows for adjusting flow that causes the ventilator to cycle from the inspiratory phase to the expiratory phase (cycle off) and for exhalation to be active.

Figure 6.8.17 illustrates the effects of changing cycle off when the ventilator begins exhalation as a function of peak inspiratory flow in a ventilator with an active exhalation system. At a cycle off set at 1%, the breath is terminated earlier than a cycle off set at 40%.

Expiratory Asynchrony

Expiratory asynchrony is due to a shortened or prolonged expiratory time and the patient attempting efforts during expiration when the ventilator is unresponsive. Shortened expiratory time creates the potential for hyperinflation secondary to air trapping and induces PEEPi.

Until recently, the expiratory valve, in the ventilators were not responsive to the patients efforts during exhalation. Recently, manufacturers have introduced active exhalation valves that continue to sense the patient's effort during exhalation and respond to it. In Figure 6.8.18, the response of an active exhalation valve is illustrated. In this example, the ventilator continues to sample for exhalation at a rate of 2,000 per second. If the patient generates an effort during exhalation, the ventilator can terminate exhalation and respond to the patient's effort. This is in contrast with systems that allow the patient to only attempt to pull flow from the system, but the patient would have to wait for expiration to terminate before another ventilator breath could be generated or triggered.

LUNG RECRUITMENT MANEUVERS

Mechanical ventilation is an essential tool for saving the lives of critically ill children, but it can also increase morbidity and mortality if applied inappropriately. An understanding of harmful and beneficial practices to the lung during positive pressure mechanical ventilation can assist with the application of "protective lung strategies."

Volutrauma versus Barotrauma

Many investigators have not made a distinction between volume- and pressure-induced injury. Evidence implicating mechanical ventilation with high PIP or lung volume in the progression of lung pathology is largely the result of experimental studies. However, the evidence is substantial and clinically relevant. Tsuno et al. ventilated healthy adult sheep with initially high tidal volumes (30 mL per kg), a clinically relevant value in light of the findings with initially high tidal volumes (30 mL per kg) with a $P_{plateau}$ of 30 cm H_2O. Over the first few hours, the measured compliance improved but progressive deterioration followed. Chest

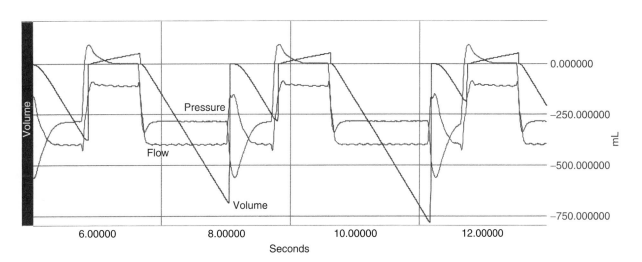

Figure 6.8.18 The illustration of two ventilators, one with an active exhalation valve and one without ventilating a lung model. The ventilator, with the active exhalation valve, is set at a rate of 10 bpm, and the other ventilator is set at 20 bpm. The second ventilator is able to trigger the ventilator with the active exhalation valve during exhalation. Adult test lung, Pressure Control, peak Inspiratory pressure 20, positive end-expiratory pressure 5 cmH$_2$O, frequency 10 breaths per minute, 3 second Inspiratory time on Servo-I; Servo 300 settings are Volume Control, Set tidal volume 70 mL, frequency 20 breaths per minute, positive end-expiratory pressure 0 cmH$_2$O. (See color Figure 6.8.18.)

radiographs suggested acute respiratory distress syndrome (ARDS), and at necropsy, the lungs were edematous and structurally damaged. The exposure of rats to high-volume ventilation with a PIP of 45 cm H_2O for just 2 minutes resulted in a significant increase in protein permeability of the pulmonary microvasculature and evidence of structural endothelial damage.

The increase in protein permeability of the pulmonary vasculature resulting from high PIP or lung volume appears to be a threshold phenomenon that is reversible when periods of high-volume ventilation are short. The duration of the exposure is an important consideration. Replicating a lung-injury model established by Kolobow et al., Borelli et al. ventilated healthy adult sheep with a PIP of 50 cm H_2O, resulting in initial tidal volumes of 50 to 70 mL per kg. Following 18 hours of ventilation, two groups of sheep were randomized to conventional ventilation (with tidal volumes of 10/15 mL per kg) or extracorporeal carbon dioxide (CO_2) removal. Three of 11 survived in the conventional ventilation group, compared to 9 out of 11 in the extracorporeal CO_2 removal group. Subsequently, after 27 hours of mechanical ventilation with a PIP of 50 cm H_2O, two additional groups were again randomized to either conventional ventilation or extracorporeal CO_2 removal. None of the animals survived.

Evidence is increasingly demonstrating that volumes that result in overdistension, rather than pressure, are implicated in contributing to iatrogenic lung injury. An increase in pulmonary vascular permeability has been observed in two studies of spontaneously breathing humans with increased lung volume. Dreyfuss et al. compared the development of lung pathology in healthy rats ventilated with a high V_T (40 mL per kg) and low PIP (induced by negative pressure ventilation) and that of rats ventilated with high PIP (45 cm H_2O) and low V_T (achieved by thoracoabdominal strapping) to a control group, ventilated with a V_T of approximately 13 mL per kg and PIP of 13 cm H_2O. Rats in the high PIP–low V_T group had lungs that were normal and comparable to controls at necropsy. The lungs of the high V_T–low PIP group exhibited marked protein permeability and microvascular structural abnormalities.

These findings are supported by subsequent studies. Hernandez et al. ventilated young rabbits with closed chests, those with full-body plaster casts placed around the chest and abdomen, and the isolated, excised lungs of young rabbits. The capillary filtration coefficient, a reflection of microvascular permeability, was evaluated. They found an increase by 850% after ventilating the isolated, excised lungs with a PIP of just 15 cm H_2O. In the closed-chest group, ventilation with a PIP of 45 cm H_2O resulted in an increase in the capillary filtration coefficient of 430%. No change in the capillary filtration coefficient occurred at any PIP which had used in the study in the subjects with body casts applied to limit inflation volume of the lungs.

Hyperinflation induces pulmonary edema by both permeability and filtration mechanisms. Pulmonary overdistension causes longitudinal tension in the thin pulmonary capillary wall and subsequent stress failure. Indeed, breaks in capillary endothelium and alveolar epithelium provide a pathophysiologic basis for the increase in pulmonary microvascular protein permeability seen with volutrauma. West described the functional relationship of alveolar surface tension to pulmonary capillaries as "... iron hoops supporting a barrel of beer." In the condition in which transpulmonary pressure is increased to 25 cm H_2O, the mean width of the pulmonary capillaries is markedly decreased, increasing filtration out of the capillary. Parker et al. observed a significant increase in pulmonary lymph flow in subjects during ventilation with high PIP when compared to ventilation with low PIP, suggesting a contributory role for increased microvascular filtration pressure in overinflation edema.

Overinflation during mechanical ventilation also causes alterations in the function of surfactant in the lung. Lung biopsy of previously healthy dogs 24 hours after a 2-hour period of ventilation, with values of PIP between 26 and 32 cm H_2O, revealed atelectasis and significantly increased surface tension when compared to dogs ventilated at low PIP or not mechanically ventilated at all. The authors subsequently performed selective ventilation-induced overinflation of the left lung, whereas the right lung was ventilated with low PIP. Atelectasis and increased surface tension were present in the left lung only on inflation, confirming their earlier findings. Faridy et al. demonstrated that increases in surface tension are directly related to increases in tidal volume and duration of ventilation. The observed increase in surface tension was reversed with subsequent delivery of CPAP. However, this reversibility was not seen in the presence of either hypothermia or tissue anoxia, leading the authors to suggest that the production of new surfactant is necessary for recovery. Surfactant deficiencies may augment protein permeability in the lung.

Deleterious effects of volutrauma are greater if preexisting pulmonary disease is present. A comparison of salt-perfused rabbit lungs ventilated with a V_T of 6 mL per kg and another group ventilated with a V_T of 18 mL per kg after oleic-acid injury revealed a significant increase in lung edema in the lungs ventilated with high V_T. Hernandez et al. compared the effects of mechanical ventilation alone (PIP of 25 cm H_2O) on excised lungs of young rabbits to the effects of oleic-acid injury alone (airway pressure maintained at 3 cm H_2O, with periodic sighs to prevent atelectasis) and to the effects of both mechanical ventilation and oleic-acid injury. The lungs that received mechanical ventilation and those that received oleic acid were not significantly different from each other. However, the lungs exposed to mechanical ventilation and oleic-acid injury had a significantly greater increase in wet-to-dry lung-weight ratio than the other two groups.

Special Considerations in Pediatric Patients

Pediatric patients may be predisposed to increased risks of iatrogenic injury from mechanical ventilation because they differ anatomically and developmentally from adults. Postnatal age is inversely related to alveolar epithelium permeability. Microvascular protein permeability in 4- to 6-week-old rabbit lungs was compared to lungs of three groups of adult rabbits after ventilation with PIPs of either 15, 30, or 45 cm H_2O for 1 hour. The pulmonary capillary filtration coefficient of the young rabbit lungs was increased by 91% at a PIP of 15 cm H_2O and by 440% at a PIP of 45 cm H_2O. The authors postulated that the amplified injuries seen in the younger lungs were attributable to their measured higher chest wall compliance. The inverse relationship of chest wall compliance and risk of microvascular damage with mechanical ventilation is supported by a lack of edema when the chest wall is restricted compared to progressively increasing edema in the unimpaired chest wall and in excised lungs. With the higher chest wall compliance of infants and small children, less protection is provided against iatrogenic lung injury. Elastic recoil of the lung and lung collagen are related to the concentration of lung elastin. Considered a good model of postnatal lung growth, lung elastins are slow to reach adult levels in rats and are associated with the structural integrity of the lung.

Techniques to Facilitate Lung Recruitment

Increased Positive End-Expiratory Pressure

Although pulmonary overinflation is a source of iatrogenesis in the intensive care unit, the maintenance of an appropriate lung volume is equally important in the application of mechanical ventilatory support in ARDS. Indeed, Dreyfuss et al. characterize this challenge of maintaining lung volume which is neither "too much" nor "too little" with the analogy of the Homeric voyage between Scylla (the rock on the Italian side of the Strait of Messina) and Charybdis (a whirlpool in the strait) or, alternatively, being "between a rock and a hard place." Suter found that total static compliance is suboptimal if PEEP is set either too low or too high.

Increasing PEEP is the most common method utilized to prevent lung derecruitment and improve lung recruitment. In pediatric patients, the selection of optimal PEEP is problematic. Sivan observed in pediatric patients with ARDS that the level of clinician-determined PEEP failed to normalize FRC in most patients. PEEP levels that did normalize FRC were up to 200% higher than in those clinically chosen.

Katz et al. demonstrated that the effects of PEEP on lung volume in patients with acute respiratory failure are complex. By measuring breath-to-breath V_T changes following the application of PEEP, they found that the initial (one to four breaths) increase in volume occurs at constant compliance, indicating an increase in the volume of already ventilated alveoli. A further increase in volume (approximately 10% of the ultimate volume change in that particular patient population) occurred at the same end-inspiratory pressure, indicating recruitment of newly opened alveoli over a 3- to 4-minute period. From the study of Katz et al., the compliance, calculated using the end-expiratory P_{AO} difference (chord compliance), did not

change at various levels of PEEP. However, when the compliance was measured at FRC after achieving steady state, it increased, with each increase in PEEP indicating that PEEP recruited alveoli, whereas tidal ventilation did not.

In another classic study of respiratory mechanics in ARDS, Matamis discerned different patterns of lung recruitment, depending upon the progression of the ARDS. They found evidence of large hysteresis early in the course of the disease with the potential for recruitment. Later in the course of the fibroproliferative phase, there was no substantial hysteresis, indicating a lower potential for recruitment.

The evidence for PEEP as a protective tool is ample. Webb and Tierney found that pulmonary edema resulting from ventilation with a PIP of 45 cm H_2O could be prevented with the addition of a PEEP of 10 cm H_2O. However, PIP was held constant in this study, and therefore, the degree of cyclic inflation was reduced when PEEP was added. With end-inspiratory pressure and volume being constant during a comparison of mechanical ventilation strategies in a canine acid-aspiration model, a large tidal volume–low PEEP approach resulted in significantly more pulmonary edema than a low tidal volume–high PEEP design. The pattern of lung injury seen in the two groups was distinctly different. Edema was primarily located in the dependent regions of the lung in the low tidal volume–high PEEP group, whereas a more uniform edema was present in the large tidal volume–low PEEP group. Although a similar type of lung injury was observed in rats ventilated with high volumes and PEEP, the degree of pulmonary injury was markedly decreased when compared to rats ventilated with high volumes without PEEP. Surfactant function remains intact with the application of PEEP. In surfactant-deficient lungs, PEEP applied at or above the inflection point on the inflation limb of the pressure–volume curve helps prevent hyaline membrane formation.

Applying the proper amount of PEEP is essential to ensure protection. In a recent study by Muscedere et al. isolated, nonperfused lungs excised immediately after surfactant washout were (i) ventilated at zero end-expiratory pressure (ZEEP); (ii) ventilated, with 4 cm H_2O PEEP (below the inflection point of the inflation pressure–volume curve); (iii) ventilated, with a PEEP above the inflection point on the inflation limb of the pressure–volume curve; or (iv) not ventilated, with a set PEEP (i.e., CPAP) of 4 cm H_2O. Their work demonstrated that the level of PEEP could influence both the degree and site of lung injury. Lung-injury scores were significantly worse when the PEEP was set below the inflection point on the inflation limb of the pressure–volume curve, with the worst lung-injury score occurring at ZEEP. The location of injury with the ZEEP group was significantly higher in the respiratory bronchioles, whereas the percentage of alveolar ducts with hyaline membranes was significantly greater in the group ventilated with a set PEEP of 4 cm H_2O. The lung-injury score for the group ventilated with PEEP set above the inflection point of the inflation limb of the pressure–volume curve was not significantly different from the group that was not ventilated. Opening and closing of small airways may cause shear stress and lung injury during mechanical ventilation. PEEP may act to splint the airways, thereby reducing shear stress.

The protective function of PEEP may be related to a reduction in shear stress, recruitment of FRC, maintenance of surfactant function, and a hemodynamic effect. Dreyfuss et al. demonstrated that overinflation-induced pulmonary edema suppressed by PEEP returned when an infusion of the inotropic agent dopamine was started.

End-inspiratory volume is the main determinant of ventilator-induced lung injury (VILI). Clinically important pulmonary protein permeability during mechanical ventilation can occur both with low PEEP and high tidal volumes and with high PEEP (and presumably high FRC) and low tidal volumes. Egan applied a static pressure of 40 cm H_2O to both lobes *in situ* and the whole lungs. A six- to 12-fold increase in gas volume and an increase in pulmonary permeability to albumin were seen with the lungs *in situ*. With inflation of the whole lung, only a three- to four-fold increase in gas volume without permeability to albumin was observed.

Sustained Inflation

A sustained inflation is a maneuver in which a high pressure is applied to the airway. A common method to this approach is to utilize CPAP, where there are no mandatory breaths. The CPAP is increased to 30 to 40 cm H_2O for 30 to 40 seconds. During this maneuver, it is essential to monitor for adverse effects such as hemodynamic compromise secondary to the dramatically increased intrathoracic pressure. This maneuver can also be obtained by placing the patient in pressure control and by choosing an ideal PEEP level. The peak pressure is then increased stepwise till a predetermined outcome is reached. Examples of the outcome are measures of lung recruitment. Classically, lung recruitment has occurred when there is an improvement in the PaO_2, ventilation (some measure of $PaCO_2$), and pulmonary compliance (change in delta ΔP or pressure for same V_T or dynamic compliance).

Sigh

Although low V_T ventilation has become the standard approach for positive pressure mechanical ventilation, there is still interest in procedures to reduce or reverse atelectasis. One method is to maintain the PEEP at a level adequate to maintain FRC. However, if alveolar collapse occurs, some investigators have recommended the incorporation of sigh breaths in ventilator modes such as Bilevel, Bivent, and PCV+. A study utilizing sigh breaths was performed by Pelosi; the study involved application of three consecutive breaths per minute at a plateau of 45 cm H_2O. The authors concluded that the application of sigh during lung-protective strategy may improve recruitment and oxygenation. A concern with this approach is the ability of the patient to breathe during a high-pressure

setting when the approach is utilized during the maintenance phase of mechanical ventilation. However in Bivent and PCV+, the manufacturers utilize an active exhalation system to improve comfort and synchrony.

PRESSURE–VOLUME CURVES

West points out that lung ventilation occurs essentially while they are "... hidden in a box." Although the best means for ascertaining optimal PEEP and tidal volume during mechanical ventilation of patients with ARDS has probably not yet been developed, perhaps the most effective tool is the static inflation pressure–volume curve. Sykes et al. demonstrated that setting PEEP at or above the inflection point on the inflation limb of the pressure–volume curve reduced the formation of hyaline membranes in surfactant-deficient lungs.

Gattinoni et al. found that the ratio of inflation compliance (slope of the curve in the most linear segment on the inflation limb of the curve) to starting compliance (the ratio between initial inflation volume and pressure) reflects the amount of lung recruitment after the application of PEEP. The inflection point (the point of intersection between starting compliance and inflation compliance) that occurs at low lung volumes represents the closing volume. Hysteresis is indicative of air trapping and can be computed as the difference in volume seen on the deflation limb and on the inflation limb of the curve at 10 cm H_2O pressure. However, an underestimation of deflation-limb compliance can occur because of endotracheal tube leaks and gas exchange and changes in temperature and humidity. As a result, the calculation of hysteresis is exaggerated. The inflation limb of the pressure–volume curve is easier to obtain and, perhaps, more valuable in the clinical setting.

Evaluation of static pressure–volume curves of 19 patients with ARDS led Matamis to conclude that the shape of the curve correlates with the evolving pathologic and radiographic stages of ARDS. An inflection point and abnormal hysteresis was seen only in patients in an early phase of ARDS. The addition of PEEP resulted in an increase in FRC and a decrease in intrapulmonary shunting in these patients. PEEP does not improve intrapulmonary shunting and may cause overdistension when there is no evidence of an inflection point or marked hysteresis. This occurs in both patients with normal compliance and those in end-stage ARDS with diffuse pulmonary fibrosis. Milic-Emili et al. observed that FRC increases with PEEP in patients whose static pressure–volume curves have an upward concavity, whereas PEEP causes overdistension in patients whose curves have an upward convexity.

Static pressure–volume curves are obtained conventionally by disconnecting the patient from the ventilator and by using a calibrated syringe to incrementally inflate and deflate the lung. Volume history is standardized and the patient is placed on ZEEP and relaxed, sedated, or paralyzed. Fernandez showed validation for a technique that does not require disconnecting the patient from the ventilator or the use of additional equipment. Recently, the dynamic pressure–volume curve measurements were found to correlate well with curves measured under static conditions. Limitations to clinical use of the pressure–volume measurements include having to place patients on ZEEP and the need to use a mode with constant flow.

HIGH-FREQUENCY OSCILLATORY VENTILATION

High-frequency ventilation is commonly used in pediatric patients who have failed conventional mechanical ventilation. High-frequency ventilatory techniques theoretically allow alveolar recruitment with the application of a high mean airway pressure while minimizing the risk of overdistension with V_T at or below dead space at frequencies of 180 to 600 ppm.

Rationale for Using High-Frequency Oscillatory Ventilation in Patients with Acute Hypoxemic Respiratory Failure

In many respects, high-frequency oscillatory ventilation (HFOV) is an extension of an "open lung approach" as

part of a lung-protective strategy of mechanical ventilation. Many animal and clinical studies have reinforced the concept that repetitive, cyclic distension and closing of injured lung results in a spectrum of VILI, including *volutrauma* (induced by overdistension of lung units), *atelectrauma* (caused by repetitive opening–closing of lung units), and *biotrauma* (induction and potentiation of pulmonary and systemic inflammatory response associated with *volutrauma* and *atelectrauma*). Recent studies in adults with ARDS have demonstrated a mortality benefit for patients ventilated with a lung-protective ventilation strategy designed to minimize VILI. More detailed discussions of VILI and lung-protective ventilatory practices utilizing conventional mechanical ventilation can be found elsewhere in this text (see Chapter 53). Because HFOV uses a constant mean airway pressure for alveolar recruitment and lung distension, utilizes a tidal volume that is in some cases smaller than anatomic dead space, and is associated with a marked attenuation of pressure from the ventilator circuit to the alveoli, it should in theory be an excellent mode for lung-protective ventilation. Here, the evidence behind HFOV is provided.

Mechanisms of Gas Exchange during High-Frequency Oscillatory Ventilation

Despite years of successful clinical use and extensive investigation, a thorough understanding of the different mechanisms of gas exchange during HFOV remains elusive.

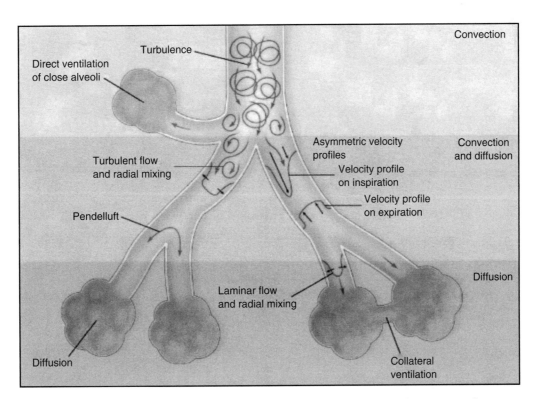

Figure 6.8.19 Different mechanisms of gas exchange active during high-frequency oscillatory ventilation. (From Slutsky AS, Drazen JM. Ventilation with small tidal volumes. *N Engl J Med.* 2002;347:631.)

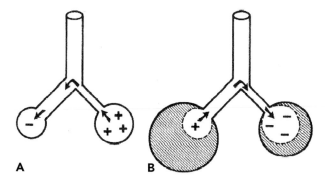

Figure 6.8.20 Illustration of time constants. (From Chang HK. Mechanisms of gas transport during ventilation by high-frequency ventilation. *J Appl Physiol.* 1984;56:555.)

Given that the tidal volume (V_T) provided during HFOV is often smaller than the anatomic dead space, bulk flow of gas cannot be the sole mechanism of gas exchange. Six distinct mechanisms of gas exchange appear to be involved in alveolar ventilation during HFOV (see Fig. 6.8.19). These six mechanisms are (i) direct bulk flow, (ii) convective mixing secondary to Pendelluft between lung units with differing time constants, (iii) convective gas transport due to asymmetric inspiratory and expiratory velocity profiles, (iv) Taylor-type dispersion caused by the interaction between axial flow velocities and radial diffusion of gases, (v) molecular diffusion near the alveolar–capillary interface, and (vi) cardiogenic oscillations.

Just as in conventional mechanical ventilation, some bulk convective gas flow occurs during HFOV and contributes to alveolar ventilation, despite the extremely small V_T being delivered. Alveolar units located proximally in the tracheobronchial tree, and only short lengths from conducting airways, receive bulk transport of gas, even when V_T is less than anatomic dead space (V_D). Various *in vivo* studies have suggested that adequate alveolar ventilation can be maintained with HFOV when V_T is in the range of 0.5x V_D to 0.75x V_D, but if V_T falls below this range, gas exchange deteriorates despite increases in frequency (f) and despite the other mechanisms of gas exchange being present.

A second mechanism of gas transport during HFOV is Pendelluft, or the exchange of gas between lung units of varying time constants. When adjacent lung units have differing time constants (tau) ($\tau = R \times C$), a "slow" lung unit will empty into a "fast" unit at end-expiration; the "slow" unit will then inspire gas from "fast" unit at end inspiration (see Fig. 6.8.20). In the setting of very high respiratory rates such as those used in HFOV, airway resistance (R) tends to dominate the rate of filling and emptying and therefore affects Pendelluft the most. In a lung with an inhomogeneous pattern of disease, as shown by computed tomography studies to be present in ARDS, Pendelluft may play a significant role in ventilation during high-frequency oscillation (HFO), particularly in peripheral lung units distal to small airways.

Gas exchange due to asymmetric velocity profiles refers to the phenomenon whereby inspiration of a high-frequency pulse creates a bullet-shaped or parabolic profile,

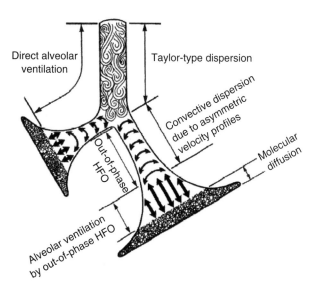

Figure 6.8.21 Possible contributions of different mechanisms of gas exchange in different lung regions. HFO, high-frequency oscillation. (From Chang HK. Mechanisms of gas transport during ventilation by high-frequency ventilation. *J Appl Physiol.* 1984; 56:555.)

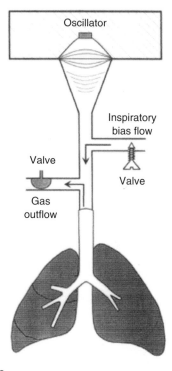

Figure 6.8.22 Diagrammatic representation of high-frequency oscillatory ventilator. (From Krishnan JA, Brower RG. High-frequency ventilation for acute lung injury and ARDS. *Chest.* 2000; 118:797.)

with molecules toward the center of the column of air moving further forward than molecules on the periphery. On exhalation, the parabolic profile is blunted so that a net dispersion inward occurs in the center of the column and a net dispersion outward occurs at the periphery (see Fig. 6.8.21). This phenomenon occurs in the setting of active inspiration and active expiration, as occurs during HFOV. In other words, a net vector of fresh gas supply streams down the center of the airway, with a net vector of exhaled gas moving out along the airway walls, providing the physiologic basis for the improvement in ventilation, which can sometimes be achieved by deflating the endotracheal tube cuff and inducing an air leak.

Another mechanism that seems to play at least some role in ventilation during HFOV is Taylor-type dispersion. Taylor, or augmented, dispersion refers to the interplay between the asymmetric flow velocity profile and radial diffusion of gas molecules produced by turbulence in highly branching airways (see Fig. 6.8.22). In other words, the concentration of a gas at a given point along an airway is related to its axial, or longitudinal, velocity and its radial, or lateral, diffusion. This phenomenon relies on turbulent flow and couples convection and molecular diffusion of gases, thereby increasing ventilatory efficiency.

Molecular diffusion of gas down a concentration gradient is the dominant mechanism of gas exchange across the alveolar–capillary membrane. This diffusion plays a major role in gas exchange during conventional mechanical ventilation and should be similar during HFOV. Finally, cardiac impulses may be transmitted to the surrounding lung tissue, probably contributing to gas mixing, although probably not to a large degree.

Although all six of these mechanisms of gas exchange collectively account for alveolar ventilation during HFOV, the precise quantitative contributions of each are unknown. Moreover, for a given set of physical conditions, the relative contributions of each of these mechanisms may vary from one lung region to the next (see Fig. 6.8.23). Despite unknown issues associated with this complex physiology, it is clear from years of clinical experience that HFOV removes CO_2 both efficaciously and efficiently.

RECOMMENDED READINGS

1. Nilsestuen JO, Hargett KD. Using ventilator graphics to identify patient-ventilator asynchrony. *Respir Care.* 2005;50(2):202–234.
2. Chao DC, Scheinhorn DJ, Stearn-Hassenpflug M. Patient-ventilator asynchrony in prolonged mechanical ventilation. *Chest.* 1997;112(6):1592–1599.
3. Tsuno K, Prato P, Kolobow T. Acute lung injury from mechanical ventilation at moderately high airway pressures. *J Appl Physiol.* 1990;69(3):956–961.
4. Dreyfuss D, Soler P, Saumon G. Spontaneous resolution of pulmonary edema caused by short periods of cyclic overinflation. *J Appl Physiol.* 1992;72(6):2081–2089.
5. Carlton DP, Cummings JJ, Scheerer RG, et al. Lung overexpansion increases pulmonary microvascular protein permeability in young lambs. *J Appl Physiol.* 1990;69(2):577–583.
6. Kolobow T, Moretti MP, Fumagalli R, et al. Severe impairment in lung function induced by high peak airway pressure during mechanical ventilation: An experimental study. *Am Rev Respir Dis.* 1987;135(2):312–315.
7. Borelli M, Kolobow T, Spatola R, et al. Severe acute respiratory failure managed with continuous positive airway pressure and partial extracorporeal carbon dioxide removal by an artificial membrane lung: A controlled, randomized animal study. *Am Rev Respir Dis.* 1988;138(6):1480–1487.
8. Marks JD, Luce JM, Lazar NM, et al. Effect of increases in lung volume on clearance of aerosolized solute from human lungs. *J Appl Physiol.* 1985;59(4):1242–1248.
9. Nolop KB, Maxwell DL, Royston D, et al. Effect of raised thoracic pressure and volume on 99mTc-DTPA clearance in humans. *J Appl Physiol.* 1986;60(5):1493–1497.
10. Dreyfuss D, Soler P, Basset G, et al. High inflation pressure pulmonary edema: Respective effects of high airway pressure, high tidal volume, and positive end-expiratory pressure. *Am Rev Respir Dis.* 1988;137(5):1159–1164.
11. Hernandez LA, Peevy KJ, Moise AA, et al. Chest wall restriction limits high airway pressure-induced lung injury in young rabbits. *J Appl Physiol.* 1989;66(5):2364–2368.
12. Dreyfuss D, Basset G, Soler P, et al. Intermittent positive-pressure hyperventilation with high inflation pressures produces pulmonary microvascular injury in rats. *Am Rev Respir Dis.* 1985;132(4):880–884.
13. Parker JC, Townsley MI, Rippe B, et al. Increased microvascular permeability in dog lungs due to high peak airway pressures. *J Appl Physiol.* 1984;57(6):1809–1816.
14. Parker JC, Hernandez LA, Longenecker GL, et al. Lung edema caused by high peak inspiratory pressures in dogs: Role of increased microvascular filtration pressure and permeability. *Am Rev Respir Dis.* 1990;142(2):321–328.
15. Fu Z, Costello ML, Tsukimoto K, et al. High lung volume increases stress failure in pulmonary capillaries. *J Appl Physiol.* 1992;73(1):123–133.

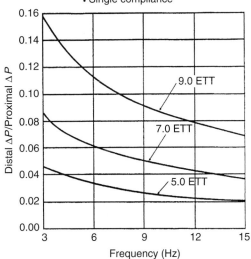

Figure 6.8.23 Pressure attenuation during high-frequency oscillatory ventilation, as reflected by the ratio of distal ΔP to proximal ΔP, demonstrating the effect of changing frequency and endotracheal tube diameter on pressure attenuation. ETT, endotracheal tube. (Copyright, SensorMedics Corporation, Yorba Linda, CA; 1998.)

16. West JB, Mathieu-Castello O. Stress failure of pulmonary capillaries: Role in lung and heart disease. *Lancet.* 1992;340(8822): 762–767.

17. Glazier JB, Hughes JMB, Maloney JE, et al. Measurements of capillary dimensions and blood volume in rapidly frozen lungs. *J Appl Physiol.* 1969;26(1):65–76.

18. Greenfiled IJ, Ebert PA, Benson DW, et al. Effect of positive pressure ventilation on surface tension properties of lung extracts. *Anesthesiology.* 1964;25:313–317.

19. Faridy EE, Permutt S, Riley RL. Effect of ventilation on surface forces in excised dogs' lungs. *J Appl Physiol.* 1966;21(5):1453–1462.

20. Wyszogrodski I, Kyei-Aboagye KK, Taeusch HW Jr, et al. Surfactant inactivation by hyperventilation: Conversation by end-expiratory pressure. *J Appl Physiol.* 1975;38(3):461–466.

21. Albert RK, Lakshminarayan S, Hildebrandt J, et al. Increased surfaces tension favors pulmonary edema formation in anesthetized dogs' lungs. *J Clin Invest.* 1978;63(5):1015–1018.

22. Bowtown DL, Kong DL. High tidal volume ventilation produces increased lung water in oleic acid-injured rabbit lungs. *Crit Care Med.* 1989;17(9):908–911.

23. Hernandez LA, Coker PJ, May S, et al. Mechanical ventilation increases microvascular permeability in oleic acid-injured lungs. *J Appl Physiol.* 1990;69(6):2057–2061.

24. Marchak BE, Thompson WK, Duffty P, et al. Treatment of RDS by high-frequency oscillatory ventilation: A preliminary report. *J Pediatr.* Aug 1981;99(2):287–292.

25. Butler WJ, Bohn DJ, Bryan AC. Ventilation by high-frequency oscillation in humans. *Anesth Analg.* 1980;59(8):577–584.

26. Amato MB, Barbas CS, Mederios DM. Beneficial effects of the "open lung approach" with low distending pressures in acute respiratory distress syndrome. A prospective randomized study on mechanical ventilation. *Am J Respir Crit Care Med.* 1995;152(6 Pt 1):1835–1846.

27. Amato MB, Barbas CS, Mederios DM, Carvalho CR. Effect of a protective-ventilation strategy on mortality in the acute respiratory distress syndrome. *N Engl J Med.* 1998;338(6):347–354.

28. Dreyfuss D, Saumon G. Ventilator-induced lung injury: Lessons from experimental studies. *Am J Respir Crit Care Med.* 1998; 157(1):294–323.

29. Tremblay LN, Slutsky AS. Ventilator-induced injury: From barotrauma to biotrauma. *Proc Assoc Am Physicians.* 1998;110(6): 482–488.

30. Ranieri VM, Suter PM, Tortorella C. Effect of mechanical ventilation on inflammatory mediators in patients with acute respiratory distress syndrome: A randomized controlled trial. *JAMA.* 1999;282(1):54–61.

31. Ricard JD, Dreyfuss D, Saumon G. Ventilator-induced lung injury. *Curr Opin Crit Care.* 2002;8(1):12–20.

32. Ferguson ND, Stewart TE. The use of high-frequency oscillatory ventilation in adults with acute lung injury. *Respir Care Clin N Am.* 2001;7(4):647–661.

33. Ventilation with lower tidal volumes as compared with traditional tidal volumes for acute lung injury and the acute respiratory distress syndrome. The Acute Respiratory Distress Syndrome Network. *N Engl J Med.* 2000;342(18):1301–1308.

34. Gerstmann DR, Fouke JM, Winter DC. Proximal, tracheal, and alveolar pressures during high-frequency oscillatory ventilation in a normal rabbit model. *Pediatr Res.* 1990;28(4):367–373.

35. Chang HK. Mechanisms of gas transport during ventilation by high-frequency oscillation. *J Appl Physiol.* 1984;56(3):553–563.

36. Priebe GP, Arnold JH. High-frequency oscillatory ventilation in pediatric patients. *Respir Care Clin N Am.* 2001;7(4):633–645.

37. Ferguson ND, Stewart TE. New therapies for adults with acute lung injury. High-frequency oscillatory ventilation. *Crit Care Clin.* 2002;18(1):91–106.

38. Ventre KM, Arnold JH. High frequency oscillatory ventilation in acute respiratory failure. *Paediatr Respir Rev.* 2004;5(4):323–332.

39. Brusasco V, Knopp TJ, Rehder K. Gas transport during high-frequency ventilation. *J Appl Physiol.* 1983;55(2):472–478.

40. Gattinoni L, Caironi P, Pelosi P What has computed tomography taught us about the acute respiratory distress syndrome? *Am J Respir Crit Care Med.* 2001;164(9):1701–1711.

41. Derdak S, Mehta S, Stewart TE. High-frequency oscillatory ventilation for acute respiratory distress syndrome in adults: A randomized, controlled trial. *Am J Respir Crit Care Med.* 2002; 166(7):801–808.

42. Fredberg JJ. Augmented diffusion in the airways can support pulmonary gas exchange. *J Appl Physiol.* 1980;49(2):232–238.

43. Slutsky AS, Drazen FM, Ingram RH Jr. Effective pulmonary ventilation with small-volume oscillations at high frequency. *Science.* 1980;209(4456):609–671.

44. Slutsky AS, Brown R. Cardiogenic oscillations: A potential mechanism enhancing oxygenation during apneic respiration. *Med Hypotheses.* 1982;8(4):393–400.

45. Derdak S. High-frequency oscillatory ventilation for acute respiratory distress syndrome in adult patients. *Crit Care Med.* 2003; 31(4 Suppl):S317–S323.

Cardiorespiratory Interactions

Cindy Sutton Barrett   Ira M. Cheifetz

The heart and lungs are anatomically and functionally interdependent. Their primary function is to provide oxygen to fuel aerobic cellular respiration. When considering the hemodynamic effects of any mode of ventilation, it is essential to consider the heart and lungs as an integral cardiopulmonary unit rather than two separate systems.[1] The relationship of the heart to the thoracic chamber has been described as a "pressure chamber within a pressure chamber." This illustration helps in understanding how changes in lung volume play an important role in altering cardiac function.

Changes in respiration, whether spontaneous or mechanical, can produce significant alterations in cardiac output and, consequently, can impact hemodynamics. Four key factors affecting cardiac function are preload, afterload, contractility, and heart rate. Positive pressure ventilation (PPV) and spontaneous respiration differ markedly, and oppositely, in their effect on intrathoracic pressure (ITP). It is the role of the pediatric intensivist to understand these interactions to minimize any associated deleterious side effects and to utilize the potential benefits for patient care.

RIGHT HEART INTERACTIONS

Preload

Venous return to the right atrium (RA) flows through the superior vena cava, inferior vena cava, and coronary sinusoids. Venous return to the RA is passive and is greatest when RA pressure is zero. Decreasing the RA pressure below zero does not further increase blood return to the atrium because of the highly compliant thoracic vasculature and the resulting venous collapse.[1]

In the absence of a left-to-right shunt, cardiac output is equivalent to the systemic venous return. For a given preload, the right heart filling is influenced by the pressure gradient between the systemic venous system and the RA.[1] Clinically, the volume of venous return to the RA (right ventricular [RV] preload) is inversely proportional to right ventricular end-diastolic pressure (RV EDP) (see Fig. 6.9.1).

During spontaneous inspiration, ITP decreases, such that right atrial pressure (P_{ra}) is lower than central venous pressure (CVP), leading to increased forward blood flow into the atrium. This increase in venous return to the RA is an important mechanism in the maintenance of maximum venous return under resting conditions and during exercise.[2]

ITP differs significantly during PPV as compared to spontaneous ventilation. During conventional mechanical ventilation, air enters the lungs through positive pressure rather than the negative pressure of spontaneous breathing. Changes in right heart function during PPV are secondary to the direct (i.e., cardiac compression) and indirect (i.e., decreased cardiac filling) effects of increased ITP on the heart.

During positive pressure inspiration, an increase in lung volume tends to parallel an increase in mean airway pressure (P_{aw}). As the lung expands, it applies pressure on the surrounding structures, distorting them and causing their surface pressures to increase.[3] Therefore, increased ITP acts directly on the heart by compressing the pericardium and decreasing the cardiac compliance. The direct effects of ITP on cardiac function are usually minimal as compared to the indirect effects.

Increased ITP acts indirectly on cardiac function through its effects on RA filling. Inspiration during PPV results in an increased ITP, which is transmitted to the RA. This, in turn, decreases the gradient between the P_{ra} and the mean CVP. The end result is decreased RA filling and, therefore, decreased RV preload. According to the Frank-Starling mechanism, decreased end-diastolic volume leads to decreased cardiac output. The most significant factor in

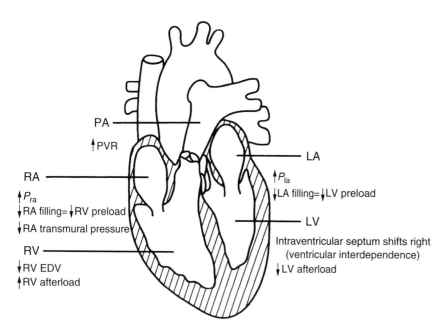

Figure 6.9.1 Relationship between intrathoracic pressure (ITP) and right atrial (RA) pressure. As ITP decreases, blood flow to the RA increases until ITP is zero or less. At this point, the compliant intrathoracic vessels collapse. If ITP is increased, as with PPV, blood flow to the RA decreases because of decreased systemic venous return. PA, pulmonary artery; PVR, pulmonary vascular resistance; LA, left atrium; P_{ra}, right atrial pressure; P_{la}, left atrial pressure; RV, right ventricle; LV, left ventricle; RV EDV, right ventricular end-diastolic volume.

depressed cardiac output associated with PPV is a decrease in systemic venous return.[4,5]

Consequently, a patient's volume status can significantly influence the hemodynamic response to increased ITP. In patients who are hypovolemic, the decrease in cardiac output secondary to decreased RV preload will be more dramatic. Increasing a patient's volume status to normovolemia can prevent or lessen the decrease in cardiac output that is seen while transitioning a patient to PPV.[6]

RV filling is determined by the difference between right atrial pressure and pericardial pressure (P_{pc}), known as *RA transmural pressure* (P_{tmRA}). Applied positive end-expiratory pressure (PEEP) that increases P_{pc} causes a reduction in P_{tmRA} and a subsequent decrease in RV preload and, therefore, RV output.[7]

Right Ventricular Afterload

The right ventricle, in a normal heart, acts as a low-pressure pump. The Laplace equation states that pressure (P) is directly proportional to the tension of the wall (T) and inversely proportional to the radius (r) of the curvature:

$$P = 2 \times \frac{T}{r}$$

RV afterload can be defined as the maximum RV systolic wall stress (i.e., tension in the Laplace equation). Therefore, using the Laplace equation, RV afterload (T) is equal to one-half the product of the radius (r) of the curvature of the right ventricle and the transmural pressure (P).[8]

Lung Volumes and Pulmonary Vascular Resistance

Functional residual capacity (FRC) is the lung volume from which normal tidal volume breathing occurs. When lung volumes are less than or greater than FRC, the pulmonary vascular resistance (PVR) increases.

The vasculature of the lung can be separated into two groups, intra-alveolar and extra-alveolar, depending on the tissue that surrounds them and the pressure that affects them. If the lung volume is less than FRC, hypoxia induces pulmonary vasoconstriction of the intra-alveolar vasculature and atelectasis distorts the extra-alveolar vessels, causing them to become more tortuous. Therefore, a reduction in lung volume increases PVR while decreasing pulmonary blood flow. Conversely, when the lung is distended beyond FRC, intra-alveolar vessels become compressed between the interstitial lung compartment and the alveolar wall. As lung distension continues to increase, extra-alveolar vessels also become compressed. Therefore, excessive lung inflation also limits capillary blood flow by increasing PVR.[9]

Additionally, increased lung volume, as occurs with PPV, can lead to increased pulmonary artery pressure (P_{pa}). Because P_{pa} is essentially systolic RV pressure, as the transmural P_{pa} is increased, RV ejection is impeded. Two factors can cause an increase in P_{pa}: (i) an increase in PVR without an increase in vascular tone, as occurs with a marked increase in pulmonary blood flow, or a passive increase in outflow pressure and (ii) an increase in PVR by either active changes in vasomotor tone or passive lung inflation.[3] Therefore, during PPV, RV afterload is often increased.

PEEP during PPV can significantly affect FRC and ITP. PEEP has several beneficial uses, which include recruiting atelectatic regions of the lung, increasing end-expiratory lung volume, improving ventilation–perfusion matching, and reducing right-to-left intrapulmonary shunting.[10] "High" levels of PEEP may result in overexpansion of normal lung units, reduced compliance, increased PVR,

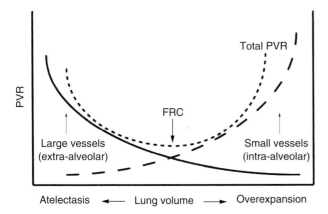

Figure 6.9.2 Illustration of the relationship between pulmonary vascular resistance (PVR) and functional residual capacity (FRC). Optimum PVR occurs at FRC. If lung volume is increased above FRC, leading to lung overexpansion, intra-alveolar vessels are compressed and PVR is increased. If the lung volume is less than FRC, hypoxia induces pulmonary vasoconstriction of the intra-alveolar vasculature, and atelectasis distorts the extra-alveolar vessels, causing them to become more tortuous. Therefore, a reduction in lung volume also increases PVR.

increased dead space ventilation, and ventilation–perfusion mismatch because of shunting of blood away from normal, yet overexpanded, alveoli to abnormal alveoli.[5,10] The amount of PEEP required to overdistend the lung is directly related to the pulmonary compliance of the individual patient (see Fig. 6.9.2).

Right Ventricular Coronary Blood Flow

Two primary factors affect coronary blood flow and, therefore, myocardial oxygen delivery: coronary artery perfusion pressure and coronary artery resistance. Myocardial oxygen delivery is a major determinant of ventricular contractility. In a normal RV, coronary blood flow occurs during both systole and diastole. However, coronary flow predominates during systole because the difference between RV systolic and aortic systolic pressures is greater than the difference between RV diastolic and aortic diastolic pressures. Therefore, the difference between aortic and RV systolic pressures primarily determines the driving pressure of coronary blood flow to the right ventricle. As ITP increases with inspiration during PPV, the P_{pa} (i.e., RV pressure) may increase. Subsequently, the systolic pressure gradient between the aorta and the right ventricle is decreased, potentially resulting in a reduction in coronary blood flow.

Myocardial perfusion pressure and, therefore, myocardial blood flow depends on ITP, aortic pressure, and RV pressure. Increases in ITP or decreases in aortic pressure will cause a decrease in myocardial blood flow, which may or may not be clinically significant. In most patients, the systolic pressure of the aorta is significantly higher than that of the RV, pulmonary artery, and ITP. Therefore, in

most patients, PPV will not adversely affect RV coronary blood flow. However, if a patient has RV dysfunction, low aortic pressure, and/or significantly increased ITP, myocardial blood flow to the RV may be severely jeopardized with resultant RV dysfunction/failure.

VENTRICULAR COMPLIANCE

While considering heart–lung interactions, pulmonary, vascular, and ventricular compliance are significant. Compliance is defined as the change in volume divided by the change in pressure. Therefore, a compartment's steady state vascular volume is related to its compliance and to the difference between inflow and outflow pressure. In understanding ventricular chamber compliance, it is easiest to start with a constant inflow pressure. Ventricular compliance, with a constant inflow pressure, may be decreased by intrinsic stiffening of the chamber walls or extrinsic compression due to the pericardial sac and/or increased lung volumes.

When one ventricle is distended, the intraventricular septum is pushed toward the other ventricle. Because the heart is surrounded by the pericardium, a fixed space, an increase in the volume of one ventricular compartment leads to a decreased compliance of the other ventricle. This concept is referred to as *ventricular interdependence*. The extreme case of this physiology is seen in cardiac tamponade—a decrease in systolic arterial pressure during inspiration, with a narrowing of the pulse pressure.

LEFT HEART INTERACTIONS

Left Ventricular Preload: Pulmonary Venous Return

Pulmonary venous return to the left atrium is analogous to systemic venous return to the RA in that the left atrial pressure affects the volume of blood return. Pulmonary venous return is also affected by changes in the mean airway pressure (P_{aw}) and lung volume.[7] Physiologic variables that affect pulmonary venous return during ventilation include RV output, lung volume, pulmonary arterial pressure, pulmonary venous (i.e., left atrial) pressure, and ventricular interdependence.

Diastolic modification of left ventricle (LV) preload during ventilation may be influenced by ventricular interdependence, pericardial constraint, heart–lung mechanical interactions, and LV contractility. According to the Frank-Starling mechanism, increases in left ventricular enddiastolic volume (LV EDV) should increase cardiac output. LV EDV may be altered by varying either systemic venous return or LV diastolic filling. During spontaneous ventilation, RV filling is transiently increased.[3] This increase in volume consequently increases blood volume in the pulmonary vasculature and blood return to the left heart. However, large increases in RV distension, or a restrictive pericardial sac, can decrease left ventricular filling because of septal shift to the left (ventricular interdependence).

Therefore, PPV can positively or negatively affect LV function, depending upon the clinical scenario. Negative interactions occur when PPV decreases blood flow to the LV by impeding systemic vascular return to the RA; decreasing RV preload; and, therefore, decreasing LV preload. Direct compression to the LV from increased ITP may further decrease LV preload. Conversely, PPV may be beneficial to the LV by decreasing right ventricular end-diastolic volume and, thereby, by allowing the LV to be more compliant through ventricular interdependence.

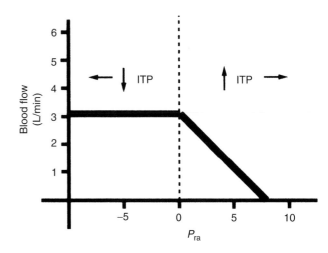

Figure 6.9.3 Summary of changes in cardiac function secondary to increased intrathoracic pressure (ITP). P_{ra}, right arterial pressure.

Left Ventricular Afterload

Left ventricular afterload can be equated with systolic wall tension. Using the Laplace equation, systolic wall tension is found to be equal to one-half the product of the radius of the curvature of the LV and the LV transmural pressure (P_{tmLV}). Left ventricular ejection pressure represents transmural pressure during systole. LV transmural wall pressure generated by the ventricle during systole can be approximated by examining the difference between LV systolic pressure and ITP ($P_{tmLV} = P_{LV} -$ ITP). P_{tmLV} and, therefore, left ventricular ejection pressure can be reduced by either decreasing aortic pressure or increasing ITP. Therefore, PPV decreases LV afterload and increases left ventricular output. In contrast, PPV can adversely affect LV performance secondary to a decrease in systemic venous return, as previously discussed. Therefore, the hemodynamic status of the patient must be monitored closely because the effects of PPV on LV function can be variable.

Changes in LV function because of PPV may not be dramatic in patients with normal left ventricular function. However, the failing LV is acutely sensitive to changes in afterload. Therefore, attempting to wean patients with LV failure from PPV to spontaneous respiration can increase LV afterload, resulting in a clinically significant decrease in cardiac output. Weaning a patient with LV failure from PPV is akin to a cardiac stress test.[11] Alternatively, initiating PPV in a patient with LV dysfunction/failure can greatly augment cardiac output.

Left Ventricular Coronary Blood Flow

As the LV systolic pressure is similar to the aortic systolic pressure, coronary resistance is high during systole. Therefore, most LV coronary blood flow must occur during diastole. With the rapid decrease in ventricular wall stress during diastole, the myocardial blood flow increases. Any process that significantly increases LV EDP or reduces systemic diastolic pressure would reduce coronary perfusion

pressure and may adversely affect LV function. Additionally, any condition that significantly decreases diastolic filling time (e.g., extreme tachycardia) could decrease LV myocardial blood flow.

CONCLUSION

Spontaneous ventilation and PPV have profound effects on cardiac function. This chapter has provided an overview of the intricate relationship between the respiratory and cardiac systems (see Fig. 6.9.3). The cardiorespiratory effects from spontaneous breathing and positive pressure breathing in an individual patient require consideration of the underlying pathophysiology and close hemodynamic monitoring.

REFERENCES

1. Shekerdemian LS, Bush A, Lincoln C, et al. Cardiopulmonary interactions in healthy children and children after simple cardiac surgery: The effects of positive and negative pressure ventilation. *Heart.* 1997;78:587–593.
2. Naughton MT, Rahman MA, Hara K, et al. Effect of continuous positive airway pressure on intrathoracic and left ventricular transmural pressures in patients with congestive heart failure. *Circulation.* 1991;5:1725–1731.
3. Pinsky MR. The hemodynamic consequences of mechanical ventilation: An evolving story. *Intensive Care Med.* 1997;23:493–503.
4. Pinsky MR. Determinants of pulmonary arterial flow variation during respiration. *J Appl Physiol.* 1984;56:1237–1245.
5. Schuster S, Erbel R, Ludwig SW, et al. Hemodynamics during PEEP ventilation in patients with severe left ventricular failure studied by transesophageal echocardiography. *Chest.* 1990;97:1181–1189.
6. Biondi JW, Schulman DS, Soufer R, et al. The effect of incremental positive end-expiratory pressure on right ventricular hemodynamics and ejection fraction. *Anesth Analg.* 1988;67:144–151.
7. Klinger JR. Monitoring cardiac function and tissue perfusion: Hemodynamics and positive end-expiratory pressure in critically ill patients. *Crit Care Clin.* 1996;12:841–864.

8. Sibbald WJ, Driedger AA. Right ventricular function in disease states: Pathophysiologic considerations. *Crit Care Med.* 1983;11:339–345.

9. Cheifetz IM, Craig DM, Quick G, et al. Increasing tidal volumes and pulmonary overdistention adversely affect pulmonary vascular mechanics and cardiac output in a pediatric swine model. *Crit Care Med.* 1998;26:710–716.

10. Tyler DC. Positive end-expiratory pressure: A review. *Crit Care Med.* 1983;11:300–308.

11. Pinsky MR, Matuschak GM, Klain M. Determinants of cardiac augmentation by elevations in intrathoracic pressure. *J Appl Physiol.* 1985;58:1189–1198.

Acute Lung Injury

Ronald C. Sanders Jr.   *K. Alex Daneshmand*

Acute lung injury (ALI) is a sudden change in the alveolar wall integrity associated with diminished gas exchange and an increased work of breathing. The severity of ALI ranges from molecular alterations without clinical manifestations to the markedly abnormal gas exchange properties and increased pulmonary hypertension of acute respiratory distress syndrome (ARDS). Differentiating the self-limited forms of ALI from those with increased morbidity and mortality has been unsuccessful. Pathologic findings in ALI can be divided into three stages on the basis of light microscopic findings: the acute stage, early proliferative stage, and the remodeled stage.

ACUTE OR EXUDATIVE PHASE

The acute or exudative phase of lung injury begins with arterial hypoxemia and a need for supplemental oxygen. It is characterized by alveolar edema, hyaline membrane formation, alveolar epithelial and endothelial cell damage, and a denuded epithelial basement membrane (see Fig. 6.10.1). In addition, the hyaline membrane contains fibrin and cellular debris and macromolecules such as IgG, fibrinogen, and fibronectin. Collagen is present in the interstitium, with the quantity of collagen type III exceeding that of collagen type I, early in lung injury, with a reversal occurring later in the course. Pneumothorax is an infrequent event early in ARDS and does not appear to be related to airway pressures. However, pneumothorax does occur late in ARDS during remodeling, when marked regional differences in compliance occur. Alveolar capillaries contain fibrin microthrombi, platelet, and neutrophil infiltration. These events may result in intravascular coagulation and endothelial damage, which leads to pulmonary hypertension and right ventricular failure. Furthermore, the combined damage to the alveolar epithelium and pulmonary endothelium interferes with effective solute, water, and gas exchange.

The host's response to lung injury is complex and mediated by a number of mechanisms that are more fully described in the section on Acute Inflammatory Phase. The extracellular matrix is a source of important information for cellular responses to injury. Communication with the extracellular environment occurs mainly with the integrin family of adhesion receptors. For example, fibroblasts migrate into sites of injury by organizing newly formed extracellular matrix and by assembling secreted matrix proteins in response to signals from the extracellular matrix.

Integrins are the largest and best-characterized family of receptors that can be used to detect changes in the extracellular milieu. The proteins known to be ligands for integrins, including basement membrane components, fibronectin, and tenascin-C among others, are plentiful in the airway lumen in association with tissue injury.

ACUTE INFLAMMATORY PHASE

Inflammation is a significant component of the acute phase of lung injury. Inflammation in the lung triggers cell-to-cell contact and the release of cytokines. Proinflammatory cytokines, namely *interleukin-1* (IL-1) and tumor necrosis factor-α (TNF-α), are released early from macrophages and lymphocytes. These mediators have several effects on endothelial cells including expression of adhesion molecules on leukocytes, production of IL-8, release of plasminogen-activator inhibitor, and activation of neutrophils for phagocytosis (see Chapter 3.2). In a lipopolysaccharide (LPS) lung injury model, IL-1 and TNF-α are released along with a neutrophilic cellular response that peaks in 6 to 12 hours. This is followed by a monocytic predominance at 24 hours and a lymphocytic infiltration at 48 hours.

The inflammatory process starts with the activation of cytokines, specifically TNF-α, IL-1, IL-6, and IL-8. These mediators are produced by alveolar macrophages,

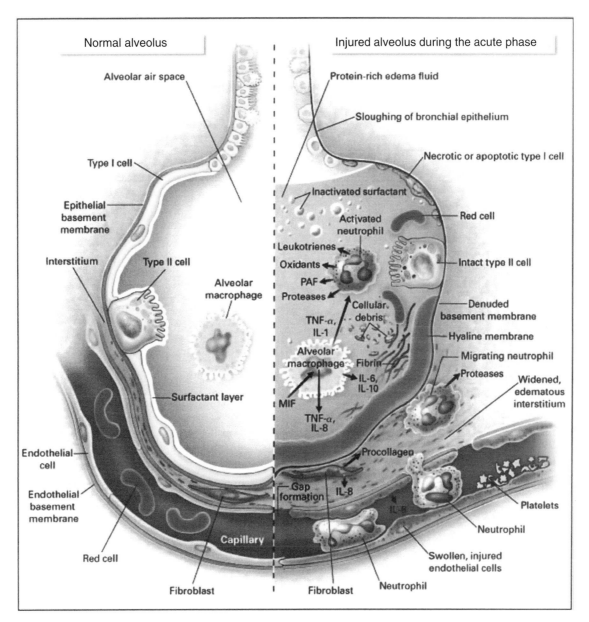

Figure 6.10.1 The normal alveolus **(left)** and the injured alveolus in the acute phase of acute lung injury and the acute respiratory distress syndrome **(right)**. In the acute phase of the syndrome **(right)**, there is sloughing of epithelial cells, with the formation of protein-rich hyaline membranes on the denuded basement membrane. Neutrophils are shown adhering to the injured capillary endothelium and marginating through the interstitium into the air space, which is filled with protein-rich edema fluid. In the air space, an alveolar macrophage is secreting cytokines. Neutrophils can release oxidants, proteases, leukotrienes, and other proinflammatory molecules. The influx of protein-rich edema fluid into the alveolus has led to the inactivation of surfactant. PAF, platelet-activating factor; TNF, tumor necrosis factor; IL, interleukin; MIF, macrophage inhibitory factor. (With permission from, Ware LB, Matthay MA. The acute respiratory distress syndrome. *N Engl J Med.* 2000;342(18):1334–1349. Copyright © 2000 Massachusetts Medical Society.) (See color Figure 6.10.1.)

fibroblasts, type II pneumocytes, and endothelial cells. A major distinguishing feature between pneumonia and ARDS is the robust endothelial activation that occurs with ARDS. Endothelial activation is not homeostatic but instead becomes deregulated during ARDS. This deregulated activation promotes the amplification of other proinflammatory responses, such as the production of nitric oxide and activation of platelet-activating factor (PAF) (see Chapter 3.2). In addition, activation of local coagulation causes tissue factor to be produced, which can inhibit fibrinolysis. This procoagulant environment results in excessive fibrin deposition.

Leukocyte Recruitment

Leukocytes are summoned by the signals delivered by other leukocytes, parenchymal cells, and endothelial cells. These include cytokines, cellular and extracellular adhesion molecules, and chemokines. Specific receptors for chemokines operate through GTP-binding proteins of the G_i subtype. In the early stages of ALI, epithelial cells express CXC chemokines in response to IL-1 and TNF-α. In turn, IL-1 and TNF-α can act further in either an autocrine or a paracrine manner to propagate further CXC chemokine release.

Microvascular endothelium activation occurs immediately in ALI and is similar to inflammation in other parts of the body. Consequently, the endothelium expresses E selectin, P selectin, and intercellular adhesion molecule-1 (ICAM-1). Neutrophils express L selectin, which facilitates attachment and subsequent "rolling" on endothelial cells. CXC chemokines activate neutrophils and downregulate L selectin expression while simultaneously up-regulating β_2-integrins. Neutrophil β_2-integrin anchors to ICAM-1 on the endothelium. Diapedesis is mediated through a CXC chemokine–driven chemotactic gradient.

Clinically, bronchoalveolar lavage (BAL) levels of IL-8 have been correlated with the development and increased mortality of ARDS. In cultured human endothelial cells, hypoxia has been shown to lead to increased IL-8 production. In addition, human monocytes subjected to hypoxia/hyperoxia (ischemia–reperfusion model) produce increased levels of IL-8.

CELLULAR INJURY AND THE EXTRACELLULAR MATRIX

Fibroproliferative Stage

Many patients recover shortly after the acute phase of lung injury, but a subset will progress with worsening lung compliance, increased dead space ventilation, and an escalated ventilatory support. The evidence for the progression of lung injury arises from both animal models and detailed autopsy examinations of patients dying after ALI and ARDS. Fibrosing alveolitis is a distinct pathologic state that occurs as early as 48 hours to 7 days after initial lung injury. The accumulation of mesenchymal cells, their extracellular products, and myofibroblasts contribute to fibrosis within the alveolar and pulmonary interstitium, the so-called acute fibroproliferative response.

Mesenchymal cell replication is controlled by growth factors released by both alveolar macrophages and mesenchymal cells themselves. The growth factors of importance are platelet-derived growth factor (PDGF), fibronectin, epidermal growth factor (EGF), and transforming growth factorα (TGFα), which facilitate the recruitment of mesenchymal cells.

The proliferative phase starts 1 to 2 weeks after the original insult. Alveolar macrophages phagocytose the hyaline membranes and cellular debris. Alveolar type II cell proliferation and fibroproliferation are important steps in the lung's attempt at repair. The fibrotic response is stimulated by mediators such as TNF-α and IL-1, which cause local fibroblasts to migrate, replicate, and produce excessive connective tissue. The fibrosis tends to localize to both the interstitial area and the intra-alveolar space.

Fibrogenesis

In extreme cases of lung injury, effective repair is supplanted by abnormal wound healing with excessive fibrin deposition. This process, which begins several days after lung injury, leads to severe damage of the pulmonary infrastructure and a "honeycomb" lung is seen on x-ray. Irreversible damage is certain, and mortality is increased in this condition. Fibrosis begins as early as 48 hours to 7 days. Precursors of fibrosis, such as procollagen III peptide, are found early during the course of the injury in the BAL fluid of patients with ALI, with higher concentrations of these peptides correlating with mortality.

The principal cell involved in fibrogenesis is the myofibroblast, which is a fibroblastlike cell that contains a contractile apparatus commonly found in muscle cells. Evidence suggests that peribronchial and perivascular adventitial fibroblasts are the progenitors of myofibroblasts after cytokines activation. Myofibroblasts participate in the formation of the collagen meshwork, particularly through type I collagen gene expression. This results in scar formation and the creation of an extracellular matrix. Physiologically, excessive scar tissue results in restrictive pulmonary mechanics and function.

Mediators—Fibrosis

TGFβ1 is one of the best-studied mediators implicated in the fibrotic response. It is a peptide produced by alveolar macrophages and other cells, which regulates the growth and differentiation of many tissues, including those involved in matrix production, and may regulate apoptosis. In the lung, TGFβ1 regulates branching morphogenesis, the accumulation of extracellular matrix, and the generation of tissue fibrosis. Fibrogenesis is the result of direct activation of target gene transcription, including collagens, fibronectin, and plasminogen-activator inhibitor-1, by TGFβ1. The observation of myofibroblasts traversing gaps in the epithelial basement membrane supports the concept of guided migration as an important aspect of healing after ALI. Several mediators such as fibronectin and TGFβ may provide a means of recruiting lung myofibroblasts to regions of injury, such as occurs early in the evolution of intra-alveolar fibrosis, where the alveolar airspaces and the surface of "hyaline membranes" contain abundant amounts of both TGFα and fibronectin.

The signals in the pulmonary microcirculation that initiate myofibroblast and primordial cell migration and replication remain undefined. However, PDGF and TGFβ are potent mediators that may play a role in the process of muscularization of the pulmonary vascular system after ALI. In addition, TGFβ stimulates endothelial PDGF production, providing a method by which the response to injury may be amplified by local growth factor synthesis. Furthermore, TGFβ can induce myofibroblasts to synthesize connective tissue proteins. Clinically, increased TGFα levels in BAL washings is associated with the fibroproliferative phase.

REMODELING STAGE

The resolution phase of ARDS has been least clearly documented. This phase is the continuation of the fibroproliferative phase. Typically, the resolution of the inflammatory phase triggers a cytokine cascade that facilitates cellular derecruitment, attenuation of proinflammatory mediators, decreased extracellular matrix production, and the disappearance of myofibroblasts by apoptosis (see Fig. 6.10.2). The persistence of the myofibroblast is the hallmark of pathologic pulmonary fibrosis. Unhalted

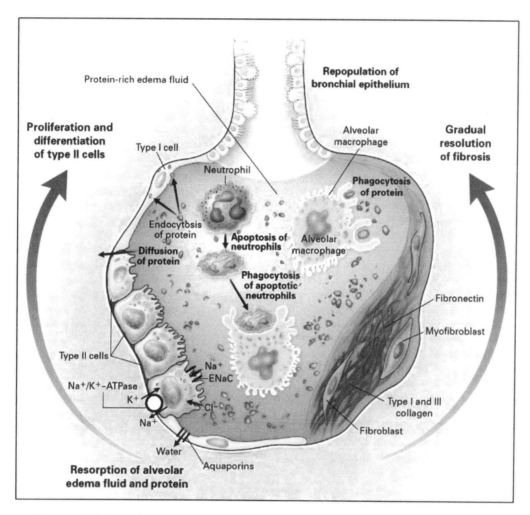

Figure 6.10.2 Mechanisms important in the resolution of acute lung injury and the acute respiratory distress syndrome. On the left side of the alveolus, the alveolar epithelium is being repopulated by the proliferation and differentiation of alveolar type II cells. Resorption of alveolar edema fluid is shown at the base of the alveolus, with sodium and chloride being transported through the apical membrane of type II cells. Sodium is taken up by the epithelial sodium channel (ENaC) and through the basolateral membrane of type II cells by the sodium pump (Na+/K+-ATPase). The relevant pathways for chloride transport are unclear. Water is shown moving through water channels, the aquaporins, located primarily on type I cells. Some water may also cross by a paracellular route. On the right side of the alveolus, the gradual remodeling and resolution of intraalveolar and interstitial granulation tissue and fibrosis are shown. ATPase, adenosine triphosphatase. (With permission from, Ware LB, Matthay MA. The acute respiratory distress syndrome. *N Engl J Med.* 2000;342(18):1334–1349. Copyright © 2000 Massachusetts Medical Society.) (See color Figure 6.10.2.)

fibroproliferation results in extensive fibrotic remodeling of the lung parenchyma. This phase of fibrocellular proliferation continues not only at the level of small arteries but also at the veins and lymphatics surrounding the alveolar structures. Specific vascular changes include arterial medical hypertrophy and intimal fibrosis with obliteration of the vascular bed. Long-term survivors of ARDS have been found to have decreased pulmonary capillary blood volumes, which may help explain the impairment in gas exchange noted in these patients during exercise.

TYPES OF LUNG INJURY

This section reviews some of the major insults to the lung and the responses that lead to repair and restoration of the body's original function. The body's response to different types of insults is similar regardless of the specific stimulus. These responses are mediated by a number of pathways that are highly integrated.

Hypoxia

Pulmonary system injury interferes with the ability of the body to participate in gas exchange, fight infection, clear debris, and detoxify certain substances. In humans, the lungs are principally involved in extracting oxygen and eliminating carbon dioxide. It is not surprising that hypoxemia is one of the hallmarks of lung injury. Acutely, hypoxia can result in pulmonary hypertension, especially at the level of the small muscular resistance arteries ($<300 \mu$m). In regions of the lung that are hypoxic, the vasoconstriction occurring in the pulmonary vessels directs blood away from these areas to minimize ventilation–perfusion mismatch and improve systemic oxygenation. Chronically, hypoxia results in the migration and proliferation of vascular smooth muscles and vascular remodeling, which is the deposition of extracellular matrix in the arterial wall.

Both the smooth muscle cell and the endothelium contribute to hypoxic pulmonary vasoconstriction. Hypoxia causes an inhibition of K^+ flux, resulting in membrane depolarization and a subsequent rise in intracellular Ca^{2+} by influx through Ca^{2+} voltage-gated channels. Smooth muscle contraction occurs, leading to enhanced vasomotor tone and increased pulmonary pressures. The endothelium releases mediators that facilitate vasoconstriction and vasodilation, thereby modulating vasomotor tone by increasing the sensitivity of the smooth muscle contractile apparatus to Ca^{2+}.

Endothelium-derived nitric oxide causes vasodilation in the pulmonary vascular bed and function to prevent pulmonary vasoconstriction. Hypoxia may inhibit the normal endothelial production of nitric oxide. However, the exact role of endothelial mediators, such as nitric oxide, in maintaining basal pulmonary vascular tone and in mediating the response to hypoxia is not yet clear. In the research setting, prostacyclin and 20-hydroxyeicosatetraenoic acid (20-HETE) attenuate pulmonary vasodilation, whereas endothelin-1 facilitates vasoconstriction. In alveolar cells, hypoxia enhances both nuclear factor-kappa β (NF$\kappa\beta$) and activator protein-1 (AP-1) translocation as well as monocyte chemoattractant protein-1 (MCP-1) expression are enhanced after hypoxia and subsequent reoxygenation, which may trigger the release of proinflammatory mediators.

Hypoxia also causes matrix metalloproteinase-2 (MMP-2) expression in human pulmonary fibroblasts, which are important in the establishment and support of the extracellular matrix. In addition, hypoxia is a potent stimulant of fibrosis.

Hypoxia-induced pulmonary hypertension and increased inflammatory cell infiltration in the lungs (neutrophils and macrophages) are both attenuated by heme oxygenase-1 (HO-1). HO catalyzes the oxidation of heme to carbon monoxide and biliverdin, with the release of chelated iron. Three isoforms of HO have been identified: the inducible HO-1 and the constitutively expressed HO-2 and HO-3.

Medications such as calcium channel blockers, vasodilators, β-agonists, and anesthetics may inhibit hypoxic vasoconstriction. In lung injury, the loss of hypoxic vasoconstriction may increase ventilation–perfusion abnormalities. Propanolol, dopamine, and almitrine (a ventilatory stimulant) can enhance pulmonary vasoconstriction. Acidosis also increases hypoxic vasoconstriction, whereas alkalosis decreases vasoconstriction.

Hyperoxia

Despite 30 years of research, hyperoxia is still not well understood. Many theories exist on how hyperoxia injures the lung. Basic science research indicates that hyperoxia induces a large influx of oxygen at the cellular level, which overwhelms the antioxidant systems in many pulmonary cell types including the alveolar type II cells. Pulmonary cells convert the large influx of oxygen to superoxide. Reactive oxygen species (ROS) are also formed under normal respiratory physiology. Most of the oxygen radicals, which include superoxide anion ($O_2^-\bullet$), hydrogen peroxide (H_2O_2), hydroxyl radical ($OH\bullet$) and peroxynitrite ($ONOO^-$), are normally degraded by the cytochrome oxidase system. When the balance between the body's defense system and these formed radicals is overcome, oxidative stress can cause damage to various cellular components and cell death. The exact mechanism of this type of cell death is still being debated. It is believed that ROS react with proteins, lipids, and nucleic acids to induce cellular and tissue damage. It is further thought that ROS effects cell death by two modes, either apoptosis or necrosis. Necrosis is unregulated cell death and is due to an acute injury. An example of necrosis is when the oxygen radicals react with the lipid component of cell membranes, causing lipid peroxidation, which results in an increased permeability to cell lysis. Another mode of cell death is apoptosis or programmed cell death. These cells are genetically regulated to die. Most of the cellular injury by ROS results in this form of cell death. Exposure of the lungs to high oxygen levels will gradually lead to increased muscularization of alveolar arterioles, as well as to decreased density of vessels.

Ischemia/Reperfusion

Ischemic-reperfusion injury (IRI) is often seen in lung transplantation. The pathophysiology of IRI involves the complement system, ROS, leukocytes, and the endothelium. IRI cascade starts at the time of surgery. The surgical stress and reperfusion to the ischemic organs begins at the time of transplantation. Proinflammatory mediators, including TNF-α, IL-1, and IL-6, up-regulate adhesion molecules found on the endothelium, which attract leukocytes, particularly neutrophils, to the site of injury. Activated neutrophils migrate through the endothelium, degranulate, and release proteolytic enzymes such as proteases, collagenases, and lipoxygenases. This inflammatory reaction disrupts the integrity of the endothelium and parenchymal tissue, leading to edema, thrombosis, and, ultimately, ischemia of the lung and cell death. When the blood flow to the ischemic graft is reestablished, cellular vitality is further compromised through the production of ROS (see section on "Hyperoxia"). Ischemia-reperfusion causes increased lung permeability, neutrophil accumulation, increased pulmonary levels of IL-1β and TNF-α. In addition, reactive nitrogen compounds, such as peroxynitrite, are known to mediate the deleterious effects of IRI (see section on "Acute Inflammatory Phase").

Drug Toxicity

Drug-associated lung injury in the pediatric intensive care unit (PICU) is a complex state to disentangle given the multiple drugs that most patients receive. More than 150 agents from a number of drug classes, including antimicrobials, anti-inflammatory agents, cancer chemotherapeutic agents, cardiovascular drugs, and recreational drugs can cause direct or indirect pulmonary reactions. Alveolar and bronchial epithelial cell injury from inhaled drugs constitutes a direct injury. These injuries may result from unregulated inflammation or oxidative damage. An indirect injury occurs when the response of another body system to a drug leads to pulmonary injury. For example, drug-induced thrombocytopenia can lead to pulmonary hemorrhage or drug-induced immunosuppression can lead to a pulmonary opportunistic infection. Several defense mechanisms exist to protect against ROS. These systems consist of enzymatic and nonenzymatic antioxidants. The enzymatic antioxidant systems include superoxide dismutase, catalase, and glutathione peroxidase. The nonenzymatic systems includes vitamins (A, E, and C), selenium, and other nutritional

molecules. Oxidative stress arises when nonscavenged oxygen radicals overwhelm these normal defense mechanisms. An example of a drug-associated oxidative stress in the lung is paraquat, a herbicide that creates oxygen radicals while simultaneously depleting nicotinamide adenine dinucleotide phosphate (NADP), which overwhelms the antioxidant defense system. Nitrofurantoin provides an example of how a drug can affect the lung indirectly. The indirect effects associated with nitrofurantoin include diffuse alveolar damage, granulomatous inflammation, and chronic interstitial pneumonia. These events may lead to fibrotic changes in the lungs and may ultimately interfere with gas exchange. A proposed mechanism for these indirect affects on gas exchange is through the long-term use of nitrofurantoin. Over time, these drugs can cause eosinophilia, proliferation of smooth muscle mass, or amyloid deposits in the alveolus and the alveolar–capillary membrane. Most of these observed mechanisms are due to chronic inflammation caused by the use of these drugs.

Some drugs may have both direct and indirect effects on the lung. Amiodarone and bleomycin cause an indirect hypersensitivity pneumonitis through T-cell–mediated mechanisms and lead to direct toxicity to the lung parenchymal cell. Both injuries result in fibrosis.

Transfusion-Related Acute Lung Injury

Transfusion-related acute lung injury (TRALI) is a concept initially described by Popovsky in 1983. It is defined as ALI caused by the transfusion of blood products. TRALI is commonly seen with the transfusion of blood products that contain plasma. This includes fresh-frozen plasma, platelets, whole blood, and packed red blood cells. Clinically, TRALI appears as an acute hypoxemic insult that causes bilateral pulmonary infiltrates, fever, and hypo- or hypertension. Symptoms associated with TRALI can develop within 30 minutes of the onset of transfusion. Resolution usually occurs within 96 hours. There are several hypotheses about the pathogenesis of TRALI. The "two-hit" hypothesis is the most accepted theory. The first "hit" is the underlying condition of the patient, whereas the second "hit" occurs with the injury caused by the blood products themselves.

The initial insult results in priming of neutrophils in response to injury related to generalized inflammation such as trauma, surgery, or sepsis. The second phase, which may be antibody-mediated, consists of the activation of those primed neutrophils and degranulation, with the subsequent release of preformed mediators and the formation of activated oxygen species. Capillary leak and pulmonary edema are end results of this cascade.

Donor antibodies are passively transferred with plasma-containing blood products at the time of transfusion. These antibodies may attach to the pulmonary endothelium and directly or indirectly activate neutrophils and monocytes, leading to increased pulmonary permeability and subsequent pulmonary edema. In addition, biologically active lipids found in transfused blood products may activate the host neutrophils.

Older blood products may contain higher concentrations of lipid breakdown products and place the patient at greater risk for lipid-induced injury. Lysophosphatidylcholine is an example of these lipid by-products. This compound primes neutrophils through the PAF receptors in in vitro studies. The mechanism of injury of TRALI may involve several pathways, which include antibody-mediated activation and activated lipid moieties.

PLEURAL RESPONSE TO INJURY

In healthy individuals, the pleural space is between 10 and 24 μm long and contains a small amount of fluid that facilitates movement of the lungs within the thoracic cage. It is enclosed by the visceral pleura, which covers the outer lung surface, and the parietal pleura, which lines the inner surface of the thorax. The parietal pleura, but not the visceral pleura, is important in pleural fluid absorption. The pleura's role in fluid removal has been discussed previously. The parietal pleura in the intercostal regions and at the periphery of the diaphragm is richly innervated with nerves originating from the intercostal nerves, making it sensitive to pain, which can be localized to the distribution of the overlying surface. In contrast, the parietal pleura near the central portion of the diaphragm and mediastinum is innervated by the phrenic nerve. Discomfort in these areas will be transmitted to the neck, shoulder, and armpit. The visceral pleura does not transmit pain. Therefore, an important point is that the presence of pleuritic chest pain always indicates a process affecting the parietal pleura. Pleuritic chest pain is classically characterized as a "pins and needles" sensation.

Both pleura are lined by a single layer of mesothelial cells that lie over a layer of connective tissue. The mesothelial cells are shaped differently, depending on the area evaluated. Microvilli and hyaluronic acid–rich glycoproteins cover the surface of the mesothelial cells. Mesothelial cells are metabolically active and respond quickly to insults within the pleura. Normally, mesothelial cells are shed into the pleural space.

In healthy individuals, the pleural fluid volume is held constant because of a balance between production and absorption. Capillaries from the parietal pleura form the major source of pleural fluid under normal conditions. However, with pulmonary edema, severe pneumonia, or left-sided heart failure, pleural fluid originates from the increased pulmonary interstitial fluid that seeps through the visceral pleura. Pleural fluid usually contains fewer than 1,500 white blood cells per μL and a few red cells. The bicarbonate level, and resulting pH, tends to be slightly higher than the serum. The stomata and lacuna will respond promptly and efficiently to absorb the excess production of pleural fluid. Therefore, any accumulation of fluid in the

TABLE 6.10.1
LIGHT CRITERIA TO DETERMINE WHETHER PLEURAL FLUID IS AN EXUDATE

Parameter	Exudate	Transudate
Absolute value of pleural fluid LDH is greater than two-thirds the upper limit of serum level	Yes	No
Ratio of pleural fluid:serum LDH concentration is >0.6	Yes	No
Ratio of pleural fluid:serum protein concentration is >0.5	Yes	No

LDH, lactate dehydrogenase.

pleural space is the result of a combination of increased fluid production and decreased fluid absorption. Pleural fluid can be categorized into two types, transudates or exudates, on the basis of chemical analysis. Changes in oncotic or hydrostatic forces that lead to pleural fluid formation usually create a transudate. In contrast, altered capillary permeability, which allows proteins, lactate dehydrogenase (LDH), and other substances to leak into the pleural fluid, leads to the formation of exudates. Light criteria comparing pleural fluid and serum proteins and LDH provide an accurate method of determining whether the fluid is an exudate or a transudate in approximately 95% of the cases (see Table 6.10.1).

Common causes of transudative pleural effusions include nephrotic syndrome due to the loss of oncotic pressure, left-sided heart failure caused by elevated pulmonary hydrostatic pressures, and cirrhotic liver disease from the inability to produce proteins for maintaining oncotic pressure. Exudative pleural effusions result from a wide variety of diseases and conditions that increase capillary permeability. The most common form of exudative pleural effusions are parapneumonic effusions. A parapneumonic effusion is a pleural effusion associated with bacterial pneumonia, lung abscess, or bronchiectasis. In contrast, an empyema is described when the concentration of leukocytes becomes macroscopically evident as a thick, highly viscous, whitish yellow, opaque, and turbid fluid (pus). It contains debris, dead cells, and bacteria. Similar to ALI, parapneumonic pleural effusions evolve through stages (see Table 6.10.2). The reader is referred to an excellent review on parapneumonic effusions and their management developed by the consensus of the American College of Chest Physicians.

VENTILATOR-INDUCED LUNG INJURY

As mechanical ventilation became established to treat patients with ARDS, a clinical entity characterized by declining pulmonary compliance, increased work of breathing, and

TABLE 6.10.2
PHASES OF PARAPNEUMONIC EFFUSIONS

Pleuritic phase	Pleuritic chest pain "pins and needles"
	No pleural effusion
Exudative phase	Little free-flowing pleural fluid (<10 mm)
	No increased leukocytes or LDH levels
	Lasts 48 h
Fibrinopurulent phase	Increased viscosity of pleural fluid
	Fibrin synthesis
	Increased leukocytes and LDH (>500 IU) levels
	Decreased pH (<7.2) and glucose level (<60 mg/dL)
	Lasts 14 d
Organizing phase	Purulent fluid
	Increased leukocytes and LDH (>1,000 IU) levels
	Decreased pH (<7.0) and glucose level (<40 mg/dL)
	Pleural peel

LDH, lactate dehydrogenase.
Adapted from Bouros D, Plataki M, Schiza SE. Parapneumonic pleural effusions and empyema. In: Bouros D. ed. *Lung biology in health and disease.* New York: Marcel Dekker; 2004;186: 353–389; Massard G and Thomas P. Therapeutic use of thoracoscopy. In: Bouros D. ed. *Lung biology in health and disease.* New York: Marcel Dekker; 2004;186:218.

worsening hypoxemia occurred. This constellation of signs was called the *respirator lung* syndrome. Studies investigating mechanical ventilation using moderate peak inspiratory pressures (PIP) cast uncertainty on ventilator-induced harm and instead refocused attention on the many different aspects of a supported breath. For example, early studies on supportive care determined that high concentrations of oxygen led to lung injury. In patients with ARDS, delivering PIP between 40 to 80 cm H_2O to achieve "normal" tidal volumes caused increased air leak syndromes. In the laboratory, interstitial perivascular edema was observed in animals subjected to high PIPs, especially near the hila, and the same group reported both alveolar flooding and perivascular edema with extraordinarily high levels of positive pressure. The proposed mechanism of this injury was lung interdependence: As pressure in the distal intra-alveolar compartment increased, the central perivascular area responded with a decreased pressure, leading to edema accumulation. However, the application of positive end-expiratory pressure (PEEP) attenuates perivascular edema, which argues against elevated mean airway pressure (MAP) as a major contributor of lung injury.

The awareness of two major factors associated with ventilator-induced lung injury dramatically improved the understanding of this entity. The first factor is alveolar overdistension and the second is direct shear injury from cyclic collapse and reopening of alveoli. Both mechanisms are associated with the induction of an inflammatory response. In an animal study looking at the effects of increased positive pressure and elevated minute ventilation, enhanced atelectasis, pleural effusions, and air leak occurred. Pulmonary edema also occurred by using negative-pressure ventilation to create hyperinflation. Similar lung pathology was observed in spontaneously breathing animals that experienced chemically induced hyperventilation and lung overexpansion although they were not subjected to mechanical ventilation. Interestingly, the deleterious effects of high PIPs in an animal model were eliminated with a thoracoabdominal strap that limited lung expansion and tidal volume. In contrast, the use of high PIPs and associated high tidal volumes resulted in increased pulmonary edema in open-chest compared to intact-chest animals.

Lymphatic Response to Mechanical Ventilation

An increased pulmonary vascular volume results in enhanced lymphatic flow in mammals, particularly in the small afferent tracheobronchial lymphatics. Carlton et al. demonstrated that lung lymph flow and protein content increased once the administered tidal volume reached a certain threshold in a lamb model. This effect occurred independent of PIP and indicated that microvascular permeability was triggered at a specific level of tidal volume. When the chest wall and abdomen were restricted to prevent overexpansion with high PIPs, lymph flow did not increase (more details of ventilator-induced lung injury are provided in Chapter 43).

RECOMMENDED READINGS

1. Warburton D, Schwarz M, Tefft D, et al. The molecular basis of lung morphogenesis. *Mech Dev.* 2000;92(1):55–81.
2. Merkus PJ, Ten Have-Opbroek AA, Quanjer PH. Human lung growth: a review. *Pediatr Pulmonol.* 1996;21(6):383–397.
3. Shannon JM, Hyatt BA. Epithelial-mesenchymal interactions in the developing lung. *Annu Rev Physiol.* 2004;66:625–645.
4. Warburton D, Zhao J, Berberich MA, et al. Molecular embryology of the lung: Then, now, and in the future. *Am J Physiol.* 1999;276(5 Pt 1):L697–L704.
5. Sadler T. Chapter 13 Respiratory system. *Langman's Medical Embryology.* 5 ed. Baltimore: Williams & Wilkins; 1985:215–223.
6. Cutz E. Cytomorphology and differentiation of airway epithelium in developing human lung. In: McDowell EM, ed. *Lung carcinomas.* Edinburgh: Churchill Livingstone; 1987:1–41.
7. Maeda S, Suzuki S, Suzuki T, et al. Analysis of intrapulmonary vessels and epithelial-endothelial interactions in the human developing lung. *Lab Invest.* 2002;82(3):293–301.
8. Crapo JD, Barry BE, Gehr P, et al. Cell number and cell characteristics of the normal human lung. *Am Rev Respir Dis.* 1982;126(2):332–337.
9. Meyrick B, Reid L. The alveolar wall. *Br J Dis Chest.* 1970;64(3):121–140.
10. Snyder LS, Hertz MI, Harmon KR, et al. Failure of lung repair following acute lung injury. Regulation of the fibroproliferative response (Part 1). *Chest.* 1990;98(3):733–738.
11. Ware LB, Matthay MA. The acute respiratory distress syndrome. *N Engl J Med.* 2000;342(18):1334–1349.
12. Uhal BD. Cell cycle kinetics in the alveolar epithelium. *Am J Physiol.* 1997;272(6 Pt 1):L1031–L1045.
13. Bitterman PB, Rennard SI, Crystal RG. Environmental lung disease and the interstitium. *Clin Chest Med.* 1981;2(3):393–412.

14. Ali MH, Schlidt SA, Chandel NS, et al. Endothelial permeability and IL-6 production during hypoxia: Role of ROS in signal transduction. *Am J Physiol.* 1999;277(5 Pt 1):L1057–L1065.

15. Zapol WM, Jones R. Vascular components of ARDS. Clinical pulmonary hemodynamics and morphology. *Am Rev Respir Dis.* 1987;136(2):471–474.

16. Fukuda Y, Ishizaki M, Masuda Y, et al. The role of intraalveolar fibrosis in the process of pulmonary structural remodeling in patients with diffuse alveolar damage. *Am J Pathol.* 1987;126(1):171–182.

17. Tomashefski JF Jr, Davies P, Boggis C, et al. The pulmonary vascular lesions of the adult respiratory distress syndrome. *Am J Pathol.* 1983;112(1):112–126.

18. Shoemaker CT, Reiser KM, Goetzman BW, et al. Elevated ratios of type I/III collagen in the lungs of chronically ventilated neonates with respiratory distress. *Pediatr Res.* 1984;18(11):1176–1180.

19. Raghu G, Striker LJ, Hudson LD, et al. Extracellular matrix in normal and fibrotic human lungs. *Am Rev Respir Dis.* 1985;131(2):281–289.

20. Schnapp LM, Chin DP, Szaflarski N, et al. Frequency and importance of barotrauma in 100 patients with acute lung injury. *Crit Care Med.* 1995;23(2):272–278.

21. Weg JG, Anzueto A, Balk RA, et al. The relation of pneumothorax and other air leaks to mortality in the acute respiratory distress syndrome. *N Engl J Med.* 1998;338(6):341–346.

22. Hudson LD. Protective ventilation for patients with acute respiratory distress syndrome. *N Engl J Med.* 1998;338(6):385–387.

23. Pierson DJ, Horton CA, Bates PW. Persistent bronchopleural air leak during mechanical ventilation. A review of 39 cases. *Chest.* 1986;90(3):321–323.

24. Jones R, Langleben D, Reid L. Patterns of remodeling of the pulmonary circulation in acute and subacute lung injury. In: Said S, ed. *The pulmonary circulation and acute lung injury.* Mount Kisco, NY: Futura Publishing; 1985:137–188.

25. Meduri GU. The role of the host defence response in the progression and outcome of ARDS: Pathophysiological correlations and response to glucocorticoid treatment. *Eur Respir J.* 1996;9(12):2650–2670.

26. Ager A. Inflammation: Border crossings. *Nature.* 2003;421(6924):703–705.

27. Pittet JF, Mackersie RC, Martin TR, et al. Biological markers of acute lung injury: Prognostic and pathogenetic significance. *Am J Respir Crit Care Med.* 1997;155(4):1187–1205.

28. Strieter RM, Kunkel SL, Keane MP, et al. Chemokines in lung injury: Thomas A. Neff Lecture. *Chest.* 1999;116(1 Suppl):103S–110S.

29. Millar AB, Foley NM, Singer M, et al. Tumour necrosis factor in bronchopulmonary secretions of patients with adult respiratory distress syndrome. *Lancet.* 1989;2(8665):712–714.

30. Ulich TR, Watson LR, Yin SM, et al. The intratracheal administration of endotoxin and cytokines. I. Characterization of LPS-induced IL-1 and TNF mRNA expression and the LPS-, IL-1-, and TNF-induced inflammatory infiltrate. *Am J Pathol.* 1991;138(6):1485–1496.

31. Speer CP. Inflammation and bronchopulmonary dysplasia. *Semin Neonatol.* 2003;8(1):29–38.

32. Zhang H, Slutsky AS, Vincent JL. Oxygen free radicals in ARDS, septic shock and organ dysfunction. *Intensive Care Med.* 2000;26(4):474–476.

33. Vasudevan A, Lodha R, Kabra SK. Acute lung injury and acute respiratory distress syndrome. *Indian J Pediatr.* 2004;71(8):743–750.

34. Piantadosi CA, Schwartz DA. The acute respiratory distress syndrome. *Ann Intern Med.* 2004;141(6):460–470.

35. Baggiolini M. Chemokines in pathology and medicine. *J Intern Med.* 2001;250(2):91–104.

36. Kennedy J, Kelner GS, Kleyensteuber S, et al. Molecular cloning and functional characterization of human lymphotactin. *J Immunol.* 1995;155(1):203–209.

37. Luster AD. Chemokines–chemotactic cytokines that mediate inflammation. *N Engl J Med.* 1998;338(7):436–445.

38. Bacon K, Baggiolini M, Broxmeyer H, et al. Chemokine/chemokine receptor nomenclature. *J Interferon Cytokine Res.* 2002;22(10):1067–1068.

39. Miller EJ, Cohen AB, Nagao S, et al. Elevated levels of NAP-1/interleukin-8 are present in the airspaces of patients with the adult respiratory distress syndrome and are associated with increased mortality. *Am Rev Respir Dis.* 1992;146(2):427–432.

40. Donnelly TJ, Meade P, Jagels M, et al. Cytokine, complement, and endotoxin profiles associated with the development of the adult respiratory distress syndrome after severe injury. *Crit Care Med.* 1994;22(5):768–776.

41. Karakurum M, Shreeniwas R, Chen J, et al. Hypoxic induction of interleukin-8 gene expression in human endothelial cells. *J Clin Invest.* 1994;93(4):1564–1570.

42. Metinko AP, Kunkel SL, Standiford TJ, et al. Anoxia-hyperoxia induces monocyte-derived interleukin-8. *J Clin Invest.* 1992;90(3):791–798.

43. Busse W, Elias J, Sheppard D, et al. Airway remodeling and repair. *Am J Respir Crit Care Med.* 1999;160(3):1035–1042.

44. Sheppard D. Airway epithelial integrins: Why so many? *Am J Respir Cell Mol Biol.* 1998;19(3):349–351.

45. Schnells G, Voigt WH, Redl H, et al. Electron-microscopic investigation of lung biopsies in patients with post-traumatic respiratory insufficiency. *Acta Chir Scand Suppl.* 1980;499:9–20.

46. Snyder LS, Hertz MI, Harmon KR, et al. Failure of lung repair following acute lung injury. Regulation of the fibroproliferative response (Part 2). *Chest.* 1990;98(4):989–993.

47. Phan SH. Role of the myofibroblast in pulmonary fibrosis. *Kidney Int Suppl.* 1996;54:S46–S48.

48. Martin C, Papazian L, Payan MJ, et al. Pulmonary fibrosis correlates with outcome in adult respiratory distress syndrome. A study in mechanically ventilated patients. *Chest.* 1995;107(1):196–200.

49. Pugin J, Verghese G, Widmer MC, et al. The alveolar space is the site of intense inflammatory and profibrotic reactions in the early phase of acute respiratory distress syndrome. *Crit Care Med.* 1999;27(2):304–312.

50. Clark JG, Milberg JA, Steinberg KP, et al. Type III procollagen peptide in the adult respiratory distress syndrome. Association of increased peptide levels in bronchoalveolar lavage fluid with increased risk for death. *Ann Intern Med.* 1995;122(1):17–23.

51. Chesnutt AN, Matthay MA, Tibayan FA, et al. Early detection of type III procollagen peptide in acute lung injury. Pathogenetic and prognostic significance. *Am J Respir Crit Care Med.* 1997;156(3 Pt 1):840–845.

52. Phan SH. The myofibroblast in pulmonary fibrosis. *Chest.* 2002;122(6 Suppl):286S–289S.

53. Desmouliere A, Geinoz A, Gabbiani F, et al. Transforming growth factor-beta 1 induces alpha-smooth muscle actin expression in granulation tissue myofibroblasts and in quiescent and growing cultured fibroblasts. *J Cell Biol.* 1993;122(1):103–111.

54. Zhang K, Flanders KC, Phan SH. Cellular localization of transforming growth factor-beta expression in bleomycin-induced pulmonary fibrosis. *Am J Pathol.* 1995;147(2):352–361.

55. Zhang K, Gharaee-Kermani M, Jones ML, et al. Lung monocyte chemoattractant protein-1 gene expression in bleomycin-induced pulmonary fibrosis. *J Immunol.* 1994;153(10):4733–4741.

56. Massague J. TGFbeta signaling: Receptors, transducers, and Mad proteins. *Cell.* 1996;85(7):947–950.

57. Dennler S, Itoh S, Vivien D, et al. Direct binding of Smad3 and Smad4 to critical TGF beta-inducible elements in the promoter of human plasminogen activator inhibitor-type 1 gene. *Embo J.* 1998;17(11):3091–3100.

58. Heldin CH, Miyazono K, ten Dijke P. TGF-beta signalling from cell membrane to nucleus through SMAD proteins. *Nature.* 1997;390(6659):465–471.

59. Bousquet J, Vignola AM, Chanez P, et al. Airways remodelling in asthma: No doubt, no more? *Int Arch Allergy Immunol.* 1995;107(1–3):211–214.

60. Chesnutt AN, Kheradmand F, Folkesson HG, et al. Soluble transforming growth factor-alpha is present in the pulmonary edema fluid of patients with acute lung injury. *Chest.* 1997;111(3):652–656.

61. Stossel TP. On the crawling of animal cells. *Science.* 1993;260(5111):1086–1094.

62. Madtes DK, Rubenfeld G, Klima LD, et al. Elevated transforming growth factor-alpha levels in bronchoalveolar lavage fluid of

patients with acute respiratory distress syndrome. *Am J Respir Crit Care Med.* 1998;158(2):424–430.

63. Desmouliere A, Redard M, Darby I, et al. Apoptosis mediates the decrease in cellularity during the transition between granulation tissue and scar. *Am J Pathol.* 1995;146(1):56–66.

64. Buchser E, Leuenberger P, Chiolero R, et al. Reduced pulmonary capillary blood volume as a long-term sequel of ARDS. *Chest.* 1985;87(5):608–611.

65. Motley H, Cournand A, Werko L, et al. The influence of short periods of induced acute anoxia upon pulmonary artery pressures in man. *Am J Physiol.* 1947;150:315–320.

66. Aaronson PI, Robertson TP, Ward JP. Endothelium-derived mediators and hypoxic pulmonary vasoconstriction. *Respir Physiol Neurobiol.* 2002;132(1):107–120.

67. Minamino T, Christou H, Hsieh CM, et al. Targeted expression of heme oxygenase-1 prevents the pulmonary inflammatory and vascular responses to hypoxia. *Proc Natl Acad Sci U S A.* 2001;98(15):8798–8803.

68. Wilson HL, Dipp M, Thomas JM, et al. Adp-ribosyl cyclase and cyclic ADP-ribose hydrolase act as a redox sensor. A primary role for cyclic ADP-ribose in hypoxic pulmonary vasoconstriction. *J Biol Chem.* 2001;276(14):11180–11188.

69. Ward JP, Aaronson PI. Mechanisms of hypoxic pulmonary vasoconstriction: Can anyone be right? *Respir Physiol.* 1999;115(3):261–271.

70. Furchgott RF. Endothelium-derived relaxing factor: Discovery, early studies, and identification as nitric oxide. *Biosci Rep.* 1999;19(4):235–251.

71. Weissmann N, Voswinckel R, Tadic A, et al. Nitric oxide (NO)-dependent but not NO-independent guanylate cyclase activation attenuates hypoxic vasoconstriction in rabbit lungs. *Am J Respir Cell Mol Biol.* 2000;23(2):222–227.

72. Farivar AS, Woolley SM, Fraga CH, et al. Proinflammatory response of alveolar type II pneumocytes to in vitro hypoxia and reoxygenation. *Am J Transplant.* 2004;4(3):346–351.

73. Leufgen H, Bihl MP, Rudiger JJ, et al. Collagenase expression and activity is modulated by the interaction of collagen types, hypoxia, and nutrition in human lung cells. *J Cell Physiol.* 2005;204(1):146–154.

74. Stenmark KR, Davie NJ, Reeves JT, et al. Hypoxia, leukocytes, and the pulmonary circulation. *J Appl Physiol.* 2005;98(2):715–721.

75. McCoubrey WK Jr, Huang TJ, Maines MD. Heme oxygenase-2 is a hemoprotein and binds heme through heme regulatory motifs that are not involved in heme catalysis. *J Biol Chem.* 1997;272(19):12568–12574.

76. Varsila E, Pesonen E, Andersson S. Early protein oxidation in the neonatal lung is related to development of chronic lung disease. *Acta Paediatr.* 1995;84(11):1296–1299.

77. Mantell LL, Horowitz S, Davis JM, et al. Hyperoxia-induced cell death in the lung–the correlation of apoptosis, necrosis, and inflammation. *Ann N Y Acad Sci.* 1999;887:171–180.

78. de Perrot M, Liu M, Waddell TK, et al. Ischemia-reperfusion-induced lung injury. *Am J Respir Crit Care Med.* 2003;167(4):490–511.

79. O'Reilly MA. DNA damage and cell cycle checkpoints in hyperoxic lung injury: Braking to facilitate repair. *Am J Physiol Lung Cell Mol Physiol.* 2001;281(2):L291–L305.

80. Jones R, Zapol WM, Reid L. Pulmonary arterial wall injury and remodelling by hyperoxia. *Chest.* 1983;83(5 Suppl):40S–42S.

81. Ardehali A, Laks H, Russell H, et al. Modified reperfusion and ischemia-reperfusion injury in human lung transplantation. *J Thorac Cardiovasc Surg.* 2003;126(6):1929–1934.

82. Hart ML, Walsh MC, Stahl GL. Initiation of complement activation following oxidative stress. In vitro and in vivo observations. *Mol Immunol.* 2004;41(2–3):165–171.

83. Krishnadasan B, Naidu BV, Byrne K, et al. The role of proinflammatory cytokines in lung ischemia-reperfusion injury. *J Thorac Cardiovasc Surg.* 2003;125(2):261–272.

84. Naidu BV, Fraga C, Salzman AL, et al. Critical role of reactive nitrogen species in lung ischemia-reperfusion injury. *J Heart Lung Transplant.* 2003;22(7):784–793.

85. Flieder DB, Travis WD. Pathologic characteristics of drug-induced lung disease. *Clin Chest Med.* 2004;25(1):37–45.

86. Higenbottam T, Kuwano K, Nemery B, et al. Understanding the mechanisms of drug-associated interstitial lung disease. *Br J Cancer.* 2004;91(Suppl 2):S31–S37.

87. Ben-Noun L. Drug-induced respiratory disorders: Incidence, prevention and management. *Drug Saf.* 2000;23(2):143–164.

88. Popovsky MA, Abel MD, Moore SB. Transfusion-related acute lung injury associated with passive transfer of antileukocyte antibodies. *Am Rev Respir Dis.* 1983;128(1):185–189.

89. Looney MR, Gropper MA, Matthay MA. Transfusion-related acute lung injury: A review. *Chest.* 2004;126(1):249–258.

90. Silliman CC, Bjornsen AJ, Wyman TH, et al. Plasma and lipids from stored platelets cause acute lung injury in an animal model. *Transfusion.* 2003;43(5):633–640.

91. Wyman TH, Bjornsen AJ, Elzi DJ, et al. A two-insult in vitro model of PMN-mediated pulmonary endothelial damage: Requirements for adherence and chemokine release. *Am J Physiol Cell Physiol.* 2002;283(6):C1592–C1603.

92. Kopko PM, Popovsky MA, MacKenzie MR, et al. HLA class II antibodies in transfusion-related acute lung injury. *Transfusion.* 2001;41(10):1244–1248.

93. Silliman CC, Dickey WO, Paterson AJ, et al. Analysis of the priming activity of lipids generated during routine storage of platelet concentrates. *Transfusion.* 1996;36(2):133–139.

94. Silliman CC, Clay KL, Thurman GW, et al. Partial characterization of lipids that develop during the routine storage of blood and prime the neutrophil NADPH oxidase. *J Lab Clin Med.* 1994;124(5):684–694.

95. Nash G, Blennerhassett JB, Pontoppidan H. Pulmonary lesions associated with oxygen therapy and artificial ventilation. *N Engl J Med.* 1971;276:368–374.

96. Nash G, Bowen JA, Langlinais PC. "Respirator lung": A misnomer. *Arch Pathol.* 1971;21:234–240.

97. Webb HH, Tierney DF. Experimental pulmonary edema due to intermittent positive pressure ventilation with high inflation pressures. Protection by positive end-expiratory pressure. *Am Rev Respir Dis.* 1974;110(5):556–565.

98. Dreyfuss D, Soler P, Basset G, et al. High inflation pressure pulmonary edema. Respective effects of high airway pressure, high tidal volume, and positive end-expiratory pressure. *Am Rev Respir Dis.* 1988;137(5):1159–1164.

99. Dreyfuss D, Saumon G. Role of tidal volume, FRC, and end-inspiratory volume in the development of pulmonary edema following mechanical ventilation. *Am Rev Respir Dis.* 1993;148(5):1194–1203.

100. Slutsky AS, Tremblay LN. Multiple system organ failure. Is mechanical ventilation a contributing factor? *Am J Respir Crit Care Med.* 1998;157(6 Pt 1):1721–1725.

101. Tremblay LN, Miatto D, Hamid Q, et al. Injurious ventilation induces widespread pulmonary epithelial expression of tumor necrosis factor-alpha and interleukin-6 messenger RNA. *Crit Care Med.* 2002;30(8):1693–1700.

102. Tsuno K, Prato P, Kolobow T. Acute lung injury from mechanical ventilation at moderately high airway pressures. *J Appl Physiol.* 1990;69(3):956–961.

103. Mascheroni D, Kolobow T, Fumagalli R, et al. Acute respiratory failure following induced hyperventilation: An experimental study. *Intensive Care Med.* 1988;15:8–14.

104. Hernandez LA, Peevy KJ, Moise AA, et al. Chest wall restriction limits high airway pressure-induced lung injury in young rabbits. *J Appl Physiol.* 1989;66(5):2364–2368.

105. Carlton DP, Cummings JJ, Scheerer RG, et al. Lung overexpansion increases pulmonary microvascular protein permeability in young lambs. *J Appl Physiol.* 1990;69(2):577–583.

106. Woo SW, Hedley-Whyte J. Macrophage accumulation and pulmonary edema due to thoracotomy and lung overinflation. *J Appl Physiol.* 1972;33:14–21.

107. Martin DJ, Parker JC, Taylor AE. Simultaneous comparison of tracheobronchial and right duct lymph dynamics in dogs. *J Appl Physiol.* 1983;54(1):199–207.

108. Weinacker A. Chapter 11 Pleural disease. In: Ali J, Summer WR, Levitzky MG, eds. *Pulmonary pathophysiology.* New York: McGraw-Hill; 1999:239–267.

109. Antony VB, Mohammed KA. Chapter 6 cytokines and pleural disease. In: Nelson S, Martin TR, eds. *Cytokines in pulmonary disease infection and inflammation.* New York: Marcel Dekker, Inc; 2000.

7

Neurosciences

Michael J. Bell   *JoAnne E. Natale*

The nervous system consists of the brain, spinal cord, and cranial and peripheral nerves. An estimated 100 billion cells form an estimated 100 trillion connections to allow us to interact with our environment, learn mathematic problems, listen to music, remember important events, and keep our organs functioning properly, among many other tasks. At the start of the 21st century, advances in the care of critically ill children have progressed to maintain or replace the function of virtually all of the organs of the body. The brain, however, remains an organ that cannot be replaced, transplanted, artificially supported, or regenerated to any significant degree. Understanding how (i) the brain and spinal cord develop, (ii) the main cellular elements of the brain function, (iii) the brain interacts with the muscles to allow physical motion and activity, (iv) its cells can be damaged, killed, or protected, (v) pathologic conditions can be managed, (vi) pain and discomfort are sensed and alleviated, and (vii) it can be monitored clinically are vitally important for pediatric intensivists. The initial sections outline these processes in detail, with particular emphasis on how these processes are relevant to pediatric critical care medicine. In subsequent sections, some of the most common neurologic conditions that occur in critically ill children are reviewed to give the reader a thorough perspective of the neuroscience relevant to pediatric intensive care medicine.

STRUCTURE AND DEVELOPMENT OF THE CENTRAL NERVOUS SYSTEM

To understand the central nervous system (CNS) diseases that confront intensivists daily, a detailed knowledge of the overall brain structure and development is essential. This section outlines the basic embryology of the nervous system, the processes required for proper neuronal development, the characteristics of glial cells and their development, and the organization of the autonomic nervous system. Understanding these aspects of development are essential for understanding the subsequent sections that outline the dysfunction/diseases of these structures or cellular elements.

Basic Nervous System Embryology

The first events in the development of the brain and CNS are evident approximately 3 weeks after conception. At this time, the embryo is divided into three distinct layers: endoderm, mesoderm, and ectoderm. The ectodermal layer will develop into the structures that interact directly with the environment: (i) the central and peripheral nervous system; (ii) the sensory epithelium of the ear, nose, and eye; and (iii) the epidermis. The endodermal layer will develop into the gastrointestinal (GI) tract, and the mesoderm will develop into the other organs within the body. The neural plate, a slipper-shaped plate of thickened ectoderm, becomes evident at this time. This plate becomes raised off the rest of the embryo, leading to two neural folds in the areas adjacent to the rest of the embryo. These neural folds grow and become more and more elevated, until they reach each other in the midline, forming the neural tube (see Fig. 7.1). The neural tube fuses first in the cervical region and then both in the cephalic and caudal directions. The neural tube forms the building block of the development of the mature nervous system. The cephalic portion of the neural tube shows three dilatations called the *primary brain vesicles* (see Fig. 7.2). The first primary brain vesicle, the prosencephalon is the most cephalic in location and will eventually develop into the cerebral hemispheres (from a portion of the prosencephalon termed the *telencephalon*) and the midbrain (from the portion called the *diencephalon*). The second primary brain vesicle, the mesencephalon, will eventually become the structures of the midbrain. The mesencephalon is separated from the third primary brain vesicle, the rhombencephalon, at a deep furrow called the *rhombencephalic isthmus*. The rhombencephalon consists of two parts. The more rostral portion, the metencephalon,

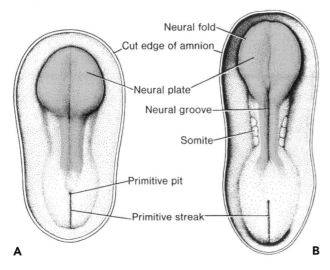

A   **B**

Figure 7.1 Formation of the early neural tube. Dorsal view of early embryo (**A:** 18 days' gestation, **B:** 20 days' gestation) showing formation of neural plate from neural folds. (From Sadler T. *Langman's medical embryology.* 7th ed. Baltimore, MD: Williams & Wilkins; 1995:375.)

will become the pons and cerebellum while the more caudal portion, the myelencephalon, will become the medulla and the start of the spinal cord.

The mature spinal cord is similar in organization to the primitive neural tube formed in the first days after conception. As the neural tube closes, a zone, called the *mantle plate*, develops whereby neural stem cells reside and begin to proliferate. As the nervous system matures, the mantle plate (which will eventually become the gray matter of the spinal cord) is separated into an alar plate in the dorsal region and a basal plate in the ventral region. The alar plate cells become the ascending projection neurons of the dorsal spinal cord, relaying the sensations of touch and pain into the CNS through the dorsal columns. The basal plate

cells become the motor neurons and interneurons of the ventral horn. A subset of basal plate cells within the thoracic and lumbar regions differentiate into autonomic neurons of the sympathetic nervous system. Similarly, basal cells in the brain stem and sacral regions form the autonomic neurons of the parasympathetic system.

Neuronal Development

Neuronal development involves ultrastructural changes that occur while complex interactions of several processes are occurring within the developing embryo to form normal neurons. These processes are (i) genetic patterning and neural induction, (ii) neurulation and neural crest separation, (iii) neuroepithelial cell proliferation and differentiation, (iv) apoptosis (programmed cell death), (v) neuroblast migration, (vi) axonal growth and pathfinding, and (vii) dendritic sprouting and synaptogenesis. These processes and commonly observed aberrations are outlined in the subsequent text (see Table 7.1).

Genetic Patterning and Neural Induction

The early development of the nervous system requires differentiation of the neuroectoderm from other ectodermal structures, establishment of rostral–caudal and dorsal–ventral polarity, bilateral symmetry, segmentation, growth gradients, and differentiation of neural cell lineages. These rudimentary features of a body plan are termed *patterning* and result from cell–cell signals. These signals are produced by several families of regulatory genes that are expressed within the embryonic structures at specific times and in specific distributions.

Induction is the influence of one embryonic tissue on another that causes induced cells to differentiate in a direction different from the fate of the inducer itself. Induction is often between germ layers, as with the notochord (mesoderm) inducing the floor plate of the neural tube (ectoderm). However, induction may also

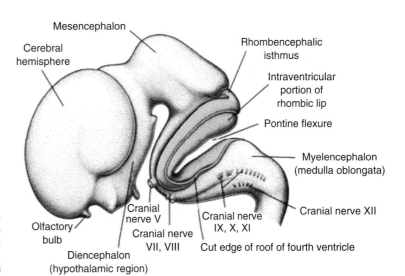

Figure 7.2 Organization of the early nervous system. Lateral view of the brain vesicles of the human embryo at approximately 6 weeks' gestation. (From Sadler T PhD. *Langman's medical embryology.* 9th ed. Image Bank, Baltimore, MD: Williams & Wilkins; 2003.)

TABLE 7.1
PROCESS OF NEUROGENESIS

Genetic patterning and neural induction
Neurulation and neural crest separation
Neuroepithelial cell proliferation and differentiation
Apoptosis (programmed cell death)
Neuroblast migration
Axonal growth and pathfinding
Dendritic sprouting and synaptogenesis

occur within a germ layer, such as when the optic cup (neuroepithelium) induces the overlying surface ectoderm to form a lens placode and cornea rather than simply more epidermis. Neural induction is the maturation of structures of the nervous system in response to inductive molecules secreted in the vicinity of these structures by other tissues of either mesodermal or ectodermal origin. The primary specificity of induction is not the inductive molecule but rather the receptors in the membrane of the induced cell during a precise time of responsiveness known as the *competence* of the induced cell. These membrane receptors also are under specific genetic control. The gene *Notch* regulates competence of response to more specific inductive cues in the CNS and in many other embryonic tissues.

The genes that program the development of the neural tube can be divided into two categories: organizer and regulatory genes. Organizer genes are those that provide for the establishment of the fundamental architecture of the CNS, including the dorsoventral, rostrocaudal, and mediolateral axes; segmentation of the neural tube; mitotic proliferation; and initial differentiation of the neuroepithelium. Regulator genes operate at a later stage in ontogenesis to program the specific identity of different types of neurons and their maturation. The same gene may serve at one stage of development as an organizer gene and at a later stage as a regulator gene, so that these two categories are not entirely different genes.

Each gene of the developing nervous system has a specific site of expression along the rostrocaudal and dorsoventral axes. Some determine particular segments of the neural tube such as the midbrain. A dorsal or ventral gradient of expression may or may not be associated with influence on adjacent regions. A dorsalizing gene not only has a dorsal distribution of expression but also causes ventral regions of the neural tube to differentiate as more dorsal regions. This principle is well demonstrated in the development of the somite, in which the sclerotome normally lies ventral to the myotome and dermatome. Ectopic floor plate cells implanted next to the somite in chick embryos cause ventralization of the somite so that excessive sclerotome (cartilage and bone) and deficient myotome (muscle) and dermatome (dermis) are formed. The floor plate in this case is a ventralizing inductor of the mesodermal somite, and

the probable gene product responsible is the *Sonic hedgehog* (*Shh*), which is also ventralizing in the neural tube.

Disturbances of proper patterning and induction can cause a wide range of disorders. The mutation of one of these regulatory genes generally results in a defective translation product without cell-signaling capability. If the function of the gene is unique, this may lead to a non-viable fetus. However, if other genes overlap in their distribution of expression, one gene may compensate for loss of the other so that the nervous system develops normally.

Whether certain midline malformations of the nervous system, such as holoprosencephaly and septo-optic dysplasia, are due to defective neural induction is unknown at this time. However, a model of holoprosencephaly in the zebrafish lacks a floor plate; the notochord is however present and secretes *Shh*, but *Shh* transcripts of RNA are not detectable in the neural plate of such mutant zebrafish embryos. This may be an example of a mutation in a regulatory gene that cannot be compensated for effectively. Conversely, consider the mouse gene *Hox 1.5*; this is also an important gene that regulates cell patterning within the CNS. Mice with defective *Hox 1.5* die shortly after birth but not because of improper CNS functioning. In an example of other genes taking over the regulatory functioning of a mutant gene, *Hox 1.5* knockout mice are born with malformation of the heart, and without thymus and parathyroid glands. The CNS is formed normally, probably because of compensation by another *Hox* gene. This condition is the murine counterpart of DiGeorge syndrome in humans.

Neurulation and Neural Crest Separation

Neurulation is the process whereby the newly formed neural tube bends and shapes itself into the primitive structures that will ultimately form the cerebrum, midbrain, brain stem, cerebellum, and spinal cord. As mentioned in the preceding text, the neural tube becomes divided into the three primary brain vesicles, and this process is under complex control. This bending of the neural plate to form the neural tube requires both extrinsic and intrinsic mechanical forces. Extrinsic forces are generated in part by the growth of mesodermal tissues flanking the neural plate, which will form the somites. Removal of this mesoderm does not prevent neural tube formation, but the neural tube is rotated toward the side of the removed tissue. Therefore, the mesoderm is important for maintaining the orientation of the neural tube, but the expansion of the surface epithelium provides the major extrinsic force for bending of the neural plate. Intrinsic forces of neurulation begin with the notochordal induction of floor plate differentiation, which establishes the longitudinal axis of the neural plate. The floor plate cells assume the shape of a wedge. The shaping of neuroepithelial cells during neurulation may be important at certain hinge points within the neural tube. Adhesion molecules probably contribute additional intrinsic factors, promoting neurulation. The selective expression of some regulatory genes, such as *WNT1*, at the lateral margins of the neural plate during neurulation probably plays a yet undefined role in the intrinsic curling of the neural plate.

Neural crest cells arise from the dorsal midline of the neural tube at the time of closure or shortly thereafter. These cells migrate extensively throughout the developing embryo and form the autonomic nervous system described later in this section. In their early development, patterns of gene expression in the hindbrain probably contribute to the segmental arrangement of neural crest cells, but their migratory paths are guided by attractant and repulsive molecules secreted by surrounding tissues such as the otic capsule, somites, and the vertebral neural arches. In addition, neural crest cells possess integrin receptors for interacting with extracellular matrix molecules. Changes in the distribution of extracellular matrix components during neural crest migration impose migratory guidance limits as well.

The most common human disorders of neurulation are the family of spinal dysraphisms known as *meningomyeloceles*, occurring most commonly in the lumbosacral region. Whether aganglionic megacolon (Hirschsprung disease) is a disturbance of the segmental neural crest formation or a peripheral disturbance of cell migration within the gut is still being debated. Some hereditary diseases of peripheral nerves and sympathetic and dorsal root ganglia are considered neurocristopathies, the most common of which is familial dysautonomia (Riley-Day syndrome).

Neuroepithelial Cell Proliferation and Differentiation

The process of increasing cell number (proliferation) is an ongoing process from the earliest times in embryogenesis. Immediately after conception, all of the cells are totipotent—able to form all of the tissues of the body. When the endoderm, mesoderm, and ectoderm are formed within the first weeks of conception, the cells would have developed a more limited number of potential fates and are now described as pluripotent. The ectoderm, for example, can form either the skin or the nervous system. Once the primitive streak and the neural plate are formed, these cells become committed to the neural fate and will only form the cells of the nervous system. These cells are termed *neural stem cells*. These stem cells proliferate and form all the cells within the nervous system—neurons, astrocytes, oligodendrocytes, Schwann cells, and neural crest cells. These are discussed in subsequent parts of this section. Microglia, the phagocytic cells within the brain, are not derived from these neural stem cells. Instead, hematopoietic stem cells produce monocytes that invade the CNS and become resident microglia.

Throughout embryonic development, neural stem cells are located near the lining of the ventricular cavity. The first layer of cells adjacent to the ventricle is the ventricular zone (VZ). In neuronal development, neural stem cells in the VZ are attached to the ventricular surface and undergo mitosis to produce either two identical cells (symmetric cell division) or a single stem cell and a committed neuron (asymmetric cell division). In mitosis, chromosomes within the cell align themselves into a cleavage plane. The cytoskeleton of the cell then contracts and the chromosomes are pulled apart in a well-orchestrated manner to ensure that each daughter cell receives identical contents of DNA. In neural stem cell mitoses, the term symmetric cell division refers not to the DNA content but to the content of receptors located in the plasma membrane at the ventricular surface. In symmetric cell division, the daughter cells are divided along an axis perpendicular to the ventricular surface, and each daughter cell receives an identical amount of plasma membrane that is attached at the ventricular surface. Conversely, in asymmetric cell division, the cleavage plane of the chromosomes is not perpendicular to the ventricular surface. In this case, the daughter cell that receives most of the plasma membrane from the ventricular surface remains a progenitor cell, whereas the other daughter cell becomes detached and differentiates into a neuron.

Many aspects of this process are only incompletely understood. Receptors responsible for the orientation of the cleavage plane have been proposed but remain speculative at this time. Similarly, it is known that neural stem cells differentiate into more committed precursor cells that are still capable of cell division. These cells are called *neuronal progenitors* and *glial progenitors*. Previous dogma held that neural stem cells could differentiate into either of these two more committed cell lines. Recently, investigators have challenged this assertion with findings that glial progenitors can be directed to become neurons, given the proper cell-culture conditions.

Currently, there are no clinical syndromes associated with faulty or aberrant stem cell proliferation and differentiation. This likely represents our limited knowledge about these complex processes and not the accuracy with which these processes occur in the developing brain. Advances in the knowledge of how stem cells function and differentiate have enormous potential clinical uses. Future applications may include the replacement of degenerated cells with stem cells and enhancement of the endogenous stem cells already located within the brain to take over the function of the injured or dead cells.

Apoptosis—Programmed Cell Death

The number of cells generated in the fetal nervous system is between 30% and 70% more than the requirement at maturity. Surplus cells survive for a finite period, usually days to weeks, and then spontaneously begin a cascade of degenerative changes and die. This process is termed *apoptosis* or programmed cell death because the cells die in an organized, programmed manner. Although this topic is discussed in detail later in this section, a few aspects of apoptosis in the development should be emphasized. During development, apoptosis seems to be programmed into every nervous system cell. Cells seem to be prevented from dying by the secretion of trophic factors from neighboring cells. Two trophic factors, nerve growth factor (NGF) and basic fibroblast growth factor, seem to be most effective at blocking cell death in the various cell lineages in the nervous system. As pointed out later in this section, not all programmed cell death is an early embryonic event. Motor neurons of the cervical spinal cord of the rat continue to show apoptosis in the early postnatal period and apoptosis occurs in many neurodegenerative diseases.

Neuroblast Migration

Neurons in the mature human brain are not located in the same site where they begin their differentiation. Neurons must shift position and migrate long distances to establish a three-dimensional relationship and synaptic circuits with other neurons that are required for proper functioning. The migration of neuroblasts is a precise and orderly process guided by specialized glial cells. These radial glial cells possess long processes, which span the distance from the VZ to the pial surface. Evidence suggests that neurons use these processes as a tract that guides them to their ultimate destination within the layers of the cortex. The signals that mediate this migration process are not fully known. Cell surface proteins, including glycoproteins and adhesion molecules, have been implicated in this process. Migration of most neurons is complete within the first 34 weeks' gestation. The invaginations of the cerebral cortex, gyri, and sulci form as the surface area of the brain continues to enlarge without a change in brain volume. By 20 weeks' gestation, only the rudimentary primary fissures are formed. The mature configuration of convolutions of the cerebral cortex is not complete until gliogenesis is complete after birth. Intense study is under way to determine whether these radial glial cells can also develop into neurons.

Nearly all major cerebral malformations are disturbances of neuroblast migration. Some may leave heterotopic, abnormally migrated neuroblasts to mature in aberrant sites where they cannot become integrated with the rest of the nervous system. In disorders of neural induction, such as holoprosencephaly, the cortical architecture is abnormal because of disturbances in migration of the neurons into the cortical plate. In agenesis of the corpus callosum, a small foci of dysplastic neurons (that may be epileptogenic) are found in the periventricular region. Throughout the cortex, neurons that have abnormally migrated may form nodules that can either be silent or disturb normal neuronal function.

Some malformations appear to be primary genetically determined disorders of neuroblast migration and of the development of cerebral convolutions, for example, lissencephaly (smooth brain without gyri) and pachygyria (a few large abnormal convolutions). Genetic disorders with specific metabolic defects can also produce malformations because of disturbed neuroblast migration (Zellweger syndrome, Menkes syndrome, and aminoacidurias).

Pathologic processes during development can also lead to disturbed neuronal migration. Hemorrhages or infarcts may interrupt or destroy the radial glial cell, thereby interrupting the migration of neuroblasts. Disturbances of the normal architecture of the pial surface, such as contusions, meningitis, or subarachnoid hemorrhages, may cause the end-foot of the radial glial process to retract and may also adversely affect migration of developing neurons.

Axonal Growth and Pathfinding

Axons innervating the lower limbs from the spinal cord must grow progressively throughout development and reach up to 1 m in length. A single axon will grow from developing neurons and must find its appropriate target (muscle cell, interneuron, or secretory gland) for proper functioning. The tip of the growing axon is called the *growth cone*. This structure is a constantly changing complex of cytoplasmic fingers, called *filopodia*, which are formed by microtubules, filaments, and mitochondria and serve as a sensor for the axon to achieve its appropriate target. Three mechanisms are involved in axonal guidance. Molecular signals between the axon and the target cell are called *cell–cell interaction*. The target cell releases factors that are sensed by the growth cone and induce the growth cone to form a synapse. This mechanism is only effective when the axon is very close to the target cell (within 1 to 2 mm). Adhesion proteins within the growth cone can also interact with proteins in the extracellular matrix. These cell–substrate interactions involve integrins of the growth cone interacting with fibronectin and laminin in the extracellular space and serving as attractants or repellents for the axon. Lastly, growth cones are very sensitive to chemicals secreted from cells along the projected path of the axon. These chemotaxic interactions can ensure the tract of the axon by attracting or repelling the growth cone.

Aberrant axons can produce faulty synaptic circuits that cannot perform their intended function. Many times, these abnormalities are random and unpredictable. However, in the syndrome of agenesis of the corpus callosum, misguided axons form the predictable pathologic fiber tracts called the *bundle of Probst*.

Dendritic Sprouting and Synaptogenesis

Once the axon has begun its migration, the other connections of the neurons, dendrites, sprout to receive input from other cells. The number of dendrites and their pattern of distribution (called *dendritic arborization*) are specific for each neuron. In the cerebrum, synaptogenesis occurs only after the neuron has migrated to its final position. However, in the cerebellum, synapses are projected as parallel fibers before the final migration of the neurons in the external granule cells.

Inputs from afferent nerves begin to innervate cortical neurons before the final architecture of the cortex is completed. These first synapses are between axons and dendrites of specialized cells within the pyramidal layer and the cells of the molecular zone (Cajal-Retzius cells). More and more synapses are formed as the development of the nervous system progresses, with most of the dendritic arborization occurring in late gestation and in early infancy. Because of this, disturbances in brain function during these relatively late developmental periods (e.g., decreased blood flow from nuchal cord at delivery and metabolic disturbances of the brain) can lead to abnormal synaptic connections required for optimal functioning.

Redundant and unnecessary synapses are generated, only to be later deleted and retracted by the axons. Using this pruning technique, optimal circuitry can be ensured. The electroencephalogram (EEG) is probably the most reliable and clinically available measure of the synaptogenesis of the cerebral cortex. In preterm infants, the waveforms generated will have increasing amounts of activity as the infant's dendritic arborization progresses. The maturation of the EEG is a precise temporal progression of predictable changes with increasing conceptional age and includes the development of sleep–wake cycles. The EEG is discussed in greater detail in the section on "Electrophysiologic Monitoring".

The major malformations mentioned earlier in this section, holoprosencephaly and lissencephaly, have been found to cause extensive abnormalities in dendritic morphology and synapses. Specialized staining techniques disclose similar abnormalities in chromosomal diseases such as Down syndrome, in inborn metabolic errors, fetal alcohol syndrome, and in some forms of infantile epilepsy. Children with tuberous sclerosis exhibit abnormal dendrites and abnormal synapses, as well as the more easily demonstrated cytologic alterations of the nerve cell body.

Glial Cell Development

The term "neuroglia" was coined over a century ago and is translated as "nerve glue." This term aptly describes the neuroglia, or just glia, as the connective tissue that supports the neurons and their processes. Estimates show that there are ten times more glia within the brain than in the neurons, indicating that understanding their biologic activity is vital to discern CNS function. There are four types of cells that make up the glia—astrocytes, oligodendrocytes, and microglia—within the CNS, and Schwann cells in the peripheral nervous system (see Table 7.2). Astrocytes, oligodendrocytes, and Schwann cells are all formed from similar glial-restricted precursor cells, as stated in the preceding text, while microglia are derived from hematopoietic cells.

Gliogenesis is the process by which glial cell precursors are formed from the neural stem cells. Whereas neurogenesis begins virtually as the neural plate is formed, gliogenesis begins much later in gestation. In rodents, it is estimated to occur at approximately 60% of gestation and continues throughout the first several weeks of postnatal life. Glial progenitors are derived from the VZ in embryonic life and from the subventricular zone (SVZ) at later periods. The choice between developing into a glial precursor or a neuronal precursor appears to be based on localized factors within these two zones of brain. Although much of the details of these pathways are currently being determined, several conditions have been described. Secretion of the growth factor neuregulin-1 induces stem cells in the neural crest to adopt a glial cell precursor fate. Similarly, localized secretion of growth factors such as platelet-derived growth

TABLE 7.2
GLIAL CELL LOCATIONS, FUNCTIONS, AND PROPERTIES

	Place of Origin	Location in Mature Nervous System	Main Functions
Astrocytes	SVZ	CNS	Contribution to blood–brain barrier, uptake of metabolic products near synapses, regulation of ion homeostasis, scar formation in response to injury
Oligodendrocytes	SVZ	CNS	Formation of myelin in CNS, saltatory nerve conduction, axonal guidance
Microglia	Blood monocytes that migrate within the brain	CNS	Inflammatory response within the CNS, production of cytokines and other markers, phagocytosis of debris
Schwann cells	SVZ of spinal cord	PNS	Formation of myelin in PNS, saltatory nerve conduction, axonal guidance

SVZ, subventricular zone; CNS, central nervous system; PNS, peripheral nervous system.

factor (PDGF) and neurotrophin-3 is needed to induce an oligodendrocyte fate. Understanding of the molecular clues to these processes is required for stem cell transplantation studies to be successful.

Astrocytes

Astrocytes are star-shaped cells (hence the term *astro-*) that serve to support neurons and other glial cells. It is believed that astrocytes constitute up to 50% of the total cell mass in many regions of the brain. There are several different astrocyte cell types. Radial glial cells, mentioned in the preceding text as cells that serve as a scaffolding for the migration of neurons, are astrocytes that serve varied functions during development. Protoplasmic astrocytes are located within the gray matter, whereas fibrous astrocytes make up most of the cells within the white matter. Characteristic proteins within the cell identify astrocytes. In particular, the proteins glial fibrillary acidic protein (GFAP) and S-100β are astrocytic markers. Ultrastructurally, gap junctions formed by proteins called *connexins* are an important distinguishing feature of astrocytes and are integral to their functioning.

Astrocytes function to wall off neurons and oligodendrocytes from the rest of the body. They achieve this by extending out processes from the outer limits of the nervous system (the pia mater) to the inner most layers (the ependyma). These processes cover the blood vessels, capillaries, synapses, dendrites, and cell bodies of neurons to insulate them from the external environment. Astrocytes are responsible for the formation of the "blood–brain barrier," which prevents the entry of cells and diffusion of molecules into the CNS from the bloodstream. In lower species, the attachment of astrocytes to themselves is by gap junctions, which form the mechanical blood–brain barrier. In humans, however, astrocytes are responsible for maintaining the tight junctions of endothelial cells, which is the blood–brain barrier. Other functions of astrocytes include production of growth factors, removal of neurotransmitters (NTs) from synapses, and regulation of ion concentrations in the interstitial space.

In pathologic states, such as traumatic injury, viral infections, inflammation, and dementia, astrocytes respond to injury by becoming hypertrophic. This process, called *reactive gliosis*, causes a rapid increase in the production of filaments within the astrocyte, which then migrates to the site of injury. At the site of injury, the astrocyte forms a scar in an attempt to wall off the CNS from the external environment. Despite this beneficial effect, reactive gliosis is blamed as a reason for failure of growth cones to refind their target tissues after an injury to the neuron.

Oligodendrocytes and Schwann Cells

As the diameter of axons becomes larger, the rate at which action potentials can be propagated also increases. In the most extreme example, the diameter of the axon of the giant squid is approximately the size of a fountain pen. This axon conducts impulses at remarkable speeds. As species evolve and develop more complex brains that require faster transmission of information, the size of the axon cannot always be increased to meet this need. Oligodendrocytes and Schwann cells have evolved to address this problem by wrapping axons in a proteolipid membrane called *myelin*. Myelin sheaths allow cell action potentials to propagate faster by a mechanism termed *saltatory conduction*. This form of conduction is discussed in detail in the following section of this text. However, the end result of myelin is the increased efficiency of action potential propagation, and this is accomplished by oligodendrocytes in the CNS and by Schwann cells in the peripheral nervous system.

Oligodendrocytes make up approximately 15% of the mass of the brain in adults and arise from precursor cells. Glial-committed precursors will produce oligodendrocytes in response to appropriate growth factors, as outlined in the preceding text. The maturation of oligodendrocytes can be described on the basis of a variety of cellular markers. Oligodendrocyte-committed precursors (OCP) exhibit the cell surface marker NG2, a proteoglycan of unknown function at this time. OCPs are bipolar cells with a limited number of cellular processes surrounding the cell body. Immature oligodendrocytes have a more complex ultrastructure, with many more complex processes extending from the cell body. Immature oligodendrocytes express the cellular marker O1. Further maturation to mature oligodendrocytes results in the complex morphology of many processes that can wrap around axons up to a dozen times and express the markers GalC and myelin basic protein (MBP). The maturation and function of Schwann cells are similar in the peripheral nervous system. An important exception to this is that an individual Schwann cell will only myelinate a single axon. In contrast, oligodendrocytes can form myelin sheaths around dozens of axons.

Myelin is a complex structure that includes a lipid bilayer overlapping itself along with proteolipids interspersed. Such proteins, MBP, cyclic nucleotide phosphodiesterase (CNP) and proteolipid protein (PLP) help compact myelin by allowing adjacent lipid bilayers to lie in close apposition by equally distributing the electric charges within the membrane. Deposition of myelin occurs at varying paces, depending on the brain region. As examples, the medial longitudinal fasciculus of the brain stem begins myelination at 24 weeks' gestation and completes it by 28 weeks. The corticospinal tract starts to be myelinated at 38 weeks' gestation and is fully myelinated by 2 years of age. The corpus callosum begins at 4 months postnatally and finishes in mid adolescence.

Delay in the normal myelination process is a nonspecific feature common to many chromosomal diseases, metabolic disorders, endocrinopathies of early infancy such as hypothyroidism, chronic systemic illness, and often intrauterine growth retardation from placental insufficiency or placental infarction. Abnormal myelin can be formed by inborn errors of metabolism that interfere with oligodendrocytes and their function. Immunologic processes, such as multiple sclerosis or acute demyelinating encephalomyelitis, can also target myelin, leading to neurologic symptoms. In these conditions, activated lymphocytes are sensitized to a cell surface component of oligodendrocytes, leading to the destruction of myelin and death of the oligodendrocyte.

Microglia

Microglia are the smallest cells within the CNS and have been called the *tissue macrophages* on the basis of their functions. As stated earlier, they are recruited from hematopoietic cells that migrate into the CNS during development. Discovered in 1899, microglia remain the least understood cells in the CNS. They represent between 5% and 20% of the total number of cells in mouse brain, although they represent a much smaller proportion of brain volume because of their size. Microglia have rod-shaped cell bodies with numerous processes that extend symmetrically around the cell.

The main function of microglia within the CNS is to phagocytose degenerating cells that are undergoing cell death. They maintain the immunologic ability as antigen-presenting cells in the immune system and are capable of secreting a host of cytokines in response to injury. Because of their structure and number, the microglia form a network throughout the CNS that seems capable of responding to environmental cues. This has led some to hypothesize a role for microglia in cellular homeostasis, but this role remains speculative at this time.

Microglia become "activated" in response to a host of pathophysiologic processes. Activated microglia change in morphology to have more ramified processes extending from the cell body. Additionally, immunologic markers of monocyte–macrophage activation are upregulated in activated microglia. These processes culminate in an increased ability to phagocytose cellular debris within the CNS.

Autonomic Nervous System

The autonomic nervous system describes the system of nerves that controls smooth muscles, cardiac muscles, and various glandular systems within the body. The term *autonomic* was coined because these functions are generally performed unconsciously. The response to stress, overall body homeostasis, cardiovascular function, GI secretions, urinary regulation, and many other metabolic functions are under the direction of this system. Dysfunctions of this system can cause dramatic symptoms and can lead to death if left untreated.

Structure of the Autonomic Nervous System

There are several differences between the structure of the autonomic nervous system and the rest of the CNS. The autonomic system is organized in relative proximity to the visceral organs they innervate. This seems symbolic of the relative independence of this system relative to the somatic nerves. Moreover, two efferent neurons carry the response from the brain to these visceral organs (preganglionic nerves arising from the brain stem or spinal cord and postganglionic nerves arising from specialized ganglia) instead of the single motor neuron of the spinal neurons.

The autonomic nervous system is divided into two parts: parasympathetic and sympathetic. Functionally, the two parts are complementary in maintaining a balance in the tonic activities of many visceral structures and organs. There are two branches of the parasympathetic nervous system: the cranial and the sacral. The cranial branch originates in the visceral nuclei of the midbrain, pons, and medulla. These nuclei include the Edinger-Westphal nucleus, superior and inferior salivatory nuclei, dorsal motor nucleus of the vagus, and adjacent reticular nuclei. The preganglionic fibers from these nuclei course through the oculomotor, facial, glossopharyngeal, and vagus nerves and regulate pupillary size, salivary gland function, and heart function. The sacral branch of the parasympathetic system originates in the lateral horn cells at the second, third, and fourth sacral spinal cord. The preganglionic fibers traverse through the sacral nerves and synapse in ganglia that lie within the walls of the distal colon, bladder, and other pelvic organs. Therefore, the sacral autonomic neurons, like the cranial ones, have long preganglionic and short postganglionic fibers.

The sympathetic system consists of neurons that originate in the gray matter from the eighth cervical to the second lumbar spinal cord (preganglionic fibers) and nerves that innervate the various visceral organs (postganglionic fibers). Preganglionic axons synapse with the cell bodies of the postganglionic neurons in two large chains on each side of the vertebral column (paravertebral ganglia) or in several single prevertebral ganglia. The postganglionic fibers travel through spinal nerves of T5 to L2, supplying blood vessels, sweat glands, and hair follicles, and also form plexuses that supply the heart, bronchi, kidneys, intestines, pancreas, bladder, and sex organs.

The sympathetic innervation of the adrenal medulla is unique in that its secretory cells receive preganglionic fibers directly, through the splanchnic nerves. This is an exception to the rule that organs innervated by the autonomic nervous system receive only postganglionic fibers. This special arrangement can be explained by the fact that cells of the adrenal medulla are the morphologic homologs of the postganglionic sympathetic neurons and secrete epinephrine and norepinephrine (the postganglionic transmitters) directly into the bloodstream. In this way, the sympathetic nervous system and the adrenal medulla act in unison to produce diffuse effects—as one would expect from their role in emergency reactions.

Structures within the brain stem and cerebrum are responsible for the integration of the functions of the autonomic nervous system. In the brain stem, the main visceral afferent nucleus is the nucleus tractus solitarius (NTS). Cardiovascular, respiratory, and GI afferents, carried in the vagus and glossopharyngeal nerves, terminate on specific subnuclei of the NTS. The hypothalamus serves as the integrating mechanism of the autonomic nervous system. The regulatory activity of the hypothalamus is accomplished in two ways—through direct pathways that descend to particular groups of cells in the brain stem and spinal cord and through the pituitary and from there to other endocrine glands. Many areas of the cortex including the prefrontal, cingulated, and insular cortices, as well as the hippocampus and amygdala, are important in coordinating the autonomic response to stimuli.

Normal Functioning of the Autonomic Nervous System

The function of the autonomic nervous system is, in many ways, homeostatic and not one of survival. The autonomic nervous system is independent of the other systems of control within the body. Except in cases of complete inactivation or complete activation, disruptions of the autonomic system lead only to diminished homeostatic control of the visceral organs and not to problems of mortality. Once autonomic control is disrupted, the body is no longer capable of adapting to internal or external stresses of the environment. Both sympathetic and parasympathetic nerves innervate most of the organs. In general, the actions of each branch of the autonomic nervous system complement each other. Sympathetic nerves to the bronchi in the lung cause bronchodilation, whereas parasympathetic nerves cause bronchoconstriction. Some structures, including the adrenal gland, are only innervated by sympathetic fibers.

Disorders of the Autonomic Nervous System—Toxins and Sympathetic Storm

Perhaps the most relevant disorders of the autonomic nervous system for the pediatric intensivist are acute intoxications of agents related to the autonomic nervous system and the disorders called *sympathetic storm*. Several toxic and pharmacologic agents, such as cocaine, are capable of producing abrupt overactivity of the sympathetic and parasympathetic nervous systems. This leads to the combination of severe hypertension and mydriasis, coupled with signs of CNS excitation. Overdoses of tricyclic antidepressants produce autonomic effects including arrhythmias and cardiovascular instability. However, because of cholinergic blockade, the symptoms also include flushing, mydriasis, and dryness of the mouth. Organophosphate insecticides cause a combination of parasympathetic overactivity and motor paralysis.

Sympathetic storms have been described as paroxysms of hypertension, intense diaphoresis, flushed skin, and mydriasis, and their causes can be epilepsy or cerebral tumor, or they can be of unknown etiology. These attacks increase sweat secretion, and often the bed sheets are soaked. These attacks are thought to result from the removal of inhibitory influences on the hypothalamus, creating, in effect, a hypersensitive decorticated autonomic nervous system. Morphine and bromocriptine have been helpful in suppressing the syndrome, and β-adrenergic blockers reduce the hypertension and tachycardia.

During episodes of intense sympathetic discharge, there are alterations in the electrocardiogram (ECG), mainly in the ST segments and T waves; in extreme cases, evidence of myocardial damage can be observed. The role of direct sympathetic innervation of the heart in producing these myocardial abnormalities is unclear, but the surge in circulating norepinephrine and cortisol consequent to subarachnoid hemorrhage and trauma is postulated as the cause. A similar hyperadrenergic mechanism has been proposed to explain sudden death from fright, asthma, status epilepticus, and cocaine overdose. Recent investigations have suggested that sustained sympathetic overactivity is responsible for the hypertension of preeclampsia, which may be considered in some ways as a dysautonomic state.

The mature spinal cord is similar in organization to the primitive neural tube formed in the first days after conception (see Fig. 7.3). As the neural tube closes, a zone called the *mantle plate* develops, where neural stem cells reside and begin to proliferate. As the nervous system matures, the mantle plate (which will eventually become the gray

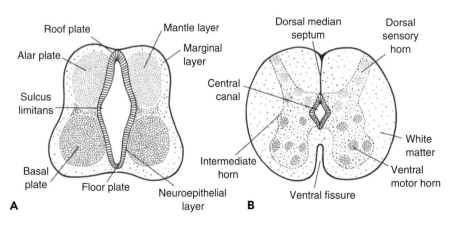

Figure 7.3 Spinal cord development and organization. Diagrams to show two successive stages of development of the spinal cord. Note the formation of the ventral motor and dorsal sensory horns. (From Sadler T. *Langman's medical embryology.* 9th ed. Baltimore, MD: Williams & Wilkins; 1995:381.)

matter of the spinal cord) is separated into an alar plate in the dorsal region and a basal plate in the ventral region. The alar plate cells become the ascending projection neurons of the dorsal spinal cord, relaying the sensations of touch and pain into the CNS through the dorsal columns. The basal plate cells become the motor neurons and interneurons of the ventral horn. A subset of basal plate cells within the thoracic and lumbar regions differentiate into autonomic neurons of the sympathetic nervous system. Similarly, basal cells in the brain stem and sacral regions form the autonomic neurons of the parasympathetic system.

NEURONAL FUNCTION

The capacity to respond to a vast array of environmental cues with complex behavioral, regulatory, and autonomic responses is dependent upon the fundamental biologic process of neurotransmission within specific anatomic circuits. In postnatal development, the neuroanatomic circuitry is refined by processes that include alterations in neuronal and glial populations, establishment of proper intercellular communications, and modification of neuronal connections by experience. During this critical period, integrated neurologic function is shaped and influenced by a broad range of factors including genetic composition, environmental exposures, life experience, toxins or pharmacologic agent exposure, and behavior. CNS injury and disease during this vulnerable phase can produce neurologic dysfunction by transiently or permanently disrupting neuroanatomic organizational structure at the micro- and/or macroanatomic level, leading to long-term consequences for the developing brain.

The purpose of this section is to review the functional cytology of neurons, mechanisms of interneuronal communication, and the patterns of neuronal connections that relate to consciousness and become relevant to infants and children with critical illness. Please refer to the section on "Structure and Development of the Central Nervous System" for a review of developmental neuroscience and details of glial cell biology.

Functional Cellular Anatomy

Although neurons are among of the most morphologically diverse cell types in the body, they share four functional compartments: a cell body, dendrites, an axon, and presynaptic terminal. In common with all cells, the neuronal cell body or soma contains structures such as the nucleus, mitochondria, and endoplasmic reticulum, as well as the Golgi apparatus (GA), ribosomes and polysomes, lysosomes, peroxisomes, microtubule-organizing center (MTOC), and a variety of transport vesicles (see Fig. 7.4). When neurons are stained with cresyl violet or other basic aniline dyes, the Nissl substance, or rough endoplasmic reticulum, becomes a prominent feature in the soma. The MTOC serves as the site of microtubule nucleation and synthesis in the

soma. Microtubules synthesized here are transported to the dendrites and axon. As discussed in subsequent text, some dendritic microtubules are synthesized in the dendrite, rather than in the soma. Regardless of the location of production of the microtubules, proper placement of microtubules and other cytoskeleton are vital to both the structure and function of the neuron.

Dendrites are specialized neuronal structures designed to receive and integrate incoming signals from numerous other neurons (Fig. 7.4). The expansion of dendritic branching is essential for synaptogenesis during postnatal development. All messenger ribonucleic acid (mRNA) is synthesized within the nucleus of the cell; however, it may be transported along the neuronal cytoskeleton to the dendritic processes that branch out from the soma through an energy-dependent process. Delivery of mRNA to the polysomes in the dendrite permits the translation of the proteins critical for synaptogenesis, including the microtubular component MAP2, at the site of synapse formation. Events that disrupt either the maturation of arborization or dendritic translation, such as hypoxia/ischemia and hypoglycemia, can have lasting effects on dendritic structure and synapse formation. Furthermore, dendrites also contain spines that are short extensions found most abundantly on the dendritic shaft of large pyramidal neurons. Each spine generally receives a single excitatory input; therefore, the number of spines is directly related to the magnitude of excitatory input to a particular neuron. Alterations in dendritic spine number and distribution have been recognized in diverse neurologic conditions, such as Alzheimer disease, traumatic brain injury, cerebral ischemia, mental retardation, and Down syndrome, and have been linked to cognitive disability. Experimental data suggest that spine pathology is a consequence of reduced excitatory input to the dendrite rather than a primary manifestation of neurologic disease.

Axons, the major signal-conducting feature of the neuron, are morphologically distinct from dendrites by their regular, nonbranching outline and by the uniform diameter throughout their length (Fig. 7.4). Many axons are much longer than dendrites, reaching up to 3 m in length. Microtubules within the axonal cytoskeleton provide the track for fast anterograde axonal transport of vesicles and organelles from the soma to the presynaptic terminal.

Loss of the axon leads to cell death, and many clinical conditions produce either a structural or functional axotomy, with resulting neurologic degeneration. For example, diffuse axonal injury is a well-recognized pathology associated with traumatic brain injury, and damage of axonal pathways contributes to functional morbidity after head injury. However, the pathogenic mechanisms contributing to traumatic axonal injury are complex, involving both axonal disruption caused by shearing at the time of the injury and delayed axotomy. Such delayed loss of the axon appears to result from disruption of the axonal membrane, which leads to increased concentrations of Ca^{2+}, accumulation of

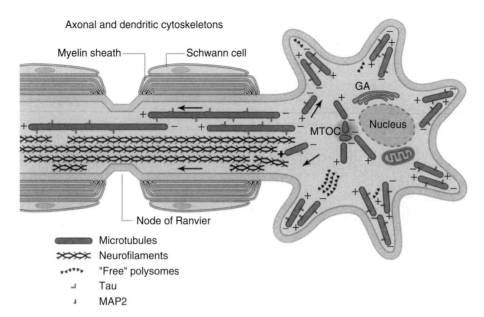

Axonal and dendritic cytoskeletons

Myelin sheath — Schwann cell

GA

MTOC Nucleus

Node of Ranvier

- ▬▬ Microtubules
- ⋙ Neurofilaments
- ⸽⸲ "Free" polysomes
- ⌐ Tau
- J MAP2

Figure 7.4 Cross-sectional structure of the neuronal cell body, with dendrites and the proximal region of the axon highlighting major organelles and cytoskeletal composition. In the cell body (structure in the right side of figure), the major cell organelles illustrated include the nucleus, mitochondria, Golgi apparatus (GA), the microtubule-organizing center (MTOC), and ''free'' polysomes. Microtubules dominate the cytoskeleton of the cell body, whereas the axonal structure is maintained by both microtubules and the longer, more organized neurofilaments. Microtubules have polarity, as indicated by + and − signs. In the dendrite, microtubules are oriented in opposite directions, whereas in the axon the negative end of the microtubule is oriented toward the cell body, with the positive end toward the synapse. MAP2 and tau are two of the many microtubular-associated proteins found in neurons. The wrapping of Schwann cells around the axon forms the myelin sheath. Regions of the axon devoid of Schwann cells are the nodes of Ranvier. (From Siegel GJ, Agranoff BW, Alberts RW, et al. (eds.) *Basic neurochemistry.* 6th ed. Philadelphia, PA: Lippincott-Raven Publishers; 1999.)

neurofilaments and amyloid precursor protein in the damaged axons, disruption of retrograde axonal transport, and ultimately to compromised functional recovery. However, in other situations, delayed axotomy has been observed in the absence of axolemma disruption. As suggested by this important example, elucidating the mechanisms of neurologic disease requires the integration of cellular anatomy with molecular processes.

The presynaptic terminal is the portion of the axon that makes contact with other cells. This structure is discussed with regard to individual NT systems in the section on "Neurotransmitter Biochemistry".

Basic Electrophysiology

Electric and chemical signals transmit information rapidly within and between neurons, often over considerable distances. In this section we discuss how ion compartmentalization establishes and maintains the resting membrane potential and describe how electric signals, called *action potentials*, are rapidly propagated along neurons by the activity of voltage-gated ion channels. The integration of electric and chemical signaling is illustrated by the examination of synaptic transmission.

Membrane Potential

At rest, the neuronal plasma membrane separates an excess of positive charges in the extracellular side from the excess negative charges on the intracellular side (see Fig. 7.5). This charge separation gives rise to a voltage across the neuronal membrane called the *resting membrane potential* (V_m). By convention, the potential on the outside of the membrane is 0, making the $V_m = -40$ to -70 mV. Sodium and chloride ions are found in high abundance in the extracellular environment, whereas potassium ions dominate inside the neuron. When these positively charged (cations) or negatively charged (anions) ions move down their concentration gradient across the membrane, an electric current is generated. The voltage required to prevent the movement of an ion across a cell membrane is known as the *equilibrium potential*. The equilibrium potential, also known as the *Nernst potential* (E_{ion}), is determined by (i) the temperature of the neuronal environment, (ii) the valence of the ion, and (iii) the concentration of the ion inside and outside the neuron. This relationship is defined by the Nernst equation:

$$E_{ion} = (RT/zF) \ln \frac{[ion]_o}{[ion]_i}$$

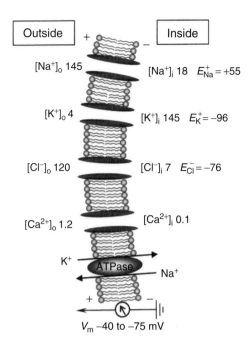

Figure 7.5 Determinants of the resting membrane potential (V_m): electrochemical and concentration differential driving forces. Ion-specific protein channels in the membrane act as pores for the movement of ions across the semipermeable lipid membrane. The membrane separates excess positive charge outside the neuron from negative charges inside. This creates an electrochemical driving force for cations to flow into the neuron, whereas the driving force for anions is outward. Concentration gradients for Na^+, K^+, and Cl^- also determine the direction of ion movement. Equilibrium potentials (E_{Na}^+, E_K^+, E_{Cl}^-) are listed. The ionic balance across the membrane is maintained by a transmembrane protein pump that hydrolyzes ATP to ADP (ATPase) to move Na^+ out of the neuron in exchange for one K^+. Ion concentrations are in millimolar units.

where R is the gas constant (8.315 J/K/mol), T is the temperature in Kelvin ($T_{kelvin} = 273.16 + T_{celsius}$), z is the valence of the ion, F is Faraday constant (96,485 C per mol), ln is the natural log, $[ion]_o$ is the extracellular concentration of the ion, and $[ion]_i$ is the intracellular concentration of the ion.

Although lipid bilayer plasma membranes are impermeable to ions, channels and pumps provide portals through which ions pass across membranes creating ion currents. These transmembrane ion currents or conductances cause changes in the resting membrane potential and are the basis for electric signaling in neurons. Therefore, controlling the opening and closing of ion channels and the activity of ion pumps is critical to the maintenance of the resting membrane potential, as well as to the generation of the action potential.

Similar to the equilibrium potential, the resting membrane potential of a neuron is determined by the *membrane permeability* and *concentration gradients* of the three most abundant ionic species across the neuronal membrane, Na^+, K^+, and Cl^-. This relationship is defined by the

Goldman equation:

$$V_m = (RT/F) \ln \frac{P_K[K^+]_o + P_{Na}[Na^+]_o + P_{Cl}[Cl^-]_i}{P_K[K^+]_i + P_{Na}[Na^+]_i + P_{Cl}[Cl^-]_o}$$

where R is the gas constant (8.315 J/K/mol); T is the temperature in Kelvin ($T_{kelvin} = 273.16 + T_{celsius}$); F is Faraday constant (96,485 C per mol); ln is the natural log; P_{Na}, P_K, and P_{Cl} are the relative permeability of the membrane to each ion; o is the concentration of the ion outside the neuron; and i is the concentration of the ion inside the neuron. At rest, the neuron is most permeable to potassium ion ($P_K:P_{Na}:P_{Cl}$ is 1:0.04:0.45). At 37°C, the equation can be simplified to:

$$V_m = 61.5 \log_{10} \frac{P_K[K^+]_o + P_{Na}[Na^+]_o + P_{Cl}[Cl^-]_i}{P_K[K^+]_i + P_{Na}[Na^+]_i + P_{Cl}[Cl^-]_o}$$

where $V_m = -73$ mV.

The flux of an ion across the membrane is the product of the electrochemical driving force (ion concentration gradient + electrostatic forces) and the membrane permeability or conductance, as defined by the Goldman equation (Fig. 7.5). For example, in the mammalian neuron, the electrochemical force would drive Na^+ into the more negatively charged cell. However, because there are few Na^+ channels open at rest, Na^+ permeability, or conductance, is low, making overall Na^+ influx small. On the other hand, the concentration gradient for K^+ would direct it out of the cell, whereas the negative membrane potential inside the cell works to stabilize intracellular K^+ and, therefore, almost balances the efflux. Thus, the net electrochemical force for K^+ produces a small efflux. This small K^+ efflux is equal to the previously described small Na^+ influx.

The movement of cations into, or anions out of, a neuron causes the membrane potential to become more positive (or less negative) and is referred to as *depolarization* (see Fig. 7.6, upper panel). Conversely, a more negative (or less positive) membrane potential is called *hyperpolarization*. When the depolarization voltage reaches a threshold level, voltage-gated ion channels open to produce the *action potential*.

Action Potential Dynamics

The action potential is a propagating, nondegrading (only when myelination is complete and uncompromised), regenerative electric signal characteristic of neurons. Sodium and potassium currents through voltage-gated channels are responsible for the specialized features of action potentials.

Using the voltage-clamp technique, Alan Hodgkin and Andrew Huxley were able to elucidate the specific ionic conductances that underlie the action potential (Fig. 7.6, upper panel). They found that when the resting membrane potential depolarizes to a threshold level, voltage-gated Na^+ channels open to facilitate a rapid influx of Na^+ ions. As Na^+ enters the cell, the membrane becomes increasingly depolarized (less negative inside), more Na^+ channels open, the Na^+ conductance increases further, and net membrane

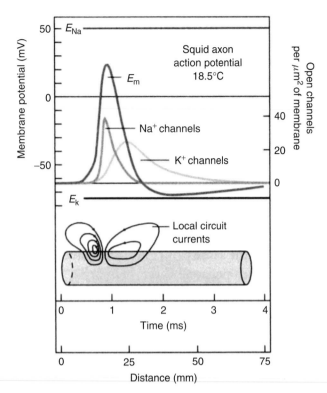

Figure 7.6 Hodgkin-Huxley model of action potential propagation in neurons. **Upper:** Action potential (E_m), where the membrane is depolarized to +25 mV from a resting membrane potential of −62 mV. Depolarization starts out slowly until a threshold potential is reached (approximately −50 mV), when voltage-gated Na^+ channels open, and Na^+ rushes into the neuron to produce the rapid depolarization potential that is characteristic of the E_m. At the threshold potential, voltage-sensitive K^+ channels also open, and K^+ moves more slowly out of the neuron to repolarize the membrane. K^+ conductance leads to a more negative V_m (approximately −75 mV) called *membrane hyperpolarization*. During the period of hyperpolarization, the neuron is refractory to the generation of another action potential. **Lower:** Propagation of the action potential in an unmyelinated fiber by local circuit currents. (From Siegel GJ, Agranoff BW, Alberts RW, et al. (eds.) *Basic neurochemistry.* 6th ed. Philadelphia, PA: Lippincott-Raven Publishers; 1999.)

potential finally becomes positive. At the peak of the action potential, the membrane is 500 times more permeable to Na^+ than K^+ (P_K:P_{Na}:P_{Cl} is 1.0:20:0.45). Using the Goldman equation again, V_m = +44 mV. When Na^+ current is maximal, voltage-sensitive K^+ channels are also activated, allowing an outward K^+ current that causes the membrane to repolarize. During this period, Na^+ channels are inactivated.

In unmyelinated axons, such as those found in early postnatal life, the action potential is propagated by local circuit currents along the length of the axon (Fig. 7.6, lower panel). In the CNS, mature oligodendrocytes produce myelin that insulates the axon. Similarly, in the PNS, Schwann cells serve the same function as they wrap themselves around axons, leaving short segments of the axons exposed (nodes of Ranvier). Action potentials in

myelinated fibers can be generated only at the nodes of Ranvier. Therefore, an action potential generated in one node will induce the depolarization of its neighboring node. This results in the rapid propagation of the action potential from node to node, called *saltatory conduction*. Therefore, axonal myelination increases the speed of action potential propagation, and demyelination of axons in neurologic diseases such as multiple sclerosis results in slowed action potential conduction.

Synaptic Transmission

The synapse is a structure formed by the interaction of two neurons (or a neuron and a muscle fiber) for communication. Synapses can be either electric or chemical; our discussion here focuses only on chemical synapses between two neurons (see Fig. 7.7). The neuromuscular junction (NMJ), a specialized synapse, is discussed in a later section.

At a chemical synapse, a rapidly propagated electric signal is converted to a graded chemical signal. Although this special structure can amplify a neuronal signal and produce excitatory or inhibitory actions, chemical synapses slow signal propagation. The prototypical chemical synapse involves the vesicular release of a chemical neurotransmitter from a presynaptic neuron, thereby transmitting the signal to the postsynaptic neuron. Signal transmission requires close proximity of the pre- and postsynaptic neurons and involves a stereotyped series of steps coupling an action potential to the release of chemical neurotransmitters. When an action potential arrives at the presynaptic terminal or bouton, the voltage-gated Ca^{2+} channels open to allow Ca^{2+} to influx. The increased [Ca^{2+}] in the terminal rapidly causes specific proteins in the neurotransmitter-containing vesicle membrane, including synaptobrevin and synaptotagmin, to dock to proteins (syntaxin and synaptosome-associated protein 25 kDa [SNAP-25]) in the presynaptic membrane. Synaptobrevin, syntaxin, and SNAP-25 are targets for cleavage by tetanus toxin and seven types of botulinum toxin. Acting as endopeptidases, these neurotoxins effectively inhibit transmitter release. The clinical manifestations of these toxins, such as infantile botulism and tetanus, are discussed more fully in Chapter 46.

Once the vesicle docks, its membrane fuses with the presynaptic membrane, releasing a discrete quantity of neurotransmitter into the synaptic cleft, called a *quantum*. These neurotransmitters can then bind directly to ion channels called *inotropic receptors* or to *metabotropic receptors* that are linked to ion channels by a second messenger, such as cAMP. The result, alteration in ionic conductance in the postsynaptic neuron, is the same whether the neurotransmitter binds to inotropic or metabotropic receptors. However, ion fluxes in the postsynaptic neuron can be either excitatory or inhibitory.

Removal of a neurotransmitter from the postsynaptic receptor will turn off this neurochemical signal. Neurotransmitter activity is terminated by three mechanisms:

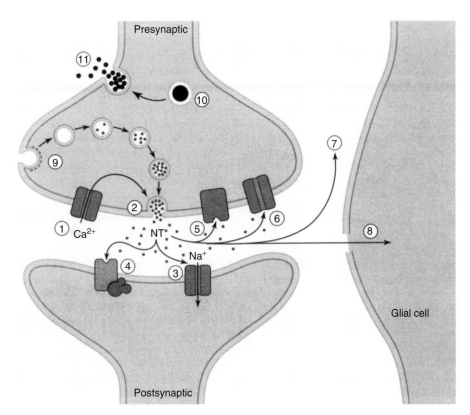

Figure 7.7 Schematic representation of a synapse with a classical neurotransmitter. The space between the presynaptic nerve terminal (upper neuron) and the postsynaptic nerve (lower neuron) is the synapse. The glial cell on the *right* represents a typical astroglia. Synaptic transmission is initiated when an action potential reaches the presynaptic nerve terminal and opens voltage-sensitive Ca^{2+} channels (*1*). Ca^{2+} flows into the terminal, resulting in the binding of synaptic vesicles, containing the neurotransmitter (NT), to the presynaptic membrane. NT is released into the synaptic cleft by exocytosis (*2*). The released NT binds to postsynaptic membrane receptors that are coupled to ion channels either directly (*3*) or indirectly through second messenger systems (*4*). NT receptors in the presynaptic membrane either inhibit or enhance further release of NT, which is removed from the synaptic cleft by (a) enzymatic degradation (*5*), (b) reuptake by a transport protein coupled to a Na^+ gradient (*6*), (c) diffusion from the cleft (*7*), or (d) uptake and metabolism by glial cells (*8*). The synaptic vesicle membrane is recycled (*9*). Neuropeptides are stored in dense granules that are distinct from the synapse (*10*) and are released after repetitive stimulation (*11*). (From Siegel GJ, Agranoff BW, Alberts RW, et al. (eds.) *Basic neurochemistry*. 6th ed. Philadelphia, PA: Lippincott-Raven Publishers; 1999.)

(i) diffusion away from receptor sites, (ii) enzymatic inactivation, and (iii) transport (reuptake) into the presynaptic terminal or surrounding glial cells. Diffusion, is the simplest method of stopping continuous stimulation of postsynaptic receptors; however, it is also unpredictable and inefficient. Enzymatic inactivation is the most efficient method of neurotransmitter inactivation. As highlighted later, specific pharmacologic agents have been developed to enhance or inhibit such enzymatically based systems to modulate neuronal signaling. The third method for terminating the process of neurotransmitter activity, reuptake, exhibits the properties of active membrane transport systems, including agonist specificity, saturability, and directionality. In the next section, we discuss the specific aspects of synaptic transmission as related to the major neurotransmitters in the CNS.

Neurotransmitter Biochemistry

Neurotransmitters are chemicals that convey information between neurons. In this section, we consider the major steps of chemical neurotransmission for select neurotransmitters that play a role in pediatric critical illness: acetylcholine, catecholamines (norepinephrine and dopamine), γ-amino butyric acid (GABA), glutamate, nitric oxide, and serotonin (5-HT).

Acetylcholine

Cholinergic projection neurons and interneurons are widely distributed in the forebrain and brain stem. Basal forebrain cholinergic neuron groups innervate the cerebral cortex, as well as the hippocampus and amygdala. Pontine cholinergic neurons send descending projections to the brain stem reticular formation and provide extensive cholinergic innervation to the thalamus. These cholinergic neurons are important in a variety of physiologic and disease states. During rapid eye movement (REM) sleep, ascending pontine projections activate thalamic GABAergic neurons, causing asynchronous firing of cortical projection neurons detected as low-voltage waves in the EEG. Two acetylcholine-containing neuronal populations have been intensively studied because of their relationship to neurodegenerative diseases. A cluster of cholinergic neurons that project from the basal forebrain to the cortex undergoes degeneration in Alzheimer disease. Degeneration of the nigrostriatal dopamine pathway in Parkinson disease leads to increased activity of cholinergic interneurons in the striatum and, subsequently, to increased basal ganglia output to the thalamus. Cholinergic receptor antagonists can be used to downregulate basal ganglia overactivity.

Biosynthesis and Storage of Acetylcholine in the Presynaptic Neuron

Acetylcholine is synthesized by the one-step transfer of the acetyl group from acetyl-CoA, generated by glucose metabolism, to choline (Fig 7.14). Choline is present in the plasma and is transported into cholinergic neurons by a low-affinity choline transporter. The cytosolic enzyme choline acetyltransferase (ChAT) catalyzes the synthesis of acetylcholine in the synaptic terminal. Once synthesized in the cytosol, acetylcholine is transported into the vesicles by the vesicular cholinergic transporter, where it is stored.

Release of Acetylcholine into the Synaptic Cleft and Binding of Acetylcholine to Synaptic Receptors

Acetylcholine is released by exocytosis, diffuses across the synaptic cleft, and binds to its postsynaptic receptor. There are two major classes of cholinergic receptors on the basis of agonist- and antagonist-binding profiles: nicotinic and muscarinic. The plant alkaloid, nicotine, is an agonist for a subclass of acetylcholine receptors (AChR), called *nicotinic acetylcholine receptors* (nAChR). The nAChR is a transmembrane structure composed of five cylindrical protein subunits oriented parallel through the membrane to form a pore. These receptors are composed of two types of subunits, α and β; to date, nine distinct α and five β subunits have been cloned. With 14 different subunits available to assemble in any combination to form nAChRs, a myriad of pentameric structures with a wide diversity of functions are possible. When two acetylcholine molecules bind to an nAChR, the receptor conformation changes to open an ion channel. Negatively charged amino acids, oriented toward the central pore, allow only cations, including Na^+, K^+, and Ca^{2+}, to pass through the channel down their respective concentration gradients.

Muscarinic receptors (mAChRs) are found in both presynaptic and postsynaptic membranes. In the CNS, binding of acetylcholine to presynaptic AChR typically inhibits the further release of acetylcholine. Of the five members of the mAChR family, M1, M3, and M4 are the major subtypes localized to the brain. Muscarinic AChRs mediate the effects of acetylcholine indirectly through modulation of three different G protein–signaling systems (see Fig. 7.8). Typical of metabotropic receptors, M1 and M3 mAChRs are coupled to G proteins that activate phospholipase C, leading to the generation of inositol-1,4,5-triphosphate (IP_3) and diacylglycerol (DAG). Acetylcholine binding to M4 mAChR in some neurons will cause the dissociation of the α from $\beta\gamma$ G protein subunits, thereby inhibiting adenylyl cyclase (AC). In the third biochemical response mediated by mAChR, the M4 subtype regulates the activation of a G protein–coupled, inwardly rectifying potassium channel, producing hyperpolarization.

Inactivation of Released Acetylcholine

Acetylcholine inactivation is primarily by enzymatic processes, with diffusion playing a minor role in its removal from the synapse. Acetylcholinesterase (AChE), the enzyme that hydrolyzes acetylcholine to choline, is a secretory enzyme located at the plasma membrane of the presynaptic and postsynaptic neurons. Therefore, acetylcholine hydrolysis to choline and acetic acid takes place extracellularly, with the released choline being recycled back into the presynaptic neuron by the low-affinity choline transporter.

Nerve agents, such as sarin, V agents, and organophosphates, bind irreversibly to the active site of AchE and prevents the hydrolysis of acetylcholine. The resulting persistent activation of AChR causes uncontrolled acetylcholine stimulation, leading to fatigue of the AChR. The depolarizing neuromuscular blocker, succinylcholine, acts by the same principle, but in this case, serum cholinesterases can hydrolyze succinylcholine and therefore prevent acetylcholine-receptor fatigue. Once inactivated, AChE cannot be reactivated, so clinical improvement occurs only after new AChE is synthesized.

Catecholamines

Catecholamines serve as neurotransmitters in the central and peripheral nervous system, and may modulate hormonal functions. This discussion focuses on the synthesis and release of these transmitters from central dopaminergic, noradrenergic, and adrenergic neurons.

Dopamine neurons are localized in four cell groups: (i) the midbrain, including the substantia nigra pars compacta; (ii) the dorsal and periventricular hypothalamus; (iii) the olfactory bulb; and (iv) the retina. The midbrain dopaminergic cells provide major ascending pathways to the striatum, frontotemporal cortex, and limbic system. The nigrostriatal pathway likely participates in the initiation of movement because degeneration of these dopaminergic neurons forms the neurobiologic basis of Parkinson disease. Mesocortical and mesolimbic dopaminergic pathways have been implicated in memory, cognition, and emotion. Dopamine-releasing neurons in the dorsal hypothalamus project to the lower brain stem and spinal cord

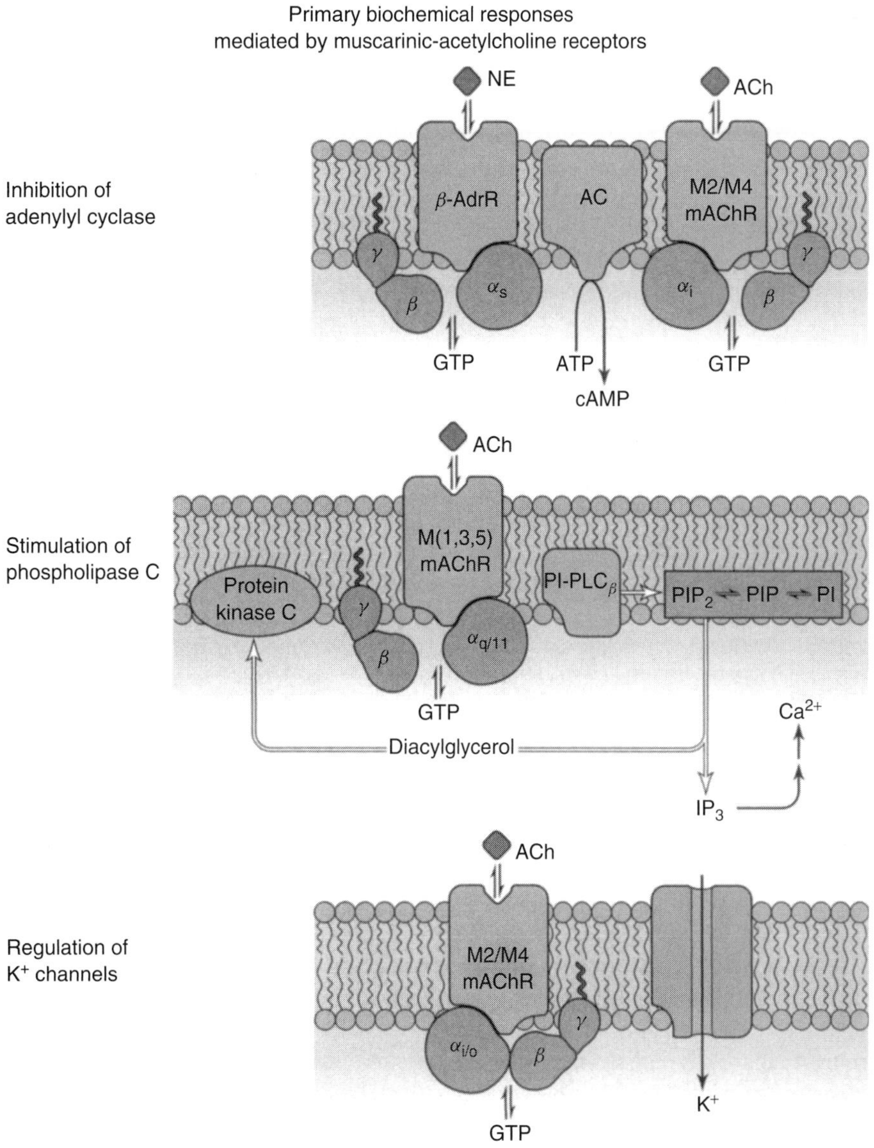

Primary biochemical responses
mediated by muscarinic-acetylcholine receptors

Inhibition of
adenylyl cyclase

Stimulation of
phospholipase C

Regulation of
K$^+$ channels

Figure 7.8 Three primary biochemical responses mediated by muscarinic acetylcholine receptors. Acetylcholine (ACh) interacts with five types of muscarinic acetylcholine receptors (mAChRs). The biochemical response of ACh binding depends upon the second messenger system that is linked to receptor subtype. (a) Inhibition of adenylyl cyclase (AC): When ACh binds to M2/M4 mAChR, subunits of the guanosine triphosphate (GTP)-binding protein dissociate and inhibit AC, leading to decreased production of the second messenger, cAMP. (b) Stimulation of phosphoinositide-specific phospholipase C$_\beta$ (PI-PLC$_\beta$): When ACh binds to M1/M3/M5 mAChR, subunits of the GTP-binding protein, G$_q$, dissociate and activate PI-PLC$_\beta$ to produce the second messengers inositol-1,4,5-triphosphate (IP$_3$) and diacylglycerol (DAG). (c) Regulation of K$^+$ channels: When acetylcholine binds to M2/M4 mAChR, a K$^+$ channel in the $\beta\gamma$ subunit of G$_i$ opens, allowing inward K$^+$ conductance that hyperpolarizes the cell. β-AdrR, β-adrenergic receptor; NE, norepinephrine; PI, phosphatidylinositol; PIP, phosphatidylinositol-4-phosphate; PIP$_2$, phosphatidylinositol-4,5-bisphosphate. (From Siegel GJ, Agranoff BW, Alberts RW, et al. (eds.) *Basic neurochemistry.* 6th ed. Philadelphia, PA: Lippincott-Raven Publishers; 1999.)

to regulate sympathetic preganglionic neurons. The second dopaminergic hypothalamic cell group, composed of neurons in the periventricular and arcuate nuclei, are part of the tuberoinfundibular hypothalamic neuroendocrine system. Dopamine released from these cells into the hypophyseal portal circulation inhibits prolactin release. Groups of dopaminergic neurons are also found in the olfactory system and the retina.

Noradrenergic cell bodies are located only in the pons and medulla. The pontine locus ceruleus, which maintains responsiveness to unexpected environmental stimuli, provides extensive ascending output to the thalamus, hypothalamus, hippocampus, and cerebral cortex, as well as the descending projections to the brain stem, cerebellum, and spinal cord. Norepinephrine-containing neuronal cell bodies in the medulla ascend to the supraoptic and paraventricular hypothalamic nuclei to contribute to the control

of cardiovascular and endocrine functions. Descending projections to the spinal cord modulate autonomic reflexes and pain sensation.

Epinephrine-synthesizing neurons are limited to two clusters in the medulla. The neurons in the dorsal medulla contribute to the nucleus of the solitary tract. The dorsal medulla adrenergic neurons descend to the sympathetic preganglionic column to provide tonic input to vasomotor neurons, whereas the ventrolateral medulla neurons ascend to the hypothalamus, where they modulate cardiovascular and endocrine responses.

Biosynthesis of Catecholamines in the Presynaptic Neuron

The synthesis of norepinephrine begins with the accumulation of L-tyrosine in the presynaptic neurons. L-tyrosine is hydroxylated by tyrosine hydroxylase to produce L-dopa, which is rapidly converted to dopamine by L-aromatic amino acid decarboxylase (also called *DOPA decarboxylase*). Dopamine is then transported into the vesicles by the vesicular monoamine transporter (VMAT). In dopaminergic neurons, this is the final step in transmitter synthesis. In noradrenergic neurons, dopamine is oxidized to norepinephrine within the vesicle by dopamine β-hydroxylase. Specific pharmacologic interventions can affect the biosynthesis of catecholamines and can therefore exert their CNS effects. One example is reserpine, an early antipsychotic agent that inhibits VMAT, leading to depletion of vesicular stores of dopamine.

Synthesis of catecholamines is controlled at several levels. Under basal conditions, tyrosine hydroxylase is the rate-limiting enzyme for norepinephrine synthesis. When neuronal activity is increased, the rate-limiting enzyme is dopamine β-hydroxylase.

Storage of Catecholamines in the Presynaptic Nerve Terminal

In the synaptic environment, most norepinephrine is stored in presynaptic vesicles, whereas a small portion is free within the terminal. The compartmentalization of norepinephrine in synaptic terminal vesicles provides three key advantages over unbound neurotransmitter: (i) the neurotransmitter is in close proximity to the synapse, (ii) it cannot diffuse out of the synaptic terminal, and (iii) it is protected from exposure to degrading enzymes.

Release of Catecholamines into the Synaptic Cleft

Norepinephrine and other catecholamines are released from synaptic vesicles through calcium-mediated exocytosis, as described in the preceding text. In addition, nonvesicular norepinephrine in the synaptic terminal can enter the synaptic cleft by the reversal of catecholamine reuptake transporters found in the synaptic terminal; this is discussed more fully in the subsequent text.

Binding of Catecholamines by Synaptic Receptors

In the nervous system, norepinephrine binds to two subclasses of adrenergic receptors: α_2 and β_1. The predominant presynaptic receptor, the α_2-adrenergic receptor, acts generally by inhibiting the release of norepinephrine through inhibition of adenylyl cyclase. β_1-Receptors, on the other hand, stimulate adenylyl cyclase to increase cAMP. At present, five dopamine receptor subtypes have been recognized in the CNS. Although two of these stimulate adenylyl cyclase, the remainder inhibits adenylyl cyclase.

Inactivation of Released Catecholamines

Removal of the neurotransmitter from its postsynaptic receptor will turn off the neurochemical signal. In common with all neurotransmitters, norepinephrine synaptic signaling is terminated by diffusion, enzymatic inactivation, and reuptake into the presynaptic terminal. Diffusion is the least efficient method for termination of norepinephrine signaling. Catabolism of catecholamines, including norepinephrine, is a major means of neurotransmitter inactivation. The two mitochondrial enzymes, monoamine oxidase (MAO) and catechol-O-methyltransferase (COMT), act in concert to catabolize catecholamines. In the CNS, the isoform MAO_A has a high affinity for norepinephrine and is inhibited by tranylcypromine.

The active transport of catecholamines into the synaptic terminal is the primary means of terminating the activity of this class of neurotransmitters. The norepinephrine transporter is a high-affinity, saturable, transmembrane protein. When norepinephrine accumulates in the synaptic terminal, it can be either transported back into a synaptic vesicle to be released again or can be metabolized by MAO and COMT in the outer mitochondrial membrane to an inactive metabolite. As norepinephrine transport is dependent on Na^+ cotransport, inhibition of the Na^+/K^+-ATPase will reduce the Na^+ concentration gradient, thereby inhibiting norepinephrine reuptake. Pharmacologic manipulation of synaptic catecholamines and serotonin, as discussed later, have been the mainstay of therapy for clinical depression. Increasing norepinephrine levels with MAO_A inhibitors had been a mainstay for treatment of depression. Despite their therapeutic effects, MAO inhibitors require a diet low in tyramine to prevent hypertensive crisis and a careful attention to drug interactions. Therefore, newer agents that increase extracellular norepinephrine by inhibiting reuptake have essentially replaced MAO inhibitors for the treatment of clinical depression. Tricyclic antidepressants achieve the same therapeutic effect by inhibiting the norepinephrine transporter.

γ-Amino Butyric Acid

GABA is the principal inhibitory neurotransmitter in the brain. Until recently, it was thought that GABA was localized predominately to cortical interneurons. However, it is now recognized that long-axoned GABA neurons project from the striatum to the midbrain, superior colliculus, and thalamus. The biochemistry of the GABAergic synapse follows the broad themes described in the preceding text.

Biosynthesis and Storage of γ-Amino Butyric Acid in the Presynaptic Neuron

Glucose is the primary precursor of GABA. α-Ketoglutarate, formed by the Krebs cycle, is transaminated to glutamate by GABA α-oxoglutarate transaminase (GABA-T) in the mitochondria. Glutamate is exported from the mitochondria to the cytosolic compartment, where, by the action of glutamic acid decarboxylase, it is converted to GABA. Because glutamic acid decarboxylase is found only in cells that use GABA as a neurotransmitter, antibodies raised against glutamic acid decarboxylase are used as a marker for GABAergic neurons. Once synthesized, GABA is concentrated in synaptic vesicles.

Release of γ-Amino Butyric Acid into the Synaptic Cleft and Binding of γ-Amino Butyric Acid to Synaptic Receptors

Similar to other inotropic receptors, GABA binding produces a conformational change that permits Cl^- to flow into the neuron, producing a hyperpolarization and moving the membrane potential away from the threshold potential. Therefore, GABA serves to stabilize the neuronal membrane by making it less likely to reach the threshold potential. There are two distinct classes of synaptic GABA receptors: $GABA_A$ and $GABA_B$. The $GABA_A$ receptor is a heteropentameric complex with four different subunits. In addition, the $GABA_A$ receptor is a Cl–channel, with positively charged amino acids located near the pore opening to provide electrostatic specificity.

$GABA_B$ receptors localized to the presynaptic membrane participate in feedback loops to inhibit further release of GABA. Unlike their postsynaptic counterparts, presynaptic $GABA_B$ receptors are ionotropic in nature. Binding of GABA to this ionotropic receptor opens the channel to permit K^+ conductance. In the postsynaptic membrane, activation of $GABA_B$ receptors opens K^+ channels indirectly through a G protein that inhibits adenylyl cyclase to produce a slow inhibitory potential.

Inactivation of Released γ-Amino Butyric Acid

A distinguishing characteristic of amino acid neurotransmitters, such as GABA and glutamate, is their removal from the synaptic cleft by uptake into glial cells. At least three presynaptic membrane GABA transporters also participate in the termination of the GABA signal by reuptake and storage of GABA into synaptic vesicles. Vigabatrin, an antiepileptic drug currently in the market, specifically inhibits glial GABA transport and metabolism.

Glutamate

Glutamate is the major excitatory neurotransmitter in the brain. Glutamatergic neurons are widely distributed in the brain. As an amino acid neurotransmitter, many of its biochemical characteristics are shared with GABA and are discussed briefly in the subsequent text.

Biosynthesis and Storage of Glutamate in the Presynaptic Neuron

Glutamate is synthesized locally in the brain because it cannot cross the blood–brain barrier (see Fig. 7.9). As mentioned in the preceding text, glutamate is formed from glucose through the Krebs cycle. In glial cells, glutamate can also be formed directly from glutamine through the action of glutamate synthase. Glutamine diffuses out of the glial cell and into the neuron, where it is converted back

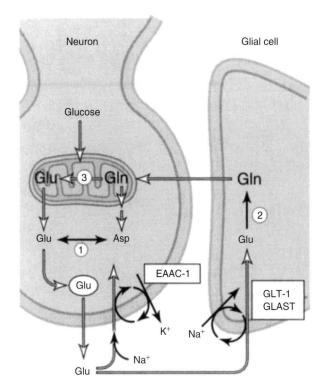

Figure 7.9 Glutamate synapse. Glutamate (Glu) is synthesized in the nerve terminal by transamination ① of aspartate (Asp) or conversion of glutamine (Gln) by glutaminase ③ in the mitochondria. Once synthesized, glutamate is stored in vesicles in the presynaptic terminal. The glutamate neurotransmitter signal is terminated by the active transport of glutamate back into the nerve terminal by the excitatory amino acid carrier-1 (EAAC-1). However, glial cells take up most of the glutamate using the glutamate transporter-1 (GLT-1) and the glutamate aspartate transporter (GLAST). In the glial cell, glu is converted to gln by glutamine synthetase, which diffuses back into the nerve terminal for conversion again to glutamate. (From Siegel GJ, Agranoff BW, Alberts RW, et al. (eds.) *Basic neurochemistry*. 6th ed. Philadelphia, PA: Lippincott-Raven Publishers; 1999.)

to glutamate, and is then concentrated through a vesicular transporter into secretory granules.

Release of Glutamate into the Synaptic Cleft and Binding of Glutamate to Postsynaptic Receptors

Two molecular families of glutamate receptors, inotropic and metabotropic, mediate most of the excitatory signaling in the brain and spinal cord (see Fig. 7.10). Within these classes of glutamate receptors, the subunit composition present on the postsynaptic neuron governs the quality, magnitude, and direction of the response to a neurotransmitter. Given the diversity of its postsynaptic receptors, a single class of neurotransmitters, such as glutamate, can produce a wide array of effects.

Glutamate binding to an inotropic receptor induces a conformational change in the five transmembrane receptor subunits, increasing the diameter of the ionic pore and

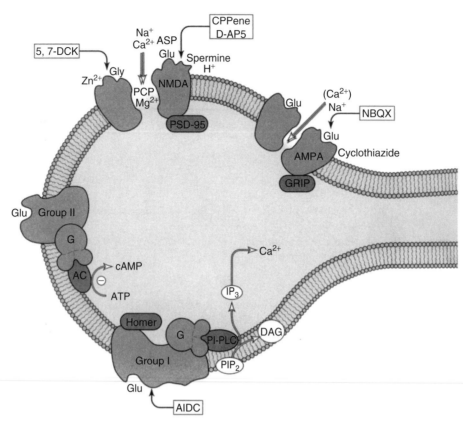

Figure 7.10 Schematic views of four types of glutamate receptors. Two ionotropic receptors, *N*-methyl-D-aspartate (NMDA) and α-amino-3-hydroxy-5-methyl-4-isoxazole propionic acid (AMPA) receptors, as well as group I and group II metabotropic receptors are shown. Competitive antagonists of each receptor are boxed. The NMDA receptor channel is blocked by Mg^{2+} and phencyclidine (PCP). Cyclothiazide removes desensitization of AMPA receptors. Both classes of metabotropic receptor are coupled through G proteins (*G*) to intracellular enzymes, phosphoinositide-specific phospholipase C (PI-PLC) for group I receptors and adenylyl cyclase (AC) for group II receptors. PI-PLC catalyzes the production of inositol-1,4,5-triphosphate (IP_3) and diacylglycerol (DAG) from phosphatidylinositol-4,5-bisphosphate (PIP_2). The resulting increase in cytoplasmic IP_3 triggers release of Ca^{2+} from intracellular stores. Activation of group II metabotropic glutamate receptors typically results in inhibition of AC. The cytoplasmic proteins PSD-95, GRIP, and Homer anchor the receptors to synaptic membranes by forming a bridge between the receptor and cytoskeletal structures. AIDC, 1-aminoindan-1,5-dicarboxylate; 5,7-DCK, 5,7-dichlorokynurenic acid; D-AP5, D-2-amino-5-phosphonopentanoic acid; CPPene, 3-(2-carboxypiperazin-4-yl)1-propenyl-1-phosphoric acid; NBQX, 6-nitro 7-sulfamobenzo[f] quinoxaline-2,3-dione. (From Siegel GJ, Agranoff BW, Alberts RW, et al. (eds.) *Basic neurochemistry.* 6th ed. Philadelphia, PA: Lippincott-Raven Publishers; 1999.)

directly allowing the influx of calcium into the postsynaptic neuron. The ionotropic glutamate receptors have been pharmacologically classified into NMDA and non-NMDA subtypes on the basis of agonist binding. Activation of NMDA receptors is associated with processes critical to brain development, learning, and memory. On the other hand, in the setting of epilepsy, hypoxia, ischemia, and traumatic brain injury, activation of NMDA receptors contributes to neuronal degeneration. Because of the pivotal role of NMDA receptors in both normal and pathologic CNS function, the regulation of these receptors is described in fuller detail in the subsequent text. Kainite and α-amino-3-hydroxy-5-methyl-4-isoxazole propionic acid (AMPA)

receptors are the two classes of non-NMDA receptors generally responsible for fast excitatory synaptic transmission mediated by glutamate.

Binding of glutamate to a seven-subunit, metabotropic family receptor activates a G protein–coupled second messenger system that indirectly gates ion channels. As seen in AChR, both adenylyl cyclase and phosphoinositide-specific phospholipase C participate in intracellular signal transduction when glutamate binds to metabotropic receptors.

The NMDA receptor possesses unique properties of a neurotransmitter receptor (Fig. 7.10). First, the NMDA receptor requires the binding of two agonists for activation. Both glycine (or serine and alanine) and glutamate (or NMDA) must simultaneously occupy their respective binding sites on the extracellular domain for receptor activation to occur. Second, when the membrane is depolarized, Mg^{2+} is released from its binding site within the ion channel of the NMDA receptor, permitting the influx of Ca^{2+} and Na^+ into the postsynaptic neuron in exchange for potassium. Therefore, both coordinate glycine and glutamate binding and membrane depolarization are required for receptor activation. Third, numerous binding sites for regulator molecules have been identified on NMDA receptors to tightly control ion-channel opening. For example, binding of H^+ to the NMDA proton-binding site will allosterically inhibit ion flux. Conversely, occupation of the polyamine-binding site with spermine or spermidine relieves the proton inhibition and, therefore, potentiates NMDA activation at lower pH. In addition to the Mg^{2+}-binding site within the ion pore, there are binding sites for Zn^{2+}, dizocilpine (MK-801), ketamine, and phencyclidine (PCP). The NMDA channel must be open for the latter three agents to reach their binding sites, but once bound with the pore, it is difficult to remove these antagonists.

In the setting of hypoxia/ischemia, traumatic brain injury, and stroke, glutamate release is increased in the brain. As more glutamate is available in the synapse, activation of postsynaptic NMDA receptors increases, causing an excessive and damaging Ca^{2+} influx into the postsynaptic neuron. Therefore, modulation of Ca^{2+} flux through the NMDA receptor channel has been proposed and investigated as a neuroprotective strategy for brain injury.

Inactivation of Released Glutamate

The efficient removal of glutamate from the synaptic cleft is required to prevent prolonged stimulation of the postsynaptic receptors with excessive flux of Ca^{2+} into the postsynaptic neuron (Fig. 7.9). Such persistent or excessive stimulation of glutamate receptors is an important mechanism of neuronal death in neurodegenerative disorders such as ischemia, traumatic brain injury, and amyotrophic lateral sclerosis (ALS). Because glutamate cannot diffuse across cell membranes, neuronal and glial-based active transporter systems have an important role in regulating extracellular glutamate concentrations. A family of glutamate transporters moves glutamate into astroglia and neurons, thereby providing the major mechanism by which glutamate is inactivated. Diffusion of glutamate away from the postsynaptic receptors and enzymatic degradation likely play a minor role in glutamate inactivation.

Nitric Oxide

Nitric oxide can be considered an unconventional neurotransmitter. Unlike the more classic neurotransmitters described in the preceding text, nitric oxide is synthesized by the postsynaptic cell and effects the presynaptic cell; it is not stored, nor is it released in a quantal, exocytotic manner. Furthermore, it does not bind to specific postsynaptic receptors, and it lacks an active process to terminate its action. Despite these somewhat untraditional features, nitric oxide freely diffuses across cell membranes, influencing both presynaptic neurons and other cells, including other neurons and glia that surround the nitric oxide–producing neuron. In this way, nitric oxide fulfills the fundamental requirement of a neurotransmitter, serving as a chemical signal between neurons.

Biosynthesis and Storage of Nitric Oxide in the Presynaptic Neuron

Nitric oxide is formed by the one-step conversion of L-arginine into nitric oxide and citrulline through the catalytic activity of nitric oxide synthase (NOS). There are three isoforms of NOS: (i) neuronal NOS (nNOS), (ii) endothelial NOS (eNOS) found in blood vessel endothelial cells, and (iii) inducible NOS (iNOS) expressed in microglia. Because NOS is controlled by regulation of NOS isoforms, nitric oxide activity is intermittent rather than tonic. As a small, uncharged molecule, nitric oxide freely passes thorough cell membranes and therefore cannot be compartmentalized to secretory vesicles.

Release of Nitric Oxide into the Synaptic Cleft and Binding of Nitric Oxide by Postsynaptic Receptors

Confounding the traditional dogma that neurotransmitters have effects downstream of the neuron releasing the molecule, nitric oxide acts as a retrograde messenger. Nitric oxide does not bind to membrane-bound receptors on postsynaptic target cells; rather, it stimulates guanylyl cyclase to increase cyclic guanosine monophosphate (cGMP) levels in the target cells. In this way, nitric oxide can modulate the release or the activity of other neurotransmitters released from presynaptic terminals. This association is illustrated by the enhanced release of glutamate by nitric oxide upon NMDA stimulation.

Inactivation of Released Nitric Oxide

Nitric oxide, with a half-life of <30 seconds, is inactivated passively by two processes. Nitric oxide can decay spontaneously to nitrite or combine with iron-containing molecules such as hemoglobin to form methemoglobin.

Serotonin

The cell bodies of serotonergic neurons are localized along the midline of the brain stem in the raphe nuclei. Clusters in the caudal medulla send descending projections to the motor and autonomic systems in the spinal cord, including the dorsal horn where they modulate pain perception. Serotonergic neurons in the pons and midbrain project to the forebrain to regulate hypothalamic cardiovascular and thermoregulatory control, and cortical neuronal responsiveness. The biochemistry of the serotonergic neuron is similar to that of catecholamines, and this discussion focuses on the unique features of serotonin neurotransmission.

Biosynthesis and Storage of Serotonin in the Presynaptic Neuron

Analogous to the synthesis of catecholamines, the biosynthesis of serotonin in a serotonergic neuron begins with an amino acid, tryptophan. Dietary changes that alter plasma levels of tryptophan will effect serotonin production in the brain. The initial and rate-limited step is the hydroxylation of tryptophan by tryptophan hydroxylase. This intermediate, 5-hydroxytryptophan, is then rapidly decarboxylated by the L-aromatic amino acid decarboxylase, the same enzyme found in catecholamine neurons, to produce serotonin. Once synthesized, serotonin is concentrated into vesicles by a vesicular transporter in the synaptic terminal that is identical to the catecholamine vesicular transporter.

Release of Serotonin into the Synaptic Cleft and Binding of Serotonin by Postsynaptic Receptors

Serotonin is released into the synaptic cleft by exocytosis, and it then activates G protein–coupled receptors on the postsynaptic membrane. Although there is overlap in the distribution of the subfamilies of serotonin receptors, each has a unique effector system. Clinically, numerous psychoactive drugs effect serotonergic neurotransmission by altering these effector systems (see Fig. 7.11). The receptors in the 5-HT$_1$ subfamily can inhibit adenylyl cyclase, hyperpolarize the neuron by opening potassium channels, or both. 5-HT$_1$ receptors act as both somatodendritic autoreceptors and as postsynaptic receptors. This subfamily of receptors densely populates components of the limbic system, neocortex, and basal ganglia. Anxiolytic drugs such as buspirone and the antimigraine drug sumatriptan are both agonists at 5-HT$_1$ subfamily receptors. The 5-HT$_2$ subfamily stimulates phosphoinositide-specific phospholipase C

and can depolarize neurons by closing potassium channels in the cortex and some parts of the limbic system. Hallucinogenic drugs, such as lysergic acid diethylamide (LSD), are agonists at the 5-HT$_{2A}$ and 5-HT$_{2C}$ receptors, whereas antipsychotic drugs, such as clozapine and olanzapine, are antagonists at the same receptors. A third metabotropic serotonin receptor subfamily, consisting of 5-HT$_4$ and 5-HT$_7$, stimulates adenylyl cyclase.

A clinically important subgroup of serotonin receptors, the 5-HT$_3$ family, is an inotropic receptor. When activated by serotonin, this ligand-gated ion channel becomes permeable to Na$^+$ and K$^+$, but not to Ca^{2+}. In the CNS, the 5-HT$_3$ receptor has been localized to the area postrema, nucleus tractus solitarii, nucleus accumbens, cingulate cortex, and structures in the limbic system including the amygdala, hippocampus, and entorhinal cortex. Related to their localization, 5-HT$_3$ receptors are involved in sensory transmission, regulation of autonomic functions, integration of the vomiting reflex, pain processing, and control of anxiety. Antagonists of 5-HT$_3$ receptors, including ondansetron, granisetron, dolasetron, and palonosetron, have clinical efficacy as antiemetics, particularly in the setting of chemotherapy-induced, radiotherapy-induced, and postoperative nausea and emesis.

Inactivation of Released Serotonin

Like norepinephrine, the primary method for termination of the serotonergic signal is through the transport of serotonin from the synaptic cleft back into the presynaptic neuron (Fig. 7.11). The plasma membrane serotonin transporter, in common with the catecholamine transporter, requires Na$^+$ cotransport. Inhibition of presynaptic serotonin transporters is a mechanism of action of the selective serotonin reuptake inhibitors, the most commonly

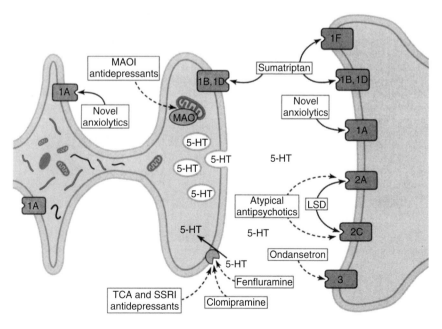

Figure 7.11 Serotonergic drugs bind to specific subfamilies of receptors in the pre or postsynaptic neuron (designated by numbers in rectangle symbols) or to transporters in the presynaptic neuron (represented by pie shaped symbol). Serotonin transporters as psychotherapeutic targets. Drugs that act as agonists are indicated by *solid-line arrows*, whereas antagonists or inhibitors are shown with *broken-line arrows*. Presynaptic neuron **(left)**, postsynaptic neuron **(right)**. The enzyme responsible for the catabolism of serotonin, monoamine oxidase (MAO), is inhibited by a class of antidepressants. 5-HT, 5-hydroxytryptamine; LSD, lysergic acid diethylamide; MAO, monoamine oxidase; TCA, tricyclic antidepressant; SSRI, selective serotonin reuptake inhibitor. (From Siegel GJ, Agranoff BW, Alberts RW, et al. (eds.) *Basic neurochemistry*. 6th ed. Philadelphia, PA: Lippincott-Raven Publishers; 1999.)

prescribed class of drugs to treat clinical depression. Enzymatic degradation accounts for a portion of serotonin signal regulation. In a two-step process involving MAO, serotonin is catabolized to its primary metabolite, 5-hydroxyindole acetic acid (5-HIAA).

Implications for Critical Care

Pediatric intensivists face the consequences of disrupted neuronal structure and function as part of routine care of critically ill children. A goal of pediatric intensive care is to ameliorate neuronal injury caused by critical illness, including those "secondary" injuries that occur as a complication of critical care, such as prolonged neuromuscular blockade. Recognizing the vulnerability of developing neurons to critical illness is an important step in promoting the neurologic recovery of critically ill infants and children.

MUSCLE SYSTEMS

Children with muscle weakness most often require critical care because of respiratory or cardiovascular compromise produced by their underlying neuromuscular disorder. Care of these children benefits from the integration of skeletal muscle pathophysiology with cardiopulmonary mechanics. This section reviews the physiology of the motor unit, describes signal transmission at the NMJ, and discusses critical care issues relevant to children with neuromuscular disorders.

Although muscle comprises 40% of body weight, its influence on the critically ill child (and adult) is frequently overlooked. Conditions that accompany critical illness, such as the systemic inflammatory response, catecholamine release, and pharmacologic agents, can all contribute to muscle protein breakdown, weakness, and atrophy. Acquired neuromuscular disorders of critical illness, including critical illness polyneuropathy and myopathy (CIPNM), prolonged neuromuscular blockade, and acute quadriplegic myopathy (AQM), can all affect patients in the intensive care unit (ICU). The pathophysiology of such acquired neuromuscular disorders of critical illness is also discussed in this section. Physiology of cardiac muscle is discussed in Chapter 5.1.

Organization of Movement

The forebrain, brain stem, spinal cord, motor neuron, and skeletal muscle comprise the motor system. Despite traveling as far as 2 m, the pathways in the motor system are composed of only two (one upper motor neuron and one lower motor neuron) or three (one upper motor neuron, an interneuron, and one lower motor neuron) neurons connected in series. Neurons that originate from the cerebral cortex or brain stem and initiate or modify movement are

known as *upper motor neurons* (UMN). Cortical UMN are involved in voluntary movement while brain stem UMN are primarily involved in posture. Motor neurons in the primary motor area, known as the *homunculus*, have a somatotopic organization. The primary motor cortex of the precentral gyrus controls *contralateral* motor neurons in the spinal cord through the lateral corticospinal tract. Clinical findings suggestive of UMN damage in the brain stem or cortex include contralateral hyper-reflexia, Babinski sign, and contralateral hemiparesis.

Motor pathways from the cortex and brain stem are integrated. When the cortical descending tracts are interrupted in the midbrain or pons, the postural reflexes mediated by the brain stem are exaggerated, producing extension of all four limbs and pronation of the hands and feet, a process called *decerebrate rigidity*. In humans with brain stem lesions, rigid limb extension may be intermittent, or it can be elicited by stimulation. Provoked limb extension is called *decerebrate posturing*. If the descending cortical motor tracts are disrupted above the midbrain, *decorticate rigidity* results. Here, the legs are extended while the arms are flexed and adducted.

Lower motor neurons arise in the ventral horn of the spinal cord to innervate the muscle fiber at the NMJ. Similar to the homunculus, the motor neurons are also somatotopically organized in the ventral horn. A motor neuron divides into branches when it enters the muscle, and each branch makes a synaptic connection with one muscle fiber (see Fig. 7.12). A motor neuron and all

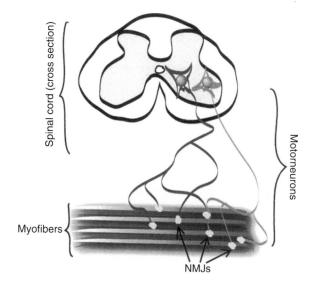

Figure 7.12 Structure of the motor unit. Two motor units are shown. The lower motor neuron cell bodies are located in the ventral horn of the spinal cord. Motor neuron axons travel from the spinal cord to innervate the muscle. Each motor unit is composed of one lower motor neuron, and the myofibers each innervates. At maturity, each myofiber is innervated by one neuron. Motor neurons join the muscle fiber at the neuromuscular junction (NMJ). (Figure contributed by Javad Nazarian.)

the muscle fibers innervated by it are referred to as a *motor unit*. Neuromuscular transmission activates all muscle fibers equally in a motor unit, except in conditions such as fatigue. In general, each muscle fiber is innervated by a single motor neuron. However, at birth, a muscle fiber is often innervated by more than one motor neuron. During the first few postnatal weeks, all but one input is eliminated by each muscle fiber. This occurs by the removal of an axonal branch and its associated synapse from the muscle fiber, a process called *divergence*, rather than by motor neuron death. The process of divergence is recapitulated following reinnervation in the mature muscle. For example, denervation of skeletal muscle occurs with neuropathies, such as CIPNM. The recovery process involves the growth of axons back to the denervated muscle, along with the sprouting of axons to innervate most muscle fibers. Single innervation of each muscle fiber is achieved by the elimination of synapses in about 3 weeks. This reinnervation process facilitates the recovery of muscle strength in neuropathic diseases.

Of the disorders of lower motor neurons, spinal muscular atrophy (SMA) and Guillain-Barré syndrome are the two diseases encountered most often by the pediatric intensivist. Both these disorders are introduced in this section; however, more extensive discussion of these important disorders is found in Chapter 46. The SMAs are diseases of the motor neurons of the spinal cord and medulla. The triad of hypotonia, weakness, and cranial nerve palsies characterizes SMA. Guillain-Barré syndrome is a postinfectious demyelinating disorder of the peripheral sensory and motor nerves. The clinical features include acute, progressive weakness and areflexia.

Skeletal muscle, the final element in the motor system, is discussed in detail in the next section.

Functional Anatomy of Skeletal Muscle

Muscle Fiber

Skeletal muscle is composed of bundles of *myofibers*. Wrapped in sarcolemma, each myofiber contains the elements required for mechanical contraction, including mitochondria to produce ATP, sarcoplasmic reticulum to store and release calcium, and bundles of slender filaments called *myofibrils* that contain the contractile apparatus. The sarcolemma has three areas of specialization: (i) the NMJ (described fully in subsequent text), (ii) the myotendinous junction, and (iii) the T tubules. The myotendinous junction is the region of muscle where the bone connects to the muscle. This region plays a role in development of contractures in the setting of muscle atrophy. Most muscle growth (in length) takes place at the myotendinous junction. Individuals with muscle weakness, such as those with CIPNM, develop contractures because of the restriction on muscle growth induced by atrophy. T tubules are invaginations of the sarcolemma that facilitate propagation of depolarizing waves deep into the myofiber and serve to link the muscle membrane action potential to calcium release from the sarcoplasmic reticulum (see Fig. 7.13). Sarcolemmal depolarization produces a conformational change in the T tubule voltage-gated Ca^{2+} channels (L-type) that then causes the opening of the Ca^{2+} channels in the sarcoplasmic reticulum, a muscle-specific network of membranous vesicles that concentrates, stores, and releases Ca^{2+}. The calcium ions are then actively transported into

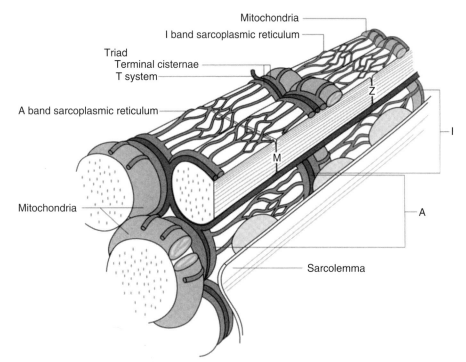

Figure 7.13 Schematic drawing of part of a mammalian skeletal muscle fiber showing the relationship of the sarcoplasmic reticulum, transverse tubule (T) system, and mitochondria to a few myofibrils. This figure shows a myofiber that is <1 sarcomere in length. A, A band; I, I band; M, M band; Z, Z line. (From Siegel GJ, Agranoff BW, Alberts RW, et al. (eds.) *Basic neurochemistry*. 6th ed. Philadelphia, PA: Lippincott-Raven Publishers; 1999.)

the sarcoplasmic reticulum by Ca^{2+}-ATPase. Mutations in the Ca^{2+} channel in the sarcoplasmic reticulum, leading to prolonged calcium release, have been associated with malignant hyperthermia (discussed later in this section).

Sarcomere

When viewed through an electron microscope, the myofibril contains dark bands alternating with light bands bisected by a Z line, giving a striated appearance. The segment from one Z line to the next, called the *sarcomere*, is the functional unit of the skeletal muscle. The sarcomere is the unit of muscle contraction because it contains all the proteins responsible for generating a contractile force. When actin filaments slide over myosin filaments by the movement of the myosin head (also known as a *cross bridge*), the sarcomere shortens. As the sarcomeres within the myofibril shorten in series, the myofibril shortens and force is produced.

Excitation–Contraction Coupling

An action potential generated at the NMJ of the sarcolemma initiates sarcomere shortening. This process, called *excitation–contraction coupling*, is unique to muscle. Briefly, an action potential in the sarcolemma stimulates the release of Ca^{2+} from the sarcoplasmic reticulum. Ca^{2+} enters the cytosol of the myofibril and binds to troponin, a protein that is part of the actin filament. Calcium binding to troponin elicits a conformational change, allowing a second protein of the actin filament, tropomyosin, to bind to the myosin head, forming a cross bridge. Powered by an ATPase in the myosin head, the cross-bridge cycles, producing sarcomere shortening. Relaxation occurs by active reuptake of Ca^{2+} by the sarcoplasmic reticulum that lowers cytosolic $[Ca^{2+}]$, causing the release of Ca^{2+} from the troponin-binding site. The troponin conformational change releases tropomyosin from the myosin head, thereby disrupting cross-bridge structures.

Degenerative Muscle Disorders

Muscular dystrophies are a clinically heterogeneous family of degenerative hereditary disorders. The pediatric intensivist usually encounters patients with muscular dystrophy when their muscle disorder limits their ability to recover from surgery or from respiratory or cardiovascular complications of their muscle disease. Critical care treatment of children with neuromuscular disease is discussed later in this section. For a summary of the muscular dystrophies, see the articles by Wagner, Mathews, and Riggs listed in the Suggested Readings at the end of this chapter.

Metabolism in Skeletal Muscle

Overview of Carbohydrate and Fatty Acid Metabolism in Muscle

Muscles requires ATP for contraction. A variety of energy-producing fuels are used by skeletal muscle, depending on the conditions. Fatty acids are the primary energy source at rest, but during bursts of activity, glucose is the fuel of choice. The liver furnishes glucose to the contracting skeletal muscle as substrate for glycolysis. The lactate produced during anaerobic glycolysis is then taken up by the liver and converted to glucose through the process of gluconeogenesis. This process of substrate transfer, the *Cori cycle*, shifts a part of the metabolic burden of the active muscle to the liver. In a similar cycle, protein catabolism in skeletal muscle generates the amino acid alanine that is also converted to glucose in the liver. Because of this metabolic interdependency of the liver and skeletal muscle, hepatic failure can significantly alter the flow of metabolic substrates to the skeletal muscle. See Chapter 2 for a more detailed discussion.

Hormonal Regulation of Muscle Metabolism

The hormones insulin and epinephrine have opposing influences on fuel utilization by the skeletal muscle. Insulin has anabolic effects on skeletal muscle. Stimulation of glucose and branched-chain amino acid transport into muscle is a fundamental component of the physiologic response to insulin. Insulin also promotes glycogenesis by stimulating the activity of glycogen synthase, the rate-limiting enzyme in glycogen synthesis, and by inhibiting phosphorylase, the rate-controlling enzyme in glycogen degradation. On the other hand, epinephrine's effects in the skeletal muscle are generally catabolic in nature. Epinephrine mobilizes glycogen and triacylglycerol in muscle. In addition, epinephrine inhibits the uptake of extracellular glucose by effectively directing muscle metabolism toward fatty acids rather than glucose.

Impact of Critical Illness on Muscle Metabolism

Acute critical illness or serious injury is associated with hyperglycemia. Release of counter-regulatory hormones, such as catecholamines, cortisol, glucagon, insulinlike growth factor–binding protein 1, and growth hormone, as well as inhibition of insulin release from pancreatic β cells and end-organ insensitivity to insulin ("insulin resistance"), lead to elevations in blood glucose concentrations. The endocrine effects of critical illness are further discussed in Chapter 2.

It is clear from this brief review of metabolism that critical illness–induced insulin resistance would impact energy substrate utilization in the skeletal muscle. In the insulin-resistance characteristic of critical illness, there is an impairment of skeletal muscle amino acid and glucose uptake, glycogen synthesis, and glycogenolysis. This leads to the question whether altered muscle metabolism contributes to the development of acquired neuromuscular disease in critical illness. Results from a randomized trial of glucose control with insulin in adult patients in a cardiothoracic surgery ICU suggest that intensive insulin therapy to achieve euglycemia may protect the skeletal muscle. In patients requiring intensive care for more then 5 days, strict adherence to normoglycemia was associated with reduction in critical illness polyneuropathy (CIPN) and muscle weakness, as well as in improved mortality. A more detailed discussion of CIPN and other acquired neuromuscular disorders recognized in the critically ill is provided later in this section.

Functional Anatomy of the Neuromuscular Junction

The NMJ is a specialized cholinergic synapse with general characteristics similar to neuron–neuron synapses. The cholinergic synapse has been reviewed in the previous section. The motor neuron terminal and the sarcolemma have morphologic features that facilitate the transmission of the neuronal action potential to the muscle fiber. As previously mentioned, the postnatal development of NMJ requires interaction between the nerve terminal and the

muscle fiber. In this section, we highlight the unique features of the NMJ and emphasize how abnormalities in NMJ function leads to muscle weakness that requires critical care.

Presynaptic Structure and Transmitter Release: Motor Neuron

The axon of a lower motor neuron broadens to form a nerve terminal, or presynaptic bouton, at the NMJ (see Fig. 7.14). A Schwann cell covers each bouton. Membrane-bound vesicles containing approximately 5,000 acetylcholine molecules occupy the terminal. When the terminal membrane is depolarized by an action potential, voltage-gated Ca^{2+} channels (P channels) open, increase cytosolic Ca^{2+} concentration, and initiate the process of exocytosis to release acetylcholine into the synaptic cleft.

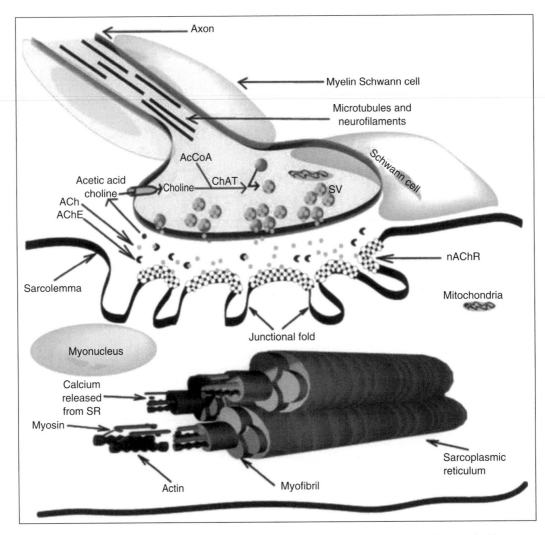

Figure 7.14 Neuromuscular junction (NMJ). Motor neuron communicates with the muscle fiber at the NMJ. Synaptic vesicles (SV) contain the neurotransmitter acetylcholine (ACh). When released from the SV, ACh binds to nicotinic ACh receptors (nAChR) that are clustered close to the synapse. Diseases and pharmacologic agents have effects at various levels of the NMJ complex. AchE, acetylcholinesterase; AcCoA, acetyl-CoA; ChAT, choline acetyltransferase; SR, sarcoplasmic reticulum. (Figure contributed by Javad Nazarian.)

As introduced in the previous section, the two *Clostridium* toxins botulinum and tetanospasmin prevent transmission at the NMJ by proteolytic cleavage of synaptic proteins, although the former presents as weakness and the latter as tetany. Both neurotoxins enter the presynaptic neuron by endocytosis. The light chain of botulinum toxin and tetanospasmin are translocated from the endocytotic vesicle into the cytosol. In the synaptic bouton, botulinum toxin types A, C, and E cleave SNAP-25; types B, D, F, and G cleave synaptobrevin; and type C cleaves syntaxin. Tetanospasmin migrates by retrograde axonal transport to the cell bodies of inhibitory interneurons in the spinal cord and brain stem. Similar to botulinum, the light chain causes proteolytic cleavage of synaptobrevin/vesicle-associated membrane protein in GABAergic synaptic vesicles. Prevention of GABA release leads to uncontrolled excitatory discharges in motor neurons, resulting in muscle rigidity and spasms.

Weakness can be caused by insufficient calcium flux into the motor neuron terminal. In individuals with Lambert-Eaton myasthenic syndrome, antibodies against the voltage-gated calcium channel block calcium flux into the terminal, producing muscle weakness. Other bivalent cations such as Mg^{2+} block P channels and account for the muscle weakness observed in pregnant women receiving infusions of magnesium sulfate or their magnesium-exposed newborns. An important point to note on the specificity of P-type calcium channels in motor neurons is that calcium-channel blockers (e.g., verapamil, diltiazem, and nifedipine) that affect L channels do not affect P channels.

Calcium is not only required for vesicle exocytosis but also acts as a stabilizer for the nerve membrane. In the setting of calcium deficiency, spontaneous depolarization of the nerve membrane causes muscle contraction. However, if the frequency of depolarization does not permit calcium reuptake into the sarcoplasmic reticulum, tetany occurs. Therefore, tetany is a cardinal clinical manifestation of low serum ionized calcium concentrations.

Postsynaptic Structure and Transmitter Action: Muscle Fiber

Synaptic boutons overlay a specialized region of the muscle fiber sarcolemma called the *end plate*. In the end-plate region, the sarcolemma invaginates to form a *junctional fold* that contains a high density of inotropic nAChR at their crests and voltage-sensitive Na channels along their walls (Fig. 7.14). Binding of two acetylcholine molecules to an nAChR opens the ion pore to permit the inflow of Na^+ and outflow of K^+. These conductances produce a net depolarization of the sarcolemma, known as the *end-plate potential*. Unlike the neuronal action potential, the end-plate potential is a local, graded, slow potential rather than an all-or-none response. The end-plate potential, usually 50 to 70 mV, is large enough to spread electrotonically to the depths of the junctional fold to trigger the opening of voltage-dependent Na^+ channels. Na^+ flows through these open pores into the muscle to further depolarize the

sarcolemma, and an action potential is generated when the threshold potential is reached. As described in the preceding text, the action potential travels along the muscle fiber length in the sarcolemma and causes Ca^{2+} release from the sarcoplasmic reticulum to initiate excitation–contraction coupling.

During normal conditions, the magnitude of the end-plate potential is more than sufficient to reach the threshold potential required for action potential generation in the muscle fiber. The difference between the end-plate–generated membrane potential and the threshold potential for initiating an action potential is called the *safety factor*. The safety factor permits effective neuromuscular transmission under various conditions. However, inherited and acquired autoimmune diseases of the NMJ, such as myasthenia gravis, can reduce the safety factor, leading to transmission failure. There are many physiologic abnormalities of the postsynaptic element present in individuals with myasthenia gravis: (i) the presence of antibodies against the α subunit of the nAChR, (ii) a reduction in the number of nAChR in the end plate, (iii) more shallow junctional folds, and (iv) a widened synaptic cleft. Taken together, these postsynaptic alterations result in lower amplitude end-plate potentials that may fail to reach threshold levels, particularly with repeated stimulation. Congenital and acquired forms of myasthenia gravis are discussed more fully in Chapter 46.

Synapse and Termination of Transmitter Action

Signaling at the NMJ is terminated by the rapid hydrolysis (<1 ms) of acetylcholine to choline through the action of AChE. In addition, a small fraction of acetylcholine is removed from the synapse by diffusion. The half-life of acetylcholine in the synapse is shorter than the decay of the end-plate potential or the refractory period of the muscle. Therefore, each nerve action potential gives rise to a single wave of depolarization in the muscle.

Pathology, drugs, or toxins can alter the catalytic activity of AChE. Denervation causes a decrease in junctional and extrajunctional acetylcholinesterase. Drugs that inhibit acetylcholinesterase are called *anticholinesterase agents*. In the presence of these agents, acetylcholine accumulates in the cholinergic synapse and has the potential to create excessive stimulation of the cholinergic receptors. In view of the widespread distribution of cholinergic synapses, these agents have broad neurologic effects. This discussion focuses on the effects of anticholinesterase inhibitors that have therapeutic value at the NMJ.

Autoimmune myasthenia gravis has characteristic clinical features including ophthalmoplegia, fatigability, and weakness of skeletal muscles without sensory abnormalities. Nonetheless, many disorders of neuromuscular transmission, metabolic or toxic syndromes, or neurogenic weakness may mimic myasthenia gravis. Edrophonium is a noncovalent anticholinesterase agent administered as a diagnostic test for myasthenia gravis. A positive response to a rapid intravenous injection of edrophonium chloride (Tensilon) consists of brief improvement in strength, although false positives and false negatives can both occur. Detection of acetylcholine-receptor antibodies in the serum should be used in conjunction with the Tensilon test to improve diagnostic accuracy.

Pyridostigmine, neostigmine, and ambenonium are the standard anticholinesterase drugs used in the symptomatic treatment of myasthenia gravis. All of these agents increase the response of myasthenic muscle to repetitive nerve impulses by preservation of endogenous acetylcholine.

Acquired Neuromuscular Disorders in Critical Illness

Patients who require intensive care for >5 days often acquire severe neuromuscular dysfunction characterized by muscle wasting and weakness that delays recovery, increases risk for hospital-acquired infections, and in some cases compromises survival. Even less severe neuromuscular disorders, such as nerve entrapment syndromes, have significant impact on recovery and quality of life after critical illness. The economic impact of ICU-acquired neuromuscular disorders may be substantial, but there are no recent estimates of hospital charges attributed to these disorders.

Limited development of such neuropathies will enhance recovery from critical illness. Failure to wean from mechanical ventilation often prompts an evaluation for possible neuromuscular weakness. However, assessing muscle strength only when a patient is unable to separate from mechanical ventilation misses an opportunity to ameliorate muscle weakness.

Acquired profound muscle weakness was first reported in a young woman with status asthmaticus who developed severe myopathy after receiving corticosteroids and neuromuscular blocking agents (NMBAs). The onset of weakness is often difficult to pinpoint because of concurrent use of sedation; presence of encephalopathy; and, particularly in infants and young children, the inability to reliably test muscle strength because of their inability to follow commands. Determining the incidence of this disorder is complicated by the diversity of clinical and diagnostic findings, incomplete application of diagnostic testing, and inconsistent terminology. Because it is often difficult to differentiate between myopathic and neuropathic causes of acquired weakness in the ICU, the term CIPNM is used here to encompass the entities described elsewhere as critical illness polyneuropathy (CIP or CIPN), critical illness myopathy (CIM), and ICU-acquired paresis (ICUAP). This section focuses on the pathogenic features of three causes of severe weakness in critically ill patients: CIPNM, AQM, and prolonged NMJ blockade. The pathophysiology of two additional muscular disorders that develop in ICU patients, atrophy and malignant hyperthermia, are also discussed.

Neurogenic and Myopathic Diseases of the Motor Unit

Clinical Criteria Distinguishing Neurogenic and Myopathic Conditions

Neurogenic disease, caused by loss of innervation to a muscle, is characterized by fasciculations, absent tendon reflexes, and occasionally sensory loss. In myogenic disorders in which primary muscle disease leads to muscle fiber degeneration, muscle wasting is prominent, whereas tendon reflexes and sensory perception are maintained. Because both neurogenic and myogenic diseases are characterized by muscle weakness and wasting, laboratory and neurophysiologic testing are often required to distinguish these conditions (see Table 7.3).

Laboratory and Neurophysiologic Criteria Distinguishing Neurogenic and Myopathic Conditions

Creatine kinase (CK) is the single most useful blood test for the evaluation of weakness in neuromuscular disease. Muscles require rapid mobilization of high-energy phosphate for contraction. Similarly, in the brain, ATP must be conveniently stored and released promptly when needed. Creatine phosphate provides a form of intracellular energy transfer that meets the needs of both muscle and brain. CK catalyzes the release of phosphate from creatine phosphate to generate ATP for excitation–contraction coupling. When the muscle fiber or neuronal membranes are disrupted by injury, inflammation, or necrosis, CK is released and can be measured in the serum.

Elevation in serum CK concentration is neither a specific nor a sensitive marker for neuromuscular disease. A normal CK is expected in steroid myopathy, thyroid myopathy, mitochondrial myopathy, and channelopathies. CK can also be transiently elevated in the absence of neuromuscular disease, such as after weight-bearing exercise, muscle trauma, surgery, or convulsive seizure. Men and African American individuals have higher CK serum levels than women and non–African American individuals. Published normal ranges for serum creatine often do not account for gender or racial influences.

The three isoforms of CK (BB, MB, and MM) are found in varying proportions in brain, skeletal muscle, and myocardium. CK-BB is the predominant (>99%) isoform of CK in the brain, and the presence of CK-BB in serum is suggestive of CNS damage. Similarly, CK in skeletal muscle is 97% to 99% MM, with the MB isoform contributing only 1% to 3%. In the myocardium, MM is again the dominant isoform, making up 75% to 80% of the total CK composition, with the balance from the MB form. Therefore, the presence of CK-MM in the serum suggests damage to either skeletal or cardiac muscle, whereas CK-MB in the serum is specific for myocardial damage. Serum CK-MM levels >100 times above normal levels suggest active muscle fiber necrosis such as inflammatory myopathy, dystrophinopathy, rhabdomyolysis, malignant hyperthermia, neuroleptic malignant syndrome, or polymyositis. An elevated CK-MM

TABLE 7.3

CHARACTERISTICS DISTINGUISHING NEUROGENIC FROM MYOPATHIC DISEASES

	Neurogenic Disease	Myopathic Disease
Associated disease	SIRS	Asthma, sepsis
Risk factors		
Corticosteroids	±	+
NMBA	−	+
Aminoglycosides	+	?
Hyperglycemia	+	?
Clinical findings		
Fasciculations	+	0
Sensory loss	+	0
Tendon reflexes	0	+
Wasting	+	+
Laboratory findings		
Creatine kinase (serum)	±	+ + + +
Cerebral spinal fluid protein	+	0
Electromyography		
Motor amplitude	↓	↓
Sensory amplitude	↓ or normal	Normal
Fibrillation, fasciculation	Widespread	Common
recruitment	↓	Variable
Nerve conduction velocity	+	0
Motor unit action potential	Polyphasic	Short duration, low amplitude, polyphasic
Muscle biopsy	Group atrophy, fiber type grouping	Necrosis and regeneration

SIRS, systemic inflammatory response syndrome; NMBA, neuromuscular blocking agent; ?, not known; ↓, less than normal.

level is also seen in ALS, SMA, and other neuropathic disorders, but the levels are much lower than that observed in muscle disorders in which necrosis is a more prominent feature.

Electromyography (EMG) and nerve conduction studies can distinguish neuropathic from myogenic causes of muscle weakness. Details of EMG testing are presented later in this chapter (see section on "Monitoring of the Nervous System"). Although electrophysiological studies are useful for the identification of neuromuscular disease, these tests often are unable to distinguish neuropathy from myopathy. Therefore, muscle biopsy is recognized as the diagnostic gold standard. Although both tests are uncomfortable to patients and they may require sedation, the comparative risks of the more invasive muscle biopsy will need to be weighted against its benefits in light of each child's specific clinical condition.

Commonly Recognized Intensive Care Unit–Acquired Neuromuscular Abnormalities

Entrapment Neuropathies

Immobility due to illness severity, developmental status, or sedatives limits the assessment of peripheral nerve function in critically ill children. Although entrapment neuropathies, caused by nerve compression due to patient positioning or intravenous infiltrates, have been described, the incidence in children is not known. However, in adult acute respiratory distress syndrome (ARDS) survivors, peripheral nerve entrapment syndromes have been recognized, with peroneal nerve palsy, foot drop, and long-term functional limitations found in 3%.

Critical Illness Polyneuropathy and Myopathy

Clinical Characteristics. A disease characterized by a diffuse axonal polyneuropathy was initially described in patients with ICU-acquired weakness. However, it is becoming increasingly clear that non-neuropathic myopathy is a dominant feature, leading to the recent understanding of CIPNM as a combined acute axonal neuropathy with myopathy. Therefore, the electrophysiologic picture of CIPNM shares both neuropathic and myopathic features.

The incidence of ICU-acquired neuromuscular disorders in adult patients ranges from 25% to 70%, depending on characteristics of the study population and criteria used to define the presence of a disorder. Well-defined incidence rates for development of CIPNM were determined in a prospective study of 98 ICU patients who were ventilated for at least 4 days, had not received NMBAs in the previous 3 days, and did not have preexisting polyneuropathy or myopathy. Patients were repeatedly evaluated during their hospital stay, using both clinical and electrophysiological tests to identify the presence of CIPNM. Clinical criteria included evidence of motor deficit, muscle wasting, and decreased or absent deep tendon reflexes. Presence of axonal polyneuropathy constituted the required electrophysiological criteria. In this sample of critically ill adults, the incidence of CIPNM was 33% (95% CI 24% to 43%). In another study using the Medical Research Council (MRC) score—a previously validated clinical measure that assesses strength in three muscle groups—25.3% (95% CI 16.9% to 35.2%) of the awake adult patients who had been ventilated for at least 6 days were found to have CIPNM.

Descriptions of muscle weakness in critically ill children were limited to case reports until a cross-sectional study of infants and children aged 3 months to 17 years without preexisting neuromuscular disease admitted to a pediatric intensive care unit (PICU) for >24 hours was performed. In this study, weakness was diagnosed in any patient meeting one of the following criteria: MRC grade ≤4, reduced or absent deep tendon reflexes, or inability to wean from mechanical ventilation in the absence of pulmonary disease. Electrophysiologic studies were available for a limited number of patients. Overall, acquired weakness was identified in 1.7% of all patients, with 5.1% of children older than 9 years being affected. The marked differences between adult studies of CIPNM and this pediatric study remain unexplained but may reflect differences in selection criteria and outcome definition, and the incidence of specific physiologic insults and/or the differential vulnerability of adults and children.

Etiology and Conditions Favoring Critical Illness Polyneuropathy and Myopathy.

Severity of illness, presence of systemic inflammatory response syndrome (SIRS), and the use of aminoglycosides have been shown to be risk factors for the development of CIPNM. Hyperglycemia has recently been added to the list of risk factors for CIPNM. On the other hand, NMBAs, glucocorticoids, and benzodiazepines have not been consistently shown to be risk factors for CIPNM. However, as discussed in the subsequent text, NMBAs are risk factors for the development of AQM. Independent risk factors for development of CIPNM include APACHE-III score >85 and the presence of SIRS. In adult patients, when both factors were present, the risk for development of CIPNM was found to be 72%.

Pathology and Pathogenesis.

Given the diversity in clinical and electrophysiological findings in CIPNM, it is not surprising that a spectrum of pathologic characteristics is present. Although muscle fiber atrophy is almost universally present, the expression of fetal myosin and desmin are evidence of regeneration and suggest a myopathic rather than a neuropathic cause for this atrophy. Loss of myosin thick filaments is characteristic of CIPNM; however, other muscle structural proteins such as titin, nebulin, and actin are also somewhat reduced.

Although the pathogenesis of CIPNM is unclear, evidence suggests possible explanatory models for the development of CIPNM. Identification of SIRS as a risk factor for CIPNM suggests that immune activation likely contributes to the pathogenesis of CIPNM. It has also been suggested that cytokines and free radicals may compromise blood flow in the axonal microvasculature, although there is no convincing pathologic evidence for endoneurial ischemia as a cause of axonal degeneration. On the other hand, interleukin-1 (IL-1) and tumor necrosis factor (TNF) do influence muscle metabolism by promoting proteolysis.

Single-fiber EMG demonstrates abnormalities related to altered end-plate potentials in disuse states. The up-regulation of glucocorticoid receptors seen in disuse states increases the vulnerability to corticosteroid myopathy. Similarly, administration of NMBAs in denervation conditions augments expressions of nAChR and increases the risk of NMBA toxicity. In addition, enormities in sarcolemma Na^+ channels with reduction in Na^+ currents have been observed in CIPNM.

Treatment and Prevention.

There are no randomized trials assessing interventions to treat CIPNM. However, the Leuven study of critically ill patients showed that tight glycemic control with insulin titration was associated with a decrease in the development of CIPNM (odds ratio 0.4, 95% CI 0.28, 0.57). Glycemic control likely prevents the combination the toxic effects of hyperglycemia while conferring the anti-inflammatory and metabolic benefits of insulin on muscles.

Avoidance or limitation of known risk factors for CIPNM is an obvious strategy for prevention. In patients with SIRS/multiorgan dysfunction syndrome (MODS), who are at highest risk for CIPNM, it makes sense to limit exposure to NMBAs, aminoglycosides, and glucocorticoids, as well as to aggressively monitor drug effectiveness and dosing to limit toxicity. Careful monitoring of renal and hepatic function is also essential so that required adjustments in drug dosing can be provided.

The association between sepsis and CIPNM also suggests prevention of sepsis as a potential strategy to prevent CIPNM. There is yet no evidence to support this strategy. Development of CIPNM may be an important outcome in evaluating new therapies for sepsis. It also makes sense to implement patient care strategies to prevent complications of critical illness that prolong ICU stay, such as semirecumbent positioning and oral hygiene to prevent ventilator-associated pneumonia; interruption of sedative infusions to titrate administration of the lowest required dose; and implementation of ventilator weaning strategies to reduce the duration of mechanical ventilation, which can prevent complications of critical illness, prolong ICU stay, and increase the risk of CIPNM.

Acute Quadriplegic Myopathy

Etiology and Conditions Favoring Acute Quadriplegic Myopathy. AQM presents with profound muscle weakness in patients with respiratory failure who receive intravenous glucocorticoids, often in combination with prolonged neuromuscular blockade. This acquired muscle disorder is characterized by generalized muscle weakness, quadriplegia, and progressive atrophy. The development of AQM may occur in the absence of SIRS or MODS, a characteristic that helps distinguish this disease from CIPNM. Nonetheless, there is clinical overlap between AQM and CIPNM.

Pathology and Pathogenesis. Myofiber atrophy without necrosis is the predominant finding on muscle biopsy in AQM. Focal myosin loss occurs in nonatrophic fibers, whereas, unlike CIPNM, titin, nebulin, and actin are generally spared. Evidence of regeneration can be seen.

The molecular events leading to AQM are beginning to be elucidated. Gene profiles obtained from muscle biopsies of five ICU patients with severe muscle weakness, myofiber atrophy, and EMG findings consistent with myopathy were compared with profiles from individuals without weakness and normal muscle histology. Muscle from patients with AQM showed strong induction of transforming growth factor-β (TGF-β)/mitogen-activated protein kinase (MAPK) pathways. In this setting, the TGF-β pathway is activated by oxidative or osmolar stress. In addition, glucocorticoids activate Ras intracellular signaling pathway. The TGF-β and the Ras pathways converge at MAPK, which initiates an intracellular cascade, leading to apoptosis, cell cycle arrest, and atrophy of the muscle. New targets for therapies to inhibit muscle atrophy can be proposed from this pathogenic model of AQM.

Diagnosis. In AQM, weakness frequently involves both proximal and distal muscle in all four extremities, and diaphragmatic weakness is common. Deep tendon reflexes may be present or absent. CK is usually at least mildly elevated. The typical EMG pattern reveals low-amplitude compound action potentials, short polyphonic motor unit potentials, but with normal nerve conduction.

Treatment and Prevention. The risk of myopathy is directly related to the duration of corticosteroid and NMBA administration. Therefore, the use of these agents should be limited and they should be administered with careful monitoring of the depth of the neuromuscular blockade with train-of-four (TOF) and assessment of deep tendon reflexes. Drug holidays should be considered as a means to prevent inadvertent overblockade. In many situations,

deep sedation without the use of neuromuscular blockade may more safely achieve the intended therapeutic goal.

Prolonged Neuromuscular Junction Blockade

Etiology. Prolonged NMJ blockade tends to occur in patients when NMBAs have an extended duration of action. Most NMBAs are metabolized in the liver and rely on renal elimination for termination of effect. Therefore, administration of vecuronium or pancuronium by continuous infusion in the presence of renal or hepatic failure places a patient at risk for prolonged blockade. In addition, female gender, acidosis, and hypermagnesemia have been reported as risk factors.

Treatment and Prevention. Although pharmacologic reversal with a cholinesterase inhibitor can briefly restore NMJ function and is often diagnostically useful, the effects are short-lived in the presence of NMBAs or their metabolites. Therefore, treatment consists of allowing the clearance of the NMBAs. Efforts to improve renal function should facilitate NMBA elimination.

As with all the myopathies associated with critical illness, limiting the administration of NMBAs is the keystone for prevention of prolonged neuromuscular blockade. However, in the rare situation in which continuous neuromuscular blockade is required, such as when high-dose sedation is ineffective or not tolerated, every effort should be made to titrate the dose of NMBAs down as far as possible while still achieving the therapeutic goal. The optimal method for monitoring neuromuscular blockade in the ICU is less obvious than in the operating room, and this controversy is discussed later in this chapter. Nonetheless, clinical assessment, peripheral nerve stimulation to monitor TOF response, and drug holidays will help the intensivist in protecting against prolonged neuromuscular blockade.

Muscle Atrophy

Critically ill patients are at risk for development of muscle atrophy. It is well recognized that muscle inactivity is associated with loss of muscle mass and with weakness. Denervation, seen with CIPNM, causes loss of protein from myofibrils. The hormonal milieu of critical illness also supports muscle wasting. Insulin and insulinlike growth factor 1 (IGF-1) are anabolic hormones whose actions tend to inhibit muscle proteolysis. The resistance to insulin and IGF-1 effects that occurs in critical illness therefore tends to promote muscle wasting. Furthermore, cortisol and epinephrine, present in high concentrations during critical illness, are catabolic and promote muscle atrophy. Drugs used in critically ill patients, such as corticosteroids, have long been known to cause muscle wasting.

Regardless of the initiating event, muscle atrophy primarily results from accelerated protein breakdown. Three major protein degradative systems are found in muscle—ubiquitin (Ub)–proteasome complex, lysosomal acid proteases (cathepsins), and calcium-activated proteases (calpains)—and of these the Ub pathway is the most significant. In spite of the fact that muscle atrophy would be interpreted as detrimental, intuitively beneficial effects of muscle atrophy have been suggested. For example, in periods of starvation, degradation of muscle protein provides substrate for gluconeogenesis to synthesize glucose for brain metabolism. Despite these benefits, for the critically ill patient, particularly with sepsis and subacute respiratory failure, prevention of atrophy is an important, yet often-overlooked therapeutic goal. Advances in the understanding of the pathways that control muscle atrophy can highlight targets for antiatrophy therapy.

Molecular Mechanisms Leading to Atrophy.

Although the catabolic effects of muscle by corticosteroids are well known, the underlying mechanism of this action has been elusive. In an experiment comparing the transcriptional response of atrophic muscle, Goldman identified two ubiquitin ligases, atrogin-1 and muscle ring finger-1 as critical factors contributing to loss of muscle protein. Dexamethasone, a glucocorticoid used commonly in the ICU, promotes muscle breakdown and induces atrogin-1 and muscle ring finger. In a study using myotubes in culture, IGF-1 and insulin blocked dexamethasone-induced atrophy by inhibiting the induction of atrogin-1 and muscle ring finger-1, thereby suppressing protein breakdown. The results of this study suggest that the effects of glucocorticoids on muscle wasting may be ameliorated by insulin administration.

Malignant Hyperthermia

Malignant hyperthermia (MH) is a syndrome usually precipitated by anesthesia and is characterized by rapid rise in body temperature, muscle rigidity and spasms, tachycardia, acidosis, hypoxemia, myoglobinuria, elevated serum CK level, hyperkalemia, and hypermetabolism with rising end-tidal carbon dioxide. MH occurs in 1 out of every 15,000 children who receive anesthesia, and some of these children will have an autosomal dominant inheritance of vulnerability to MH. In addition, malignant hyperthermia can occur sporadically in association with certain neuromuscular diseases.

Pathogenesis.

MH is caused by a mutation in the *RYR1* genes that codes for the voltage-sensitive Ca^{2+} channel in the sarcoplasmic reticulum. In MH-susceptible individuals, the RYR1 receptor is activated by lower levels of calcium from the T tubule. In addition, higher than normal levels are required to close the channel. The open RYR1 channel permits excessive calcium release from the sarcoplasmic reticulum into the cytosol of the myofibril, causing persistent occupation of Ca^{2+} on troponin and continuous cross-bridge cycling. Depletion of ATP stores by the myosin ATPase limits ATP availability for the active reuptake

of calcium into the sarcoplasmic reticulum, resulting in further increase in intracellular calcium, which eventually produces membrane damage and cell lysis. Potassium, phosphate, CK, myoglobin, and uric and lactic acid flow from the ruptured myofiber into the blood, leading to the laboratory characteristics of MH.

Differential Diagnosis.

Rapid elevation in body temperature and muscle rigidity during or following anesthesia should prompt an evaluation for MH. Myoglobinuria is frequently seen in the postoperative setting, particularly in patients exposed to cardiopulmonary bypass or in those experiencing a transfusion reaction. Osteogenesis imperfecta is also associated with a perioperative hyperthermia syndrome that is not associated with muscle hypermetabolism.

Treatment and Prevention.

Management of MH includes removal of any precipitating agents, administration of oxygen, treatment of hyperkalemia, rapid cooling, and administration of sodium bicarbonate to alkalinize the urine and protect the myocardium from hyperkalemia. In addition, it is important to maintain adequate hydration and administer dantrolene, the mainstay of pharmacologic therapy for MH. This muscle relaxant reverses the pathologic cycle of excessive calcium release from the sarcoplasmic reticulum and produces muscle relaxation.

Muscle weakness and atrophy are recognized consequences of prolonged critical illness. Nonetheless, the muscular system is often overlooked when caring for critically ill patients. The purpose of this section has been to draw attention to the importance of skeletal muscle metabolism and function in critical illness. For the child with prolonged critical illness, designing patient care strategies to shift the balance of skeletal muscle size away from atrophy will likely lead to fewer days of mechanical ventilation, more rapid return to baseline motor function, and perhaps improved quality of life.

CELL DEATH IN THE CENTRAL NERVOUS SYSTEM

The study of cell death within the nervous system has become a focal point of neuroscience research and clinical medicine. Cell death occurs throughout the development of the nervous system and because of CNS injuries. There are two predominant forms of cell death: necrosis and apoptosis. Aberrancies of apoptotic cell death regulation during development can lead to pathologic conditions; brain cancer, SMA type I in infancy, and amyotrophic lateral sclerosis in later years are but a few examples. A comprehensive understanding of the developmental processes related to cell death is essential to develop successful interventions for these diseases. Furthermore, injuries to the CNS cause cell death by either necrotic or apoptotic mechanisms. Mitigating the amount of cell death in the brain or spinal cord after injury is of paramount importance to clinicians attempting to maximize clinical outcome. Therefore, therapeutic strategies that either antagonize pathways leading to cell death or enhance endogenous neuroprotective mechanisms may be effective in limiting the nature of these injuries. For these reasons, detailed understanding of cell death in the CNS is essential for the intensivist.

Forms of Cell Death—Necrosis and Apoptosis

Necrotic cell death occurs after an overwhelming stimulus, such as trauma or complete ischemia, is applied to the cells within the brain or spinal cord. Necrosis has been compared to cellular "explosion" because of the nature of the reactions within the cell (see Table 7.4). Biochemical collapse of the cell begins as the cells utilize the remaining energy stores. With this loss of energy, the cell can no longer maintain ionic gradients, and the cellular membrane integrity becomes compromised. As the process evolves, histologic markers of necrotic cell death become manifest. The mitochondria and nucleus swell, the cellular organelles swell and dissolve, and the chromatin within the nucleus condenses. At a critical period, the cellular swelling results in the bursting of the cell membrane and in the release of reactive oxygen species, cytokines, excitatory amino acids, and cellular contents into the interstitial space around the cell. These molecules lead to the recruitment of phagocytic and inflammatory cells into the region of damage and result in escalation of the damaged area. Ultimately, the nuclear and cytoplasmic membranes dissolve, and the DNA is degraded nonspecifically by random cuts in the molecule. The end result is a localized inflammatory reaction surrounding the injured region, with a wide variety of mediators locally released into the tissue. The entire process takes only several minutes to occur and, therefore, is extremely difficult to treat.

Apoptotic cell death, also called *programmed cell death*, occurs during normal development, as well as in response to injurious stimuli. During development, it has been hypothesized that apoptosis may be necessary to:

- Remove cells that appear to have no function.
- Remove cells of an inappropriate phenotype (precursors that have migrated to regions not populated by these cells in adults).
- Correct errors (death of neurons with inappropriate synaptic connections).
- Remove guiding cells (death of neurons or glia that were required for guidance of axons that become unnecessary).
- Remove cells with only transient function (death of neurons that served a transient function at one period of development that are now irrelevant).
- Provide neuroprotection (death of cells with defective DNA or infected with viruses).

The overall extent of apoptosis is difficult to quantify in human brain development. In rodents, however, up to 70% of cells that develop in certain brain regions undergo this form of cell death. In contrast to the "explosion" of cells after necrosis, apoptotic cell death appears to be more of an "implosion." These intracellular processes, outlined in detail in the subsequent text, are complicated cascades of events, with multiple proteins activating one another,

TABLE 7.4
COMPARISON OF NECROSIS AND APOPTOSIS

	Necrosis	Apoptosis
Ultrastructural characteristics	Dissolution of plasma membrane, increased cellular water, cellular swelling and increased cell size, decreased Na^+/K^+-ATPase activity, decreased ATP, nonspecific DNA fragmentation	Chromatin condensation, nucleosomal DNA fragmentation, increased gene expression, mitochondrial swelling, intact plasma membrane and shrinking cell size, increased energy expenditure
Timing	Within several minutes	Hours to longer
Triggers	Energy failure, mediators of injury, trauma	Normal development, mediators of injury, activation of intracellular signals
Mechanism of cell dissolution	Generalized protease activation	Coordinated activation of caspase enzymes
Prompt an inflammatory reaction?	Yes	No

ATP, adenosine triphosphate; ATPase, adenosine triphosphatase.

much like those of the complement or coagulation systems. Eventually, the end result of this process is the histologic findings of apoptosis: chromatin condensation; breakdown of intracellular proteins; DNA fragmentation at nucleosomal sites; and, most importantly, cell surface alterations leading to the rapid phagocytosis of the dead cell debris by neighboring cells. Evolutionarily, this seems quite advantageous. Consider brain regions with >50% of apoptotic cell death occurring at a given stage of development. If these cells underwent necrotic cell death, the interstitial spaces between cells would be inundated with inflammatory cells and mediators that would continually escalate the response. By undergoing apoptosis, this cell death is mostly silent except for the given cell.

It is becoming increasingly clear that apoptosis is extremely important in pathologic conditions as well. Several decades ago, most of the cell death in stroke was believed to be related to necrotic mechanisms. With improved markers to detect apoptosis and with a better understanding of the apoptotic processes, we now know that a considerable portion of the cells dying after global cerebral ischemia are undergoing apoptosis. Most importantly, because the apoptotic processes take several hours to more than a day to become activated, interventions to protect these critically injured cells might have the greatest therapeutic potential. For these reasons, an in-depth understanding of apoptosis is a necessary component of the pediatric intensivist's armamentarium.

Pathways in Apoptosis

The Role of Caspases

Caspases (or cysteinyl aspartate-specific proteases) are the effector proteins in the apoptotic cascade of cell death. Caspases are proteases that use cysteine as the nucleophilic group for substrate cleavage and cleave peptide bonds on the carboxyl side of aspartic acid residues. Caspases were initially discovered in the development of the nematode worm, *Caenorhabditis elegans*. Because *C. elegans* has a relatively small number of total somatic cells (1,090 in the adult) and the organism is transparent, it has been invaluable in studying the ultimate fate of cells in neural differentiation. Initial studies in the early 1970s established that 131 of these cells died during development and were phagocytosed by adjacent cells. The timing of these cell death events was precise between different individual worms, leading to the hypothesis that this cell death was somehow genetically "programmed." A mutagenesis gene screen revealed that 14 different mutant worms (named *ced-1* to *ced-10, nuc-1, ces-1, ces-2, egl-1*) exhibited defects in this programmed cell death process. Three of these genes seemed to play a central role in the programmed cell death pathway. Mutant worms lacking functional *ced-3* and *ced-4* showed virtually no programmed cell death during development and, therefore, had a large number of extra cells. This suggested that *ced-3* and *ced-4* were positive regulators of the programmed cell death pathway. Perhaps,

these genes encoded proteins that were lethal to cells or were responsible for the breakdown of the cell after an activating stimulus was applied. By contrast, worms lacking functional *ced-9* genes were killed embryonically because of the death of normally unaffected cells. The finding that this gene was a negative regulator of programmed cell death was supported further by studies showing that mutant *ced-9* worms were restored to normal phenotype when a gain-of-function mutation was reinserted into the genome.

Proteins from genes homologous to these are also found in the human genome. To date, 11 human caspases have been identified and appear to act in concert with one another. Caspases are synthesized as inactive proenzymes that require proteolytic cleavage at internal aspartate (Asp) residues for full functional activity. Caspase proteins are organized into three distinct regions, the prodomain, a large subunit, and a small subunit. Either an external stimulus or another activated caspase breaks the Asp bond between the prodomain and the other subunits. Another cleavage, at an Asp residue between the large and small subunit, occurs to allow the caspase to acquire its full functional activity. Most of the caspases function as tetramers (two small subunits and two large subunits are joined), revealing two active sites of enzymatic activity.

Human caspases are divided into two main groups: those related to apoptosis (caspases-2, 3, 6, 7, 8, 9, and 10) and those related to cytokine processing (caspases-1, 4, 5, and 11). Of those related to apoptosis, there are several that initiate the process (initiator caspases-2, 8, 9, and 10) and others that ultimately kill the cell (effector caspases-3, 6, and 7). The prodomains of initiator caspases are considerably longer than those of effector caspases, ultimately allowing initiator caspases to interact and recruit other molecules that are required for signaling the pathway within the cell. The effector caspases do not require such an interaction with other intracellular modulating proteins for their activity.

Activation of Caspases by Intrinsic and Extrinsic Stimuli

Two distinct processes within the cell activate caspases, termed the *intrinsic* and *extrinsic cascades*. In the intrinsic cascade, the cellular organelles responsible for oxidative homeostasis of the cell, the mitochondria, are the initiating elements (see Fig. 7.15). Mitochondria within the cell act as a sensor of cellular damage. Cellular stresses such as ionizing radiation, DNA damage, heat shock, or oxidative stress lead to an increase in the permeability of the outer mitochondrial membrane. This allows proteins from within the mitochondria, particularly cytochrome C of the respiratory transport chain, to be released within the cytosol. In the presence of ATP, cytochrome C binds to Apaf-1 (the mammalian homolog of *ced-4* from *C. elegans*), which leads to a conformational change in Apaf-1 structure, promoting oligomerization of Apaf-1 molecules. Once this occurs, procaspase-9 can bind to each of the

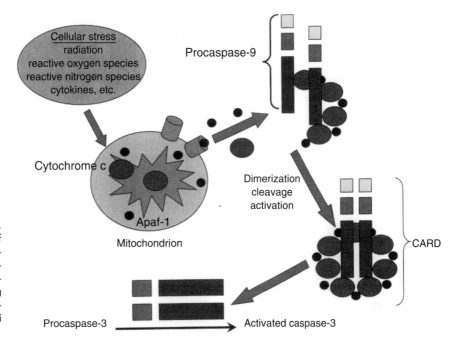

Figure 7.15 Intrinsic caspase cascade. Internal cellular stressors cause loss of mitochondrial membrane potential and release of cytochrome C and Apaf-1. Dimerized procaspase 9 forms the caspase recruitment domain (CARD) complex, leading ultimately to the activation of the effector caspase 3. (Figure contributed by Aditi Sharangpani.)

Apaf-1 monomers using interactive motifs on each protein. This complex of Apaf-1/caspase-9 proteins is called the *apoptosome*. The formation of the apoptosome leads to the activation of caspase-9, which leads to the activation of the effector caspases (particularly caspase-3), along with a rapid escalation of the activation of the nonbound caspase-9 and the destruction of the cell from within.

The extrinsic caspase pathway involves binding of various ligands with transmembrane receptors (see Fig. 7.16). For instance, members of the TNF superfamily of receptors (TNF, Fas/Apo/CD 95, DR4 [TRAIL-R1], DR5 [TRAIL-R2]) have been called *death receptors* because of this function. Binding of a ligand, FasL, for example, to its receptor starts a complex series of intracellular reactions. The Fas receptor contains a highly conserved motif called the *death domain* (DD). This site becomes bound by procaspase-8 protein after FasL is bound to its receptor. Once the Fas receptor is bound with procaspase-8 and the death-effector protein, Fas-associated death domain (FADD), these interactions lead to the activation of caspase-8. This activation again

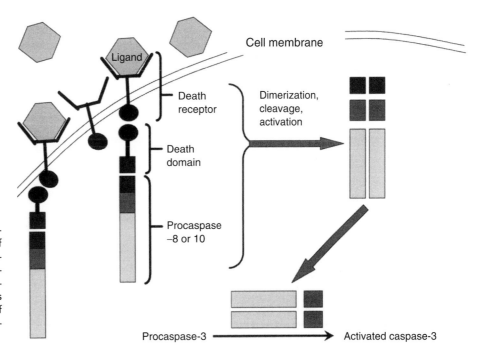

Figure 7.16 Extrinsic caspase cascade. Diagram showing activation of the extrinsic caspase cascade requiring ligand–receptor interaction, recruitment of intracellular death domains, cleavage of initiator caspases (−8 or 10), and ultimately cleavage of the effector caspase-3. (Figure contributed by Aditi Sharangpani.)

leads to activation of the effector caspase-3 and ultimately to cell death.

How Caspases Ultimately Cause Cell Death

Activated caspases are responsible for the histologic findings of apoptosis described in the previous sections. Individual caspases recognize specific four-peptide regions within the structural proteins of the cells and cleave the protein at that site. Caspases require an Asp residue in the first position of the four-peptide sequence and cleave the protein between the first and second residue. It is the residue at the fourth position that is the most critical in determining the substrate specificity of the individual caspases. All proteins within the cell containing these sequences are cleaved and dismantled. The cleavage of the cytoskeleton proteins (gelsolin, fodrin, nuclear laminins A and B, keratin 18, β-catenin) that form the framework of the cell leads to dramatic reorganization of the cellular contents and retraction of the cellular membrane typically seen in apoptosis. DFF45 (DNA fragmentation factor 45 kDa) is a well-studied substrate for caspase activation. Once caspase activation occurs, DFF45 is cleaved and acts to cleave DNA in patterns (internucleosomal pattern) characteristic of apoptotic cell death.

Regulators of Apoptosis—The Bcl-2 Family

The Bcl-2 family of proteins are key regulators of the intrinsic caspase pathway of cell death and their role in human disease is becoming clearer. In this family of proteins, there are members that augment apoptosis and others that are neuroprotective. The proapoptotic proteins serve as sensors to death signals and executors of the death program, whereas the antiapoptotic proteins inhibit the initiation of the program.

Bcl-2 is the prototype of the Bcl-2 family. Bcl-2 was first identified as a protein expressed from genes at the breakpoint in a human follicular lymphoma, a proto-oncogene that functions to prevent apoptotic cell death (hence the term *B cell lymphoma type 2*). One of the key features of the Bcl-2 family proteins is that the members share sequence homology in four regions (labeled BH1 to 4). The BH1 and BH2 domains are required for the antiapoptotic properties of these proteins, whereas the BH3 domain is present in those with proapoptotic properties (such as Bax). These proteins are located within the matrix of the mitochondria and are regulated at multiple levels, including at protein transcription, protein translation, and after translation. It appears that the proapoptotic members of the Bcl-2 family translocate from the mitochondrial matrix to the outer mitochondrial membrane. These proteins then form channels within the outer membrane and lead to the release of cytochrome C into the cytosol of the cell. This process, of course, is the first step in the activation of the intrinsic caspase pathway. Antiapoptotic proteins seem to function by binding to the proapoptotic proteins, thereby inhibiting them from binding to the membrane and not allowing these permeability channels to form.

Role of Necrosis, Apoptosis, Caspases, and Bcl-2 in Critical Illness

Cell death of neurons or glia is the pathologic process behind all the injuries described in the Neurologic Disorders section (Chapters 45 to 53). Our current therapies, as well as possible new advances, are all dependent on mitigating the death of these cells. Although never successfully proven, the current hypothesis in neurologic critical care is as follows: Stopping cells from dying in a critical illness will necessarily allow for improved mortality, greater degrees of clinical functioning, and a better quality of life for the surviving person.

Cell death and recovery are intricately related to global and regional ischemia, as described in Chapter 54. Ischemia is a trigger for both necrotic and apoptotic cell death. Although necrotic cell death was first recognized, it is becoming clear that the apoptotic cell death related to these disorders may be the pathway most amenable to treatment. Apoptotic cell death takes many hours to several days to become manifest histologically, whereas necrotic cell death is determined within minutes of the injury. The role of apoptosis in ischemic injuries is becoming clearer. Ischemic stroke was the first neurologic condition to demonstrate activation of any caspase (caspase-1), and inhibition of this caspase was associated with improvement in stroke volume in animal models. Furthermore, activation of caspases-3, 8, 9, 10, and 11 and release of cytochrome c have been shown in humans following cerebral ischemia. Mice deficient in caspase-1 or 11 are protected from regional ischemic injuries. And most recently, pharmacologic treatment with caspase inhibitors has shown promise in animals after strokes.

Disorders of muscles and the NMJ are discussed in Chapter 46. Although some of the conditions are related to abnormal metabolites of muscle cells themselves, some of these conditions are directly related to abnormal cell death in the motor neurons. Consider the disorder called *SMA type I* (Werdnig-Hoffman disease). SMA is inherited in an autosomal recessive manner and leads to weakness and decreased movement after apoptosis of anterior motor horn neurons. *SMA type I* presents in the first few months of life and is the most severe subtype of the disease, with death occurring from respiratory failure by 2 years of age. More than 97% of patients with SMA have mutations in the survival motor neuron gene (*SMN1*) on chromosome 5q13. The loss of function of this gene leads to apoptotic cell death in spinal motor neurons through mechanisms that are still unclear. However, the amount of the gene product that is expressed does correlate well with clinical outcome. Further investigation will be needed to determine how this protein interacts with others in the apoptotic cell death pathway outlined in the preceding text.

Chapter 47 outlines both the impact of cancer on the CNS and the result of cord compression on the spinal cord. In the case of cancer, abnormal activation of oncogenes, genes that normally lead to cell proliferation and growth, can lead to an unchecked cell growth and damage to normal structures. Many cancer therapies are based on augmenting the cell death response to kill these invading cells. In the case of spinal cord compression, spinal neurons and glial cells are damaged by a mass that impairs the blood flow to healthy regions. These healthy regions then undergo cell death by either necrotic or apoptotic pathway.

Coma and alterations in mental status caused by metabolic diseases of the brain that result in either accumulation of toxic products within brain cells or altered cellular function after exposure to a drug are discussed in Chapter 48. The goal in treating these conditions is to intervene before either apoptotic or ischemic cell death occurs. Similarly, Chapter 49 discusses CNS infections in which cell death from infectious agents is sometimes necrotic (in the case of bacterial meningitis when the organisms either directly invade brain tissue or cause venous strokes from invasion of organisms into the vascular lumen) and sometimes apoptotic (activation of the extrinsic caspase cascade through the TNF superfamily of receptors and activation of the intrinsic pathway after viral infection of cells). Chapter 50 reviews the therapies for status epilepticus and intractable seizures. The reasons for treating this disorder as aggressively as is recommended is (i) to minimize the risk of ischemic injury from cells utilizing more energy than can be supplied by the blood stream and (ii) to decrease the production of excitatory amino acids and other metabolites that will be toxic to neuronal elements and cause their cell death. Chapter 51 contains a review of the criteria for brain death, a process that obviously occurs after cell function is no longer detectable within the CNS. In Chapter 52, we review brain trauma, and all of the therapies and concepts of clinical management that are aimed at minimizing secondary injury and secondary cell death.

Neuroprotection—Cerebral Preconditioning

There is evidence for the participation of excitotoxins, free radicals, activated endothelium, leukocytes, cytokines, platelets, platelet-activating factor, eicosanoids, endothelin, altered gene expression, edema, nitric oxide, poly(ADP-ribose) polymerase (PARP), growth factors, apoptosis, matrix metalloproteinases, and mitochondrial permeability pore transition in evolving brain injury and secondary cell death. Clinical trials of a host of agonists and antagonists of these mediators of brain injury have yielded disappointing results. Before 1996, results of >80 clinical trials on >30 different neuroprotective agents for the treatment of stroke were published. None showed clear evidence of a benefit until recombinant tissue plasminogen activator was tested (which acts by restoring blood flow and not by any of the mechanisms of cell death outlined in the preceding text).

The juxtaposition of this clinical futility along with the breadth of understanding of the cell death pathways led to the hypothesis that studying endogenous neuroprotective processes may be a more effective method of developing clinical therapies. There are several examples of endogenous neuroprotection that can be studied (including those used by hibernating animals and others) but cerebral preconditioning is the most clinically relevant and is extensively studied. This is reviewed in the following section. Also, an exogenous neuroprotective strategy that has shown promise, hypothermia, is reviewed.

Preconditioning is the phenomenon by which a nonlethal stimulus sets in motion a cascade of biochemical events that renders cells, tissues, or the whole organism tolerant to a future, more lethal stimulus. This process was initially studied using ischemia as a primary stimulus within the myocardium but now has been extensively studied in the brain as well. There are several clinical syndromes that have been recognized as preconditioning paradigms. For instance, angina pectoris and transient ischemic attacks (TIAs) may involve preconditioning of the heart and brain, respectively. Patients with angina pectoris have been shown to have a decreased infarct size compared to those with a single ischemic event. Similarly, several studies suggest that patients who have TIAs have smaller subsequent strokes than patients without such symptoms. These observations have spurred efforts to understand the biochemical mechanisms responsible for this protection and led to the studies outlined in the subsequent text.

Myocardial Preconditioning as a Model for Neuroprotection

Myocardial preconditioning has been studied since the mid-1980s after the clinical experience cited in the preceding text was first noted. Animal models were developed to study this phenomenon, and Murry et al. were among the first to develop a preconditioning paradigm. This paradigm was performed in dogs and involved four episodes of brief ischemia, each consisting of a 5-minute occlusion of circumflex artery followed by 5 minutes of reperfusion. A longer ischemic insult was imposed immediately thereafter for varying amounts of time (40 minutes or 3 hours). Preconditioned dogs had a 75% reduction in infarct size compared to shams. This suggested that several brief episodes of ischemia created a brief period of protection from more lethal ischemia but that this protection was not complete if the subsequent episode was overwhelming.

Further study demonstrated that the protection achieved from brief episodes of ischemia was biphasic. A second "window" of protection from ischemia was found 24 hours after the initial preconditioning stimuli. Marber et al. found that a similar preconditioning stimulus of four episodes of 5-minute coronary artery occlusion provided approximately 30% protection from a 30-minute ischemic insult given 24 hours after the preconditioned stimulus. This phenomenon was termed *late* preconditioning in contrast to *classic* or *early* preconditioning described in the preceding text. Initial hypotheses were formulated suggesting that products of metabolism immediately released after ischemia may mediate "early" preconditioning, whereas newly synthesized proteins may be required for "late" preconditioning cardioprotection.

Early Preconditioning Mechanisms in the Heart

The rapidity with which the early protection was afforded in the study suggests that substances released from the ischemic myocardium are likely responsible for the cardioprotection observed rather than the *de novo* synthesis of protein (which generally takes several hours). Adenosine, bradykinin, and opioid peptides were identified as agents that could independently substitute as the preconditioning stimulus. Adenosine was found to exert its effects by binding to its A1 or A3 receptors within the myocardium in studies involving isolated cardiac myocytes, animal, and humans cardiac tissue. Binding of bradykinin to its B2 receptor leads to protection in cardiac myocytes, although its marked hemodynamic effects make it very difficult to exclude effects not related to preconditioning. Opioid peptides trigger the preconditioning cascade by binding to their δ-receptor subtype, and selective δ-opioid receptor agonists have been shown to induce cardioprotection in experimental models.

With these mediators having been identified, efforts to define the intracellular events responsible for cardioprotection continue. Currently, the working theory of cardiac preconditioning involves the ATP-sensitive potassium channel (K_{ATP}). This channel, thought to link myocardial metabolism to membrane electrical activity, is present in the sarcoplasmic reticulum membrane (sarc K_{ATP}) and the mitochondrial membrane (mt K_{ATP}). Evidence for a role of these channels in preconditioning was furnished by a series of studies. First, selective K_{ATP} antagonists (glibenclamide and sodium 5-hydroxydecanoate) block the protection, whereas a K_{ATP} opener (aprikalim) augments the protection of preconditioning. Also, multiple mediators associated with ischemic preconditioning, including adenosine, regulate K_{ATP} channel function. Most convincingly, the development of specific openers of mt K_{ATP} channels, specifically diazoxide, demonstrated that opening of mt K_{ATP} channels can confer cardioprotection without the involvement of sarc K_{ATP} channels. This work has culminated in clinical trials using nicorandil, a K_{ATP} channel opener with nitratelike hemodynamic properties. Nicorandil improves left ventricular wall motion in ischemic heart disease and has improved electrocardiogram (ECG) findings in patients undergoing angioplasty.

Late Preconditioning Mechanisms in the Heart

Examination of the mechanisms involved in late preconditioning is in its infancy in comparison to the detailed delineation of the key processes in early preconditioning. Although some have suggested release of adenosine leading to protein kinase C activation as a potential mechanism of late preconditioning, the heat shock response, which involves the production of novel proteins in response to a stress, has been most often implicated. First described as a

response of cells to thermal injury, this response has been shown to be elicited by many other stimuli including ischemia and oxidative stress. It has been conserved through evolution in species as diverse as fruit flies, yeast, plants, and mammals. Marber et al. found that the cardioprotection of preconditioning was coincident with the up-regulation of an inducible 70-kDa heat shock protein (HSP 70) and that the overexpression of HSP 70 in transgenic mice also increased resistance to myocardial ischemia.

Brain Preconditioning

Perhaps, because the brain and myocardium are uniquely sensitive to ischemia or because of the other similarities between the organs, study groups attempted to replicate in neurologic models the preconditioned responses to ischemia observed in the myocardium. The similarities between the organs include the necessity of ion channels for functioning, the need for high-energy substrates to maintain homeostasis, and a commonality of mediators known to alter the organ's function (e.g., adenosine and nitric oxide). But important differences exist as well, such as the heterogeneity of cell types within the CNS (i.e., neurons, astrocytes, oligodendrocytes, and microglia, in addition to blood vessels) compared to the relatively homogeneous population of myocardial myocytes within the heart. In work spanning more than a decade, groups of investigators have successfully demonstrated that the principles of preconditioning can be applied within the CNS and that ischemia need not be the sole stimulus that starts the process in motion.

Ischemic Preconditioning—Clinical Experience to Animal Models

The clinical evidence of preconditioning neuroprotection from TIAs is relatively scarce. Recently, a small retrospective study showed that prior TIAs were associated with milder stroke symptoms after controlling for other cardiovascular risk factors, yet most studies still list the occurrence of TIAs as a risk factor for the development of stroke.

The paucity of definitive clinical evidence of preconditioning notwithstanding, a number of animal models demonstrated that sublethal doses of ischemia could protect against a future, more lethal dose. As in the myocardium, multiple, small preconditioning stimuli were found to be more effective than a single stimulus, and the interval between the preconditioned stimulus and the subsequent insult was found to be critical. However, brain models of preconditioning found key differences. Mainly, the interval between the preconditioning and the lethal stimuli needed to be longer, and the duration of the neuroprotection was increased relative to the observations in the myocardium. Furthermore, global and focal preconditioning stimuli were found to have protection against both global and focal lethal insults. These findings have led investigators to postulate novel mechanisms of protection within the brain.

Global preconditioning stimuli can protect against both global and focal injuries. Kitigawa et al. showed that a

5-minute episode of bilateral carotid artery occlusion in gerbils caused selective damage to the CA1 region of the hippocampus, a region of the brain selectively vulnerable to ischemia. They demonstrated that two episodes of sublethal ischemia (2-minute duration) performed at 24-hour intervals for 2 days before the lethal ischemic injury provided almost complete protection of this vulnerable region. They also found that a single dose of the preconditioning stimulus was partially effective in providing protection, but multiple smaller doses of preconditioning ischemia (1-minute duration) were ineffective. Simon et al. found that 48 hours after a global ischemia, rats were protected against permanent middle cerebral artery (MCA) occlusion, a focal injury, manifested as a decrease in the overall infarct size.

Similarly, focal preconditioning stimuli can protect against both focal and global injuries. Chen et al. used three 10-minute episodes of MCA occlusion (separated by 45 minutes of reperfusion) as a preconditioning stimulus and showed decreased infarct size after a subsequent 100-minute occlusion of the MCA in rats. Interestingly, the protection was only elicited 2 to 5 days after the preconditioning stimulus. At day 1 and day 7 after preconditioning, the protective effects of the preconditioning were not observed. Glazier et al. demonstrated that a focal preconditioning stimulus could protect against a global injury. Using rats, the MCA was occluded for 20 minutes followed by 24 hours of reperfusion. The rats were then subjected to bilateral common carotid artery occlusion with hemorrhagic hypotension, and the preconditioned animals showed decreased damage in ipsilateral and contralateral hippocampi. Others have observed essentially the same results using gerbils.

Alternative Preconditioning Stimuli can Confer Neuroprotection

Because administration of intentional periods of ischemia is impractical clinically, the study of preconditioning in animals has expanded to include models using alternative preconditioning stimuli. Hypoxia, defined as decreased oxygen delivery with no alteration in blood flow, is distinct from ischemia in which blood flow is reduced. Using neonatal rats, 4 hours of hypoxia (8% oxygen environment) administered 24 hours before a hypoxic–ischemic insult (left carotid artery occlusion and 8% oxygen environment for 2 hours) led to decreases in infarct volume and in hippocampal cell loss. Inflammatory mediators, particularly TNF, can also serve as a preconditioning stimulus in animal models. Systemic injection of lipopolysaccharide (LPS) induced protection from permanent MCA occlusion in spontaneously hypertensive rats, and pharmacologic blockade of the effects of TNF nullified this protection. In a follow-up study, preconditioning with intracisternal injection of TNF 24 hours before ischemia decreased infarct size in mice after secondary permanent MCA occlusion in a dose- and time-dependent manner.

Mechanisms of Ischemic Preconditioning in Animal Models

Several mechanisms have been postulated for preconditioning neuroprotection. Some evidence suggests that mediators released coincident with ischemia, such as excitatory amino acids and adenosine, may be involved in the ischemic preconditioning. Excitatory amino acids, specifically glutamate, through the interaction with their receptor, NMDA, are released after ischemic injury. An NMDA receptor antagonist (MK-801) administered before the ischemic preconditioning stimulus blunts the neuroprotective response in gerbils. However, others have failed to show a difference between interstitial brain concentrations of glutamate in preconditioned and sham animals using ischemic preconditioning models. Adenosine A1 antagonists blunt the neuroprotection of ischemic preconditioning, whereas A1 agonists have failed to show the degree of neuroprotection induced by ischemia alone.

Brain preconditioning follows a time course similar to the "late" form of cardiac preconditioning. By far, the most common response noted in animal models of preconditioning involves the heat shock response. Both global and focal preconditioning stimuli increased heat shock protein expression. HSP 72 was detected in some models, whereas HSP 70 was detected in others. Competitive inhibition of HSP 70 gene expression has blocked thermotolerance. Additional evidence for the heat shock response in preconditioning includes demonstration of a dose–response relationship between the dose of preconditioning stimuli and the expression of heat shock proteins. Kitigawa et al. found that 2- or 5-minute doses of preconditioning stimuli increased HSP 72 protein level and afforded protection, whereas 1-minute stimulation was insufficient for expression of the protein, and protection was not observed. Furthermore, the timing of HSP expression coincides with the period of protection from subsequent ischemia. Expression of HSP 70 in the cortex was noted between 1 and 5 days after preconditioning at a time when protection was noted. Yet the expression was undetectable by 7 days, and protection was no longer afforded at this delayed period.

Other proteins, including the apoptosis-regulating proteins Bcl-2 and Bcl-x-long, have been implicated in preconditioning, but these proteins have been reviewed previously. Bcl-2 is overexpressed in neurons that survive either focal or global ischemia, is increased in a time course consistent with the induction of preconditioning, and inhibition of Bcl-2 protein exacerbates neuronal injury after ischemia. It is possible that nonlethal stimuli cause a protective release of Bcl-2 that can then protect against the larger stimulus to come. This currently remains speculative.

Mechanisms of Ischemic Preconditioning in Cell-Culture Systems

Cell-culture systems can offer several advantages over whole animal models in discerning molecular mechanisms of preconditioning. Cell-culture systems allow the study of isolated cell types within the CNS because differences might exist between neurons and glial cells with respect to responses to ischemia. The exposure of these cells to either preconditioning stimuli or therapeutic agents can be carefully controlled in these systems to enhance the validity of the studies. Cell cultures also allow the completion of multiple experiments in a short period, eliminate the need for blood–brain barrier penetration of novel agents, and eliminate the potential bias caused by unknown systemic side effects in pilot studies. Of course, results from cell-culture studies need to be replicated in animal models before human trials can be considered.

Ischemia cannot be precisely replicated in cell-culture models, but hypoxia with deprivation of glucose has most often been used as an effective surrogate. Bruer et al. developed a model of hypoxic preconditioning in neuronal cell culture, which used a preconditioning stimulus of 1.5 hours of oxygen–glucose deprivation (OGD) consisting of a humidified atmosphere with a Po_2 of 2 to 4 mm Hg, 5% CO_2/95% N_2, and without glucose in the medium. This stimulus was applied 48 to 72 hours before a more lethal (3 hours) dose of OGD. Controls (3 hours OGD without preconditioning) showed an increase in lactate dehydrogenase (LDH) release, had 70% to 90% neuronal degeneration noted by phase contrast microscopy, and showed a DNA fragmentation pattern consistent with apoptotic cell death. Preconditioned neurons showed decreased LDH release (attenuation between 30% and 60% compared to controls) and increased cell viability, with many culture plates showing no signs of damage. In addition, the authors found that ouabain, a potent Na^+/K^+-ATPase inhibitor, given as a preconditioning stimulus offered similar degrees of neuroprotection. Recent studies have suggested a role for alterations in NMDA receptor properties; upregulation of adenosine A3 receptors and hypothermia in preconditioning have not added to the intracellular mechanisms involved.

In a novel approach, Ginis et al. have suggested that the plethora of stresses that can initiate preconditioning argues for a single common denominator underlying the protective mechanisms. They suggest that TNF may be that agent because of its pleiotropic effects outside and inside the CNS. In this multifaceted study, neurons were exposed to 20 minutes of hypoxia as a preconditioning stimulus. No morphologic changes were noted with this treatment alone, and ethidium fluorescence revealed no cell death after this insult. Pretreated cells were protected against exposure to 2.5 hours of hypoxia or 2.5 hours of OGD at 24 hours, with cell loss inhibited by 50% in both sets of experiments, thereby demonstrating the classical preconditioning response. The authors then showed that neurons exposed to TNF for 24 hours as a preconditioning stimulus had a similar degree of protection as those preconditioned with hypoxia and that the addition of an antibody against TNF in the culture medium abolished the protective response. Immunostaining showed that the number of TNF

receptors was not increased in preconditioned compared to naïve cells. These findings suggested that the TNF released from neurons during preconditioning initiates a cascade of intracellular events that leads to neuroprotection.

Using this data, the authors suggested that ceramide, a sphingolipid known to mediate TNF effects in other cellular models, may be a mediator of TNFs preconditioning effects. The authors tested this theory by determining (i) whether the presence of ceramide is protective, (ii) whether ceramide level is increased at the appropriate time for preconditioning, and (iii) the effects of blocking ceramide synthesis on preconditioning. Ceramide C2, a cell-permeable ceramide, was added to cell cultures, and the cells were then subjected to the lethal hypoxic insult (2.5 hours). The presence of ceramide C2 decreased cell death by >50% in this paradigm. Secondly, after a 20-minute hypoxic stimulus, ceramide levels within neurons were increased to 120% to 140% of the control by 16 hours and were further increased to 180% to 200% by 24 hours, which is the time course when protection against hypoxia is observed. This data was replicated by substituting TNF as the preconditioning stimulus. Lastly, cells that were preconditioned with 20 minutes of hypoxia in the presence of fumonisin B1, a ceramide synthesis inhibitor, lacked the protection from subsequent insults observed in cells treated without fumonisin B1. These results implicate TNF and the newly synthesized ceramide as potential mediators of the preconditioning response, but more study is needed to fully define the intracellular processes involved.

Another provocative strategy to achieve neuroprotection involves preconditioning with brain structural proteins to alter the inflammatory response to brain injuries. This form of preconditioning, also known as *cerebral tolerance*, can be achieved by feeding doses of MBP to rats before an ischemic insult. Animals had up to 30% smaller infarct measured throughout the first week after the stroke. Immunohistochemistry revealed TGFβ1 T cells in lesions of tolerant animals but not in shams, whereas the systemic levels of TGFβ1 were unchanged between the two groups. TGFβ1 is an anti-inflammatory cytokine that acts by diminishing the actions of a variety of other cytokines, including TNF and IL-1. Because this anti-inflammatory strategy is localized within the brain, fewer systemic complications would be expected. This approach has led to clinical trials involving administration of both selectin and integrin to populations at high risk for stroke. However, data from these trials are not currently available.

Several clinical situations can be considered as preconditioning stimuli within the brain, including TIAs and reperfusion after stroke with recombinant tissue plasminogen activator (rTPA). The mechanisms currently under study may show clinical promise in minimizing damage to the brain during these clinical situations. Because the antagonism of a single putative mediator has been ineffective in protecting the brain from injury, the study of preconditioning may lead to novel therapeutic strategies. A myriad of mediators including adenosine, excitatory amino acids, and newly synthesized proteins may be associated with preconditioning within the brain. At present, intracellular events related to the development of the heat shock response; the synthesis of genes from the Bcl-2 family; and the relationship between hypoxia, TNF, and ceramide are interesting potential mediators of neuroprotection. Unraveling the intracellular mechanisms of this important protective response may offer hope in clinical situations in the future.

Hypothermia—The Exogenous Neuroprotectant

Investigators have experimented with hypothermia to protect the brain for >50 years. In 1950, Bigelow et al. reported that decrease in temperature to 20°C in dogs extended the safe time of cerebral ischemia from only a few minutes to >15 minutes. Beginning in the 1970s, the protective effects of profound hypothermia (8°C to 10°C) in global cerebral ischemia were exploited in the repair of congenital heart disease in infants. Primarily on the basis of these findings, the advent of the use of therapeutic hypothermia after global ischemia and severe brain injury began. One hundred and twenty-one patients with brain injury were treated with moderate hypothermia, and cases were reported in the medical literature from 1958 to 1989 with temperatures from 28°C to 34°C and for durations of 2 to 10 days. The benefit was not clearly established, and complications (such as severe cardiac arrhythmia) were relatively infrequent.

In the 1980s, additional information about hypothermia was gleaned while laboratories began testing the protective effects of various drugs thought to be pivotal in the evolution of brain injuries. During these experiments (many of which were testing the efficacy of NMDA receptor antagonists and antioxidants administered both before and after global ischemia, stroke, and brain injury), investigators reported that the differences in intraischemic brain temperature were highly protective. The effect of hypothermia was found to be much greater than the effect of any of the cytoprotective drugs under study. This work also demonstrated that hypothermia had an incremental effect. Small changes in temperature, as small as 1°C to 2°C, were protective, and larger changes showed an additive benefit. These findings led to the clinical case series in the 1990s that were not powered to determine benefit but did demonstrate that surface cooling to moderate levels (32°C) were not associated with significant cardiovascular toxicities.

On the basis of the strength of these studies, a multicenter, randomized, prospective phase III study of moderate systemic hypothermia in severe brain injury was completed. Three hundred and ninety-two adults with Glasgow Coma Score (GCS) <8 after traumatic brain injury were recruited from multiple centers. A target temperature of 33°C was reached by 8.4 hours after injury, and this temperature was maintained for 48 hours before rewarming was initiated. Outcome at 6 months was poor (defined as severe disability, vegetative state, and death) in 57% of patients in both groups, with a mortality rate of 28%

in the hypothermia group and 27% in the normothermia group. The only positive finding of the study was decreased intracranial pressure (ICP) in the hypothermia group compared to controls. Variability among the centers in the management of hypotension, fluids, electrolytes, and medications were suggested as possible explanations responsible for the negative result. But enthusiasm for the routine use of hypothermia after traumatic injury was significantly diminished. It remains as a therapeutic option in many centers when uncontrollable ICP is encountered.

More promising results were recently published in the use of hypothermia after cardiac arrest. In two studies, moderate hypothermia (32°C to 34°C) induced for either 12 or 24 hours resulted in significantly improved neurologic outcomes. Hypothermia was instituted very early in these studies (within 4 and 8 hours, respectively), and this relatively minor difference between these studies and the unsuccessful trials in trauma may be important. In many animal models, the induction of hypothermia must occur within 1 hour after the brain injury to afford neuroprotection. For this reason, it appears that hypothermia might be most effective when applied to patients after a witnessed cardiac arrest within a hospital or in communities in which hypothermia can be induced outside the hospital. Because of their smaller size, achieving the goal temperature within these strict time limits might be less problematic in children than in adults.

The mechanisms by which hypothermia may exert its neuroprotective effects are incompletely understood. Various investigators have implicated the following mediators and have shown that hypothermia modulates their activity: aspartate, glutamate, hydroxyl radicals, taurine, IL-1β, NGF, E selectin, intracellular adhesion molecule-1 (ICAM-1), neutrophil adhesion, and TNF. It appears that hypothermia acts on the multiple pathways responsible for cell death simultaneously, giving the cellular protective responses the time to absorb injurious stimuli without causing cell death. It is clear that hypothermia will continue to be investigated in severe brain injury in the coming years, and studies in children with various head injuries are likely to advance our knowledge significantly.

PHYSIOLOGIC PRINCIPLES IN THE MANAGEMENT OF THE NEUROLOGICALLY INJURED CHILD

The maintenance of maximal organ function during critical illness is a basic tenet in pediatric critical care medicine. The relative success of this process is critical for obtaining optimal clinical functioning after the injury or disease has subsided. In treating children with critical neurologic illnesses, both systemic and organ-specific physiologic and pathophysiologic principles need to be understood. The goal of this portion of the text is to outline the broad physiologic concepts that are central to the care of children with critical neurologic injuries. Understanding (i) the mechanical principles within the cranial vault, (ii) the regulation of cerebral blood flow (CBF), and (iii) the basic tenets involved in cerebral metabolism is essential to optimize clinical outcomes. These concepts are described in the subsequent text because they are essential to managing the diseases outlined in Chapters 45 to 53.

State-of-the-art care of the brain during a critical illness is useless unless the rest of the organs of the body are optimally maintained. Children with neurologic injuries require optimization of the respiratory system. Dysfunction of the reticular-activating system or brain stem can cause sudden loss of airway reflexes, leading to the need for intubation. In cases with cerebral swelling, minimization of intrathoracic pressure is essential to ensure adequate venous return, lower cerebral blood volume, and lower ICP. The cardiovascular system is essential because of the relationship between blood pressure and CBF, delivery of oxygen to the brain, and the avoidance of hypotensive episodes that might extend to secondary injuries. Fluid balance is critical to the care of neurologically injured children. Excessive fluid can cause increases in cerebral blood volume, whereas hypovolemia can lead to shock and inadequate substrate delivery to neurons. Inadequate renal function can cause uremia, a condition that leads to altered consciousness. Severe anemia can cause acute decreases in oxygen delivery to the brain, and polycythemia can lead to increased blood viscosity, sludging in capillaries, and ultimately to strokes. Finally, optimal nutrition is required to account for catabolic losses, as well as to provide substrates for damaged neural elements to heal. Application of the principles and strategies outlined in the remainder of this section is most effective as a part of a comprehensive plan for the management of critical illness.

Physiology of the Intracranial Compartment

Contents of the Intracranial Vault and the Munro-Kellie Doctrine

There are three main constituents in the cranial vault under normal conditions: the brain, the cerebrospinal fluid (CSF), and the cerebral blood. The brain is a soft, malleable organ that constitutes up to 80% of the total intracranial volume. This malleability of the brain changes a great deal during normal development. The water content in the brain of the newborn is significantly higher (up to 85% in infants, 78% in adults) and the myelin content significantly lower than in later periods of life. Because of this, the brain of a newborn is much more liquid in structure and is less compressible than in later times of development.

Despite these developmental changes, the mass of the brain is relatively static under normal conditions. Many serious injuries to the brain lead to cellular swelling and brain edema. Two differing forms of edema have been proposed: vasogenic and cytotoxic. Vasogenic edema is thought to develop because of extravasation of protein-rich fluid from the intravascular space. This fluid accumulates in the interstitial tissue of the brain because of the breakdown of the blood–brain barrier. This barrier, as mentioned previously, is formed because of the tight junctions of endothelial cells in humans and is further supported by the multiple processes of astrocytes. Cytotoxic edema is thought to be due to the intracellular accumulation of fluid following dysfunction of the normal ionic gradients. As mentioned in the section on "Cell Death in the Central Nervous System", loss of high-energy compounds leads to dysfunction of Na^+/K^+-ATPase channels as a first step in the process of necrotic cell death. As this occurs, cell swelling begins and can lead to increases in overall brain volume. Therefore, the brain mass may increase after injuries and must be managed.

The average adult has approximately 90 to 150 mL of CSF within the cranium at any given time, whereas children have a slightly lesser volume (estimated to be 65 to 140 mL in 4- to 13-year olds). It is produced (approximately 20 mL per hour) by the choroid plexus, with additional contribution to the total volume by the bulk flow of interstitial water from the brain into the ventricular system. It is produced at a relatively constant rate in physiologic and pathophysiologic conditions by a two-step process. Hydrostatic pressure within the choroid plexus produces a plasma ultrafiltrate, and this fluid is subsequently modified by the secretion of substances from the choroidal epithelium. CSF flows from the choroid plexus of the lateral ventricle through the third and fourth ventricles within the brain stem (see Fig. 7.17). It exits through the foramens of Luschka and Magendie and overflows into the perimesencephalic cisterns at the level of the tentorium cerebelli. It then travels around the convexity of the brain in the subarachnoid space around the brain and spinal cord and is absorbed into the venous system at the subarachnoid villi. This process, although not well understood, involves the villi acting as a one-way valve into the sagittal sinus when CSF pressures exceed 5 mm Hg.

CSF production or absorption can affect the amount of CSF within the cranium at any given moment. Its production can be decreased by several mechanisms. Furosemide can lead to decreased total body water and intravascular water, limiting the production of CSF in the choroid plexus. Acetazolamide is a carbonic anhydrase inhibitor that can lower CSF production in the choroid plexus by increasing the bicarbonate concentration in the CSF. Increased ICP may suppress CSF production to a small degree, but this effect appears to be minimal. The only clinical situation in which CSF production is supranormal occurs in children with papillomas of the choroid plexus. Decreased absorption of CSF occurs when anatomic obstructions of the flow of CSF within the brain prevent CSF from reaching the areas of absorption in the subarachnoid space. In particular, obstruction at the various foramen causes dilatation of the proximal ventricle and accompanying symptoms. These obstructions can be congenital or can result from infections (meningitis), hemorrhages, or neoplastic processes. Blood within the subarachnoid space can

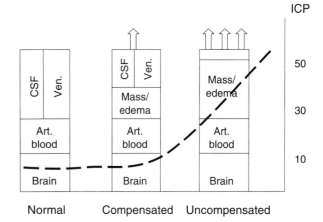

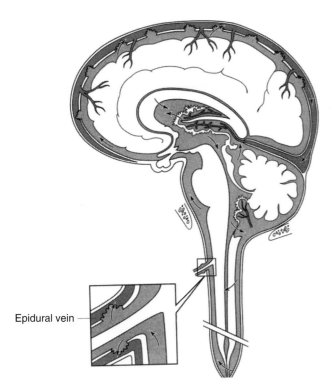

Figure 7.17 Circulation of cerebrospinal fluid (CSF). CSF (*gray*) is secreted by the choroid plexus present in the lateral ventricles. It circulates from the lateral ventricles, through the third ventricle and into the brain stem through the fourth ventricle. CSF exits into the perimesencephalic cisterns and circulates around the convexity of the brain within the subarachnoid space. Absorption into the venous blood (*dark gray*) occurs through the arachnoid villi in the superior sagittal sinus and along the optic, olfactory, and spinal nerve sheaths (*inset*). (From Siegel GJ, Agranoff BW, Alberts RW, et al. (eds.) *Basic neurochemistry*. 6th ed. Philadelphia, PA: Lippincott-Raven Publishers; 1999.)

Figure 7.18 Munroe-Kellie doctrine. **Left:** Total brain volume is the sum of the volume of the components that comprise the total volume. **Middle:** When the volume of one component increases (e.g., mass/edema), the volume of other components must decrease (cerebrospinal fluid [CSF], venous). Intracranial pressure (ICP) (*dashed line*) does not change at this point. **Right:** When component volumes cannot decrease to accommodate increasing volume of another component (mass/edema), ICP rises dramatically. Ven., venous; Art., arterial.

also lead to decreased absorption from the subarachnoid villi and result in increased CSF content within the cranium.

Cerebral blood constitutes the final compound within the cranial cavity under normal conditions. Cerebral blood volume reflects the sum of the blood within the cerebral arteries, veins, and capillaries and must be distinguished from CBF. CBF is the amount of blood delivered to a given amount of brain tissue within a given time. Cerebral blood volume is affected by both CBF and cerebral vasomotor tone. Consequently, when vasomotor tone decreases, cerebral blood volume increases if CBF is maintained.

The Munro-Kellie doctrine states that because the brain, CSF, and cerebral blood volume are encased in a rigid skull, any increase in volume in any of the compartments must be met with either (i) a decrease in volume of the other compartments or (ii) an increase in the pressure within the brain. In pathologic conditions, the increased volume may represent cerebral edema, hemorrhages, hematomas, meningitis, tumors, or other space-occupying lesions (see Fig. 7.18). Pivotal to the complete understanding of the Munro-Kellie doctrine is the concept of intracranial compliance. Intracranial compliance is similar to the compliance calculated within the respiratory system and is defined as:

$$\text{Compliance} = \frac{\text{Change in volume}}{\text{Change in pressure}}$$

$$C = \frac{dV}{dP}$$

In older children with calcified skulls, the volume of the cranial vault cannot significantly change in the acute setting. In this population of children, when an additional mass begins to accumulate, substances within the cranium that are under the least pressure are excluded from the cavity. Initially, CSF from the cranium is forced downward to the subarachnoid space around the spinal cord. As the mass increases in size, the brain constituent with the next lowest pressure, the venous blood, is forced out as much as possible. Further increases in the abnormal mass lead to progressive increases in ICP until arterial blood flow is compromised. Finally, once these compensatory mechanisms are exhausted, pressure increases lead to cerebral herniation syndromes.

In certain circumstances, the Munro-Kellie doctrine can be slightly modified. Before calcification of the skull, the cranium of an infant can expand in response to an abnormal mass collection. The unfused sutures can widen and the various fontanelles can bulge to accommodate this acute increase in cranial volume. Also, the calcified skulls of children and adults can accommodate masses if these grow slowly over time. In this instance, the slow increase in intracranial volume is compensated for by all the mechanisms stated in the preceding text, along with the osteoclastic thinning of the bones of the cranium. This remodeling leads to small but not insignificant increases in overall cranial volume and compensates for the growing volume of the mass. Of course, this compensatory mechanism is as limited as the others, eventually being overcome as the mass grows to a critical size.

Regulation of the Cerebral Vasculature

The brain receives 15% of the total cardiac output and utilizes up to 20% of the oxygen of the entire body. Anatomically, blood reaches the brain through either of the two internal carotid arteries and the vertebral artery. These form a web of connections at the base of the brain, the circle of Willis, ultimately leading to separate arteries that supply the brain with oxygenated blood. The blood circulates through capillaries, leading progressively to veins that converge on another web of structures, cerebral sinuses. The sinuses then convey the blood back to the internal jugular vein and the right atrium.

Because of these anatomic considerations, interruptions of blood flow are minimized. As an example, complete occlusion of a carotid artery does not necessarily lead to cerebral ischemia. While instituting venoarterial extracorporeal membrane oxygenation, the right carotid artery is ligated and used as a conduit for blood to return to the aorta. In children with an intact circle of Willis, CBF continues from the other contributing arteries, and immediate brain ischemia is avoided. Similarly, when individual sinuses within the venous system are occluded, cerebral blood return may be accomplished using the other sinuses. However, occlusion of a vessel that does not have such collateral circulation, such as the MCA or any of the many penetrating arteries or veins, will lead to cerebral infarction in a matter of minutes.

Cerebral Autoregulation

The "normal" CBF of an adult has been measured at approximately 50 mL per 100 g brain tissue/minute. This value assumes that the adult is in a relative resting state, with normal ventilation and normal cerebral metabolism. CBF in neonates has been estimated at between 25 to 30 mL/100 g/minute, and children during development have intermediate values. CBF can be measured using a variety of methods. The currently used clinical methods are outlined in the section on "Monitoring of the Nervous System".

Under normal conditions, CBF is tightly linked to the metabolic requirements of the brain. The mechanisms of this coupling are complex but likely involve the local effects of metabolic products (K^+, adenosine, ATP, and pH) and neural regulation of vasomotor tone. During periods of seizures or fever, brain metabolic activity increases, and CBF increases in a linear manner. This response occurs by vasodilatation of the cerebral vasculature in response to a decrease in ATP or other local factors. The end result of this process is an overall increase in cerebral blood volume and a consequent increase in ICP. Similarly, when

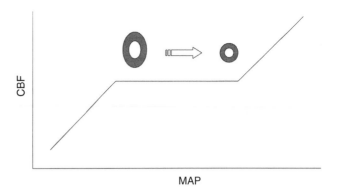

Figure 7.19 Cerebral autoregulation. Cerebral blood flow (CBF) remains constant across a wide range of mean arterial blood pressures (MAPs). This phenomenon of cerebral autoregulation is accomplished by reflex regulation of cerebral arteriolar diameter.

administering drugs to induce coma for therapy, decreases in cerebral metabolism lead to decreases in CBF. This leads to an overall decrease in cerebral blood volume.

CBF is also maintained over a wide range of blood pressures (see Fig. 7.19). When mean arterial blood pressure is maintained in a middle range (thought to be between 50 mm Hg and 150 mm Hg in adults), CBF remains constant. The mechanism for this process, termed *cerebral autoregulation*, involves the cerebral vascular resistance. As blood pressure within cerebral arteries increases, baroreceptors within the vessels sense this event and cerebral arterioles vasoconstrict. The net effect of this action is maintenance of CBF, but with a decreased amount of cerebral blood volume. In contrast, as blood pressure decreases, cerebral arterioles dilate to maintain CBF and overall cerebral blood volume increases.

This relationship between blood pressure and CBF is lost in normal circumstances at the lowest and highest blood pressure ranges and in pathologic states. Although the actual limit is unclear and probably varies for each individual, CBF decreases linearly in relationship to MAP below the autoregulatory range. This leads to ischemia of regions of brain, such as occur in strokes and after cardiac arrest. Similarly, above the upper limit of this range, CBF increases linearly as MAP increases. In this state, hypertensive encephalopathy develops as cerebral blood volume and ICP increase. Lastly, in pathologic states, autoregulation can be lost at all blood pressures. After brain trauma, cardiac arrest, or many other processes, CBF increases and decreases with MAP. This "pressure-passive" circulation may be localized to a given region of the brain or may be generalized to the entire brain.

Mediators of Cerebral Blood Flow

There are several local and global mediators of CBF and metabolism that are important. Among the most important are hypoxia and pH. The relationship between oxygen and CBF is relatively straightforward and is linked to local oxygen content. Globally, arterial oxygen content (CaO_2) is measured by:

$$CaO_2 = 1.34 \times ([\text{hemoglobin}] \times O_2 \text{ saturation}) + (PaO_2 \times 0.003)$$

Because oxygen is readily diffusible in tissue, local oxygen content is closely linked to arterial oxygen content and oxygen delivery. Therefore, local CBF increases linearly as the local brain oxygen content decreases. During times of hemorrhage and acute anemia, CBF increases, and oxygen delivery to the brain (CBF $\times$ CaO_2) is maintained. Because of the oxyhemoglobin dissociation curve, CaO_2 changes very little until PaO_2 decreases below 50 mm Hg. Therefore, CBF is relatively constant over a wide range of arterial oxygen pressures.

CBF is affected by pH and its surrogate, the carbon dioxide tension PCO_2, over its physiologic range. Changes in pH that occur as PCO_2 decreases from 40 to 20 mm Hg lead to a 40% decrease in CBF. Changes in pH that occur as PCO_2 increases from 40 to 80 mm Hg almost double the CBF. This relationship has been intensely studied as a therapeutic option in the cases of pathologic conditions. In particular, intentional hyperventilation was used as a therapy for increased ICP because the lower CBF led to a decrease in cerebral blood volume and ICP. These maneuvers are discussed in the Neurologic Disorders section.

Brain Metabolism

As mentioned in the preceding text, the brain uses a disproportionate amount of oxygen compared to the rest of the body. In fact, the brain represents only 2% of the total body weight and consumes 20% of the total systemic oxygen delivered. In the resting state, cerebral oxygen consumption is 3.5 mL/100 g brain/minute. As mentioned in the preceding text, in situations when cerebral metabolism increases, such as with fever or seizures, CBF increases in parallel to maintain a constant cerebral oxygen delivery.

The organ most sensitive to hypoxia and/or ischemia is the brain. With normothermic circulatory arrest, brain oxygen stores are depleted, producing unconsciousness within 20 seconds. By 3 to 5 minutes, brain glucose and ATP stores are depleted. Coupled with energy failure, numerous pathologic cascades proceed to irreversible neuronal degeneration and ultimately to brain death. Therefore, the brain is vitally dependent on the uninterrupted delivery of oxygen and glucose to meet cerebral metabolic needs.

To provide for its critical dependence on oxygen, the brain tightly couples its blood flow with its metabolic demands. In normal conditions when CBF and metabolism are coupled, extraction of oxygen from the blood as it flows through the cerebral vasculature is a reflection of the cerebral metabolic rate. The cerebral extraction of oxygen (CEO_2) is defined as the difference between arterial oxygen saturation (SaO_2) and the jugular venous oxygen saturation ($SjvO_2$). Normal range for $SjvO_2$ in children is 55% to 70%, whereas CEO_2 normally ranges from 24% to 42%. The

cerebral extraction ratio for oxygen ($CERO_2$) is defined as the ratio of cerebral consumption of oxygen ($CMRO_2$) to cerebral oxygen delivery (CCO_2), but more practically, it can be calculated using the more readily available measures of arterial and jugular venous oxygen saturations: ($SaO_2 - SjvO_2$)/SaO_2. The expected range for $CERO_2$ is 25% to 45%. In the setting of traumatic brain injury in adults, cerebral consumption of oxygen is directly related to GCS, with levels of $CMRO_2$ being 10% to 15% of normal in patients with GCS <5. $CMRO_2$ in children with a GCS of 3 was 20% to 30% of the levels observed in children with a GCS of 4 to 7.

$CERO_2$ may show one of three patterns in children when $CMRO_2$ is low. The first pattern, a lower cerebral metabolic rate, is matched with a decline in CBF. In this situation, a decrease in cerebral metabolic rate leads to a reduction in neuronal carbon dioxide production, causing cerebral vasoconstriction and a proportional reduction in CBF. Cerebral autoregulation and the typical balance between cerebral oxygen consumption and delivery are intact. Moderate hypothermic cardiopulmonary bypass is an example of flow–metabolism coupling. In this case, CBF is provided by the bypass pump, and the redirection of blood to the brain due to systemic vasoconstriction is produced by the moderate (25°C to 28°C) hypothermia. Cooling also lowers the cerebral metabolic rate; cooling from 37°C to 27°C lowers $CMRO_2$ by 3.6 fold. Cerebral autoregulatory mechanisms remain intact during moderate hypothermic cardiopulmonary bypass.

The second pattern, which if prolonged leads to ischemia, is referred to as *oligemic CBF*. Here, there is a loss of coupling between $CMRO_2$ and CBF; the cerebral metabolic rate is low, but CBF is even lower. Like the heart, the brain responds to a reduction in oxygen delivery caused by anemia, hypoxemia, intracranial hypertension, cerebral vasospasms, or severe hypocarbia by increasing the $CERO_2$, measured by a fall in $SjvO_2$. In a study by Skippen et al. of children with severe traumatic brain injury, the CBF, cerebral oxygen consumption, cerebral perfusion pressure, and oxygen extraction ratio were estimated using xenon-enhanced computed tomography scans, jugular venous bulb oxygen saturation, and arterial oxygen saturation. Cerebral oxygen consumption decreased disproportionately with the decrease in CBF. During stepwise lowering of PCO_2, the frequency of cerebral ischemia (defined as CBF of <18 mL/minute/100 g) was 28.9% during normocapnia, with an increase to 73.1% when $PaCO_2$ was <25 mm Hg. Clinical interventions to improve cerebral oxygen delivery, such as transfusion of packed red blood cells, increased inspired oxygen concentration, less severe hypocapnea, lowering of ICP with osmotherapy or craniectomy, are indicated emergently to prevent cerebral infarction. Additionally, interventions to further lower the cerebral metabolic rate such as administering sedatives, imposing a pharmacologic coma with barbiturates, treating seizures, and preventing fever may help match $CMRO_2$ to

CBF. Despite these efforts, a rise in $Sjvo_2$ after a period of levels in the ischemic range suggests that tissue ischemic changes are irreversible.

The third pattern is cerebral hyperperfusion, or oligemic intracranial hypertension. In this case, the coupling between the cerebral metabolic rate and CBF is again lost; however, CBF exceeds the cerebral metabolic need. $Sjvo_2$ rises in this situation as $CERO_2$ falls. Such hyperperfusion syndromes have been observed in children after severe traumatic brain injury, characterized by an increase in CBF, with a subsequent increase in cerebral blood volume. On the basis of the Munro-Kellie doctrine, without a concomitant change in either brain or CSF volume, this rise in cerebral blood volume will cause ICP to rise.

Development of hepatic encephalopathy produces pathologic changes in CBF as autoregulation fails. Initially, there is elevation in CBF at normal arterial blood pressures that leads to hyperemic intracranial hypertension. Cerebral edema then develops, producing oligemic intracranial hypertension and ultimately leading to loss of CBF and brain death. Because of hyperperfusion syndrome, CBF should be held within the normal physiologic range by manipulation of arterial blood pressure in order to avoid hypertension-induced cerebral edema.

A third clinical condition in which cerebral hyperperfusion occurs is during deep hypothermic cardiopulmonary bypass. Deep hypothermia is used to preserve organ function, primarily the brain, when circulatory arrest is required to correct congenital heart defects. At deep levels of hypothermia ($15°C$ to $18°C$), cerebral pressure/flow autoregulation is lost and $CMRO_2$:CBF is 75:1. Therefore, if adequate cerebral oxygen delivery is supplied, low-flow bypass could indefinitely meet the metabolic demands during deep hypothermic bypass.

Implications for Critical Care

In conclusion, a thorough understanding of the physiologic properties of the intracranial vault, the regulation of CBF, and the determinants of cerebral metabolism are essential for the clinical management of children with severe brain injuries. These concepts will be discussed in the Neurologic Disorders section.

CENTRAL NERVOUS SYSTEM REGULATION OF ANALGESIA, ANESTHESIA, AND PAIN

Pain is the sensory experience of a noxious stimulus. Because tissue damage may be associated with pain, the perception of, and response to, pain can serve a critical protective function. Critically ill patients are bombarded by noxious stimuli in the ICU, and sources of pain are numerous and often persistent. Furthermore, the ability to communicate pain location is limited in infants and young children, as well as in intubated patients. Therefore, the goals of chronic pain management in the ICU are to recognize and minimize sources of pain and to safely and effectively respond to unpreventable discomfort.

It is important to distinguish the experience of pain from the neural mechanisms of nociception. Nociception is the process in which specialized sensory receptors in peripheral tissues detect sensations generated during tissue damage such as burning, prickling, aching, or stinging. However, nociception alone does not necessarily lead to the experience of pain. Pain perception requires the integration of sensory, affective, and cognitive components.

Perception of pain provokes a broad range of physiologic responses. For example, post-thoracotomy pain causes an increase in local skeletal muscle tension that not only compromises pulmonary mechanics but also intensifies the pain. The objective of this section is to discuss the neurobiology of pain perception and to review the pharmacology of subacute and chronic pain modulation and sedation administered to limit pathophysiologic consequences that arise from pain in critically ill children. Aspects of short-term sedation and analgesia are not addressed in this section.

Functional Anatomy of Pain Perception

Receptors and Primary Afferents

Pain perception results from the balance of noxious signals from nociceptors and modulating input from non-nociceptive afferents. Nociceptors responsive to noxious mechanical, thermal, and polymodal stimuli are widely distributed in the peripheral nerve endings of the skin and deep tissues. To demonstrate how input from afferent nociceptive fibers is perceived as being painful, we use the example of touching a hot pan, then reflexively shaking the burned finger. Mechanical and thermal nociceptors are stimulated on touching a hot pan and a sharp pain is felt immediately, followed by a more prolonged burning or aching pain. The initial pain stimulus is transmitted rapidly from thermal and mechanical nociceptors to the CNS by myelinated Aδ fibers. Signals from polymodal nociceptors are transmitted by unmyelinated C fibers, resulting in the longer-lasting perception of aching pain. Myelinated, large-diameter, non-nociceptive afferents, known as *Aβ fibers*, modulate the nociceptive signal. The observation that shaking or vibration attenuates pain leads to development of the gate control theory of pain. This theory states that activity of Aβ mechanoreceptors inhibits discharges of projection neurons (that transmit nociceptive signals to the CNS) through an inhibitory neuron in the dorsal horn. The gate control theory forms the basis of pain relief by transcutaneous electrical nerve stimulation (TENS), which predominantly stimulates Aβ fibers.

It is important to distinguish between nociceptive pain, as discussed in the preceding text, and neuropathic pain. In the latter, pain is caused by damage to neural structures.

Stimulus-induced neuropathic pain is often divided into allodynia and hyperalgesia, however, in clinical practice these states often coexist. Hyperalgesia and allodynia are abnormal pain states produced by pathologic activation of nociceptors. In allodynia, pain results from stimuli that are not normally perceived as noxious, such as light touch. On the other hand, individuals with hyperalgesia exhibit an exaggerated response to a noxious stimulus.

Dorsal Horn and Central Projections

Nociceptive afferent fibers synapse to neurons in specific layers within the dorsal horn of the spinal cord. Projection neurons in the most superficial layer of the dorsal horn, called the *marginal layer* or *lamina I*, receive input from Aδ fibers and project to the thalamus through the contralateral spinothalamic tract. Whereas C fibers synapse to interneurons in lamina II or the substantia gelatinosa, Aβ fibers terminate in the more ventral layers, lamina III and IV. Lamina V contains neurons that receive direct input from Aδ, C, and Aβ fibers, as well as nociceptive input from visceral structures. Like projection neurons in the marginal layer, lamina V neurons ascend along the contralateral spinothalamic tract.

A brief discussion of nociceptive afferent fiber termination in the dorsal horn is important in understanding referred pain. Referred pain is a phenomenon in which pain is perceived at the skin in response to organ tissue injury. A well-recognized example of referred pain is left arm pain occurring with myocardial infarction. It has been suggested that convergence of somatic and visceral afferent nociceptive fibers on the same projection neuron in lamina V of the dorsal horn can account for referred pain.

Central Modulation of Nociception and Processing of Pain

Thalamic nuclei process nociceptive information and relay afferent information to the somatosensory and association cortices. However, because pain perception is a process that integrates nociceptive input in the context of prior experiences and behavioral reactions, it would be expected that additional cortical brain regions would participate in the process. Positron emission tomography (PET) studies have identified the cingulate gyrus and insular cortex as regions that are specifically activated in humans exposed to noxious heat or cold.

Pathophysiology of Pain

Physiologic responses to pain perception may be detrimental in a critically ill child. When an individual perceives pain, the sympathetic nervous system is activated, leading to increased heart rate, tachycardia, cardiac work, and cardiac oxygen consumption. Pain also triggers a hypothalamic neuroendocrine response characterized by the augmented release of catabolic hormones and inhibition of anabolic hormone secretion. Taken together, uncorrected pain can exacerbate physiologic derangements common in critically ill patients.

Endogenous Pain Control Systems

The brain contains three major classes of opioid receptors (μ, δ, and κ) that bind the endogenous opioid peptides, enkephalins, β-endorphin, and dynorphins, to produce analgesia. The two enkephalins, leucine and methionine enkephalin, are pentapeptides cleaved from the polypeptide precursor preproenkephalin. Dynorphin A, dynorphin B, and neoendorphin are also derived from a precursor polypeptide, preprodynorphin, and are selective agonists of the κ receptor. Proenkephalin and prodynorphin are distributed in areas of the CNS that are related to pain perception (such as laminae I and II of the dorsal horn and the periaqueductal gray), and response to pain (such as the limbic system, the cerebral cortex, and caudate and globus pallidus of the motor system), and regulation of the autonomic nervous system. Enkephalins bind to both μ and δ opioid receptors. Pro-opiomelanocortin (POMC) is the precursor polypeptide whose cleavage gives rise to β-endorphin and adrenocorticotropic hormone (ACTH). With stress, both β-endorphin and ACTH is released into the bloodstream. POMC-producing neurons are limited to areas of the human brain where electrical stimulation can relieve pain, specifically, the arcuate nucleus, NTS and spinal cord.

Nociceptin/orphanin FQ (N/OFQ) is a novel endogenous opioid peptide that shares significant sequence homology with dynorphin A. N/OFQ binds to the opioid receptor–like (ORL1) receptor, a specific G protein–coupled receptor. The N/OFQ-ORL1 receptor system appears to play an important role in pain, anxiety, appetite regulation, stress responsiveness, effects of drug reward and reinforcement, and learning and memory processes. The ORL1 receptor therefore represents a new molecular target for the design of novel agents for anxiety, analgesia, and drug addiction. The replacement of tyrosine with phenylalanine in the amino-terminal eliminates interaction of N/OFQ with the classical opioid receptors.

Opioid Receptor Signaling

The three classical endogenous opioid receptors are coupled through G proteins for the inhibition of adenylyl cyclase activity, activation of ligand-gated K^+ currents, and closure of voltage-sensitive Ca^{2+} currents, thereby producing membrane hyperpolarization. There is evidence that opioid receptors may be coupled to phospholipase C–mediated cascades, leading to the generation of IP_3 and DAG. As discussed in the subsequent text, the development of tolerance, sensitization, and withdrawal result in adaptations at multiple levels within these receptor/second messenger cascades.

Pharmacologic Modulation of Pain

The fundamental pharmacologic approach to pain management includes (i) the administration of regularly scheduled dosing rather than p.r.n. dosing for control of persistent pain, (ii) the titration of analgesics on the basis of pain severity as measured by validated scales, and (iii) the use of adjuvant medications to improve the efficacy of analgesics while minimizing harmful side effects. This section highlights the mechanisms of action of analgesic agents; a more detailed clinical discussion of these agents, including dosing ranges and toxicity, is found in Chapter 53.

Nonopioid analgesics

Nonsteroidal Anti-inflammatory Drugs

Nonsteroidal anti-inflammatory drugs (NSAIDs) and acetaminophen are the primary nonopioid analgesics used in children. They produce analgesia without producing ventilatory depression, a change in sensorium, or the risk of dependency. These drugs reduce tissue nociceptive stimulation, thereby reducing prostaglandin synthesis by the inhibition of nonselective cyclooxygenase-1 and 2 (COX-1 and COX-2). The antipyretic activity of these agents is also related to inhibition of hypothalamic cyclooxygenases. Analgesic efficacy can be attained with lower doses of opiates when used in combination with acetaminophen. The lack of antiplatelet effects and the wide therapeutic window makes acetaminophen an attractive agent in the setting of critical illness. Unlike acetaminophen, NSAIDs have potent anti-inflammatory properties. Concerns about complications from antiplatelet and GI effects of NSAIDs have traditionally limited NSAID use in the ICU. However, ketorolac tromethamine, an NSAID available in parenteral form, has been used widely and safely for the short-term management of postoperative pain despite its potential for prolonging bleeding time. The development of selective COX-2 inhibitors that lack antiplatelet effects have brought new agents for short-term use in the critical care environment.

Ketamine

NMDA excitatory glutamate receptors participate in nociception in humans. NMDA receptor antagonists, such as ketamine, inhibit the excitability of the spinal cord nociceptive neurons induced by C-fiber stimulation, producing analgesia. Ketamine is also effective in treating hyperalgesia and allodynia after trauma or other peripheral injury. Increased dorsal horn excitability, and therefore, the development of hyperalgesia and allodynia, involves cellular modulation linked to NMDA receptor activity. Ketamine inhibits these spinal cord NMDA receptors and is an effective therapeutic agent for pain generated by tissue injury.

Other CNS effects, such as memory impairment, ataxia, motor dyscoordination, and hallucinations, limit the long-term use of ketamine as a single agent for sedation in critically ill patients. However, combining ketamine administration with other analgesic agents, such as opioids, has attractive therapeutic potential. For example, in a common situation encountered in an ICU patient, and as discussed in the subsequent text, ketamine used in low doses decreases tolerance to opioids.

Dexmedetomidine

Binding of agonists to α_2-adrenergic receptors in the brain leads to inactivation of sympathetic activity, whereas in the spinal cord α_2-adrenergic agonists produce analgesia. In the periphery, rapid intravenous administration of α_2-adrenergic agonists leads to vascular smooth muscle contraction, producing hypertension and reflex bradycardia. Clonidine is the major α_2-adrenergic agonist in clinical use today. Although the analgesic effects of clonidine are not clinically significant, it has found favor as a sedative during the less acute phase of illness in ICU patients. In addition, clonidine is often administered to patients as long-term opioids are being weaned. In this setting, it may help ameliorate some of the adverse sympathetic activity associated with withdrawal.

Dexmedetomidine is a highly selective α_2-adrenergic agonist recently approved by the U.S. Food and Drug Administration for short-term infusion as a sedative agent in critically ill adult patients. Its effects are related to tissue-specific α_2-adrenergic activation, including sedation brought on by receptor binding in the locus ceruleus and analgesia due to supraspinal, spinal cord, and peripheral sites of action. Further, dexmedetomidine produces bradycardia because of sympatholytic and reflex vagomimetic action and hypertension because of vasoconstrictive effects predominating over vasodilatory effects on vascular smooth muscle. Dexmedetomidine also treats shivering but the mechanism unknown. In addition to having some direct analgesic effects, dexmedetomidine appears to increase the effectiveness of other analgesic agents. Therefore, dexmedetomidine has sedative, analgesic-sparing, and sympatholytic effects that may benefit select PICU patients. Unfortunately, information on the safety and efficacy of dexmedetomidine in critically ill children is extremely limited.

Opioid Analgesics

Opioids are the mainstay of pain treatment, exerting their action by mimicking the action of endogenous opioid peptides. Despite the existence of endogenous agonists, the opioid receptors were originally classified on the basis of their affinity to exogenous agonists. Opiate alkaloids such as morphine, methadone, fentanyl, and sufentanil are agonists of the μ receptor, found at high concentrations in the ascending pain pathways. These pathways include the periaqueductal gray matter, the medulla, and the superficial lamina of the spinal cord dorsal horn, although μ receptors are also found more widely distributed throughout the central and peripheral nervous systems. The affinity of binding to the μ receptor directly correlates to the analgesic potency. A discussion of the clinical pharmacology of the therapeutic opioids, including selection of appropriate agents for particular indications, is found in Chapter 53.

Opioid Tolerance; Physical and Psychological Dependence

Three major problems are associated with chronic medical use of opiates: tolerance, physical dependence, and addiction. Tolerance is the requirement for escalating doses of a drug to achieve the same level of effectiveness. At a cellular level, development of tolerance involves opioid receptor internalization and/or alterations in second messenger signaling following chronic exposure to an opioid. Whereas μ and δ receptors undergo agonist-mediated internalization through endocytosis, κ receptors do not. Interestingly, certain agonists such as enkephalins, cause rapid internalization of the μ receptor, whereas internalization does not occur when morphine is bound. Chronic treatment with μ receptor agonists causes superactivation of adenylyl cyclase that functionally inhibits signal transduction at this receptor.

Chronic opioid use can produce physical dependence, manifested by irritability, nausea/vomiting, diarrhea, chills, fever, diaphoresis, yawning, papillary dilation, piloerection, rhinorrhea, and insomnia when opioids are withdrawn. The time course and severity of these withdrawal symptoms depend upon the characteristics of the opioid. For example, because of the differing half-life of the opioids, the onset of acute withdrawal symptoms is 6 to 12 hours after stopping treatment with morphine, but 36 hours after stopping methadone.

Parents of critically ill children who are receiving long-term administration of opioids sometimes express the fear that their child will develop drug dependence. It is important to explain that an expected physiologic response to opioids is tolerance and dependence, and opioids can be discontinued in a manner that prevents the development of withdrawal. Furthermore, it is essential to distinguish tolerance and dependence from addiction. Addiction, or psychological dependence, is a behavioral pattern characterized by the compulsive use of a drug and the overwhelming involvement with its procurement and use. Addiction does not occur in the setting of critical illness.

Glutamate Receptor Antagonists Reduce Opioid Tolerance

In spite of escalating opioid dosing, opioid tolerance can lead to inadequate pain control, patient discomfort, and potential exacerbation of the patient's medical condition. Addition of a glutamate NMDA antagonist, such as ketamine or dextromethorphan, has been shown to block or reverse opioid tolerance. There is growing evidence that adjunctive use of low-dose ketamine can successfully reduce opioid tolerance and improve analgesia in the ICU setting. Clinical aspects of this strategy to overcome tolerance are discussed in Chapter 53.

Opioid Agonist/Antagonists

The stimulus for development of opioid agonist/antagonists agents was the need for analgesics with less respiratory depression and addictive potential. However, side effects including respiratory depression often occur in doses required to achieve adequate analgesic responses. The agonist/antagonist opioids, nalbuphine and butorphanol, exert their analgesic effects by acting as κ receptor agonists. Nalbuphine is a competitive μ receptor antagonist, whereas butorphanol is a partial agonist at the μ opioid receptor.

Sedative/Hypnotic Agents

Agitation, evidenced by inadvertent removal of endotracheal tubes and intravascular catheters, ventilator dyssynchrony, sleep deprivation, or augmentation of the stress response, can have deleterious effects on critically ill children. Relief from anxiety and reduction in agitation are therapeutic goals in almost every critically ill patient. Sedatives and hypnotic agents, prescribed to ameliorate anxiety and agitation, are therefore among the most commonly used drugs in the ICU. Nonetheless, identification and removal of physiologic causes for agitation or anxiety, as well as adequate analgesia, must be considered before administration of sedatives in critically ill children. This section reviews the mechanism of action and pharmacology of sedative and hypnotic agents used commonly in the ICU and discusses dependence and withdrawal as related to these agents. Guidelines and practice parameters for the sustained use of sedatives in the adult critical ill patient, developed by the American College of Critical Care Medicine, is highlighted, although no such consensus has been developed for pediatric patients. Detail of drug dosing and side effects are found in Chapter 53.

Benzodiazepines

Mechanism of Action. Structurally, benzodiazepines are composed of a benzene ring fused to a seven-member diazepine ring. Various modifications in the structure of the ring systems yield compounds with qualitatively similar clinical effects but variable pharmacokinetic and pharmacodynamic characteristics. An exception is flumazenil, in which substitutions in the ring structures produce a compound that acts as a benzodiazepine antagonist.

Benzodiazepines exert their effects by binding to a site on the GABA$_A$ receptor/ion-channel complex (see Fig. 7.20). In the presence of GABA, benzodiazepines enhance GABA-induced chloride currents, thereby potentiating inhibitory synaptic transmission.

The enzymes of the cytochrome P-450 system, particularly CYP3A4, metabolize benzodiazepines extensively. Coadministration of the CYP2A4 inhibitors erythromycin, clarithromycin, ketoconazole, or itraconazole can affect benzodiazepine metabolism. Particularly for midazolam, compromised renal function may delay elimination and prolong clinical effects because of accumulation of the active metabolite α-hydroxymidazolam. Because of the formation of active metabolites, the duration of clinical effects of diazepam and midazolam cannot be predicted from the half-life of the parent compounds. Furthermore, when

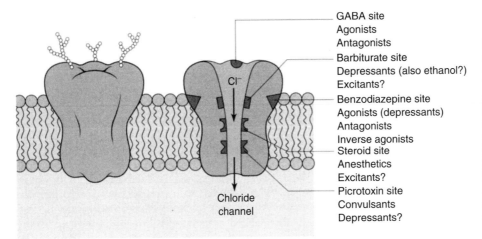

GABA site
Agonists
Antagonists
Barbiturate site
Depressants (also ethanol?)
Excitants?
Benzodiazepine site
Agonists (depressants)
Antagonists
Inverse agonists
Steroid site
Anesthetics
Excitants?
Picrotoxin site
Convulsants
Depressants?

Cl⁻

Chloride
channel

Figure 7.20 Structural model of the GABA$_A$ benzodiazepine receptor chloride (Cl⁻) ionophore complex. The cutaway view demonstrates targets for a variety of compounds that influence the receptor complex. No specific drug receptor location is implied. The "?" indicates that there is some evidence that these ligands bind at the indicated sites, but the evidence is certain at this time. (From Siegel GJ, Agranoff BW, Alberts RW, et al. (eds.) *Basic neurochemistry.* 6th ed. Philadelphia, PA: Lippincott-Raven Publishers; 1999.)

administered as an infusion, the accumulation of the parent drug or its active metabolites may produce inadvertent oversedation. Daily interruption of midazolam infusions was associated with a reduction in the duration of mechanical ventilation and length of ICU stay in adult patients. In the PICU, the risk of inadvertent extubation or removal of other devices during a daily awakening session must be balanced with the beneficial effects noted by Kress et al.

Tolerance to benzodiazepines has been described, and the risk for withdrawal is directly related to the rate of medication weaning. Signs and symptoms of benzodiazepine withdrawal include seizures, delirium, anxiety, agitation, headache, tremor, nausea, sweating, paresthesias, myoclonus, and muscle cramps. Systematically tapering daily dosing can successfully prevent withdrawal symptoms.

Barbiturates

Mechanism of Action. Barbiturates also exert their sedative effects at the GABA$_A$ receptor but bind to a site distinct from the GABA or benzodiazepine site on the receptor/ion-channel complex. In addition to activation of the inhibitory GABA$_A$ receptor, barbiturates also inhibit the excitatory AMPA receptor. Taken together, the effects on these postsynaptic receptors account for the sedative effects of barbiturates.

Although barbiturates had been used extensively for sedation in critically ill patients, the more attractive side effect profile and increased safety margin of benzodiazepines has reduced the long-term use of barbiturates. However, the short-term use of barbiturates is appropriate in situations such as rapid sequence intubation or sedation for procedures. In addition, pentobarbital is administered as a constant intravenous infusion to induce barbiturate coma.

Propofol

Propofol (2, 6-diisopropylphenol) is an intravenous sedative–hypnotic agent used widely in pediatric medicine for the induction and maintenance of anesthesia and as a sedative for procedures such as endoscopy. Similar to benzodiazepines and barbiturates, the sedative activity of propofol is attributed to the direct activation of GABA$_A$ receptors. In addition, propofol inhibits the NMDA receptor, which leads to reduced calcium influx across the postsynaptic membrane. Onset of action is rapid; however, an attractive property of propofol not shared by other sedative–hypnotic agents is rapid recovery even after prolonged infusion.

Propofol has other effects that makes it an attractive sedative–hypnotic agent in the ICU environment. Rapid elimination allows the evaluation of a patient's neurologic status within minutes after discontinuing the infusion. As a potential cerebral protective agent, propofol decreases cerebral oxygen consumption, reduces ICP, has antioxidant and anti-inflammatory properties, and has anticonvulsant properties. Furthermore, in critically ill adults, dose-related hypotension is the most common side effect, whereas hypertriglyceridemia and pancreatitis are uncommon complications. Given these effects, propofol is used widely for ICU sedation in adults.

However, the safety of propofol administration for long-term (>24 hours) sedation in critically ill children has not been established. Propofol infusions have been associated with the "propofol infusion syndrome" in children. This potentially fatal complication is characterized by severe metabolic acidosis, lipidemia, rhabdomyolysis, bradycardia, hypotension, and asystole. This rare complication is believed to be due to decreased transmembrane electrical potential and alteration of electron transport across the inner mitochondrial membrane. Nonetheless, although the current data have not established a causal relationship between protocol and the syndrome of metabolic acidosis with cardiovascular collapse, data from case reports are sufficient to justify significant concern. Although propofol may provide systemic benefits beyond its sedative effects, currently, the risks of morbidity and mortality outweigh these potential benefits. Therefore, the manufacturers of propofol have emphasized that it is not currently approved for sedation in PICU patients.

Muscle Relaxants

Neuromuscular blockade is commonly used in the ICU to achieve muscle relaxation when other modalities have been tried without success. Although these agents have particular indications, their major limitations must be recognized, particularly when prolonged use is considered. Here, we briefly review the site of action of the neuromuscular blocking drug (the NMJ), focus on the mechanism of action of the two major classes of NMBAs, and discuss the application of muscle relaxation in the ICU, with particular emphasis on the balance between their benefits and hazards. Similar to the discussion of sedatives, guidelines and practice parameters for the use of sustained neuromuscular blockade in the adult critical ill patient, developed by the American College of Critical Care Medicine, is highlighted, although no consensus has been developed for pediatric patients. Details of drug dosing and side effects are found in Chapter 53.

Mechanisms of Action

The NMJ is discussed in detail in the section on "Functional Anatomy of the Neuromuscular Junction". Briefly, the NMJ is a specialized cholinergic synapse composed of the terminal of a motor neuron and a motor end plate in the muscle. When an action potential in the motor neuron reaches the nerve terminal, acetylcholine is released from synaptic vesicles. Acetylcholine then diffuses across the synapse to the postsynaptic muscle end plate, where it binds to nAChR to open an ion channel, leading to depolarization of the muscle membrane. NMBAs bind to the nAChR and either partially depolarize the end plate, rendering it unresponsive to acetylcholine (known as *depolarizing agents*), or competitively inhibit the actions of acetylcholine at the nAChR (known as *nondepolarizing agents*).

Depolarizing Neuromuscular Blocking Agents. Succinylcholine is the most widely used depolarizing NMBAs in clinical practice. In the NMJ, depolarizing NMBAs open the nAChR ion channel, causing membrane depolarization from -80 mV to -55 mV. Because succinylcholine is not eliminated by AChE, a brief period of repeated excitation usually elicits transient muscle fasciculations. Although acetylcholine continues to be released into the junction, the partially depolarized state of the muscle membrane prevents further depolarization, resulting in a block of neuromuscular transmission and flaccid paralysis. During prolonged membrane depolarization, the nAChR ion channel remains open, allowing K^+ efflux and Na^+, Cl^-, and Ca^{2+} influx. Because serum potassium concentration rises approximately 0.5 mEq per L with a 1 mg per kg dose, succinylcholine-induced hyperkalemia can be a life-threatening complication of succinylcholine administration. As discussed in Chapter 53, succinylcholine is contraindicated in patients with select conditions.

Nondepolarizing Neuromuscular Blocking Agents. Nondepolarizing NMBAs are competitive antagonists at the nAChR. These agents bind at the postjunctional membrane and prevent the generation of an end-plate potential. The nondepolarizing NMBAs have been classified into three groups: (i) the natural alkaloids (D-tubocurarine), (ii) the benzylisoquinolines (atracurium, mivacurium) and (iii) the aminosteroids (pancuronium, rocuronium, vecuronium). The benzylisoquinolines have a slight propensity for release of histamine but have the benefit of degradation by plasma cholinesterases. The prototype aminosteroid, pancuronium, blocks muscarinic receptors to produce vagal blockade and tachycardia. However, pancuronium and the other aminosteroids do not release histamine.

Indications for Use of Muscle Relaxants in the Intensive Care Unit

Administration of NMBAs can provide protection for the patient or can facilitate procedures, but these shorter-term benefits are often the onset of longer-term complications. Muscle relaxation, or "therapeutic paralysis," is commonly applied to critically ill patients when sedation and analgesia fail to meet therapeutic goals. Facilitation of ventilation, decrease in oxygen consumption, treatment of muscle spasm, reduction in intracranial hypertension, protection of wound or tracheal anastomoses, or alleviation of shivering are the frequently cited indications for long-term use of NMBAs. There is, however, little evidence supporting use of NMBAs for these indications. Furthermore, there have been no studies comparing clinical outcomes when ICU patients are randomizing to receive NMBAs or placebo.

On the other hand, challenges to safe use of NMBAs include adequate monitoring of the depth of blockade, interactions between muscle relaxants and other pharmacologic agents, muscle weakness and atrophy following long-term treatment, and lower respiratory tract infections due to compromised airway mucociliary activity and suppression of the cough reflex. Monitoring the depth of neuromuscular blockade allows for the lowest NMBA dose with the potential for minimizing adverse effects. Peripheral nerve stimulation is the standard for monitoring the depth of neuromuscular blockade in the operating room. TOF is the most commonly used mode of peripheral nerve stimulation (see Fig. 7.21). Four electrical stimuli are provided, and the motor response of the fourth stimulus is compared to the magnitude of the response to the first stimulus. If the magnitude of the motor response cannot be quantified, counting the number of motor responses to the four stimuli will provide a measure of the degree of neuromuscular blockade. Specifically, zero twitches out of four stimuli (one TOF test) corresponds to approximately 100% blockade of the nAChR in the NMJ. One twitch corresponds to 90% blockade, two twitches to 80% blockade, and three twitches to 75% blockade; with four twitches the extent of nAChR blockade cannot be predicted. Therefore,

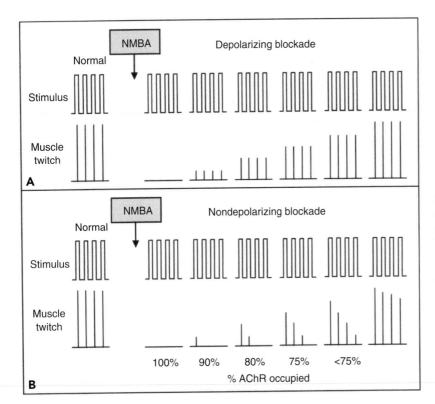

Figure 7.21 Results of peripheral nerve stimulation with train-of-four (TOF) stimulation. **A:** TOF stimulus to a peripheral nerve produces four uniform muscle twitches. TOF stimulation in the presence of a depolarizing neuromuscular blocking agent (NMBA) produces four muscle twitches. The magnitude of the muscle twitch corresponds to the depth of neuromuscular blockade. **B:** TOF stimulus to a peripheral nerve produces four uniform muscle twitches. With TOF stimulation in the presence of a nondepolarizing NMBA, the number of muscle twitches elicited directly relates to the percentage of acetylcholine receptors (AChR) occupied in the neuromuscular junction.

with the use of TOF, the effects of muscle relaxants are carefully titrated to safely intubate to maintain immobility during surgery, and to allow for rapid extubation of patients when the surgery is complete.

Titration of neuromuscular blockade in the ICU should include both clinical assessment and TOF by peripheral nerve stimulation. The goal of monitoring is to avoid 100% blockade of nACh receptors. Adequate neuromuscular blockade is achieved when the ventilator synchrony is maintained and when clinical movement is minimal. Patellar deep tendon reflex can also be used as a clinical assessment of neuromuscular blockade. Attenuation or loss of patellar deep tendon reflex with NMBA administration suggests 90% to 100% blockade and a reduction in dosing. Using the TOF, at least two twitches is the level of neuromuscular blockade to be targeted in ICU patients. Objective monitoring of neuromuscular blockade is recommended whenever a nondepolarizing NMBA is used.

In most situations, provision of adequate levels of sedation and analgesia will reduce the need for muscle relaxants. Feelings of helplessness and anxiety, leading to distress, can be seen in individuals who are muscle relaxed, with inadequate anxiolysis and/or analgesia. Hypertension and tachycardia in a muscle-relaxed patient requires an evaluation of the adequacy of the underlying sedation.

Implications for Critical Care

The environment of the intensive care exposes patients to persistent noxious stimuli including tracheal suctioning, immobilization, sensory overload or deprivation, noise, light, and sleep deprivation. Sedative–hypnotics are used in combination with analgesics to improve patient comfort by providing pain control and sedation.

MONITORING OF THE NERVOUS SYSTEM

The overall goal of monitoring the nervous system of critically ill children is to detect injurious processes at a time when they can be corrected. There is a growing number of monitoring systems available to clinicians to perform this vital task. There are monitors that are readily available at the child's bedside, whereas others require machinery that must be located at a central location. There are monitors that use simple observation or are relatively basic, whereas others require advanced physics and computer analysis to generate data. The monitors currently available can assess the clinical condition, the brain structure, ICP, electrophysiology, CBF, or cerebral metabolism. The physiologic principles of these monitors along with the relative strengths and weaknesses of each device are discussed in this section.

Assessing the Clinical Condition

Physical Examination

The most fundamental method to monitor the CNS of critically ill children is by consistent, repetitive physical examinations performed by caregivers. Changes in cranial nerve function, muscular tone, strength, sensation, and levels of consciousness can be observed virtually continuously without undue harm to the child. These regular, frequent assessments are a cornerstone of neurocritical care, and their importance cannot be overestimated. Detection of new neurologic abnormalities is dependent on the experience of the examiner and the care in which the examination is performed; training of bedside caregivers is critical to the early detection of correctable neurologic injuries.

In critically ill children, a focused assessment of cranial nerve function is extremely important. Children may be sedated for mechanical ventilation, may have hemodynamic instability, or may be administered agents that will affect the overall neurologic examination. However, there are relatively few agents that can confound an assessment of the cranial nerves (with the exception of various pupillary responses and sympathomimetic agents or high-dose barbiturates). Some cranial nerves (CN I [olfactory] and CN XI [spinal accessory]) are almost never assessed. Injuries to these nerves are rarely associated with critical illness and may not herald severe intracranial pathology. CN II (optic) transmits signals sensed by the retina to the occipital cortex. Because of the decussation of the nerves, damage to a single nerve will cause a visual field defect, often difficult to ascertain in a critically ill child. However, deficit in CN II will also lead to the pupil not constricting in response to light, but does constrict when light is shone in the other eye (consensual response). CN III (oculomotor) innervates all of the extraocular muscles of the eye except the superior oblique and lateral rectus and mediates pupillary constriction and accommodation. Failure of a pupil to constrict to light is a sign of CN III lesion, often heralding cerebral herniation (see preceding text). CN IV (trochlear) innervates the superior oblique muscle. Damage to this nerve causes diplopia and leaves the affected eye rotated slightly outward (because of unopposed actions of the inferior rectus). CN VI (abducens) innervates the lateral rectus, and lesions produce a deviation of the eye medially. CN V (trigeminal) senses stimuli from the face and innervates the muscles of mastication. CN VII (facial) innervates the muscles of facial expression, as well as sensory input from the tongue. CN V and VII can be tested by eliciting a corneal reflex (blinking action [motor VII] in response to touching the sclera of the eye with a cotton swab [sensory V]). CN VIII (vestibulocochlear) is responsible for hearing and balance. CN VIII is tested using calorics to elicit nystagmus. CN IX (glossopharyngeal) mediates sensation from the palate in response to swallowing, whereas CN X (vagus) mediates swallowing in response to such a stimulus. Autonomic fibers from CN X innervate the heart, blood vessels, trachea, bronchi, stomach, and intestines, so disruptions in these functions can cause bradycardia, hypotension, and many other symptoms. Lastly, CN XII (hypoglossal) innervates the muscles of the tongue. Lesions can be detected by observing the wasting of the musculature or the deviation of protrusion of the tongue laterally.

The remainder of the clinical examination is dependent, to some degree, on the clinical condition of the child. Muscular tone and strength should be assessed in all extremities in a child to attempt to discern any deficits. NMBAs (or other medications that might decrease muscular strength) or the inability to follow the instructions of the examiner can confound this examination. Similarly, a sensory examination should be performed to determine any decrement in sensation to pinprick or other painful stimuli. Assessments of fine motor functioning (vibration, cold, etc.) are usually not feasible in the unconscious child. But these can be carried out in some children and can provide valuable information. Deep tendon reflexes should be elicited from muscle groups of all extremities as a part of a complete examination.

A standardized tool to assess the level of consciousness in critically ill children is the GCS score (see Table 7.5). Initially developed for adults after traumatic brain injury, this simple scale can provide a rapid, objective assessment of a child's level of consciousness (as measured by eye opening, verbal responses, and motor responses) that is relatively reproducible between caregivers. Eye opening is scored on a 1 to 4 point basis (4 = eyes open spontaneously, 3 = eyes open to voice, 2 = eyes open to painful stimuli, 1 = eyes never open). Verbal response is scored on a 1 to 5 point scale (5 = speaking using clear words, 4 = speaking in words that are intelligible, but not appropriate for the situation, 3 = speaking in unintelligible words, 2 = sounds in response to painful stimuli, 1 = no verbal response to stimuli). Motor response is scored on a 1 to 6 point scale (6 = obeys commands, 5 = localizes a painful stimulus, 4 = withdraws from a stimulus but is not a localized response, 3 = abnormal flexion movements, 2 = abnormal extensor movements, 1 = no response). The

TABLE 7.5
GLASGOW COMA SCALE SCORE

Eye opening	4 = Eyes open spontaneously
	3 = Eyes open to command
	2 = Eyes open to painful stimuli
	1 = Eyes closed
Verbal response	5 = Speaks clearly and understandably
	4 = Speaks in comprehensible words, but not appropriate
	3 = Speaks in unintelligible words
	2 = Sounds in response to painful stimuli
	1 = Does not speak
Motor response	6 = Obeys commands
	5 = Localizes a painful stimulus
	4 = Withdraws to pain, but does not localize response
	3 = Abnormal flexion movements
	2 = Abnormal extension movements
	1 = No movements

GCS has proved to be relatively reliable in predicting neurologic injury in adults after trauma, but it has never been fully evaluated in this role for children. Perhaps, more importantly, it serves as a reasonably reliable method of assessing the overall level of consciousness of a child when assessed serially during their hospitalization. The GCS has been used as a marker of neurologic deterioration after trauma. For instance, a decrease of more than three points over an observational period is indicative of a significant clinical change according to published guidelines. Because of the relative ease and replicability of the GCS, it has become an integral part of neurocritical care.

Neuroimaging

The ability to image the brain and spinal cord has revolutionized medicine over the last two decades. In the past, meticulous examination of a child was required for an accurate determination of the location of a mass lesion or a reasonable assessment of traumatic injuries. Today,

assessments of these problems are routinely performed in minutes in institutions of varied expertise. The basic modalities to image the brain, computerized tomography (CT) and magnetic resonance imaging (MRI), are described in the subsequent text (see Table 7.6). Variations in these modalities that allow for the study of CBF or metabolism are outlined later in this section.

Computerized Tomography

In CT scan, a series of narrow, highly restricted beams of radiation are projected from within an x-ray tube onto scintillation crystals (detectors much more sensitive than standard x-ray film). Both the x-ray source and the detectors are rotated, and a series of transmission images are generated. The radiodensity of a single region of the brain, skull, or fluid space is calculated by summing up the readings of all the beams passing through that region. The resulting data from each brain region is a matrix of attenuation coefficients determined from thousands of measurements

TABLE 7.6
THE BASIC MODALITIES FOR IMAGING THE BRAIN

Disease	Magnetic Resonance Imaging	Computed Tomographic Scanning	Metrizamide-Enhanced Computed Tomographic Scanning
Tumors			
Low-grade			
Supratentorial	+++	++	—
Infratentorial	++++	++	—
High-grade			
Supratentorial	++++	++++	—
Infratentorial	++++	++	—
Metastases			
Supratentorial	+++	++	—
Infratentorial	+++	+	—
Demyelinating diseases	++++	++	—
Trauma			
Craniocerebral	++	+++	—
Spinal	+++[a]	+++	+++
Vasculitis (systemic lupus erythematosus)	+++	±	—
Cervicomedullary junction and cervical spinal cord			
Congenital anomalies	++++	+	++
Tumors (intra-axial)			
Brain stem	++++	+	++
Cerebellopontine angle	+++	++	+++
Cervical spine	++++	±	++
Tumors (extra-axial)			
Brain stem	++++	+	++
Cervical spine	++++	±	+++

++++, Preferred initial approach; +++, of definite value; ++, of value, but should not be considered as the initial diagnostic approach; +, of some value, but other procedures are superior; ±, of questionable value.
[a]Radiographic computed tomographic scanning is superior in visualizing bone abnormalities, whereas magnetic resonance imaging may be superior in demonstrating blood and spinal cord injury.
Adapted from Council of Scientific Affairs. Report of the panel on magnetic resonance imaging. Magnetic resonance imaging of the central nervous system. *JAMA.* 1988;259:1211, with permission.

and is displayed in dark and light regions on the x-ray film. By using these techniques, blood, CSF, brain, skull, and all of the intracranial contents can be resolved with machines currently in use.

CT scanning has revolutionized the monitoring of the critically ill child. Because it has become a routine procedure within most institutions:

- Mass lesions can be identified before catastrophic events have occurred.
- Strokes can be identified expediently to allow for the institution of therapies such as rTPA.
- Traumatic injuries can be diagnosed in a patient within minutes of his/her arrival to the hospital for surgical intervention.
- White matter injuries, such as demyelinating diseases, can be easily identified.
- The spinal cord can be evaluated for integrity, mass lesion, and adequacy of the supporting bones structure.

There are very few disadvantages of CT scanning of the brain apart from very mild radiation exposure and lack of portability. CT scan is superior to other imaging systems in determining bone structure and in detecting extra-axial fluid collections, particularly in the subarachnoid space. Currently, all CT scans require the transportation of critically ill children to a separate location within an institution for examination. There have been attempts to make CT scanners mobile such that they can be used at the bedside. Currently, no such capability exists. Increased resolution has been achieved with newer generations of scanners. However, ultrastructural resolution of tracts within the brain is still not possible with CT scan.

Magnetic Resonance Imaging

When objects of odd atomic weights (such as H^+ in water, with an atomic weight of 1) are exposed to a strong, homogeneous magnetic field, the nuclei of these atoms behave as spinning magnets and adopt an orientation along the magnetic field. The images in MRI are generated by applying brief pulses of radio waves to these atoms that are oriented in this field and by then measuring the energy released from the atoms as the radio wave pulses are turned off. When the pulses are turned off, the nuclei "resonate" at a given frequency and reveal their presence to detectors from the scanner. The rate at which the nuclei return to their baseline energy level is called *relaxation* and is described as a time constant (T). Individual atoms have different relaxation time constants in the two most common relaxation parameters currently used (T1: spin–lattice relaxation and T2: spin–spin relaxation). It is beyond the scope of this chapter to fully analyze the methods of MRI detection. It would suffice to say that hydrogen atoms have a different relaxation time in fat compared to water and that these differences are noted on T1- and T2-weighted MRI images.

These differences in relaxation time between protons in the gray matter, white matter, CSF, and bone give MRI its powerful ability to resolve very subtle changes in the architecture of structures within the brain and spinal cord. MRI does not expose the child to ionizing radiation and can be performed as often as needed to obtain the images required. MRI scanning is currently quite expensive and requires significant financial and technical investment for the institution. Metallic objects must be removed because of the large magnetic field required for the functioning of the scanner, making children with metal devices ineligible for this process. As with CT scanners, there are no portable MRI machines for bedside monitoring, and children must be transported for this relatively time-consuming examination.

Intracranial Pressure Monitoring

Measurement and management of abnormal increases in ICP have been a mainstay of medical care of children and adults for decades. In the 1960s, ICP monitors were used to manage severe traumatic brain injury in adults. In the 1970s, this technology was used in children for trauma, as well as for metabolic diseases (Reye syndrome, in particular). The scientific rationale for using this monitoring system involves (a) prevention of cerebral herniation and (b) prevention of secondary injuries related to decreased brain perfusion because of increased pressure within the cranial cavity. The overall management of intracranial hypertension is outlined in Section F. Options for different monitoring systems are outlined in the subsequent text.

Measuring ICP can be accomplished using monitors in a variety of locations (see Fig. 7.22). Currently, ICP monitors are placed either in the brain parenchyma or in the ventricular space. Although monitors in each location can drift (by up to 1 mm Hg per day, depending on the type), intraventricular monitors can be recalibrated as needed. Intraparenchymal monitors cannot be recalibrated, and first-generation intraparenchymal monitors were thought to have significant drift. This problem has been corrected in newer intraparenchymal monitors. The main advantage of intraventricular monitors is the ability to withdraw CSF as a therapy for increased ICP. Intraventricular monitors may be more technically challenging to place (especially when significant cerebral swelling has already occurred), and there have been anecdotal reports of increased infection risk. No systematic reviews of this complication are available at the time of writing this chapter. The main advantage of intraparenchymal monitors is the ease of placement, with only a burr hole and reflection of the dura being required.

Electrophysiologic Monitoring

Electrophysiologic monitoring in the PICU has become more common over the last decade. The various monitoring systems outlined in the subsequent text can serve one or more of four vital functions (detection of epileptiform activity, monitoring of depth of sedation or drug-induced coma, early detection of neurologic deterioration, and

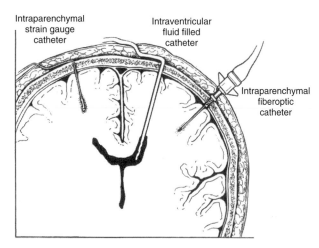

Figure 7.22 Intracranial pressure monitor devices. Intracranial pressure is most accurately measured with (i) intraventricular or (ii) intraparenchymal devices. An intraventricular catheter is placed through a burr hole in the skull and is advanced into the lateral ventricle. Intracranial pressure is directly related to the pressure of the cerebrospinal fluid (CSF) in the catheter. An intraparenchymal catheter is also inserted into the brain through a skull burr hole but is inserted a few centimeters into the cerebral cortex. Using fiberoptic technology, measurements from the brain tissue directly reflect intracranial pressure.

prognostication of overall clinical outcome) in critically ill children. These monitors have similar strengths and weaknesses. All of the monitors discussed in the subsequent text are noninvasive, can be used effectively at the patient's bedside, and can be used serially to follow interval changes in the child's condition. However, most of the monitors require relatively advanced training in interpretation (all except for the bispectral (BIS) index monitor) and can be adversely affected by the relatively hostile electric environment within ICUs. Nevertheless, electrophysiologic monitoring is a mainstay in the care of children with neurologic disorders.

Bispectral Index Monitoring

Because most critically ill children require sedation for procedures (mechanical ventilation, in particular), an objective assessment of the depth of sedation is critical. Several physical examination scores (e.g., the COMFORT score and the Ramsey scale) have been used, but a more objective measure of sedation depth has been sought. The BIS index is derived from two surface EEG electrodes placed over the frontal cortex, and it generates numerical values that correlate with levels of sedation from a wide variety of anesthetics (0 = isoelectric; 100 = fully awake). The mathematical computations from the EEG signal used to generate the BIS index involve artifact filtering, suppression detection, fast Fourier transformation, and estimation of signal quality. Intraoperative studies have demonstrated that adequate anesthesia, as assessed by movement at incision, correlates well with BIS values <60 and that

BIS values of 40 to 60 are typical during maintenance of general anesthesia.

Most relevant to pediatric intensivists are studies that suggest that amnesia reliably occurs at BIS values <64 to 80. Ideally, sedative medications could be administered to critically ill children and titrated to given BIS scores to maintain an adequate, but not an overdose, of medication. At present, several small series have attempted to correlate BIS values with both clinical sedation scores and signs of drug withdrawal. The correlations have been relatively weak, and because of this, the BIS monitor has not yet become standard at this time.

Electroencephalography

EEGs are surface tracings of brain's electrical activity. The traces are generated by measuring amplified electric potential differences between two EEG electrodes (represented as an EEG channel) placed in designated locations on the child's skull. An almost unlimited number of EEG channels can be obtained, but most centers use either 16 or 32 channels on the basis of international standards. Rhythmicity, amplitude, and location of the waves are determined and can be indicative of normal or abnormal function of the relevant brain structures. For instance, waves of 8 to 13 Hz over the posterior portions of the head during wakefulness are termed as α *waves*, whereas waves of any frequency over 13 Hz are designated as β activity. Young children have greater amounts of θ activity (defined as waves of 4 to 7 Hz), but focal or lateralized θ activity is indicative of CNS pathology. Overall, much can be gleaned from careful interpretation of EEG. However, more detailed examination of these waves is beyond the scope of this chapter.

EEGs can be performed as a single examination (intermittent EEG [iEEG]) or on a continuous basis (continuous EEG [cEEG]). Provocative stimuli or commands (eye opening and closing, loud auditory stimuli, induced hyperventilation, photic stimuli) are routinely used in iEEG to elicit characteristic wave changes. With the advent of digital monitors to record and sometimes interpret data, cEEG has become more common in neurologic intensive care. The detection of status epilepticus is one of the most common indications for EEG monitoring in the PICU. Recent studies have suggested that a significant percentage of patients undergoing cEEG monitoring were found to have nonconvulsive status epilepticus. In children, cEEG is commonly needed to monitor the depth of drug-induced coma because the duration of burst suppression is highly correlative with tissue concentrations of these agents. In adults, cEEG has also been used to detect impending cerebral ischemia caused by vasospasm after subarachnoid hemorrhage, although this complication is less common in children.

EEG monitoring is noninvasive and gives immediately available data at the bedside. However, there are a few limitations to EEG monitoring, including the requirement for trained staff for lead placement, the necessity of expert interpretation of waveforms, and the difficulties in obtaining clear signals in an electrically noisy intensive care environment. Despite these limitations, EEG monitoring is the mainstay of neurologic monitoring, and advances in technology will likely lead to an increased use of these monitors in the future.

Evoked Potentials

Evoked potentials are measurements of electrical activity of relevant brain regions after a peripheral stimulus has been applied. Stimuli are applied to sensory nerves (normally the median or posterior tibial nerve), visual fields, or auditory pathways, and the conduction of the impulses to the cortex is measured. Characteristic waves are generated, and amplitudes and latencies can implicate regions of damage to sensory nerves or nuclei within the CNS.

Somatosensory (SSEP), brain stem auditory (BAEP), and visual (VEP) evoked potentials serve predominantly as prognosticators of outcome in critically ill children. After traumatic brain injury, the absence of SSEP was associated with universally poor outcome in a relatively large series. Similarly, BAEP and VEP combined predicted poor outcome in a series of children following hypoxic coma. Abnormal SSEP latencies have also been correlative with encephalopathy from sepsis in adults. The main advantage of evoked potentials is that these waves are unaffected by sedatives. The tests are relatively labor intensive, require technical expertise, and can only be performed intermittently. These monitoring modalities are less frequently used than conventional EEG but are still quite useful in select patient populations within the ICU.

Electromyography

EMG refers to methods of studying the electric activity of muscles. The overall goal of this monitoring system is to determine the level of the muscular dysfunction: neural or muscular. Normally, needle electrodes are placed within the muscle and potential changes are measured and displayed relative to a reference electrode. Surface electrodes may be used, but spontaneous electric activity (fibrillations and positive sharp waves) can be observed only with needle electrodes. Diagnostic information includes the type and amount of spontaneous activity, evaluation of motor unit form with minimal volitional activity, and the density of motor units during maximal activation.

Information from EMG can be discerned both at rest and during voluntary muscle contraction. In denervation of nerves, muscle fibers discharge spontaneously. These potentials are called *positive sharp waves* and *fibrillation potentials*. Muscle fibrillation potentials can also be observed at rest and are (i) biphasic or triphasic, (ii) of short duration, and (iii) generated by discharges of single muscle fibers. Positive sharp waves are thought to have the same implications as fibrillation potentials but are differently shaped because the traveling wave terminates at the point of needle recording, so there is no upward negative phase. Fasciculations are spontaneous discharges of an entire motor unit (defined as all the muscle fibers innervated by a single axon). The amplitude and duration of the fasciculation potential are therefore greater than that of the fibrillation. In contrast to fibrillations, fasciculations are of neurogenic origin and are most often associated with proximal diseases, such as anterior horn cell disease or radiculopathy.

If the child is co-operative enough, more information can be generated by instructing the child to contract a given muscle maximally. Motor unit configuration during voluntary contraction depends on the particular disease. In neurogenic disease, the motor unit territory increases, and the motor unit potentials increase in duration and amplitude. In myogenic disease, motor unit potentials decrease in amplitude and duration. The recruitment pattern refers to the electrical activity generated by all activated motor units within the recording area of a maximally contracting muscle. Normally, the recruitment pattern on maximal effort is dense with no breaks in the baseline. The amplitude of the envelope is normally 2 to 4 mV. In neurogenic disease, the density of the recruitment is reduced, and the firing frequency of the remaining units increases. In myogenic disease, the number of motor units is unchanged by the disease, but the amplitude and duration of the motor units are reduced. Therefore, the recruitment density is normal, but the overall amplitude is reduced. This leads to the characteristic EMG in myopathy (full neural recruitment in a weak wasted muscle).

These monitoring tools of muscular and neural functioning are used selectively in children with critical illness. They are invaluable in discriminating between muscular and neural processes that are often indistinguishable clinically. They can often allow diagnosis that otherwise may only be made by muscle biopsy and can thereby prevent unnecessary procedures. However, considerable skill is required in performing the tests and in their interpretation.

Assessments of Blood Flow and/or Metabolism

Because of the brain's large requirement for oxygen and its dependence on aerobic respiration for optimal neuronal functioning, it has been widely accepted that measures of CBF, metabolism, and oxygenation are useful indicators of local or global cerebral function. A variety of monitors have been developed to assess these parameters either locally or globally, and those that are in widespread use are summarized in the subsequent text. Some of the monitors directly measure one or more of these parameters, whereas others use inferences to derive data that can be used by clinicians. Monitoring techniques that are available at specialized centers for research purposes (such as PET) will not be discussed in this review.

Near-infrared Spectroscopy

Near-infrared spectroscopy (NIRS) takes advantage of biochemical properties of the brain and hemoglobin to estimate cerebral oxygenation. Because oxyhemoglobin and deoxyhemoglobin have different light absorbances, the Beer-Lambert law (stating that the attenuation of an absorbing compound in a nonabsorbing solvent is directly proportional to the product of the concentration of the compound and the optical path length) can be used to determine the concentrations of the compounds. Newer generation machines can estimate the oxidation state of various cytochrome c enzymes, and inferences can be drawn about the state of these critical enzymes in the electron transport chain.

NIRS has been used in small studies to assess cerebral oxygenation in children with coma, during heart surgery, and after cardiac arrest, but its reliability and validity have not been conclusively determined in children. Because NIRS is noninvasive, it can be measured continuously, and both trends and absolute values of cerebral oxygenation can be followed. NIRS assumes that forms of hemoglobin other than oxy- and deoxy-hemoglobin are not present within the blood in significant quantities and would be unreliable in these situations. Furthermore, the penetration of light from NIRS is limited to several centimeters under normal conditions. Therefore, the calculated oxygenation index will not reflect the deep structures of the brain in older children. For these reasons, its clinical utility is relatively limited at present.

Transcranial Doppler Ultrasonography

Transcranial Doppler (TCD) ultrasonography is a noninvasive technique to determine the cerebral blood velocity in large intracranial arteries. TCD measures mean cerebral blood flow velocity (MCBFV) using the principles of ultrasound and Doppler shift of blood cell flow through these large vessels and can (i) determine the presence or absence of flow; (ii) calculate systolic, diastolic, and mean velocities; and (iii) determine the direction of flow. With these determinations graphically represented, a pulsatility index (PI) can also be calculated ([peak velocity − diastolic velocity]/mean velocity) that represents downstream resistance to blood flow. Another commonly determined parameter is the ratio between the mean velocity within the MCA to that in the internal carotid artery ($MCBFV_{MCA}/MCBFV_{ICA}$), called the *hemispheric index* or Lindegaard ratio. When this ratio is <3, it is indicative of cerebral vasospasm, whereas ratios >3 indicate hyperemia.

The main clinical indications for TCD in children are determination of vessel patency, detection of focal areas of vasospasm after intracerebral hemorrhage, and confirmation of the clinical diagnosis of brain death (criteria involve severely diminished $MCBFV_{ICA}$, absent diastolic flow, reverberating flow, and severely elevated PI). TCD is readily available at the bedside but does require a relatively high level of technical expertise.

Jugular Venous Oxygen Saturation

Measurement of the oxygen saturation in the blood leaving the brain ($SjvO_2$) is not a measure of CBF or metabolism.

Instead, its function is to identify periods in which CBF is inadequate for metabolic demands. Under ideal conditions, the blood returning to the body from the brain can be sampled for oxygen saturation. At times when the saturation is suboptimal (defined by most investigators as <50% saturated), there are areas of the brain where CBF and metabolism are mismatched and represent a potential period of ongoing cerebral ischemia. Using this information, clinicians can act to determine the cause of the abnormality, be it excessive hyperventilation, anemia, impaired oxygen content of arterial blood, or intracranial hypertension. Today, $SjvO_2$ monitoring is used in children after traumatic brain injury and during extracorporeal membrane oxygenation. In the past, it was also used to monitor cerebral function in children with Reye syndrome.

Despite the advantages of $SjvO_2$ monitoring (ease of placement and interpretation, relatively basic technology required for use, and real-time data generation), its use is currently limited by its questionable reliability and potential complications. Although commercially available monitors can accurately measure $SjvO_2$, the reliability of these devices to accurately sample all of the blood leaving the brain has been questioned. In a series of 32 adults in traumatic coma, both jugular vein saturations were measured simultaneously, and a difference of at least 15% between each monitor was noted in almost half of the patients during the study. In addition to this unreliability, catheter thrombosis and infection have been reported as complications in adults. Although these complications are relatively rare, they may be more important in children with decreased caliber of jugular vein diameter. These factors have proven to be significant impediments to the widespread use of this monitor in children.

Brain Oxygen Monitoring and Cerebral Microdialysis

Although $SjvO_2$ may detect global disturbances in CBF and metabolism, newer monitors have emerged to assess the adequacy of some of these parameters in very localized areas of the brain. Specifically, the partial pressure of oxygen of brain parenchymal tissue ($PbtO_2$) and cerebral microdialysis can assess substrate delivery or metabolic conditions within the brain parenchyma. These devices are similar in that both require a neurosurgical procedure (either with or without placement of an ICP monitor) and both can be performed with relative ease at the bedside.

$PbtO_2$ is measured using a small electrode embedded at the end of a catheter. This electrode senses oxygen concentration, and the results are displayed on a screen in real time. The clinical team can determine the location of the electrode, but it usually is placed within the cortex in a region at risk for secondary injury. Normative values of $PbtO_2$ can vary quite widely, depending on arterial oxygen tension and other factors. However, the depth and duration of low $PbtO_2$ was found to be an independent risk factor for mortality in a series of 101 adults after traumatic injury. Others have suggested that Pbto$_2$ <15 mm Hg indicates potential areas of cerebral ischemia, and this threshold has been found to correlate with increased mortality. Pbto$_2$ monitoring has the obvious advantage of providing minute-to-minute assessment on the adequacy of CBF for metabolic needs. However, critics of this type of monitoring point out that these readings reflect sampling from a relatively small volume of cerebral cortical tissue and do not reflect changes occurring elsewhere within the brain. The monitor is also reasonably invasive, although there are no published reports of significant damage to brain tissue from this device. Overall, its use in children is just beginning, and time will determine whether this monitor can play a role in monitoring critically ill children.

Cerebral microdialysis has been performed over the last two decades and serves as a device to measure mediators of interest directly from the brain parenchyma. Microdialysis catheters are constructed with an inflow port, an outflow port, and a semipermeable membrane (see Fig. 7.23). Artificial cerebrospinal fluid is perfused as a dialysate through the inflow port and into the semipermeable membrane within the brain parenchyma. Solutes from the brain tissue can diffuse into the membrane and are recovered from the outflow port. The recovery of solutes depends upon the dialysate flow rate, the pore size of the membranes, and the solute concentration within the brain. Assuming that the dialysate flow rate is unchanged and that the pore size remains the same (as is the case except as the membrane becomes epithelialized), the relative change in dialysate concentration represents the relative change of the solute of interest within the brain parenchyma. Samples are collected over a given period (30 minutes to 1 hour normally), and a wide variety of mediators can be measured from the dialysate, including glucose, pyruvate, lactate, glycerol, excitatory amino acids,

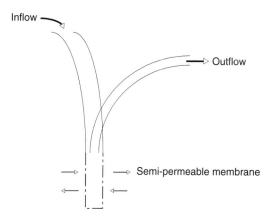

Figure 7.23 Microdialysis probe. A microdialysis probe contains two ports connected by a common region containing the semipermeable membrane. Dialysate fluid is continuously infused into the inflow port to the membrane region. As dialysate moves across the membrane, molecules diffuse into and out of the surrounding tissue on the basis of their concentration gradients. The continuous dialysate flow takes fluid away from the membrane area that contains the analytes of interest (outflow).

purines, and nitric oxide metabolites. Bedside analyzers can provide almost real-time analysis of cerebral glucose metabolism, lactate/pyruvate ratios (increases in lactate or the ratio are indicative of ischemia), and glycerol changes (released after phospholipid breakdown of the cell membrane). Cerebral microdialysis has limited use so far in neurointensive care, mainly because of its invasiveness as a monitor. There are also controversies about which brain region should be sampled and the optimal metabolites to be used for the study.

Xenon Computerized Tomography Scan

Xenon (Xe)-133 is a diffusible, inert, lipid-soluble gas that can be used as a tracer for CBF. After inhalation (although previous monitors used intravenous administration), Xe rapidly crosses the blood–brain barrier and is distributed in proportion to CBF. With the use of specialized software and CT imaging, Xe is detected in the brain, and a color map is generated for the brain. CBF is quantified in mL/100 g tissue/minute, and local, regional, and global regions of interest can be identified.

This technique has many clinical applications. It can be used to detect focal areas of ischemia or hyperemia, leading to clinical decisions about lobectomy for unrecoverable regions of the brain. Adjusting pH or arterial blood pressure during sequential examinations can assess cerebral autoregulation in regions of interest in the brain. Confirmation of the clinical diagnosis of brain death can also be accomplished without the artifactual contribution from extracerebral blood sources that occurs with nuclear medicine techniques. The main disadvantages of xenon computerized tomography (Xe-CT) blood flow determinations are the relatively high cost in CT infrastructure technology and the requirement for transportation of a critically ill child to a CT scanner. In centers with this capability, Xe-CT blood flow determinations can significantly impact clinical care.

Perfusion Magnetic Resonance Scanning

CBF can also be directly measured by MRI (described in the preceding text) after injection of gadolinium contrast. After injection, rapid sequential MR images are generated to detect the intravenous contrast as it passes through the brain. CBF and cerebral blood volume can be determined with relatively high resolution, often with superior detail compared to Xe-CT scan. Perfusion MR scanning can perform all of the functions of Xe-CT scan; the contrast agent is not nephrotoxic, making perfusion MR scanning a valuable clinical tool. However, its expense remains considerable, and scanning times remain relatively long for children with even mild hemodynamic instability.

Magnetic Resonance Spectroscopy

Magnetic resonance spectroscopy (MRS) is performed using the same equipment as conventional MRI. MRS can be performed using protons or ^{31}P as the ion of detection. MRS provides information on the cerebral metabolites and some neurotransmitters in one or more small regions of interest. The major metabolites that can be detected by proton MRS include *N*-acetyl compounds, primarily *N*-acetylaspartate (NAA); creatinine (including phospho-creatine and its precursor, creatine); and choline-containing compounds, including free choline and phosphoryl and glycerophosphoryl choline. NAA is a neuronal marker, whereas the choline compounds are released as membranes are damaged. Proton MRS also can be used to determine the concentration of lactate, which accumulates because of tissue damage and consequent anaerobic metabolism. Neurotransmitters, such as GABA and glutamate, also can be estimated using proton MRS. Concentrations of ATP, phosphocreatine, and some of the other high-energy phosphates involved in cellular energetics can be assessed using ^{31}P-MRS.

Spectra can be acquired within 1 hour, and changes in intracellular pH and metabolites can be followed. Proton MRS and ^{31}P-MRS have been used in the evaluation of muscle diseases; localization of epileptic foci; evaluation of the extent of post-traumatic lesions; classification of brain tumors; and diagnosis of the various mitochondrial disorders, leukodystrophies, and other demyelinating disorders. These techniques have also been used to determine the extent, timing, and prognosis of asphyxia. Their main limitation in intensive care is the relatively long scanning time that is required. Care must be taken to ensure patient safety during the time the spectra are being generated.

Positron Emission Tomography

PET scanning provides important information about the metabolism of substrates within the brain. PET combines the principles of nuclear imaging with CT. Whereas CT rotates an x-ray source and detector around the brain to form images, PET rotates detectors around the head to detect emissions of radioactive material from within the brain to determine the rate of utilization of these substances as they decay. Since glucose utilization is linked closely to neuronal activity, the general activity of brain regions can be deduced by studying the decay of radiolabeled glucose as it is metabolized.

PET scanning is available in only a limited number of centers, primarily because generating the required isotopes requires specialized equipments and operators. For this reason, PET scanning is not commonly used clinically in critically ill children. Certain centers have used PET scanning for critically ill adults after head injuries and have added to the literature in this field.

Implications for Critical Care

Clinical neuromonitoring is a rapidly advancing field in pediatric critical care medicine. It is clear that no single monitor can effectively perform all the functions demanded by clinicians caring for critically ill children. Developing the proper combination of techniques appropriate for given populations of children is the challenge of the coming years to improve neurologic outcomes from the wide variety of critical illnesses.

RECOMMENDED READINGS

1. Banwell BL, Mildner RJ, Hassell AC, et al. Muscle weakness in critically ill children. *Neurology.* 2003;61(12):1779–1782.
2. Blanpied TA, Ehlers MD. Microanatomy of dendritic spines: Emerging principles of synaptic pathology in psychiatric and neurological disease. *Biol Psychiatry.* 2004;55(12):1121–1127.
3. Brand-Saberi B, Ebensperger C, Wilting J, et al. The ventralizing effects of the notochord on somite differentiation. *Anat Embryol.* 1993;188:239–245.
4. Brosseau L, Milne S, Robinson V, et al. Efficacy of the transcutaneous electrical nerve stimulation for the treatment of chronic low back pain: A meta-analysis. *Spine.* 2002;27(6):596–603.
5. Cohen G. Caspases: The executioners of apoptosis. *Biochem J.* 1997;326:1–16.
6. Coursin DB, Maccioli GA. Dexmedetomidine. *Curr Opin Crit Care.* 2001;7(4):221–226.
7. Craig AD, Bushnell MC. The thermal grill illusion: Unmasking the burn of cold pain. *Science.* 1994;265(5169):252–255.
8. Cruz J, Miner M, Allen S, et al. Continuous monitoring of cerebral oxygenation in acute brain injury: Assessment of cerebral hemodynamic reserve. *Neurosurgery.* 1991;29:743–749.
9. Dabeney P, Pilkington S, Daubeney JE, et al. Cerebral oxygenation measured by infrared spectroscopy: Comparison with jugular bulb oximetry. *Ann Thorac Surg.* 1996;61:930–934.
10. De Jonghe B, Sharshar T, Lefaucher JP, et al. Paresis acquired in the intensive care unit: A prospective multicenter study. *JAMA.* 2002;288(22):2859–2867.
11. de Letter MA, Schmitz PI, Visser LH, et al. Risk factors for the development of polyneuropathy and myopathy in critically ill patients. *Crit Care Med.* 2001;29(12):2281–2286.
12. Di Giovanni S, Molon A, Broccolini A, et al. Constitutive activation of MAPK cascade in acute quadriplegic myopathy. *Ann Neurol.* 2004;55(2):195–206.
13. Eriksson LI. Evidence-based practice and neuromuscular monitoring: It's time for routine quantitative assessment. *Anesthesiology.* 2003;98(5):1037–1039.
14. Farber L, Haus U, Spath M, et al. Physiology and pathophysiology of the 5-HT3 receptor. *Scand J Rheumatol Suppl.* 2004;119:2–8.
15. Feen E, Zaidat O, et al. Principles of Neurointensive Care. In: Bradley W, Daroff R, Fenichel G, et al., eds. *Neurology in clinical practice.* Philadelphia, PA: Elsevier; 2004:941–962.
16. Fiala JC, Spacek J, Harris KM, et al. Dendritic spine pathology: Cause or consequence of neurological disorders? *Brain Res Brain Res Rev.* 2002;39(1):29–54.
17. Fitzpatrick MO, Maxwell WL, Graham DI, et al. The role of the axolemma in the initiation of traumatically induced axonal injury. *J Neurol Neurosurg Psychiatry.* 1998;64(3):285–287.
18. Glanzer JG, Eberwine JH. Mechanisms of translational control in dendrites. *Neurobiol Aging.* 2003;24(8):1105–1111.
19. Gupta A, Daggett C, Drant S, et al. Prospective randomized trial of ketorolac after congenital heart surgery. *J Cardiothorac Vasc Anesth.* 2004;18(4):454–457.
20. Hallett M. One man's poison–clinical applications of botulinum toxin. *N Engl J Med.* 1999;341(2):118–120.
21. Hentgartner M, Horvitz H. C. elegans cell survival gene ced-9 encodes a functional homolog of the mammalian protooncogene Bcl-2. *Cell.* 1994;76:665–676.
22. Jacobi J, Fraser GL, Coursin DB, et al. Clinical practice guidelines for the sustained use of sedatives and analgesics in the critically ill adult. *Crit Care Med.* 2002;30(1):119–141.
23. Jacobson M, Weil M, Raff M, et al. Programmed cell death in animal development. *Cell.* 1997;88:347–354.
24. Kress JP, Pohlman AS, O'Connor MF, et al. Daily interruption of sedative infusions in critically ill patients undergoing mechanical ventilation. *N Engl J Med.* 2000;342(20):1471–1477.
25. Lecker SH, Jagoe RT, Gilbert A, et al. Multiple types of skeletal muscle atrophy involve a common program of changes in gene expression. *Faseb J.* 2004;18(1):39–51.

26. Lewis S, Myburgh J, Thornton E, et al. Cerebral oxygenation monitoring by near-infrared spectroscopy is not clinically useful in patients with severe closed head injury: A comparison with jugular venous bulb oximetry. *Crit Care Med.* 1996;24:1334–1338.

27. Li P, Nijhawan D, Budihardjo I, et al. Cytochrome c and dATP-dependent formation of Apaf-1/caspase-9 complex initiates an apoptotic protease cascade. *Cell.* 1997;91:479–489.

28. MacFarlane IA, Rosenthal FD. Severe myopathy after status asthmaticus. *Lancet.* 1977;2(8038):615.

29. Martin S, Green D. Protease activation during apoptosis: Death by a thousand cuts. *Cell.* 1995;82:349–352.

30. Mathews KD. Muscular dystrophy overview: Genetics and diagnosis. *Neurol Clin.* 2003;21(4):795–816.

31. Matsuzaki M, Honkura N, Ellis-Davies G, et al. Structural basis of long-term potentiation in single dendritic spines. *Nature.* 2004;429(6993):761–766.

32. Maxwell WL, Povlishock JT, Graham DL, et al. A mechanistic analysis of nondisruptive axonal injury: A review. *J Neurotrauma.* 1997;14(7):419–440.

33. Menkes J, Sarnat H. Neuroembryology, genetic programming and malformations of the nervous system. In: Menkes J, Sarnat H, eds. *Child neurology.* Philadelphia, PA: Lippincott Williams & Wilkins; 2000:277–305.

34. Murphy B, Martin S. Caspases: Structure, activation, pathways and substrates. In: Yin X, Dong Z, eds. *Essentials of apoptosis: A guide for basic and clinical research.* Totowa, NJ: Humana Press; 2003:1–12.

35. Murray MJ, Cowen J, DeBlock H, et al. Clinical practice guidelines for sustained neuromuscular blockade in the adult critically ill patient. *Crit Care Med.* 2002;30(1):142–156.

36. Nagdyman N, Fleck T, Ewert H, et al. Cerebral oxygenation measured by near infrared spectroscopy during circulatory arrest and cardiopulmonary resuscitation. *Br J Anaesth.* 2003;91:438–442.

37. Nicholson D. Caspase structure, proteolytic substrates and function during apoptotic cell death. *Cell Death Differ.* 1999;6:1028–1042.

38. Nilsson O, Brandt L, Ungerstedt U, et al. Bedside detection of brain ischemia using intracerebral microdialysis: Subarachnoid hemorrhage and delayed ischemic deterioration. *Neurosurg.* 1999;45:1176–1185.

39. O'Rahilly R, Muller F. Bidirectional closure of the rostral neuropore in the human embryo. *Am J Anat Path.* 1989;184:259–268.

40. Okamoto MP, Kawaguchi DL, Amin AN, et al. Evaluation of propofol infusion syndrome in pediatric intensive care. *Am J Health Syst Pharm.* 2003;60(19):2007–2014.

41. Petrenko AB, Yamakura T, Baabe H, et al. The role of N-methyl-D-aspartate (NMDA) receptors in pain: A review. *Anesth Analg.* 2003;97(4):1108–1116.

42. Pigula FA, Siewers RD, Nemoto EM, et al. Hypothermic cardiopulmonary bypass alters oxygen/glucose uptake in the pediatric brain. *J Thorac Cardiovasc Surg.* 2001;121(2):366–373.

43. Rakic P. Radial versus tangential migration of neuronal clones in the developing cerebral cortex. *Proc Natl Acad Science.* 1995;92:11323–11327.

44. Renatus M, Stennicke H, Scott FL, et al. Dimer formation drives the activation of the dell death protease caspase-9. *PNAS.* 2001;98:14250–14255.

45. Riggs JE, Bodensteiner JB, Schechet SS, et al. Congenital myopathies/dystrophies. *Neurol Clin.* 2003;21(4):779–94,v–vi.

46. Robertson C, Narayan R, Gokastan Z, et al. Cerebral arteriovenous oxygen difference as an estimate of cerebral blood flow in comatose patients. *J Neurosurg.* 1989;70:222–230.

47. Rudis MI, Sikora CA, Angus E, et al. A prospective, randomized, controlled evaluation of peripheral nerve stimulation versus standard clinical dosing of neuromuscular blocking agents in critically ill patients. *Crit Care Med.* 1997;25(4):575–583.

48. Sacheck JM, Ohtsuka A, McLary SC, et al. IGF-I stimulates muscle growth by suppressing protein breakdown and expression of atrophy-related ubiquitin ligases, atrogin-1 and MuRF1. *Am J Physiol Endocrinol Metab.* 2004;287(4):E591–E601.

49. Sadler T. *Langman's medical embryology.* Baltimore, MD: Williams & Wilkins; 1985:334–367.

50. Schiavo G, Benfenati F, Poulain B, et al. Tetanus and botulinum-B neurotoxins block neurotransmitter release by proteolytic cleavage of synaptobrevin. *Nature.* 1992;359(6398):832–835.

51. Segredo V, Caldwell JE, Matthay MA, et al. Persistent paralysis in critically ill patients after long-term administration of vecuronium. *N Engl J Med.* 1992;327(8):524–528.

52. Shah N, Marchionni M, Isaacs I, et al. Glial growth factor restricts mammalian neural crest stem cells to a glial fate. *Cell.* 1994;77:349–360.

53. Shapiro BA, Warren J, Egol AB, et al. Practice parameters for sustained neuromuscular blockade in the adult critically ill patient: An executive summary. Society of Critical Care Medicine. *Crit Care Med.* 1995;23(9):1601–1605.

54. Skippen P, Seear M, Poskitt K, et al. Effect of hyperventilation on regional cerebral blood flow in head-injured children. *Crit Care Med.* 1997;25(8):1402–1409.

55. Slee E, Harte M, Kluck RN, et al. Ordering the cytochrome-c initiated caspase cascade: Hierarchical activation of caspases- 2, -3, -6, -7, -8 and -10 in a caspase -9 dependent manner. *J Cell Biol.* 1999;144:281–292.

56. Strange C, Franklin C, et al. Comparison of train-of-four and best clinical assessment during continuous paralysis. *Am J Respir Crit Care Med.* 1997;156(5):1556–1561.

57. Tavernier B, Rannou JJ, Vallet B, et al. Peripheral nerve stimulation and clinical assessment for dosing of neuromuscular blocking agents in critically ill patients. *Crit Care Med.* 1998;26(4):804–805.

58. Thomas L, Gates M, Steindler D, et al. Young neurons from the adult subependymal zone proliferate and migrate along an astrocyte, extracellular enriched pathway. *Glia.* 1996;17:1–14.

59. Trujillo KA, Akil H. Inhibition of morphine tolerance and dependence by the NMDA receptor antagonist MK-801. *Science.* 1991;251(4989):85–87.

60. Tsujimoto Y, Finger L, Yunis J, et al. Cloning of the chromosome breakpoint of neoplastic B cells with the t(14;18) chromosomal translocation. *Science.* 1984;226:1097–1099.

61. Van den Berghe G, Wouters P, Weekers F, et al. Intensive insulin therapy in the critically ill patients. *N Engl J Med.* 2001;345(19):1359–1367.

62. Vitale MG, Choe JC, Hwang MW, et al. Use of ketorolac tromethamine in children undergoing scoliosis surgery. An analysis of complications. *Spine J.* 2003;3(1):55–62.

63. Wagner KR. Genetic diseases of muscle. *Neurol Clin.* 2002;20(3):645–678.

64. Wood SJ, Slater CR. Safety factor at the neuromuscular junction. *Prog Neurobiol.* 2001;64(4):393–429.

65. Wyllie A, Kerr J, Currie A, et al. Cell death: The significance of apoptosis. *Int Rev Cytol.* 1980;68:251–306.

66. Yin, X, Ding W-X, et al. Bcl-2 family proteins: Master regulators of apoptosis. In: Yin X, Dong Z, eds. *Essentials of apoptosis: A guide for basic and clinical research.* Totowa, NJ: Humana Press; 2003:13–18.

67. Yin X, Oltvai Z, Korsmeyer S, et al. BH1 and BH2 domains of Bcl-2 are required for inhibition of apoptosis and heterodimerization with bax. *Nature.* 1994;369:321–323.

68. Yuan J, Shaham S, Ledoux S, et al. The C. elegans cell death gene ced-3 encodes a protein similar to mammalian interleukin 1beta converting enzyme. *Cell.* 1993;75:641–652.

69. Zeilhofer HU, Calo G. Nociceptin/orphanin FQ and its receptor-potential targets for pain therapy. *J Pharmacol Exp Ther.* 2003;306(2):423–429.

70. Zhong W, Jiang M-M, Weinmaster G, et al. Differential expression of mammalian Numb, Numblike and Notch1 suggests distinct roles during mouse cortical neurogenesis. *Development.* 1997;124:1887–1897.

Nephrology

8

Robert E. Lynch

This chapter provides a detailed description of many aspects of renal physiology. It occasionally delves into pathophysiology; however, it is mainly about understanding renal processes in the healthy individual. Intensivists need not know everything presented here. But investing in a deeper insight into renal physiology will facilitate a better understanding of its disturbances.

The chapter starts with fetal development and circulation, then moves to glomerular filtration and tubular function and renal acid–base mechanisms, and finally to acute renal failure and some issues of dialysis materials and complications.

Fetal development links molecular biology to gross anatomy and touches everything in between. The macro- and microcirculations of the kidney are the most basic of functions but are not without vulnerabilities and subtleties.

Once perfused, the glomerulus filters, giving the nephron material to work with. And work it is, as renal oxygen consumption and metabolic activity reflect a wealth of active transport processes, many driven by Na^+/K^+-ATPase. Tubular fluid constituents are individually reabsorbed and secreted as needed. Systemic messengers and local systems modify and regulate homeostasis, and renal products act at distant sites to maintain it. It is a fragile set of interdependencies, and although the organ is resilient, it can be stunned into lethal dysfunction. Recovery is frequent but often delayed, during which time the multidisciplinary critical care and nephrology teams must buy the time needed to recover renal function.

The understanding that we have of renal physiology comes from studies of a variety of animal species. In some ways, the kidney in humans is studied much less compared to that in dogs, cats, rabbits, and other species. Transference of the knowledge obtained from invasive studies of other mammals, fishes, and reptiles to humans needs to be done with some skepticism. Physiologic processes described in this chapter do occur, probably almost all occur in humans, and they are presented as though that is the case. Some caution while interpreting the processes is always advisable.

The list of references at the end of this chapter is an under-representation of the true number of contributing sources. For further reading, there are excellent nephrology texts,[1–3] as well as cited papers.

BASIC FETAL RENAL AND RENOVASCULAR DEVELOPMENT AND FUNCTION

From the near-term newborn to the young adult, the management of critical illness is impacted by a spectrum of renal functions and dysfunctions. On occasion, renal dysfunction itself is the central issue, although a secondary role is most common. Understanding developmental renal anatomy and physiology provides an initial intellectual framework that is adequate to support and organize the many details of critical renal pathophysiology.[4]

In the human fetus, a lengthy paraspinous region of intermediate mesoderm runs from areas that are destined to be the cervical portion to the most caudad portion of the early embryo. A common duct extends through three zones in this tissue, each associated with differentiation of excretory structures of varying potential (see Fig. 8.1).

At approximately 3 weeks, the pronephros can be identified in the cervical zone and consists of epithelial tubular structures that may or may not connect to the pronephric duct. Glomerular structures may appear but do not directly connect to the pronephric tubules. In humans, the pronephric glomerulus and tubule regress and disappear.

The pronephric duct continues caudally and enters the mesonephric zone, where buds from the duct connect to the differentiating tubules, which specifically relate to glomerular structures. Although most of this mesonephric

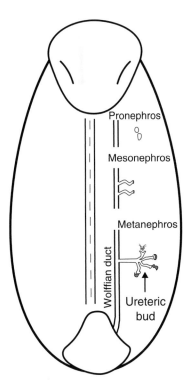

Figure 8.1 Fetal renal structures.

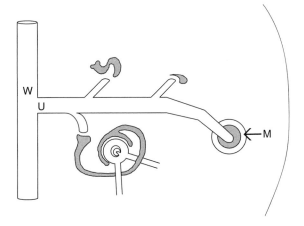

Figure 8.2 Nephron induction. W, wolffian duct; U, ureteric bud; M, reactive mesenchyme.

kidney also disappears, the pronephric duct, renamed the wolffian duct, persists in the male fetus as the vas deferens. Gonadal differentiation occurs in this same region, and mesonephric tissues contribute to gonadal structure. Mutations of transcription factors expressed in the wolffian duct may be associated with renal and reproductive anomalies.

By gestational day 28, tissue signaling in the most caudad or metanephric zone initiates events that lead to the formation of kidneys that will mature into adult organs.[5]

Metanephric areas differentiate into three tissues. The ureteric bud is an epithelial tubular diverticulum arising from the wolffian duct. A mesenchymal condensate develops around the invading tip of the ureteric bud. Finally, a subregion of the cellular condensate is invaded by a blood vessel and begins a complex transformation into the glomerular capillary tuft covered by the glomerular epithelial cells. Nephron formation in this process appears to result from an ongoing process of biochemical cross talk from cellular subregions, resulting in progressive and multidirectional inductive processes.

The ureteric bud invades the predestined metanephric mesenchyme, subdivides, and arborizes into legions of ducts extending centrifugally from the renal hilum toward the renal capsule. Side branches participate in the induction of generations of deep nephrons followed by what will be more and more superficial generations of nephrons. In each human kidney, 600,000 to 1,000,000 branching ureteric buds collaborate, each with a small mass of mesenchymal cells, which are at first globular, then comma-shaped, and

then S-shaped, as one portion of the S-shaped mesenchyme develops a lumen, extends, and differentiates into the renal tubule (see Fig. 8.2). The other portion of the S-shaped mesenchyme surrounds the vascular capillary tuft with two layers of epithelial cells, one layer being directly below the basement membrane forming around the vascular endothelial cells. The bowman space lies outside this epithelial layer and is surrounded by a second epithelial layer, the Bowman capsule, creating a luminal space continuous with that of the renal tubule. The proximal tubule (PT), loop of Henle, and distal tubule developing from the metanephric mesenchyme then connect to the closest portion of the ureteric bud. The cortical collecting tubule (CCT) and collecting duct originate from the ureteric bud sharing embryologic history with the renal pelvis, ureter, and bladder trigone (see Fig. 8.3).

Renal tubule formation occurs in such a way that an early portion of the distal tubule lies between and in apposition to the afferent and efferent arterioles of the same nephron's glomerulus. This portion of the tubule becomes the macula densa (MD), and the related arteriolar cells also develop special functions as the juxtaglomerular apparatus (JGA).

The centrifugal pattern of nephron formation results in the earliest nephrons having larger glomeruli and loops of Henle that extend into the deeper portions of the renal medulla. Nephrons formed during the latest stage of this nephronogenesis process will have relatively short loops of Henle, which will not extend into the medullary regions of highest solute concentration. Therefore, anatomic heterogeneity exists as a consequence of progressively more superficial nephronogenesis. However, the functional significance of this heterogeneity remains uncertain. For instance, species with an increased proportion of either short or long loops do not necessarily demonstrate reduced or exaggerated urine-concentrating ability.

Factors disrupting the coordination of mesenchymal differentiation and ureteric bud branching may result in multicystic, dysplastic kidneys. These are nonfunctional,

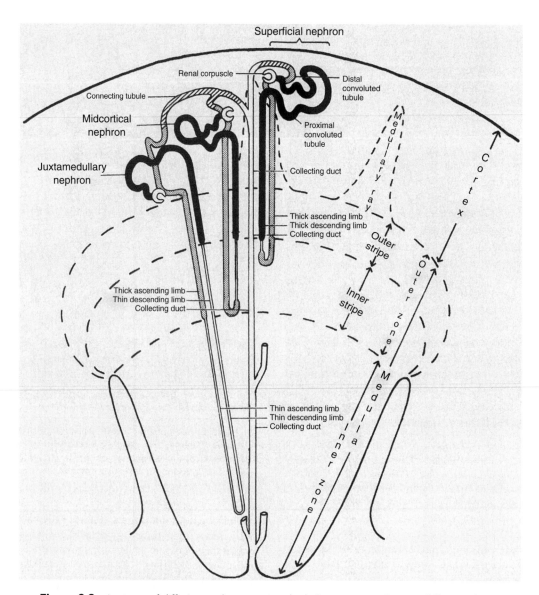

Figure 8.3 Anatomy of differing nephron types and tubular segments. Juxtamedullary nephrons are those induced earliest in fetal development. (From Schrier RW. *Diseases of the kidney and urinary tract.* 7th ed. Philadelphia, PA: Lippincott Williams & Wilkins; 2001.)

may be unilateral or bilateral, and tend to occur more often in individuals with chromosomal abnormalities.

Abnormal Nephronogenesis

Although their products and roles are incompletely understood, many individual genes and gene combinations have been shown to play critical roles in renal embryology. Wilms tumor gene 1 (*WT1*) provides mesenchymal-ureteric bud signaling. Glial-derived neurotropic factor (GDNF) is also involved, as are *PAX2*, *Lim 1*, and the *formin* genes. Targeted deletion of *PAX2* in animals results in the absence of both the mesonephric and metanephric kidneys.[6] Multiple deletions in the *HOX* gene clusters can result in renal agenesis. c-Ret interacts with GDNF, and the mutation

of c-Ret is associated with anomalies. Inactivation of the angiotensin II receptor gene results in anomalies of the collecting system, as well as renal hypoplasia–dysplasia.

Many more genetic influences over renal development are known. Continuing molecular studies will clarify hierarchies and inter-relationships, as well as identify many more critical factors.[7]

Nephronogenesis in the metanephric kidney continues until 34 to 35 weeks' of gestational age. Its progress may be hindered by intrauterine growth retardation or maternal consumption of certain drugs,[8] resulting in a reduction in the total number of nephrons. Particularly damaging is the gestational exposure to angiotensin-converting enzyme (ACE) inhibitors, nonsteroidal anti-inflammatory drugs, or cocaine. Renal failure and stillbirth may result, but oligohydramnios and pulmonary hypoplasia can result from a lesser injury that causes a significant reduction in fetal urine output. Renal agenesis, of course, may cause the fatal Potter sequence, but less severe global and pulmonary defects are frequently lethal when combined with neonatal severe renal failure. Unfortunately, several patients have already been treated with extracorporeal-membrane oxygenation (ECMO) for pulmonary failure when poor renal function leads to the discovery of severe renal hypoplasia–dysplasia. Survival with failure of both organ systems is most unlikely.

Severe oligohydramnios present during weeks 16 to 25—canalicular phase of lung development—is particularly prohibitive to lung growth. If oligohydramnios occurs after the second trimester, there may still be adequate lung development.

If an embryologic failure results in unilateral renal agenesis or unilateral severe hypoplasia–dysplasia, the contralateral normal kidney undergoes compensatory hypertrophy. The infant is born with an enlarged unilateral kidney and near normal renal function. This does not appear to confer a statistically detectable decrease in survival, although the risk of late hypertension may be increased.

Loss of a kidney beyond the neonatal period still results in hypertrophy of the remaining normal kidney. Overall renal mass may be detectably increased in 48 to 72 hours and results mostly from cellular hypertrophy rather than hyperplasia. The control system regulating renal mass and stimulating this hypertrophy is poorly understood. Evidence exists for the effects of circulating growth factors whose levels or activities may be altered, regulators that sense and react to increases in filtered load of sodium or other solute, and perhaps a permissive role of growth hormone or testosterone. Factors controlling renal blood flow would be interesting candidates, but renal innervation does not seem to be a major contributing factor.

An additional fetal renal concern occurs in twinning when placental vascular malformations result in a twin–twin transfusion. The donor twin may be stressed in terms of both intravascular volume and hematocrit. High angiotensin levels and perhaps effects of renal vascular innervation may result in significantly decreased renal perfusion and function. An increased incidence of renal dysfunction occurs in infants who have been twin–twin donors. In our experience, one infant was born with renal cortical necrosis, severe hypertension, and total renal failure. Fortunately, a cadaver transplant provided during infancy is still functioning well more than 18 years later.

Fetal Kidney Function

Early in pregnancy, placental function provides most of the homeostatic regulation for which the kidneys will ultimately assume responsibility. At approximately 20 weeks, it begins to make sense to refer to fetal kidney function.

From this time onward, urine output accounts for approximately 90% of the production of amniotic fluid, which is vital for multiorgan system development. The fetal kidneys are receiving only approximately 5% of the cardiac output and are reabsorbing only 85% to 95% of the filtered sodium, as compared to 98% to 99% in adults. In those nephrons that have been formed, the expression of Na^+/K^+-ATPase and aquaporin-1 (AQP-1) and 2 is limited. Nephron formation will continue into the 34th to 36th week but it is susceptible to quantitative disruptions, such as dexamethasone-induced oligonephronia, or a qualitative maturational failure, such as the global loss of proximal tubular function secondary to genetic absence of hepatocyte nuclear factor-1 (HNF-1).

Although a specific glomerular initiating event remains uncertain, platelet-derived growth factor and hepatic hepatoma-derived growth factor appear to have a renal developmental role.[9] Renin starts being detectable at approximately 8 weeks of gestational age. Subsequent exposure to ACE inhibitors may be teratogenic or may result in fetal death.

THE KIDNEY OF THE TERM OR NEAR-TERM NEWBORN

Term infants should have a full complement of nephrons, nephronogenesis having been completed by approximately 36 weeks. However, a great deal of nephron growth and maturation must still occur. Neonatal glomeruli are approximately half the diameter of adult glomeruli, and the basement membrane is approximately one third the thickness of the adult. The basement membrane is also more permeable and the tubules less efficient. The tubules must eventually grow to three to four times their neonatal mass.

In the first few weeks of postnatal life, a remarkable transformation in renal function occurs (see Fig. 8.4). The cardiac output and systemic blood pressure of the newborn increase over the first few weeks of life and renal vascular resistance decreases. The result is that the kidneys' share of an increasing cardiac output nearly doubles to approximately 10% by the end of the first week of life. Absolute renal blood flow doubles and triples over the first several weeks, as does the glomerular filtration rate (GFR). The typical kidney volume of 10 mL at birth becomes more than 20 mL by the third week. In the glomerulus, there is an increase not only in the capillary hydrostatic pressure but also in the hydraulic permeability and surface area, which contribute to increasing glomerular filtration. All these changes affect the renal pharmacology and contribute to the dosage adjustments needed for drugs such as digoxin, vancomycin, and aminoglycosides during the early infant period.

The decreased renal vascular resistance may have a neural component but it certainly has contributions from prostaglandins (PGs) and atrial natriuretic peptide (ANP), levels of which are elevated in neonates. Nitric

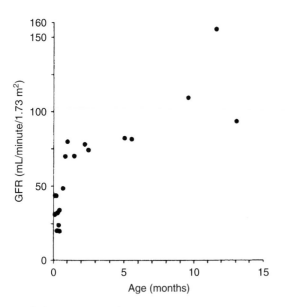

Figure 8.4 Glomerular filtration rate (GFR) transition and development during the first year of life. (From Aperia A, Broberger O, Thodenius K, et al. *Acta Paediatr Scand.* 1975;64:393, as reproduced in Avner ED, Harmon WE, Niaudet P. *Pediatric nephrology.* 5th ed. Philadelphia, PA: Lippincott Williams & Wilkins; 2003.)

oxide is present and is active. Endothelin, ordinarily a vasoconstrictor, may actually contribute to vasodilation in the neonate. Angiotensin II preferentially constricts the efferent arteriole of the glomerulus, thereby tending to raise glomerular capillary hydraulic pressure.

In addition, the kallikrein–kinin system may be important in renal transition.[10] Kallikrein may be detected in the urine within a few days of birth and its level in the urine increases parallel to the increase in the renal blood flow. Studies on newborn animals demonstrate significant decreases in renal blood flow when the animals undergo bradykinin blockade. Kinins are clearly acting as vasodilators and have been proposed as an actual growth stimulant during this period of rapid renal enlargement.

The profound sensitivity of the newborn's kidney to ACE inhibition persists in early infancy. Although it is known that ACE inhibition interferes with the metabolism of kinins and could result in bradykinin accumulation, the profound hypotension occurring in infants following captopril dosing does not appear to be bradykinin-dependent. Blockade of kinin receptors does not prevent ACE-inhibitor toxicity.

The rapid increase in renal capability during transition is dependent on the complex interaction of many mechanisms. For infants born before 34 to 36 weeks of gestational age, these interacting systems have not yet matured in some important ways, resulting in delayed and somewhat slower transition. Even in the term newborn, critical illness including ventilator-dependent respiratory failure, hypoxemia, asphyxia, metabolic acidosis, hyper or hypothermia, and congestive heart failure may disrupt the transition process, significantly delaying the expected doubling and tripling of the GFR during the newborn period.

In the normal kidney of the newborn, tubular function also undergoes postnatal maturation. Although the newborn may dilute urine well and a urine osmolarity as low as 40 mmol per L can be achieved, the urine concentrating ability is limited at birth. It typically increases rapidly, with the ability to produce a urine osmolarity of 400 mmol per L in approximately 1 week, increasing to approximately 600 mmol per L at 6 weeks. These changes are mediated in part by increases in medullary solute accumulation and the density of the antidiuretic hormone (ADH) receptors as well as the maturation of intracellular mechanisms.

Recovery of the filtered HCO_3^- by the PT is incomplete in the term newborn and more so in the premature infant. The expected serum HCO_3^- levels are lower (16 to 20 mEq per L) in the preemie than in the term infant (19 to 21 mEq per L). This value continues to increase during infancy, with young children achieving adult values.

At birth, hydrogen ion transporter systems and carbonic anhydrase resources in the PT are immature and contribute to the lower PT HCO_3^- threshold. Proximal tubular glutamine-dependent ammoniagenesis is also limited. However, the distal segments are more effective at acid secretion, helping to maintain acid–base balance.

RENAL VASCULAR ANATOMY AND FUNCTION

Under reasonably normal conditions, the kidneys receive approximately 20% of cardiac output. Although their tissue mass is a smaller percentage of the body mass, the kidneys are metabolically quite active, with the occurrence of many energy-requiring transport processes. Nevertheless, whole-organ oxygen extraction under baseline conditions is relatively low, and renal venous oxygen content is relatively generous. It is tempting to speculate that the evolution of this circumstance represents a protective buffer so that temporary reductions in cardiac output do not result in acute renal failure. Increasing appreciation of the importance of the renal medullary microcirculation provides an alternative rationale.[11] Medullary oxygenation under normal conditions is metabolically marginal. Perhaps, the seemingly luxuriant oxygen delivery is required for the preservation of renal medullary function.

As a concept, renal vascular function begins at the left ventricle. Acute or chronic hypertension involves cardiorenal, neural, and endocrine interactions.[12] Severe acute hypertension can cause end-organ damage in the kidney.

The more common problem in the pediatric intensive care unit (PICU) is that of decreased left ventricular function in relative or absolute terms. Autoregulation of renal blood flow is discussed in the subsequent text and does compensate for some of the excesses or deficiencies of cardiac output as perceived by the kidneys. However, sodium and water retention, oliguria, decreasing clearance, and acute renal insufficiency can result from left ventricular failure. Renal perception of heart failure may be mediated through the sympathetic nervous system, endocrine mediators, and intrarenal vascular and tubular function regulators. The sympathetic nervous system may be more active, the renin–angiotensin system may be highly activated, and intrarenal blood flow and function may be highly dependent on the compensatory mechanisms of major significance only in times of such physiologic crisis. Downstream from the left ventricle, aortic coarctation provides another challenge to the renal function. Similarly, bilateral renal artery stenosis or unilateral stenosis in a solitary kidney results in diminished renal perfusion pressure. Absolute renal blood flow may be preserved in part by the increase in systemic blood pressure and in part by intrarenal compensatory mechanisms. Preservation of glomerular filtration requires afferent arteriolar dilatation and efferent arteriolar constriction. If the systemic hypertension is severe enough to cause congestive heart failure, the resultant fall in renal perfusion may lead to significant functional loss. The hypertension of renal artery stenosis or aortic coarctation is sustained by both elevated renin–angiotensin activity and by increased sympathetic nervous system activity. Significant sodium retention may also contribute a volume component. The glomerular filtration in these patients is dependent upon angiotensin activity, so that the use of an ACE inhibitor may relax the efferent arteriole, decrease the glomerular hydraulic perfusion pressure, and result in acute renal failure.

Renal blood flow may be totally interrupted during aortic cross clamping for surgical procedures including cardiac bypass, liver transplantation, and trauma reconstruction. In addition, renal homotransplantation or autotransplantation requires vascular interruption. The consequence on kidney function depends upon tissue temperature, duration of ischemia, and coexisting morbidities.

Renal Vascular Anatomy

Fetal kidneys begin forming near the bladder in what will become the pelvic zone. Normal fetal development will result in an internal rotation of the renal organs along with a relative ascension of the kidneys to their usual mid-abdominal location. At this site, the renal arteries depart from the aorta at approximately the level of the first lumbar vertebra. Anomalies of development can result in failure of rotation or ascension, resulting in malrotated or pelvic kidneys. This change is most likely to be unilateral. Much less commonly, the ascension of kidneys fails to cease at the usual location. The kidney may continue to migrate into a lower thoracic location.

Normally located kidneys usually have a single main renal artery. However, multiple renal arteries, usually

two, are not uncommon. Dual renal arteries may be of similar size, but a normal-sized main renal artery may be supplemented by a smaller accessory artery, usually at the renal lower pole. This accessory artery may provide the blood supply for parts of the renal pelvis and ureter.

Before penetrating the renal tissue, the main renal artery branches into segmental arteries, each supplying one of four to six rather discrete kidney segments. It is reasonably accurate to consider the cortical segments to be supplied by end arteries; that is, obstruction of a segmental artery leads to virtually no flow in any of the structures of that renal segment. As they cross the renal hilum and enter the renal tissue, the segmental arteries give rise to multitudes of interlobar arteries moving between columns of deep kidney tissue and reaching centrifugally outward toward the renal capsule. These interlobular arteries then make a 90-degree turn, becoming the arcuate arteries that run parallel to the renal capsule, but at the level of the inner cortex margin. From these arcuate arteries, a forest of intralobular arteries again turn directly toward the overlying capsule, carrying the blood flow directly away from the renal hilum. These interlobular arteries may branch, but the branches pursue a rather straight course toward the capsule. As they grow from the arcuate artery toward a slightly subcapsular terminus, these intralobular arteries give off right-angled generations of afferent arterioles with their associated glomeruli, tubules, and capillary complexes. Nephrons formed early in fetal life will branch from the interlobular arteries very near the arcuate arteries. Those formed later will be successively farther away from the arcuate arteries and nearer to the capsule region. The last generation of glomeruli in humans and many species lies several tubule diameters below the capsular surface, with the outermost subcapsular region being made up of tubules and their adjacent capillaries.

Cortical blood flow moves from the interlobular arteries through the afferent arterioles into the glomeruli and emerging through the efferent arterioles. These vessels then arborize into extensive capillary beds that gradually coalesce into venules and the renal venous drainage system.

Quantitatively, renovascular resistance is particularly dependent upon that of the interlobular arteries, afferent arteriole, and efferent arteriole (see Fig. 8.5). Control of afferent arteriolar resistance occurs through both systemic and intrarenal regulatory mechanisms. Likewise, the efferent arteriole is sensitive to both systemic and intrarenal mechanisms. However, these two distinct periglomerular arteriolar populations may behave independently, reacting in opposite directions to the same stimulus. These mechanisms are discussed later in the chapter.

The postglomerular vasculature is functionally critical not only for the control of efferent arteriolar resistance but also for the effect on tubular reabsorption that is exerted by the postglomerular blood traversing the peritubular capillary bed. In a nonquantitative sense, the hydraulic pressure contributing to the glomerular filtration has been

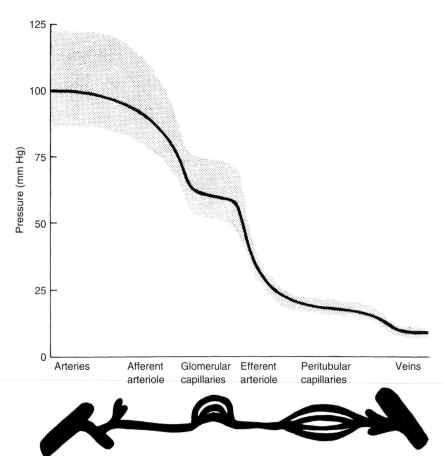

Figure 8.5 Pressure drop indicative of segmental vascular resistance in the kidney. (From Schrier RW. *Diseases of the kidney and urinary tract.* 7th ed. Philadelphia, PA: Lippincott Williams & Wilkins; 2001.)

converted into oncotic pressure, favoring reabsorption of tubular fluid into the peritubular capillaries.

Peritubular capillary beds do not bear a constant relationship to the tubule associated with their glomerular origin. They are more likely to supply a neighboring tubule and are universally interconnected with other efferent capillary beds within their renal segment.

The deepest and earliest glomerular generations have a particularly specialized postglomerular circulation. The efferent arterioles of these juxtamedullary glomeruli dive deeper in vascular bundles directed toward the deep medullary tissue. In the outer medullary region, capillary beds provide oxygen and substrate to the metabolically active ascending limb of Henle loop segments that lie in this region. In this region, the juxtamedullary efferent arterioles also give rise to straight vessels, the vasa rectae, consisting of a few endothelial lining cells and interspersed pericytes, which provide contractile function. These thin vessels descend into the medulla and papilla. They are essential for the function of the countercurrent concentrating mechanisms of the deep medullary tissue. At the tip of the medulla, a small capillary network arises but once again coalesces into ascending vasa rectae, whose interactions with the descending medullary vessels is described further in the subsequent text.

The renal venous circulation arising from the venules of the various renal tissue beds appears to have many segmental interconnections. Renal veins probably participate in systemic capacitance vein phenomena; however, it is not clear that the venous tone or other characteristics are regulated for intrarenal purposes.

Control of Overall Renal Blood Flow

The intensivist is usually concerned about conditions that threaten to decrease renal blood flow, although some chronic conditions with a relative excess of flow are known. Changes in renal vascular resistance and renal blood flow can result from vasoconstrictors, failure of vasodilators, or changes in vascular resistance in other major organ systems.[13]

Cardiac failure and various forms of shock have the potential to overcome renal compensatory mechanisms and decrease renal blood flow. These physiologic challenges are usually associated with increased sympathetic nerve activity, release of endogenous catechols, increased angiotensin II levels, and increased activity of other potential vasoconstrictors such as thromboxane products or endothelin. The shifts in blood volume that occur in distributive shock and hepatorenal syndrome complicate therapeutic maneuvers that seek adequate overall hemodynamics while balancing systemic and local organ needs.

Renal vascular control systems also include endogenous vasodilators, with significant roles in regulation being played by nitric oxide,[14] adenosine,[15] PGs, and bradykinin. As in pulmonary hypertension, conditions of increased renal vascular resistance leave the intensivist wishing for a selective and organ-specific vasodilator. Renal vasodilators certainly have been identified and include dopamine, fenoldopam, ANP, brain natriuretic peptide (BNP), other members of the natriuretic peptide family, and vasopressin receptor antagonists. Development of an effective therapeutic strategy for the use of renal vasodilators remains an appropriate and elusive goal.

The renin–angiotensin system of the kidney responds to and influences systemic hemodynamics. It is now appreciated that ACE is present in various sites in the renal tissue and that this system contributes to local, intrarenal regulation of vascular and tubular events.

Various forms of nitric oxide synthase have been identified in many renal locations, and additional sites of synthetic function appear when conditions favor synthase stimulation. Renal blood flow decreases when nitric oxide's inhibitor is infused systemically at levels too low to cause systemic blood pressure effects. Larger doses affect renal vascular resistance disproportionately compared to changes in systemic perfusion pressure. Clearly, nitric oxide is involved in the physiologic control of renal vascular resistance. Inhibition not only causes increased renal vascular resistance but also causes exaggerated responses to other vasoconstrictive stimuli.

Autoregulation of Renal Blood Flow

Preserving renal blood flow in a functional range despite excursions of blood pressure to the physiologic margins clearly has a survival and, therefore, evolutionary value. Blood flow autoregulatory mechanisms are genetically present in several organs.

The effect of renal autoregulation is illustrated in Figure 8.6. Overall renal blood flow across a wide range of blood pressures is maintained relatively constant. This

requires progressive vasodilation as the perfusion pressure falls and vasoconstriction as the perfusion pressure rises toward the physiologic margins. Clearly in contrast to the intuitive baroreceptor neural control, this phenomenon requires local control mechanisms. Autoregulation, of course, can be overcome by extremes of perfusion pressure or extremes of other agents with renal vascular activity.

Renal blood flow autoregulation has been described in many species and circumstances. The fact that similar mechanisms occur in many vascular beds suggests that at least partial control may reside in the vasculature itself. The persistence of autoregulation in the presence of inhibition of angiotensin II formation or nitric oxide synthesis also argues for a basic system. However, the concomitant autoregulation of GFR seems to require some complex interacting control systems.

Current evidence supports major roles for an intrinsic myogenic mechanism, acting in concert with a tubuloglomerular feedback (TGF) loop, in autoregulation (see Fig. 8.7). For the myogenic component, some function of pressure is sensed in the vascular wall of arcuate, interlobular, and afferent arterioles. A characteristic such as transmembrane pressure gradient causes depolarization of the vascular smooth muscle cell with calcium entry through L-type voltage-dependent calcium channels (VDCCs). This phenomenon can be largely disrupted by calcium channel blockers and modified somewhat by a variety of vasoactive

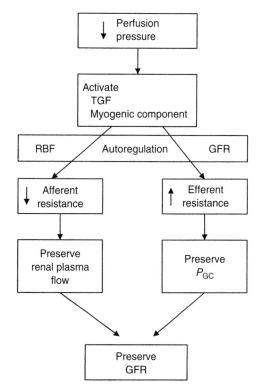

Figure 8.7 Mechanisms of autoregulation. TGF, tubuloglomerular feedback; P_{GC}, glomerular capillary pressure; GFR, glomerular filtration rate; RBF, renal blood flow.

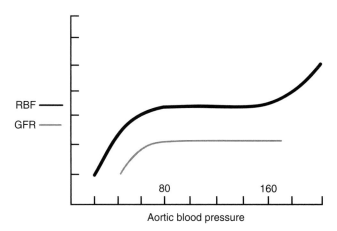

Figure 8.6 The effect of autoregulation: renal blood flow (RBF) and glomerular filtration rate (GFR).

agents. Nevertheless, a myogenic control system is a potent regulator of glomerular perfusion pressure.

The nephron forming with a given glomerulus includes an association of the distal tubule of that nephron with the glomerular hilar region of the same glomerulus such that the tubule lies in near apposition to the cells of the afferent and efferent arterioles. This JGA provides an anatomic basis for tubular events to signal changes in preglomerular or glomerular circumstance. More information on this system is provided later in the chapter; however, the basic feedback loop is involved in the autoregulation of glomerular blood flow. The cells of the distal tubule lying next to the arterioles are referred to as the *MD*. These cells are capable of sensing the delivery of solute to the distal portion of the tubule. In brief, increases in sodium delivery to this site may reflect an increase in glomerular filtration. Sensing this increase, the MD may signal the afferent arteriole through mediators that increase afferent arteriolar resistance, thereby decreasing glomerular perfusion pressure and returning the MD tubular delivery to some physiologic set point.

Considerable evidence supports a central role for adenosine as the preglomerular vasoconstrictor in TGF, whereas nitric oxide and PGE_2 seem to contribute to the vasodilatory limb of the system, as well as act to modulate vasoconstrictor actions. These actions and interactions are discussed later in the chapter.

Autoregulation of renal blood flow has a developmental aspect, which is largely uninvestigated. Newborn and juvenile animals demonstrate autoregulation but do so around mean blood pressures that are significantly lower than that in adults.

Additional uninvestigated aspects include the relationship of pulse pressure to other potential sensed pressures. For instance, if systolic pressure is increased but mean pressure is decreased, autoregulatory vasoconstriction still occurs.

Structural Renovascular Pathology

Renovascular compromise is relatively common in the geriatric population and relatively uncommon in the pediatric population. However, several such conditions should be noted by the pediatric intensivist.

Partial or complete vascular occlusion includes the rare occurrence of congenital renal artery stenosis, as well as its acquired forms. Renal artery emboli from a patent ductus or, more commonly, from an umbilical artery catheter can cause severe hypertension, heart failure, and even total renal failure. Traumatic injury may cause kidney loss. However, even with major blood flow interruption, there appears to be an approximately 4-hour window during which period revascularization may result in kidney salvage.[16] Neurofibromatosis and necrotizing vasculitis of large arteries may compromise renal perfusion.

In the renal transplantation population, particular attention should be paid to any renal graft whose arterial supply includes a lower pole accessory artery. The presence of compromised perfusion from such an artery may result in ureteral or renal pelvic necrosis and a urinary leak.

Grossly bloody urine seldom signifies an underlying critical illness; however, there are a few exceptions. An arterial–venous malformation may produce a life-threatening hemorrhage. These may occur, for instance, at a previous renal biopsy site. Direct connections from the renal artery to the renal pelvis can develop, again with impressive hemorrhagic potential. Patients with sickle cell disease and sickle trait are at risk for major hemorrhage and papillary necrosis.

Venous occlusion is not likely to produce sudden, severe hypertension and may be more amenable to renal salvage management. Renal vein thrombosis tends to occur in the setting of a hypercoagulable state, such as nephrotic syndrome, as well as in circumstances of dehydration. Renal tumors may also invade and essentially occlude the renal vein. The role of renal venous flow compromise in the abdominal compartment syndrome continues to be investigated.

GLOMERULAR AND MEDULLARY CIRCULATIONS

Glomerular Structure

Interlobular arteries coursing centrifugally toward the renal capsule give off afferent arterioles as right-angled, short branches leading to the glomerular hilum, where the arteriolar internal elastic layer ceases and specialized granular cells surround the vascular endothelium (see Fig. 8.8). Believed to be of smooth muscle origin, these cells form the vascular component of the JGA. Additional agranular specialized cells can be seen in the hilar mesangium and efferent arteriole.

The afferent arteriole then branches into a capillary tuft made of several individual convoluted channels lined by fenestrated endothelial cells. Basement membranes surround the endothelial surface toward the Bowman space, and mesangial cells and matrix material contact the medial surface of the capillary endothelial cells in a stalklike or mesenterylike arrangement.

At their efferent end, the glomerular capillaries coalesce suddenly into the sinuslike beginning of the efferent arteriole. This critical resistance vessel will subsequently divide into peritubular capillaries for cortical glomeruli or dive into the medulla as vasa rectae from the juxtamedullary glomeruli.

The glomerular capillary basement membrane is covered by the foot process projections of the glomerular visceral epithelial cells. This multilayer capillary wall is described further in the subsequent text.

A single cell layer of squamous epithelial cells forms the parietal layer or Bowman capsule. Roughly opposite the glomerular hilum, the capsule opens into the origin of the PT with a sudden transition to tubular epithelial cells with their brush-bordered luminal surface.

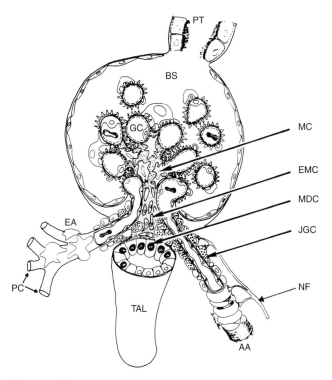

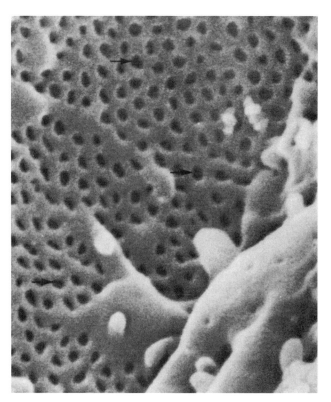

Figure 8.8 Glomerular and juxtaglomerular structure. MC, mesangial cell; EMC, extraglomerular mesangial cell; MDC, macula densa cell; JGC, juxtaglomerular apparatus cell; NF, nerve fiber; AA, afferent arteriole; TAL, thick ascending limb; PC, peritubular capillaries; EA, efferent arteriole; GC, glomerular capillary; BS, Bowman space; PT, proximal tubule. (From Casellas D, Navar LG. *Am J Physiol.* 1984;15:F349; reproduced from Schrier RW. *Diseases of the kidney and urinary tract.* 7th ed. Philadelphia, PA: Lippincott Williams & Wilkins; 2001.)

Figure 8.9 Fenestrated glomerular capillary. (From Schrier RW. *Diseases of the kidney and urinary tract.* 7th ed. Philadelphia, PA: Lippincott Williams & Wilkins; 2001.)

Juxtaglomerular Apparatus Substructure

The walls of the afferent and efferent arterioles contain specialized cells with both smooth muscle and epithelial characteristics. While retaining their vascular smooth muscle characteristics, these myoepithelial cells have regions packed with secretory granules and have well-developed endoplasmic reticulum and Golgi apparatus. The granules clearly contain renin and smaller amounts of precursors and derivatives such as angiotensin II. The local and systemic effects of renin released from this site appear to depend on receptor physiology.

The JGA also includes mesangial cells interposed between MD and juxtaglomerular granular cells. These may serve as communication channels, as well as structural components. They are continuous with the glomerular mesangial region.

Glomerular Substructure

The capillaries of the glomerulus appear as though they are made to leak but do so in a very selective manner.[17] Their lining endothelial cells represent not a solid surface but more of a netlike veil separating the basement membrane and capillary lumen (see Fig. 8.9). These cells

are submicroscopically thin and are perforated throughout by 100-Å fenestrae, providing controlled exposure to the basement membrane. The cell surface is negatively charged, similar to other components of the capillary wall. Nitric oxide and endothelin are both produced by capillary endothelial cells, as are a variety of cell surface receptors.

The formation of specialized fenestrae occurs under the influence of vascular endothelial growth factor (VEGF) synthesized by the visceral epithelial cells lining outside the glomerular capillaries. Therefore, the endothelial cells provide a barrier to the larger elements of circulating blood, prevent direct exposure of thrombogenic collagen sites, yet allow a large surface area of nearly direct access to an ultrafiltering membrane.

Electron microscopy (EM) shows the capillary endothelial cells attached to the inner layer, lamina rara interna, of the trilaminar glomerular basement membrane (GBM) (see Fig. 8.10). The central lamina densa underlies the lamina rara externa, which directly contacts the projections of the glomerular visceral epithelial cells.

Type IV collagen is a major GBM component, as are the heparan sulfate–containing glycosaminoglycans. Collagen not only imparts structural integrity, along with laminin and fibronectin, but also has genetic variability, resulting in the mutational pathology of Alport syndrome leading to progressive renal destruction.

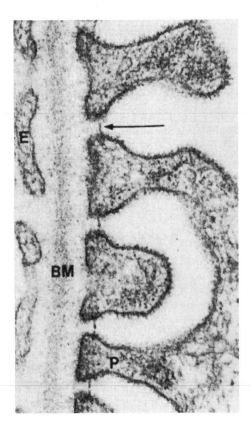

Figure 8.10 Glomerular capillary basement membrane detail. E, endothelial cell; BM, trilaminar basement membrane; P, epithelial podocyte; ←, filtration slit membrane. (From Schrier RW. *Diseases of the kidney and urinary tract.* 7th ed. Philadelphia, PA: Lippincott Williams & Wilkins; 2001.)

Glycosaminoglycans contribute to the negative charge of the glomerular filtration barrier. Although both endothelial and epithelial negativity contribute to the repulsion of albumin and other negatively charged plasma components, the charge density of the trilaminar GBM itself may be the major barrier. Loss of this charge profoundly alters the barrier and results in heavy proteinuria, which may be relatively selective for small, negatively charged albumin or may be a part of more extensive GBM damage, resulting in leakage of larger, nonselective proteins.

Glomerular filtration integrity is also critically dependent upon the visceral epithelial function. These cells interdigitate frondlike projections onto the lamina rara externa, producing the "foot process" appearance in the EM cross-section.

The cytoplasm of these cells is complex, and the cell membrane of the foot processes or podocytes appears to be an active component of glomerular filtration regulation. An epithelial-derived slit membrane extends between foot processes. A negatively charged material, referred to as *glycocalyx,* is present on the surface of these podocytes and is now being characterized at the molecular level. Podocin, nephrin, and CD2-associated protein normally contribute to the barrier function of the foot processes and

the filtration slits between them. Genetic deficiencies are associated with forms of nephrotic syndrome.

In addition to these barrier functions, evidence suggests that the actual synthesis of GBM material is an activity of the visceral epithelial cells. Damage to these cells is evident in many forms of acute and chronic renal disease.

The Mesangium

The mesangial region of the glomerulus consists of mesangial cells and extracellular matrix material arranged as a stalklike supporting mesentry based at the glomerular hilum. For an individual capillary loop, the GBM does not totally encircle the capillary endothelial cells but rather leaves a medial region of direct endothelial–mesangial attachment with no interposed GBM. Attractive consequences of this direct connection could include the traffic of macromolecules for phagocytosis or perhaps the sensing of physical properties in the glomerular capillary.[18]

Mesangial cells elaborate extracellular mesangial matrix material that is rich in negatively charged glycosaminoglycans and proteins. Therefore, to some extent, a negative charge barrier still exists in this region. The transit of large molecules into the mesangium is well documented, however.

Mesangial cells contain many actin and myosin microfilaments and have contractile capabilities. In addition, these cells produce and respond to a variety of vasoactive substances.[19] Therefore, their position and physiology could influence glomerular capillary pressures and filtration. Direct observation of glomeruli *in vivo* does not suggest cyclic or major dynamic mesangial contractile activity. However, contractile elements could also exist to respond to physical changes in a way that would tend to maintain glomerular stability rather than movement.

Glomerular Filtration

For a patient with an acute, critical illness, glomerular filtration is most pertinent in terms of the quantity of water and small solutes entering the nephron. Adequate filtration of these is needed for the nephron to regulate the balance of Na^+, K^+, H^+, HCO_3^-, and water.

These small solutes move with water, and the following discussion on glomerular filtration forces relates to the movement of water and these solutes from the glomerular capillary to Bowman's space.

Single-nephron glomerular filtration rate (SNGFR) is primarily the result of the effects of glomerular capillary surface area (S) and hydraulic permeability (k), as well as the balance between transmembrane hydraulic pressure (ΔP) and colloid osmotic pressure ($\Delta \pi$).

$$\Delta P = P_{GC} - P_{BS}$$

where P_{GC} is glomerular capillary hydraulic pressure and P_{BS} is pressure in the Bowman space. Transmembrane pressure is "meaned" because capillary pressure is pulsatile. Osmotic pressure ($\Delta\pi = \pi_{GC} - \pi_{BS}$) is "meaned" or averaged because it changes over the length of the filtering capillary.

Surface area and permeability can be conceptually aggregated as the glomerular ultrafiltration coefficient, K_f, yielding the relationship: $SNGFR = K_f(\Delta P - \Delta\pi)$. Therefore, the net transmembrane pressure ($\Delta P - \Delta\pi$) acts over a given surface area with a given hydraulic permeability. At first glance, it would seem that hydraulic pressure might be the only dynamic variable. Certainly, capillary hydraulic pressure is a regulated variable. Afferent arteriolar relaxation may increase P_{GC} and constriction may decrease P_{GC}. Also, efferent constriction may raise or sustain P_{GC} and relaxation might significantly diminish P_{GC}. Note, however, that changes in hydraulic pressure that speed filtration also speed the resulting rise in capillary colloid osmotic pressure, thereby modulating any overall increase in SNGFR. Changes in other variables may also be important. Colloid osmotic pressure can vary over a limited range, and hydraulic permeability may vary in pathologic conditions. Potential changes in glomerular capillary filtration surface area are of more interest and perhaps of more physiologic significance.

As the process of filtration occurs with flow through the glomerular capillary, hydraulic pressure changes little, but osmotic pressure rises as the nonfiltered plasma proteins become more concentrated (see Fig. 8.11). Therefore, a balance between ΔP and $\Delta\pi$ may occur, and filtration may cease before flow reaches the efferent end of the capillary. The capillary surface area up to this point of filtration equilibrium is the total surface area that will contribute to the ultrafiltration coefficient. However, if renal blood flow increases even without a change in P_{GC}, this point of equilibrium may be moved further downstream in the glomerular capillary. A higher plasma volume per unit time enters the capillary, and a higher volume of filtration will have to occur before hydraulic and osmotic pressure equilibrium is achieved. Assuming little change in capillary diameter, the equilibrium occurs more distally in the capillary; therefore, a greater capillary surface area actively filters, such that K_f increases. Decreases in K_f can occur because of the action of certain vasoconstrictors. The concept of glomerular capillary filtration equilibrium emphasizes the importance of renal blood or plasma flow rate in determining GFR through altered K_f.

Filtration equilibrium could also occur if the hydraulic pressure in the Bowman space rises because of tubular obstruction. Some models of acute tubular injury (ATI) predict this event, although some filtration would persist at a rate similar to the back leak of tubular fluid from the lumen of the damaged tubule into the peritubular capillaries.

Glomerular Filtration Rate and Vasoactive Compounds

In the human kidney, angiotensin II acts by binding to AT_1 receptors found in the arterioles and mesangium.[20]

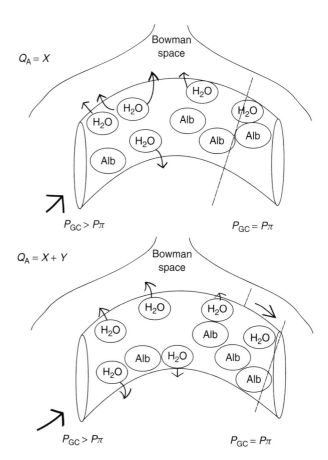

Figure 8.11 Increased glomerular capillary plasma flow, Q_A, shifts the location of filtration equilibrium downstream, increasing the filtering capillary surface area. P_{GC}, glomerular capillary pressure; P_π, glomerular capillary oncotic pressure; Alb, albumin; Q_A, glomerular capillary plasma flow; *dashed line*, site of filtration equilibrium.

Systemic administration of pressor doses results in an increased afferent arteriolar resistance and an even larger increase in efferent arteriolar resistance, resulting in increased glomerular capillary pressure. Despite decreases in renal plasma flow and K_f, the single-nephron GFR tends to be preserved. In subpressor doses, the afferent arteriole changes little and the efferent arteriole constricts, further illustrating its sensitivity. It is then not surprising that inhibition of angiotensin II generation or receptor binding could result in exaggerated efferent arteriolar relaxation and acute renal failure because of decrease in glomerular filtration pressure.

Angiotensin receptors in the mesangial cells are undoubtedly physiologically active. Isolated glomeruli demonstrate contraction in response to angiotensin II, and this contraction is reduced by the presence of nitric oxide. Experimental models demonstrate decreased K_f following angiotensin II administration, but a consistent mechanistic explanation remains elusive. In addition to nitric oxide, PGs and other vasodilators contribute to the counterbalancing of angiotensin II, thereby preserving renal blood flow.

Norepinephrine likewise increases afferent and efferent arteriolar resistance and decreases renal plasma flow in the intact animal. However, the net effect on renal blood flow when norepinephrine is administered as an inotrope and pressor in critical illness is not so easily predicted. Net changes in renal blood flow will depend upon relative effects of norepinephrine on perfusion pressures and renal vascular resistance, factors influenced by volume therapy, and administration of other inotropic and vasoactive drugs.

The glomerular ultrafiltration coefficient, K_f, is decreased by endothelin, ADH, and leukotriene D_4, all of which can constrict mesangial cells. Endothelin and ADH, however, can have variable effects on renal blood flow. Vasoconstrictive leukotrienes or thromboxane derivatives may be particularly pertinent to both gram-positive and gram-negative septicemia. Overall renal vascular resistance and segmental resistances are controlled by the physiologic tension between tonic but variable effects of vasoconstrictors and vasodilators. In this later category, nitric oxide, bradykinin, and PGs are particularly noteworthy. In addition to humoral regulation, renal nerves play a direct role in regulating vasomotor tone. Increased neural activity stimulates renin release and angiotensin generation, further contributing to vasoconstriction. This effect is expected in cardiac failure and other critical illness.

Glomerular filtration is also affected by a family of natriuretic peptides including ANP, BNP, urodilatin (URO), and C-type ANP. These very similar compounds act through cyclic guanosine 3′,5′-monophosphate (cGMP) and directly impact both glomerular and tubular events. ANP is released from atrial tissue with increasing stimulation of atrial stretch receptors. ANP and BNP are elevated in volume-expanded states and congestive heart failure. The natriuretic peptides act to decrease salt and water reabsorption in the tubule and increase GFR despite little change in glomerular blood flow. As might be expected, afferent arteriolar resistance is decreased and efferent arteriolar resistance is increased or remains little changed. Cortical efferent arterioles appear to constrict more than juxtamedullary efferents in response to these peptides. Pharmacologic use of brain natriuretic peptide, in particular, appears to have some promise in the treatment of critical illness.

Many counterbalancing systems act to control and preserve glomerular filtration. Quantitative protection of renal plasma flow and glomerular capillary pressure have been repeatedly demonstrated. The role of mesangial contractility and ultrafiltration coefficient, K_f, in this process is less clear. Additional understanding of the impact of critical illness on these systems will hopefully provide new therapeutic windows.

TUBULAR OVERVIEW

The PT is made up of elongated cuboidal epithelial cells, with different cell surfaces specialized to facilitate function.

The luminal or apical surface of the cell is densely covered with the microvillus brush border, greatly increasing the surface area for contact with the luminal fluid. The basal and lateral cell membranes fold extensively and have projections that interdigitate with surrounding cells. Cell nuclei tend to have a basilar location, as do the numerous mitochondria.

The first tubular segment, pars convoluta or proximal convoluted tubule (PCT), contains epithelial cells whose basilar surfaces are quite complex and reminiscent of the projections of the glomerular visceral epithelial cells. Overall, of course, the basilar cell surface is convex in the PT versus the concave, capillary surrounding surface in the glomerulus. The lateral cell surfaces are functionally similar to the basal surface. Near the lumen, the lateral intercellular space is relatively sealed at the apex by an almost continuous tight junction structure, the zona occludens. Desmosomes and intermediate junctions lie slightly deeper in the intercellular space and provide cell–cell adhesion. This region of luminal exposure of cell borders is not totally permeable to water and solute, but it does contribute to reabsorption and is discussed further in the subsequent text.

PCT cells appear metabolically primed (see Fig. 8.12). Elongated mitochondria are densely packed into the basolateral regions, endoplasmic reticulum and Golgi are prominent, and many microtubules traverse the cytoplasm. In addition to energy-producing enzyme systems and a variety of transport systems, apical endocytosis also plays a variable role in removing tubular fluid constituents.

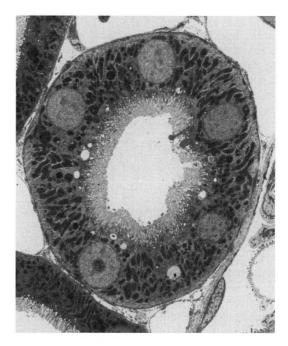

Figure 8.12 Proximal convoluted tubule with prominent mitochondria and brush border. (From Schrier RW. *Diseases of the kidney and urinary tract*. 7th ed. Philadelphia, PA: Lippincott Williams & Wilkins; 2001.)

The base of the proximal tubular cell adheres to basement membrane material through structural proteins. This region abuts the peritubular capillaries and some renal lymphatics, providing egress of material reabsorbed. This region also allows hormones, drugs, and metabolic products to traffic from blood to receptors on the tubular cells.

Pars Recta

The character of the tubular cells changes as they become the straight portion or pars recta of the PT. Overall, these cells suggest much less intense metabolic activity, largely transport, compared to earlier proximal cells. Basolateral membrane architecture is simpler, with fewer, nonglobular mitochondria. The brush border does persist, as does endocytotic activity, but animal studies suggest that less reabsorption activity is occurring in this segment.

Thin Limb

The pars recta of the PT begins the nephron's drive toward the medulla and transitions into the thin limb (TL) of the loop of Henle at the outer medulla. As previously noted (Fig. 8.3), the loop of Henle from cortical nephrons will reach only the outer medulla while the loops extending into the inner medulla originate from the larger juxtamedullary nephrons.

In humans, the vascular bundles of the vasa rectae are associated only with the long loops from the juxtamedullary nephrons.

In contrast to the PT epithelia, the cells of the TL are flattened and lose the brush border. Four types of cells are separable in animal studies and vary in terms of their surface and basolateral complexity. Type II appears most complex and makes up the descending TL lining of juxtamedullary long loops.

Thinner, less complex cells appear in the deep medulla and in the thin ascending limb as it rises to the transition zone in the outer medulla, where the thick ascending limb begins.

Thick Ascending Limb

The cells of the TAL return to an appearance of being metabolically action-packed. The cell height increases, basolateral complexity returns, elongated mitochondria are packed in, endoplasmic reticular and Golgi apparatus are prominent, and other cytoplasmic structures are common. Luminal cell surfaces become more irregular with increased area as the TAL approaches the beginning of the distal convoluted tubule (DCT). Although relatively impermeable to water, basolateral ATPases provide for the prominent active solute transport of this diluting nephron segment.

Macula Densa

The MD are the specialized cells of the TAL that lie next to the arteriolar JGA at the glomerular hilum (see

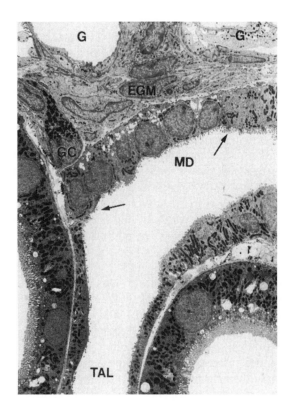

Figure 8.13 Macula densa structure. MD, macula densa; TAL, thick ascending limb; EGM, extraglomerular mesangium; G, glomerulus. (From Schrier RW. *Diseases of the kidney and urinary tract.* 7th ed. Philadelphia, PA: Lippincott Williams & Wilkins; 2001.)

Fig. 8.13). This is discussed further in the section on "Tubuloglomerular Feedback". The MD occurs in the distal nephron at or near the transition point from TAL to DCT.

The cells of the DCT appear abruptly and are taller than those of the TAL. Their apical nuclear placement and lack of a brush border distinguish them from PCT cells. Their basolateral projections and elongated mitochondria resemble PCT cells, as do their tight and intermediate junctions.

The DCT in the human is followed by a transitional, connecting tubule distinguished in part by histology and by the varying distribution of the four cell types—distal, intercalated, principal, and connecting tubule—of this region. Connecting tubules may connect one DCT to an initial collecting tubule (ICT) or may connect more than one DCT to a single ICT.

The ICT is part of the cortical collecting duct (CCD), the diameter of which grows as more ICTs join together and gather in the medullary rays between cortical areas. Intercalated cells and principal cells make up the CCD and display a growing array of subtypes. Histologically defined, these cells continue as the outer medullary collecting duct (OMCD) segment, although nephron functions tend to shift with differing segments.

The MCDs become the inner medullary collecting ducts (IMCD) that, amazingly enough, can be further subdivided in regions of differing functional properties—as mentioned in the subsequent text. MCDs are not only important for plumbing but are also important for "polishing" the final nephron product, a product regulated to a very high degree.

Tubular Function

The glomerulus has provided the tubule with a selective ultrafiltrate of plasma. Molecules within an effective radius of <20 Å, an elongated shape, a neutral or positive charge, and a molecular weight less than approximately 6,000 Da will pass through the GBM largely unrestricted. Under normal conditions, the tubule fluid (TF) will contain only very small amounts of much larger molecules.

The kidney is often thought of, appropriately, as an excretory organ. However, most of the nephron's energy expenditure is in its role as a conservationist, recovering most of the glomerular filtrate for return to the intravascular space. In simplistic terms, it is the PT that carries the major portion of this large, volume-reabsorptive load. Approximately 60% of filtered sodium and water and even higher percentages of solutes will be reabsorbed in the PT. These solutes include chloride; HCO_3^-; potassium; glucose; amino acids; acids; and many macromolecules, such as albumin, that are present in small quantities.[21] The PT, of course, is also a secretory tissue, a site of molecular degradation and metabolism, and an active synthetic site for molecules such as ammonia. Mannitol as a nonreabsorbable solute diuretic is active in the PT.

The straight portion of the PT is not as metabolically active as the PCT but contributes to the overall volume of reabsorbate. It leads to the descending limb of the loop of Henle, referred to as the *TL*. This segment should be thought of as a concentrating segment where water is relatively free to move from the lumen into the increasingly hyperosmolar medullary interstitium. The TL turns and becomes the ascending TL before abruptly transitioning into the TAL of the loop of Henle.

In contrast to the TL, the TAL is relatively water-impermeable. Because it is very active in transporting particularly sodium and chloride out of the tubular lumen, the TAL now becomes a diluting segment with decreasing luminal concentrations of sodium chloride as it ascends into the cortex. The TAL active transport is the target of the potent loop diuretics.

Having traversed an isotonic, volume-reabsorptive unit, the PT, a concentrating TL segment, and a diluting TAL, the tubular fluid now passes by the specialized cells of the MD.[22] This structure samples the fluid and provides feedback to the glomerular hilum, which is described further in the subsequent text. Just beyond the MD, the DCT and connecting tubule constitute an important reabsorptive and secretory site. Under the control of mineralocorticoids, tubular fluid flow rate, and intracellular metabolic circumstances, fine-tuning of sodium, potassium, and hydrogen

excretion occurs in this region. Thiazide diuretics are active here.

The collecting tubule still has a regulatory role to play, particularly in terms of variable water permeability affecting the final urine concentration.

Tubuloglomerular Feedback

TGF has been mentioned in earlier sections; it represents a mechanism of significance to virtually all nephron functions (see Fig. 8.14). The fetal apposition of the early distal tubule to the cleft between the same nephron's afferent and efferent arterioles and extraglomerular mesangium allows for feedback control of SNGFR, depending on the delivery of NaCl to the MD.

Apical transport of luminal NaCl into the MD cells is a key step in sensing distal delivery. Approximately 80% of this entry is facilitated by the $Na^+/K^+/2Cl^-$ cotransporter of the apical membrane. This cotransporter is saturable, with maximal transport occurring when the luminal NaCl concentration reaches approximately 60 mmol per L.

The remaining 20% of Na^+ entry is facilitated through the NHE_3 Na^+/H^+ exchanger, which does not show concentration saturation.

Unlike most renal tubular cells, those of the MD do not have a major basolateral membrane ATPase to transport NaCl out of the cell. Therefore, changes in luminal delivery should be quickly reflected in the intracellular NaCl content.

Basolateral egress channels have been identified for Cl^- and adenosine triphosphate (ATP) transport, as well as VDCC for Ca^{2+} transport. ATP, described further in the subsequent text, can be metabolized to vasoactive adenosine.

Increases in intracellular Cl^- level feed basolateral channel-mediated egress and membrane depolarization. The resultant opening of VDCCs increases cytosolic Ca^{2+} and stimulates the release of additional paracrine mediators.[23] These messengers appear to traverse the extraglomerular mesangium and directly or indirectly act on the afferent and efferent arteriolar tone to change SNGFR.

The GFR-reducing limb of this control system releases ATP, which may act directly at P2X receptors to liberate Ca^{2+} and cause afferent vasoconstriction.

Alternatively or in addition, local enzymes appear to adequately metabolize ATP to adenosine, which can bind to afferent AT_1 receptors, constricting the afferent arteriole, and efferent AT_2 receptors, dilating the efferent arteriole.

The sensitivity of this control limb is increased by angiotensin II, which binds to apical and basolateral AT_1 receptors, causing increased Na^+/H^+ exchange and increased $Na^+/K^+/2Cl^-$ cotransport for a given amount of NaCl delivery.

The expected preglomerular vasodilatory limb is less defined, but PGE_2 is synthesized in the MD cells through

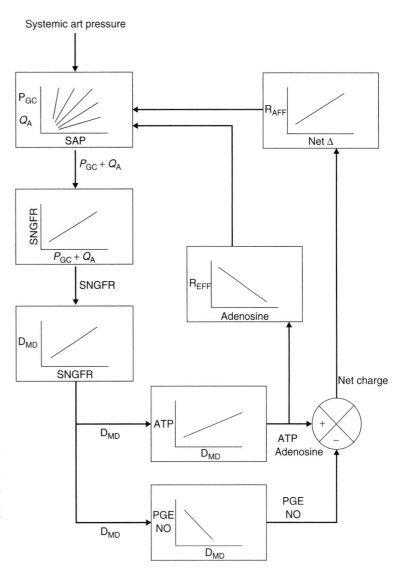

Figure 8.14 Systems diagram—tubuloglomerular feedback. P_{GC}, glomerular capillary pressure; D_{MD}, delivery to macula densa; R_{EFF}, efferent arteriolar resistance; R_{AFF}, afferent arteriolar resistance; SNGFR, single-nephron glomerular filtration rate; PGE, prostaglandin E; ATP, adenosine triphosphate; Q_A, glomerular capillary plasma flow; NO, nitric oxide; SAP, systemic arterial pressure; NetΔ, net change.

cyclooxygenase-2 (COX-2), which in turn responds to NaCl delivery.

Nitric oxide is also a candidate vasodilator or modulator of vasoconstriction and probably plays a role in the local events of TGF.

TGF response occurs rapidly and appears best suited for short-term adjustments, perhaps around variable set points. Obviously, the renin–angiotensin system is subject to other strong stimuli, as are all preglomerular arterioles, and a simple overall control system is unlikely.

SEGMENTAL TUBULAR FUNCTION

Segmental nephron physiology has been mostly studied using the techniques of micropuncture, isolated tubule perfusion, cell culture, and complex histology. A simplified overview of segmental function is presented in Table 8.1. More details are provided in the text of this section.

Proximal Tubule

Na^+ reabsorption is isotonic in the PT, that is, Na^+ and water are reabsorbed proportionately so that the Na^+ concentration in TF all along the PT is similar to that in plasma and glomerular filtrate.[24]

In the early PT, Na^+ is reabsorbed not only with Cl^- but also with amino acids, glucose, and HCO_3^-, resulting in a small Cl^- excess and a negative potential in the TF. The next segment of the PCT tends to rebalance these factors through passive paracellular Cl^- reabsorption and active apical NaCl reabsorption. The diffusive reabsorption of Cl^- and Na^+ through paracellular pathways probably represents more than half the total NaCl reabsorption in the late PCT.

TABLE 8.1
SEGMENTAL NEPHRON REABSORPTIVE ACTIVITY

| | Segment | | | | |
Solute	PT	TL	TAL	DCT/CCT	CD
NaCl	++++	—	++	+	+
HCO_3^-	++++	—	++	±	±
H_2O	++++	+	—	++	++
K^+	++++	—	++	±	—
Ca^{2+}	++	—	++	±	—
Mg^{2+}	–	—	++++	+++	—
PO_4^{3-}	+++++	—	—	+	—
Glucose	++++++	—	—	—	—
Organic acids	++++++	—	—	—	—

PT, proximal tubule; TL, thin limb; TAL, thick ascending limb; DCT, distal convoluted tubule; CCT, cortical collecting tubule; CD, collecting duct.

Transcellular reabsorption of solute requires crossing the apical cell membrane into the cell in one step and exiting the cell through the basolateral cell membrane in a second step that then allows re-entry into blood of the peritubular capillary. The transport systems differ at each membrane site.

The apical membrane contains the NHE_3 Na^+/H^+ exchange transporter that, with carbonic anhydrase, contributes to the net HCO_3^- reabsorption, leaving a negative potential difference (PD) in the tubular lumen. This negative PD also derives from coupled reabsorption of Na^+ and neutral solutes from early PT and helps drive paracellular Cl^- reabsorption.

A major driving force for the apical inward Na^+ transport is the basolateral Na^+/K^+-ATPase pump that extrudes three Na^+ for two entering K^+, thereby leaving an intracellular gradient favoring apical Na^+ entry (see Fig. 8.15).

Other contributors probably include a basolateral Cl^- channel that may have variable conductance, an apical Cl^-/base exchanger linked with H^+ recycling, some basolateral K^+/Cl^- cotransport, and basolateral Cl^-/HCO_3^- exchange.

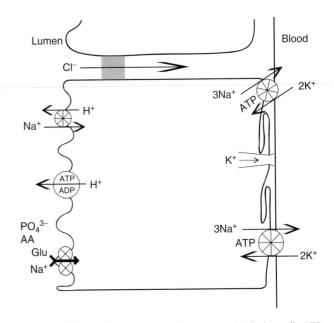

Figure 8.15 Sodium reabsorption, proximal tubular cell. ATP, adenosine 5'-triphosphate; ADP, adenosine 5'-diphosphate; AA, amino acid; Glu, glutamic acid.

Proximal Na^+Cl^- Reabsorption Regulation
Given all these potential effector mechanisms for proximal Na^+Cl^- reabsorption, the control of these systems would seem potentially chaotic. There certainly are many adjustments being made simultaneously but the dominant mechanism is clearly that reabsorption is roughly proportional to the delivery of filtrate from the glomerulus. The term *glomerulotubular balance* (GTB) encompasses intra- and extracellular mechanisms that increase or decrease reabsorption with increases or decreases in the filtered load of solute and water, respectively.[25]

Such an overall mechanism in the "mass reabsorption" tubule segment tends to reduce fluctuations of TF delivery to the loop of Henle. This recurrent theme of load-dependent reabsorption is seen in subsequent tubule segments.

In the PT, the effect of peritubular colloid osmotic pressure could account for some of this modulation; that is, if an increased fraction of a stable renal plasma flow is filtered, an increase in postglomerular, peritubular colloid osmotic force would be expected for reabsorption. This should lead to an increase in absolute TF reabsorption in the PT. Other circumstances seem to require additional tubular mechanisms. Other factors known to be capable of affecting proximal Na^+Cl^- reabsorption include parathyroid hormone (PTH), angiotensin II, renal nerves, and acute hypertension.

Thin Limb

The TL, as mentioned in the preceding text, is a site of water efflux in excess of solute. Na^+/K^+-ATPase activity is limited in short loops and in the lower portion of long loops, and passive NaCl permeability is reduced. The result is progressively increasing concentration of Na^+ and Cl^- as the loop approaches the bend.

As it goes round the deep bend, the TL becomes the ascending TL, still with very little Na^+/K^+-ATPase activity, but now with high solute permeability and low water permeability. Transcellular solute escape predominates and net dilution occurs, even before reaching the TAL.

Thick Ascending Limb

Roughly 30% of filtered Na^+ can be reabsorbed in the TAL. Quantitative reabsorption tends to increase as solute delivery to this segment is increased. Reabsorption is also influenced by humoral mediators, probably in part through changes in cyclic adenosine monophosphate (cAMP)-dependent phosphorylation providing active transport energy.

On the apical membrane, cell entry of Na^+Cl^- is facilitated by the $Na^+/K^+/2Cl^-$ cotransporter also present in MD cells. K^+ enters these cells, then returns to the lumen through a separate K^+ channel, and continues to recycle, thereby multiplying the effect of a relatively low luminal K^+ concentration (see Fig. 8.16).

The acquired intracellular load of Na^+Cl^- leaves the cell through egress toward the peritubular capillary, Na^+/K^+-ATPase pump, Cl^- channels, and a K^+/Cl^- cotransporter for egress, toward the peritubular capillary. A positive luminal voltage aids additional cation transfer in this region through paracellular pathways.

Loop diuretics target the apical $Na^+/K^+/2Cl^-$ cotransporter and probably indirectly decrease Ca^{2+} and Mg^{2+} reabsorption in this region also.[26]

Note that the effectiveness of a natriuretic drug targeting a segment depends on events in any preceding tubule segment, as well as in any following tubular segment. The depression of proximal reabsorption loads the TAL, which may increase compensatory reabsorption. Alternatively, depression of reabsorption in two segments should synergistically increase downstream flow.

Distal Collecting Tubule

The distal tubule drives Na^+Cl^- reabsorption with the familiar basolateral Na^+/K^+-ATPase, but apical Na^+Cl^- reabsorption differs, being linked through a thiazide-sensitive cotransporter (see Fig. 8.17). Inhibition of this cotransporter by thiazides results in decreased Na^+Cl^- reabsorption but increased Ca^{2+} reabsorption through a mechanism that remains unclear.

An apical K^+ channel is present, but K^+ transport is not directly linked to Na^+/Cl^- cotransport into the cell, as it was in the TAL (Fig. 8.17).

There are multiple cell types and subtle transitions in the distal tubule and connecting segment. The collecting duct will also have some functional overlap, as might be expected because it is the fine-tuning segment for solute and acid–base excretion.

Cortical Collecting Tubule

Having completed some transition of histology and function through the connecting tubule, the CCT of the distal nephron as the CCT acquires aldosterone responsiveness.[27] Aldosterone increases inward Na^+ traffic through luminal epithelial Na^+ channels (ENaC) while facilitating K^+ or H^+ secretion into the TF. The exact link between the known nuclear gene activation of aldosterone and the apical events remains arguable. Na^+ reabsorption in excess of needed H^+ or K^+ secretion may be made electroneutral by paracellular Cl^- transport.

Although aldosterone is the most potent natural mineralocorticoid, other steroid drugs variably stimulate Na^+ retention. Interestingly, intact animals escape from the acute Na^+-retaining action of mineralocorticoids after a few days despite being continuously administered. This phenomenon is accompanied by elevated ANP levels,[28] but

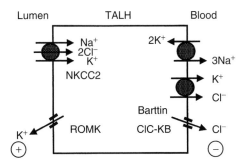

Figure 8.16 Sodium reabsorption, thick ascending limb of Henle. NKCC2, $Na^+/K^+/2Cl^-$ cotransporter; ROMK, potassium channel; ClC-KB, chloride channel; Barttin, subunit of chloride channel; TALH, thick ascending limb of Henle. (From Avner ED, Harmon WE, Niaudet P. *Pediatric nephrology.* 5th ed. Philadelphia, PA: Lippincott Williams & Wilkins; 2003.)

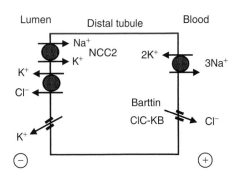

Figure 8.17 Sodium reabsorption on distal tubule. NCC2, cotransporter. ClC-KB, chloride channel. (From Avner ED, Harmon WE, Niaudet P. *Pediatric nephrology.* 5th ed. Philadelphia, PA: Lippincott Williams & Wilkins; 2003.)

it seems inoperative or obscured in severe Na^+-retaining states such as congestive heart failure, cirrhosis, and nephrosis. Basolateral Na^+/K^+-ATPase generates a driving force for apical Na^+ entry.

As previously mentioned, the late distal nephron has some specific cell types and tends to follow a specific pattern of distribution. Type A intercalated cells secrete H^+ through a H^+-ATPase driver upregulated in hypokalemia. Type B intercalated cells provide net HCO_3^- secretion. Principal cells become more and more predominant in the OMCD. The IMCD includes virtually all the principal cells. Functionally, principal cells can reabsorb Na^+ and secrete K^+, in addition to their critical regulatory role in water excretion, which is discussed further later in this chapter.

Collecting Duct

The OMCD can secrete H^+ and appears to exchange Cl^- and HCO_3^-. The inner medullary principal cells participate

in the final regulation of the excretion of Na^+, H^+, and K^+, as well as of water and urea.

Renal Potassium Management

The mammal's store of potassium is large and is mostly intracellular. It is closely regulated, acutely and chronically, both intracellularly and in the extracellular fluid (ECF). Shifting a very small fraction of total body potassium from the intracellular space to the extracellular space can have catastrophic consequences for cardiac myocyte function.

Hyperkalemia is a critical care issue, but hypokalemia is much more common in our ICUs. Potassium disturbances are largely renal, adrenal, and iatrogenic processes. The basic tubular physiology is described in the subsequent text (see Fig. 8.18).

As a quick overview, potassium is freely filtered and is reabsorbed in the PT in proportion to Na^+ and water. Roughly two third of the filtered potassium is reabsorbed

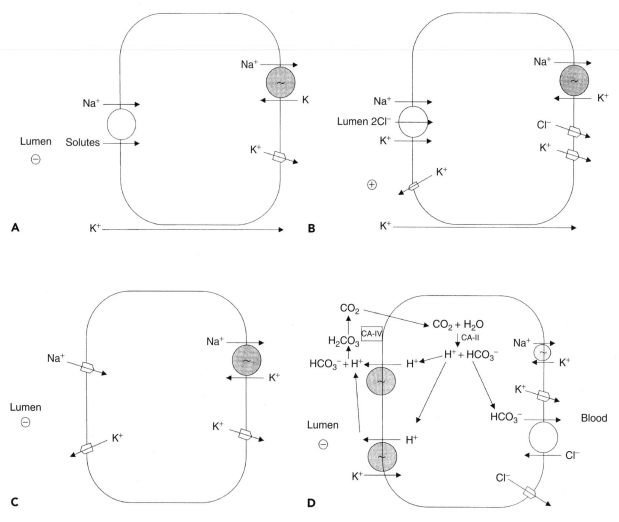

Figure 8.18 Potassium reabsorption and secretion. **A:** Proximal tubule. **B:** Thick ascending limb. **C:** Principle cell. **D:** Intercalated cell. "$\sim$," active transporter. Channels, pentagonal directional figures. CA IV, carbonic anhydrase IV; CA II, carbonic anhydrase II. (From Avner ED, Harmon WE, Niaudet P. *Pediatric nephrology.* 5th ed. Philadelphia, PA: Lippincott Williams & Wilkins; 2003.)

near the end of the PT, although the concentration of K^+ remains similar to that of the filtrate. Through the descending TL, K^+ concentration rises as it diffuses into the tubule from MCD reabsorbate in the interstitium. In the TAL, K^+ is again reabsorbed, producing a very low TF K^+ concentration at the beginning of the DCT. Final urine K^+ concentration is then determined by significant K^+ secretion into the TF of the distal nephron, modified somewhat by the medullary duct reabsorption mentioned in the preceding text. The distal nephron is capable of profound K^+ conservation in conditions of depletion. Major contributors to the control of K^+ excretion include mineralocorticoid activity, Na^+ delivery to a tubular segment, intracellular pH, and Na^+/K^+-ATPase pump integrity.

Although most K^+ reabsorption occurs in the PT, the cellular driving force and pathways are unclear. At the basolateral membrane, the Na^+/K^+-ATPase provides Na^+ exit and K^+ entry. The K^+ then returns to the peritubular interstitium through regulated K^+ channels and through K^+/Cl^- cotransport. Reabsorptive apical paths for TF K^+ are less defined. In fact, paracellular reabsorption in the later PCT may be very important because factors in this segment favor paracellular diffusion, which may be assisted by pumping of K^+ from the lateral intercellular space into the cell followed by basal channel or cotransport toward the capillary.

The TL at the papillary bend may contain K^+ at a concentration in excess of that in the plasma. Although significant water egress from TF occurs, the net K^+ entry from the medullary interstitium is likely required. Therefore, a limited K^+ recycling scenario exists, with the MCD supplying K^+ reabsorbate to the interstitium by diffusion or channel entry into the TL lumen for transit through the reabsorptive and secretory sites of the TAL and the distal nephron.

Cells of the deep TAL appear to be robust reabsorbers of K^+, having a high basolateral K^+ conductance for its exit. Apical $Na^+/K^+/2Cl^-$ cotransport out of the TF is prominent and is the target of furosemide-induced K^+ loss. Multiple apical and basolateral K^+ channels and potential regulators influence net reabsorption. Under homeostatic conditions, the TF reaching the early DCT has a very low K^+ content.

From the early DCT to the initial cortical collecting tubule (iCCT), there is a significant increase in K^+ secretory capacity. Secretory transport of K^+Cl^-, multiple apical K^+ channels, mineralocorticoid stimulation, and a negative luminal potential contribute to this increase. Among the intercalated cells and principal cells in these segments, the latter appear to have predominant secretory capacity. The potential for reabsorption of K^+ in these same cells is suggested by the action of the IMCD, which is populated by principal cells but appears to reabsorb K^+ for recycling into the descending thin limb (DTL), as described in the preceding text.

Stimulation of Na^+ reabsorption and K^+ secretion by mineralocorticoids and increased K^+ secretion by the distal nephron in exchange for increased delivery of Na^+ both seem relatively straightforward.

The increase in K^+ secretion occurring when distal flow is increased independent of Na^+ load is intriguing. Specialized, apical, flow-dependent K^+ channels have been described. Normally resistant, these channels become generous K^+ secretory channels when stimulated by increased tubular fluid flow.

Tubular Calcium Handling

Human bone contains approximately 98% of the total body calcium. ECF content and a small amount of intracellular calcium complete the picture. Calcium in the ECF may be protein-bound, complexed to inorganic ions, or present as calcium ions (ιCa^{2+}). Ionized calcium is tightly regulated and is crucial for critical organ function.

Acute pH changes alter Ca^{2+} binding and can have important consequences, particularly for cardiac, neural, and neuromuscular function. PTH secretion responds to acute changes in ιCa^{2+} and mobilizes Ca^{2+} stores if needed to restore ECF ιCa^{2+}. PTH also acts at the kidney tubule, preserving Ca^{2+} stores by a more gradual action.

The renal cortex metabolizes 25-(OH) vitamin D to a more active form, 1,25-$(OH)_2$ vitamin D, crucial for intestinal calcium absorption. The renal osteodystrophy of chronic renal failure results from phosphate ($P\iota$) retention and the deficiency of 1,25-$(OH)2$ vitamin D production.

The glomerular filtrate contains both free ιCa^{2+} and Ca^{2+} complexed to small anions. Calcium reabsorption by the PT parallels that of Na^+ and water under many conditions. As water reabsorption occurs in the early PT, Ca^{2+} concentration rises, providing a driving force for diffusion down a concentration gradient through paracellular, regulated channels. Transcellular active transport of Ca^{2+} at best seems very limited in the PT.

Loop of Henle

Net reabsorption of calcium does not again become significant until the fluid enters the TAL (see Fig. 8.19). As in the PT, paracellular channels account for most of the net reabsorption here, although a PTH-responsive active component has been described. Active transport of Ca^{2+} in the DCT and connecting segment includes a basolateral PTH-sensitive pump by inference, and likely apical channels potentially subject to other regulatory factors.[29] Urinary Ca^{2+} excretion is dependent upon regulation in these segments because later CDs are not known to have important roles.

Control of Tubular Calcium Ion Reabsorption

Proximal GTB occurs with Ca^{2+}, tending to modulate distal Ca^{2+} delivery. PTH is able to decrease glomerular capillary K_f, as well as increase Ca^{2+} reabsorption, protecting ECF Ca^{2+} content. Calcitonin and vitamin D analogs have primary roles at extrarenal sites. Loop diuretics inhibit $Na^+/K^+/2Cl^-$ cotransport and decrease lumen electropositivity, decreasing the gradient favoring Ca^{2+} diffusion. In contrast, thiazides decrease Na^+ reabsorption but increase Ca^{2+} reabsorption, a quality exploited

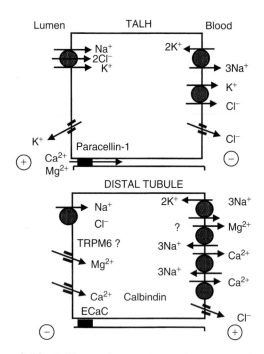

Figure 8.19 Calcium and magnesium reabsorption in the thick ascending limb and distal tubule. ECaC, epithelial calcium channel; TRPM6, magnesium channel. (From Avner ED, Harmon WE, Niaudet P. *Pediatric nephrology.* 5th ed. Philadelphia, PA: Lippincott Williams & Wilkins; 2003.)

in the management of hypercalciuria, which is probably frequently present in critically ill patients.

Renal Magnesium Handling

Mg^{2+} is approximately 50% localized to the bone and is also a vital participant in soft-tissue intracellular metabolic activities. The intracellular component accounts for most of the remaining 50% of total body magnesium, with only approximately 1% present in the ECF. Like calcium, magnesium exists in its free, ionized form, complexed to a variety of anions, and 20% to 30% is protein-bound. Plasma levels of ionized magnesium are important to many organ functions, but the relatively tight control systems for plasma magnesium are not understood.

Ionized and complexed magnesium are relatively freely filtered. More than 95% of the filtered magnesium is recovered by tubular reabsorptive mechanisms that can be up-regulated or down-regulated as needed.

In a PT, measurements of tubular fluid magnesium increase as one proceeds down the tubule, similar to nonreabsorbable inulin. It would seem that very little magnesium recovery occurs in this site.

In the TAL, however, avid sodium reabsorption drives a positive luminal voltage, resulting in paracellular Mg^{2+} reabsorption amounting to approximately two third of filtered Mg^{2+} (Fig. 8.19). Loop diuretics decrease this pivotal, sodium-dependent PD and profoundly reduce magnesium reabsorption.

Further magnesium recovery occurs in the DCT and connecting segment.[30] Here, active Mg^{2+} transport occurs. Magnesium-wasting syndromes have been described in association with defective genes for apical divalent ion channels.[31] Further understanding of gene products may clarify magnesium controllers.

Overall control of Mg^{2+} depends greatly on the control of sodium reabsorption, particularly in the TAL. Loop diuretics and calcineurin-inhibitor immunosuppressive agents can affect Mg^{2+} homeostasis and hence their use is a major issue in the ICU.

Phosphorus

As for magnesium, <1% of total body phosphorus is located in the ECF. Most of the remainder resides in bone, but critical soft-tissue cell structures and functions are phosphorus-dependent. Phosphorus participates in cell and organelle membranes and structures, as well as in energy storage and transfer processes.

Univalent or divalent $P\iota$ ions can be free, complexed, or protein bound. As with calcium and magnesium, the protein-associated fraction is not filtered at the glomerulus.

Critical care interest in $P\iota$ most often relates to hypophosphatemia, usually secondary to poor intake, osmotic diuresis, or a genetic syndrome. Renal failure is commonly associated with hyperphosphatemia but more critical $P\iota$ elevations occur with certain lymphoid malignancies and tumor lysis syndrome.

Tubular Reabsorption of Phosphorus

Various studies have suggested that anywhere from 80% to almost 99% of tubular $P\iota$ reabsorption occurs in the PT.

Apical active transport is facilitated by Na^+ cotransporters, particularly type IIa. A greater proportion of $P\iota$ reabsorption occurs early in the PT, but the apical mechanisms of the late PT bind $P\iota$ more avidly, thereby continuing effective transport even as its concentration declines.

PT cells are capable of bidirectional basolateral $P\iota$ transport and appear to have both Na^+-dependent and independent sites.

$P\iota$ reabsorption also occurs in the DCT. Although limited in quantity, this capability may be very important in conserving $P\iota$ during an active growth phase or a period of restricted intake.

Phosphorous balance is influenced by a variety of factors, some being currently elucidated. The most clear-cut actual control system, however, remains the PTH—ιCa^{2+}-$P\iota$ axis. Although PTH receptors were first characterized on the basolateral margin, they have now been demonstrated on the apical brush border as well. It is likely that both regions are biologically active PTH targets and that adenylyl cyclase and protein kinases are active messengers.

Increasing levels of PTH decrease tubular $P\iota$ reabsorption. Increased serum $P\iota$ may stimulate counterregulatory PTH secretion directly or by decreasing ιCa^{2+} concentration.

As was true for calcium, 1,25-$(OH)_2$ vitamin D is important for intestinal Pi absorption. Renal conversion of 25-(OH) vitamin D to 1,25-(OH) vitamin D is stimulated by decreased plasma Pi. The more active metabolite of vitamin D then not only acts to increase intestinal Pi absorption, but also acts directly and indirectly to decrease potentially phosphaturic PTH secretion.

Renal conservation or excretion of Pi can be quite effective, but changes occur more slowly than with some other cations.

Glucose Recovery

Well-functioning kidneys recover filtered glucose essentially completely in the PT. The exception is the small group of patients with kidneys that leak small amounts of glucose—renal glycosuria—on a genetic basis, the exact mechanism of which remains undefined.

For early PT glucose reabsorption, a major driving force emanates from the basolateral Na^+/K^+-ATPase pump (see Fig. 8.20). This pump generates a net Na^+ and charge transfer that favors luminal entry of Na^+. Therefore, apical Na^+/glucose cotransport through the sodium-dependent glucose cotransporter (SGLT-2) transporter is facilitated, luminal negativity is generated, and paracellular Cl^- reabsorption is also facilitated.

Having entered the cell, glucose must be transferred across the basolateral membrane. The glucose transporter (GLUT) gene family of high-affinity sugar transporters also includes GLUT-2, a low-affinity, high-capacity basilar transporter in the early PCT, as well as in the organs of the gastrointestinal (GI) system. Basolateral glucose exit depends largely on this transporter.

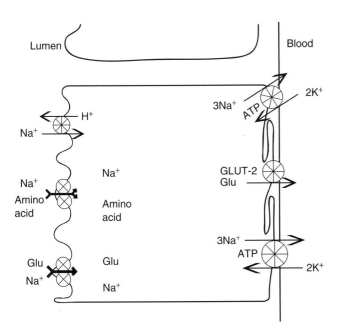

Figure 8.20 Proximal tubule reabsorption of glucose and amino acids. Glu, glutamic acid; ATP, adenosine triphosphate.

Hyperglycemic glucosuria usually occurs at blood sugar levels of 180 to 200 mg per dL but may develop at lower levels in infants and younger children. The stress of critical illness usually leads to minor abnormalities in urinalysis that should not be overinterpreted. Current data suggest that blood sugar levels for many critically ill patients should be targeted well below the glycosuria range.

Amino Acid Reabsorption

Transmembrane movement of amino acids is a ubiquitous, nutritive, cellular requirement. Transtubular reabsorption of amino acids across both apical and basolateral membranes is a more specialized epithelial function.

The classic concept of genetically determined apical transporters shared by similar amino acids appears to be valid (Fig. 8.20). As more detailed investigations are possible, more distinctions within transporter groups and more mutational specificities are being described.

In an oversimplified scheme, neutral, acidic, and basic amino acids are efficiently internalized by the PCT cell with a variable requirement for Na^+ cotransport. Amino acid conservation is efficient, although some normal amino acid excretion can be measured. Derivations from expected patterns are very difficult to interpret in the presence of critical illness, with the exception of a few specific syndromes associated with profound amino acid excretion.

RENAL WATER MANAGEMENT

Total body water as a percentage of body mass varies from 75% to 80% in the premature infant to 55% to 60% in the senior citizen. After allowing for a decreasing relative ECF percentage in infancy, one can generalize that approximately 35% to 40% of body mass is intracellular water and that 20% to 25% is ECF, including 6% to 7% that is intravascular fluid (IVF).

Although not obvious, body water volume is controlled largely by the systems that control Na^+ balance. At the same time, Na^+ and other solute concentration is more directly controlled by arginine vasopressin (AVP). True homeostasis requires that both these interacting systems work well.

Autoregulation of renal blood flow and GFR help modulate potential swings in renal water loss by tending to normalize the amount of filtrate presented for tubular action. Because proximal tubular reabsorption of Na^+ and H_2O are proportional, it is apparent that this segment serves as a bulk reabsorber, recovering approximately two thirds of the filtered tubular fluid. Peritubular capillary oncotic pressure has been increased above arterial pressure by glomerular filtration and serves as a major driving force for reabsorption. Water continues to leave the tubular lumen in the DTL as part of the generation of the hypertonic medullary interstitium. The solute reabsorption of the TAL is key to this function, which then allows control of the permeability of the collecting duct to be variable, regulated by AVP activity. This variable permeability next to a hypertonic interstitium allows control of the final process, water excretion.

Because the human kidney has limitations in terms of its maximal urinary concentration and, in general, has an obligate amount of solute to excrete, it follows that the kidney has an obligate amount of water containing the solute that must be excreted. For an average solute intake, the needed urine output is approximately 1.0 mL/kg/hour. Water intake in excess of the obligate urinary excretion becomes a volume to be regulated in terms of metabolic needs and water loss at other sites—skin, respiratory tract, and GI tract. In the ICU, specific drainage of cerebrospinal fluid (CSF), pleural fluid, ascites, and others are added.

In addition to AVP, which is discussed in detail in subsequent text, it is clear that other factors affect the integrity of the water excretion control system. Adrenal glucocorticoid effect is permissive for normal water excretion. The mechanism may involve a change in some quality of cardiovascular tone as sensed by afferent volume receptors, but glucocorticoid effect at a nephron site involved in AVP response has not been totally excluded.

Similarly, hypothyroidism has been associated with hyponatremia. One might again suspect a role for a change in cardiovascular integrity, but more evidence suggests inappropriately increased AVP-dependent water reabsorption as the cause.

Of particular note for the ICU patient is the lengthy list of drugs that perturb the physiologic control of H_2O excretion and osmoregulation.

Proximal Water Reabsorption

Both peritubular capillary oncotic pressure and basolateral Na^+ pumping may provide reabsorptive force. With two potential water reabsorptive drivers affecting the basal and the lateral interstitial spaces, it might seem that the major reabsorptive route could be either transcellular or paracellular. A variety of studies have concluded that the transcellular route predominates. Therefore, dissolved solute is subject to the specific solute permeability and transport characteristics of the cell membrane.

Facilitative water channels, now called *AQP-1*, are generously distributed in both apical and basolateral membranes of mammalian PTs and TLs of the Henle loop. Water is relatively free to follow this transcellular path in these regions.[32]

In the PT, solute transport is quite active, resulting in relatively balanced salt and water reabsorption. As TF enters the DTL, a different circumstance is encountered. Water permeability remains high, resulting in easy egress to the interstitium. However, solute permeability is greatly diminished, and the descending fluid becomes more and more concentrated as the solvent leaves and solute remains.

The interstitial hypertonicity driving DTL water egress is derived from the solute-only reabsorptive character of the countercurrent TAL. Because the TL is a concentrating segment, the TAL is a diluting segment, lowering the TF salt concentration while maintaining an interstitial solute concentration that rises progressively toward the papillary tip. This basic countercurrent multiplier system provides a driving force for eventual MCD water reabsorption.[33] Movements of urea, NH_3, and other solutes affect and depend on this system. A most puzzling aspect, however, is that deep juxtamedullary nephrons have long loops of Henle, such that their TLs actually make the turn at the papillary tip and ascend partly toward the outer medulla, where transition to the TAL and solute-only reabsorption occurs. How this deepest region of TL and thin ascending limbs maintain the maximal interstitial concentration gradient is unclear.

What is clear is that water egress through AQP-1 channels in the PT and the TL is crucial to mammalian water conservation, not only because of PT bulk reabsorption but also because of the crucial concentrating segment role of the TL. At least ten distinct AQP channels are known, but none are demonstrable in the water-impermeable TAL. AVP does, however, have a specific receptor, V_2R, on the basolateral membrane.

$AVP–V_2R$ binding stimulates adenylyl cyclase, cAMP, and protein kinase A (PKA) activity. In the TAL, this results in some stimulation of Na^+Cl^- reabsorption but has no effect on water permeability because AQP channels cannot be generated.

AQP-2 channels are increased by AVP binding to V_2R receptors.[34] In the late distal tubule or connecting segment, both V_2R receptors and AQP-2 channels are found, and vasopressin-induced water reabsorption occurs. Their availability increases in the outer and inner MCDs, where principal cells predominate.[35]

Binding of basilar $AVP–V_2R$ complexes and subsequent activation of PKA in these tubules results in phosphorylation and luminal exposure of AQP-2 channels, increasing water transport out of the tubule lumen and toward the hypertonic interstitium (see Fig. 8.21). Following an AVP surge, the newly exposed AQP-2 channels are endocytosed, moving intracellularly as a vesicular reservoir of potential channels awaiting phosphorylation and a return to the apical membrane.

A dysfunctional mutation in V_2R interrupts the system. This is the classic lesion of X-linked congenital nephrogenic diabetes insipidus.[36] Additional patterns of concentrating defects have been described with AQP-2 mutation.

Following apical water entry, basolateral water exit is facilitated by additional AQP channels, AQP-3 and AQP-4. The regulated step, however, appears to be intracellular AQP-2 phosphorylation.

Arginine Vasopressin Control

The primary control system for blood AVP levels is osmoregulation through hypothalamic sensors. When serum osmolality is below approximately 284 mOsm per L,

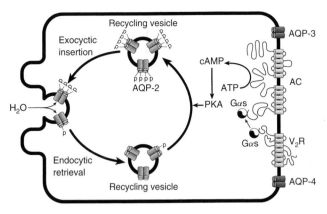

Figure 8.21 CT/CD cell. V_2R, arginine vasopressin (AVP) receptor; AQP, aquaporin; cAMP, cyclic adenosine monophosphate; PKA, protein kinase A; ATP, adenosine triphosphate; AC, adenylyl cyclase; CT, collecting tubule; P, phosphorus. (From Schrier RW. *Diseases of the kidney and urinary tract.* 7th ed. Philadelphia, PA: Lippincott Williams & Wilkins; 2001.)

pituitary AVP secretion is basal and V_2R stimulation is minimal. As osmolality rises to approximately 1% above that of the threshold, AVP secretion rises along a steep, nearly linear curve, resulting in V_2R binding, increased water conservation, and a return of osmolality toward the set point (see Fig. 8.22).

In reality, other factors complicate the simple feedback system. A volume-depleted individual might best conserve water more aggressively, and, indeed, volume receptors sense atrial stretch and other hemodynamic parameters and appear to increase the slope of the osmolality—serum AVP curve in hypovolemia. The slope is decreased in hypervolemia (see Fig. 8.23).

Surges in AVP secretion and even prolonged hypersecretion can result from anesthesia, respiratory dysfunction, nausea, psychosis, and central nervous system inflammation.

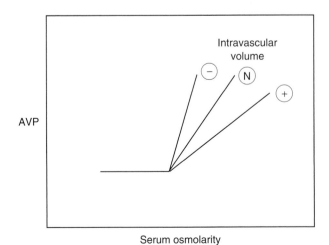

Figure 8.22 Plasma arginine vasopressin (AVP) as a function of osmolality and intravascular volume. N, normal volume status.

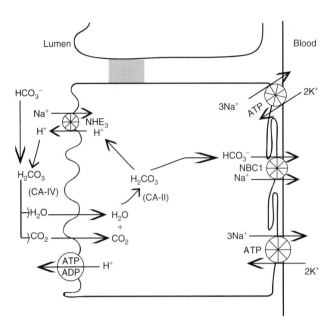

Figure 8.23 Sodium bicarbonate reabsorption, proximal tubule cell. ATP, adenosine triphosphate; ADP, adenosine 5'-diphosphate.

Congestive heart failure, cirrhosis, and nephrosis have long been associated with the concept of decreased "effective" arterial blood volume. Despite normal or even increased total blood volume, hemodynamic and oncotic forces in these conditions signal both the Na^+ and water regulatory systems to conserve and retain water, at least transiently improving the sensed hemodynamic parameters. Activation of the renin–angiotensin system and many other factors are involved, but the overall result is the expansion of the ECF in the form of edema and closed-space collections such as ascites. Mild hyponatremia often occurs consistent with the somewhat shifted osmo–AVP relationship.

Polyuric dehydration is associated with antipsychotic lithium treatment or intoxication and derives, at least in part, from inhibition of AQP-2 and AQP-3 formation. An accompanying Na^+ transport injury causes coincident Na^+ wasting.

RENAL ACID–BASE PROCESSES

The internal mammalian environment tolerates nanomolar concentrations of H^+ compared to millimolar quantities of many other ions. Virtually all cells contribute to compartmental pH control, but crucial roles are played by the lungs for CO_2 excretion, bones and other biochemical buffering systems for damping of potential pH excursions, the liver for metabolic conversions, and the kidneys for accepting a large potential loss of base as HCO_3^- and converting it into a small, regulated net acid excretion.

The clinical evaluation and management of acid–base disturbances is a large topic. The more limited goal of this chapter is to provide a discussion of the major intrarenal processes at work in the conservation of filtered HCO_3^- and the excretion of the usual net ingestion and metabolic production of a daily acid load.

Much of that task is accomplished through two basic mechanisms. First is the carbonic anhydrase–facilitated conversion of filtered HCO_3^- to CO_2 and H_2O for transcellular recovery, and the second is the release of net H^+ into the tubular fluid to become excretable acid. In the Bowman space, HCO_3^- concentration and pH are very similar to that of plasma. In the bladder, HCO_3^- concentration is usually negligible and H^+ concentration has increased by at least a couple of log units. The major intervening tubular steps are described in the subsequent text.

Proximal Tubule Acid–Base

As with other luminal anions, the active transport of Na^+ out of the cell by the basolateral Na^+/K^+-ATPase (Na^+:K^+ is 3:2) generates an initial driving force that facilitates HCO_3^- reabsorption from the tubular fluid (Fig. 8.23). A low-sodium, negatively charged cell interior favors apical luminal Na^+ for intracellular H^+ exchange through the NHE_3 Na/H$^+$ exchanger. This secreted H^+ can then bind to filtered HCO_3^- and enter the $H^+ + HCO_3^- \leftrightarrow H_2CO_3 \leftrightarrow H_2O + CO_2$ relationship. The biologic requirement to move to the right-sided $H_2O + CO_2$ products is greatly facilitated by the generous presence of carbonic anhydrase, isoform IV, on the early proximal epithelial brush border.

Carbonic anhydrase is a family of metalloenzyme catalysts distributed selectively in mammalian tissue. Type IV is bound to both luminal and basolateral early proximal tubular and TAL cell membranes.

After carbonic anhydrase–dependent conversion to CO_2 and water, these products can move relatively freely into the epithelial cell, where the reaction equilibrium shifts back, under the influence of type II carbonic anhydrase (CAII) to the dissociated $H^+ + HCO_3^-$ stage. This frees the H^+ to return to the apical Na^+/H^+ exchanger to cycle again through reabsorption of HCO_3^-. The HCO_3^- released intracellularly by CAII can move in the opposite direction toward the basolateral membrane for eventual transport to the peritubular capillary.

A second apical H^+ secretary mechanism operates independent of Na^+ transport. This vacuolar H^+-ATPase also occurs in the collecting tubule cells.

At the basolateral membrane, HCO_3^- must again cross the cell membrane for peritubular capillary recovery. The NBC1 Na^+ HCO_3^- cotransporter facilitates Na^+ and HCO_3^- egress at a ratio of either 1:3 or 1:2, tending to balance the charge effect of the basilar 3:2 Na^+/K^+ exchange.[37]

In addition to HCO_3^- recovery, proximal H^+ secretion can occur when the previously mentioned recycling H^+ encounters a filtered weak acid, most notably HPO_4^{2-}. A decreasing luminal pH will favor $H_2PO_4^-$ formation and

preservation in the flowing TF as opposed to potential reabsorption.

Ammonium Ion Excretion

Net H^+ excretion can also be achieved in the form of NH_4^+, leaving behind conserved HCO_3^-.[38] This system accelerates in response to acidosis. It depends largely on the proximal epithelial metabolism of the amino acid glutamine, although the capability is present in multiple nephron segments. The ability to ramp up glutamine metabolism during acidosis implies a surplus substrate supply or an increasable supply. Acidosis may increase plasma glutamine, increasing both filtered and peritubular glutamine available for cell entry. Once inside the cell, glutamine metabolism may be further stimulated.

Glutamine breakdown begins after mitochondrial entry (see Fig. 8.24). It sequentially yields glutaminate and α-ketoglutarate while releasing two NH_4^+ ions to the cytoplasm. α-ketoglutarate can be further metabolized to produce HCO_3^- for basolateral reabsorption.

Cytoplasmic NH_4^+ may become NH_3 for luminal or basilar diffusion with H^+ entering luminal Na^+/H^+ exchange, or NH_4^+ may enter the exchanger and be transported to the lumen. Other exchangers accepting Na^+ or K^+ may also transport small quantities of NH_4^+. Therefore, ammoniagenesis may feed both TF NH_3 and capillary plasma NH_3 content.

TF NH_3 content leaving the PT is variable but consistently rises as the TF descends to the bend of Henle loop. The rise in total content is due to TAL NH_4^+ reabsorption, medullary recycling, and a countercurrent concentrator

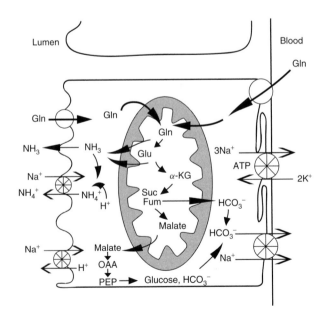

Figure 8.24 Proximal tubule ammoniagenesis. Gln, glutamine; Glu, glutamic acid; α-KG, α-ketoglutarate; OAA, oxaloacetate; ATP, adenosine triphosphate; PEP, phosphoenolpyruvate, Suc, succinate; Fum, fumarate.

mechanism that results in a high NH_3 content in the deep medullary interstitium. A gradient is formed that favors movement of NH_3 into the IMCD for excretion. As previously noted, multiple steps in nephron NH_4^+ excretion are stimulated by systemic metabolic acidosis.

In addition to ammoniagenesis, other PT acid–base processes respond to acute or chronic metabolic acidosis, in part by increasing the activity or exposure of apical and even basolateral exchangers and transporters.

Depletion of the intravascular or the previously mentioned effective circulating volume stimulates increased HCO_3^- reabsorption. Hypokalemia is a frequent contributor but activation of renin-angiotensin is a major contributor. Angiotensin II stimulates apical Na^+/H^+ exchange and basolateral Na^+/HCO_3^- cotransport. Aldosterone is also stimulated but acts in the more distal nephron.

Glucocorticoids appear to stimulate proximal tubular NHE_3 and $NBC1$ activity. Endothelins acting on the ET_B receptor likewise seems to increase apical Na^+/H^+ exchange. Both glucocorticoid and endothelin levels increase with metabolic acidosis.

Thin Limb and Thick Ascending Limb Acid–Base

The descending and ascending TL of Henle loop participate in the NH_3 recycling and its concentration described in the preceding text. The HCO_3^- concentration also rises in the TL but only because of water loss. The more concentrated $Na^+HCO_3^-$ solution is then presented to the TAL. The apical $Na^+/K^+/2Cl^-$ cotransporter, as well as carbonic anhydrase–dependent HCO_3^- reabsorption, is active here. Hydrogen for recycling is available through Na^+/H^+ apical exchange, and apical NH_4^+ reabsorption is facilitated by substitution of NH_4^+ in K^+ cotransport or luminal K^+ channels.

Intracellular HCO_3^-, reformed from luminal CO_2 and water, may exit the basolateral membrane through Na^+ or K^+ cotransport or Cl^- exchanger.[39] Therefore, this segment reabsorbs most of the 10% to 20% of filtered HCO_3^- that escapes the PT.[40]

Systemic metabolic acidosis stimulates transporter function and exposure as in the PT. Transport also increases as a function of HCO_3^- delivery into this tubular segment. Increasing Na^+ reabsorption in the TAL favors more HCO_3^- reabsorption, and adrenal steroids are permissive, at least, in supporting this function.

Distal Nephron Acid–Base

Beyond the TAL, a small amount of HCO_3^- may be reabsorbed or secreted, and additional net H^+ is secreted to be excreted as inorganic acids or NH_4^+.[41]

In the distal tubule, apical H^+ secretion occurs through the Na/H exchanger and an H^+-ATPase. Carbonic anhydrase is present, as is the potential for HCO_3^- to move out of or into the TF (see Fig. 8.25).

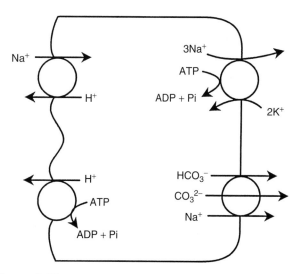

Figure 8.25 Distal tubular acid–base mechanisms. ATP, adenosine triphosphate; ADP, adenosine 5′-diphosphate. (From Schrier RW. *Diseases of the kidney and urinary tract.* 7th ed. Philadelphia, PA: Lippincott Williams & Wilkins; 2001.)

As previously noted, the cortical and medullary collecting tubules are segments made up of multiple cell types, which transition predominantly to principal cells in the deepest IMCD. In the cortical and medullary collecting tubules and ducts, the intercalated cells are the primary sites of acid–base regulation.[42] Particularly, type A intercalated cells have an apical H^+-ATPase secretory transporter providing a major portion of H^+ secretion. A luminal membrane H^+/K^+-ATPase also contributes to the secretion. On the basolateral membrane, cytosolic HCO_3^- can be conserved by being exchanged for extracellular Cl^- through the AE1 anionic exchanger. Chloride channels are also available. Type B intercalated cells can exchange cytosolic HCO_3^- at the apical membrane for luminal Cl^-, resulting in HCO_3^- secretion in conditions of metabolic alkalosis (see Fig. 8.26).

As in other tubule segments, the distal nephron responds to metabolic acidosis with increased HCO_3^- reabsorption and H^+ secretion. Increased Na^+ delivery to the distal nephron usually drives increased H^+, as well as increased K^+ secretion. This is also stimulated by increasing levels of circulating mineralocorticoids.

In summary, ingested nutrients and metabolism provide a net acid load while huge quantities of HCO_3^- are lost from plasma through glomerular filtration. The kidney acts to conserve HCO_3^- and excrete H^+ combined with ammonia and inorganic anions. Ammoniagenesis is particularly available for stimulation during metabolic acidosis, but HCO_3^- reabsorption and direct H^+ secretion also respond. Likewise, H^+ secretion can be curtailed and a small amount of HCO_3^- can even be secreted during metabolic alkalosis. Conditions of kidney failure, then, will usually impose an increased acid load on body buffers because H^+ secretion will be severely impaired although HCO_3^- loss will be

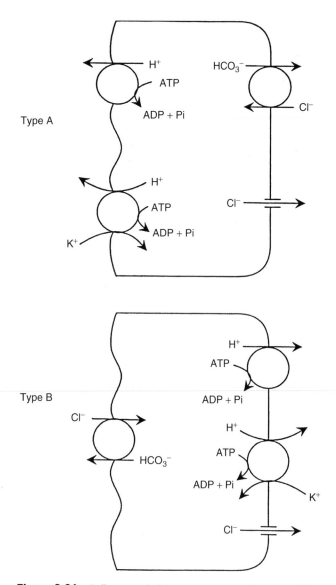

Figure 8.26 Collecting tubule intercalated cells. Type A, HCO_3^- reabsorption. Type B, capable of HCO_3^- secretion. ATP, adenosine triphosphate; ADP, adenosine 5'-diphosphate. (From Schrier RW. *Diseases of the kidney and urinary tract.* 7th ed. Philadelphia, PA: Lippincott Williams & Wilkins; 2001.)

minimal. That load is usually on the order of 1 to 2 mEq/kg/24 hours but will appear increased during times of multiorgan failure.

ACUTE RENAL FAILURE

Acute kidney failure occurs in a variety of etiologic categories and to varied extents.[43] Clinically, this refers to renal insufficiency that develops over a period of hours to weeks and that, in general, has potential for reversibility. Some obviously irreversible causes are mentioned in the subsequent text. As a general rule, severity of renal failure is proportional to the loss of GFR. When GFR falls below approximately 10% of normal, many homeostatic mechanisms fail. If renal failure occurs abruptly, physiologic disturbance is more pronounced and less compensated. The degree of renal failure is most often estimated from changes in the serum creatinine level. Although very useful, one must keep some caveats in mind . First, serum creatinine level in the presence of stable renal function varies with the supply of creatinine, which is proportional to muscle mass. Patients with severely diminished muscle mass will have lower serum creatinine levels than normal muscle mass patients with identical clearances do. Second, the normal range for creatinine is somewhat wide, in part related to the muscle mass. This means that creatinine clearance can be significantly diminished, whereas a single creatinine determination may remain in or very near the normal range. Therefore, serial determinations and knowledge of baseline creatinine are helpful in evaluating renal insufficiency. Lastly, as function deteriorates severely, the portion of creatinine excretion that occurs through tubular secretion becomes a larger contributor to creatinine clearance estimates, leading to underestimation of functional compromise.

In addition to serum creatinine, a common clinical index of renal function is urine output. As mentioned earlier in this chapter, normal solute clearance requires approximately 1 mL/kg/hour of concentrated urine output. Oliguria is defined by urine outputs less than this level, and severe oliguria might be considered if urine output is <0.5 mL/kg/hour. The term anuria implies zero urine output. This, in fact, is a very uncommon occurrence. Anuria implies that either there is no glomerular filtration occurring in continuity with the urinary drainage system or there is total obstruction of the urinary drainage system. Anuria should always prompt a focused search for a potentially reversible cause. The commonest forms of acute renal failure are unlikely causes of true anuria.

Vascular Causes of Acute Renal Failure

Preserving intact renal blood flow is basic to the preservation of renal function. Compromise of large vessel integrity relative to renal blood flow can occur in several ways. Traumatic injury can lacerate aortic or renal artery vascular walls or create endothelial flaps that can occlude flow. Significant recovery of function is most likely if flow can be restored within approximately 4 hours; however, if the kidney can be cooled or has partial preservation of flow, one might anticipate recovery after even longer interruptions.

The quality of renal blood flow is altered by aortic coarctation or renal artery stenosis. In the latter case, the most vulnerable individual has bilateral renal artery stenosis or has stenosis of an artery to a solitary kidney. These conditions produce activation of the renin–angiotensin–aldosterone system (RAAS), as well as increased sympathetic nervous tone. Compensatory vasodilators preserve renal blood flow, whereas efferent arteriolar vasoconstriction secondary to angiotensin II activity preserves glomerular filtration. Patients with these lesions are at particular risk for acute renal failure, usually reversible, if angiotensin I conversion is inhibited or angiotensin II receptors are blocked. The effect is to relax the efferent arteriole, drop glomerular perfusion pressure, and sustain inadequate glomerular filtration. As in many pathologies involving somewhat compromised renal blood flow, pharmacologic interference with preglomerular vasodilators may disrupt renal autoregulation processes and result in ischemic tubular injury.

Renal artery embolization is of particular concern in neonates. Many such emboli originate in association with umbilical artery catheters. However at least two other sources are possible. It should be remembered that very little flushing volume is needed for a peripheral arterial catheter to return a peripheral clot to the aorta for embolization to any organ. The other source is not iatrogenic but is the ductus arteriosus. Rarely, a ductal luminal clot can dislodge, perhaps with ductal opening stimuli, with resultant embolization to other arteries. These emboli may present in a very young infants as episodes of unexplained congestive heart failure. In the classic example, as the heart failure is treated, the blood pressure becomes elevated and the hypertensive etiology of the heart failure leads to the diagnosis of renal perfusion deficits.

As more attention has been paid to *in situ* thrombosis, the hypercoagulable states have been appreciated more. The occurrence of renal venous thrombosis is associated with some known, as well as some unknown, coagulopathies. More rarely, aortic, including renal artery, *in situ* thrombosis can lead to acute renal failure. Such patients do not frequently survive but require thrombotic investigation as rapidly as possible.

Small vessel disease within the kidney can also be a dramatic form of acute renal compromise. In the younger pediatric age-group, hemolytic uremic syndrome is well appreciated. This process, which occurs in virtually all age-groups, is usually associated with toxin-producing *Escherichia coli* or *Streptococcus pneumoniae*, although other contributors exist and are discussed in Chapter 57. Vascular occlusion, particularly of glomerular capillaries, occurs, with thrombi being made up largely of platelets and plasma proteins. A component of tubular ischemia likely contributes to renal compromise. The overall mechanism involves endothelial injury and disruption of the normal controls of clotting mechanisms. Although virtually any organ can be involved, the kidneys are particularly likely targets, apparently related to the distribution of critical receptors on vascular endothelial cells.

Intrinsic renal failure on a microvascular basis also occurs in the older pediatric population in the form of rapidly progressing glomerulonephritis. A variety of immunological etiologies are known, most resulting in glomerular disruption with the formation of epithelial crescents. These processes may be associated with remote organ dysfunction, such as pulmonary hemorrhage, or may be relatively limited to the kidney, as in aggressive, poststreptococcal glomerulonephritis. Patients may become dependent on dialysis in a matter of a few days in addition to frequently developing severe hypertension and other organ damage.

Acute Tubular Injury

Acute renal failure associated with a variety of systemic hemodynamic disruptions has been referred to as *ischemic acute tubular necrosis*. This term remains relevant but does not describe the spectrum of etiologies or pathologic presentations observed. ATI is more inclusive but potentially undervalues the contribution of vascular endothelial injury, which is described further in the subsequent text. Nevertheless, because the vascular lesion contributes to tubular dysfunction, the term ATI is used in this section.

Two general settings can be described for ATI. In the first, a discrete drop in perfusion pressure and blood flow to the kidney is associated with subsequent tubular dysfunction. In the second, the deficiency may be more subtle, may be more prolonged, may occur in the setting of multiorgan failure, and certainly appears to involve mechanisms other than simple failure of perfusion.[44] Examples might include bacterial sepsis, which is not always associated with severe compromise of blood flow, or primary myocardial failure, in which prolonged, moderate hypoperfusion associated with endocrine and neural reaction can eventually lead to frank renal decompensation.

It is useful to describe the course of the resulting clinical entity in terms of four phases—initiation, extension, maintenance, and recovery. The initiation phase includes the insulting process and its immediate consequences. In some patients, this phase may be difficult to recognize. During the extension phase, the process, as set in motion with initiation, amplifies and extends its impact, evolving into a more or less stable degree of renal insufficiency. In many patients, events that could initiate ATI occur; however, no current early index of substantial injury has been fully validated. Such an index or marker would be of particular assistance when therapeutic intervention becomes possible. It might also help in terms of timely arrangement of appropriate care resources for patients who would eventually require renal replacement therapy. It is apparent that serum creatinine is limited in its rate of rise following even total nephrectomy. It is not very definitive as an early indicator of the severity of a recent insult.

The maintenance phase of ATI refers to a period during which renal function is compromised and changes very little. Although some evidence of ongoing cellular insult can be found, this phase usually appears to be the period when systemic and local events take place, which rather silently develop the milieu in which recovery can occur. The recovery phase refers to the period during which functional improvement occurs. However, recovery at the cellular level clearly predicts clinical recovery.

Histologic evidence of ATI is not universally observed. In general, patchy areas of apoptosis or cell necrosis accompanied by exposure of the tubular basement membrane and the presence of intraluminal debris is demonstrable. Much of the histologic information about these processes comes from mammalian experiments rather than human tissue biopsy. At this point, therapy for such patients is not biopsy driven, rendering the procedure an unnecessary risk in most cases. Histologic data suggest that the last segment of the PT and the portion of the TAL of Henle loop that lies in the outer medulla are major sites of tubular cell injury. In addition to tubular cell injury, congestion and occasional inflammatory change in the peritubular capillaries and vasa rectae are noted.

Renal Tubular Cell Injury Events

Epithelial cells can sustain reversible amounts of injury, probably accounting for some of the clinical cases of ATI of very short duration (see Fig. 8.27). It seems particularly true in infants. More severe injury is likely to end in cell deaths of either of the two types. It is increasingly recognized that tubular cells may die the programmed death of apoptosis or may undergo classic cellular necrosis.

Mitochondrial work must cease eventually when deprived of oxygen. Cells with generous glycolytic cycle potential may be more resistant to depletion of ATP, but their reserve can be exhausted. As ATP Ps are liberated to adenosine monophosphate (AMP), some reversible potential persists (see Fig. 8.28). Once AMP is broken down to constituents, the molecule is unlikely to regenerate as an energy resource.

Accompanying mitochondrial swelling and disruption is an increase in free calcium level in the cytosol, as well as the generation and reactions of the usual variety of reactive oxygen species. Stimulation of catabolic enzymes including proteases and phospholipases occurs and irreparable nucleic acid damage develops.

The unique message or degree of injury that directs a cell to utilize its final energy in the process of apoptosis is unclear. The caspase enzymes are crucial to this process, in which nuclei condense, fragmented cells of the DNA shrink and blebs and brush-border disruption occur, and mitochondria disintegrate. This process generates little in the way of inflammatory stimulation, perhaps limiting the tissue damage in the presence of death of selected cells.

PT cells undergoing necrosis demonstrate mitochondrial swelling and displacement, disruption of the apical brush border, as well as loss of cell polarity. This results in migration and misplacement of transporters and pumps away from their scripted locations. In addition to the loss of the internal cytoskeleton, basilar integrins, and other adhesives are disrupted, cells are shed, and basement membrane is exposed (Fig. 8.28).

Shed cells stimulate inflammatory mediators and combine with luminal proteins to form tubular casts and tubular obstruction in many models.

Unfortunately, there is another degree of cortical injury possible. If ischemic necrosis is so severe as to disrupt basement membranes and vascular structures, recovery of function is not possible. However, this process can be patchy; therefore, biopsy histology is not necessarily prognostically reliable. In the instances in which severe

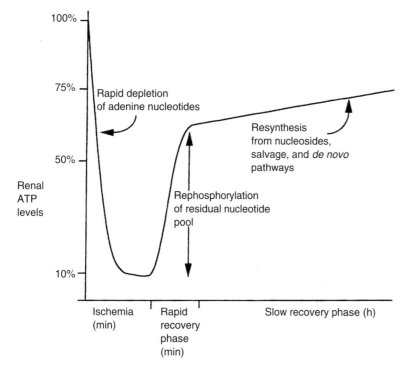

Figure 8.27 Adenosine triphosphate (ATP) depletion and recovery, ischemia, and reperfusion. (From Avner ED, Harmon WE, Niaudet P. *Pediatric nephrology*. 5th ed. Philadelphia, PA: Lippincott Williams & Wilkins; 2003.)

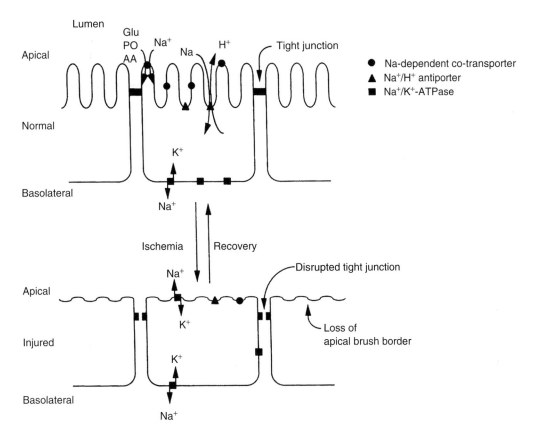

Figure 8.28 Ischemic proximal tubule (PT) cell injury, including loss of cell polarity, migration of active transporters, loss of brush border, and potential loss of basement membrane adhesion. ATP, adenosine triphosphate; AA, amino acid; Glu, glutamic acid. (From Avner ED, Harmon WE, Niaudet P. *Pediatric nephrology.* 5th ed. Philadelphia, PA: Lippincott Williams & Wilkins; 2003.)

ATI occurs with patchy cortical necrosis, recovery of some function is likely to be accompanied by severe hypertension, probably because of areas of compromised perfusion and excessive renin release. Widespread bilateral cortical necrosis is a cause of end-stage kidney disease.

In less severe ATI, the maintenance phase is usually associated with pronounced oliguria, although polyuria with poor function is certainly possible.

Injury Mechanisms

Several mechanisms appear to contribute to the common oliguric maintenance phase.

As indicated in the preceding text, sloughing of cellular debris can result in tubular obstruction, an increase in tubular pressure conducted retrograde to the Bowman space, and compromise of the filtration pressure gradient. Some of the increased resistance to downstream flow is dissipated by back leak of tubular fluid across denuded basement membranes into the peritubular capillaries. Therefore, obstruction and back leak of filtrate limit urine output.

Compromised renal plasma flow is another potential contributor to GFR limitation. Autoregulation of renal blood flow may be lost either by extreme perfusion pressure or by humoral or pharmacologic disruption. In the face of

decreased preglomerular perfusion pressure, efferent arteriolar constriction may be unable to compensate, resulting in negligible net filtration pressure. Theoretically, tubuloglomerular feedback may aggravate glomerular perfusion pressure. If tubular injury prevents proximal tubular reabsorption of sodium chloride, its increased delivery to the ascending limb and the MD might be expected to signal increased preglomerular constriction and limitation of filtration. Whether the right mix of intact and disrupted mechanisms in human ATI actually results in TGF-mediated aggravation of filtration is not totally clear.

Another theoretic concern involving TGF relates to postglomerular perfusion and the constriction of the efferent arteriole that becomes pronounced at the lower autoregulatory perfusion pressure range. For juxtamedullary nephrons, the increased efferent vascular resistance may further compromise blood flow to the outer medullary tissue, a region of ischemic vulnerability.

The outer medulla is a metabolically active, oxygen-dependent region that under normal circumstances has a very small margin between oxygen supply and demand. As noted earlier, tubular segments here include the late, descending straight portion of the PT and the TAL of Henle loop. These segments show early histologic signs of injury when renal perfusion is compromised. In addition, the endothelial cells of the vasa rectae in this region are susceptible to inflammatory injury, vascular congestion, and resultant further compromise of perfusion. Tenuous oxygenation in this region no doubt contributes to medullary and papillary necrosis secondary to sickling in the diseased condition.

Endothelial cell injury, particularly in the vasa rectae, may be the key to some models of ATI. Exposure of kidneys to injury mechanisms associated with endothelial damage is more likely to result in prolonged functional compromise than is a similar exposure to ischemia alone.

An additional issue difficult to explore in human disease is the change in the ultrafiltration coefficient, K_f, that occurs in some ATI models, particularly associated with severely increased activity of the RAAS or with calcineurin-inhibitor toxicity. Contractile elements in the mesangium cause changes in the perfused glomerular surface area, but qualitative changes in the endothelial surface may also contribute to the alterations.

Renal dysfunction associated with early septic shock illustrates one of the poorly understood circumstances in which a change in K_f or other nephron characteristics seem to be needed to explain the degree of GFR compromise. In the early septic state, hyperdynamic cardiac function and systemic vasodilatation tend to preserve renal blood flow. Autoregulation of GFR, however, is shown to be disrupted in some models, with resultant renal dysfunction being disproportionate to changes in renal blood flow. Local and systemic effects of inflammatory mediators may contribute to dysfunction, as discussed in the subsequent text.

Inflammation and Acute Tubular Injury

As previously indicated, tubular cell injury can activate inflammatory systems. Proinflammatory cytokines, interleukin (IL-1), tumor necrosis factor (TNF), and others, contribute to cellular detachment, leukocyte activation, and secondary inflammatory mediator release. Leukocyte activation contributes to degradative enzymes and reactive oxygen species activity. It is interesting that ATI protection is conferred in animals with genetic manipulation to provide overexpression of antioxidant activity. Tubular cell injury may be amplified by inflammation but vascular endothelial cells may also be an important target. Compromise of prostacyclin or nitric oxide availability may further limit perfusion, as may increased activity of endothelin or other vasoconstrictors. Endothelial cell adhesion molecules such as intercellular adhesion molecule-1 (ICAM-1) or vascular cell adhesion molecule (VCAM) may be upregulated, contributing to vascular congestion and decreased perfusion.

Acute Tubular Injury and Interorgan Cross Talk

In addition to remote influences of the endocrine and neural systems on ATI, there exists evidence of potential inflammatory modulation of evolving renal injury.[45] It has been pointed out that IL-6 production is stimulated from renal injury. In the serum, IL-6 is bound to soluble IL-6 receptors, which can react with cell surfaces on which a specific gp130 receptor is found. Apparent target cells would include hepatic macrophages, which can subsequently release IL-10, an anti-inflammatory cytokine perhaps capable of modulating further renal injury. IL-10 receptors do appear to be present in the target renal tissue.

Another proposed mechanism includes injury-induced enzyme release, resulting in the activation of hepatic growth factor (HGF) precursor to HGF. A specific receptor (c-MET) is expressed on injured kidney cells and binds HGF. Theoretically, it may confer some benefit to these cells.

Acute Tubular Injury Protection

Many interventions can be shown to protect against ATI, provided they are delivered before the insult. Delivery after the insult has usually proved to be clinically futile. Avoidance of poor perfusion and oliguria prior to an insult is helpful. However, many attempts to use diuretics, energy sources, or vasodilators have been disappointing.

One interesting protective maneuver that appears helpful in dissecting injury mechanisms is that of ischemic preconditioning. This maneuver involves exposure to a limited bout of ischemia with recovery and a subsequent decreased susceptibility to a standard ischemic challenge. A variety of factors are altered by this preconditioning, including increases in inducible nitric oxide synthase, heat shock proteins, and some potentially injurious kinases. Increased levels of some factors appear to be protective, but in the kinase situation, a second ischemic insult causes significantly less activation and potentially less injury.

Melanocyte-stimulating hormone (MSH), an IL-10 inducer, also protects against ischemic ATI. IL-10, mentioned in the preceding text in terms of interorgan cross talk, is an anti-inflammatory cytokine. MSH mitigates renal injury even when given after the insult. In addition to anti-inflammatory responses, MSH inhibits inducible nitric oxide (iNOS) expression. Although nitric oxide vasodilatation may have a protective effect before or at the time of insult, its ongoing stimulation in ATI is a source of further damage, probably related in part to the generation of reactive oxygen species.

Acute Tubular Injury Recovery

Not surprisingly, histologic evidence of recovering epithelial activity may precede the recovery of urine output and adequate clearance. Although many epithelial cells may be shed from the tubular basement membranes, many remain attached and viable. Subpopulations of the epithelial cells may then be responsible for regenerative behavior. Observations include spreading of the epithelial cells over uncovered basement membrane, resulting in a thin cell layer with some characteristics of dedifferentiated mesenchymal stem cells. Differentiation of these cells into renal tubular cells occurs under the complex influence of intracellular systems and is apparently aided by a variety of growth factors including epidermal growth factor, hepatocyte growth factor, endothelial growth factor, and insulinlike growth factor.

In the mostly futile search for vasoactive potential protectors, the family of natriuretic peptides has been examined. Only one, the vasodilator peptide, has so far shown potential of particular interest.

Facilitating recovery of injured renal tubules and vessels certainly has therapeutic potential. However, being able to intervene before some anticipatable insults or to mitigate consequences during the initiation–extension early phase would seem even more desirable. The concept of ATI has grown much more complex than the concept of simple ischemia leading to oxygen deprivation, cell necrosis, and tubular obstruction. It seems very appropriate to expect that the evolving understanding of multiple mechanisms will eventually lead to effective therapeutic interventions.

Vasoconstrictive Mechanisms of Renal Failure

A variety of clinical scenarios result in renal vasoconstriction and impaired renal function. Outer medullary blood flow, particularly in times of renal hemodynamic stress, is critically dependent on PG-mediated vasodilation. Administration of nonsteroidal anti-inflammatory drugs interferes with the COX synthase, resulting in inhibition of PG synthesis and vasoconstriction severe enough to cause renal failure.

In patients with sepsis and hypotension, a variety of therapeutic vasoconstrictors are used particularly as a means of counteracting decreased systemic vascular resistance. The net effect of a drug such as norepinephrine in this setting is difficult to predict. However, it is clear that renal injury can occur with excessive doses. Vasopressin may offer a less renally toxic alternative in some situations, but information is still being accumulated. Of note is the difficulty encountered in showing beneficial affects of theoretic renal-protective drugs such as dopamine and fenoldopam. Further study is clearly called for.

Particularly in the setting of hypotension, poor perfusion, and metabolic acidosis, the presence of free hemoglobin or myoglobin in the serum results in globin filtration and renal tubular damage related in part to the scavenging of nitric oxide by these proteins. This may result in vasomotor imbalance and vasoconstrictive ischemia.

Radiocontrast dyes continue to present a frustrating clinical challenge. Despite being able to anticipate the insult and recognize the high-risk patients, renal vasoconstriction and tubular injury are difficult to avoid.

Solid organ and bone marrow transplantation patients are frequently treated with calcineurin inhibitors. High levels of these drugs are associated with acute vasoconstriction, including a decreased glomerular ultrafiltration coefficient, and tubular dysfunction.

In the population of renal transplantation patients, renal vascular insufficiency is associated with the inflammatory congestion and disruption of aggressive vascular rejection.

Severe hypercalcemia increases systemic vascular resistance including renal vascular compromise.

Hepatorenal syndrome combines significant renal vasoconstriction in response to angiotensin and renal nerve activity at the same time such that splanchnic vascular resistance is unusually low.[46] This leads to shunting of volume and flow away from the kidney. Tubular function is usually preserved in terms of potential because transplantation of an affected kidney results in immediate function in a more normal donor. Truly excellent therapy awaits specific vasodilators for the renal circulation and vasoconstrictors for the splanchnic circulation. Currently, increasing overall intravascular volume while slightly constricting the splanchnic and peripheral circulation tends to improve renal function for a certain time.

Acute Tubular Injury from Direct Tubular Toxicity

A variety of pharmaceuticals and toxins reach renal tubular cells and create injury directly without depending upon vascular reactivity. Most need to reach an intracellular site, as illustrated by antibiotics including aminoglycosides and amphotericin B, which are reabsorbed, as well as by secreted antibiotics such as vancomycin. While the toxicity of these drugs is less than what was initially believed, it remains a well-established threat that is particularly pertinent when two or more nephrotoxic drugs are used together.

The family of nephrotoxins includes antivirals, antibacterials, and chemotherapeutic agents. Intracellular disruption occurs at Na^+/K^+-ATPase pumps, mitochondria, and protein synthesis processes, and through lipid peroxidation. There has been an increased appreciation for renal injury associated with immunoglobin infusions. As one might expect, this varies with products and product batches, depending to a certain extent on the distribution of components.

Volatile solvents continue to be ingested with systemic and renal consequences. Ethylene glycol and methanol are of particular note.

Much more extensive lists of potential nephrotoxins are available through regional poison control centers and other resources.

Interstitial Nephritis

Cell-mediated immune systems and inflammatory processes are key to the development of most forms of interstitial nephritis. This lesion can produce renal failure within days. Many pharmaceuticals have this potential, particularly antibiotics and antiepileptiform drugs. Both bacterial and, more commonly, viral infections may provoke a significant interstitial nephritis and functional compromise. Likewise acute, cell-mediated renal transplant rejection predominantly presents histologically as an interstitial inflammatory lesion.

Noncellular Tubular Obstruction

Luminal obstruction is significant in many models of ischemic ATI. It is also a primary mechanism in other forms of acute renal failure. Uric acid accumulation in TF during tumor lysis is at risk of precipitating at low pH. Similarly, high doses of methotrexate can lead to diffuse intratubular deposition, obstruction, and renal failure. Acyclovir and indinavir present a similar risk, particularly in underhydrated patients. Calcium oxylate in genetic oxalosis and tubular protein in paraproteinemias represent more unusual causes of obstruction. In patients with severe tumor lysis syndrome, calcium phosphate deposition has been implicated but not proved to have a potential similar to uric acid. Hypoxanthine, a precursor of urate, can clearly accumulate in a manner similar to that of uric acid in patients aggressively treated with allopurinol.

A variety of inherited metabolic disorders are associated with periodic, severe episodes of decompensation. During these episodes, renal function may deteriorate and become insufficient for metabolic needs. McArdle syndrome is associated with episodic rhabdomyolysis. In others, such as maple syrup urine disease or methylmalonic acidemia, metabolic acidosis and accumulation of extremely high levels of intermediary metabolites may contribute to renal dysfunction.

Postrenal Obstruction

One might think that obstruction of the macrourinary drainage system occurs gradually over time as stones accumulate. However, acute renal failure is possible with obstructions that can move acutely from a tolerable position to an obstructive position or when a mass undergoes a sudden change for other reasons.

A basic rule for interpreting possible postrenal obstruction requires that, in the presence of only a unilateral kidney, renal failure results from obstruction occurring at the level of the urethra, bladder, or ureter. In the presence of two good kidneys, bilateral ureteral obstruction is necessary to cause clinically obvious renal insufficiency.

Normal and immunocompromised infants are at risk for candidal or other fungal masses obstructing the renal pelvis and ureters. Urinary stones can obstruct bilaterally or can obstruct in the bladder or urethra. Hemorrhage in the urinary tract related to trauma, biopsy, or papillary necrosis may result in obstructive clots. Sickle cell disease, SS or SA, may be associated with severe hemorrhage, although clotting is uncommon.

Tumors such as teratomas or rhabdomyosarcomas may gradually impinge until obstruction occurs rather acutely. Urinary anomalies such as ureteroceles can be associated with sudden obstruction, although the structural abnormality has obviously been developing over time.

Trauma or transverse myelitis can result in a neurogenic bladder. Although not likely to be a cause of total renal failure, this form of obstruction does have significant implications on renal function.

A patient with a significant urinary tract anomaly may develop a urinary tract infection with resultant mucosal swelling that obstructs the urinary system. Rarely, a suture may be placed around a ureter during an unrelated surgical procedure. In the presence of two kidneys, this should not result in total renal failure. However, in the case of the renal transplant recipient, ureteral obstruction immediately affects total renal function. This obstruction can occur through postoperative hemorrhage and thrombosis in the ureter. A ureteral leak due to a small area of ureteral necrosis is more common. In this case, urine may form a perinephric collection or may empty directly into the peritoneal cavity.

Summary

Acute renal failure can result from a variety of mechanical processes, mostly prerenal vascular and postrenal urinary drainage issues. Direct tubular toxicity is another relatively common mechanism.

Although ischemic injury and cell necrosis have classically been denoted by the acute tubular necrosis label, it is suggested that the kidney has a variety of scalable responses to insults. In addition, there may be multiple damaging mechanisms potentially contributing. Of particular interest is the role of inflammatory processes and their possible therapeutic manipulation.

ARTIFICIAL MEMBRANES AND DIALYSIS

Dialysis procedures for acute renal failure provide a means of normalizing extracellular fluid constituents of small molecular weight at times when renal function is inadequate. In addition, dialysis treatments can remove small molecules that are potentially toxic in the amounts that accumulate during renal failure. Finally, dialysis procedures allow removal of fluid accumulating in the absence of adequate urine output.

Although medical correction of many isolated electrolyte abnormalities may be possible, dialysis procedures have the advantage of correcting multiple abnormalities simultaneously. These may include issues such as metabolic acidosis in the presence of hypocalcemia in which the correction of the acidosis alone may exacerbate the hypocalcemia.

The ability to remove fluid from the ECF using dialysis techniques allows for administration of additional fluid-containing medication and nutrition. ECF volume adjustments through dialysis may be essential for managing pulmonary edema, congestive heart failure, or volume-dependent hypertension. Hemodialysis techniques, particularly continuous forms of hemodialysis, are becoming more common in the ICU setting. Issues involved in these procedures are the primary subject of the discussions in the subsequent text.

Intermittent Hemodialysis and Continuous Renal Replacement Therapy

In general, hemodialysis techniques may be divided into intermittent hemodialysis treatments, usually provided for $2\frac{1}{2}$ to 4 hours, and continuous renal replacement therapy (CRRT). Assertions of the superiority of one technique over the other do not appear particularly productive, especially in pediatrics, because adequate, scientifically solid comparison data do not exist. Even more important is the patient's differing qualities that should affect the choice of therapy. Each technique has distinct advantages. As usual, the most appropriate therapy should be chosen to match the needs of the individual patient.

In patients who are hemodynamically stable, the relative short exposure to treatment of intermittent hemodialysis allows a longer period when the patient is free from a technologic tether, providing more opportunity for other diagnostic or therapeutic events. This statement presumes that the dialysis treatments are expertly prescribed and administered because it is possible to destabilize particularly small pediatric patients.

For patients who are hemodynamically unstable or tenuous in terms of oxygenation, CRRT may be much more appropriate. Spreading out the needed adjustments in fluid balance and solute concentrations over the course of 24 hours, as opposed to 3 hours for intermittent hemodialysis, may allow for much more stability in a patient. There is a price to be paid in terms of complex technology, meticulous monitoring, and nursing workload. However, in the unstable patient, that price may be well worth paying.

It is appropriate at this point to recognize peritoneal dialysis as a valid alternative therapy for some patients. Difficulties with vascular access, startup urgency, technical limitations, and other issues may make peritoneal dialysis the best choice on occasion. Once again, expertise and experience will often be the critical issues for success of this therapy.

RISKS OF HEMODIALYSIS/CONTINUOUS RENAL REPLACEMENT THERAPY PROCEDURES

Several of the risks of hemodialysis/CRRT procedures are shared and to some extent concentrated toward the beginning of the procedure (see Table 8.2).

Extracorporeal circulation requires that a certain percentage of the child's blood volume be in the tubing and dialyzer cartridge. Although pediatric-specific tubing sets and cartridges are available, more than 10% of the

---

TABLE 8.2
RISK OF EXTRACORPOREAL RENAL REPLACEMENT THERAPY

Vascular access
 Clotting and embolization
 Site loss
 Infection
 Complication of placement

Hypotension
 Extracorporeal volume loss
 Bradykinin syndrome
 Acetate vasodilation
 Air embolism

Inflammatory mediator activation
 Bradykinin syndrome
 Pulmonary V/Q mismatch
 Possible ARF prolongation

Blood product exposure
 Immune reaction
 Communicable disease

Thermal
 Hypothermic (CRRT > HD)
 Hyperthermic (HD > CRRT)

Anticoagulation
 Hemorrhage
 Citrate—electrolyte, acid–base imbalance

Procedural errors
 Manufacturing
 Compounding
 Prescription
 Monitoring

V/Q, ventilation/perfusion; ARF, acute renal failure; CRRT, continuous renal replacement therapy; HD, hemodialysis.

---

child's blood volume can easily be taken for extracorporeal circulation. When 10% or more of the child's blood volume is in the circuit, it is difficult to remove ECF fluid using ultrafiltration because of the tendency to precipitate hypotension. Use of intravascular colloid or inotrope/pressor infusions may be successful but scrupulous attention to extracorporeal volume is preferred. At times, all of these measures will be required.

Another useful technique for the potentially unstable patient is to prime the extracorporeal circuit with blood or colloid. This has the obvious disadvantage of exposing the patient to transfusion risk. These risks must be weighed against the need for dialysis and the risks of using other techniques.

The need for volume compensation early during the initiation of a hemodialysis procedure will sometimes support the use of CRRT, because the risk will not be repeatedly faced with each intermittent treatment.

Despite the miracles that artificial membranes have provided in terms of multiple life-saving procedures, these membranes remain foreign and capable of varying the degrees of interaction with the patient's blood components. The results may be mild, local effects but may also produce systemic, life-threatening anaphylactoid reactions. These are discussed further in the subsequent text (Table 8.2).

As for other forms of central venous access, vascular catheter complications appear underappreciated. The blood flow requirements of hemodialysis/CRRT attract generous-sized venous catheters. Careful ultrasound studies suggest local thrombosis as an essentially universal complication, with its clinical significance being variable. Site sclerosis, remote embolization, and life-threatening infection are additional complications.

Finally, the risk of these procedures include the risk of procedural errors. These can be manufacturing errors, errors in compounding dialysate or other solutions, errors in technical decisions or execution, and errors of inadequate monitoring. Expertise, vigilance, double checking, and a high index of suspicion are our patients' best defense.

Common Elements of Extracorporeal Circuits

In addition to a membrane-containing cartridge or other critical separation elements, extracorporeal circuits consist of complex tubing sets in arrangements that have common elements. Although single-lumen, push–pull dialysis techniques are known, most procedures are done with a dual-lumen cannulae or multiple cannulae. Therefore, an aspiration lumen leads to the initial connection to the tubing set. Further down from this connection is a T-connection entry port, where fluid or medication can be administered before the tubing reaches at a roller pump, which provides the negative pressure for aspirating blood from the patient. In most systems, an anticoagulant may be administered before the blood pump.

Post blood pump, there is positive pressure in the tubing system that usually goes directly to the critical dialysis cartridge, oxygenator cartridge, or separation bowl in the case of pheresis. Because the extracorporeal circuit causes thermal loss, a warming mechanism is usually incorporated in the dialysis cartridge in the form of warm dialysate or further down from the oxygenator as a separate warmer in an ECMO circuit. Temperature control of pheresis bowls provides a similar function.

At variable locations downstream from the pump, there are monitoring sites for pressure, hematocrit, oxygen saturation, or other variables. Dialysis systems typically have an air bubble trap and safety occlusion clamp, which is activated if a malfunction is sensed in the system. Tubing access for medication administration downstream of the pump is also typical. In the case of CRRT, anticoagulation may be provided before the pump and reversal may be provided just before returning the blood to the patient, thereby limiting anticoagulant activity in the patient. Tubing outflow

into the return lumen of the access catheter is a critical function because increased resistance to flow at this site is common and very deleterious to circuit function.

Dialysis/CRRT and ECMO circuits have parallel, usually countercurrent channels, for dialysate or gas exposure to the external surface of the critical membrane. The permeability characteristics of the membranes become critical as movement of solute, fluid, or gas depends upon the gradients at the boundary layers of membrane contact.

Manipulated Variables

Dialysis/CRRT is adjusted to the needs of the individual patients. Adjustments are possible in a limited number of variables that determine the characteristics, particularly of the transmembrane processes (see Table 8.3).

Blood flow rate is a basic variable, influencing both pressures within the system and the rate of change of fluid exposure to diffusion-critical boundary layers next to the membrane surface. Curves characteristic of individual dialysis cartridges or materials can be drawn, indicating the relationship between blood flow rates and potential diffusion of individual solutes. Because diffusion over time determines the efficiency of clearance and also the risk of osmolar shifts, choosing an appropriate blood flow is critical.

Clearance is also affected by the surface area of the exposed membrane, the number of pores per unit surface area, and the average size of the pores, usually measured in angstroms.

A critical and adjustable force is the pressure gradient from one side of the membrane to the other. This transmembrane pressure is determined by the hydraulic force applied against the membrane, the permeability characteristics of which allow a predictable amount of fluid per unit of time to move from the blood compartment to the

---

TABLE 8.3
DIALYSIS VARIABLES

Diffusion—efficiency
    Membrane pore size and density
    Membrane thickness
    Membrane surface area
    Blood flow rate
    Specific solute

Ultrafiltration—flux
    Membrane water permeability
    Membrane surface area
    Transmembrane hydrostatic pressure

Blood chamber volume
    Membrane compliance
    Device architecture
    Transmembrane hydrostatic pressure

dialysate and removal compartment. In addition to determining ultrafiltration, changes in transmembrane pressure can alter the size of the blood compartment, thereby altering the amount of extracorporeal blood volume. The blood compartment demonstrates compliance and expands if its pressure increases. The compliance of modern dialyzers is not large compared to the plate dialyzers of the past; however, when dealing with small patients, small changes in extracorporeal blood volume can become significant.

Obviously, the composition of the dialysate is important in determining diffusion gradients and the transmembrane movement of molecules in both directions. Manipulation of concentrations of sodium and potassium are common. Magnesium is less often varied but is included in the dialysate. Most treatments are now provided with HCO_3^- as the base. Because many of these patients have metabolic acidosis secondary to failure of H^+ excretion, the HCO_3^- concentration in the dialysate will be higher than the normal plasma level to guarantee the transfer of the buffering base into the patient. In addition, glucose and calcium are usually provided at concentrations in excess of that of the typical serum, again to ensure adequate levels in the patient at the end of dialysis.

Dialysate temperature control is critical in hemodialysis procedures. Fatal hemolytic reactions have occurred from exposure to hyperthermic dialysate. At the other extreme, achieving adequate warming of the returning blood in CRRT has been somewhat problematic, but the technology continues to improve. Finally, anticoagulation is critical in patients without severe coagulopathy. Heparin and citrate represent the most common choices, although there are other options. Regardless of the choice, careful monitoring of coagulant parameters and therapeutic adjustment is critical.

Solute clearance is affected by membrane characteristics, as indicated in the preceding text, but it is also augmented by convection in some conditions. Adding dilutional fluid before the dialysis cartridge not only decreases clotting within the cartridge but also allows greater ultrafiltration. This may result in more transmembrane movement of larger molecules, although the decreased concentration gradients will decrease the diffusion of smaller molecules.

Ultrafiltration depends upon transmembrane pressure, which is manipulated on the dialysate side of the membrane, thereby maintaining relative independence from blood flow or pressure in the blood compartment. As previously mentioned, very high resistance to blood flow returning to the patient can increase pressures in the blood compartment beyond the ability of the circuit to compensate.

An additional process, that of adsorption, also removes material from circulation. Complement, erythropoietin, and some anticoagulant and coagulation factors can be adsorbed in quantitatively significant amounts, which vary depending on membrane characteristics. It is probably less critical for acute renal failure management than for chronic

dialysis, where the adsorption of β_2-microglobulin may diminish the toxicity of these materials that accumulate in chronic renal failure.

Artificial Membrane Characteristics

The chemical composition and structure of artificial membranes determine their physical behavior, as well as their biocompatibility. Biocompatibility can be loosely defined as the quality of being exposed to blood without inducing deleterious activation or degradation of blood components.

Commercial artificial membranes usually fall into one of three broadly defined categories.[47] The first category, regenerated cellulose, was used in early dialyzer membranes and continues, with refinements, to play a role. This material has a surface exposure of hydroxyl groups that react with blood components. In the second category, substituted or partially synthetic cellulose, the exposed groups are modified by chemical substitutions during manufacture, resulting in less reactivity and, therefore, increased biocompatibility.

Finally, increasing use is being made of totally synthetic membranes whose characteristics are quite variable. These materials can be designed for specific biocompatibilities, such as decreased thrombogenicity, although other unexpected incompatibilities, such as bradykinin activation, can result.

Artificial Membrane Primary Characteristics

The movement of water through an artificial membrane is characterized by an ultrafiltration coefficient (K_f) and is usually denoted by the term *flux*. Therefore, a high-flux membrane allows increased ultrafiltration at a given transmembrane pressure and surface area. This characteristic is dependent upon pore density and is proportional to the fourth power of the mean pore radius in the material.

The diffusion of molecules across artificial membranes results in mass transfer and is referred to as *dialyzer efficiency*. This diffusion is also dependent upon the number of pores available; the size of the pores relative to the solute of interest; and, particularly, the thickness of the membrane and, therefore, the length of the pore channel. Dialysis membranes have become thinner with manufacturing refinements, allowing the production of high-efficiency dialyzers. The characteristics of ultrafiltration and diffusion, flux and efficiency, can be disassociated. Therefore, individual dialyzers can be characterized as low- or high-flux and as standard or high-efficiency.

Matching patient needs with a dialysis plan then involves consideration of materials, extracorporeal volume, anticoagulation, blood flow rate, transmembrane pressure settings, choice of continuous versus intermittent therapy, and a variety of other subtleties[48] (Table 8.3).

Artificial Membranes Secondary Characteristics

The biocompatibilities of artificial membranes can be examined on the basis of several individual characteristics.[49]

Early in hemodialysis, it was noted that a transient but striking leukopenia occurred in the first hour of the procedure. Total leukocyte counts tended to return toward normal by the end of the 6-hour dialysis procedure that was standard at that time. Subsequently, this leukopenia was shown to be associated with the activation of complement through the alternate complement pathway. Generation of C5a was associated with leukocyte sequestration in pulmonary capillaries and was felt to be a cause of the decrease in arterial oxygenation frequently seen early in dialysis. A decrease in respiratory drive, with mild hypoventilation related to acid–base changes, seen early in dialysis also contributes to relative hypoxemia in some patents.

Although complement activation is virtually universal, it varies in degree and clinical significance. Other early reactions with anaphylactoid, life-threatening consequences do occur on an infrequent basis.

Such a response has been particularly associated with polyacrylonitrile (PAN) membranes and the generation of bradykinin, leading to vasodilatory hypotension through increased nitric oxide synthesis.[50] In fact, various degrees of this response occur with many membranes, and its clinical severity is probably very much patient-dependent. An additional variable affecting the event's severity is the coincident use of ACE inhibitors in the exposed patient. Bradykinin is normally metabolized through ACE. Inhibition of ACE results in increased and prolonged bradykinin exposure. Although it would be uncommon for patients with acute renal failure to be simultaneously on ACE inhibitors, should that situation arise, consideration should be given to alternative drug groups or angiotensin receptor blockers.

Membrane characteristics and other dialyzer materials determine the sterilization procedure that may be applied to an individual product. Retention of sterilizing solutions or manufacturing process chemicals can result in their infusion into the patient, resulting in life-threatening consequences. The classic example is that of ethylene oxide, a common sterilant that must be flushed from the system to prevent severe reactions.

In addition to plasma proteins, circulating macrophages are exposed to foreign material on initiation of extracorporeal circulation. Release of primary cytokines such as TNF-α and IL-1, as well as the generation of more downstream proinflammatory products, have been demonstrated. These may contribute to immediate symptomatology and may have currently unknown effects on longer-term immune functions. Of particular concern, however, is the possibility that cytokine activation may increase renal inflammation, one of the contributors to ongoing renal failure. There is some evidence that such cytokine activation may be associated with prolonged courses of acute renal failure, a phenomenon worthy of further study.

As alluded to previously, the artificial membrane surfaces are thrombogenic. Anticoagulation is required in most instances. However, an additional concern results from this quality. Increased deposition of coagulants on the membrane traps additional red blood cells, resulting in an increased amount of blood loss from the membrane for each procedure. This is of particular concern for the youngest patients and may contribute to transfusion risks.

Whereas the classic cellulose dialysis membranes have increasingly restricted diffusion of molecules from 300 to 1,500 Da and very little passage of molecules above 2,000 Da, newer high-efficiency membranes may pass molecules whose molecular size exceeds 2,000 Da. When membranes are permeable to relatively large molecules, endotoxin from dialysate water may also cross the membrane in the opposite direction, from the dialysate into the patient. The hydraulic pressure maintained in the blood compartment is in excess of that in the dialysate compartment. Nevertheless, some reverse diffusion may be possible. The obvious potential for patient reaction has prompted increased attention to dialysate water quality.

Additional Techniques

Plasmapheresis for known or suspected deleterious antibodies has a small but slowly growing number of clinical indications. This procedure is performed in intensive care settings on occasion. Three basic issues are of note. The equipment commonly available may or may not be adaptable to small volumes of pediatric patients. As previously raised, the issue of extracorporeal blood volume and hemodynamic stability is crucial. In addition, because citrate is a commonly used anticoagulant for these procedures and is present in relatively high concentrations in fresh frozen plasma, the induction of hypocalcemia is occasionally significant. This phenomenon may influence the choice of fresh frozen plasma versus albumin as partial or complete volume replacement for removed serum. This choice must also consider the effect of adding the antibody spectrum of the fresh frozen plasma product to the pathologic process of the patient.

Additional extracorporeal procedures continue to be developed on a larger experimental basis. It is possible to use immune characteristics to adsorb specific circulating blood constituents can possibly cause damage. It is also possible to prepare cell cultures that can be selectively exposed to the circulation to provide desired metabolic replacement therapy.

Nonspecific hemadsorption cartridges containing activated charcoal or synthetic resins have been used for some time for removal of drugs or toxins that are not susceptible to dialysis removal. Current clinical wisdom dictates very limited use of this approach.

ACKNOWLEDGMENTS

The author is deeply grateful for assistance, tolerance, and inspiration from GCM, EGW, FGK, SMM, EBO, and JMN. The original illustrations are by John P. Lynch.

REFERENCES

1. Avner ED, Harmon WE, Niaudet P. Pediatric nephrology. In: Avner ED, Harmon WE, Niaudet P, eds. Philadelphia, PA: Lippincott Williams & Wilkins; 2004.
2. Brenner BM. *Brenner & Rector's the kidney.* 7th ed. In: Brenner BM, ed. Philadelphia, PA: WB Saunders; 2004.
3. Rose BD, Post TW. *Clinical physiology of acid-base and electrolyte disorders.* 5th ed. In: Wonsciewicz M, McCullough K, Davis K, eds. McGraw-Hill; 2001.
4. Guignard JP. *Renal and genitourinary systems. Chapter in Avery's disease of the newborn.* 8th ed. R Ballard, I Seri, eds. Philadelphia, PA: Elsevier; 2005.
5. Burrow CR. Regulator molecules in kidney development. *Pediatr Nephrol.* 2000;14:240–253.
6. Brophy PD, Ostrom L, Lang KM, et al. Regulation of ureteric bud outgrowth by Pax2-dependent activation of the glial derived neutrotrophic factor gene. *Development.* 2001;128:4747–4756.
7. Quaggin SE. A "molecular toolbox" for the nephrologist. *J Am Soc Nephrol.* 2002;13:1682–1685.
8. Vanderheyden T, Kumar S, Fisk NM. Fetal renal impairment. *Semin Neonatol.* 2003;8:279–289.
9. Abrahamson DR, Robert B, Hyink DP, et al. Origins and formation of microvasculature in the developing kidney. *Kidney Int Suppl.* 1998;67:S7–S11.
10. Tóth-Heyn P, Guignard JP. Bradykinin in the newborn kidney. *Nephron.* 2002;91(4):971–575.
11. Pallone TL, Zhang Z, Rhinehart K. Physiology of the renal medullary microcirculation. *Am J Physiol Renal Physiol.* 2003;284: F253–F266.
12. Suzuki H, Saruta T. An overview of blood pressure regulation associated with the kidney. *Contrib Nephrol.* 2004;143:1–15.
13. Schetz M. Vasopressors and the kidney. *Blood Purif.* 2002;20: 243–251.
14. Baylis C, Qiu C. Importance of nitric oxide in the control of renal hemodynamics. *Kidney Int.* 1996;49:1727–1731.
15. Hansen PB, Schnermann J. Vasoconstrictor and vasodilator effect of adenosine in the kidney. *Am J Physiol Renal Physiol.* 2003; 285:F590–F599.
16. Barsness KA, Bensard DD, Partrick D, et al. Renovascular injury: An argument for renal preservation. *The J Trauma Inj, Infect, Crit Care.* 2004;57:310–315.
17. Deen WM, Lazzara MJ, Myers BD. Structural determinants of glomerular permeability. *Am J Physiol Renal Physiol.* 2001; 281(4):F579–F596.
18. Buschhausen L, Seibold S, Gross O, et al. Regulation of mesangial cell function by vasodilatory signaling molecules. *Cardiovasc Res.* 2001;51:463–469.
19. Sorokin A, Kohan DE. Physiology and pathology of endothelin-1 in renal mesangium. *Am J Physiol Renal Physiol.* 2003;285: F579–F589.
20. Arima S. Role of angiotensin II and endogenous vasodilators in the control of glomerular hemodynamics. *Clin Exp Nephrol.* 2003;7:172–178.
21. Wright SH, Dantzler WH. Molecular and cellular physiology of renal organic cation and anion transport. *Physiol Rev.* 2004;84: 987–1049.
22. Komlosi P, Fintha A, Bell PD. Current mechanisms of macular densa cell signaling. *Acta Physiol Scand.* 2004;181:463–469.
23. Schnermann J, Levine DZ. Paracrine factors in tubuloglomerular feedback: Adenosine, ATP, and nitric oxide. *Annu Rev Physiol.* 2003;65:501–529.
24. Greger R. Physiology of renal sodium transport. *Am J Med Sci.* 2000;319:51–62.
25. Kiil F. Mechanism of glomerulotubular balance: The whole kidney approach. *Ren Physiol.* 1982;5:209–221.
26. Shankar SS, Brater DC. Loop diuretics: From the Na-K-2Cl transporter to clinical use. *Am J Physiol Renal Physiol.* 2003;284: F11–F21.
27. Meneton P, Loffing J, Warnock DG. Sodium and potassium handling by the aldosterone-sensitive distal nephron: The pivotal role of the distal connecting tubule. *Am J Physiol Renal Physiol.* 2004;287:F593–F601.
28. Beltowski J, Wojcicka G. Regulation of renal tubular sodium transport by cardiac natriuretic peptides: Two decades of research. *Med Sci Monit.* 2002;8:RA39–RA52.
29. Hoenderop JGJ, Willems PHGM, Bindels RJM. Toward a comprehensive molecular model of active calcium reabsorption. *Am J Physiol Renal Physiol.* 2000;278:F352–F360.
30. Dai LJ, Ritchie G, Kerstan D, et al. Magnesium transport in the renal distal convoluted tubule. *Physiol Rev.* 2001;81:51–84.
31. Ellison DH. Divalent cation transport by the distal nephron: Insights from Bartter's and Gitelman's syndromes. *Am J Physiol Renal Physiol.* 2000;279:F616–F625.
32. Verkman AS. Aquaporin water channels and endothelial cell function. *J Anat.* 2002;200:617–627.
33. Pallone TL, Turner MR, Edwards A, et al. Countercurrent exchange in the renal medulla. *Am J Physiol Regul Integr Comp Physiol.* 2003;284:R1153–R1175.
34. Brown D. The ins and outs of aquaporin-2 trafficking. *Am J Physiol Renal Physiol.* 2003;284:F893–F901.
35. Inoue T, Nonoguchi H, Tomita K. Physiological effects of vasopressin and atrial natriuretic peptide in the collecting duct. *Cardiovasc Res.* 2001;51:470–480.
36. Bichet DG. Nephrogenic diabetes insipidus. *Am J Med.* 1998; 105:431–432.
37. Soleimani M. $Na^+{:}HCO_3^-$ cotransporters (NBC): Expression and regulation in the kidney. *J Nephrol.* 2002;15(suppl. 5):S32–S40.
38. Karim Z, Attmane-Elakeb A, Bichara M. Renal handling of NH_4^+ in relation to the control of acid-base balance by the kidney. *J Nephrol.* 2002;15(suppl. 5):S128–S134.
39. Alper SL, Darman RB, Chernova MN, et al. The AE gene family of Cl^-/HCO_3^- exchangers. *J Nephrol.* 2002;15(suppl. 5):S41–S53.
40. Capasso G, Unwin R, Rizzo M, et al. Bicarbonate transport along the loop of Henle: Molecular mechanisms and regulation. *J Nephrol.* 2002;15(suppl. 5):S88–S96.
41. de Mello-Aires M, Malnic G. Distal tubule bicarbonate transport. *J Nephrol.* 2002;15(suppl. 5):S97–S111.
42. Wagner CA, Geibel JP. Acid-base transport in the collecting duct. *J Nephrol.* 2002;15(suppl. 5):S112–S127.
43. Lamiere N, Van Biesen W, Vanholder R. Acute renal failure. *Lancet.* 2005;365:417–430.
44. Schrier RW, Wang W. Mechanism of disease acute renal failure and sepsis. *N Engl J Med.* 2004;351:159–169.
45. Bonventre JV. Pathophysiology of ischemic acute renal failure. inflammation, lung-kidney cross-talk, and biomarkers. *Contrib Nephrol.* 2004;144:19–30.
46. Cardenas A. Hepatorenal syndrome: A dreaded complication of end-stage liver disease. *Am J Gastroenterol.* 2005;100:460–467.
47. Clark WR, Gao D. Properties of membranes used for hemodialysis therapy. *Sem Dial.* 2002;15:191–195.
48. Clark WR, Hamburger RJ, Lysaght MJ. Effect of membrane composition and structure on solute removal and biocompatibility in hemodialysis. *Kidney Int.* 1999;56:2005–2015.
49. Opatrny K. Clinical importance of biocompatibility and its effect on haemodialysis treatment. *Nephrol Dial Transplant.* 2003; 18(Suppl. 5):41–44.
50. Stoves J, Goode NP, Visvanathan R, et al. The bradykinin response and early hypotension at the introduction of continuous renal replacement therapy in the intensive care unit. *Artif Organs.* 2001;25:1009–1013.

Gastroenterology

9

David M. Steinhorn   Jonathan S. Evans

The gastrointestinal (GI) tract represents a major set of organs comprising a significant amount of tissue mass primarily contained within the abdominal cavity. It is composed of the alimentary tract, which includes all hollow viscera from the oral cavity to the anus; the liver and the gall bladder forming the hepatobiliary tract; and the pancreas. Diseases of the GI and hepatobiliary tracts are frequent causes of admission to the pediatric intensive care unit (PICU). Additionally, dysfunction of the GI tract is common in the PICU and requires expert management to avoid further complications or organ failures. The GI tract plays vital roles in a wide range of functions beyond simple digestion. These roles involve immunologic, endocrinologic, and microbiologic functions.[1,2] Normal function of the gut is so central to health that a thorough understanding of this organ system is critical for clinicians caring for hospitalized children. Interactions between the liver and lung and between the liver and kidneys have demonstrated the central nature of the GI tract as a major contributor to multiple organ dysfunction.[3] A wide range of responses by the various components of the GI tract are seen during critical illness in patients with the same apparent clinical disease, suggesting subtle individual differences in their response to illness. Current work on genetic polymorphism may further illuminate the sources of individual differences.

THE ALIMENTARY TRACT

The alimentary tract serves several integrated purposes involving the mechanical and enzymatic digestion of nutrients, absorption of biochemical substrates, hormonal regulation of substrate flow, separation of the external environment from the internal, and excretion of waste. The process of digestion alters food to make it compatible with the internal aqueous environment of the body.

The basic functional unit of the small intestine consists of villi and crypts (see Fig. 9.1). The cells (enterocytes) of the small intestine are separated from one another by specialized junctions that serve as gaskets to prevent the back-diffusion of material into the intestinal lumen. A layer of mucus secreted by the goblet cells residing in the crypts separates the enterocytes from coming into direct contact with the luminal contents. Stem cells in the crypts produce enterocytes and other specialized epithelial cells that migrate up the crypt–villous axis as they become differentiated. The migratory process from the crypts to the villous apex takes 48 to 72 hours. Mature villar cells (typical life span 6 days) have microvilli (brush border) containing digestive enzymes and membrane-bound transport systems for nutrients and electrolytes (see Fig. 9.2). The villous tip has a predominantly absorptive function, in contrast to crypt cells that are primarily secretory. Conditions such as rotavirus infection cause villous loss, resulting in a small intestinal mucosa composed largely of crypts and immature villi. A net secretory state arises, leading to malabsorption and osmotic diarrhea. Other clinical manifestations of villous injury include malabsorption of nutrients.

The epithelial surface area and the integrity of intercellular junctions are major determinants of water and solute flux across the intestinal mucosa. The transport of solute and water across the epithelium occurs by active or passive transport, or by facilitated diffusion, as outlined in Table 9.1.[4] In the small and large bowel, the surface area is greatly amplified through the mucosal folds that form the villi and microvilli (Fig. 9.2). Loss of mucosal surface area through disease or surgical resection greatly alters the net flux of solute and water in the GI tract. In addition, the loss of specialized absorptive function may occur following loss of specific areas of the gut, for example, *short-bowel syndrome* resulting from resection of the terminal ileum (see section on "Enterohepatic Circulation").

The alimentary tract must conserve large volumes of endogenously secreted material associated with digestion. Up to 5 L of fluid per m² of body surface area enters the GI tract daily, with only 100 mL per m² being lost through the

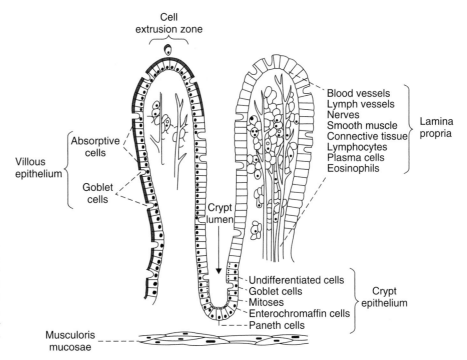

Figure 9.1 Structure of intestinal villi. The epithelial cells organize into villi. Their life span is 4 to 6 days following their formation in the crypt regions and migration to the villous tips. (From Feldman M, Friedman SL, Slesinger HM, et al. *Slesinger & Fordtran's gastrointestinal and liver disease.* 7th ed. Elsevier; 2002.)

feces under normal conditions. Therefore, the gut possesses an enormous reserve capacity for handling solute and fluid loads. Therefore, diminished absorptive capacity may lead to life-threatening loss of fluid and electrolytes.

During the process of digestion, different components of the ingested food are handled through different mechanisms. It is therefore useful to consider the disposition of nutrients by considering the macronutrients, which consist of carbohydrates, proteins, and lipids, and micronutrients, which consist of minerals, electrolytes, trace elements, vitamins, and other metabolic cofactors such as biotin and carnitine. Critical illness leads to a reduction in the intake of all nutrients, as well as to important alterations in substrate requirements and utilization. It is useful to contrast the

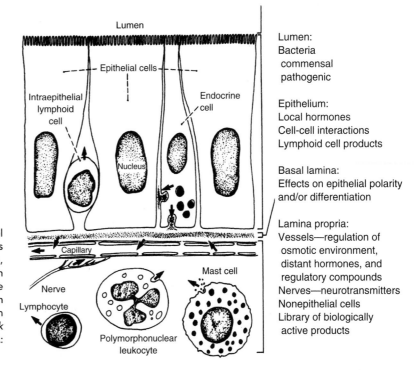

Figure 9.2 Cellular organization of epithelial surface. The brush border of the epithelial cells is adjacent to the lumen. At the abluminal surface, the epithelial cells lie in close association with vascular, lymphatic, and immune tissue in the submucosa, creating a dynamic interface between the external and internal environments. (From Yamada T, Alpers DH, Laine L, et al. eds. *Textbook of gastroenterology.* 4th ed. Philadelphia, PA: Lippincott Williams & Wilkins; 2003.)

TABLE 9.1
INTESTINAL TRANSPORT MECHANISMS

Active	Against electrochemical gradient
	Saturable kinetics
	Requires ATP
Passive	Ionic specificity
	May be associated with transport of a nonelectrolyte
	Proceeds down the electrochemical gradient
	Steady state based upon concentration differences
	Displays first-order kinetics
	May occur by convection through osmotic or hydrostatic gradient
Facilitated diffusion	Saturable kinetics
	Substrate-specific
	Depends on carrier molecules (e.g., glucose and amino acid)

ATP, adenosine triphosphate.

responses seen during fasting in a healthy person with those seen during periods of increased physiologic stress, which are summarized in Table 9.2. During prolonged fasting or starvation in otherwise healthy individuals, compensatory responses lead to a decrease in overall metabolic rate, a decrease in gluconeogenesis from amino acids, and an increase in reliance on ketone bodies derived from fatty acid oxidation for energy as the body attempts to conserve energy and protein stores. This state is characterized by depressed levels of insulin, glucagon, cortisol, and catecholamines[5] and leads gradually to chronic malnutrition.

TABLE 9.2
COMPARISON OF NUTRIENT METABOLISM IN STARVATION VERSUS SEPSIS/TRAUMA

	Starvation	Sepsis/Trauma
Protein breakdown	+	+++
Hepatic protein synthesis	+	+++
Ureagenesis	+	+++
Gluconeogenesis	+	+++
Energy expenditure	Reduced	Increased
Mediator activity	Low	High
Hormone counter-regulatory capacity	Preserved	Poor
Utilization of ketones	+++	+
Loss of body stores	Gradual	Rapid
Primary fuels	Fat	Amino acids, glucose, triglycerides

+, increased; +++, very increased.
Adapted from Barton R, Cerra FB. The hypermetabolism, multiple organ failure syndrome. *Chest.* 1989;96:1153–1160.

In contrast to the fasting state, prolonged physiologic stress, as seen during critical illness, leads to increased metabolic rate, gluconeogenesis in excess of that needed to maintain serum glucose levels, proteolysis, and peripheral oxidation of amino acids with increased ureagenesis.[5] This state leads rapidly to malnutrition as a result of autocannibalism of lean tissue mass and is characterized by elevations of glucagon levels in excess of endogenous insulin response and by elevated catecholamine and cortisol levels that drive the relentless breakdown of peripheral proteins. Our understanding of the pathogenesis of the stress state remains incomplete, although the biologic mediators include cytokines, such as tumor necrosis factor (TNF); interleukin-1 (IL-1); free radicals derived from superoxide anion and nitric oxide;[6,7] and activation of the vascular endothelium, leukocytes, platelets, and tissue macrophages. The overall systemic process associated with the stress response forms an important part of the systemic inflammatory response syndrome. The stress response is considered in more detail in Chapter 2.

During periods of high physiologic stress, the relative proportions of macronutrients delivered to the patient must be changed to allow for the decreased reliance on fat and carbohydrate for energy production. Proteins are utilized increasingly for energy production and must be replaced with additional amino acids to support the ongoing synthesis of proteins and immunoglobulins by the liver and immune system. Depressed plasma levels of the branched-chain amino acids have been found in many critically ill children, paralleling those seen in critically ill adults. Unfortunately, it has been difficult to demonstrate a convincing benefit of specialized feeding formulations in critically ill children in spite of the tremendous enthusiasm for their use a decade ago. Recent work in critically ill adults has demonstrated benefit from extensively modified enteral feeding regimens.[8,9] Currently, a multicenter study is under way to evaluate similar formulas containing modified fatty acids and antioxidants in critically ill children.

Carbohydrate Digestion

Commonly ingested carbohydrates in the diet may be classified as monosaccharides and disaccharides (simple sugars), polysaccharides (complex sugars), and fiber. Glucose and fructose are the principal dietary monosaccharides and are abundantly present in fruits, sweet corn, corn syrup, and honey. The disaccharides include lactose (glucose and galactose), the principal mammalian sugar; sucrose (glucose and fructose); and maltose (glucose and glucose). Polysaccharides are polymers of glucose, for example, starch, which is a complex carbohydrate of plant origin abundantly present in wheat, grains, potatoes, dried peas, beans, and vegetables. Fiber consists of nondigestible complex polysaccharides of plant origin. Fibers may be further classified as water-insoluble, for example, celluloses, hemicelluloses, and lignins (e.g., in cereal brans from wheat, rye, and rice), or water-soluble, for example, pectins, gums, and mucilages (e.g., pectins from fruits and vegetables, β-glucan from oats and barley, gums from vegetables, mucilages from outer surface of plants such as sea weeds), with the average ratio of soluble to insoluble fiber in the American diet being 3:1. Insoluble fibers affect fecal bulk, whereas soluble fibers have viscous effects in the upper GI tract, resulting in delayed gastric emptying, decreased postprandial glycemic response, and a constipating effect. Carbohydrates are a major source of calories in healthy children, with their metabolism being primarily through the glycolytic (Embden-Meyerhof) and tricarboxylic acid (Krebs cycle) pathways.

Carbohydrates may be stored as glycogen and lipids when ingested beyond the momentary energy needs or converted to structural materials. In general, a person's requirement for energy is highly dependent on activity level or, in the case of hospitalized patients, the state of convalescence and the degree of hypermetabolism accompanying acute illness. In addition, the maximal ability to utilize carbohydrates may be limited during periods of high physiologic stress as a result of the complex effects of hormonal mediators of the stress response.

The process of chewing initiates carbohydrates digestion by decreasing the size of food particles and increasing the total surface area for action by digestive juices. Saliva is necessary for lubrication and contains salivary amylase (ptyalin), an endoenzyme that cleaves the α-1 to α-4 links of the polysaccharide chain, resulting in short, linear oligosaccharides with maltotriose and maltose. Salivary amylase is rapidly inactivated by gastric acid, resulting in most of the starch digestion occurring in the duodenum under the action of pancreatic amylase and the intestinal brush-border disaccharidases. The amylase contained in human milk facilitates starch digestion in breast-fed infants because they have low levels of endogenous salivary and pancreatic amylase. Pancreatic amylase is the major enzyme of starch digestion, resulting in short oligosaccharides, maltotriose, maltose, and α-limit dextrins; however, the enterocyte is incapable of absorbing carbohydrates more than monosaccharides. Therefore, further hydrolysis to monosaccharides is performed by the intestinal brush-border disaccharidases, which include lactase (lactose $\rightarrow$ glucose and galactose), glucoamylase (hydrolysis of 1- to 4-linked oligosaccharides liberating glucose monomers), sucrase (sucrose $\rightarrow$ glucose and fructose), and isomaltase ("debrancher enzyme" hydrolyzing the 1 to 6 glycosidic linkage in α-limit dextrins). These enzymes are synthesized in the rough endoplasmic reticulum of the enterocyte and are subsequently inserted into the apical brush-border membrane. With the exception of lactase and, occasionally, sucrase, the disaccharidases are rarely rate-limiting for complete carbohydrate digestion. Deficiencies (acquired or hereditary) of any of the disaccharidase enzymes may result in carbohydrate malabsorption, leading to osmotic diarrhea (with elevated levels of fecal reducing

sugars), abdominal distension, and flatulence secondary to fermentation of undigested oligosaccharides by colonic bacteria.

Although simple diffusion of monosaccharides occurs during periods of high luminal carbohydrate concentration, two transport mechanisms exist in the brush border for the absorption of monosaccharides.[4] Glucose, galactose, and xylitol are transported with sodium by the Na^+/glucose cotransporter. A low intracellular sodium concentration is created by the sodium–potassium–adenosine triphosphatase (Na^+/K^+-ATPase) pump located on the basolateral membrane. The concentration gradient leads to movement of luminal sodium across the apical membrane, taking with it glucose or galactose in a 1:1 molar ratio. The second mechanism is a non–energy-dependent facilitated transport system for fructose. The basic intestinal transport mechanisms are summarized in Table 9.1.

Clinical conditions that lead to loss of the epithelium and brush-border system, such as rotavirus gastroenteritis, inflammatory bowel disease, celiac disease, sprue, ischemia/hypoxia, bacterial overgrowth of the proximal gut as a result of stasis or use of antacids, and malnutrition, may lead to symptoms of carbohydrate malabsorption (i.e., osmotic diarrhea, abdominal pain, gaseous discomfort, and flatus). Severe mucosal damage requires 7 to 10 days for recovery of brush-border function. Several infant and enteral formulas rely on starch as a carbohydrate source to minimize reliance on lactase. The digestion of carbohydrates is generally very efficient, ranging from almost complete absorption of rice starch to 80% absorption of starch from beans. Bacterial fermentation of fiber and undigested carbohydrates produces short-chain fatty acids, which are used as a fuel by the enterocytes, and gaseous hydrogen, hydrogen sulfide, and methane, contributing to the flatulence associated with increased dietary fiber and malabsorption syndromes.

Protein Digestion

Given the central role of protein in growth, maintenance of structural integrity and enzyme systems, repair of injured tissue, and immune defenses, the alimentary tract has developed efficient mechanisms for processing exogenous peptides and complex proteins. Endogenous proteins such as digestive enzymes, mucus, sloughed cells, and plasma proteins that leak into the alimentary tract are also reutilized to efficiently conserve nutrients. The recommended dietary protein intake in healthy children range from 2.5 to 3.5 g/kg/day during early infancy to 1.2 g/kg/day during childhood and 0.8 to 0.9 g/kg/day during adolescence.[10] The enteral processing of proteins may be divided into digestive and transport phases. Gastric acid secretion initiates denaturation of complex proteins, making them more susceptible to the actions of proteolytic enzymes. The chief cells of the stomach release pepsinogens that are converted to active pepsins under the influence of gastric acid. In addition to initiating protein digestion in the mature individual, pepsins act as milk-clotting factors, which are important in the neonate for curd formation, and provide bulk to the infant's stool. The pepsins are endopeptidases that release relatively large peptides and are inactivated when the pH rises above 4 as the food enters the duodenum. Interestingly, patients with achlorhydria or those receiving antacids, H_2 blockers, or both agents have no evidence of impaired protein digestion ability.

Digestion of proteins proceeds in the small intestine and is mediated by five pancreatic peptidases secreted by the pancreatic acinar cells as proenzymes and activated by enterokinase and trypsin. Each peptidase possesses proteolytic activity at specific internal or external peptide bonds. Proteins are degraded typically into mixtures of one-third free amino acids and two-third peptides containing two to six amino acid residues,[11] which are suitable substrates for the brush-border peptidases. These brush-border peptidases convert the oligopeptides into monopeptides, dipeptides, and tripeptides that are suitable for transport into the enterocyte.

Specific membrane-associated transport mechanisms exist for the uptake of amino acids and dipeptides.[12] They involve *simple diffusion, facilitated transport,* and *carrier-mediated active transport* (Table 9.1). Na^+-coupled active transport is an energy-dependent process associated with the uptake of luminal Na^+ and an amino acid (or glucose) and with the exchange of Na^+ and associated molecules for K^+ through the basolateral membrane on the abluminal side.[13] An important characteristic of these transporters is that many amino acids are absorbed more rapidly as dipeptides than as free amino acids. This fact has been capitalized on in the development of enteral nutrition formulas. Mixtures of oligopeptides have a lower osmolarity and are more efficiently absorbed than single amino acid solutions of equal nitrogen content. Because of the efficient GI absorption of dipeptides, patients with specific amino acid transport defects, for example, Hartnup disease (defective tryptophan transport) and lysinuric protein intolerance (defect in dibasic amino acid transport—lysine, arginine), infrequently have GI symptoms related to dietary protein malabsorption and instead more commonly manifest with non-GI symptoms, for example, aminoaciduria. Once inside the enterocyte, peptides are quickly degraded into their constituent amino acids by cytoplasmic peptidases that complement the activity of the brush-border peptidases. Beyond early infancy, only minute quantities of intact peptide and protein gain access to the systemic circulation. The cytoplasmic amino acids derived from digested proteins are a major source of free amino acids used directly by the enterocyte. When absorbed beyond immediate cellular needs, the free amino acids are released to the portal venous circulation for hepatic and systemic use. Only 23% of absorbed amino acid nitrogen passes to the periphery without modification.[14] Of the remaining nitrogen, 57% is converted to urea, with the carbon skeleton being salvaged for synthesizing other substances, and 20% of the total ingested amino acids is used directly for hepatic protein synthesis. During periods of fasting, the enterocyte derives most of its nourishment from the mesenteric arterial vascular supply, whereas during digestion, the enterocyte derives a significant part of its nutrient requirements from the luminal contents. Experience with mucosal recovery and adaptation after injury reveals that an enteral route of nutrition permits optimal intestinal recovery.

In the premature infant and the neonate, the small intestine is capable of absorbing intact milk proteins by pinocytosis. These proteins may include secretory immunoglobulins from breast milk, as well as food antigens.[15] Peptidase inhibitors have been demonstrated in colostrum and breast milk, partially explaining the failure of normal digestive mechanisms to degrade some of these complex dietary proteins. Both antibodies and antigens ingested with maternal milk form an important part of the immune repertory developed during early infancy.[16] Although the exact time of "closure" of the intestinal mucosa to the uptake of macromolecules has not been defined in human infants, other mammals demonstrate marked intestinal impermeability to foreign proteins by the time of weaning[17] from breast feeding.

Fat and Lipid Digestion

Dietary fat accounts for approximately 50% to 70% of the nonprotein calories consumed by infants and for approximately 34% of nonprotein calories consumed after the age of 2 years.[18] Dietary fat is ingested principally in the form of triglycerides containing the fatty acids palmitate and oleate (C16:0 and C18:1, respectively). Dietary triglycerides of animal origin predominantly contain long-chain (i.e., longer than C14 chain length) saturated fatty acids. Polyunsaturated fatty acids are mostly of vegetable origin and include linoleic and linolenic acid, also referred to as *essential fatty acids* because of absent *de novo* synthesis in humans. Other dietary lipids include fat-soluble vitamins, cholesterol, prostaglandins, waxes, and phospholipids. In healthy adults, digestion and absorption of fat is complete, with only 5% to 7% of ingested fat escaping absorption. Under normal physiologic conditions, healthy infants up to the age of 9 to 12 months fail to absorb 15% to 35% of dietary fat. Digestion and absorption of dietary fat is generally completed by the middle third of the jejunum; however, the presence of dietary fiber may reduce the rate and extent of absorption. Dietary fat is an important macronutrient substrate for children, and its deficiency places children at significant risk for calorie and fat-soluble vitamin malnutrition.

The assimilation of fat appears to have been a far greater challenge in the evolution of digestion, requiring a significantly greater proportion of the alimentary tract than proteins or carbohydrates do. The digestion of fat begins with formation of emulsions, which increase the surface area for enzyme interaction. Emulsification begins with the release of fat by mastication and gastric "milling" of chyme. Coating by phospholipids derived from the diet and bile salts produced by the liver results in a stable emulsion droplet with a hydrophobic center consisting of triglyceride, cholesterol esters, and diglyceride in a hydrophilic envelope. Mammary, lingual, and gastric lipases play an important role in direct lipolysis of long- and medium-chain triglycerides (MCTs) that are present in maternal milk.[19] Lingual and gastric lipases are active at pH <5 and begin digestion of fat in the stomach; however, overall, they only play a limited role in the digestion of lipids. Most of the enzymatic degradation of dietary lipids to fatty acids and monoglyceride is by the action of pancreatic lipase and colipase and requires an alkaline environment (pH 6 to 8). Colipase is an essential cofactor for lipase action. The role of colipase is to displace the bile salt–triglyceride interaction in emulsion droplets and micelles to facilitate lipase hydrolysis of the triglyceride. Triglyceride hydrolysis occurs at the interface between the emulsion droplet and aqueous phase within the lumen. It involves two major steps: The first is the enzymatic hydrolysis of long-chain triglycerides and the liberation of fatty acids from the glycerol backbone and the second is the formation of fatty acid micelles with the aid of bile salts, which traffic the fatty acids across the unstirred water layer to the mucosa for absorption.

When not limited by bile salt concentration or pancreatic insufficiency, the transit through the unstirred layer adjacent to the epithelial surface (see Fig. 9.3) is considered the rate-limiting step in lipid absorption; however, there are intrinsic gut brush-border lipases as well. The milieu of the unstirred water layer is acidic (pH 5 to 6) owing to the activity of the brush-border membrane sodium/hydrogen (Na^+/H^+) exchanger. The acidic environment facilitates dissociation of fatty acids from micelles, resulting in a high concentration of fatty acids necessary for diffusion across the mucosal membrane.[20] Once inside the enterocyte, long-chain fatty acids and monoglycerides are resynthesized into triglycerides and packaged as chylomicrons. Lipoproteins (e.g., apo-A, apo-B) and cholesterol are attached to the intestinal chylomicrons and confer important properties for the subsequent systemic uptake and metabolism of the chylomicrons. They are exported into the intercellular space and transported through the intestinal lacteals to become part of the intestinal lymph. On entering the bloodstream through the thoracic duct, the chylomicrons are associated with other apolipoproteins that allow them to be recognized by specific peripheral tissues.

Dietary lipids containing short-chain triglycerides (C1 to C5) and MCTs (C6 to C12) are handled differently from those of long-chain triglycerides. As much as 30% of MCTs may be absorbed intact by enterocytes by passive diffusion and enter the portal venous blood directly. In addition, MCTs are hydrolyzed by pancreatic and mammary lipases to fatty acids and monoglycerides and rapidly enter the enterocytes, where they emerge into the portal venous

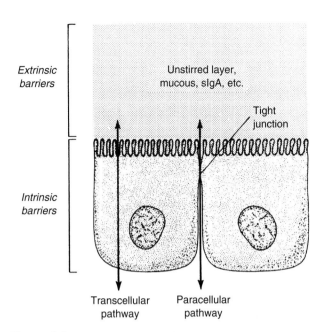

Figure 9.3 Epithelial barrier at the luminal interface. The figure demonstrates the "unstirred" layer separating the enterocytes from the lumen consisting of mucous, secretory antibodies, and digestive enzymes secreted in the proximal alimentary tract. Lipid micelles and nutrients must traverse the unstirred layer for absorbance by the enterocyte. (From Yamada T, Alpers DH, Laine L, et al. eds. *Textbook of gastroenterology.* 4th ed. Philadelphia, PA: Lippincott Williams & Wilkins; 2003.)

system without re-esterification, as occurs with long-chain fatty acids.

Lymph Formation Through the Alimentary Tract

The intestinal lymph, *chyle* is composed of chylomicrons and lipoproteins[21] secreted by the intestinal epithelium in the postprandial state together with nonresorbed interstitial fluid. Chyle follows the intestinal lymphatic channels along the mesentery and enters regional lymph nodes from where it flows cephalad through the thoracic duct and ultimately enters the central circulation. In the fasting state, intestinal lymph production is relatively low. It increases 20-fold during the active absorption of a typical meal. The intestinal chyle is joined by lymphatic drainage from other organs including liver and pancreas. The protein content of chyle is 2.2 to 5.9 g per dL, with a triglyceride content of 0.4 to 6.0 g per dL and a lymphocyte count of 400 to 6,800 per μL. During digestion of a meal containing long-chain fatty acids, chyle has a typical milky white appearance because of the presence of chylomicrons. The rate of formation of chyle depends on several factors such as the state of nutrient absorption, portal venous pressure, and the rate of lymphatic uptake. Factors that increase portal pressure (e.g., cirrhosis, congestive heart failure) or impair the flow of lymph back to the central circulation (e.g., increased central venous pressure, superior vena cava syndrome) predispose to the collection of chylous ascites in the abdomen.

Regulation of Electrolyte and Water Movement

Although mechanisms for regulating free water balance in the body exist at the systemic level, the movement of water at the cellular level and in epithelial tissues is closely linked to the movement of solute in the form of electrolytes and nutrients. The movement of solute and nutrients often depends on energy or on the electrochemical gradients that are costly to maintain from an energetic point of view. Although solute flux across tissue and cell membranes is highly regulated, water tends to move in conjunction with the controlled solute movement. As in many circumstances in nature, water tends to move toward regions of high solute concentration. A three-compartment model has been proposed for the absorption of fluid in the GI tract. In this model, the luminal contents are isolated from the vascular space by three compartments separated by two semipermeable membranes of differing porosities.[2,22,23] Electrolytes are taken up by the enterocytes and extruded through the basolateral membrane into the paracellular space. The relatively hypertonic paracellular fluid pulls water into this space, increasing the hydrostatic pressure locally. Because the tight junction between enterocytes is more impermeable to fluid flux than the capillary membranes are, fluid and electrolytes are preferentially driven in the direction of the vascular space.

Effects of Systemic and Hormonal Factors on Fluids and Electrolytes

The co-ordination of digestion, solute transport, and gut motility is under the control of a regulated system involving both systemic and local stimuli.[24] A wide range of substances have been identified such as muscarinic receptor agonists, serotonin, substance P, and similar agents that probably work through increased adenyl cyclase activity or increased cytosolic Ca^{2+} concentration to induce active chloride secretion. The complex role of signaling mechanisms on electrolyte homeostasis is illustrated in Table 9.3 for chloride ion regulation.

Systemic acidosis increases Na^+ and Cl^- absorption in the ileum and colon, whereas alkalosis has the opposite

TABLE 9.3
FACTORS AFFECTING CL⁻ FLUX

Substance	Second Messenger	Notes
Endogenous Stimuli (Hormones, Neurotransmitters, and Immune/Inflammatory Mediators)		
Acetylcholine	Calcium	Acts through M3 muscarinic receptor on epithelial cells
Histamine	Calcium	Histamine-1 receptor on epithelium; indirect effects are also possible[a]
5-Hydroxytryptamine	Calcium, cAMP	Indirect effects are also possible[a]
Prostaglandins	cAMP	E-series prostaglandins are particularly potent
Bradykinin	Calcium	Bilateral BK2 receptors; indirect effects are also possible[a]
Reactive oxygen species, hydrogen peroxide	Calcium, cAMP	Effects are likely to be largely indirect[a]
Platelet-activating factor	cAMP	Indirect effects[a]
Vasoactive intestinal polypeptide	cAMP	Direct effect through basolateral receptors
Guanylin, uroguanylin	cGMP	Apical receptor
Adenosine, 5′ AMP	cAMP? Other effectors?	Bilateral adenosine A2B receptors on epithelium
Lipoxygenase metabolites of arachidonic acid	Unknown	Effects are largely indirect
Exogenous Stimuli (Bacterial Products and Luminally Active Agents)		
Cholera toxin	cAMP	—
Escherichia coli heat-labile toxin	cAMP	—
E. coli heat-stable toxin (STₐ)	cGMP	Binds to apical guanylin receptor
Clostridium difficile toxins A and B	Calcium, other effectors?	Indirect effects and effects on paracellular pathway likely important
Bile acids	Calcium, cAMP?	Indirect effects also likely contribute[a]
Pharmaceutical agents (e.g., laxatives)	Largely unknown	—

cAMP, cyclic adenosine monophosphate; AMP, adenosine monophosphate; cGMP, cyclic guanosine monophosphate; ?, suspected, not proven.
[a]Indicates agonists that may mediate at least a portion of their effects through stimulation of mucosal prostaglandin production of activation of enteric nerves, which, in turn, can alter epithelial cAMP or calcium levels.
From Yamada T, Alpers DH, Laine L, et al. eds. *Textbook of gastroenterology.* 4th ed. Philadelphia, PA: Lippincott Williams & Wilkins; 2003.

effect. As seen in other epithelial tissues, aldosterone increases ileal and colonic absorption of Na^+, and spironolactone blocks this effect. The terminal ileum and colon are particularly important in this respect, and the presence of an ileostomy increases the risk of excessive sodium losses, dehydration, and electrolyte abnormalities. Glucocorticoids play a role in intestinal maturation[25] and increase sodium and water absorption in the distal colon. Opiate receptor stimulation increases active sodium and chloride absorption in the ileum, and opiate antagonists decrease basal absorption of water and electrolytes. The primary antidiarrheal effect of opiates, however, is mediated through a slowing of transit time. Vasoactive intestinal peptide (VIP) mediates the increased secretion of electrolytes and water by increased cyclic adenosine monophosphate production that stimulates active chloride secretion and inhibits sodium chloride absorption. Certain arachidonic acid metabolites, especially prostaglandins (e.g., prostaglandin E_1), have been shown to increase active chloride secretion, leading to increased loss of electrolytes and fluid.

Many laxatives and antacids may affect fluid and electrolyte balance by stimulating active electrolyte and fluid secretion in the terminal ileum. In addition, these agents may increase mucosal permeability and stimulate motility. Hyperosmolality of the ileal and colonic contents leads to an osmotic diarrhea. This state is seen when unabsorbed nutrients enter the distal alimentary tract and are broken down by enteric bacteria, resulting in increased luminal osmotic activity and osmotic diarrhea.

Neuroendocrine Factors Affecting the Alimentary Tract

Control over secretion and motility depends on a complex series of neurohormonal mechanisms frequently referred to as the *paracrine immunoneuroendocrine system* of the gut, frequently referred to as *PINES*. Its detailed discussion is beyond the scope of this text and interested readers should consult one of the standard textbooks on gastroenterology for greater detail;[2,24] however, a list of commonly encountered hormonal signaling agents are listed in Table 9.4.

Secretion and motility are mediated through typical agonist membrane receptor mechanisms or by local autocrine and paracrine action, or they may demonstrate remote endocrine and neurocrine actions. The peptides are secreted by endocrine or nerve cells of the gut and influence a wide range of functions throughout the gut including control of cell proliferation, motility, secretion, and mesenteric perfusion.[25] Regulation of intestinal motility is critical for keeping the chyme in contact with the epithelial surface long enough for efficient absorption of nutrients and yet permitting removal of unusable material and bacteria from the alimentary tract on a regular basis. GI smooth muscle demonstrates phasic and tonic patterns of contraction. The frequency of contractions may be affected by (i) changes in autonomic tone, (ii) stimulation of the gut by neurohormonal peptides and pharmacologic agents, or (iii) noxious stimuli associated with infectious or inflammatory processes. Hypoxia and ischemia decrease motility, frequently leading to paralytic ileus.

Electrolyte Transport

Several basic mechanisms have evolved for the transport of electrolytes by the epithelia. Sodium is transported by (i) a Na^+/H^+ exchange mechanism present throughout the intestine, resulting in a 1:1 exchange of luminal sodium for protons (a critical system for maintaining intracellular pH, cell volume, and sodium content); (ii) coupled sodium/chloride absorption, (iii) sodium/chloride cotransport; (iv) sodium/potassium/chloride cotransport; and (v) moving down its electrochemical gradient. The Na^+/H^+ exchanger plays a role in the regulation of intracellular pH, regulation of cell volume, initiation of cell growth in response to various trophic factors, and metabolic response to insulin. To maintain electrical neutrality, the epithelium simultaneously exchanges Na^+ for H^+ and Cl^- for HCO_3. In the colon, active absorption and secretion of K^+ occurs in a manner consistent with K^+/H^+ exchange. It is electroneutral and independent of Na^+/Cl^- exchange. The presence of glucose in the lumen of the small intestine stimulates increased sodium absorption through coupled transport. The uptake of glucose is carrier-mediated; however, the coupled transport of glucose with sodium is electrogenically driven by the Na^+ gradient across the cell membrane.[26] After the ion has entered the enterocyte at the luminal surface, extrusion occurs through the basolateral membrane into the paracellular spaces. It is generally agreed that the process of sodium extrusion depends on the function of the Na^+/K^+-ATPase pump located at the basolateral membranes. Extrusion of Cl^- is probably along an electrochemical potential difference.[27] The intraluminal secretion of water and other electrolytes appears to follow active secretion of Cl^- from the crypt cells of the jejunum, ileum, and colon. This physiologic pattern, that is, water following the secretion of an osmotically active molecule, is common in the liver (e.g., bile salt–dependent bile flow), pancreas, and kidney.

Because a major task for the GI tract is sodium conservation, backflow of sodium into the lumen is generally only a passive process. Disruption of normal Na^+/K^+-ATPase activity results in the net secretion of fluid and electrolytes. This mechanism is the final common pathway in a number of secretory diarrheal states such as cholera and enterotoxigenic *Escherichia coli*, *Salmonella*, *Campylobacter jejuni*, and *Clostridium perfringens*.[28] In addition, the effects of various paracrine and endocrine mediators alter intestinal adenyl cyclase activity and lead to changes in electrolyte and water balance.[27]

Zinc

Zinc is an important cofactor with increased requirement seen during wound healing. Large intestinal losses of zinc

TABLE 9.4

GASTROINTESTINAL HORMONES

Location	Hormone	Cell Type
Endocrine Cells		
Stomach	Gastrin	G
	Somatostatin	D
Duodenum/jejunum	Secretin	S
	CCK	I
	GIP	K
	Somatostatin	D
	Motilin	M
Ileum/colon	Enteroglucagon	L
	PYY	L
	Neurotensin	N
	Somatostatin	D
Pancreas	Insulin	B
	Glucagon	A
	PP	D_1
	Somatostatin	D

Neuropeptides

Calcitonin gene–related peptide
CCK
Dynorphin
Enkephalins (Leu and Met)
Galanin
GRP
Motilin
NPY
PHM
PYY
Somatostatin
Substance K (neurokinin A)
Substance P
VIP

Locally Secreted Growth Factors (Fibroblasts, Endothelial Cells, Epithelial Cells, Hematopoietic Cells)

EGF
FGF
IGF
PDGF
Transforming growth factor-α and β

Structurally Similar Families

Gastrin–CCK family
   Gastrin, CCK
PP family
   PP, PYY, NPY
Tachykinin family
   Substance P, GRP
Somatostatin family
   Somatostatin
Motilin family
   Motilin, ghrelin
Secretin family
   Secretin, VIP, PACAP, GIP, glucagon, glucagonlike peptide-1
Tyrosine kinase receptor family
   EGF, FGF, IGF, PDGF

CCK, cholecystokinin; GIP, glucose-dependent insulinotropic peptide; PYY, peptide YY; PP, pancreatic polypeptide; GRP, gastrin-releasing peptide; NPY, neuropeptide Y; PHM, peptide HM; VIP, vasoactive intestinal polypeptide; EGF, epidermal growth factor; FGF, fibroblast growth factor; IGF, Insulin-like growth factor; PDGF, platelet-derived growth factor; PACAP, pituitary adenylate cyclase–activating polypeptide.
From Yamada T, Alpers DH, Laine L, et al. eds. *Textbook of gastroenterology.* 4th ed. Philadelphia, PA: Lippincott Williams & Wilkins; 2003.

with and without complexed proteins often occur in association with high intestinal fluid losses through GI stomas and fistulae. Zinc levels should be checked periodically in critically ill patients who fail to respond to nutritional support with adequate protein and calorie intake.

Hydrogen Ion

The creation of an acidic milieu in the stomach is necessary for pepsinogen activation (pH <5.0) and to control bacterial colonization in the proximal alimentary tract. The main stimuli for gastric acid secretion are histamine, gastrin, and acetylcholine.[29] Through stimulation of histamine, pituitary adenyl cyclase–activating polypeptide plays a major role in nocturnal acid secretion.[30] Histamine release by gastric enterochromaffinlike cells is the dominant physiologic stimulus for acid secretion by the gastric parietal cells. Gastric distension and dietary amino acids and amines stimulate gastrin hormone secretion by G cells located in the antrum of the stomach. Gastrin stimulates the enterochromaffinlike cells, in close proximity to parietal cells to release histamine. Histamine then binds to histamine-2 (H_2) receptors on parietal cells, leading to acid secretion along with chloride (170 mEq per L) and potassium (8 to 20 mEq per L). The carbon dioxide derived from this process is converted to blood bicarbonate, producing a transient postprandial metabolic alkalosis referred to as the *alkaline tide* and thought by some to be responsible for the somnolence that follows ingestion of a large meal. Prostaglandins and somatostatin have an inhibitory effect on gastric acid secretion through specific receptors located on the parietal cell.[31] H_2 receptor antagonists (e.g., ranitidine, famotidine, and cimetidine) block histamine-mediated gastric acid secretion, that is, postprandial acid secretion, Zollinger-Ellison syndrome, and other disorders associated with hypergastrinemia. Proton pump inhibitors (PPIs) (e.g., omeprazole, lansoprazole and pantoprazole) block H_2-, gastrin-, and cholinergic-mediated gastric acid secretion by inhibiting the parietal cell H^+/K^+ ATPase (the proton pump [PP]), which is the final common pathway for gastric acid secretion. Furthermore, because PPIs bind irreversibly to ATP, subsequent secretion of acid can occur only with the synthesis of new PP enzyme, a process that takes >12 to 24 hours. For these reasons, PPIs have revolutionized gastric acid suppression therapy.[32,33]

THE PANCREAS

Embryogenesis of the pancreas begins at 4 weeks' gestation with the appearance of ventral and dorsal outpouchings of the foregut. As a result of duodenal development and axial rotation, these two buds will fuse forming the uncinate process (former ventral bud) and the body and tail (former dorsal buds) of the pancreas. Dysembryogenesis involving this complex process may result in well-recognized clinical entities such as pancreas divisum or annular pancreas.

The pancreas has both endocrine and exocrine functions. Through the endocrine function, the pancreas together with the liver serves as a major regulator of blood glucose levels (see Chapter 2). Endocrine-secreting cells of the pancreas are aggregated in the islets of Langerhans. Four distinct cell types that serve the endocrine function include B cells secreting insulin, A cells secreting glucagon, D cells secreting somatostatin, and PP cells secreting pancreatic polypeptide.[34] Functional ectopic pancreatic tissue may be found commonly throughout the upper GI tract but most frequently in the pylorus, duodenum, and Meckel diverticulum. The blood supply to the pancreas is derived from branches of the celiac, superior mesenteric, and splenic arteries (see Fig. 9.4). The venous drainage from the pancreas is through the pancreaticoduodenal veins, the splenic veins, and ultimately the portal vein, which provides direct hormonal influence over hepatic metabolism. Both parasympathetic and sympathetic innervation of the pancreas occurs by means of the vagi and abdominal plexuses, respectively. The vagal innervation of acini, islets, and ducts facilitates secretory function, whereas sympathetic innervation occurs primarily to vascular structures.

Exocrine Function of the Pancreas

The exocrine function is derived from specialized cells containing secretory granules and arranged in an acini that drain into ductules, which coalesce to form the pancreatic duct. Ultimately, the pancreatic duct joins with the common bile duct and drains into the duodenum through the ampulla of Vater. Ductal cells must be differentiated from acinar cells because each plays different physiologic roles. Each acinar cell is capable of secreting all the pancreatic digestive enzymes including lipase, amylase, and peptidases. Stimulation of the vagus nerves or the administration of acetylcholine induces digestive enzyme secretion, whereas these effects may be blocked with atropine. Peptidases are synthesized as inactive propeptidases and include mainly the endopeptidases trypsinogen, chymotrypsinogen, and proelastase. These propeptidases require activation in the gut lumen. Enterokinase, an intestinal brush-border enzyme, converts trypsinogen into trypsin, which in turn activates chymotrypsinogen, proelastase, and any remaining trypsinogen.[35]

Zymogen (secretory) granules can be recognized within the acinar cell as early as 9 weeks' gestation, but exocrine function continues to mature long after birth. For example, pancreatic amylase is measured at low levels in the newborn, resulting in functional maldigestion of complex carbohydrates. Adult levels are achieved between 2 and 3 years of age.

The final composition of pancreatic effluent is determined by the ductular epithelium, which regulates water and inorganic ion secretion. It is characteristically an isotonic, aqueous fluid containing Na^+, K^+, HCO_3^-, and Ca^{2+} in concentrations similar to extracellular fluid. Along

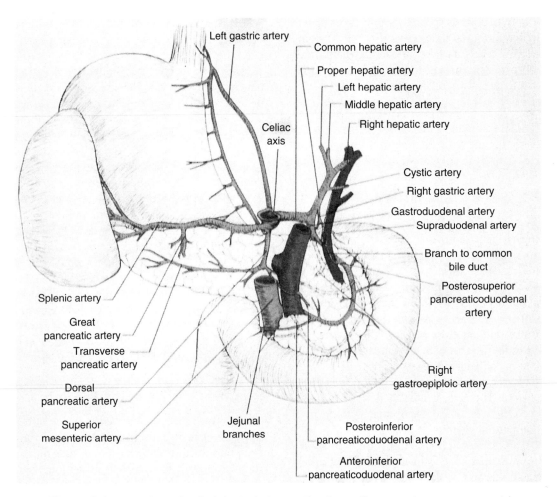

Figure 9.4 Arterial supply of abdominal viscera. The figure illustrates the common arterial relationships to the major abdominal organs. (From Yamada T, Alpers DH, Laine L, et al. eds. *Textbook of gastroenterology.* 4th ed. Philadelphia, PA: Lippincott Williams & Wilkins; 2003.)

with traces of Mg^{2+}, Zn^{2+}, and HPO^{2-}, its concentration is approximately 150 mEq per L. The contribution of each anion varies reciprocally, depending on the rate of secretory flow. Secretion of bicarbonate and water is mediated through the actions of the gut hormones secretin, cholecystokinin, and VIP.

The processes affecting pancreatic secretion have been divided into four interrelated phases, depending upon the primary stimuli and pathways eliciting exocrine function. *Basal secretion* represents approximately 2% of the potential maximum HCO_3^-. The *cephalic phase* is mediated by the vagal nerves in response to the sight and smell of food. Distention of the stomach either artificially or after the ingestion of food evokes a *gastric phase*, consisting of secretion of a protein-rich pancreatic juice of low volume and HCO_3^-. The *intestinal phase* is characterized by marked output of digestive enzymes, fluid, and HCO_3^-. The presence of HCO_3^- is essential to achieve an optimal pH (pH >5) for pancreatic digestive enzyme activity and to ensure solubility of bile salts. In addition to bicarbonate, the primary secretory products of the exocrine pancreas are amylase, lipase, and the proteases. The secondary digestive enzymes consist of nucleases, colipase, and lecithinase. The roles of the pancreatic digestive enzymes are discussed in the sections on "Carbohydrate Digestion" (amylase), "Fat and Lipid Digestion" (lipase), and "Protein Digestion" (proteases).

Inhibitors of exocrine pancreatic secretion include somatostatin, pancreatic polypeptide, and peptide YY. Somatostatin inhibits release of secretin from duodenal mucosa and is also a competitor at secretin receptor sites, resulting in decreased pancreatic secretion of both bicarbonate and enzymes.[36] Pancreatic polypeptide hormone present in the islets of Langerhans also has an inhibitory effect on pancreatic secretion of water, bicarbonate, and enzymes. Peptide YY, released from the distal ileum and colon in response to intraluminal fat, exerts its inhibitory effect by decreasing pancreatic responses to cholecystokinin and secretin. Octreotide, a somatostatin analog has been used for its antisecretory effect in the clinical management of pancreatic- pseudocysts and fistulae.[37] Inflammation of the pancreas both from infectious and noninfectious causes can produce a dramatic systemic inflammatory response, resulting in generalized permeability changes and acute lung injury. The inflammatory and healing response of the pancreas is documented in a recent review by Bentrem and Joehl.[38]

Pancreatitis occurs when propeptidases, and trypsinogen in particular, are prematurely activated before they can reach the gut lumen. This results in autodigestion in the gland. Premature trypsinogen activation is normally prevented by protective mechanisms that occur at the ductular and acinar levels. Ductular secretion of high-volume bicarbonate-rich fluids flushes the pancreas of digestive enzymes produced by the acinar cells. Cystic fibrosis transmembrane conductance regulator (CFTR) is an important regulator of duct cell fluid secretion. Mutations of the CFTR gene results in defective duct cell fluid secretion, stasis, and premature trypsinogen activation within the pancreas, leading to the acute and chronic pancreatitis of cystic fibrosis.[39] The first protective mechanism within the acinar cell is the production of an inactive form of trypsin (trypsinogen). Mutations in the cationic trypsin gene, such as those seen in certain familial forms of pancreatitis, can lead to premature activation.[40] If trypsinogen becomes activated within the acinar cell, a protective mechanism of trypsin autolysis becomes effective. Autolysis, however, can be inhibited by high intracellular calcium level, which has been recognized as a potent trigger for pancreatitis. Also, a secondary protective mechanism involving the serine protease inhibitor, Kazal type 1 (SPINK-1) can inhibit activated trypsin within the acinar cell. Mutations of the SPINK-1 gene have been associated with certain forms of familial and tropical pancreatitis.[41]

HEPATOBILIARY SYSTEM

Examination

It is axiomatic that all patients undergo a complete screening physical examination upon admission to the PICU. Although the clinician's attention will quickly focus on areas of primary concern, careful inspection, palpation, and auscultation of the abdomen must be a standard part of the evaluation. Particular attention should be paid to hepatic or splenic enlargement, distended superficial venous channels, abdominal masses, the characteristics of the bowel sounds, and finally visual inspection of the perianal region for signs of trauma, fistulae, and venous distension. Palpation of the liver provides information not only about the hepatobiliary tract but also about the function of the right side of the heart. In healthy individuals, the liver is palpable by no more than 1 to 3 cm below the right costal margin in the midclavicular line except during deep inspiration; however, assessment of liver *span*, and not palpation alone, is the only reliable nonradiologic method for determining liver size. Liver span is determined by percussion, palpation, and

auscultation along the right midclavicular line with the patient supine and breathing quietly. Percussion is employed to define the upper border, and palpation or "scratch" auscultation is used to establish the lower border.[42] The average liver span is 4 to 5 cm in preterm infants, 5 to 6.5 cm in healthy term infants, 6 to 7 cm between ages 1 to 5 years, 7 to 9 cm between ages 5 to 10 years, and 8 to 10 cm between ages 10 to 16 years.[43] Conditions associated with downward displacement of a normal liver include hyperinflated lungs, pneumothorax, retroperitoneal mass, and subdiaphragmatic abscess. Tenderness over the liver suggests inflammation or stretching of the fibrous capsule through rapid enlargement. End-stage liver disease and cirrhosis are associated with a reduced liver span, corresponding to decreased hepatic cell mass and hepatic sclerosis. The spleen tip may be palpable normally in children, especially during inspiration. Enlargement of the spleen generally represents portal venous hypertension or invasive processes such as sequestration, malignancies, extramedullary hematopoiesis, or hyperplasia of the reticuloendothelial system.[44]

Hepatic Microanatomy and Structure

The liver is the largest organ in the body and is composed of 60% hepatocytes, approximately 17% to 20% endothelial cells and Kupffer cells (reticuloendothelial cells), 3% to 5% bile ducts, and 1% Ito cells and oval cells. The liver has a dual vascular supply derived from the hepatic artery branches of the celiac axis and the portal vein. Innervation of the liver is by the parasympathetic branches derived from both vagi and sympathetic branches, which also carry afferent fibers derived from thoracic segments.

The functional unit of the liver is the "liver lobule," which is composed of interconnected hepatocytes (hepatic plates) 1 to 2 cells thick and 20 to 25 cells in length separated by a venous sinusoidal space and radiating around the central veinlike spokes in the wheel (see Fig. 9.5). The hepatic "acinus" is a conceptual description of the hepatocytes that organize into three zones (zones of Rappaport): (i) periportal (zone 1), which includes the limiting plate; (ii) midzone (zone 2); and (iii) perivenular (zone 3), with the terminal hepatic venule at its outer lateral margin. There is no discrete boundary separating these zones from one another. The watershed areas occur at the periphery of the acini, where blood derives from the smallest arteriolar branches and portal venules from adjacent acini. Biliary drainage runs parallel to the vascular sinusoidal circulation. Endothelial cells form a porous lining between the venous sinusoidal space and hepatic plates.

The microcirculatory "path" within the lobules leads along a declining hydrostatic pressure gradient from the terminal hepatic arterioles and portal venules toward the terminal branch of the hepatic vein, further defining the three hepatocyte zones (Fig. 9.5). Depending upon the substrate availability in a given zone, for example, oxygen tension and substrate or metabolite concentrations in the

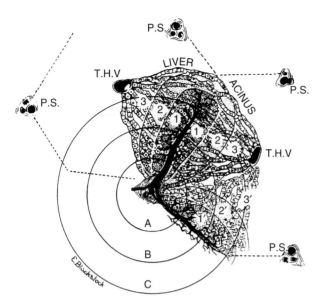

Figure 9.5 Microanatomy of the liver depicting the hepatic acinus and microcirculatory zones of Rappaport. Arrangement of simple liver acinus form zones centered around portal triads. The designated regions A, B, C, represent relative distance from the portal triad (highest oxygen and substrate concentrations) forming functional zones 1,2 and 3. Zone 3 forms the microcirculatory periphery because its cells are the farthest from afferent vessels. Cell damage in the area surrounding the terminal hepatic venule, which extends into zone 3 produces a typical stellate pattern of fibrosis. Extensive fibrosis in zone 3 produces "bridging necrosis." PS, preterminal portal tract, which contains terminal afferent vascular branches, bile ductules, lymph vessels, and nerves; THV, terminal hepatic venule. (From Schiff ER, Sorrell MF, Maddrey WC. eds. *Schiff's diseases of the liver.* 9th ed. Lippincott Williams & Wilkins; 2003.)

TABLE 9.5

SPECIALIZATION OF METABOLIC FUNCTION IN HEPATIC ZONES

Zone 3 (Perivenular)	Zone 1 (Periportal)
Glycolysis	Gluconeogenesis
Glycogen synthesis from glucose	Glycogen synthesis from lactate
Lipogenesis	β-Oxidation of fatty acids
Removal of ammonia from blood by glutamine	Amino acid catabolism
Detoxification, biotransformation of most drugs and toxins[a]	Urea synthesis
	Cholesterol synthesis
Ketogenesis	Bile acid secretion
Bile acid synthesis	Bile salt–dependent fraction of bile formation; bile acid uptake (sodium-dependent)
Bile salt–independent fraction of bile formation; bile acid uptake (sodium-independent)	
Glucuronidation	
Mixed-function oxidase	
Increase in Kupffer cell phagocytic activity	

[a]Note that certain drugs and toxins (e.g., allyl formate, phosphorus) are metabolized and may cause liver cell injury in zone 1 because of different pathophysiologic mechanisms.

sinusoidal blood, each of the zones is associated with different hepatocyte function. A description of regional specialization in hepatic zones is illustrated in Table 9.5.

The narrow tissue space between the endothelial cells and hepatic plates is called the *space of Disse*, which in turn connects with lymphatic vessels in the interlobular septa. The space of Disse lies between the hepatocyte and the endothelial cells, measures 0.2 to 1.0 μm in width, and forms a space that is not appreciated on routine light microscopy on biopsy material but that can sometimes be seen in livers during autopsy, secondary to liver cell shrinkage from autolysis. Numerous microvilli can be seen projecting from the liver cell membrane into the space of Disse. The discontinuity of the adjacent endothelial cells enables plasma to have easy permeability to the liver cell membranes. The space of Disse contains reticulin fibers, which can best be appreciated on special reticulin stains and which are easily seen on electron microscopy. Ito cells, also known as *stellate cells*, also lie within the space of Disse. These cells serve as the hepatic storage site of vitamin A, are effectors of fibrogenesis, and play a role in extracellular matrix remodeling after recovery from injury. Chronic activation and proliferation of Ito cells may lead to noncirrhotic portal hypertension, fibrosis, and cirrhosis.[45,46] The endothelial lining has large

pores that facilitate bidirectional exchange of solutes into the sinusoidal space, for example, bilirubin, bile salts, and other protein-bound solutes can easily transfer from the sinusoid to the space of Disse and, subsequently, to the hepatocyte. And likewise, movement of products secreted by the hepatocytes (e.g., lipoproteins) is facilitated from the space of Disse to the sinusoid. In between adjacent hepatocytes are bile canaliculi that drain into small terminal bile ducts, which successively drain into larger bile ductules, intralobular bile ducts, and eventually extrahepatic bile ducts. In addition to passive diffusion, several different carriers, receptors, and transport proteins facilitate movement of compounds across the sinusoidal, hepatocyte, and canalicular membranes. ATP-binding cassette (ABC) proteins are expressed in the canalicular membrane and play an important role in transport of organic ions. The ABC proteins of interest include the multidrug resistance, or MDR 1 gene product, which plays a role in the canalicular secretion of organic cations; MDR 2, which is thought to play a role in the secretion of biliary phospholipids; and multispecific organic anion transporter (MOAT) gene product, which is important in the secretion of bilirubin. The CFTR gene product is also expressed in biliary cells and appears to be an important determinant of biliary secretion and bile flow.[47] Alkaline phosphatase (ALK), leucine aminopeptidase, and γ-glutamyl transpeptidase are transaminase enzymes selectively localized in the bile canaliculi.

Most hepatic lymph is derived from the space of Disse, whereas approximately 10% is obtained by the capillary leakage from the peribiliary plexus. Its main function is to drain the excess proteinaceous fluid from the interstitial hepatic spaces. The hepatic lymph drainage within the space of Disse travels into the smallest lymphatic vessels within the portal tracts by way of "endothelial massaging" by circulating erythrocytes and leukocytes within the sinusoids. The terminal branches form plexuses lined by endothelial cells and are accentuated around the hepatic arterioles in the smaller portal structures, although lymphatics are also seen adjacent to portal veins and bile duct tributaries in larger portal tracts. Small branches can also be seen along the hepatic venous outflow branches. A lymphatic plexus is also identified within the Glisson capsule and communicates with the intrahepatic lymphatics through anastomotic channels. Most lymphatics leave the liver at the porta hepatis, although lymphatic drainage is prominent through the Glisson capsule when the hepatic venous drainage is impaired (e.g., acute and chronic hepatic venous outflow obstruction, cirrhosis). The larger lymphatic channels have an identifiable wall and are valved.

Macrophage-derived Kupffer cells are the resident phagocytes of the liver residing downstream in the portal circulation from the bacteria- and endotoxin-laden intestines. The Kupffer cells are sinusoidal lining cells that function as phagocytes and represent >75% of fixed macrophages throughout the body. These cells are ideally situated to counter invasion by intestinal bacteria through the portal circulation. They play a major role in mediating the liver's inflammatory response to local and systemic invasion, as well as in clearing particulate material, clearing endotoxins and degenerating cellular components, synthesis and catabolism of lipids, clearing senescent erythrocytes, sequestering of antigens, and clearing immune complexes. Kupffer cells represent the intrahepatic portion of the reticuloendothelial system. Their role along with the hepatocytes in setting the stage for the multiple organ dysfunction syndrome (MODS) has become apparent in recent years.[48–50] Both the intestine- and the hepatic-based macrophages can serve as a major source of nitric oxide following injury or stimulation.[51–53] The recently recognized role of nitric oxide in immune function further emphasizes the role of the GI tract in systemic responses.[54] The frequent association of hepatic dysfunction with the acute respiratory distress syndrome has led to intensive investigation of the lung–liver axis during critical illness.[48,52] A major unifying theme in these organ interactions is the regional activation of macrophages and platelets and damage to the endothelium after injury, leading to both localized and remote organ function disturbance.[49,52,55] For the pediatric intensivists, observations made in mature human or animal subjects provide only partial insights into the effects of life-threatening illness in very young children. As previously mentioned, *in vitro* work using isolated hepatocyte and Kupffer cell cocultures demonstrated decreased responsiveness of the cocultures in newborns to lipopolysaccharide stimulation compared with mature cells, suggesting a greater reserve capacity against inflammatory stimuli.[56]

Portal Circulation

The portal venous system drains the intestines, pancreas, and spleen, with numerous collateral anastomoses to other venous beds of the abdomen. The portal vein delivers approximately 70% of the hepatic blood flow. Portal and systemic blood circulation mix within the sinusoids, and all the blood eventually drains from the liver through the hepatic veins to the inferior vena cava. The liver has a high blood flow (approximately 27% of the resting cardiac output) and low vascular resistance, with an average portal venous pressure of 9 mm Hg and a hepatic vein pressure of 0 to 5 mm Hg. A rise in hepatic venous pressure of up to 3 to 7 mm Hg results in increased hepatic vascular pressure and, ultimately, a transcapsular fluid transudation containing a protein level of 80% to 90% as much as plasma protein. Obstruction of the portal venous drainage at any level leads to portal hypertension. Inferior vena caval pressures of 10 to 15 mm Hg result in gross ascites.[57] Ascites may be classified as prehepatic, intrahepatic, or posthepatic, according to the level at which the obstruction to flow occurs. The determination of the location of obstruction is critical for instituting appropriate therapy. The "classic theory" of ascites formation implicates an increased resistance to blood flow through the liver resulting from cirrhosis. Impaired portal drainage leads to a decrease in circulating blood volume, which stimulates the renin–angiotensin–aldosterone system and releases the antidiuretic hormone. This process induces sodium and water retention, leading to plasma volume expansion and further portal hypertension. The "overflow theory" of ascites formation invokes abnormal renal sodium and water retention resulting from liver damage as the primary defect. In association with reduced plasma oncotic pressure, the excess retained fluid "overflows," that is, exceeds the Starling forces in the vascular bed, and accumulates in the peritoneal cavity. The "classic" and "overflow" theories both operate at different stages in the pathogenesis of ascites and ultimately reconcile with each other.[58–60] Ascites may also form in the absence of portal hypertension, primarily as the result of low plasma oncotic pressure associated with malnutrition or renal or enteral protein losses, or through impaired thoracic duct lymph drainage. Rarely, arterial–portal venous malformations may lead to portal hypertension as a result of excess portal blood flow. An additional factor predisposing to ascites is an elevated central venous pressure that increases the formation and impairs the resorption of interstitial fluid often associated with generalized anasarca.

Hepatic Function

The liver plays a number of essential roles in maintaining health. Broadly viewed, the functions of the liver include

(i) production of substances uniquely made in the liver; (ii) the degradation, elimination, and detoxification of biologic materials; (iii) the maintenance of biochemical homeostasis; and (iv) the storage of nutritional materials.

Given the liver's unique position in the pathway of nutrient flow, it is not surprising that it plays a major role in maintaining nutrient and substrate homeostasis throughout the body. Hepatocytes are exposed to large quantities of absorbed nutrients after ingestion of a meal, with 20% of the total absorbed nitrogen being used for hepatic protein synthesis. Several of the proteins synthesized by the liver have a major significance for critically ill patients and deserve particular attention. Albumin, with its half-life ($t_{1/2}$) of approximately 20 days, is the most significant contributor to colloid oncotic pressure. Decreased albumin levels may predispose to edema formation and decreased binding of bilirubin, calcium, xenobiotics, and other highly protein-bound molecules. Low serum albumin levels may occur secondary to (i) impaired synthesis from protein-calorie malnutrition, chronic liver disease, cachexia, or inflammatory cytokines;[61] (ii) increased catabolism of proteins during hypermetabolism; (iii) translocation of albumin due to capillary leak syndrome; or (iv) increased losses from proteinuria, protein-losing enteropathy, burns, and other iatrogenic losses including paracentesis. Prealbumin (transthyretin) is a visceral protein with a short $t_{1/2}$ of 1.9 days. Because hepatic synthesis is exquisitely sensitive to both the adequacy and levels of protein and energy intakes,[62] it may be used as a nutritional marker and for monitoring short-term response to nutritional intervention. α_1-Antitrypsin is an important antiprotease with regulatory activity for elastase, as well as other proteases.[63] α_1-Antitrypsin may be important in regulating elastase-induced tissue injury in certain lung diseases, with its absence leading to uncontrolled proteolytic activity in the lung.[64] Because α_1-antitrypsin is an endogenous protein that is relatively resistant to hydrolysis by enteric bacteria, elevated levels detected in feces suggest protein-losing enteropathy.[65] Hepatic synthesis of transferrin facilitates iron transport in the plasma by binding two molecules of iron. Storage of iron is accomplished primarily in the form of ferritin, with each molecule storing up to 4,500 atoms of iron. Many coagulation factors are synthesized in the liver, including plasminogen; fibrinogen; and factors II, V, VII, IX, X, XI, XII, and XIII. Factors II, VII, IX, and X are the so-called vitamin K–dependent factors that require vitamin K for their synthesis and secretion in the active form.[66] In addition, the anticlotting proteins antithrombin-III, protein C, and protein S are synthesized largely in the liver and may be vitamin K–dependent. Several additional common plasma proteins are synthesized by the liver, including haptoglobin, ceruloplasmin, lipoproteins, α-fetoprotein, and the C3 component of the complement.

Alterations in plasma proteins frequently occur during acute and chronic liver disease. Although the levels of many of these proteins (e.g., ceruloplasmin and α_2-macroglobulin) may rise as part of the systemic inflammatory response (acute-phase reactants), plasma levels are generally reduced during liver disease, depending on the duration of hepatic insufficiency and the half-lives of the specific proteins. Therefore, a decrease in albumin ($t_{1/2} = 16$ to 21 days) generally represents a chronic disease state, whereas a prolonged prothrombin time (PT) may be seen within hours of acute hepatic failure because of the short $t_{1/2}$ of factor VII (approximately 6 hours).[66]

Detoxification and catabolism of ammonia, bilirubin, and xenobiotics is essential to life. Ammonia arises through bacterial degradation of nitrogenous compounds in the intestine, as well as from other physiologic sources of protein degradation, including the kidneys and peripheral tissues such as the skeletal muscle and brain. High levels of ammonia are incompatible with life; therefore the liver is endowed with a large capacity for urea synthesis from ammonia. During hepatic failure, hyperammonemia represents a life-threatening aspect of liver disease. Bilirubin elimination is another critical excretory function of the liver. The largest source of bilirubin is heme, derived from hemoglobin as a result of hemolysis, with smaller amounts being liberated through the breakdown of cytochromes and myoglobin. Heme is broken down into bilirubin in the reticuloendothelial system. Hepatic metabolism of bilirubin involves several steps, including transport to the hepatocyte and cellular uptake, cytosolic transport within the hepatocyte, conjugation, active cellular export, and elimination. Impairment at any juncture is manifested as hyperbilirubinemia and, ultimately, clinical jaundice. Bilirubin has a high affinity for elastin- and collagen-containing tissue, thereby explaining the presence of noticeable scleral and palatal icterus in patients with jaundice.

Enterohepatic Circulation

Bile acids represent a family of steroid molecules derived from cholesterol. Their primary functions are the elimination of cholesterol from the body and the solubilization of dietary fats through their detergentlike action and micelle formation. Because a minimum concentration of bile acids is required for micelle formation, an efficient mechanism has been evolved in the form of the enterohepatic circulation for the conservation of bile acids. Bile salts are secreted into the duodenum, with reuptake of 97% in the terminal ileum, and undergo recycling 4 to 12 times per day. The distal and terminal ileum have specialized transport mechanisms for absorption of bile salts and vitamin B_{12}, which are adversely affected by terminal ileal resection, jejunostomies, inflammatory bowel disease, or other acquired lesions in this anatomic region (e.g., necrotizing enterocolitis). Functional loss of the distal and terminal ileum results in malabsorption of vitamin B_{12}, bile salt deficiency, and impaired digestion and absorption of fat-soluble vitamins and long-chain fatty acids. Furthermore, unresorbed bile acids have a detergent and osmotic effect on the colonic epithelium, resulting in secretory diarrhea.[2]

The elimination of many drugs is affected by hepatic insufficiency either from immaturity or as a result of disease. A large number of commonly used drugs of all classes including aminophylline preparations, narcotics, barbiturates, H_2-blockers, vasodilators, and antidysrhythmics demonstrate significant hepatic elimination. The hepatic, microsomal P-450 system refers to membrane-bound internal enzymes that play a central role in many of the mixed-function oxidative reactions responsible for converting lipophilic compounds into more water-soluble ones. In addition, the liver may conjugate drug metabolites with sugars, amino acids, sulfates, or acetate to form products that can be more easily eliminated in bile or through the kidney. Further, hepatic enzymes—esterases, deaminases, hydrolases, and reductases—play an important role in the biotransformation of endogenous substances and xenobiotics.[67] The $t_{1/2}$ of many drugs may be prolonged during hepatic insufficiency as a result of a decrease in the total number of functioning hepatocytes. In addition, the apparent $t_{1/2}$ of many drugs may be prolonged through competitive inhibition by the presence of other drugs or, in fact, may be shortened by induction of elimination. For example, phenobarbital decreases the $t_{1/2}$ of xanthines and may increase the toxicity of acetaminophen. Adjustment of medication dosage and schedule must be considered for those drugs with significant hepatic elimination when impaired liver function exists.[67] Common drugs that must be adjusted during severe hepatic failure are listed in Table 9.6.

Hepatic regulatory function involves (i) interconversion of amino acids to maintain physiologic plasma levels, (ii) gluconeogenesis to maintain adequate serum levels for glucose-dependent tissues, and (iii) regulation of numerous plasma hormones (see Table 9.7). The direct secretion of insulin and glucagon into the portal circulation exposes the liver to much higher concentrations of these hormones than the peripheral tissues are. This relationship amplifies the hepatic influence over carbohydrate metabolism. Approximately 50% of the secreted insulin is degraded on a first-pass basis by the liver, with a large first-pass uptake of glucagon as well. Both these hormones are known to have hepatotrophic effects and are thought to be important for differentiation and regeneration of hepatocytes. The trophic effect of insulin on hepatocytes may be yet another benefit of the current move toward insulin supplementation in critically ill patients.[68,69]

The last category of hepatic function involves storage of glycogen, triglycerides, folic acid, and vitamins B_{12}, A, and D. Hepatic glycogen stores provide the most immediate source of glucose to maintain serum levels by glycogenolysis. Pathologic conditions associated with retention of excess storage material are familiar to pediatricians and include the glycogenoses and the mucopolysaccharidoses. Synthesis of vitamin D_3 (cholecalciferol) occurs in the skin, with its subsequent accumulation in the liver. Hydroxylation of vitamin D_3 in the 25-position, which occurs in the liver, results in a large pool of circulating 25-$(OH)D_3$, the precursor of the active 1,25-$(OH)_2D_3$. Defective storage and absorption of dietary vitamin D and 25-hydroxylation may be present in chronic liver failure.

Gastrointestinal Host-Defense Mechanisms: Immunology and Microbiology

Loss of normal gut function has been recognized over the last two decades as an important factor predisposing to the syndrome of MODS.[3,70] Integrity of the intestinal

TABLE 9.6
COMMON DRUGS REQUIRING ADJUSTMENT IN HEPATIC FAILURE

Analgesics
Acetaminophen
Opioids
Salicylates

Antimicrobials
Cefoperazone
Ceftriaxone
Chloramphenicol
Clindamycin
Erythromycin
Isoniazid
Metronidazole
Nafcillin
Rifampin

Antiarrhythmics
Lidocaine
Verapamil
Quinidine

Anticonvulsants
Phenobarbital
Phenytoin

Sedative–Hypnotics
Diazepam
Midazolam
Chlordiazepoxide

Antihypertensives
Hydralazine
Labetalol
Nitroprusside

Miscellaneous
Haloperidol
Theophylline

TABLE 9.7

HEPATIC REGULATORY FUNCTIONS

Catabolism Primarily by Liver

- Insulin
- Glucagon
- Growth hormone
- Glucocorticoids
- Estrogens
- Progesterone
- Parathyroid hormone
- Some gut hormones

Catabolism by Liver and Other Tissues

- Thyroid hormone
- Luteinizing hormone
- Antidiuretic hormone
- Testosterone
- Aldosterone
- Oxytocin
- Adrenocorticotropic hormone
- Thyroid-stimulating hormone
- Thyroid-releasing hormone

Adapted from Johnston DG, Alberti KGMM. The liver and the endocrine system. In: Wright R, Millward-Sadler GH, Alberti KGMM, et al., ed. *Liver and biliary disease.* 2nd ed. Philadelphia, PA: WB Saunders;1985.

epithelium is vital to maintaining the separation between the environment outside the body and the *milieu intérieur*. The epithelium of the small bowel possesses immunologic and nonimmunologic defense mechanisms serving to separate the host from the numerous microbes, antigens, and toxins present in the external environment. The normal microflora consists of more than 400 bacterial species. The average bacterial count is lowest in the stomach (10^3 per g) because of the effects of gastric acid and in the ileum (10^4 per g) because of rapid transit, and biliary and pancreatic secretions. The colon is the most densely colonized region of the GI tract, with microbial counts ranging from 10^{11} to 10^{12} per g. The microflora of the mouth and upper alimentary tract are predominantly gram-positive organisms, whereas in the distal ileum and colon, gram-negative and anaerobic organisms predominate, with *Bifidobacterium* and *Bacteroides* genera accounting for 25% and 30% of the total anaerobic counts, respectively.[71] Normal colonization of the alimentary tract proceeds rapidly after birth by means of oral inoculation.[72] Both oral and parenteral antibiotics profoundly reduce the number of anaerobic and coliform bacteria in the alimentary tract, with recolonization taking 4 to 6 days after the cessation of antibiotics.[73] In addition, pancreatic and biliary secretions have been demonstrated to play a role in inhibiting bacterial proliferation and colonization of the small intestine in infants; however, this process does not appear to be as significant in older children and adults.

Finally, protease and lipase activity lead to the destruction of antigens and viable bacteria, thereby controlling the number and species of flora in the gut.

Nonimmunologic Host-Defense Mechanisms

The nonimmunologic defense mechanisms consist of gastric acid, proteolytic enzymes, gut motility, mucus, and glycocalyx barriers over the epithelium and the microvillus membrane.[74] In the healthy neonate, the saliva and ingested breast milk provide both immunologic and non-immunologic factors that protect the gut from infectious pathogens and intact dietary antigens. Gastric acid secretion provides a mechanism for reducing the bacterial load reaching the small intestine. Considerable attention has been directed toward the routine clinical practice of H_2-blocker therapy for stress-ulcer prophylaxis in critically ill patients, following reports in adults associating alkaline gastric pH with higher rates of gastric and upper airway colonization by gram-negative organisms and with nosocomial pneumonia. A meta-analysis demonstrated that patients receiving an H_2 antagonist were at increased risk for nosocomial pneumonia compared to those receiving sucralfate.[75] Although the issue continues to be debated, the clinician must be aware of potential iatrogenic problems resulting from changes in flora when treating low gastric pH. The need to prevent GI bleeding in critically ill patients will necessitate the ongoing use of H_2 antagonists or PP inhibitors to control gastric pH.

Intestinal motility is a critical factor for clearing antigens and bacteria from the gut lumen, thereby reducing bacterial overgrowth with its resultant malabsorption of nutrients. Decreased motility leading to bacterial overgrowth may be seen in premature infants and may be associated with many disorders seen in older children, including the use of narcotics and some neuromuscular blockers (e.g., pancuronium bromide). A physical barrier composed of mucin and glycocalyx is formed over the intestinal epithelium by secretions from the goblet cells. It forms a gel that can change from a semisolid to a semifluid state under varying intraluminal conditions and therefore provides either a relatively impervious barrier protecting the epithelium from osmolar forces or a fluid medium helping to propel bacteria and antigens aborally.[2]

Mucosal blood flow appears to be an important mechanism for maintaining mucosal integrity in both the stomach and the small intestine. Inadequate microcirculation in the gastric mucosa, which provides cytoprotection, appears to be a major factor contributing to stress ulceration in critically ill patients. As submucosal and mucosal blood flow diminishes, the buffering ability of the acid that back-diffuses into the tissues is reduced and leads to tissue damage. Hypoxia, hypotension, and states of high circulating levels of catecholamines are commonly associated with altered mucosal circulation and stress-ulcer formation. Finally, the small intestine, especially the terminal ileum, of newborns and infants is more sensitive to systemic hypoxia and ischemia than that of adults, predisposing them to mucosal injury and necrotizing enterocolitis.

Bacterial Translocation

The discovery of viable bacteria, their products, or both across the intestinal barrier to the mesenteric lymph nodes, general circulation, liver, spleen, or other organs has created tremendous interest in understanding the role of gut in producing bacteremia. Known as *translocation*, this process has been recognized as a potential source of pathogens producing sepsis in a variety of premorbid disease conditions.[76,77] Translocation may occur directly through the M cells that cover the Peyer patches, or it may occur by the ingestion of viable pathogenic material by the mobile phagocytic system, with transport into the host bypassing the previously outlined barrier mechanisms. The three main mechanisms predisposing a host to bacterial translocation are disruption of the ecologic equilibrium, allowing intestinal bacterial overgrowth; deficiencies in the host immune defenses; and damage to the intestinal mucosa and vasculature that causes increased permeability.[76] Certain aerobic enteric bacteria including *E. coli, Proteus mirabilis, and Klebsiella pneumoniae* appear to be more commonly associated with translocation from the GI tract, presumably because oxygen in the blood may exert an inhibitory effect on anaerobic organisms. Intra-abdominal inflammatory foci are susceptible to invasion by translocating bacteria, suggesting one mechanism for abdominal abscess formation. Attempts to prophylactically decontaminate the gut in critically ill, but otherwise immunocompetent, adult patients have not shown an improved outcome for the multisystem organ dysfunction syndrome.

Immunologic Mechanisms of Host Defense

Of central importance to the immune function of the gut are the gut-associated lymphoid tissues (GALT), consisting of Peyer patches and single lymphoid nodules of the intestinal mucosa and appendix.[78] Migration of lymphocytes from one compartment to another provides communication of immunologic information. In addition, migration of lymphocytes to extraintestinal tissues including the mammary gland, female genital tract, and bronchus-associated lymphoid tissue may mediate immune responses in these tissues. Peyer patches consist of mononuclear cells, plasma cells, macrophages, and other antigen-presenting cells. B cells are the predominant lymphocytes. Peyer patches are covered by a specialized epithelium containing M cells, which transport luminal antigen into the patches.

Penetration of the mucosal barrier by antigenic material occurs because the epithelial barrier is not totally impermeable to macromolecules. It may be accelerated by inflammation or mucosal damage. Increased permeability and tissue damage occur with such diverse disease entities as infectious enterocolitis, idiopathic inflammatory bowel diseases, hypersensitivity diseases such as celiac sprue and food allergies, and gut ischemia or hypoxia. As barrier mechanisms fail in the injured gut, bacterial penetration is more likely to occur, producing portal and systemic bacteremia. Cell-mediated cytotoxic reactions and antibody-dependent cell-mediated cytotoxicity represent two responses of the GALT to the encounters with antigens. These processes involve the co-operative interaction of other lymphoid cells such as killer, lymphokine-activated killer, and natural killer cells. Infected or necrotic cells and noncellular antigenic materials are targeted for ultimate lysis by phagocytic cells in the circulation and reticuloendothelial system.

Kupffer cells, which account for the largest pool of mononuclear phagocytes with direct access to the blood, play a major role in clearing portal bacteria. In addition, Kupffer cells are the key participants in the response to tissue injury or organ invasion through the elaboration of cytokine mediators, such as TNF and IL-1, and the release of nitric oxide, leading to many of the systemic responses seen in sepsis. Through their intimate proximity to the hepatocyte, Kupffer cells interact directly with hepatocytes by means of cell–cell and paracrine interactions. In response to TNF and IL-1, well-documented alterations in hepatic function occur including the inhibition of albumin synthesis, gluconeogenesis, and P-450–mediated detoxification. Acute-phase reactant synthesis is also induced by TNF and IL-1.[79]

TESTING OF GASTROINTESTINAL FUNCTION IN THE INTENSIVE CARE UNIT

Diagnostic testing in the intensive care unit (ICU) permits the identification of organ system injury and dysfunction. In addition, it assists in monitoring the course of a disease and the response to therapies. Progressive deterioration of major organ function leading to the MODS has been known since the mid 1970s to be associated with poor outcome; however, the best biochemical discriminators of organ dysfunction are not universally agreed upon.

Laboratory testing is helpful in detecting and monitoring hepatocellular injury and dysfunction, which represents the common final pathway resulting from a variety of both immunologic and nonimmunologic mechanisms (see Chapter 63). In the ICU setting, impaired synthetic function is the hallmark of liver failure, which is of more immediate concern than hepatocellular injury alone. Decreased synthesis of the liver-dependent clotting factors I (fibrinogen), II (prothrombin), V, VII, IX, and X results in a prolonged PT, which in the absence of vitamin K deficiency or related inhibitors represents liver failure.[66] Furthermore, because factor VII has the shortest $t_{1/2}$ (2 to 6 hours) compared to the other factors, it becomes the rate-limiting step for conversion of prothrombin to thrombin. For this reason, the management of intractable coagulopathy in fulminant liver failure may benefit from specific replacement therapy with recombinant factor VII.[80] Other less-specific indicators of liver dysfunction include decreased serum albumin level, and elevation or depression of serum cholesterol and triglyceride levels in association with their respective carrier lipoproteins. Liver failure may also be associated with life-threatening hypoglycemia through several mechanisms including decreased hepatic synthesis and release of glucose, hyperinsulinemia (from impaired hepatic degradation), and increased glucose utilization secondary to anaerobic metabolism.[81] A frequent finding in advanced liver failure is elevated serum ammonia level, reflecting impaired deamination and/or clearance of ammonia. Ammonia elevation results primarily from fulminant hepatic failure, urea cycle defects, portal systemic shunting, and events such as a large GI hemorrhage that is a substrate for increased ammonia production by enteric bacteria, leading to hyperammonemia when liver failure is present.[81]

The biochemical tests commonly used to detect cholestasis (impaired bile flow) and hepatocellular injury are serum bilirubin and aminotransferase activities (alanine aminotransferase [ALT] and aspartate aminotransferase [AST]). Liver disease can be broadly categorized into hepatocellular, cholestatic, and infiltrative processes. Preferential elevations in the levels of serum conjugated bilirubin, bile acids, ALK, γ-glutamyltransferase (GGT), and 5'-nucleotidase (5-NT) represent cholestasis, reduced bile excretion, transport, or obstruction in the canalicular or large biliary ducts. Conjugated hyperbilirubinemia is assessed by the direct (Van den Bergh) reaction, whereas the unconjugated (indirect) fraction represents the difference between the total bilirubin and the direct fraction. Elevated levels of predominantly indirect bilirubin result from (i) increased bilirubin load to the liver (e.g., hemolysis), (ii) its diminished uptake and intracellular transport, and (iii) its reduced conjugation (e.g., immaturity, fulminant necrosis). In children, elevations in ALK level may be seen with rickets or during periods of rapid skeletal growth, necessitating the determination of isoenzymes to distinguish between bone and biliary sources. ALT (or SGPT) and AST (or SGOT) are hepatic cytosolic enzymes that catalyze the reversible transfer of the α-amino group of the amino acids alanine and aspartic acid to the α-keto group of α-ketoglutaric acid, producing pyruvic and oxaloacetic acids, respectively, along with glutamate. Elevations in serum activities of ALT and AST suggest hepatocellular injury (see Table 9.8). AST is also present in myocardial tissue, skeletal muscle, kidney, pancreas, and erythrocytes; therefore, increased serum activity is not specific for hepatocellular injury. Fortunately for the hepatologist, ALT is present in only relatively low concentrations in tissues other than liver, thereby providing greater specificity for hepatocellular injury than AST does. Elevated serum lactate dehydrogenase (LDH) activity lacks specificity and may be seen in association with hepatocellular injury, hemolysis, and myopathy; however, when in association with elevated serum levels of creatinine phosphokinase (CPK) or aldolase, it indicates myopathy or a rhabdomyolysis. In general, biochemical tests have limited discriminative value for differentiating between primarily hepatocellular and cholestatic or infiltrative liver injury; nonetheless, the differential diagnosis may be narrowed down (see Table 9.9).

Imaging of the hepatobiliary system has become easier, safer, and more reliable in the last decade. Ultrasonography is particularly useful in the ICU and allows rapid, safe, bedside evaluation of (i) hepatic vascular structures and patterns of blood flow; (ii) structural abnormalities such as tumors, abscess, hematoma, or dilated intrahepatic bile

TABLE 9.8

PATTERN OF BIOCHEMICAL TESTS BASED ON THE CATEGORY OF LIVER DISEASE

Biochemical Test	Hepatocellular Necrosis	Cholestasis	Infiltrative Process
ALT, AST	+ + to + + +	0 to +	0 to +
ALK, GGT	0 to +	+ + to + + +	+
Total/conjugated bilirubin	0 to + + +	0 to + + +	0 to +
PT	Prolonged	Prolonged; responsive to vitamin K	0
Albumin	Decreased in chronic disorders	0	0
Cholesterol	0	0 to + + +	0
Bile acids	+ to + + +	+ to + + +	0

0, normal; + to + + +, degrees of elevation.
ALT, alanine aminotransferase; AST, aspartate aminotransferase; ALK, alkaline phosphatase; GGT, γ-glutamyltransferase; PT, prothrombin time.

TABLE 9.9

DIAGNOSIS OF SELECTED HEPATOBILIARY DISORDERS

Form of Liver Injury	Supportive History/ Laboratory Data
Predominantly Hepatocellular	
Viral hepatitis	Viral serologies: hepatitis A, B, C, and E, and EBV
Drug-induced hepatitis	History of toxic/excess ingestion, ± elevated eosinophil count
Ischemia	Shock, postcardiac surgery
Autoimmune hepatitis	Increased globulin ratio, antinuclear antibody, anti–smooth muscle antibody, anti–liver antibodies microsomal antibody
Wilson disease	Serum ceruloplasmin
α-Antitrypsin deficiency	Pi typing
Cholestatic	
Bacterial sepsis	*Proteus, Escherichia coli* and UTI
Galactosemia	Urine succinyl choline
Biliary atresia	Intraoperative cholangiogram
Anatomic anomalies: choledochal cysts, biliary stricture, cholelithiasis, congenital hepatic fibrosis, Caroli disease, Alagille syndrome, cystic fibrosis	Ultrasonography, cholangiogram
GVHD, venoocclusive disease	History of bone marrow transplant, high-dose busulfan
Ischemia	ECMO
Infiltrative	
Hepatocellular carcinoma	α-Feto protein
Predominant Coagulopathy	
Neonatal hematochromatosis	Serum iron and ferritin

EBV, Epstein-Barr virus; UTI, urinary tract infections; GVHD, graft versus host disease; ECMO, extracorporeal-membrane oxygenation; Pi, protease inhibitor.

ducts; (iii) the gallbladder, extrahepatic, pancreatic, and common biliary system; (iv) the pancreas; (v) the genitourinary system; and (vi) the abdomen and retroperitoneum. In addition, ultrasonography can provide guidance for therapeutic interventions such as drainage of abscesses. Computed tomographic (CT) scan with and without contrast and magnetic resonance imaging (MRI) provide additional methods for evaluating the abdominal and retroperitoneal organs for masses, abscess, fluid collections, and so on; however, both modalities usually require a prolonged period away from the ICU, which may lead to instability in a tenuous, critically ill patient. Many of the radioisotope studies can be performed in the ICU and provide a wide range of diagnostic possibilities in critically ill patients. Technetium 99m (^{99m}Tc) acetanilidoiminodiacetic acid (IDA) compounds are handled by the hepatobiliary system much like bilirubin and provide a qualitative and semiquantitative image of function and structure. These compounds may be used diagnostically to evaluate infants with persistent jaundice and may also be used in follow-up after Kasai procedure or liver transplantation.

Of the available biochemical markers of pancreatic disease, serum amylase and lipase determinations are the most widely available. Serum lipase is elevated in approximately 87% of patients with acute pancreatitis and demonstrates fewer false-positive results than amylase testing. Transient hypocalcemia (<8.0 mg per dL) occurs in approximately 30% of patients with pancreatitis. Mild to moderate hyperglycemia as a result of islet cell damage is seen in up to 25% of cases, often necessitating the administration of exogenous insulin.

Evaluation of the alimentary tract consists of examining gastric aspirates and stool samples for gross bleeding or occult blood with the guaiac test (Hemoccult). A positive result mandates further evaluation and surveillance to determine the source and severity of GI tract blood loss. ^{99m}Tc sulfur colloid or red blood cells labeled with ^{99m}Tc may provide information about the site of active mucosal bleeding and are less invasive than arteriography. Esophageal pH probe recording to detect occult gastroesophageal reflux is indicated in the evaluation of unexplained apnea, recurrent pulmonary infections or wheezing, and unusual neck or body posturing. Multiple-site monitoring of pH in the esophagus, pharynx, and stomach is indicated when there is recurrent unexplained cough or laryngeal symptoms and suspected bile reflux, and to monitor the efficacy of gastric acid suppression therapy. The frequency and duration of episodes during which the probe pH is <4 or >8 corresponds with acid and bile exposure, respectively, and the final interpretation is based on correlation with the clinical symptoms.

Imaging studies are of primary importance in acutely ill patients in a number of circumstances. Plain radiographs can be reliably used to locate radiopaque objects and to diagnose intestinal ileus, mechanical obstruction, and perforated viscus, whereas contrast studies are required to diagnose organ and soft-tissue inflammation including appendicitis, pancreatitis and its complications; mesenteric and retroperitoneal masses; abscesses/fluid collections; intussusceptions; and anatomic anomalies.

GI bleeding from sites inaccessible to video endoscopy, that is, distal to the ligament of Treitz and proximal to the terminal ileum (e.g., Meckel diverticulum, vascular malformations and altered anatomy post-GI surgery), is best assessed using radio nuclide scans and angiography. Because of the need to perform the more sophisticated imaging studies away from the controlled environment of the ICU, the studies must be tailored to the patient's diagnostic needs according to the priorities of the initial stabilization of life-threatening illness and subsequent treatment of the underlying pathologic condition.

Video and or fiber-optic endoscopy in the hands of operators skilled in managing small children has found a place in ICU management to diagnose the source of upper GI tract bleeding, to control and sclerose bleeding varices, to place percutaneous gastrostomy tubes for feeding, and to place stents to maintain the patency of the distal biliary and pancreatic tract.

Lastly, liver biopsy may frequently be required in critically ill patients to determine the etiology of liver failure and to assess the potential need for transplantation. Correction of coagulopathy is important to minimize hemorrhagic complications following biopsy. When correction of the coagulopathy is not possible, biopsy may be performed in older children through a transjugular approach, reducing the risk of bleeding.

REFERENCES

1. Nagler-Anderson C, Terhoust C, Bhan A, et al. Mucosal antigen presentation and the control of tolerance and immunity. *Trends Immunol.* 2001;120:1372–1380.
2. Thomson A, Keelan M, Thiesen A, et al. Small bowel review. *Dig Dis Sci.* 2001;46:2555–2607.
3. Deitch E. Role of the gut lymphatic system in multiple organ failure. *Curr Opin Crit Care.* 2001;2:92–98.
4. Ganong W. The general and cellular basis of medical physiology. In: *Review of medical physiology.* McGraw-Hill; 2003, Chapter 1.
5. Shronts E, Beilman G, Cerra F. The inflammatory response, immune dysfunction, and immunonutrition. In: Irwin R, Cerra F, Rippe J, eds. *Irwin and Rippe's intensive care medicine.* Philadelphia, PA: Lippincott Williams & Wilkins; 1999, Chapter 207.
6. Das U. Critical advances in septicemia and septic shock. *Crit Care.* 2000;4:290–296.
7. Szabo G, Romics L, Frendl G. Liver in sepsis and systemic inflammatory response syndrome. *Clin Liver Dis.* 2002;6:1045–1066.
8. Gadek J, DeMichele S, Karlstad M, et al. Effect of enteral feeding with eicosapentaenoic acid, gamma-linolenic acid, and antioxidants in patients with acute respiratory distress syndrome. *Crit Care Med.* 1999;29:1409–1420.
9. Pacht E, DeMichele S, Nelson J, et al. Enteral nutrition with eicosapentaenoic acid, gamma-linolenic acid, and antioxidants reduces alveolar inflammatory mediators and protein influx in patients with acute respiratory distress syndrome. *Crit Care Med.* 2003;31:491–500.
10. JFWUE Consultation. ed. Food and Agriculture Organization/World Health Organization/United Nations University. *Energy and protein requirements,* WHO Technical Report Series 724, Geneva: WHO, 1985.
11. Silk D, Gimble G, Rees R. Protein digestion and amino acid and peptide absorption. *Proc Nutr Soc.* 1985;44:63.
12. Leibach F, Ganapathy V. Peptide transporters in the intestine and the kidney. *Ann Rev Nutr.* 1996;16:99.
13. Kekuda R, Rottes-Zamorano V, Fei Y. Molecular and functional characterization of intestinal Na(+)-dependent neutral amino acid transporter. *Am J Physiol.* 1997;272:G1463.
14. Elwyn D. The role of the liver in regulation of amino acid and protein metabolism. In: Munro H, ed. *Mammalian protein metabolism.* New York: Academic Press; 1970.
15. Jalonen T. Increased beta-lactoglobulin absorption during rotavirus enteritis in infants: Relationship to intestinal permeability. *Pediatr Res.* 1991;30:290–298.
16. Holsapple M, West L, Landreth K. Species comparison of anatomical and functional immune system development. *Birth Defects Res Part B Dev Reprod Toxicol.* 2003;68(4):321–334.
17. Udall J, Walker W. The physiologic and pathologic basis for the transport of macromolecules across the intestinal tract. *J Pediatr Gastroenterol Nutr.* 1982;1:295–302.
18. Lenfant C, Ernst N. Daily dietary fat and total food-energy intakes–NHANES III, Phase 1, 1988–1991. *JAMA.* 1994;271:1309–1311.
19. Hamosh M. The milky way: From mammary gland to milk to newborn–Macy-Gyorgy Award presentation. *Adv Exp Med Biol.* 2002;503:17–25.
20. Shiau Y. Mechanism of intestinal fatty acid uptake in the rat: The role of an acidic microclimate. *J Physiol.* 1990;421:463–474.
21. Rodriquez M, Kalogeris T, Want X, et al. Rapid synthesis and secretion of intestinal apolipoprotein A-IV after gastric fat loading in rats. *Am J Physiol.* 1997;272:R1170–R1177.
22. Madara J, Trier J. The functional morphology of the mucosa of the small intestine. In: Johnson L, ed. *Physiology of the gastrointestinal tract.* New York: Raven Press; 1994.
23. Lencer W, Desjeux J. Transport of water and ions. In: Walker W, Durie P, Hamilton JR, et al., eds. *Pediatric gastrointestinal disease.* St. Louis, MO: Mosby; 1996.
24. Sellin J. Intestinal electrolyte absorption and secretion. In: Feldman M, Friedman L, Slesinger M, eds. *Slesinger and Fordtran's gastrointestinal and liver disease.* Philadelphia, PA: Elsevier; 2002:1693–1714.
25. Murphy MS, Aynsley-Green A. Regulatory peptides of the gastrointestinal rect in early life. In: Walker WA, Durie PR, Hamilton JR, eds. *Pediatric gastrointestinal disease.* St. Louis, MO: Mosby; 1996.
26. Wright E, Loo D. Coupling between Na+, sugar, and water transport across the intestine. *Ann N Y Acad Sci.* 2000;915:54–66.
27. Holtug K, Hansen M, Skadhauge E. Experimental studies of intestinal ion and water transport. *Scand J Gastroenterol.* 1996;S216:95–110.
28. Field M. Intestinal ion transport and the pathophysiology of diarrhea. *J Clin Invest.* 2003;111:931–943.
29. Wolfe M, Soll A. The physiology of gastric acid secretion. *N Engl J Med.* 1988;319:1707–1715.
30. Zeng N, Athmann C, Kang T, et al. PACAP type I receptor activation regulates ECL cells and gastric acid secretion. *J Clin Invest.* 1999;104:1383–1391.
31. DelVale J, Lucey M, Yamada T. Gastric secretion. In: Yamada T, ed. *Textbook of gastroenterology.* Philadelphia, PA: JB Lippincott; 1995.
32. Wolfe M, Sachs G. Acid suppression: Optimizing therapy for gastroduodenal ulcer healing, gastroesophageal reflux disease, and stress-related erosive syndrome. *Gastroenterology.* 2000;118:S9–31.
33. Pisegna J. Pharmacology of acid suppression in the hospital setting: Focus on proton pump inhibition. *Crit Care Med.* 2002;30:S356–S361.
34. Kemp D, Thomas M, Habener J. Developmental aspects of the endocrine pancreas. *Rev Endocr Metab Disord.* 2003;4:5–17.
35. Yeo C, Cameron J. Exocrine pancreas. In: Townsend CM, Beauchamp RD, Evers BM, et al. ed. *Textbook of surgery: The biological basis of modern surgical practice.* Philadelphia, PA: WB Saunders; 2001:1112–1142.
36. Henderson J. Pancreatitis. In: Henderson J, ed. *Gastrointestinal pathophysiology.* Philadelphia, PA: Lippincott-Raven; 1996:185–212.
37. Uhl W, Anghelacopoulos S, Friess H, et al. The role of octreotide and somatostatin in acute and chronic pancreatitis. *Digestion.* 1999;60:S23–S31.
38. Bentrem D, Joehl R. Pancreas: Healing response in critical illness. *Crit Care Med.* 2003;31:S582–S589.
39. Cohn J, Friedman K, Noone P, et al. Relation between mutations of the cystic fibrosis gene and idiopathic pancreatitis. *N Engl J Med.* 1998;339:653–658.
40. Whitcomb D, Gorry M, Preston R, et al. Hereditary pancreatitis is caused by a mutation in the cationic trypsinogen gene. *Nat Genet.* 1996;14:141–145.
41. Whitcomb D. How to think about SPINK and pancreatitis. *Am J Gastroenterol.* 2002;97:1085–1088.
42. Boyle J. Hepatomegaly. In: Kliegman RM, Nieder ML, Super DM, et al. ed. *Practical strategies in pediatric diagnosis and therapy.* Philadelphia, PA: WB Saunders; 1996.
43. Naveh Y, Berant M. Assessment of liver size in normal infants and children. *J Pediatr Gastroenterol Nutr.* 1984;3:346–348.

44. Shurin S. Splenomegaly. In: Kliegman R, ed. *Practical strategies in pediatric diagnosis and therapy*. Philadelphia, PA: WB Saunders; 1996.
45. Hautekeete M, Geerts A. The hepatic stellate (Ito) cell: Its role in human liver disease. *Virchows Arch*. 1997;430:195–207.
46. Davis B, Kresina T. Hepatic fibrogenesis. *Clin Lab Med*. 1996; 16:361–375.
47. Feranchak A, Sokol R. Cholangiocyte biology and cystic fibrosis liver disease. *Semin Liver Dis*. 2001;21:471–488.
48. Matuschak G. Liver-lung interactions in critical illness. *New Horiz*. 1994;2:488–459.
49. Hauser C. Regional macrophage activation after injury and the compartmentalization of inflammation in trauma. *New Horiz*. 1996;4:235–251.
50. Xu D, Lu Q, Adams C, et al. Trauma-hemorrhagic shock-induced up-regulation of endothelial cell adhesion molecules is blunted by mesenteric lymph duct ligation. *Crit Care Med*. 2004;32:760–765.
51. Salzman A. Nitric oxide in the gut. *New Horiz*. 1995;33:33–44.
52. Rolla G. Hepatopulmonary syndrome: Role of nitric oxide and clinical aspects. *Dig Liver Dis*. 2004;36:303–308.
53. Grange J, Amiot X. Nitric oxide and renal function in cirrhotic patients with ascites: From physiopathology to practice. *Eur J Gastroenterol Hepatol*. 2004;16:567–570.
54. Tritto I, Ambrosio G. The multi-faceted behavior of nitric oxide in vascular "inflammation": Catchy terminology or true phenomenon? *Cardiovasc Res*. 2004;63:1–4.
55. Yegenaga I, Hoste E, Van Biesen W, et al. Clinical characteristics of patients developing ARF due to sepsis/systemic inflammatory response syndrome: Results of a prospective study. *Am J Kidney Dis*. 2004;43:817–824.
56. Steinhorn D, Cerra F. Comparative effects of lipopolysaccharide on newborn versus adult rat hepatocyte and nonparenchymal cell cocultures. *Crit Care Med*. 1997;25:121–127.
57. Guyton A, Hall J, eds. The liver as an organ. In: *Textbook of medical physiology*. Philadelphia, PA: WB Saunders; 2000.
58. Schrier R, Arroyo V, Bernardi M, et al. Peripheral arterial vasodilation hypothesis: A proposal for the initiation of renal sodium and water retention in cirrhosis. *Hepatology*. 1988;8:1151–1157.
59. Cardenas A, Arroyo V. Mechanisms of water and sodium retention in cirrhosis and the pathogenesis of ascites. *Best Pract Res Clin Endocrinol Metab*. 2003;(17):607–622.
60. Sivayokan T, Dillon J. Cirrhotic ascites: A review of management. *Hosp Med*. 2004;65:22–26.
61. Tisdale M. Biomedicine. Protein loss in cancer cachexia. *Science*. 2000;29:2293–2294.
62. Bernstein L, Ingenbleek Y. Transthyretin: Its response to malnutrition and stress injury. Clinical usefulness and economic implications. *Clin Chem Lab Med*. 2002;40:1344–1348.
63. Stockley R. Proteases and antiproteases. *Novartis Found Symp*. 2001;234:189–199.
64. Needham M, Stockley R. Alpha 1-antitrypsin deficiency. 3: Clinical manifestations and natural history. *Thorax*. 2004;59:441–445.
65. van der Sluys Veer A, Biemond I, Verspaget H, et al. Faecal parameters in the assessment of activity in inflammatory bowel disease. *Scand J Gastroenterol* Suppl. 1999;230:106–110.
66. Hedner U, Erhardtsen E. Hemostatic disorders in liver disease. In: Schiff E, Sorrell M, Maddrey W, eds. *Schiff's diseases of the liver*. Philadelphia, PA: Lippincott Williams & Wilkins; 2003.
67. Arns P, Wedlund P, Branch R. Adjustment of medications in liver failure. In: Chernow B, ed. *The pharmacologic approach to the critically ill patient*. Baltimore: Williams & Wilkins; 1988.
68. van den Berghe G, Wouters P, Weekers F, et al. Intensive insulin therapy in the surgical intensive care unit. *N Engl J Med*. 2001; 345:1417–1418.
69. Jeschke M, Klein D, Bolder U, et al. Insulin attenuates the systemic inflammatory response in endotoxemic rats. *Endocrinology*. 2004;145:4084–4093.
70. Villar J, Maca-Meyer N, Perez-Mendez L, et al. Bench-to-bedside review: Understanding genetic predisposition to sepsis. *Crit Care*. 2004;8:180–189.
71. Hao W, Lee Y. Microflora of the gastrointestinal tract: A review. *Methods Mol Biol*. 2004;268:491–502.
72. Fanaro S, Chierici R, Guerrini P, et al. Intestinal microflora in early infancy: Composition and development. *Acta Paediatr Suppl*. 2003;91:48–55.
73. Fry D, Schermer C. The consequences of suppression of anaerobic bacteria. *Surg Infect*. 2000;1:49–56.
74. Israel E, Walker W. Host defense development in gut and related disorders. *Pediatr Clin North Am*. 1988;35:1–15.
75. Messori A, Trippoli S, Vaiani M, et al. Bleeding and pneumonia in intensive care patients given ranitidine and sucralfate for prevention of stress ulcer: Meta-analysis of randomized controlled trials. *BMJ*. 2000;321:1103–1106.
76. Lichtman S. Bacterial translocation in humans. *J Pediatr Gastroenterol Nutr*. 2001;33:1–10.
77. Steinberg S. Bacterial translocation: What it is and what it is not. *Am J Surg*. 2003;186:301–305.
78. Spahn T, Kucharzik T. Modulating the intestinal immune system: The role of lymphotoxin and GALT organs. *Gut*. 2004;53:456–465.
79. Pannen B, Robotham J. The acute phase response. *New Horiz*. 1995;3:183–197.
80. Brown J, Emerick K, Brown D, et al. Recombinant factor VIIa improves coagulopathy caused by liver failure. *J Pediatr Gastroenterol Nutr*. 2003;37:268–272.
81. Whitington P. Fulminant liver failure in children. In: Suchy F, ed. *Liver disease in children*. St. Louis: Mosby; 1994.

Shock and Shock Syndromes

10

Joseph A. Carcillo **Jefferson Pedro Piva** **Neal J. Thomas** **Yong Y. Han**
John C. Lin **Richard Andrew Orr**

DEFINITION

Shock is a state of acute energy failure in which there is not enough adenosine triphosphate (ATP) production to support the systemic cellular function. ATP production is most efficient when oxygen and glucose combine to form acetyl-CoA. Each acetyl-CoA molecule that enters the Krebs cycle produces 32 molecules of ATP in the mitochondrion (see Figs. 10.1 and 10.2). Shock can be caused by lack of oxygen delivery (*anemia, hypoxia,* or *ischemia*), lack of glucose substrate delivery (*glycopenia*), or mitochondrial dysfunction (*cellular dysoxia*). Oxygen delivery is defined by the following equation: oxygen content ($1.36 \times$ % hemoglobin $\times$ oxygen saturation $- 0.0003 \times Pao_2$) $\times$ flow (cardiac index) (see Table 10.1). *Anemic* shock occurs when hemoglobin concentration is too low, *hypoxic* shock occurs when oxygen saturation is too low, and *ischemic* shock occurs when flow is too low. Glucose delivery depends on glucose levels; blood flow; and, for cells with insulin-responsive glucose transporters (e.g., cardiac), insulin. *Glycopenic* shock can be caused by hypoglycemia, as well as by extreme insulin resistance. Even when oxygen delivery and glucose delivery are adequate, shock may occur as a result of mitochondrial dysfunction. For example, cyanide poisons the oxidative phosphorylation chain preventing the production of ATP. *Cellular dysoxia* occurs when the mitochondrial DNA repair enzyme, poly(ADP-ribose) polymerase (PARP), is activated to use more nicotinamide adenine dinucleotide (NAD) and ATP than is being produced.

Although the definition of shock in the preceding text is logical and operationally sound, it is not very functional because ATP measurements are not performed in patients. Therefore, the clinical state of the art in 2005 is to use surrogate clinical signs and measures to diagnose and assess shock. These signs must identify the earliest stages of shock or preferably stages of pathology, which occur before shock ensues. *Anemia* is identifiable by pallor, early compensatory tachycardia and hemoglobin concentrations <8 g per dL. Tachycardia increases cardiac output to maintain oxygen delivery despite decreased hemoglobin. *Hypoxia* is identified by early compensatory tachypnea and decreased Pao_2 <65 mm Hg. Hemoglobin remains adequately saturated until this threshold Pao_2 is reached. Tachypnea causes a reduction in Pco_2, which according to the alveolar gas equation results in a proportional increase in Pao_2. *Ischemia* is recognized in its earliest stages by tachycardia. Decreased flow occurs if stroke volume is decreased as a result of either hypovolemia or poor cardiac function. Flow under these conditions can be maintained by increased heart rate (cardiac output = heart rate $\times$ stroke volume). *Glycopenia* is identified in its earliest stages by mild hypoglycemia or hyperglycemia. Implementation of therapies that reverse anemia, hypoxia, ischemia, and glycopenia before ATP deficiency occurs can prevent shock.

Shock can be diagnosed and assessed by the progression of these clinical signs (see Table 10.2). *Anemic* shock occurs with hemoglobin levels <6 g per dL and is recognized clinically by an increase in heart rate above 98% with age, altered mental status, and tachypnea. *Ischemic* shock is recognized as persistent tachycardia with prolongation of capillary refill to >2 seconds when the systemic vasculature "vasoconstricts" to maintain perfusion pressure and blood flow to the central organs including the brain and kidney. If flow continues to decrease, hypotension ensues with reduced blood flow to the brain and altered mental status. In its final stages, shock can be recognized by the presence

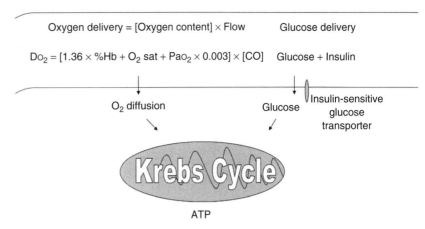

Figure 10.1 The major sources of ATP production: glucose and oxygen. ATP, adenosine triphosphate.

of anion gap acidosis. At present, the anion gap >16 mEq per L is the most commonly used surrogate marker for ATP depletion and energy failure. When oxygen delivery is inadequate, anaerobic metabolism occurs through glycolysis. Pyruvate is transformed to lactate, and lactic acid causes an anion gap. *Glycopenic* shock can be diagnosed as an anion gap of 16 mEq per L in the presence of hypoglycemia (inadequate substrate), hyperglycemia (insulin resistance), or euglycemia (inadequate substrate and insulin resistance). When glucose utilization is inadequate, an anion gap >16 mEq per L is caused by organic acid intermediates produced by catabolism of protein and/or fat to fuel the Krebs cycle.

The diagnosis of shock is confirmed by a positive response to timely therapy. Blood infusion will increase hemoglobin and should reverse tachycardia and tachypnea in patients with *anemic* shock. Fluid administration and

inotropic support should improve stroke volume, reverse tachycardia, and reduce capillary refill to <2 seconds in patients with *ischemic* shock. Glucose administration as 10% dextrose (D10) at maintenance with use of insulin to correct hyperglycemia should attain euglycemia and resolve the anion gap in patients with *glycopenic* shock.

SHOCK, SEVERITY OF ILLNESS SCORES, AND OUTCOMES

Shock commonly contributes to mortality in critically ill children. Abnormalities in physiologic parameters that represent clinical signs of shock are among the most robust predictors of death in the pediatric risk of mortality (PRISM) and pediatric logistic organ dysfunction (PELOD) scores. In the PRISM score, tachycardia (>150 bpm for children

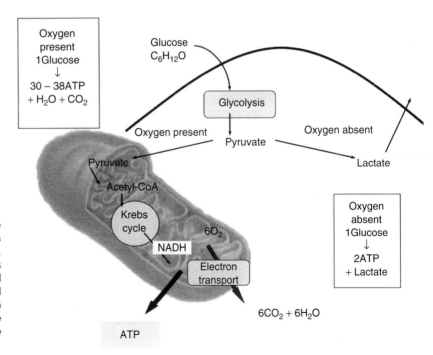

Figure 10.2 Metabolism of glucose, in the presence of oxygen, to pyruvate, which fuels the Krebs cycle. In the absence of oxygen, glucose is metabolized to pyruvate, which is metabolized to lactate. This can be recognized by an anion gap >16 mEq per L, an elevated lactate, and a wide arteriovenous oxygen saturation difference (AVDo$_2$). ATP, adenosine triphosphate, NADH, nicotinamide adenine dinucleotide (reduced form).

TABLE 10.1

HEMODYNAMIC AND OXYGEN UTILIZATION EQUATIONS

Flow and Perfusion Pressure

$Q = P/R$

$CO = MAP - CVP/SVR$ (normal $CO = 3.5-5.0$ L/min/m^2)

$MAP - CVP = CO \times SVR$ (normal $MAP - CVP$; age-specific)

$SVRI = MAP - CVP/CI \times 80$ (normal $SVRI = 70-230$ dyne sec/cm^5/m^2)

$PVRI = MPAP - PAOP/CI \times 80$ (normal $PVRI = 70-230$ dyne sec/cm^5/m^2)

Right and Left Ventricular Function

$CO = SV \times HR$

$RVSWI = SV \times MPAP$ (normal $RVSWI = 7-10$ g/min/m^2)

$LVSWI = SV \times MAP$ (normal $LVSWI = 45-55$ g/min/m^2)

Oxygen Utilization

Oxygen content $= 1.36 \times Hb \times$ % oxygen saturation $+ (0.003 \times PaO_2)$ (normal $CaO_2 = 15-20$ vol%)

$CO \times$ arterial oxygen content $=$ oxygen delivery (normal $DO_2 = 550-650$ mL/min/m^2)

$AVDO_2 =$ arterial oxygen content $-$ mixed venous oxygen content (normal $AVDO_2 = 3-5$ vol% difference)

$CO \times AVDO_2 =$ oxygen consumption (normal VO_2 range $130-190$ mL/min/m^2)

Oxygen extraction $= VO_2/DO_2$

Q, flow; P, pressure; R, resistance; Hb, hemoglobin; SV, stroke volume; HR, heart rate; CO, cardiac output; MAP, mean arterial pressure; CVP, central venous pressure; SVR, systemic vascular resistance; CI, cardiac index; SVRI, systemic vascular resistance index; PVRI, pulmonary vascular resistance index; MPAP, mean pulmonary arterial pressure; AVDO$_2$, arteriovenous oxygen saturation difference; PAOP, pulmonary artery occlusion pressure; LVSWI, left ventricular stroke work index; RVSWI, right ventricular stroke work index.

and >160 bpm for infants), tachypnea (>50 rpm for children and >60 rpm for infants), PaO$_2$/FiO$_2$<300, glucose levels <60 or >250 mg per dL, and bicarbonate concentration <16 mEq per L all predict an increased mortality. In the PELOD score, hypotension (systolic BP<65 mm Hg in neonates, <75 mm Hg infants, <85 mm Hg in children, and <95 mm Hg in adolescents) and decreased mental status (Glasgow coma scale 7 to 11) predict mortality. Abnormalities in serum creatinine (in μmol per L: <140 for

TABLE 10.2

SHOCK RECOGNITION

I do not feel good

Tachycardia (unless hypothermic) and tachypnea

Capillary refill >2 s or flash

Narrow pulse pressure or wide pulse pressure

Hypotension is a late sign

<7 days, <55 for 7 days to 1 year, <100 for 1 to 12 years, and <140 for >12 years) and prothrombin time (PT) (INR 1.5) also predict mortality. Prolonged shock and ATP depletion >1 hour causes increased serum creatinine level when renal tubular cells lose their orientation and are shed into the tubules, where tubulo-obstruction leads to acute renal dysfunction and failure. Prolonged low flow shock states also cause intravascular coagulation, with consumption of prothrombotic factors and resultant prolongation of PT.

Low cardiac output, <2 L/minute/m^2, also predicts mortality and can be assessed clinically by a capillary refill >2 seconds, a cold toe temperature, or a wide arteriovenous oxygen saturation difference (AVDO$_2$), or by more direct measures of cardiac output. Parr et al. examined cardiac output using the Fick-dilution indocyanine green dye injection technique in infants younger than 6 months who required cardiac surgery.[1] The study showed that mortality risk increased in this population when cardiac index was less then 2 L/minute/m^2. Inotropic support followed by afterload reduction with nitroprusside and volume loading was effective in improving cardiac output in these children.[2] Capillary refill <2 seconds was a clinical sign that cardiac index was >2 L/minute/m^2 in this population. Children with septic shock appear to require a higher cardiac output than children with isolated cardiogenic shock. Pollack et al. demonstrated that best outcomes are observed in these patients when the cardiac index is between 3.3 to 6 L/minute/m^2 in children with septic shock.[3] Ceneviva et al. demonstrated that children with septic shock could have any of the three cardiovascular derangements: high cardiac output (>5.5 L/minute/m^2) and low systemic vascular resistance (SVR) (<800 dynes sec per cm^5), low cardiac output (<3.3 L/minute/m^2) and low SVR, or low cardiac output and high SVR (>1,200 dynes sec per cm^5). They found that the use of vasopressors, inotropes and vasopressors, or inotropes and vasodilators returned the cardiac output to the favorable range.[4] Similar to Parr et al., they found that patients with low cardiac output had the highest risk of mortality.

Time-Sensitive Reversal of Clinical Signs of Shock Improves Outcomes

Time-sensitive early reversal of clinical signs of shock improves outcomes in patients who are critically ill. A recent adult study by Rivers et al. demonstrated the importance of early goal-directed therapies, which maintain not only blood pressure but also oxygen delivery.[5] In this study, adults presenting to the emergency department in shock were randomized to therapies directed at achieving normal blood pressure in one arm and to those directed at achieving normal blood pressure and a superior vena cava oxygen saturation, >70%, (equivalent to a mixed venous oxygen saturation of 62%) in the other arm, using packed red blood cell transfusion for patients with a hemoglobin level <10 g per dL (to reverse *anemic* shock) and then using fluids and inotropic support (to reverse *ischemic* shock) if the superior venous saturation remained <70%. Mitochondria usually extract oxygen according to the metabolic need. Oxygen delivery to mitochondria depends on the oxygen-carrying capacity (% hemoglobin), the extent of oxygen provided (oxygen saturation of hemoglobin plus oxygen dissolved in plasma), and cardiac output. If the % hemoglobin and arterial oxygen saturation are normal, then only cardiac output determines oxygen delivery. As cardiac output decreases and metabolic demands remain the same, the mitochondria extract more oxygen to maintain the same oxygen consumption and subsequent energy production. When this happens, the oxygen saturation of blood returning to the heart decreases. In a healthy child, the superior vena cava oxygen saturation is 75%. Rivers et al. observed that patients in the first arm attained a normal blood pressure but had a superior vena cava oxygen saturation of only 65%, whereas those in the second treatment arm maintained the blood pressure and had a superior vena cava oxygen saturation >70%. This was attained with more blood transfusion, fluid resuscitation, and inotrope use. This combination of blood pressure and oxygen delivery–directed therapy resulted in a 50% reduction in mortality, as well as reversal of PT abnormalities. Resuscitation efforts directed at the maintenance of blood pressure and cardiac output improved outcome and also reversed coagulopathy.

In a second analysis of the study, the authors evaluated patients who had shock (defined as tachycardia and decreased central venous oxygen saturation [$ScvO_2$]) irrespective of blood pressure. Interestingly, these patients had higher mortality rates than patients with hypotension. When patients with tachycardia, $ScvO_2$ saturation <70%, and normotension were evaluated according to treatment arms, those who received therapies directed at improving $ScvO_2$ saturation to >70% received more fluids and more inotropes. These patients had a reduction in the development of multiple organ failure and mortality compared to the patients not treated to maintain an $ScvO_2$ saturation >70%. The authors called *adult* shock without hypotension as "cryptic shock." *Ischemic* shock without hypotension can be represented by the following equation: decreased cardiac output = normal or high mean arterial pressure (MAP) − central venous pressure (CVP)/increased SVR. Reversal of normotensive *ischemic* shock reduces organ failure and mortality.

Emergency departments place central lines for measurement of superior vena cava oxygen saturations less frequently in children than in adults. Therefore, Han and Orr et al. examined early goal-directed therapy for neonatal and pediatric septic shock and all cause septic shock in community hospital emergency departments, using prolonged capillary refill >2 seconds as a surrogate marker of decreased cardiac output, according to the recommendations of Parr et al. (in the preceding text), rather than using decreased $ScvO_2$ saturation.[1,6,7] Mortality and neuromorbidity increased in ascending order with tachycardia alone, hypotension with normal capillary refill, prolonged capillary refill without hypotension, and prolonged capillary refill with hypotension. Reversal of these clinical signs in the emergency department reduced mortality and neuromorbidity by >50%. Each hour that went by without reversal of hypotension or reduction in capillary refill to <2 seconds was associated with a twofold increased odds ratio of death from multiple organ failure.

The importance of reversing glycopenia was documented by Van den Berghe et al. in the adult surgical intensive care unit (ICU) setting.[8] These investigators gave all patients D10 at maintenance dose to meet glucose requirements. They then randomized patients to strict euglycemic control with insulin to maintain glucose levels between 80 and 120 mg per dL or to usual practice. Patients treated with insulin had a decreased serum glucose/glucose infusion rate ratio (45 vs. 75) compared to those not treated with insulin, and the former experienced a 50% reduction in mortality (3% vs. 7%). All improvement in outcome was attributed to reduction in deaths from septic shock and multiple organ failure. Administration of glucose prevents hypoglycemia, and administration of insulin for hyperglycemia guarantees delivery of glucose into the organs with insulin-dependent glucose transporters, especially the cardiovascular system. Using anion gap acidosis as a surrogate marker of energy failure, Lin et al. reported that elevated serum glucose/glucose infusion rate ratio predicted anion gap acidosis in children with shock.[9] Use of insulin to decrease the serum glucose/glucose infusion rate ratio resolved anion gap acidosis in these patients.

PHYSIOLOGY AND PATHOPHYSIOLOGY

The Stress Response

The stress response is common in critical illness. Also referred to as the *fight* or *flight response*, it is dominated by central and sympathetic nervous system activation. The central nervous system releases adrenocorticotropic hormone (ACTH), which in turn stimulates the adrenal glands to release cortisol. The sympathetic system releases epinephrine and norepinephrine. Cortisol facilitates the actions of these two catecholamines. Epinephrine and norepinephrine increase cardiac output by increasing heart rate and stroke volume. These catecholamines also increase blood pressure. Epinephrine increases heart rate and contractility, whereas norepinephrine increases contractility and systemic vascular tone. To fuel these increased energy needs, glucagon is also released. It increases glucose delivery to the Krebs cycle through activation of glycogenolysis and gluconeogenesis.

The Shock Response

The shock response occurs when the stress is not from fight or flight but instead from an acute decrease in oxygen delivery and/or ATP production. Severe and acute hemorrhage; hypovolemia from diarrhea; or cardiac and vascular dysfunction from sepsis, toxins, or drugs causes the brain to orchestrate the immediate life-preserving shock response. This is somewhat similar to the stress response, but more pronounced. Catecholamine and cortisol levels are higher. For example, cortisol levels can reach 30 μg per dL during stress but 150 to 300 μg per dL during shock. The angiotensin/aldosterone–ADH/vasopressin system is also activated to preserve the intravascular fluid. The catecholamine surge induces tachycardia, and the angiotensin/aldosterone–ADH/vasopressin surge causes oliguria. Glucagon is also released. In concert with higher cortisol and catecholamine levels, this hormone induces hyperglycemia not only through gluconeogenesis but also inadvertently through insulin resistance. This shock response attains short-term survival in patients, but medical interventions are frequently needed to attain long-term survival in most cases. Understanding and use of physiologic principles is required to attain long-term survival in these patients.

Cardiovascular Physiology

Flow across a pipe depends on the difference in pressure from one end to the other (perfusion pressure), as well as on the circumference of the pipe. The greater the difference in pressure, the greater the flow. The greater the circumference, the lesser the resistance and the greater the flow. This can be viewed by the following equation: flow (Q) = change in Pressure (ΔP)/Resistance (R).

The cardiovascular system can be viewed similarly as cardiac output = MAP − CVP/SVR. This equation explains the important pathophysiologic principles of shock. First, it guides us in the management of blood pressure. MAP − CVP is more important than MAP alone. According to the equation, one can theoretically have a normal MAP but no forward flow (cardiac output = 0), for example, if CVP = MAP. When one uses fluid resuscitation to improve blood pressure, the increase in MAP must be greater than the increase in CVP. If the increase in MAP is less than the increase in CVP then the perfusion pressure is reduced. Cardiovascular agents, and not more fluid, are indicated to improve blood pressure in this scenario. Second, the equation guides us in the management of cardiac output or blood flow. Cardiac output can be decreased when MAP − CVP is decreased, but it can also be decreased when MAP − CVP is normal and vascular resistance is increased. Perfusion pressure can be maintained, even in a low cardiac output state, by increased vascular resistance. Hence, patients with normal blood pressure can have inadequate cardiac output because systemic vascular tone is high. Cardiac output can be improved in these patients with the use of inotropes, vasodilators, and volume loading.

Cardiac output = heart rate × stroke volume. Frank and Starling are given the much deserved credit for "popularizing" basic principles that influence stroke volume (see Fig. 10.3). Frank noted that cardiac muscle fibers contract more vigorously when stretched, as long as the fiber is not "overstretched." Starling illustrated Frank's important principle with a useful curve, which plots stroke volume (y-axis) against ventricular end-diastolic volume. Stroke volume moves up along the curve as end-diastolic filling increases to a point where the ventricle is overfilled, and then stroke volume falls off again. Inadequate preload is defined as

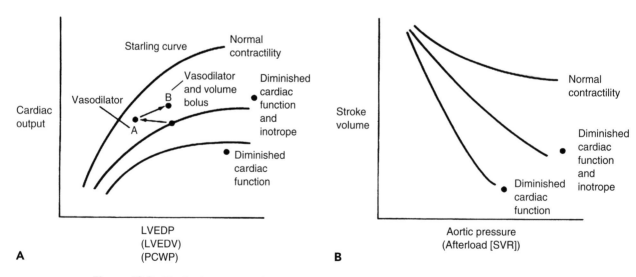

Figure 10.3 The Starling curve and ventricular compliance curve. These curves predict physiologic response to inotrope, vasopressor, and vasodilator therapies. The right side and the left side of the heart can have different Starling and ventricular compliance curves. Therapies directed at right ventricular dysfunction can be different from those directed at left ventricular dysfunction. LVEDP, left ventricular end-diastolic pressure; LVEDV, left ventricular end-diastolic volume; PCWP, pulmonary capillary wedge pressure; SVR, systemic vascular resistance.

the end-diastolic volume below which maximum stroke volume is attained. Congestive heart failure occurs when preload or end-diastolic volume goes above this optimal range. Cardiac dysfunction is represented by downward and rightward displacement of the curve. This curve can be used to demonstrate the therapeutic principles of volume loading, inotropes, and vasodilators. Patients who have inadequate stroke volume despite adequate volume loading have reduced contractility. This is represented by a flattened Starling curve. Inotropic therapy improves the Starling curve, moving it upward and to the left. Stroke volume will be greater for any given end-diastolic volume in patients treated with inotropic therapy compared to those left untreated. Patients with severe cardiac dysfunction shock require addition of a vasodilator to improve the Starling curve, moving it further upward and to the left. Concomitant volume loading is often required to move these patients up and along the new and improved Starling curve because vasodilator therapy often reduces preload.

The relationship between afterload and stroke volume is best viewed in a modified compliance curve. As afterload or aortic diastolic pressure increases, stroke volume decreases. A heart with normal function can tolerate increased aortic diastolic pressures fairly well. However, the heart with decreased contractility does not tolerate increased afterload at all. This explains the salutary effect of vasodilator therapy on the Starling curve. Afterload reduction with vasodilator therapy decreases aortic diastolic blood pressure and improves stroke volume, particularly in the poorly contracting heart. However, it is important to note that diastolic pressure is an important determinant of coronary artery perfusion pressure. Two thirds of the cardiac cycle is spent in diastole. Tachycardia, a reduced diastolic blood pressure, or increased wall stress can reduce coronary filling. The use of vasodilator therapies should be directed at reducing wall stress (afterload reduction) without causing tachycardia or diastolic hypotension.

Cardiovascular Molecular Physiology

Inotropes, vasodilators, and vasopressors work through receptors, second-messenger systems, and intracellular calcium release and sequestration (see Figs. 10.4 and 10.5). Intracellular calcium is the "currency" of the cell. Increased intracellular calcium leads to increased contraction, and decreased intracellular calcium leads to relaxation in cardiac and vascular smooth muscle cells. The cardiac cell has β-adrenergic receptors coupled by stimulatory and inhibitory G proteins to adenylyl cyclase. Interaction of β-adrenergic agonist agents (inotropes) with the β$_1$-adrenergic receptor activates adenylyl cyclase to produce cyclic adenosine monophosphate (cAMP) from adenosine monophosphate (AMP). This second messenger activates cAMP kinase, which in turn phosphorylates two important proteins, which lead to improved contractility during systole and improved relaxation during diastole. Increased

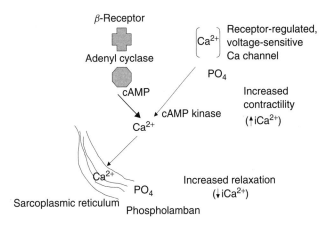

Figure 10.4 Stimulation of inotropes by β-adrenergic receptors, which increase intracellular calcium during systole and reduce intracellular calcium during diastole. This is accomplished through the cAMP second-messenger system. Type III phosphodiesterase inhibitors can potentiate these effects by preventing cyclic adenosine monophosphate (cAMP) breakdown.

contraction occurs because the calcium channel is phosphorylated in a more open position. This allows more calcium to enter the cell when the voltage-regulated calcium channel is opened by electrical depolarization. Improved relaxation occurs because the protein phospholamban is phosphorylated. This protein increases the uptake of calcium into

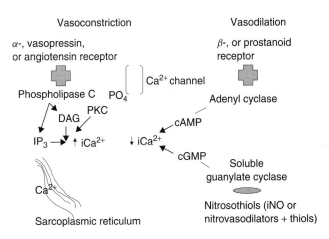

Figure 10.5 Stimulation of opposing second-messenger systems by vasoconstrictors and vasodilators. α-Adrenergic agonists, angiotensin, and vasopressin stimulate different receptors that stimulate the production of inositol tris phosphate (IP$_3$) and diacylglycerol (DAG), leading to increased iCa^{2+} and contraction. β$_2$ Agonists and vasodilator prostanoids stimulate cyclic adenosine monophosphate (cAMP) production, and nitrosovasodilators and inhaled nitric oxide (iNO) stimulate guanosine monophosphate (GMP) production. These second messengers decrease iCa^{2+} and induce vasodilation. Type III and V phosphodiesterase (PDE) inhibitors, respectively, can potentiate the effect of vasodilators. PKC, protein kinase C; cGMP, cyclic guanosine monophosphate; iCa^{2+}, ionized calcium.

the sarcoplasmic reticulum during diastole, resulting in less intracellular calcium and improved relaxation. Type III phosphodiesterases (PDEs) hydrolyze cAMP, ending the process. The type III phosphodiesterase inhibitors (PDEIs) prevent the breakdown of cAMP and prolong the effects of β agonists on contraction and relaxation.

Activation of the β-adrenergic receptor has the opposite effect in vascular smooth muscle cell. The β_2-receptor is linked to adenylyl cyclase, but the production of cAMP in this setting leads to a reduction in intracellular calcium and vasorelaxation. Intracellular calcium is also reduced and vasorelaxation caused by the second messenger cyclic guanosine monophosphate (cGMP) and guanosine monophosphate (GMP) kinase. Nitrosovasodilators can act through receptors or soluble guanylate cyclase to increase cGMP levels. Contraction of vascular smooth muscle cells is attained through the phospholipase C-mediated second-messenger system. α-Adrenergic agonists, vasopressin, and angiotensin activate phospholipase C that produces inositol tris phosphate (IP$_3$) and diacylglycerol (DAG). IP$_3$ causes release of calcium from the sarcoplasmic reticulum. DAG activates protein kinase C that phosphorylates

the calcium channel in the open position. Both second messengers lead to increased intracellular calcium and contraction.

Coagulation Physiology

During homeostasis, blood is in an endogenously anticoagulated state. However, in prolonged states of low flow shock, thrombosis and hypofibrinolysis occurs. This occurs in part because of stasis, endothelial cell ATP depletion, and endothelial cell activation mediated by systemic inflammation. The activated endothelium is procoagulant and antifibrinolytic and causes consumption of both procoagulant and anticoagulant proteins in platelet and fibrin thrombi. This is the mechanism by which patients who die from shock commonly have thrombosis and bleeding. Prolonged PT is directly related to time to resuscitation and indirectly to the amount of fluid resuscitation administered. Rapid reversal of shock with fluid resuscitation, inotropes, and vasodilators reverses and prevents systemic disseminated intravascular coagulation and bleeding. In circumstances where resuscitation is delayed, replenishment of

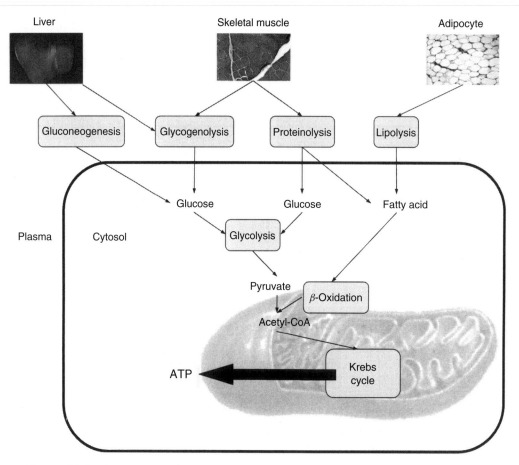

Figure 10.6 The major endogenous sources of glucose (when exogenous glucose delivery is limited) obtained by glycogenolysis and gluconeogenesis. Because children have relatively small liver and skeletal mass, they are more prone to hypoglycemia (glycopenic shock) and rely on lipolysis for energy when exogenous glucose infusion is limited. ATP, adenosine triphosphate.

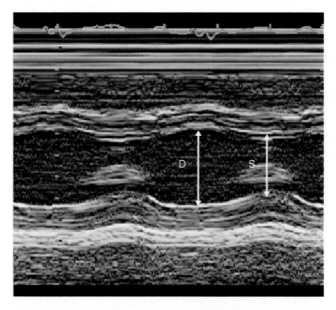

Figure 5.2.10 M-mode echocardiogram of the left ventricle from a parasternal short axis. Two cardiac cycles are depicted. The *arrows* represent the left ventricular internal cavity dimension in diastole (*D*) and systole (*S*).

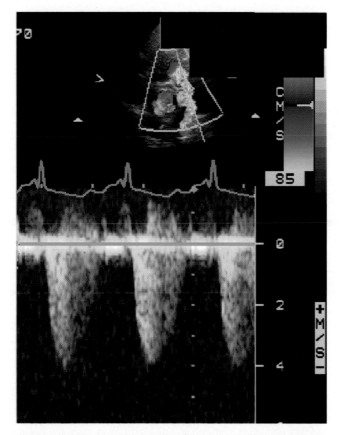

Figure 5.2.11 Doppler measurement of flow across a stenotic pulmonary valve. The velocity measures 4 m per second, which represents a pressure gradient of 64 mm Hg across the valve. $\triangle P = 4 \times (4)^2$.

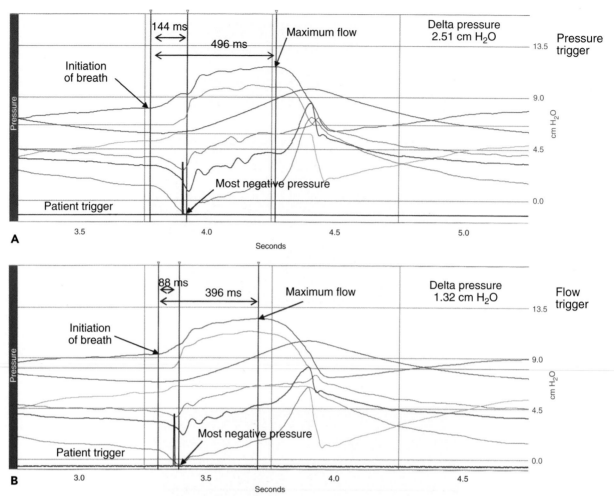

Flow pressure volume (inspiratory flow, expiratory flow, inspiratory pressure, expiratory pressure)

Figure 6.8.16 Illustration of two breaths, with ventilator set on **(A)** pressure triggering and **(B)** flow triggering. In a pressure-triggered breath, the response time and the effort necessary to trigger the ventilator (most negative pressure) are greater. PSV, pressure support ventilation.

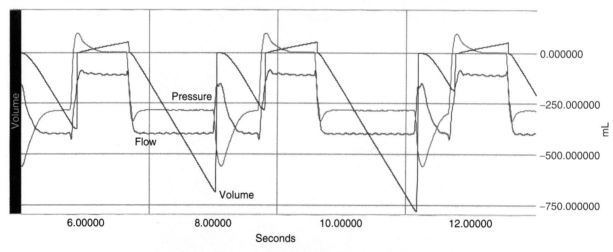

Figure 6.8.18 The illustration of two ventilators, one with an active exhalation valve and one without ventilating a lung model. The ventilator, with the active exhalation valve, is set at a rate of 10 bpm, and the other ventilator is set at 20 bpm. The second ventilator is able to trigger the ventilator with the active exhalation valve during exhalation. Adult test lung, Pressure Control, peak Inspiratory pressure 20, positive end-expiratory pressure 5 cmH$_2$O, frequency 10 breaths per minute, 3 second Inspiratory time on Servo-I; Servo 300 settings are Volume Control, Set tidal volume 70 mL, frequency 20 breaths per minute, positive end-expiratory pressure 0 cmH$_2$O.

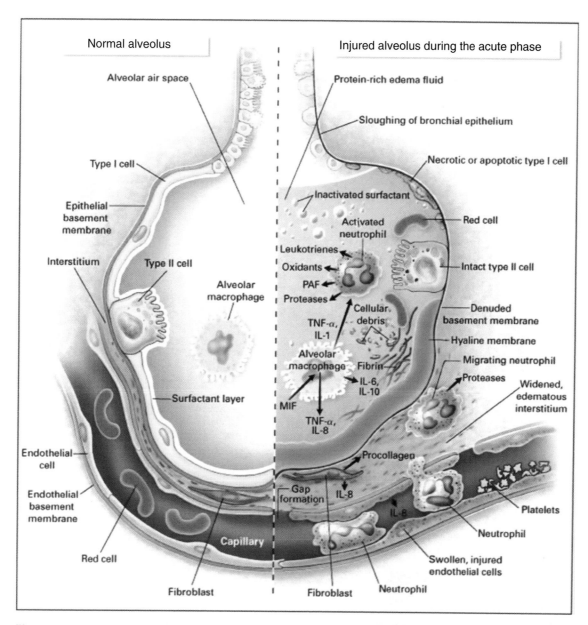

Figure 6.10.1 The normal alveolus **(left)** and the injured alveolus in the acute phase of acute lung injury and the acute respiratory distress syndrome **(right)**. (With permission from, Ware LB, Matthay MA. The acute respiratory distress syndrome. *N Engl J Med.* 2000;342(18):1334–1349. Copyright © 2000 Massachusetts Medical Society.)

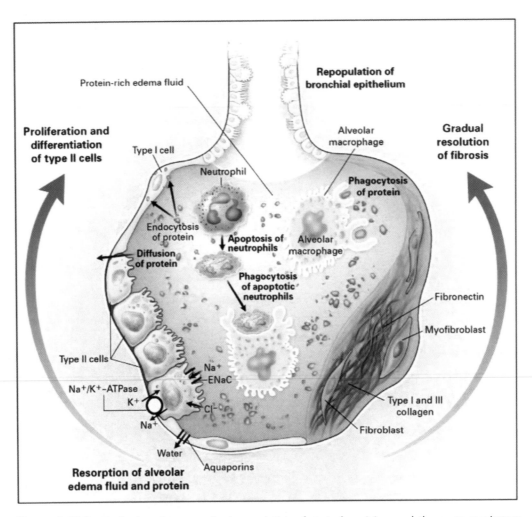

Figure 6.10.2 Mechanisms important in the resolution of acute lung injury and the acute respiratory distress syndrome. (With permission from, Ware LB, Matthay MA. The acute respiratory distress syndrome. *N Engl J Med.* 2000;342(18):1334–1349. Copyright © 2000 Massachusetts Medical Society.)

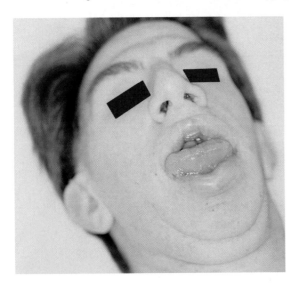

Figure 19.1 Facial swelling and airway obstruction from acute allergic reaction and anaphylaxis. (From Fleischer GR, Ludwig S, Baskin M. *Atlas of emergency medicine.* Philadelphia, PA: Lippincott Williams & Wilkins; 2004.)

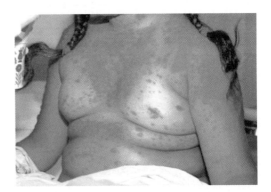

Figure 19.2b Stevens-Johnson syndrome. **B:** Same child. Note the distribution of lesions. (From Fleischer GR, Ludwig S, Baskin M. *Atlas of emergency medicine.* Philadelphia, PA: Lippincott Williams & Wilkins; 2004.)

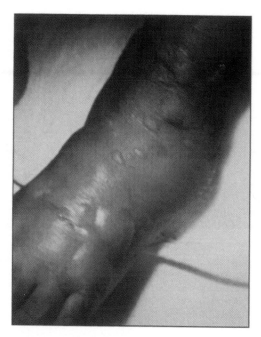

Figure 19.3 Toxic epidermal necrolysis (TEN) demonstrating the diffuse erythema and edema with overlying bullae. (From Anderson JA, Allergic drug reactions. In: Lieberman PL, Blaiss MS. *Atlas of allergic diseases*. Philadelphia, PA: Lippincott Williams & Wilkins and Current Medicine:2002:260.)

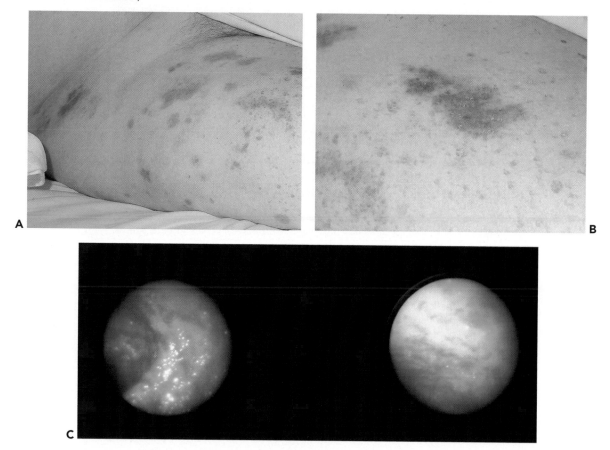

Figure 19.4 Vascular lesions of a patient with Henoch-Schönlein purpura. **A, B:** Veins of macular and papular pruritic lesions on the thigh. **C:** Endoscopic view of gastric mucosa demonstrates purpura. (From Yamada T, Alpers DH, Kaplowitz N, et al. *Atlas of gastroenterology*. 3rd ed. Philadelphia, PA: Lippincott Williams & Wilkins; 2003.)

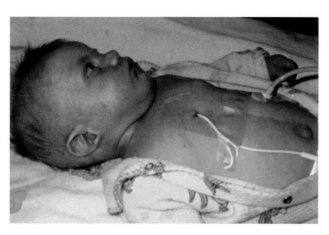

Figure 20.1 DiGeorge syndrome. A number of abnormalities that involve structures from the face to the thorax may be seen in this syndrome. (From Williams LW, Roberts JL. Immunodeficiency disorders. In: Lieberman PL, Blaiss MS, eds. *Atlas of allergic diseases*. Philadelphia, PA: Lippincott Williams & Wilkins Current Medicine; 2002.)

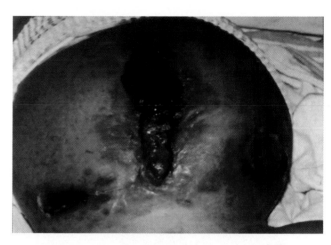

Figure 20.2 Leukocyte adhesion deficiency (LAD). In LAD, there is severe impairment of the migration of leukocytes to areas of inflammation or infection. (From Williams LW, Roberts JL. Immunodeficiency disorders. In: Lieberman PL, Blaiss MS, eds. *Atlas of allergic diseases*. Philadelphia, PA: Lippincott Williams & Wilkins Current Medicine; 2002.)

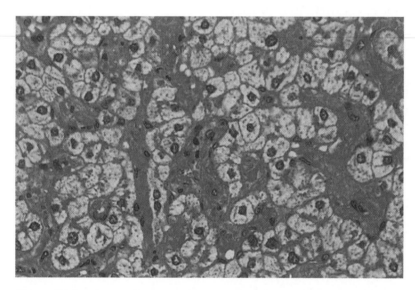

Figure 24.1 Clumps of sickled red blood cells packed in the sinusoidal spaces. (H&E stain; original magnification × 200.) (From Yamada T, Alpens DH, Laine L, et al. *Atlas of gastroenterology*, 3rd ed. Philadelphia, PA: Lippincott Williams & Wilkins; 2003:938.)

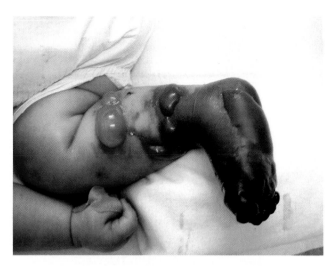

Figure 25.1 Physical findings of a child with a popliteal artery thrombosis.

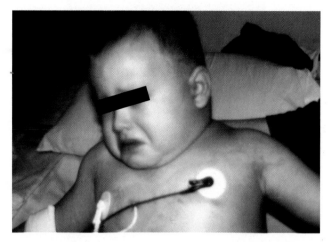

Figure 25.3 Physical findings of a child with superior vena cava syndrome.

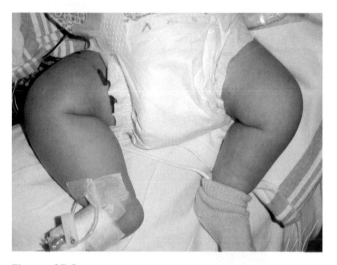

Figure 25.2 Physical findings of a child with a femoral vein thrombosis.

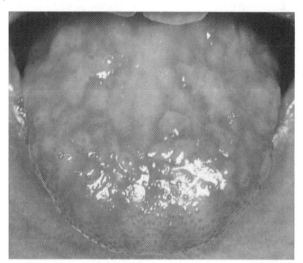

Figure 29.1 Ulcerated tongue in a patient with graft versus host disease following BMT. (From Yamada T, Alpers DH, Kaplowitz N, et al. *Atlas of gastroenterology*. Philadelphia, PA: Lippincott Williams & Wilkins; 2003.)

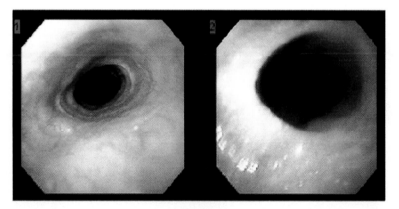

Figure 29.2 Graft versus host disease. Multiple fine mucosal webs are present in the esophagus. (From Yamada T, Alpers DH, Kaplowitz N, et al. *Atlas of gastroenterology*. Philadelphia, PA: Lippincott Williams & Wilkins; 2003:216.)

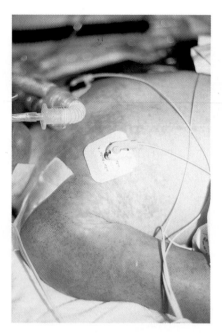

Figure 49.1 Purpura fulminans in a child with pneumococcal sepsis. (From Fleisher GR, Ludwig S, Baskin M. *Atlas of emergency medicine*. Philadelphia, PA: Lippincott Williams & Wilkins; 2004: 181.)

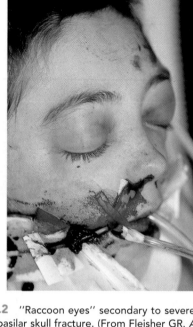

Figure 52.2 "Raccoon eyes" secondary to severe closed head injury with basilar skull fracture. (From Fleisher GR. *Atlas of emergency medicine*. Philadelphia, PA: Lippincott Williams & Wilkins; 2004:388.)

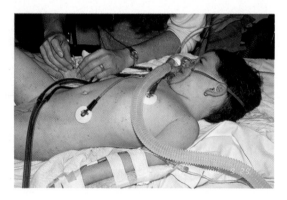

Figure 49.2 Infection with *Neisseria meningitidis*. (From Fleisher GR, Ludwig S, Baskin M. *Atlas of emergency medicine*. Philadelphia, PA: Lippincott Williams & Wilkins; 2004: 180.)

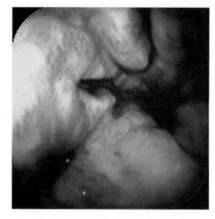

Figure 60.1 Endoscopic view of moderate-sized esophageal varices with multiple red marks. (From Yamada T, Alpers DH, Kaplowitz N, et al. Alpers DH, Laine L, et al., eds. *Atlas of gastroenterology*, 3rd ed. Philadelphia, PA: Lippincott Williams & Wilkins; 2003.)

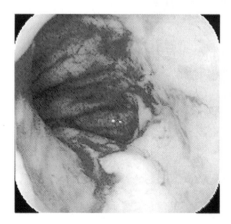

Figure 60.2 Endoscopic view of an oozing distal esophageal ulcer. (From Yamada T, Alpers DH, Laine L, et al., eds. *Atlas of gastroenterology*, 3rd ed. Philadelphia, PA: Lippincott Williams & Wilkins; 2003.)

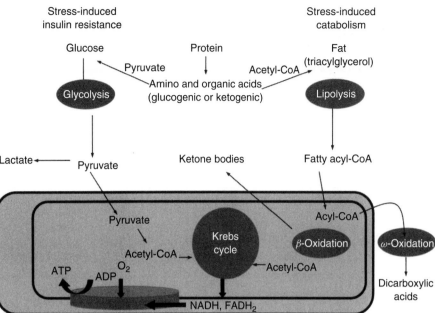

Figure 10.7 Insulin resistance occurring during stress secondary to increased glucagon, cortisol, and catecholamine. This can contribute to hyperglycemic glycopenic shock even when oxygen delivery is adequate. These patients will have an anion gap >16 mEq per L caused by some combination of metabolic acids including lactate, amino acids, organic acids, ketone bodies, and/or dicarboxylic acids generated from ω-oxidation. The combination depends on the metabolic capabilities of the child. ATP, adenosine triphosphate; ADP, adenosine diphosphate; NADH, nicotinamide adenine dinucleotide (reduced form); FADH$_2$, flavin adenine dinucleotide (reduced form).

anticoagulant proteins such as protein C may be helpful. In the face of life-threatening or limb-threatening thrombosis, fibrinolytic therapies can be effective to restore blood flow.

Energy Metabolism Physiology

The predominant pathway of energy production goes through the Krebs cycle, which produces ATP in mitochondria. Glucose or carbohydrates are the major energy substrates that fuel the Krebs cycle to produce 36 ATPs per molecule. During stress and periods of increased energy demand, glucose is produced from glycogenolysis and gluconeogenesis (see Fig. 10.6). However, in children and infants in particular, glycogenolysis and gluconeogenesis is limited because of small liver (site of glycogenolysis) and skeletal muscle (site of gluconeogenesis) mass. Fat metabolism is the secondary source of energy in this circumstance. Long-chain fatty acids are oxidized, and carnitine is utilized to shuttle acyl-CoA into mitochondria. Protein catabolism can also contribute amino acids directly into the Krebs cycle for energy production.

When oxygen delivery is limited, glycolysis becomes a major source of energy. Pyruvate cannot be converted to acetyl-CoA, so it is instead converted into lactate, which can be measured. In the presence of limited glucose delivery caused by hypoglycemia or insulin resistance, fatty acid metabolism and amino acid metabolism become the predominant sources of energy. The intermediates in these cycles are organic acids, which can be measured as well. ATP production can be increased by providing glucose to these patients. If insulin resistance is severe, then hyperglycemia will be present, and the addition of insulin will increase ATP production, increasing glucose delivery (see Fig. 10.7). Inborn errors of metabolism become quite

important when infants and children depend on fat and protein catabolism for energy. Some intermediates in these conditions are themselves mitochondrial poisons. Therapy in these children (with the notable exception of those with pyruvate dehydrogenase complex deficiency) is directed at adequate glucose delivery and the use of insulin for hyperglycemia to provide adequate energy substrates and to turn off catabolism. Cardiovascular energy metabolism function is dependent on glucose transporters II and IV, which are insulin-dependent. The use of glucose, insulin, and potassium improve contractility and cardiac function. It was initially thought that this was mediated through increased cAMP production. However, it is now accepted that therapy with insulin and glucose increases ATP stores and energy balance in myocardium.

GOAL-DIRECTED THERAPY

Clinical Goals

Resuscitation to clinical goals is the first priority (see Table 10.3). Patients should be resuscitated to normal mental status, normal pulse quality proximally and distally, equal central and peripheral temperatures, capillary refill <2 seconds, and urine output >1 mL/kg/hour. Twenty percent of blood flow goes to the brain and 20% goes to the kidney; therefore, clinical examination of function in these two organs is quite useful. These two organs control blood flow with autoregulation and are dependent on perfusion pressure (MAP − CVP) to maintain perfusion (see Fig. 10.8). Endotoxemia, cirrhosis, aminoglycosides, cisplatin, tacrolimus, and cyclosporine A induce preglomerular vasoconstriction. In these children, higher perfusion pressures (MAP − CVP) are required to perfuse the

TABLE 10.3
RESUSCITATION GOALS

I feel good
Normal heart rate and respiratory rate for age
Normal pulse pressure for age
Capillary refill <2 s
Normal perfusion pressure (MAP − CVP)
Superior vena cava oxygen saturation >70
Cardiac index >2 L/min/m^2 for cardiogenic shock
Cardiac index 3.3–6 L/min/m^2 for septic shock
AVDo$_2$ difference 3%–5%
Difference between arterial and central venous oxygen
    saturation 25%
Anion gap <16 mEq/L
Lactate <2 mmol/L
Normoglycemia (D10 at maintenance ± insulin)
PT <1.5 s
Urine output >1 mL/kg/h

MAP, mean arterial pressure; CVP, central venous pressure; AVDo$_2$,
arteriovenous oxygen saturation difference; PT, prothrombin time.

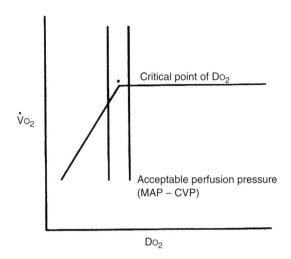

Normal MAP − CVP for age:

Infant (6 mo)	>56 mm Hg
Toddler (2 y)	>59 mm Hg
School age (7 y)	>65 mm Hg
Adolescent (15 y)	>75 mm Hg

Figure 10.9 The goal of inotrope, vasodilator, and vasopressor therapy: maintaining perfusion pressure while also maintaining a cardiac output, which provides enough oxygen delivery to meet the patient's oxygen consumption needs. MAP, mean arterial pressure; CVP, central venous pressure.

kidney and to maintain urine output. Distal pulse quality, temperature, and capillary refill reflect systemic vascular tone and cardiac output. Normal capillary refill and toe temperature assures a cardiac index >2 L/minute/m^2. Fluid resuscitation should be monitored using hepatomegaly, rales being heard on auscultation, increasing tachypnea, or a wet cough as indications to stop fluid resuscitation and begin inotrope therapy.

Hemodynamic and Oxygen Utilization Goals

Normal heart rate for age and normal perfusion pressure for age (MAP − CVP) are the initial hemodynamic goals before central access is attained (see Fig. 10.9). Fluid resuscitation

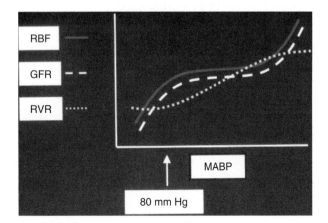

Figure 10.8 Maintenance of blood flow in the kidney and brain by perfusion pressure even if hypovolemia or reduced cardiac output is present. RBF, renal blood flow; GFR, glomerular filtration rate; RVR, renal vascular rate; MABP, mean arterial blood pressure.

can be monitored by observing effects on heart rate and MAP − CVP. The heart rate will decrease and MAP − CVP will increase when fluid resuscitation is effective. The heart rate will increase and MAP − CVP will narrow if too much fluid is given. The shock index (heart rate/systolic blood pressure [SBP]) can be used to assess the effectiveness of fluid and inotrope therapy as well. As stroke volume is increased by therapy, heart rate will decrease and SBP will increase. The shock index will decrease. If stroke volume does not improve with resuscitation, then heart rate will not decrease, SBP will not increase, and shock index will not improve.

In patients with superior vena cava central venous catheters, an oxygen saturation >70% should be used as a goal. If oxygen saturation is <70% and if anemia is present, then the child should be transfused with Hb >10 g per dL. If oxygen saturation is <70% without anemia, then inotropes and vasodilators can be used to improve cardiac output until the central venous saturation is >70%. AVDo$_2$ can also be calculated with a hemodynamic goal of 3% to 5%. If it is wider than 5% then cardiac output should be increased with therapy until the AVDo$_2$ returns to the normal range. The AVDo$_2$ is most accurate when the central venous catheter is in the pulmonary artery. Cardiac output can be measured using either the pulse-induced contour cardiac output (PICCO) or pulmonary catheters.

The goal is a cardiac index >2 L/minute/m^2 in cardiogenic shock and between 3.3 and 6 L/minute/m^2 in septic shock. In patients with pulmonary artery or left atrial catheters, the pulmonary artery occlusion pressure and left atrial pressure (LAP) should be attained at the level that assures the best cardiac output. Higher pressures are required to attain the optimal end-diastolic volume for function on the Starling curve in a noncompliant heart such as the heart of children who are recovering from cardiopulmonary bypass and cardiac surgery.

Biochemical Goals

Many use lactate as a serum measure of anaerobic metabolism; however, the lactate level can be elevated by many conditions even in the absence of shock. These include metabolic disorders, lymphoproliferative disorders, liver failure, and sepsis. Lactate is most useful in the setting of preoperative and postoperative cardiogenic shock (although its levels can be increased even in the absence of the low flow state). For these patients, mortality risk increases as serum lactate levels rise above 2 mmol per L. When used as a hemodynamic goal, a level <2 mmol per L is the target. In other instances, anion gap acidosis is used as a biochemical goal. Anion gap acidosis can be attributed to anaerobic metabolism in low flow states and to organic acids in glycopenic states; the goal is an anion gap <16 mEq per L. If patients have received bicarbonate, it will mask acidosis but not the anion gap. Non–anion gap acidosis caused by the strong ions such as Na$^+$ and Cl$^-$ is common in patients resuscitated with saline. The acidosis remains although the anion gap is resolved. It is caused by strong ion administration (NaCl) not by energy failure. Troponin I levels can be used as a therapeutic marker for cardiac injury and dysfunction. These levels are increased with myocardial injury and become normal with the resolution of myocardial injury. Creatinine clearance can be used as a therapeutic marker for renal dysfunction. Creatinine clearance improves as the renal hemodynamics improves.

THERAPY

Fluids

Fluid therapy is the hallmark of shock resuscitation in infants and children. It is used to reverse the hypovolemic state and optimize the Starling curve to provide optimal flow and cardiac output for any degree of contractility. Approximately 8% of total blood volume is in the arterial side, 70% in the venous side, and 12% in the capillary beds. The total blood volume is 85 mL per kg in a newborn and 65 mL per kg in an infant. Rapid resuscitation can restore the circulating volume. Because of significant vasoconstricting abilities, hypotension is not seen until 50% of blood volume is lost (see Fig. 10.10). Therefore, a rapid push of 30

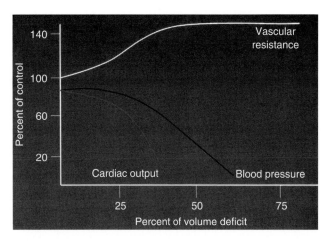

Figure 10.10 Maintenance of mean arterial pressure (MAP) and perfusion pressure by systemic vasoconstriction despite hypovolemia and reduced cardiac output.

to 40 mL per kg is required to restore intravascular volume. If the patient has capillary leak syndrome and crystalloid fluids are being used, then quite large volumes of fluid can be needed in the first hour (up to 200 mL per kg in septic shock). Crystalloids or colloids can be used to restore the intravascular volume. Less colloids are needed than crystalloids because they redistribute to the extravascular space more slowly. In a large randomized controlled trial, albumin appeared to be most effective in patients with adult sepsis/septic shock compared to crystalloids.[10] In a randomized controlled trial of children with dengue shock, crystalloid and colloids performed equally well.[11] Some use crystalloid as the first line and followed it up with colloid if needed.[12]

Providing rapid volume bolus using a pushing technique not only restores intravascular volume but also turns off the expression of inflammation and coagulation genes. Rapid and aggressive volume in the first hour with shock improves survival in animal models and humans. Fluid administration should be judicious, however, in neonates and children with cardiogenic failure from cardiomyopathy or congenital heart disease. These children may be pushed off the Starling curve if too aggressively managed. Volumes of 20 mL per kg of fluid are recommended, with monitoring of CVP/LAP/ pulmonary artery occlusion pressure (PAOP) in these patients.

Blood

Blood is required in patients with *anemic* shock. Mitochondria cannot extract the last 20% of oxygen bound to hemoglobin. Under normal conditions, the mitochondria extract 25% of oxygen bound to hemoglobin. This is seen clinically by a mixed venous oxygen saturation of 75% in a healthy patient with an arterial blood oxygen saturation of 100%. In a child with 10 g per dL of hemoglobin, only 8 g per dL is available for extraction (20% cannot be extracted), 2.5 g per dL is used for oxygen extraction, leaving a surplus of 5.5 g per dL of hemoglobin. In states of hemolysis, hemolytic shock can occur when this surplus is lost or when hemoglobin drops below 5 g per dL. Mortality rates increase when hemoglobin drops below 6 g per dL. This is also true with hemorrhagic shock. Transfusion of blood is lifesaving in these circumstances. Whole blood is available in some parts of the world, and packed red blood cells are available in other parts of the world. The usual hemoglobin concentration of packed red blood cells is 20 g per dL. Because the blood volume of a child ranges from 85 mL per kg in the newborn to 65 mL per kg in the child, 10 mL per kg of packed red cells should increase the hemoglobin concentration by approximately 2 g per dL.

Inotropes

Inotropic agents are used to increase contractility and cardiac output (see Table 10.4). *Dobutamine* is a β_1-adrenergic agonist with chronotropic and inotropic actions. It is considered to be a partial agonist. In adults, dobutamine is effective; however, there is an age-specific insensitivity to the agent in children. Perkin et al. demonstrated that children younger than 2 years have reduced response to dobutamine.[13] At a dosage >10 μg/kg/minute, dobutamine can lead to significant afterload reduction and at times to hypotension. This is thought to occur because dobutamine at this dosage has some α_2-racemer effect that inhibits release of norepinephrine from the presynaptic terminal. This in turn reduces vascular tone.

Epinephrine is the inotrope of choice for patients who fail dobutamine therapy. Adults and children who are resistant to dobutamine therapy respond to epinephrine.[14] Epinephrine is the natural circulating neurohormone that is produced to increase contractility during stress and shock. Epinephrine is a β_1-, β_2-, α_1-, and α_2-adrenergic agonist. At lower dosage (0.05 μg/kg/minute), the β_2-adrenergic effect negates the α_1-adrenergic effect, giving nearly pure inotrope qualities. The α_1-adrenergic effects become more prominent as the epinephrine dosage approaches and exceeds 0.3 μg/kg/minute. Patients with heart failure and increased SVR may be harmed by higher dosage of epinephrine unless it is concomitantly administered with a vasodilator or inodilator (see subsequent text).

Vasodilators

Vasodilators are used to reduce pulmonary vascular resistance or SVR and to improve cardiac output. The nitroso-vasodilators depend on the release of nitrosothiols, nitric oxide donors, to activate soluble guanylate cyclase and release cGMP. Nitroprusside is a systemic and pulmonary vasodilator. An accepted starting dosage is 1 μg/kg/minute. Nitroglycerin has somewhat selective dose-dependent effects. It is a coronary artery vasodilator at <1 μg/kg/minute, a pulmonary vasodilator at 1 μg/kg/minute, and a systemic

TABLE 10.4

INOTROPES, VASOPRESSORS, AND VASODILATORS

Dopamine	Inotrope (β_1 agonist) at low dose, vasopressor (α agonist at higher dose), age-specific insensitivity
T$_3$	Effective inotrope (increases cAMP) postcardiopulmonary bypass
Dobutamine	Inotrope (β_1 agonist) with some afterload reduction and chronotropy with higher dose (α_2 agonist effect)
Epinephrine	Most potent inotrope (β_1, β_2, α_1, and α_2 activity) vasopressor effect with higher dose
Isoproterenol	Potent inotrope and pulmonary vasodilator (β_1 and β_2 agonist); useful in pulmonary hypertensive crisis
Norepinephrine	Most potent vasopressor (β_1, α_1, and α_2 agonist), also potent inotrope; absent β_2 effect distinguishes it from epinephrine
Phenylephrine	Pure α agonist is a vasopressor without inotropic activity; indicated in tetralogy of Fallot "spells"
Angiotensin	Vasopressor without inotrope activity; can be used for norepinephrine resistance and vasodilator toxicity
Vasopressin	Vasopressor without inotrope activity; physiologic replacement can be used for norepinephrine resistance and vasodilator toxicity
Phentolamine	α_1- and α_2-antagonist vasodilator; can be used in combination with epinephrine or norepinephrine
Nitroglycerin	Dose-dependent venous and pulmonary artery, and systemic artery vasodilator (cGMP-mediated)
Nitroprusside	Systemic arterial vasodilator (cGMP-mediated); monitor cyanide and isothiocyanate metabolites
Amrinone	Inodilator (type III phosphodiesterase inhibitor) metabolized predominantly in the liver
Milrinone	Inodilator (type III phosphodiesterase inhibitor) metabolized predominantly in the kidney
Enoximone	Inodilator (type III phosphodiesterase inhibitor)
Prostacyclin	Good pulmonary vasodilator (cAMP mediated); also improves microcirculatory perfusion
Prostaglandin E$_1$	Maintains open ductus arteriosus (cAMP effect)
Inhaled nitric oxide	Excellent pulmonary vasodilator (cGMP effect)
Pentoxyfilline	Improves outcome in premature infants with sepsis (phosphodiesterase inhibitor)
Phenoxy benzamine	Long-acting α_1- and α_2-antagonist used in single ventricle patients after cardiopulmonary bypass

cAMP, cyclic adenosine monophosphate; T$_3$, tri-iodothyronine; cGMP, cyclic guanosine monophosphate.

vasodilator at 3 μg/kg/minute. Inhaled nitric oxide (iNO) is a selective pulmonary vasodilator, which can be started at 5 ppm. Prostaglandins are vasodilators that increase cAMP levels. Prostacyclin can be started at 3 ng/kg/minute. Prostaglandin E_1 can be started at 0.1 μg/kg/minute and is effective in maintaining an open ductus arteriosus in newborns with ductal-dependent congenital heart disease.

α-Adrenergic antagonists also have a role as vasodilators. Phentolamine is a competitive antagonist. It has been used in combination with epinephrine or norepinephrine to offset the α-adrenergic effects and to facilitate the β-adrenergic effects of these agents. Phenoxybenzamine has been used for afterload reduction in neonates with single ventricle physiology.[15] Phenoxybenzamine binds to and inhibits the α-adrenergic receptor through covalent modification. Hence, it has a very long half-life elimination. Phenoxybenzamine has also been used to reverse hypertension in patients with pheochromocytoma.

Inodilators

The PDEIs are an important class of drugs, which mediate inotropy and vasodilation by preventing hydrolysis of cAMP (type III PDEI, milrinone, amrinone, enoximone, or pentoxyfilline) and/or cGMP (type V PDEI, sildenafil, dipyridamole, or pentoxyfilline). When administered alone, the increase in cAMP improves contractility and diastolic relaxation and also causes vasodilation of pulmonary and systemic arterial vasculature. The interaction of PDEIs with concomitant inotropes, vasodilators, and even vasopressors can be used to a therapeutic advantage in patients with shock. For example, epinephrine can remain a potent, relatively pure inotrope at higher dosages. For any given dose of epinephrine, type III PDEIs prevent the breakdown of cAMP produced by β_1- and β_1-adrenergic stimulation. This increased intracellular cAMP inhibits the effects of α_1-adrenergic stimulation. Hence, vasoconstriction is less likely to occur at higher dosage of epinephrine. Norepinephrine can also become a more effective inotrope, while maintaining vasopressor effectiveness, when administered with a type III PDEI. The cAMP produced by the β_1-receptor is not hydrolyzed. Increased cardiac cAMP level leads to improved contractility and relaxation. The α_1- and α_2-adrenergic effects remain the same because, in the absence of β_2 stimulation, milrinone has a minimal effect on vasodilation compared to the norepinephrine-mediated α-adrenergic vasoconstriction. The type V PDEIs (e.g., sildenafil, dipyridamole) have also been evaluated in patients for potentiation of the pulmonary vasodilator effects of iNO.

The major problem with presently used PDE drugs is their relatively prolonged half-life compared to catecholamines and nitrosovasodilators. Although the latter agents are eliminated within minutes, PDEIs are not eliminated for hours. This half-life elimination is a more important consideration when organ failure exists. For example, milrinone is predominantly eliminated by the kidney and amrinone is predominantly eliminated by the liver. When toxicities such as hypotension or tachyarrhythmias are observed, these drugs should be discontinued. Interestingly, norepinephrine has been reported as being an effective antidote for these toxicities. As mentioned in the preceding text, norepinephrine is an α_1-adrenergic agonist with β_1- but not β_2-adrenergic activity. It increases the blood pressure (α_1-adrenergic effect) and cardiac output (β_1-adrenergic effect) but does not exacerbate the vasodilatory effect of the PDEIs (no β_2-adrenergic effect).

Isoproterenol is an important inodilator with β_1- and β_2-adrenergic activity. It is an important drug in the treatment of heart block, refractory status asthmaticus, and pulmonary hypertensive crises with right ventricular failure. Levosimendan represents a new class of inodilators, which sensitizes calcium binding in the actin–tropomyosin complex, improving contractility while also hyperpolarizing K channels, causing vasodilation.

Vasopressors

Phenylephrine is a pure α-adrenergic receptor agonist. Its main role in children is for reversal of *tetralogy of Fallot* spells. Infants and children with *tetralogy of Fallot* have a thickened infundibulum, which tends to undergo spasm and causes right-to-left blood flow through the ventricular septal defect. This spasm can be so severe that it prevents blood flow through the lung. The therapies used include oxygen and morphine to relax the infundibulum and knee-to-chest positioning to increase afterload and help generate left-to-right flow across the ventricular septal defect. When these maneuvers fail, phenylephrine is the drug of choice. Increased systemic arterial vasoconstriction leads to left-to-right shunting and perfusion of the lung. Because phenylephrine has no β-adrenergic effects, it does not increase heart rate. Hence, the heart is better able to fill, and the infundibular narrowing is also not worsened by increased contractility.

There has been a recent interest in the use of two old vasopressors, angiotensin and vasopressin. Angiotensin interacts with the angiotensin receptor and mediates vasoconstriction through the phospholipase C second-messenger system. It has a relatively long half-life compared to catecholamines. Angiotensin also mediates blood pressure effects through increased aldosterone secretion. It is prudent to determine whether the use of angiotensin reduces cardiac output in children with hypotension because it has no known inotropic effects. Vasopressin has been rediscovered as well. Unlike angiotensin, vasopressin is administered only in physiologic dosage and is thought to improve blood pressure not only through interaction with the vasopressin receptor and the phospholipase C second-messenger system but also by increasing the ACTH release and subsequent cortisol release. This vasopressor should also be used with caution because it can reduce cardiac output in children with poor cardiac function.

Inovasopressors

Dopamine is the most commonly used, dose-dependent inotrope/vasopressor. At a dosage of 3 to 10 μg/kg/minute, the β_1-adrenergic receptor is stimulated. At dosages >10 μg/kg/minute, the α_1-adrenergic receptor effect becomes predominant. As with dobutamine, there is an age-specific insensitivity to the drug. Dopamine mediates much of its β_1- and α_1-adrenergic effects through the release of norepinephrine from the sympathetic vesicles. Immature animals and infants younger than 6 months do not have the full number of sympathetic vesicles. This has been proposed as one cause of reduced effectiveness of dopamine in this age-group. Dopamine insensitivity can also be found in older children and adults, particularly in those who have exhausted their endogenous catecholamine reserves.

Norepinephrine is effective for dopamine-resistant shock. It mediates its effects through the β_1-, α_1-, and α_2-adrenergic receptors. Norepinephrine is always an inotrope, but its vasopressor properties predominate even at a low dosage of 0.01 μg/kg/minute. Dopamine and norepinephrine have their greatest role in the maintenance of adequate perfusion pressure in children with shock. Renal function in particular can be improved by using these inovasopressors to increase blood pressure to the point where renal perfusion pressure is adequate.

Hydrocortisone

Hydrocortisone has also been rediscovered. Centrally and peripherally mediated adrenal insufficiency is increasingly common in the pediatric intensive care setting. Many children are being treated for chronic illnesses with steroids, with subsequent pituitary–adrenal axis suppression. Many children have central nervous system anomalies and acquired illnesses. Some children have purpura fulminans and Waterhouse-Friderichsen syndrome. Others have reduced cytochrome P-450–activity and production of cortisol and aldosterone. Interestingly, adrenal insufficiency can present with low cardiac output and high SVR or with high cardiac output and low SVR. The diagnosis should be considered in any child with epinephrine- or norepinephrine-resistant shock. The dose of hydrocortisone recommended in the literature is 50 mg per kg of hydrocortisone succinate followed by an additional dose over 24 hours.[16] The dose recommended for stress is 2 mg per kg followed by the same dose over 24 hours. Central or peripheral adrenal insufficiency may be diagnosed in infants or children who require epinephrine or norepinephrine infusions for shock and who have a cortisol level <18 mg per dL.[17]

When considering the dose of hydrocortisone to be used in patients with shock, it is important to understand two concepts. First, hydrocortisone doses seem higher than they are because of relative glucocorticoid potency. Hydrocortisone dose must be multiplied by six to be glucocorticoid equivalent to methylprednisone and by 30 to be glucocorticoid equivalent to dexamethasone dosing. The use of methylprednisone at a dose of 2 mg per kg as a loading dose and then at 1 mg per kg q6h (total dose: 5 mg per kg) is equivalent to 30 mg per kg of hydrocortisone in glucocorticoid dosing. The use of 0.5 mg per kg of dexamethasone q6h (total dose: 2 mg per kg) is equivalent to 60 mg/kg/day of hydrocortisone in glucocorticoid dosing. Neither methylprednisone nor dexamethasone has any mineralocorticoid effect; however, hydrocortisone has glucocorticoid and mineralocorticoid effect. This is the reason for using hydrocortisone and not methylprednisone or dexamethasone. Second, cortisol levels differ during stress and shock, so efforts to treat patients with adrenal insufficiency should be directed at achieving these levels. During surgical stress, cortisol levels increase to 30 μg per dL. However, during acute shock, cortisol levels can reach 150 to 300 μg per dL. Hydrocortisone infusion at 2 mg/kg/day (50 mg/m^2/day) helps attain cortisol levels of 20 to 30 μg per dL. Hydrocortisone infusion at 50 mg/kg/day helps attain cortisol levels of 150 μg per dL.

Glucose and Insulin

Glucose and insulin are effective inotropes, which increase both cAMP and ATP production in the heart. The amount of glucose required to meet glucose delivery requirements is provided by D10 at the maintenance intravenous fluid rate. The amount of insulin required can vary from 0 to >1 U/kg/hour, with higher concentrations of insulin required with greater insulin resistance. Higher insulin infusion rates can be associated with electrolyte abnormalities. Monitoring of phosphorus, calcium, magnesium, and potassium levels with appropriate replacement is recommended when using this therapy.

Tri-iodothyronine

Tri-iodothyronine (T$_3$) is an effective inotropic agent, which has long been used to preserve myocardial function in patients who are brain dead and have low T$_3$ levels. A recent randomized controlled trial in neonates showed that use of T$_3$ as a postcardiac surgery inotrope improves outcomes.[18] Hypothyroidism should be expected in children who require epinephrine or norepinephrine and have trisomy 21, central nervous system illness, or a panhypopituitary state.

Atropine and Ketamine

Sedation for placement of invasive lines or for intubation can be required in patients with shock. Ketamine is not only the drug of choice for this indication but also an inovasopressor, which turns off IL-6 production. Ketamine induces the endogenous release of norepinephrine. In experimental studies, ketamine was found to improve survival from septic shock, possibly because, as an *N*-methyl-D-aspartate (NMDA) receptor antagonist, it turns off systemic inflammation and reverses myocardial suppression. In adults undergoing cardiopulmonary bypass surgery, ketamine infusion at 0.25 mg/kg/hour decreases systemic inflammation and improves cardiac function.[19] Ketamine allows safe anesthesia in adult septic shock. Atropine should be used in conjunction with ketamine to reduce bronchorrhea. The addition of a benzodiazepine may or may not be needed to reduce the incidence of re-emergence.

Hypothermia

Hypothermia has been used for many years to allow cardiac surgery to be performed in neonates and children under low flow or no flow states. The rationale is that reduction in temperature reduces energy demands. Lower levels of ATP are required to provide vital cell function at lower temperatures. With each degree centigrade increase above $37°C$, the energy metabolism increases by approximately 10%. With each degree centigrade reduction, the relationship is different. At $35°C$ to $36°C$, energy demands actually increase as shivering occurs. This temperature is met with a cardiovascular response that includes vasoconstriction and increased blood pressure. At $34°C$, energy demands normalize, but blood flow is increased in the brain. Below $33°C$, energy demands decrease; however, below $30°C$, ventricular arrhythmias and asystole become risk factors. During cardiopulmonary bypass, deep hypothermia, below $18°C$, is required to reduce ATP requirements to levels that allow surgery. Maintenance of adequate hemoglobin concentrations and oxygen saturations are required to maintain higher oxygen content levels, and maintenance of normal temperature-corrected pH is required to maintain optimal cerebral blood flow. Glucose must also be delivered to meet ATP production demands.

In some patients with refractory shock, mild/moderate hypothermia may be helpful as a bridge to provide extra mechanical support. If a patient is in refractory shock and the decision is made to begin extracardiac mechanical support, there is little rationale in warming him/her above $34°C$ before commencing. Once on extracardiac mechanical support, warming can be done with the understanding that vasodilation will require volume loading of the patient.

Extracardiac Mechanical Support

In patients who remain in *ischemic* shock (cardiac index <2 L/m^2/minute) despite the use of the above therapies, extracardiac mechanical support can be used to attain 50% survival in children and 80% in newborns. These forms of cardiac support include the veno–arterial or veno–veno extracorporeal membrane oxygenator, the left ventricular assist device (LVAD), and the aortic balloon counterpulsation device. Extracorporeal membrane oxygenation (ECMO) is

commonly used in smaller children. Venovenous ECMO is successful if shock is due to ventilator-associated cardiac dysfunction. Centers generally use an oxygenation index (mean airway pressure × FIO$_2$/PaO$_2$) >40 as an indication. Veno–arterial ECMO is successful when shock is due to cardiac dysfunction. Larger children require larger cannulae and oxygenators. Criteria for this use include a cardiac index <2 L/minute/m^2 or the need for >1 μg/kg/minute of epinephrine. Larger children can be managed with the LVAD or counterpulsating balloon for refractory cardiogenic shock. The LVAD can be used for prolonged support. Attention should be paid to hemolysis in all forms of cardiac assist. Hemolysis will scavenge nitric oxide and adenosine, causing vasoconstriction, thrombosis, and multiple organ failure. A free serum hemoglobin >10 g per dL is abnormal.

PRINCIPLES OF MANAGEMENT

Modern Medical History of Shock

Shock was likely first recognized by clinicians in patients who hemorrhaged to death. However, the measurement of shock became established outside laboratory investigation only after measures of blood pressure such as the sphygmomanometer were available. Clinicians noted that reductions in blood pressure below critical levels for prolonged periods were associated with inevitable death. In the 19th century, resuscitation of hypovolemia from cholera was performed with the goal of correcting urine specific gravity. However, it was not until the 20th century and World War II period that plasma or blood was rapidly infused on a large scale to reverse traumatic shock, defined as hypotension from hemorrhage. In the 1950s, cardiology textbooks described cardiogenic shock as a condition in which blood pressure could be maintained by norepinephrine infusion, but the patient nevertheless developed overwhelming acidosis, dying eventually of hypotension. The use of indocyanine green allowed these clinicians to calculate cardiac output using the Fick dye dilution principle. They derived the following formula: cardiac output = MAP − CVP/SVR, a cardiovascular derivation of the flow equation $Q = \Delta P/R$. These patients had a normal MAP but increased CVP and SVR and died because the cardiac output was too low. Using the work of Frank and Starling, cardiologists then developed a better understanding of the role of fluid, inotrope, and vasodilator therapy in aiding the failing heart and in reversing cardiogenic shock. In the 1970s, Swan and Ganz developed a catheter, which allowed bedside catheterization of the right side of the heart and measurement of cardiac output using the Fick thermodilution principle. Placed in the pulmonary artery, this catheter allowed direct measurement of the right heart pressures and indirect measurement of the LAP through the pulmonary artery occlusion pressure. The literature showed that cardiogenic shock could be caused by right side or left side heart failure, sometimes, but not always, caused by pulmonary or systemic hypertension, respectively. Treatment with vasodilators, as well as inotropes, reversed shock in these patients. In the 1970s, general surgeons began to note that infected postoperative patients dying from hypotension without hemorrhage commonly had high cardiac output, at least initially. These patients had high cardiac output, with low SVR being the cause of hypotension. Using the Swan-Ganz catheter, pulmonary artery oxygen saturation was measured and oxygen consumption and oxygen extraction was calculated. Unlike cardiogenic patients who had low or low-normal oxygen consumption with high oxygen extraction, these patients with sepsis had normal or high oxygen consumption with low oxygen consumption. From this work, septic shock was described as hypotension associated with high cardiac output, low SVR, and low oxygen extraction.

Definitions and management of shock in children followed a slightly different path. In patients with traumatic and hypovolemic shock, it was evident that delay in treatment until hypotension occurred was ill advised. Using indocyanine green, cardiovascular surgeons reported that a cardiac index <2 L/minute/m^2 was associated with mortality. Importantly, a capillary refill >2 seconds identified these at-risk children. Unlike the adult literature, the term *compensated shock* was used to describe pediatric patients with prolonged capillary refill without hypotension. It became well accepted that *pediatric shock occurs in the absence of hypotension*. In the 1980s, the Swan-Ganz catheter was developed for children. Investigators tested whether children had the same hemodynamic and oxygen utilization variables as those previously reported in adults. Surprisingly, they did not. Although patients with cardiogenic shock had increased SVR and increased oxygen extraction, many patients with septic shock also had decreased cardiac output, increased SVR, and increased oxygen extraction. Septic shock could have any hemodynamic or oxygen utilization pattern. Interestingly, the last 5 years of work on septic shock in adults in the emergency room suggests that adults are more similar to children than previously thought. Investigators have now used the term *cryptic* septic shock to characterize adult patients having septic shock with low cardiac output, high SVR, normal or high blood pressure, and increased oxygen extraction. As in children, fluids, inotropes, and vasodilators reverse shock and improve outcomes in these adults.

Hypovolemic Shock

Hypovolemic shock remains the most common form of shock in infants and children. Dr. William O'Shaughnessy is credited for one of the first accounts of fluid resuscitation of this condition in *Lancet* in 1831, when he noted that blood from patients with cholera "lost a large portion of its water" and that the suggested treatment aimed at returning blood to its "natural specific gravity" by replacing

its deficient saline; however, fluid therapy was not used universally until >100 years later.[17]

The modern era of resuscitation of hypovolemic shock occurred in the 1960s and 1970s, when intravenous therapy replaced subcutaneous therapy. Deaths associated with diarrheal disease per 100,000 infants in the United States decreased from 67 to 23 with the widespread use of metal intravenous catheters and from 23 to 2.6 by 1985 with the widespread use of plastic intravenous catheters and the establishment of critical care medicine throughout the United States. Although other public health efforts may have contributed as well, most of the US population was consuming safe water by 1965. Upon evaluating deaths from four diseases associated with hypovolemic shock (i.e., diarrheal disease, hernia and intestinal obstruction, diabetes mellitus, and septicemia), Thomas and Carcillo reported an eightfold reduction in the mortality rate from 1 per 1,000 infants in 1960 to 0.12 per 1,000 infants in 1991.[20] Of interest, the steepest decrease in mortality occurred between 1975 and 1985, coinciding with the implementation of IV fluid therapy using plastic catheters in children. This profound reduction in mortality in such a short time represents one of the great accomplishments of modern pediatric medicine (see Fig. 10.11).

Causes of hypovolemic shock in children include fluid and electrolyte losses, hemorrhage, plasma losses, or endocrine abnormalities (see Table 10.5). It is reasonable to hypothesize that depending on the cause, some fluids may be better than others. Fluids are categorized as crystalloids and colloids. Crystalloids can be provided as isotonic normal saline or Ringer lactate solution, or as hypertonic 3% or 7.5% normal saline. Colloids are purified from plasma in the form of albumin or plasma purified fraction or are synthesized in the form of dextrans or starches. Colloids can be provided as normal or iso-oncotic (e.g., 5% albumin) or hyperoncotic (e.g., 25% albumin)

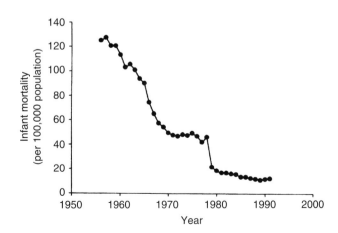

Figure 10.11 Infant mortality (per 100,000 population) in the United States from diseases associated with hypovolemic shock—1955 to 1991. Infant mortality is defined as all deaths of children younger than 1 year.

TABLE 10.5
COMMON CAUSES OF HYPOVOLEMIC SHOCK IN CHILDREN

Fluid and electrolyte losses
  Vomiting
  Diarrhea
  Renal losses (intrinsic renal dysfunction)
  Excessive sweating
  Heat stroke
  Pharmacologic (diuretics)
  Water deprivation
Hemorrhage
  Trauma
    Fractures
    Hepatic rupture
    Splenic rupture
    Major vessel injury
    Intracranial bleeding (especially in neonates)
  Gastrointestinal bleeding
  Surgery
Plasma losses
  Sepsis
  Burns
  Nephrotic syndrome
  Intestinal obstruction
  Peritonitis
  Hypoproteinemia
  Pancreatitis
Endocrine causes
  Diabetes insipidus
  Diabetes mellitus
  Adrenal insufficiency

TABLE 10.6
PHYSICAL EXAMINATION SIGNS FOR EACH PERCENTAGE OF DEHYDRATION

% Dehydration	Physical Signs
5 (mild)	Dry skin, mild tachycardia, concentrated urine
10 (moderate) greater	Lethargy, decreased skin turgor, increase in heart rate, hyperpnea, peripheral vasoconstriction (normal blood pressure), sunken eyes, sunken fontanelle, oliguria
15 (severe)	Obtundation, marked increase in heart rate, periods of apnea, ashen color, hypotension

solutions. Ngo et al. performed a randomized controlled trial by rapidly resuscitating children with dengue shock with one of four fluids—Ringer lactate solution, normal saline, dextran, or albumin.[11] All four groups had 100% survival. In the Screening for Atrial Fibrillation in the Elderly (SAFE) trial, adults were randomized to albumin or saline as the resuscitation fluid. Albumin resuscitation was nearly associated with improved survival in patients with sepsis/septic shock, whereas normal saline was associated with improved survival in patients with head trauma.[10]

Why Are Children so Susceptible to Hypovolemic Shock?
It has long been appreciated that dehydration is poorly tolerated by children. Ten percent dehydration can be associated with lethargy and 15% dehydration with obtundation, apnea, and shock (see Table 10.6). The younger the child, the greater the body water content. Because children are very small, even a small amount of fluid loss can result in catastrophe (see Tables 10.7 and 10.8). For example, a 350-mL fluid loss in a newborn causes 10% dehydration, whereas this degree of dehydration in an adult requires the loss of 7 L of fluid. Similarly, small amounts of blood loss

can result in catastrophe. A 28-mL blood loss in a newborn is equivalent to a 420-mL blood loss in an adult, with both resulting in a 10% reduction in blood volume. Children also have a diminished cardiac reserve compared to adults. The resting heart rate of an adult is 70 bpm. During shock, the heart rate doubles to 140 bpm. The newborn infant is not so capable. A doubling of heart rate from 140 to 280 bpm cannot be tolerated. Because infants are less able to use heart rate to compensate for the reduction in stroke volume associated with hypovolemia, shock occurs more readily in this age-group (see Table 10.9).

The Physiologic and Molecular Rationale for Fluid Resuscitation of Hypovolemic Shock
In the physiologic model of hypovolemic shock, a reduction in volume results in reduced preload or end-diastolic volume (see Fig. 10.12). This causes a reduction in stroke volume and cardiac output according to the Frank-Starling curve. Several compensatory mechanisms ensue. The peripheral vasculature attempts to maintain preload with vasoconstriction, and the heart attempts to maintain cardiac output with an increased heart rate. When these compensatory mechanisms are unsuccessful in maintaining oxygen delivery, the cellular mitochondria increase oxygen extraction. If oxygen delivery plummets below the point where mitochondria can keep up with the oxygen needs, then cell death occurs. Restoration of intravascular volume with fluid resuscitation reverses this process. When a normal end-diastolic volume is achieved and stroke volume and cardiac output become normal, oxygen delivery is restored and shock is reversed.

In the molecular model of hypovolemic shock, a reduction in volume causes changes in gene expression in endothelial cells, leading to inflammatory cell adhesiveness, thrombosis, and antifibrinolysis. This facilitates white blood cell, platelet, and fibrin plugging of the microvasculature. This thrombotic microangiopathy can prevent perfusion of organs because the microvasculature is no longer patent. According to this model, fluid resuscitation

TABLE 10.7
VOLUME LOSS (ML) NEEDED FOR EACH PERCENTAGE OF DEHYDRATION

Age	Weight (kg)	10% Dehydration	20% Dehydration	30% Dehydration
Newborn	3.5	350	700	1,500
6 mo	7	700	1,400	2,100
1 y	10	1,000	2,000	3,000
6 y	20	2,000	4,000	6,000
10 y	30	3,000	6,000	9,000
Adult	70	7,000	14,000	21,000

is most effective if given before gene signaling changes the phenotype of the endothelium. In support of this concept, Rivers et al. showed that emergency department resuscitation directed at maintaining the $Scvo_2$ saturation >70% prevented PT prolongation.[5] Han et al. reported that inadequate volume resuscitation in the first hour of shock is associated with an increased risk of death from multiple organ failure in children with severe sepsis.[6] These investigators found a 40% increased risk of mortality with each hour that went by without fluid resuscitation. In adults with septic shock, it has been reported that resuscitation with starch (hydroxy ethyl starch [HES]) results in reduced levels of adhesion molecules compared to resuscitation with albumin.[21] Although some fluids may be more efficient than others in preventing endothelial transition to a thrombotic and adhesive phenotype, time for adequate fluid resuscitation is most important.

For many years, investigators were unable to develop an animal model of hyperdynamic sepsis. In 1982, Carrol and Snyder reported that 60 mL per kg of fluid resuscitation was needed to achieve a hyperdynamic state in cynomolgus monkeys.[22] In 1991, three separate groups reported improved survival in animal models of toxic shock syndrome,

TABLE 10.8
BLOOD VOLUME LOSS (ML) (PERCENTAGE OF TOTAL BLOOD VOLUME) REQUIRED ON THE BASIS OF AGE DURING HEMORRHAGIC SHOCK

Age	Weight (kg)	Total Blood Volume	10%	20%	30%
Newborn	3.5	280	28	56	84
6 mo	7	560	56	112	168
1 y	10	800	80	160	240
6 y	20	1,400	140	280	420
10 y	30	2,100	210	420	630
Adult	70	4,200	420	840	1,260

TABLE 10.9
HEART RATE CHANGES (BEATS/MIN) BY PERCENT INCREASE

Age	Basal Heart Rate	20% Increase	50% Increase
Newborn	145	174	218
6 mo	120	144	180
1 y	115	138	173
5 y	95	114	143
10 y	75	90	113
Adult	70	84	105

endotoxic shock, and *Escherichia coli* septic shock.[23-25] Fluid resuscitation was found to increase stroke volume and cardiac output in these models. In 1991, Wilson et al. reported that fluid resuscitation of mice with septic shock induced by cecal ligation and puncture reduced liver tumor necrosis factor (TNF) and IL-1 mRNA expression.[26] This observation supported a role for fluid resuscitation in preventing the transition of cytokines to a proinflammatory cytokine phenotype. Fluid resuscitation also improved survival in these animals.

Other models of experimental hypovolemic shock showed similar findings in 1991.[27] O'Neill et al. reported that 65 mL/kg/hour of Ringer lactate solution with 5% dextrose was more effective than 15 mL/kg/hour in restoring blood pressure and improving outcome in an immature bowel ischemia reperfusion model.[27] Xia et al. showed that time to fluid resuscitation of shock was also important. Animals resuscitated early after burn injury had greater ATP levels in liver, heart, and kidney tissues than animals who underwent delayed fluid resuscitation of shock.[28]

Before the 1990s, there was a general hesitance in the practice of fluid resuscitation of hypovolemic shock. Before the advent of pediatric critical care medicine, there had been a great deal of fear that children developed pulmonary edema after fluid resuscitation. There was also

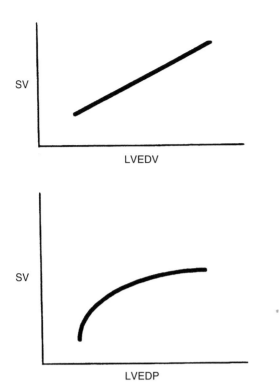

Figure 10.12 Hypovolemia and ventricular function. The relationship of stroke volume (SV) to left ventricular end-diastolic volume (LVEDV; **top**) and left ventricular end-diastolic pressure (LVEDP; **bottom**). By increasing LVEDV, SV increases proportionally. Increasing LVEDP will increase SV to a certain point but will eventually plateau because of the compliance of the left ventricle. The goal of fluid resuscitation is to maintain SV at this plateau.

a fear that children with meningitis would develop cerebral edema and herniation if fluid-resuscitated. In the late 1980s, multiple adult reports documented that aggressive fluid resuscitation did not increase extravascular water in patients who were critically ill. Then in 1990, investigators from the Harbor-UCLA Medical Center reported that children with meningitis had increased ADH levels because of fluid restriction practices and not because of meningitis itself. Fluid infusion restored ADH levels to normal values without causing clinical evidence of cerebral edema.[29] These relative "safety" studies allowed investigators to study the role of fluid resuscitation in children.

In 1991, an observational emergency department study showed that aggressive fluid resuscitation of children with septic shock was associated with improved survival without any discernible evidence of increased incidence of pulmonary edema or cerebral edema.[12] On the basis of this study, pediatric advanced life support (PALS) recommendations supporting aggressive fluid resuscitation were made, with up to and >60 mL per kg as an early goal in the management of septic shock. Two studies using 20 mL per kg of Ringer lactate solution or 4.5% albumin have shown improved stroke volume and blood pressure in premature and term newborns with shock.[30,31]

In the mid-1990s, clinical investigators began to describe patients with hypovolemic shock who were refractory to fluid resuscitation alone. Reynolds et al. described decreased left ventricular stroke work index (LVSWI) in pediatric patients with burn shock who were refractory to fluid resuscitation.[32] Dobutamine restored cardiac function and reversed shock with good outcome. Ceneviva et al. examined this question in children with fluid-refractory septic shock. Although some of these patients were refractory because of vasoplegia, most children had poor cardiac function and increased vascular tone. Persistent shock was associated with progressive cardiac failure even in those who initially presented with a hyperdynamic state.[4] Unlike patients with burn shock, most of these children required support with the direct-acting catecholamine epinephrine. There is an age-dependent response to dopamine and dobutamine, which can be overcome by use of epinephrine.

What Fluid Should One Use?

In the only randomized controlled trial on fluid resuscitation in hypovolemic shock, it was determined that crystalloid or colloid attained 100% survival in children with dengue shock if they were resuscitated aggressively and if the shock was reversed within an hour of presentation to the emergency department.[11] In adults, it has been shown that colloids (HES or albumin) maintain pulmonary capillary wedge pressure and improve colloid oncotic pressure with less volume than crystalloids require during resuscitation of hypovolemic shock.[33] The SAFE trial supports the use of albumin in patients with sepsis ($p = 0.05$) and crystalloid in patients with trauma ($p < 0.05$).[10]

The experimental literature supports the use of hypertonic saline/hetastarch and hypertonic saline/dextran solutions over isotonic solutions in resuscitation of hypovolemic shock. The accepted veterinarian approach is the use of hypertonic/hyperoncotic resuscitation in large animals. Two liters of hypertonic saline is used for adult cows and 120 to 200 mL of hypertonic saline/dextran is used in calves with hypovolemic shock.[34] There is a need to study the role of tonicity and oncotic qualities of fluid in resuscitation of humans with hypovolemic shock.

Clinical Recommendations for Resuscitation of Hypovolemic Shock

Clinical recommendations for resuscitation of hypovolemic shock begin with emergency access, attained according to PALS/neonatal resuscitation program (NRP) recommendations for the use of peripheral IV or intraosseous, or umbilical access. Because each hour that progresses without appropriate fluid resuscitation of shock is associated with increased risk of mortality,[6] resuscitation should be accomplished in an emergent manner. Boluses of 20 mL per kg of isotonic crystalloid should be pushed until the tachycardia is resolved, narrow pulse pressures are widened to normal, capillary refill is reduced to <2 seconds, and urine output is established at 1 mL/kg/hour. When a CVP catheter is in place, resuscitation can continue until the CVP of 5 to 10 mm Hg is attained. If crystalloid is not effective in reversing shock, then colloid can be used (colloid may be used as the first line when sepsis is complicated by hypovolemic shock). In patients with ongoing fluid losses, continued fluid administration will be required to prevent relapse of hypovolemic shock. In patients with fluid-refractory shock, the use of inotropes and hydrocortisone (if adrenal insufficiency is suspected) should be strongly considered.

Adrenal Shock

Many investigators have been reporting a role for adrenal insufficiency in children with fluid- and inotrope-refractory hypovolemic shock.[35] Addisonian crisis is indistinguishable from other forms of hypovolemic shock.[36] Risk factors that should induce suspicion include the presence of purpura fulminans or a history of long-term steroid use. Other pathognomonic signs include the presence of increased skin pigmentation, particularly in areas not exposed to sun, and a history of progressive fatigue. The recommended dose of hydrocortisone for adrenal shock is 50 mg per kg followed by an infusion of 50 mg per kg over 24 hours.

Hemorrhagic Shock

Similar to hypovolemic shock, hemorrhagic shock is manifested in its earliest stages by tachycardia and then by narrow pulse pressure with normal mean arterial blood pressure. It is not until there is approximately a 50% blood loss that hypotension occurs. Resuscitation should be directed at attaining normal heart rate and pulse pressure. Advanced Trauma Life Support (ATLS) guidelines call for initial resuscitation with crystalloid at 20 mL per kg followed by cross-matched blood transfusion as needed. In circumstances where cross-matched blood is not available, un–cross-matched O-type blood group can be given, particularly when shock persists. Resuscitation should proceed until restoration of normal heart rate, MAP, pulse pressure, and perfusion. Hemoglobin concentrations >6 g per dL in children and >10 g per dL in newborns are usually required to attain these goals.

The management of unresolving hemorrhagic shock is directed at hemostasis and coagulation. If fluid and blood resuscitation is not successful and hemorrhaging continues, then surgical hemostasis should be actively pursued. Patients at highest risk of postoperative bleeding include infants undergoing craniofacial frontal advancement, patients after tonsillectomy and adenoidectomy, patients undergoing burn surgery, and patients who have undergone cardiac surgery. When possible, PT, partial thrombin time (PTT), and platelet counts should be corrected with fresh frozen plasma, cryoprecipitate, and platelet infusions. Thromboelastogram can be used to direct blood component therapy and to diagnose surgical versus coagulation disorder bleeding (von Willebrand disease being

the notable exception). Activated factor VII is effective in reversing refractory hemorrhagic shock, especially when it is caused by diffuse bleeding. In patients with bleeding diatheses, such as hemophilia or von Willebrand disease, specific concentrates are needed, including factor VIII concentrate and activated factor VIII for recalcitrant bleeding. Bleeding in neonates after cardiac surgery can be caused by a transient von Willebrand disease, which can be reversed by desamino-8-D-arginine vasopressin (DDAVP) treatment, which increases endothelial production of von Willebrand factor. Hemorrhagic shock can also occur from anticoagulant therapies. Protamine is used to reverse the heparin effect after cardiopulmonary bypass. Fibrinolysis inhibitors are needed for hemorrhagic shock caused by secondary fibrinolysis. Aminocaproic acid (Amicar) is effective in stopping bleeding during ECMO. The thromboelastogram can also be used to direct antifibrinolytic therapy.

Cardiogenic Shock

Cardiogenic shock is manifested clinically by tachycardia, narrow pulse pressure, prolonged capillary refill >2 seconds, and hepatomegaly. The ductus arteriosus closes in the first days to weeks of life. The treatment of choice in neonates with "ductal-dependent" lesions, including coarctation of the aorta, transposition of the great arteries, and single ventricle pathology, is prostaglandin E_1 at 0.1 μg/kg/minute (see Fig. 10.13). Myocarditis and idiopathic cardiomyopathy are the most common causes of

---

Neonates should be started on PGE_1. If congenital heart disease is diagnosed, then surgery is required.

For neonates and children without congenital heart disease the approach is as follows:

Depending on preload, furosemide can be administered to reduce preload or 10–20 mL per kg of crystalloid may be administered to improve preload

Inotropic support should begin with dobutamine, but epinephrine should be used if needed

Concomitant use of afterload reduction with nitrosovasodilators and type III PDE inhibitors is also recommended

↓

Persistent cardiac failure after 7 days?

↓

Begin ACE inhibitor and aldactone

↓

Cardiac index <2.0 L/min/m², evidence of end-organ damage?

↓

Consider extracorporeal assist device

Figure 10.13 Suggested approach recommended by the authors for hemodynamic support of neonates and children with acute cardiac failure. PGE_1, prostaglandin E_1; PDE, phosphodiesterase; ACE, angiotensin-converting enzyme.

cardiogenic shock outside this age-group. Furosemide is standard therapy for acute congestive heart failure because patients are frequently beyond the effective range on the Starling curve. Brain natriuretic peptide has become an important therapeutic agent in furosemide-resistant patients. For the most part, therapies are based on the use of inotropes and vasodilators in the acute period. Dobutamine and nitroprusside are good first-line drugs, but type IV PDEIs (e.g., milrinone, amrinone, and enoximone) and α blockers (e.g., phentolamine, phenoxybenzamine) are becoming increasingly popular. Epinephrine is reserved for resistant heart failure.

After the first weeks of heart failure, strong consideration should be given to the addition of, or transition to, angiotensin-converting enzyme inhibitors and spironolactone (Aldactone). Both have been shown to improve long-term survival in adults with cardiomyopathy. The acute protective response of the body to shock is to increase endogenous production of catecholamines, aldosterone, and angiotensin. This response becomes deleterious over time. Digoxin can also be used to resensitize the baroceptor reflex. Although the outcome has not been influenced, digoxin reduces rate of hospitalization for pulmonary edema associated with congestive heart failure in the adult population. β Blockers are also effective in improving outcome in adults with cardiomyopathy; however, their use in the pediatric population has not yet become a standard. The acceptance of dichotomous therapy in acute and chronic heart failure occurred only after multiple studies showed that long-term use of inotropes or type III PDEIs increased mortality. Hence, acute-care medicines may be deleterious with long-term use.

Cardiogenic Shock in the Cardiopulmonary Bypass and Postoperative Cardiac Surgery Patient

Low cardiac output syndrome is common after cardiopulmonary bypass and cardiac surgery (see Fig. 10.14). The cardiac output nadir occurs at 6 hours after the surgery and recovers by 24 hours. Because of this phenomenon, the hallmark of cardiovascular support after cardiac surgery has become afterload reduction. Ischemia experienced during cardiopulmonary bypass leads to increased intracellular calcium concentrations in the heart and vasculature. This is because the Ca^{2+} extrusion pumps, which remove calcium from the cell, are more ATP-dependent than the calcium channels that bring calcium into the cell. The result is a noncompliant, poorly functioning heart and high vascular resistance. Dobutamine and nitroprusside are an effective combination, and amrinone, milrinone, and enoximone can be effective in these patients as well. Milrinone, in particular, has been shown, in a randomized controlled trial, to reduce the incidence of low cardiac output syndrome after cardiopulmonary bypass.[37,38] T_3 has also been shown, in a randomized controlled trial, to improve cardiac output and outcome in neonates after cardiac surgery as well.[18] In addition to these agents, volume loading is

As the patient becomes warm, pump blood (low or normal Hb) or colloid/crystalloid (high Hb) to maintain optimum preload (usually need higher than normal LAP)

Begin inotropic support with dobutamine and escalate to epinephrine if needed. T_3 is also indicated.

Use concomitant afterload reduction with type III PDE to prevent wide AVDo$_2$. Phenoxybenzamine can also be used.

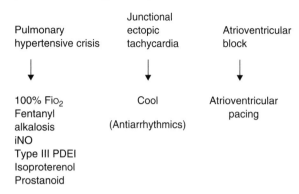

Pulmonary hypertensive crisis → 100% Fio$_2$, Fentanyl, alkalosis, iNO, Type III PDEI, Isoproterenol, Prostanoid

Junctional ectopic tachycardia → Cool (Antiarrhythmics)

Atrioventricular block → Atrioventricular pacing

Cardiac index <2 mV Pao$_2$ <30, AVDo$_2$ >5 Unremitting lactic acidosis

Consider ECMO (5–7 days) for cardiac stun

Figure 10.14 Suggested approach for use of cardiovascular support for patients after cardiopulmonary bypass (see subsequent text). LAP, left atrial pressure; T_3, tri-iodothyronine; PDEI, phosphodiesterase inhibitor; iNO, inhaled nitric oxide; AVDo$_2$, arteriovenous oxygen saturation difference; ECMO, extracorporeal membrane oxygenation.

necessary. Infants generally return from the operation room with hypothermia. As the infants become warmer and the systemic vasculature dilate, hypovolemia can be treated by transfusing the "pump" blood removed during cardiopulmonary bypass. It is not uncommon to also administer colloids, or crystalloids, in patients with hypovolemia and high hematocrits. Because the heart is noncompliant, higher left atrial filling pressures are frequently required to attain an adequate stroke volume. Heart rate is also an important consideration. Many infants will require pacing to maintain an adequate cardiac output. Epinephrine should be used when these measures do not improve the cardiac output. Hemodynamic goals include warm toes; capillary refill <2 seconds; urine output ≥ 1 mL/kg/hour; a difference between arterial and superior vena cava oxygen saturation of <25% (assuming Hb ≥ 10 g per dL); or a superior vena cava oxygen saturation >70%, an AVDo$_2$ <5, and serum lactate <2 mmol per L.

There are several special considerations in the postoperative period. In infants and children with left-to-right shunt physiology, *reactive pulmonary hypertension can be expected to contribute to cardiogenic shock for 72 hours after surgery.* Approaches to this problem include mechanical ventilation, high-dose fentanyl derivatives, oxygen, alkalinization, iNO, milrinone, and isoproterenol. *Junctional ectopic tachycardia*

(*JET*) is the most common arrhythmia causing cardiogenic shock in the postoperative period. The rapid heart rate and lack of co-ordinated atrial and ventricular contraction can lead to a life-threatening low cardiac output state because of inadequate stroke volume. This condition generally responds to volume loading and cooling. Because hypothermia obscures many of the clinical signs of normal perfusion, serum lactate level, base deficit, superior venous oxygen saturation, and AVDO$_2$ should be monitored when titrating inotrope and vasodilator therapies. Children with *septal hypertrophy* may be treated with β blockers, such as esmolol, or calcium channel blockers, such as nicardipine, to slow heart rate, reduce contractility, and improve ventricular stroke volume. Careful titration of afterload therapies is required in these children. Children with *valve replacement surgery or coarctation of the aorta repair* need afterload reduction therapy to prevent any incident of hypertension.

The *single ventricle patient with shock* presents with important challenges. In the prerepair state, shock can be caused by pulmonary overcirculation. This usually occurs when oxygen is administered to the infant for a low arterial oxygen saturation. This increases arterial saturation but simultaneously widens AVDO$_2$ because, as blood preferentially flows to the low-resistance pulmonary vascular bed, it is being "stolen" from the circulation. Despite increasing oxygen saturation, the patient becomes tachypnic, tachycardic, and cold, with a prolonged capillary refill and lactic acidosis. This can be remedied by providing room air or hypoxic gas mixtures, which increase pulmonary vascular resistance and restore systemic circulatory blood flow. Arterial oxygen saturation decreases as the AVDO$_2$ narrows and shock resolves. In the postoperative period after the first stage of correction, cardiogenic shock occurs for the most part because of increased SVR (see preceding text). Wide AVDO$_2$ can be narrowed by treating with systemic vasodilators including nitroprusside, chlorpromazine, milrinone, enoximone, or phenoxybenzamine. Vasodilator toxicity can be reversed with vasopressor; however, continued inotrope support will be required as well.[39] Attention must also be paid to the maintenance of high hemoglobin concentrations to maintain adequate oxygen delivery in the presence of arterial saturation, which normally ranges from 70% to 80%. Because oxygen saturation is reduced by 20% to 30% in these patients, hemoglobin concentrations must be increased by 20% to 30% to maintain oxygen content and oxygen delivery without demanding high output from the already ischemic heart. This point is crucial not only in single ventricle patients but also in patients with *cyanotic heart disease and shock*. After total correction, patients are left with a *Fontan* physiology. Cardiogenic shock in these patients can be precipitated by conditions that reduce preload, including dehydration, increased pulmonary vascular resistance, and increased intrathoracic pressure from positive-pressure ventilation. Because patients with Fontan or hemi-Fontan correction have no functioning atrial kick, they are completely dependent on

venous pressure–generated preload for perfusion of the right ventricle. Therapy for these patients in shock includes volume resuscitation, as little positive pressure as possible, and pneumatic devices to increase venous return. These children require high CVPs for perfusion.

Primary, Persistent, or Acquired Pulmonary Hypertension–Induced Shock

Systemic pulmonary blood pressures can be associated with right ventricular failure and shock. Right ventricular failure is usually associated with secondary left ventricular failure caused by septal bowing into the left ventricle and an inability to fill during diastole. These patients have dilated right ventricular failure and inadequate left ventricular stroke volume. The treatment strategy is to reduce the afterload in the right ventricle. The most selective pulmonary vasodilator is iNO. This gas stimulates soluble guanylate cyclase, increases cGMP, reduces calcium in the smooth muscle cell, and induces vasodilation. The nitric oxide is then absorbed by circulating hemoglobin/red blood cells and reduced to an inactive form, preventing significant systemic effects. Inhaled prostacyclin is a good second-line drug if iNO is unsuccessful. Intravenous prostacyclin (cAMP drug), milrinone (cAMP), and nitroglycerin (cGMP) also have some selectivity for the pulmonary vasculature and can be effective adjuncts. Nitroglycerin tachyphylaxis can be treated by giving *N*-acetylcysteine (Mucomyst), which replaces the sulfhydryl group to allow further production of biologically active nitrosothiols. Isoproterenol is an effective inotrope and pulmonary vasodilator as well. It improves right ventricular contractility while promoting pulmonary and systemic vasodilation. The use of α-adrenergic agents should be carefully monitored. Many believe that pulmonary hypertension can be exacerbated. Norepinephrine is advocated to improve right ventricular filling in adults with right ventricular failure due to right-sided infarction; however, these patients rarely have systemic pulmonary artery hypertension. Acute failure of the right side of the heart and cardiogenic shock caused by pulmonary embolus should be treated with tissue plasminogen activator and subsequent heparinization.

Septic Shock

Outcomes in neonatal and pediatric sepsis have improved with the advent of neonatal and pediatric intensive care. The University of Minnesota reported a 97% mortality rate from gram-negative sepsis in 1968.[40] In 1985, the National Children's Medical Center reported a 60% mortality rate in all cause septic shock.[3] By 1999, the mortality rates from severe sepsis had dropped to 9% in a US sample estimate.[41] Several reports in the 21st century suggest further improvement, with the implementation of resuscitation practices now being recommended in the American College of Critical Care (ACCM)/PALS guidelines and clinical practice parameters for hemodynamic support of pediatric and newborn sepsis. Booy et al. reported a decrease in mortality from meningococcemia from 22% to 2% when they implemented early recognition and treatment with aggressive volume resuscitation and inotrope use.[42] Ngo et al. reported 100% survival from dengue shock in Vietnamese children when aggressive fluid resuscitation was given.[11] Kutko et al. reported 100% survival in all cause septic shock in previously healthy children and 85% survival in children with chronic illness, predominantly cancer-related.[43] Lin et al. reported similar results with the implementation of the ACCM/PALS guidelines. Twenty-eight–day survival was 97% and hospital survival was 94%.[44]

The hemodynamic response to newborn and pediatric septic shock is different from the "classically" described hemodynamic response of adults. Opinion holds that the predominant cause of mortality in adult septic shock is vasomotor paralysis. Adults have myocardial dysfunction manifested as a decreased ejection fraction; however, cardiac output is usually maintained or increased by two mechanisms, tachycardia and ventricular dilation. Adults who do not develop this adaptive process to maintain cardiac output have a poor prognosis. This dogma may not be entirely correct because Rivers et al. have recently shown that adults with sepsis, normal blood pressure, and decreased superior vena cava oxygen saturation, a condition of low cardiac output and elevated SVR, have increased multiple organ failure and mortality.[5] Importantly, inotrope and fluid therapy directed at increasing cardiac output with a goal of attaining a $ScvO_2$ saturation >70% prevented multiple organ failure and improved survival.

Pediatric septic shock is associated with severe hypovolemia, and children frequently respond well to aggressive volume resuscitation; however, the hemodynamic response of fluid-resuscitated children appears diverse compared to that classically attributed to adults. Contrary to the adult experience, low cardiac output, and not low SVR, is associated with mortality in pediatric septic shock. Attainment of the therapeutic goal of cardiac index 3.3 to 6 L/minute/m^2 is associated with improved survival.[3] Also, contrary to adults, oxygen delivery, and not oxygen extraction, is the major determinant of oxygen consumption in children.[45] Attainment of the therapeutic goal of VO_2 >200 mL/minute/m^2 is also associated with improved outcome.

In 1998, investigators reported positive outcome when aggressive volume resuscitation (60 mL per kg fluid in the first hour) and goal-directed therapies[4] (the goal was a cardiac index 3.3 to 6 L/minute/m^2 and normal pulmonary capillary wedge pressure) were applied to children with septic shock. Ceneviva et al. reported 50 children with fluid-refractory ($\geq$60 mL per kg of fluid resuscitation in the first hour), dopamine-resistant shock.[4] Most children (58%) showed a low cardiac output/high SVR state and 22% had low cardiac output and low vascular resistance. Hemodynamic states frequently progressed and changed over the first 48 hours. Persistent shock occurred in 33% of the patients. There was a significant decrease in cardiac function

over time, requiring addition of inotropes and vasodilators. Although decreasing cardiac function accounted for most patients with persistent shock, some showed a complete change from a low-output state to a high-output/low SVR state. Inotropes, vasopressors, and vasodilators were directed at maintaining normal cardiac index and SVR in the patients. Mortality from fluid-refractory, dopamine-resistant septic shock in this study (18%) was markedly reduced compared to the mortality in the 1985 study (58%),[4] in which aggressive fluid resuscitation was not used.

Neonatal septic shock can be complicated by the lack of physiologic transition from fetal to neonatal circulation. *In utero*, 85% of fetal circulation bypasses the lungs through the patent ductus arteriosus and foramen ovale. Prenatally, this flow pattern is maintained by suprasystemic pulmonary artery pressures. At birth, inhalation of oxygen triggers a cascade of biochemical events that ultimately result in reduction of pulmonary artery pressure and transition from fetal to neonatal circulation, with blood flow now being directed through the pulmonary circulation. Closure of the patent ductus arteriosus and foramen ovale complete this transition. Pulmonary artery pressures can remain elevated and the ductus arteriosus can remain open for the first 6 weeks of life, whereas the foramen ovale may remain probe patent for years. Sepsis-induced acidosis and hypoxia can increase pulmonary artery pressure and maintain patency of the ductus arteriosus, resulting in persistent pulmonary hypertension of the newborn (PPHN) and persistent fetal circulation (PFC). Neonatal septic shock with PPHN is associated with increased right ventricle work. Despite *in utero* conditioning, the thickened right ventricle may fail in the presence of systemic pulmonary artery pressures. Decompensated right ventricular failure can be clinically manifested by tricuspid regurgitation and hepatomegaly. Newborn animal models of group B streptococcal and endotoxin shock have also documented reduced cardiac output and increased pulmonary resistance, mesenteric resistance, and SVR. Therapies directed at the reversal of right ventricle failure, through reduction of pulmonary artery pressures, are commonly needed in neonates with fluid-refractory shock and PPHN.

The hemodynamic response in premature, very low–birth weight infants with septic shock (<32 weeks gestation, <1,000 g) is least understood, in part because pulmonary artery catheterization is not possible in this population. Most information has been assessed from echocardiographic evaluation alone. There is a paucity of studies devoted to septic shock. Literature is available, for the most part, on the hemodynamic response in premature infants with respiratory distress syndrome or shock of undescribed etiology. Echocardiographic analysis has documented reduced right ventricle and left ventricle function in premature newborns. Premature infants with shock can respond to volume and inotropic therapies with improvements in stroke volume, contractility, and blood pressure.

Several other developmental considerations influence therapies for shock. Relative initial deficiencies in the thyroid and parathyroid hormone axes have been appreciated and can result in the need for thyroid hormone and/or calcium replacement. Hydrocortisone has been examined in this population as well. Hydrocortisone "prophylaxis" does reduce the incidence of hypotension in very low–birth weight infants.[46] Immature mechanisms of thermogenesis require attention to external warming. Reduced glycogen stores and muscle mass for gluconeogenesis require attention to the maintenance of serum glucose.

Standard practices in resuscitation of premature infants in septic shock employ a more graded approach compared to the resuscitation of term neonates and children. This more cautious approach is a response to anecdotal reports that premature infants at risk for intraventricular hemorrhage (<30 weeks gestation) can develop hemorrhage after rapid shifts in blood pressure; however, it is now agreed that long-term neurologic outcomes are related to periventricular leukomalacia (a result of prolonged underperfusion) more so than to intraventricular hemorrhage. Indeed, many lines of evidence have now linked cerebral palsy to perinatal sepsis and shock. Cerebral palsy risks are increased in offspring of mothers with chorioamnionitis, and antepartum antibiotic use is associated with a reduced risk of cerebral palsy. Intraventricular hemorrhage, periventricular leukomalacia, and infant neurodevelopmental delay have been linked to hypotension and/or ischemia rather than hypoxia. The mechanism of white matter injury in perinatal sepsis has been delineated. The developing brain experiences white matter injury when cytokine-induced glutamate production is coupled with ischemia.

Another complicating factor in very low–birth weight infants is the persistence of the patent ductus arteriosus. This can occur because the immature muscle is unable to constrict. Most infants with this condition are treated medically with indomethacin or surgically with ligation. Rapid administration of fluid may cause left-to-right shunting through the ductus, with ensuant congestive heart failure induced by ventricular overload. Studies of therapies specifically directed at very low–birth weight infants with septic shock are needed. One single-center, randomized controlled trial reported improved outcome with use of daily 6-hour pentoxifylline infusions in very premature infants with sepsis.[47]

Early Recognition and Goal-Directed Therapy

St Mary's Hospital reported a reduction in mortality from meningococcemia from 22% to 2% after implementing a time-sensitive, goal-directed inotrope and fluid therapy program for rapid restoration of perfusion.[42] Ngo et al. reported 100% survival in dengue shock when goal-directed fluid resuscitation was used to rapidly restore perfusion.[11] Investigators implementing ACCM/PALS guidelines for goal-directed therapy have reported similar results in patients with all-cause septic shock.[17,43,45] These results were accomplished with early goal-directed therapy.

Septic shock should be recognized, before hypotension occurs, by a clinical triad that includes hypothermia or hyperthermia, altered mental status, and peripheral vasodilation (warm shock) or cool extremities (cold shock).[17] Therapies should be directed at restoring normal mental status and peripheral perfusion (capillary refill <2 seconds and strong peripheral pulses).[17] Han et al. showed that each hour that progressed without restoration of normal blood pressure and a capillary refill <2 seconds increased the odds of mortality twofold.[6] Restoration of urine output can also be a reassuring measure of successful resuscitation.

Septic shock should also be evaluated and resuscitated using hemodynamic variables. Flow (Q) varies directly with perfusion pressure (dP) and inversely with resistance (R). This is mathematically represented by $Q = dP/R$. For the whole body, this is represented by cardiac output = MAP − CVP/SVR. This relationship is also evident for organ perfusion. In the kidney, for example, renal blood flow (RBF) = mean renal arterial pressure (RAP)—mean renal venous pressure (RVP)/renal vascular resistance. Some organs including the kidney and brain have vasomotor autoregulation, which maintains blood flow in low blood pressure (MAP or RAP) states (see Figs. 10.15 and 10.16). At some critical point, perfusion pressure is reduced below the ability of the organ to maintain blood flow. The purpose of the treatment of shock is to maintain perfusion pressure above the critical point below which blood flow cannot be effectively maintained in individual organs. Because the kidney receives the second highest blood flow of all organs in the body, the measurement of urine output (with the exception of patients with hyperosmolar states leading to osmotic diuresis) and creatinine clearance can be used as an indicator of adequate perfusion pressure. In this regard, maintenance of MAP with norepinephrine has been shown to improve urine output and creatinine clearance in hyperdynamic sepsis. Maintenance of supranormal MAP above this point is likely not of benefit.

Reduction in perfusion pressure below the critical point necessary for adequate organ perfusion can also occur in disease states with increased intra-abdominal pressure

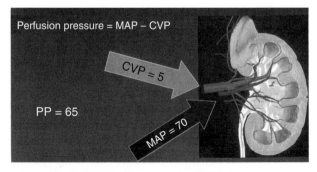

Figure 10.15 Restoration of perfusion pressure by volume resuscitation alone in hypovolemic patients. MAP, mean arterial pressure; CVP, central venous pressure; PP, perfusion pressure.

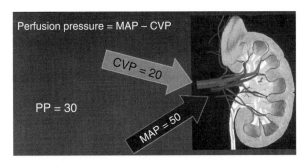

Figure 10.16 Reduced perfusion pressure in patients with poor cardiac function. MAP, mean arterial pressure; CVP, central venous pressure; PP, perfusion pressure.

(IAP), such as bowel wall edema, ascites, or abdominal compartment syndrome. Increased IAP is associated with increased CVP. If this is not compensated for by an increase in MAP, then perfusion pressure is decreased. Therapeutic reduction of IAP (measured by intrabladder pressure) results in restoration of perfusion pressure and has been shown to improve renal function in children with burn shock. Furosemide infusion can be used to relieve intra-abdominal pressures up to 15 cm H_2O. Intraperitoneal catheter drainage or surgical decompression is recommended for an intra-abdominal pressure of 30 cm H_2O and the so-called abdominal compartment syndrome.

Septic shock should also be treated according to oxygen utilization measures. Measurement of cardiac output and oxygen consumption (cardiac index × [arterial oxygen content–mixed venous oxygen content]) can be of benefit in patients with persistent shock because a cardiac index between 3.3 and 6.0 L/minute/m^2 and an oxygen consumption >200 mL/minute/m^2 are associated with improved survival. Assuming a hemoglobin concentration of 10 g per dL and 100% arterial oxygen saturation, a cardiac index >3.3 L/minute/m^2 would correlate with a mixed venous oxygen saturation of >70% in a patient with a normal oxygen consumption of 150 mL/minute/m^2 ([oxygen consumption = cardiac index × arterial oxygen content × oxygen extraction]; therefore, 150 mL/minute/m^2 = 3.3 L/minute/m^2 × [1.36 × 10 g per dL × 100 + Pao$_2$ × 0.003] × [100% − 70%]). Low cardiac output is associated with mortality in pediatric septic shock. In one study, children with fluid-refractory, dopamine-resistant shock were treated with goal-directed therapy (cardiac index >3.3 and <6 L/minute/m^2) and were found to have predictably improved outcomes compared to historical reports.[3] Low cardiac output is associated with increased oxygen extraction. In an emergency room study in adults with septic shock, maintenance of superior vena cava oxygen saturation at >70%, using blood transfusion to a hemoglobin level of 10 g per dL and inotropic support, resulted in a 50% reduction in mortality compared to the group in whom MAP − CVP was maintained without paying attention to superior vena cava oxygen saturation.[5]

Intravenous access for fluid resuscitation and inotrope/vasopressor infusion is more difficult to attain in newborns and children compared to adults. The American Heart Association and American Academy of Pediatrics have developed NRP and PALS guidelines for emergency establishment of intravascular support (see Figs. 10.17 and 10.18).

Fluid Therapy

Two clinical studies have evaluated fluid resuscitation in pediatric septic shock. The case series used a combination of crystalloid and colloid therapies.[12] There is only one randomized controlled trial comparing the use of colloid to crystalloid resuscitation (dextran, gelatin, Ringer lactate solution, or saline) in children with dengue shock.[11] All these children survived regardless of the fluid used, but the longest time to recovery from shock occurred in children who received Ringer lactate solution. Among patients with the narrowest pulse pressure, there was a suggestion that colloids were more effective than crystalloids in restoring normal pulse pressure. Fluid resuscitation with crystalloids and colloids is fundamentally important to survival from septic shock. Some promote the efficacy of exclusive colloid resuscitation. Investigators at St Mary's, who are widely considered to demonstrate the best practice in resuscitation of meningococcal septic shock, reported that they use 5% albumin exclusively (20 mL per kg boluses over 5 to 10 minutes) and intubate all patients who require >40 mL per kg.[42] The SAFE trial was recently completed in adult critical illness. There was a tendency toward improved survival in the sepsis population resuscitated with albumin ($p = 0.05$).[10] The use of blood as a fluid expander has been examined in two small pediatric studies, but no recommendations were given by the investigators.[48,49] Although there are no published studies of, or recommendations on, targeted hemoglobin concentration in children, an emergency room protocol directed at maintenance of hemoglobin at 10 g per dL in adults with a superior vena cava oxygen saturation <70% was associated with improved outcomes.[5]

Fluid infusion is best initiated with boluses of 20 mL per kg, titrated on the basis of the clinical monitors of cardiac output including heart rate, urine output, capillary refill, and level of consciousness. Large fluid deficits typically exist, and initial volume resuscitation usually requires 40 to 60 mL per kg but can be as much as 200 mL per kg.[10] Patients who do not respond rapidly to initial fluid boluses, or those with insufficient physiologic reserve, should be considered for invasive hemodynamic monitoring. Filling pressures should be increased to optimize preload to attain maximal cardiac output. In most patients, this will occur with a pulmonary capillary wedge pressure between 12 and 15 mm Hg. Increases above this range usually do not significantly enhance end-diastolic volume or stroke volume and may be associated with decreased survival. Large volumes of fluid for acute stabilization in children have not been shown to increase

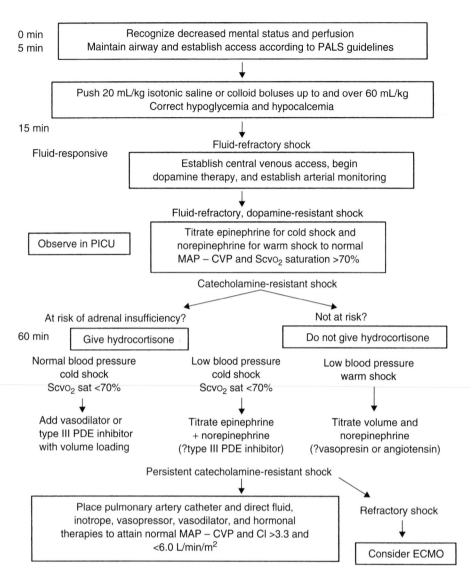

0 min
5 min

Recognize decreased mental status and perfusion
Maintain airway and establish access according to PALS guidelines

Push 20 mL/kg isotonic saline or colloid boluses up to and over 60 mL/kg
Correct hypoglycemia and hypocalcemia

15 min

Fluid-responsive

Fluid-refractory shock

Establish central venous access, begin
dopamine therapy, and establish arterial monitoring

Fluid-refractory, dopamine-resistant shock

Observe in PICU

Titrate epinephrine for cold shock and
norepinephrine for warm shock to normal
MAP – CVP and Scvo$_2$ saturation >70%

Catecholamine-resistant shock

At risk of adrenal insufficiency?

Not at risk?

60 min

Give hydrocortisone

Do not give hydrocortisone

Normal blood pressure
cold shock
Scvo$_2$ sat <70%

Low blood pressure
cold shock
Scvo$_2$ sat <70%

Low blood pressure
warm shock

Add vasodilator or
type III PDE inhibitor
with volume loading

Titrate epinephrine
+ norepinephrine
(?type III PDE inhibitor)

Titrate volume and
norepinephrine
(?vasopresin or angiotensin)

Persistent catecholamine-resistant shock

Place pulmonary artery catheter and direct fluid,
inotrope, vasopressor, vasodilator, and hormonal
therapies to attain normal MAP – CVP and CI >3.3 and
<6.0 L/min/m^2

Refractory shock

Consider ECMO

Figure 10.17 Recommendations for stepwise management of hemodynamic support, with the goals of maintaining normal perfusion and perfusion pressure (mean arterial pressure [MAP] – central venous pressure [CVP]) and a pre- and postductal oxygen saturation difference <5% in infants and children with septic shock. Proceed to next step if shock persists. PALS, pediatric advanced life support; PICU, pediatric intensive care unit; Scvo$_2$, central venous oxygen saturation; CI, cardiac index; PDE, phosphodiesterase; ECMO, extracorporeal membrane oxygenation. (Modified from the ACCM Guidelines for Hemodynamic Support of Children with Septic Shock.)

the incidence of acute respiratory distress syndrome[50] or cerebral edema.[51] Increased fluid requirements may be evident for several days. Fluid choices include crystalloids (normal saline) or colloids (dextran, gelatin, or 5% albumin). Fresh frozen plasma may be infused to correct abnormal PT, and PTT but should not be pushed because it has hypotensive effects, likely caused by vasoactive kinins. Oxygen delivery depends significantly on hemoglobin concentration (oxygen delivery = cardiac index × [1.36 × % hemoglobin × % oxygen saturation] + Pao$_2$ × 0.003). Hemoglobin should be maintained at a minimum of 10 g per dL.

Monitoring

Minimally invasive monitoring is necessary in children with fluid-responsive shock; however, central vein access and arterial pressure monitoring should be considered and used in children with fluid-refractory shock (see Fig. 10.19). Maintenance of perfusion pressure (MAP –

CVP or MAP – IAP if the abdomen is tense secondary to bowel edema or ascitic fluid) is necessary for organ (particularly renal) perfusion. Echocardiography is an appropriate noninvasive tool to rule out the presence of pericardial effusion. Superior vena cava oxygen saturation >70% is associated with improved outcome during the first 6 hours of septic shock presentation. The decision to use pulmonary artery catheter, PICCO, or femoral artery thermodilution catheter monitoring should be reserved for those who remain in shock despite therapies directed at clinical signs of perfusion, MAP – CVP, and superior vena cava oxygen saturation.

The pulmonary artery catheter, PICCO, or femoral artery thermodilution catheter should be used to attain the intended cardiac output, SVR, and oxygen utilization in these patients. In children with fluid-refractory, dopamine-resistant shock, these catheters diagnose improper cardiovascular support strategies, which had been based on incorrect assessment of hemodynamic state. This

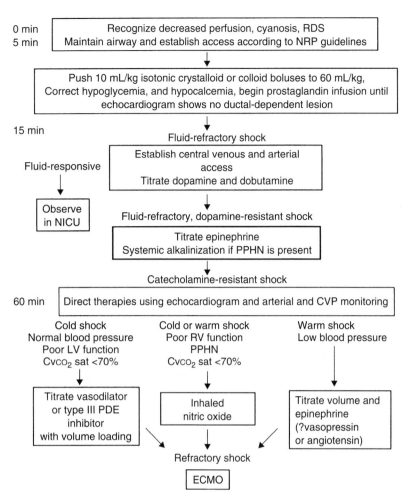

Figure 10.18 Recommendations for stepwise management of hemodynamic support, with the goals of maintaining normal perfusion and perfusion pressure (mean arterial pressure [MAP] – central venous pressure [CVP]) and pre- and postductal oxygen saturation difference <5% in near-term newborns with septic shock. RDS, respiratory distress syndrome; NRP, neonatal resuscitation program; NICU, newborn intensive care unit; PPHN, persistent pulmonary hypertension of the newborn; CVP, central venous pressure; LV, left ventricle; RV, right ventricle; $Cvco_2$, carbondioxide content of venous blood; ECMO, extracorporeal membrane oxygenation; PDE, phosphodiesterase. (Published in the ACCM Guidelines for Hemodynamic Support of Newborn patients with Sepsis.)

new information guides a change to appropriate therapies that reverses shock and improves survival.[4] Echocardiography can be used to assess pericardial effusion; ventricular filling; and, in experienced hands, afterload. Gastric tonometry can give an assessment of intestinal perfusion.

Inovasopressor Therapy
Dopamine remains the first-line vasopressor for high-output low–vascular-resistance shock in adults. Dopamine can also be used as the first-line drug for fluid-refractory hypotensive shock in the setting of low SVR in children; however, there is an age-specific insensitivity to dopamine.[52] Dopamine causes vasoconstriction by releasing norepinephrine from sympathetic vesicles. Immature animals and young humans (<6 months) may not have developed their full component of sympathetic vesicles. Dopamine-resistant shock commonly responds to norepinephrine or high-dose epinephrine. Norepinephrine may also be used as a first-line agent for warm hyperdynamic shock.[53,54] The use of phenylephrine is limited to that of a pure vasopressor because it has no β-adrenergic activity and has little role in septic shock unless accompanied by a vasopressor. Angiotensin or arginine vasopressin can be used successfully in patients who are refractory to

norepinephrine because it does not use the α-receptor and its efficacy is therefore not affected by ongoing α-receptor downregulation. However, these agents may reduce cardiac output, and addition of an inotrope may be required. Use of vasopressors can be titrated to endpoints of perfusion pressure (MAP – CVP) or SVR, which assure optimum urine output and creatinine clearance.

Inotrope Therapy
As in adults, dobutamine or mid-dosage dopamine can be used as the first line of inotropic support;[13] however, children younger than 12 months can be less responsive. Dobutamine or dopamine-refractory shock due to low cardiac output can be reversed with epinephrine infusion.[14] Epinephrine is more commonly used in children than in adults. Low-dose epinephrine can be used as a first-line choice for cold hypodynamic shock. Adults rarely receive epinephrine, in part because atherosclerosis makes epinephrine a risky drug and in part because epinephrine transiently reduces pH in adults with hyperdynamic sepsis.[55] However, infants and children rarely have atherosclerosis, and epinephrine is only used for hypodynamic, and not hyperdynamic, septic shock.

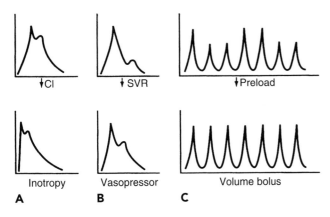

Figure 10.19 Pulse wave hemodynamic prediction of response to volume, inotropes, vasopressors. SVR, systemic vascular resistance; CI, cardiac index;.

Inodilator Therapy

When pediatric patients remain in a normotensive, low cardiac output/high vascular resistance state, despite epinephrine and nitrosovasodilator therapy, the use of milrinone (if liver dysfunction is present) or amrinone (if renal dysfunction is present) or enoximone should be strongly considered. Amrinone and milrinone are rarely used in adults because catecholamine-refractory, low cardiac output/high vascular resistance is so uncommon; however, this hemodynamic state can represent a major proportion of children with fluid-refractory, dopamine-resistant shock.[4] Type III PDEIs prevent the hydrolysis of cAMP and therefore potentiate the effect of β-receptor stimulation in cardiac and vascular tissue. Downregulation of the β_1- and β_2-receptor can be overcome by these drugs. Fluid boluses are likely to be required if amrinone, milrinone, or enoximone are administered with loading doses. Although bolus administration is recommended in the literature, many clinicians administer the drugs only as a continuous infusion, recognizing that it will take four half-lives to reach steady state effect. Because of the long half-life elimination, these drugs should be discontinued at the first sign of tachyarrhythmias, hypotension, or diminished SVR. Hypotension-related toxicity with these drugs could be potentially overcome by stopping milrinone, amrinone, or enoximone and by beginning norepinephrine. Norepinephrine counteracts the effects of increased cAMP in vascular tissue by stimulating the α-receptor. Norepinephrine accomplishes this without further β_2 stimulation.

Vasodilator Therapy

The use of vasodilators can reverse shock in pediatric patients who remain hypodynamic with a high SVR state despite fluid resuscitation and implementation of inotropic support. Nitrosovasodilators (nitroprusside or nitroglycerin have a very short half-life elimination) can be used as first-line therapy for children with epinephrine-resistant, low cardiac output/elevated systemic vascular resistance

shock because hypotension-associated toxicity can be immediately reversed by stopping the infusion. Milrinone, amrinone, or enoximone can be used for their vasodilating properties in patients with nitrosovasodilator-resistant, low-output syndrome or nitrosovasodilator-associated toxicity (cyanide or isothiocyanate toxicity from nitroprusside or methemoglobin toxicity from nitroglycerin). Other vasodilators used and reported in neonatal and pediatric septic shock include prostacyclin, phentolamine, pentoxyfilline, and dopexamine.

Glucose, Calcium, Thyroid, Hydrocortisone, and Insulin Replacement

It is important to maintain metabolic and hormonal homeostasis in newborns and children. Hypoglycemia can cause neurologic devastation when not diagonized. Hypoglycemia must be rapidly diagnosed and promptly treated. To meet glucose infusion requirements, children should be given D10 at maintenance intravenous fluid administration rates (4 mL/kg/hour for the first 10 kg, 3 mL/kg/hour for the next 10 kg, and 2 mL/kg/hour >20 kg). Patients with liver disease may require twice this glucose infusion rate. Hypocalcemia is a frequent, reversible contributor to cardiac dysfunction. Calcium replacement should be directed at normalizing ionized calcium levels. Replacement with thyroid and/or hydrocortisone is lifesaving in children with central or peripheral absolute thyroid and/or adrenal insufficiency and catecholamine-resistant shock. Hypothyroidism and hypoadrenalism are common in children with hypothalamic-pituitary abnormality. Primary thyroid insufficiency is common in children with trisomy 21. Acquired adrenal insufficiency is found in patients who have Waterhouse-Friderichsen syndrome (purpura fulminans) and in children with prior exposure to steroids (hypothalamus-pituitary-adrenal axis suppression) or etomidate (cytochrome P-450–inhibitor).

Annane et al. evaluated adrenal function in adults with dopamine-resistant shock and reported no absolute adrenal insufficiency (defined as a peak cortisol level of 18 μg per dL after a 250-μg ACTH challenge) but attributed highest mortality rates to patients with baseline cortisol levels >30 μg per dL, but with levels in response to ACTH being <9 μg per dL (relative adrenal insufficiency).[56] These same investigators then randomized patients with dopamine-resistant adult septic shock to a 7-day course of hydrocortisone and fludrocortisone, achieving serum levels of approximately 100 μg per dL. This therapy improved outcomes among patients who had a cortisol response <9 μg per dL to the ACTH stimulation test (so-called nonresponders with relative adrenal insufficiency).[57] This study has led to the recommendations that adults with dopamine-resistant shock and relative adrenal insufficiency should be treated with a 7-day steroid course. However, upon further re-examination of this study, it was found that 92 patients were intubated with etomidate, with 87 of these being nonresponders. The placebo arm of this subgroup had an extraordinarily high mortality. Etomidate is a cytochrome P-450–inhibitor that prevents adrenal synthesis and causes adrenal insufficiency even after one dose. A recent study led Annane to declare that "ICU physicians should ban the use of etomidate," a plea given once before in the 1980s when the first moratorium was called on its use.[58,59] Ketamine is the induction agent of choice for intubation of septic shock.

Absolute adrenal insufficiency occurs in 10% to 25% of children with dopamine-resistant septic shock. Hydrocortisone (not methylprednisolone) therapy should be reserved for use in children with catecholamine resistance and with suspected or proved absolute adrenal insufficiency. Patients at risk include children with purpura fulminans and associated Waterhouse-Friderichsen syndrome, children who have previously received steroid therapies for chronic illness, and children with pituitary or adrenal abnormalities. The most conservative diagnostic approach for definition of absolute adrenal insufficiency in a patient with dopamine-resistant shock is a peak cortisol level <18 μg per dL after ACTH stimulation. However, patients with centrally mediated adrenal insufficiency will have a peak response, >18 μg per dL, to ACTH but will be unable to mount this response on their own. The metapyrone test can be used to diagnose this group of patients. In the absence of the metapyrone test, a less conservative approach to the diagnosis of absolute adrenal insufficiency is a baseline cortisol level <18 μg per dL in a patient with dopamine-resistant, fluid-refractory shock.[17] This test assumes that the patient is adequately volume loaded and really dopamine-resistant rather than hypovolemic. The dose of hydrocortisone used in these patients should be titrated to effect in the same manner that catecholamine infusions are titrated to effect. The lowest dose given should be the stress dose (2 mg per kg bolus followed by 2 mg/kg/day infusion) and the highest dose give should be the shock dose (50 mg per kg bolus followed by 50 mg/kg/day infusion). Intermittent dosing can be tried, but the short half-life of hydrocortisone sometimes requires a constant infusion for optimal effect. Two randomized controlled trials of hydrocortisone in children have been performed. Both used shock-dose hydrocortisone for patients with dengue shock. The first study showed improved outcome.[60] The second study was underpowered, and, although it reduced mortality, the effect was not statistically significant.[61] One randomized controlled trial of prophylaxis stress-dose hydrocortisone in premature newborns showed a reduction in hypotension episodes in the first 2 days of life.[46]

Insulin therapy is recommended for the control of hyperglycemia. Hyperglycemia reduces immune function, causes thrombosis, and promotes microbial and fungal growth. Van den Berghe et al. showed that infusion of adequate glucose calories and strict euglycemic control with insulin prevented sepsis and reduced sepsis-induced multiple organ failure and deaths in adult surgical ICU patients.[8] Adequate glucose calories were provided by giving maintenance intravenous fluids as D10. Hypoglycemia and hyperglycemia are associated with poor outcomes in neonates and children. Glucose should be administered as D10 at maintenance fluid rates and insulin should be administered for hyperglycemia.

Persistent Pulmonary Artery Hypertension of the Newborn Therapy

iNO therapy is the treatment of choice for uncomplicated PPHN. Two randomized controlled trials show that iNO reduces the need for ECMO.[62,63] PPHN can be reversed when acidosis is corrected. For centers with access to iNO, this is the only selective pulmonary vasodilator reported to be effective in reversal of PPHN. Inhaled or intravenous prostacyclin can also be beneficial.[64] ECMO remains the therapy of choice for patients with iNO-refractory PPHN and sepsis.

Extracorporeal Membrane Oxygenation Therapy

ECMO is not routinely used in adults with septic shock because mortality caused by vasoplegia is unlikely to be helped by extracardiac mechanical support. However, ECMO is a viable therapy for refractory shock in neonates with septic shock because death occurs as a result of refractory pulmonary hypertension and cardiogenic shock. The Extracorporeal Life Support Organization (ELSO) registry suggests that neonates have a similar outcome (approximate 80% survival) regardless of whether the indication for ECMO is refractory respiratory failure or refractory shock. Although the outcome is similar, neonates with septic shock have more complications (e.g., bleeding, infection) associated with therapy. Outcomes of ECMO therapy used for refractory pediatric respiratory failure or refractory pediatric septic shock (50% survival) are also similar. Interestingly, ECMO is quite effective in patients with adult Hantavirus who have low cardiac output/high SVR shock, supporting the speculation that ECMO therapy is likely most successful in patients with refractory low cardiac output septic shock.

The diagnosis of pediatric septic shock[17] should be made in the presence of the inflammatory triad of fever, tachycardia, and vasodilation. Septic shock is suspected when children with this triad have a change in mental status, manifested as inconsolable irritability, lack of interaction with parents, or increasing inability to arouse. The clinical diagnosis of septic shock is made in children who have (i) a suspected infection manifested by hypothermia or hyperthermia and (ii) clinical signs of decreased perfusion including decreased mental status, prolonged capillary refill >2 seconds (cold shock) or flash capillary refill (warm shock), diminished (cold shock) or bounding (warm shock) peripheral pulses, mottled cool extremities (cold shock), or decreased urine output (<1 mL/kg/hour). Hypotension is not necessary for the clinical diagnosis of septic shock; however, its presence in a child with clinical suspicion of infection is confirmatory.

Goals in the first hour include (i) maintenance of airway, oxygenation, and ventilation; (ii) maintenance of threshold heart rate; and (iii) attainment of normal perfusion and blood pressure. One should strive to achieve capillary refill <2 seconds, normal pulses with no differential between peripheral and central pulses, warm extremities, urine output >1 mL/kg/hour, normal mental status, and normal blood pressure for age. Initial monitoring includes pulse oximetry, continuous electrocardiogram (EKG), blood pressure, temperature, urine output, glucose, and ionized calcium.

Airway and breathing should be rigorously monitored and maintained. Lung compliance and work of breathing may change precipitously. Patients typically manifest hypoxemia, as well as metabolic acidosis, and are at high risk for developing respiratory acidosis. The decision to intubate and ventilate is made on the basis of clinical diagnosis of increased work of breathing, hypoventilation, impaired mental status, or presence of a moribund state. Waiting for confirmatory results of laboratory tests is discouraged. Volume loading is required during intubation because of relative or absolute hypovolemia. Atropine and ketamine should be used as induction agents to maintain cardiovascular integrity.

Vascular access should be rapidly attained. Intraosseous access should be established if reliable venous access cannot be rapidly attained. Placement of central line access will usually be required for vasoactive infusions. Rapid fluid boluses of 20 mL per kg (isotonic saline or colloid) should be administered by push while observing for the development of rales, gallop rhythm, hepatomegaly, and increased work of breathing. In the absence of these clinical findings, fluid can be administered to as much as 200 mL per kg in the first hour. The average requirement is 40 to 60 mL per kg in the first hour. Fluid should be pushed with the goal of attaining normal perfusion and blood pressure.

Patients with severe shock uniformly require vasoactive support during fluid resuscitation. Vasoactive agents should be administered when a second line, preferably a central line, has been established. Dopamine can be used as the first-line agent; however, dopamine-resistant shock should be quickly recognized and epinephrine used for cold shock or norepinephrine used for warm shock to restore normal perfusion and blood pressure. Adrenal insufficiency should be suspected in catecholamine-resistant hypotensive shock in children with a history of long-term steroid use or with purpura fulminans. Use of hydrocortisone in this situation may be lifesaving. Dose recommendations vary from a bolus of 1 to 2 mg per kg for stress coverage to 50 mg per kg for shock, followed by the same dose as a 24-hour infusion. Performance of the ACTH stimulation test is usually not possible in this scenario.

After the first hour, the following goals should be attained: (i) normal perfusion, defined by a capillary refill <2 seconds, normal pulses with no differential between peripheral and central pulses, warm extremities, urine output >1 mL/kg/hour, and normal mental status; (ii) perfusion pressure (MAP − CVP or MAP − IAP), which is appropriate for age; and (iii) a superior vena cava or mixed venous oxygen saturation >70% or a cardiac index >3.3 L/minute/m^2 and <6.0 L/minute/m^2. Preload should be adjusted to increase cardiac output and perfusion. Other monitoring may be required including intra-arterial blood pressure, CVP/oxygen saturation and pulmonary artery pressure/oxygen saturation, or PICCO-derived cardiac output.

Fluid losses and persistent hypovolemia secondary to diffuse capillary leak can continue for days. Ongoing fluid replacement should be directed at clinical endpoints, including perfusion, pulmonary capillary wedge pressure, and cardiac output. Crystalloid is the fluid of choice in patients with Hb >10 g per dL. Packed red blood cell transfusion can be given to children with Hb <10 g per dL. Paradoxically, furosemide boluses or furosemide infusion is uniformly required to prevent fluid overload by transforming oliguric renal failure to nonoliguric renal failure. If furosemide alone is unsuccessful, ten sequential blockade with the distal loop diuretic hydrochorthiazide and the adenosine receptor antagonist aminophylline (low dose to attain a theophylline level of 2 mg per dL) is recommended.[65] Often, hyperoncotic salt poor 25% albumin will be required to maintain intravascular volume and diurese interstitial fluid. If this regimen is unsuccessful in reversing fluid overload, then continuous renal replacement therapy should be implemented.[66]

Hemodynamic support can be required for days in children with fluid-refractory shock. Children can present with low cardiac output/high SVR, high cardiac output/low SVR, or low cardiac output/low SVR shock. Although children with persistent shock frequently have worsening cardiac failure, hemodynamic states may completely change over time. A pulmonary artery catheter or PICCO catheter should be placed when poor perfusion, including reduced urine output, acidosis, or hypotension, persists despite the use of hemodynamic therapies guided by clinical examination, blood pressure analysis, echocardiographic analysis, and arterial and superior vena cava oxygen saturation analysis. Children can respond to a change in hemodynamic therapeutic regimen with resolution of shock. Therapies should be adjusted to maintain superior vena cava oxygen saturation >70%, cardiac index >3.3 L/minute/m^2, and a normal perfusion pressure for age (MAP − CVP) with the ultimate goal of restoration of normal perfusion. There is no benefit in increasing Do_2 beyond the point of Vo_2 plateau (critical point of oxygen delivery).

For *shock with low cardiac output*, epinephrine is the first-line drug for dopamine-resistant shock. If hemodynamics are dependent on epinephrine and the cortisol level is <18 μg per dL, consider beginning hydrocortisone. If thyroxine (T_4) or T_3 level is low and sick euthyroid syndrome has been excluded, PO levothyroxine or liothyronine can be used to restore normal values for age. For *shock with low cardiac output, normal blood pressure, and high SVR*, nitroprusside or nitroglycerin are first-line vasodilators in patients with epinephrine-resistant shock. If cyanide or isothiocyanate toxicity develops from nitroprusside or methemoglobin toxicity develops from nitroglycerin, or if there is a continued low cardiac output state, then the clinician should substitute with milrinone, enoximone, or amrinone. As noted in the preceding text, the long half-life elimination of these drugs can lead to slowly reversible toxicities (hypotension or tachyarrhythmias), particularly if abnormal renal or liver function exists. Such toxicities can be reversed in part with norepinephrine infusion. Additional volume loading is necessary to prevent hypotension when loading doses are used. For *shock with high cardiac output and low SVR*, norepinephrine is the drug of choice for age-dependent dopamine resistance. If hemodynamics are dependent on norepinephrine and cortisol level is <18 μg per dL, then hydrocortisone may be initiated. If the T_4 or T_3 level is low and sick euthyroid syndrome is excluded, then thyroxine or liothyronine can be given. For *refractory shock*, children with catecholamine-refractory shock must be suspected to have unrecognized morbidities including pericardial effusion, pneumothorax, hypoadrenalism, hypothyroidism, ongoing blood loss, intra-abdominal catastrophe, and necrotic tissue. When these morbidities have been excluded, ECMO becomes an important alternative to consider. Currently, however, the expected survival is not >50%. If the clinician suspects that the outcome will be better with ECMO, flows >110 mL per kg may be required if vasodilation exists. Calcium concentration should be normalized in the red blood cell pump prime (usually requires 300 mg $CaCl_2$ per unit of pRBCs [packed red blood cells]). Attention should be given to proper cannula size to avoid hemolysis-induced multiple organ failure. Ongoing support with inotropes and vasodilator therapy is often required to attain central venous oxygen saturations >70%.

Septic shock[17] should be suspected in any neonate with respiratory distress and reduced perfusion, particularly in the presence of a maternal history of chorioamnionitis or prolonged rupture of membranes. It is important to distinguish newborn septic shock from cardiogenic shock caused by closure of the patent ductus arteriosus in newborns with ductal-dependent complex congenital heart disease. Any newborn with shock and hepatomegaly, cyanosis, a cardiac murmur, or differential upper and lower extremity blood pressures or pulses should be started on prostaglandin E_1 until complex congenital heart disease is ruled out by echocardiographic analyses. Newborn septic shock is typically accompanied by increased pulmonary artery pressures. Persistent pulmonary hypertension can cause right ventricle failure.

Goals in the first hour are (i) maintenance of airway, oxygenation, and ventilation; (ii) attainment of neonatal circulation (difference in pre- and postductal oxygen saturation <5% with >95% arterial oxygen saturation); and (iii) maintenance of normal perfusion with capillary refill <2 seconds, normal pulses with no differential between peripheral and central pulses, warm extremities, urine output >1 mL/kg/hour, normal mental status, and normal blood pressure for age. Monitoring includes temperature, pre-

and postductal pulse oximetry, intra-arterial (umbilical or peripheral) blood pressure, continuous EKG, urine output, blood gases, glucose level, and ionized calcium level.

Airway and breathing should be rigorously monitored and maintained. The decision to intubate and ventilate is made on the basis of clinical diagnosis of increased work of breathing or the moribund state. Volume loading is necessary during intubation and ventilation because of hypovolemia. Vascular access should be rapidly attained according to NRP guidelines. Placement of an umbilical arterial and venous line is preferred. If these lines cannot be placed, a peripheral arterial and peripherally positioned central line can be placed. Rapid fluid boluses of 10 mL per kg should be administered, while observing for the development of rales, hepatomegaly, and increased work of breathing. Up to 60 mL per kg may be required in the first hour. Fluid should be pushed with a goal of attaining normal perfusion and blood pressure.

Patients with severe shock uniformly require vasoactive support during fluid resuscitation. Although dopamine can be used as the first-line agent, its effect on pulmonary vascular resistance should be taken into account. Usually, a combination of dopamine at low dosage (<8 mg/kg/minute) and dobutamine (up to 30 μg/kg/minute) is used; if the patient is not responsive to therapy, then epinephrine should be infused to restore normal blood pressure and perfusion. Hydrocortisone can be used if the patient is epinephrine-refractory. For PPHN, hyperoxygenate initially with 100% oxygen and provide metabolic alkalinization (up to pH 7.50) with $NaHCO_3$ or tromethamine if iNO is unavailable. Mild hyperventilation can also be instituted until 100% oxygen saturation and <5% difference in pre- and postductal saturations are obtained. Therapeutic narcosis with fentanyl and paralysis with neuromuscular blockers should be considered to reduce pulmonary blood pressures in intubated, ventilated patients who do not respond to the PPHN therapy outlined in the preceding text. iNO should be the first-line drug administered when available.

Beyond the first hour, the goals remain similar, including maintenance of threshold heart rate, normal perfusion and blood pressure, and neonatal circulation.

In addition, volume should be administered according to CVP. Central venous oxygen saturation should be maintained >70%. The absence of right-to-left shunting, tricuspid regurgitation, or right ventricular failure should be documented by echocardiographic analysis.

Similar to children, fluid losses and persistent hypovolemia secondary to diffuse capillary leak can continue for days, and furosemide and sequential tubule blockade may be paradoxically required to maintain a nonoliguric renal failure state. Ongoing fluid replacement should be directed at clinical endpoints, including perfusion and CVP. Crystalloid is the fluid of choice in patients with Hb >12 g per dL. Packed red blood cell transfusion can be added in newborns with Hb <12 g per dL.

The pulmonary vascular reactivity will tend to decrease after 5 days of life, although this should be evaluated carefully before stopping therapies directed at PPHN. In the patient with suprasystemic pulmonary hypertension, right ventricle failure may accompany shock. This can make inotrope and vasopressor therapies less effective in supporting cardiac output. Therapies directed at reducing pulmonary artery pressure are paramount. iNO can be given, with greatest effects usually found at 20 ppm. In newborns with poor left ventricle function and normal blood pressure, the addition of nitrosovasodilators or type III PDEIs can be effective but must be monitored for toxicities. It is important to volume load when using these systemic vasodilators.

Newborns with refractory shock must be suspected to have unrecognized morbidities including pericardial effusion, pneumothorax, ongoing blood loss, hypoadrenalism, hypothyroidism, inborn errors of metabolism, and/or cyanotic or obstructive heart disease. When these causes have been excluded, ECMO becomes an important therapy to consider. The expected ECMO survival rate for newborn septic shock is currently 80%. Most centers accept refractory shock or a $PaO_2 <40$ mm Hg after maximal therapy to be a sufficient indication for ECMO support. ECMO flows >110 mL per kg may be required when vasodilation exists. When on veno–arterial or veno–veno ECMO, persistent hypotension and/or shock should be treated with inotropes, vasodilators, or vasopressors to maintain normal blood pressure and central venous saturation $>70\%$. Persistent low flow states with normal blood pressure and decreased central venous oxygen saturation should be treated with epinephrine and milrinone or nitrosovasodilators. Having said this, the veno–arterial system provides inotropic support, and inotrope requirements frequently lessen when veno–arterial ECMO is used. Calcium concentration should be normalized in the red blood cell pump prime (usually requires 300 mg $CaCl_2$ per unit of pRBCs).

Anaphylactic Shock

Anaphylactic shock is associated with vascular failure, in part because of massive histamine and bradykinin release. High-dosage epinephrine (α-adrenergic vasoconstriction range) is considered the therapy of choice, initially in the form of an epinephrine pen. High-dose epinephrine mediated vasoconstriction offsets histamine-induced vasodilation. Epinephrine also reverses bronchospasm. Epinephrine can be continued as repeated subcutaneous or intramuscular boluses or provided as an intravenous infusion. Combined H_1 and H_2 blockers and steroids are also recommended for reducing ongoing anaphylaxis.

Drug-Induced Shock

Pentobarbital-Induced Shock
Management of severe intracranial hypertension includes intracranial pressure monitoring and the use of pentobarbital. This agent reduces cerebral metabolism, metabolism-coupled blood flow, and intracranial pressure. Unfortunately, pentobarbital is also a cardiac and vascular depressant. Children receiving pentobarbital infusions can require inotrope and/or vasopressor therapies. Some of these patients can require a pulmonary artery or PICCO catheter to determine whether decreased cardiac output or vasoplegia is contributing to hypotension. Superior vena cava oxygen saturation measurements can be misleading because pentobarbital reduces oxygen consumption. Capillary refill may also be misleading if patients are also receiving mild/moderate hypothermia therapy. The important goal in these patients is not only adequate cardiac output and systemic blood pressure but also adequate cerebral perfusion pressure (MAP – ICP). Prolonged perfusion pressure <40 mm Hg is associated with death. Most recommend age-specific perfusion pressure goals of 50 to 60 mm Hg.

Calcium Channel Blocker, β-Blocker, Type III Phosphodiesterase Inhibitor, and Nitroprusside Toxicity
In the United States, it has been suggested by the Institute of Medicine that the eighth leading cause of death is medical errors. Among these are drug errors. Some occur from overdosage; some from organ failure, which prevents elimination of drug; and some from drug interactions. It is important to understand the antidotes for these problems. *Calcium channel blockade toxicity* can be reversed in part by using agents that increase intracellular cAMP and calcium in the heart, including glucagon and type III PDEIs (milrinone, amrinone, and enoximone), and increase intracellular IP_3 and calcium in vascular smooth muscle cells, including vasopressin, angiotensin, and norepinephrine. Calcium can be given, but it is unlikely to overcome the calcium channel blockade. *β-Blocker toxicity* can be overcome with massive amounts of β-agonist drug. Antagonists have a much greater affinity for the receptor than agonists. One or more adult ampules of isoproterenol can be required to overcome β-blockade toxicity in a child. *Type III PDEI toxicity* can be reversed with norepinephrine, which stimulates vasoconstriction through the α-adrenergic receptor. Epinephrine would be less effective because β_2-adrenergic stimulation would offset the α-adrenergic effect. *Nitroprusside toxicity* leads to cyanide and isothiocyanate toxicity. The levels of these drugs should be checked regularly and the medication stopped when toxic levels occur. This is common in children with renal dysfunction or with use of the drug at dosages >1 μg/kg/minute. *Phenoxybenzamine toxicity* can be overcome by vasopressin or angiotensin infusion. These agents increase vascular smooth muscle cell IP_3, DAG, and intracellular calcium, bypassing the α-adrenergic–receptor blockade.

Status Asthmaticus–Induced Shock

Sudden death is the leading cause of death associated with β_2-agonist therapy in children with asthma. The

β_2-agonist therapy can cause systemic vasodilation. Many patients with asthma receive long-term steroids and can develop central adrenal insufficiency with a depressed pituitary/adrenal axis. The combination can lead to vasodilated shock with decreased diastolic filling pressures (vasodilation) and increased troponin levels (myocardial injury from inadequate diastolic coronary artery filling). Patients with this drug-induced pathology can be treated by reducing of β_2-agonist therapy or adding of a vasopressor such as dopamine to counteract the β_2-agonist effect. If adrenal insufficiency plays a role in diastolic hypotension, then replacement with steroids for pituitary/adrenal shock should be done with hydrocortisone or fludrocortisone. Neither methylprednisolone nor dexamethasone (steroids used for asthma) has any mineralocorticoid effect.

Death from shock can also occur when intrathoracic pressure is paradoxically increased in patients with status asthmaticus. In the earlier stages of status asthmaticus, large negative inspiratory and, therefore, intrathoracic pressures are generated. However, as air trapping becomes excessive, functional residual capacity can approach total lung capacity and cause cardiac tamponade physiology. Most of these patients require intubation. If volume loading and ketamine are used, then venous return is maintained despite high intrathoracic pressures, and intubation can be safely performed. If not used, hypotensive arrest can occur during intubation as venous return is decreased. Death from shock and cardiac arrest can still subsequently occur in the safely intubated patient with status asthmaticus if inhaled volumes remain consistently higher than exhaled volumes because intrathoracic pressure continues to increase until the development of tension pneumothorax or intrathoracic impedance of venous return. Extraordinary therapies such as inhaled anesthesia or ECMO are indicated before shock and arrest occur.

Intubation and Shock

Blood flow in the human body can be conceptualized in compartments. According to this physiologic model, blood flows from the higher pressure compartment to the lower pressure compartment. In the spontaneously breathing patient, the pressure in the intrathoracic compartment is negative during inspiration, allowing blood to flow from the extrathoracic compartment to the right side of the heart. When patients require intubation and positive-pressure ventilation, this physiologic pattern is reversed. Positive-pressure ventilation increases intrathoracic pressure above extrathoracic pressure and impedes venous return to the right side of the heart. Induction agents can exacerbate this problem if they reduce venous and arterial tone by reducing either catecholamine production (narcotics, benzodiazepines) or cortisol production (etomidate). Therefore, intubation of patients with shock, who cannot tolerate the reduction in preload associated with positive-pressure ventilation, should be preceded by volume resuscitation

and induction with atropine and ketamine (which increase catecholamine levels and maintain cortisol levels).

Anesthetic Agents and Shock

Anesthetic agents are necessary during surgical procedures. Unfortunately, this class of agents can induce vasoplegic and cardiogenic shock. Vasoplegia is quite common and should be treated with fluid resuscitation to normal CVP/pulmonary artery occlusion pressure, blood pressure, capillary refill, superior vena cava oxygen saturation, and urine output. The use of selective vasoconstrictors such as phenylephrine should be carefully evaluated because most anesthetics also reduce cardiac function. The use of a pure vasoconstrictor will increase afterload and worsen cardiac function. Mixed inovasopressors such as dopamine, epinephrine, or norepinephrine should be considered under these circumstances. Special consideration must be given if propofol is used. In some patients, particularly those with viral or bacterial infection, an acute cardiac failure syndrome with bradycardia and lactic acidosis can occur. The drug, and the surgical case if possible, should be stopped, and inotropes should be used to reverse cardiogenic shock. High levels of positive end-expiratory pressure (PEEP) can be required to oxygenate these patients because pulmonary edema from failure of the left side of the heart is common.

WHEN SHOCK DOES NOT RESPOND TO THERAPY

Despite one's best clinical hopes, agents may not be effective. It is important to think about potential reasons. First, drugs such as dopamine or dobutamine are not particularly effective in younger children. Therefore, graduation to norepinephrine (warm shock) and epinephrine (cold shock) should be quickly considered. One should next consider the question, "Am I missing something?" It should be ensured that there are no unrecognized problems such as hemorrhagic shock, tension pneumothorax, or cardiac tamponade. Catecholamine-resistant warm shock can be treated with more volume. Hydrocortisone therapy should be considered if adrenal insufficiency is suspected and/or diagnosed. Vasopressin or angiotensin therapy may be effective if warm shock continues. Catecholamine-resistant cold shock should be treated with nitroprusside and/or type III PDEIs after hypotension has been controlled. Hydrocortisone can be considered if adrenal insufficiency is suspected or diagnosed. T_3 can be considered as well, particularly in patients with central nervous system pathology or hypothyroidism. Consideration should also be given to the possibility of undiagnosed pulmonary hypertension and right ventricular failure if therapies remain ineffective. Echocardiogram, superior vena cava oxygen saturation, and pulmonary artery or PICCO catheter can be used to confirm the hemodynamic cause of refractory shock.

CONCLUSION

Shock is a major determinant of outcome in pediatric ICUs. And outcome is dependent on time-sensitive recognition and implementation of goal-directed therapies. Facility with volume resuscitation and with inotrope, vasopressor, and vasodilator therapies is one of the most important attributes of the master pediatric intensivist. Choice of therapeutic regimens should be based upon an in-depth understanding of physiologic and biochemical principles, with each patient requiring ongoing evaluation and titration of concentrations and combinations of fluids, drugs, and machines directed at attaining goals of normal perfusion (normal capillary refill, MAP − CVP, and cardiac output), normal oxygen utilization ($Scvo_2$ >70% or $AVDo_2$ between 3% to 5%), and normal glucose utilization (normal glycemia on D10 at maintenance intravenous fluid rates).

REFERENCES

1. Parr GV, Blackstone EH, Kirklin JW. Cardiac performance and mortality early after intracardiac surgery in infants and young children. *Circulation.* 1975;51(5):867–874.
2. Appelbaum A, Blackstone EH, Kouchoukos NT. Afterload reduction and cardiac output in infants after intracardiac surgery. *Am J Cardiol.* 1977;39(3):445–451.
3. Pollack MM, Fields AI, Ruttimann UE, et al. Distributions of cardiopulmonary variables in pediatric survivors and nonsurvivors of septic shock. *Crit Care Med.* 1985;13(6):454–459.
4. Ceneviva G, Paschall JA, Maffei F, et al. Hemodynamic support in fluid-refractory pediatric septic shock. *Pediatrics.* 1998;102(2):e19,1–6.
5. Rivers E, Nguyen B, Havstad S, et al. Early goal directed therapy in the treatment of severe sepsis and septic shock. *N Engl J Med.* 2001;346(19):1368–1377.
6. Han YY, Carcillo JA, Dragotta MA, et al. Early reversal of pediatric-neonatal septic shock by community physicians is associated with improved outcome. *Pediatrics.* 2003;112(4):793–799.
7. Orr RA, Kuch B, Carcillo J, Han Y, et al. Shock is under-reported in children transported for respiratory distress: A multi-center study. *Crit Care Med.* 2003;31(12):A18.
8. Van den Berghe G, Wouters P, Weekers F, et al. Intensive insulin therapy in the critically ill patients. *N Engl J Med.* 2001;345(19):1359–1367.
9. Lin JC, Karapinar B, Finegold DN, et al. Increased glucose/glucose infusion rate ratio predicts anion gap acidosis in pediatric shock. *Crit Care Med.* 2004;32(12):A5.
10. Finfer S, Bellomo R, boyce N, et al. SAFE Study Investigators. A comparison of albumin and saline for fluid resuscitation in the intensive care unit. *N Engl J Med.* 2004;350(22):2247–2256.
11. Ngo NT, Cao XT, Kneen R, et al. Acute management of dengue shock syndrome: A randomized double-blind comparison of 4 intravenous fluid regimens in the first hour. *Clin Infect Dis.* 2001;32(2):204–212.
12. Carcillo JA, Davis AI, Zaritsky A, et al. Role of early fluid resuscitation in pediatric septic shock. *JAMA.* 1991;255(9):1242–1245.
13. Perkin RM, Levin DL, Webb R, et al. Dobutamine: A hemodynamic evaluation in children with shock. *J Pediatr.* 1982;100(6):977–983.
14. Bollaert PE, Bauer P, Audibert G, et al. Effects of epinephrine on hemodynamics and oxygen metabolism in dopamine-resistant septic shock. *Chest.* 1990;98(4):949–953.
15. Motta P, Mossad E, Toscana D, et al. Comparison of phenoxybenzamine to sodium nitroprusside in infants undergoing surgery. *J Cardiothorac Vasc Anesth.* 2005;19(1):54–59.
16. *American Hospital Formulary.* www.ashp.org/ahfs/.
17. Carcillo JA, Fields AI. American College of Critical Care Medicine Task Force Committee members clinical practice parameters for hemodynamic support of pediatric and neonatal patients in septic shock. *Crit Care Med.* 2002;30(6):1365–1378.
18. Bettendorf M, Schmitt KG, Grulich Henn J, et al. Tri-iodothyronine treatment in children after cardiac surgery: A double blind, randomized placebo controlled study. *Lancet.* 2000;356(9229):529–534.
19. Roytblat L, Talmor D, Rachinsky M, et al. Ketamine attenuates the interleukin 6 response after cardiopulmonary bypass. *Anesth Analg.* 1998;87(2):266–271.
20. Thomas NJ, Carcillo JA. Hypovolemic shock in the pediatric patient. *New Horiz.* 1998;6(2):120–129.
21. Boldt J, Muller M, Heeson M, et al. Influence of different volume therapies and pentoxyfilline infusion on circulating soluble adhesion molecules in critically ill patients. *Crit Care Med.* 1996;24(3):385–391.
22. Carrol GC, Snyder JV. Hyperdynamic severe intravascular sepsis depends on fluid administration in cynomolgus monkeys. *Am J Physiol.* 1982;243(1):R131–R141.
23. Lee PK, Deringer JP, Kreisworth BN, et al. Fluid replacement of rabbits challenged subcutaneous with toxic shock syndrome toxins. *Infect Immun.* 1991;59(3):879–898.
24. Ottoson J, Davidson I, Brandberg A, et al. Cardiac output and organ blood flow in experimental septic shock: Effect of treatment with antibiotics, corticosteroids, and fluid infusion. *Circ Shock.* 1991;35(1):14–24.
25. Hoban LD, Paschall JA, Eckstein J, et al. Awake porcine model of intraperitoneal sepsis and altered oxygen utilization. *Circ Shock.* 1991;34(2):252–262.
26. Wilson MA, Chou MC, Spain DA, et al. Fluid resuscitation attenuates early cytokine mRNA expression after peritonitis. *J Trauma, Inj, Infect Crit Care.* 1996;41(4):622–627.
27. O'Neill PJ, Cobb LM, Steigman CK, et al. Prevention of secondary cardiovascular instability after intestinal ischemia reperfusion improves survival. *Am J Physiol.* 1993;264(3Pt2)R622–R629.
28. Xia ZF, He F, Barrow RE, et al. Reperfusion injury in burned rats after delayed fluid resuscitation. *J Burn Care Rehabil.* 1991;12(5):430–436.
29. Powell KR, Sugarman LI, Eskenazi AE, et al. Normalization of plasma arginine vasopressin concentration when children with meningitis are given maintenance plus replacement fluid therapy. *J Pediatr.* 1990;117(4):515–522.
30. Lambert HJ, Baylis PH, Gulthard MG, et al. Central-peripheral temperature difference, blood pressure, and arginine vasopressin in preterm neonates undergoing volume expansion. *Arch Dis Child Fetal Neonatal Ed.* 1998;78(1):F43–F45.
31. Simma B, Fritz MG, Trawagewr R, et al. Changes in left ventricular function in shocked newborns. *Intens Care Med.* 1997;23(9):982–986.
32. Reynolds EM, Ryan DP, Sheridan RL, et al. Left ventricular failure complicating severe pediatric burn injuries. *J Pediatr Surg.*30(2):264–269; discussion 1995;269–270.
33. Haupt MT, Rackow EC. Colloid osmotic pressure and fluid resuscitation with hetastarch, albumin, and saline solution. *Crit Care Med.* 1982;10(3):159–162.
34. *Constable Veterinary Clinics of North America-Food Animal Practice,* 1999, www.ashp.org/ahfs/.
35. Hatherill M, Tibby SM, Hilliard T, et al. Adrenal insufficiency in septic shock. *Arch Dis Child.* 1999;80:51–55.
36. Bouachour G, Tirot P, Varache N, et al. Hemodynamic changes in adrenal insufficiency. *Intens Care Med.* 1994;20(2):138–141.
37. Bailey JM, Miller BE, Kanter KR, et al. A comparison of the hemodynamic effects of amrinone and sodium nitroprusside in infants after cardiac surgery. *Anesth Analg.* 1997;84(2):294–8–36.
38. Hoffman TM, Wernovsky G, Atz AM, et al. Efficacy and safety of milrinone in preventing low cardiac output syndrome in infants and children after corrective surgery for congenital heart disease. *Circulation.* 2003;107(7):996–1002.
39. O'Blenes SB, Roy N, Konstantinov I, et al. Vasopressin reversal of phenoxybenzamine induced hypotension after the Norwood procedure. *J Thorac Cardiovasc Surg.* 2002;123(5):1012–1013.
40. DuPont HL, Spink WW. Infections due to gram negative organisms: An analysis of 860 patients with bacteremia at University of Minnesota Medical Center 1958–1966. *Medicine.* 1968;48(4):307.

41. Watson RS, Carcillo JA, Linde-Zwirble WT, et al. The epidemiology of severe sepsis in children in the United States. *Am J Respir Crit Care Med.* 2003;167(5):605–701.

42. Booy R, Habibi P, Nadel S, et al. Meningococcal Research Group. Reduction in case fatality rate from meningococcal disease associated with improved health care delivery. *Arch Dis Child.* 2001;85(5):380–390.

43. Kutko MC, Calarco MP, Flaherty MB, et al. Mortality rates in pediatric septic shock with and without multiple organ system failure. *Pediatr Crit Care Med.* 2003;4(3):333–337.

44. Lin JC, Kuch BA, Felmet KA, et al. Best practice outcome attained with implementation of ACCM/PALS guidelines for resuscitation of neonatal and pediatric septic shock; an UTSTEIN Style analysis. *Crit Care Med.* 2003;31(12):A70.

45. Carcillo JA, Pollack MM, Ruttimann UE, et al. Sequential physiologic interactions in cardiogenic and septic shock. *Crit Care Med.* 1989;17(1):12–16.

46. Efird MM, Heerens AT, Gordon PV, et al. Av randomized controlled trial of prophylactic hydrocortisone supplementation for the prevention of hypotension in extremely low birth weight infants. *J Perinatol.* 2005;25(2):119–124.

47. Lauterbach R, Pawlik D, Kowalczyk D, et al. The effect of the immunomodulatory agent, pentoxyfilline in the treatment of sepsis in prematurely delivered infants; placebo controlled, double blinded trial. *Crit Care Med.* 1999;27:807–814.

48. Lucking SE, Williams TM, Chaten FC. Dependence of oxygen consumption on oxygen delivery in children with hyperdynamic septic shock and low oxygen extraction. *Crit Care Med.* 1990; 18(12):1316–1319.

49. Mink RB, Pollack MM. Effect of blood transfusion on oxygen consumption in pediatric septic shock. *Crit Care Med.* 1990; 18(10):1087–1091.

50. Zadrobilek E, Hackl W, Sporn P, et al. Effect of large volume replacement with balanced electrolyte solutions on extravascular lung water in surgical patients with sepsis syndrome. *Intensive Care Med.* 1989;15(8):505–510.

51. Powell KR, Sugarman LI, Eskenazi AE, et al. Normalization of plasma arginine vasopressin concentrations when children with meningitis are given maintenance plus replacement fluid therapy. *J Pediatr.* 1990;117(4):515–522.

52. Outwater KM, Treves ST, Lang P. Renal and Hemodynamic effects of dopamine in infants following cardiac surgery. *J Clin Anesth.* 1990;2(4):253–257.

53. Meadows D, Edwards JD, Wilkins RG, et al. Reversal of intractable septic shock with norepinephrine therapy. *Crit Care Med.* 1988;16:663–666.

54. Desjars P, Pinaud M, Potel G, et al. A reappraisal of norepinephrine therapy in human septic shock. *Crit Care Med.* 1987;15:134–137.

55. Meier-Hellman A, Reinhart K, Bredle DC, et al. Epinephrine impairs splanchnic perfusion in septic shock. *Crit Care Med.* 1997; 25:399–404.

56. Annane D, Sebille V, Troche G, et al. A 3-level prognostic classification in septic shock based on cortisol levels and cortisol response to corticotrophin. *JAMA.* 2000;283(8):1038–1045.

57. Annane D, Sebille V, Charpentier C, et al. Effect of treatment with low doses of hydrocortisone and fludrocortisone on mortality in patients with septic shock. *JAMA.* 2002;288(7):862–871.

58. Annane D. ICU physicians should abandon the use of etomidate! *Intensive Care Med.* 2005;10:1454.

59. Newby DM, Edbrooke DL. Influence of sedation on mortality in trauma patients. *Lancet.* 1983;1(8338):1381.

60. Min MUT, Aye M, Shwe TN, et al. Hydrocortisone in the management of dengue shock syndrome. *Southeast Asian J Trop Med Public Health.* 1975;6(4):573–579.

61. Sumarmo S. The role of steroids in dengue shock syndrome. *Southeast Asian J Trop Med Public Health.* 1987;18(3):383–389.

62. Roberts JD Jr, Rinnai JR, Main FC III, et al. The Inhaled Nitric Oxide Study Group. Inhaled nitric oxide and persistent pulmonary hypertension of the newborn. *N Engl J Med.* 1997;336(9):605–610.

63. Inhaled Nitric Oxide Study Group. Inhaled nitric oxide in full term and nearly full-term infants with hypoxic respiratory failure. *N Engl J Med.* 1997;336:597–604.

64. Konduri GG. New approaches for persistent pulmonary hypertension of newborn. *Clin Perinatol.* 2004;31(3):591–611.

65. Bell M, Jackson E, Mi Z, et al. Low-dose theophylline increases urine output in diuretic dependent critically ill children. *Intensive Care Med.* 1998;24(10):1099–1105.

66. Foland JA, Fortenberry JD, Warshaw BL, et al. Fluid overload before continuous hemofiltration and survival in critically ill children: A retrospective analysis. *Crit Care Med.* 2004;32(8):1771–1776.

Clinical Disorders

Endocrine Disorders

Murray M. Pollack   *Paul Kaplowitz*

Endocrine Disorders of Water Regulation

11

Susan B. Nunez

CLINICAL SYNDROMES OF ABNORMAL WATER REGULATION

Manifestations of derangements in osmotic homeostasis are due to alterations in cell volume in the central nervous system (CNS), changes in effective circulating volume and local disturbances produced, that is, by an intracranial neoplasm. In the steady state, the net water balance should be zero. Hypertonicity occurs when the renal plus extrarenal water losses exceed water intake, causing the ratio of solutes to water in the body fluids to increase. In hypotonic syndromes, water intake exceeds the sum of renal plus extrarenal water losses; but in chronic hyponatremia, water intake and water output may be equal.

HYPONATREMIA

Hyponatremia, defined as a serum sodium level <135 mEq per L, is a common electrolyte imbalance in the setting of pediatric critical care. It can occur in children who are volume contracted and have lost sodium in excess of water, as in severe diarrhea, or renal sodium losses due to adrenal insufficiency with inadequate aldosterone production. This is particularly challenging in patients with acute CNS disease, especially if the sodium is low (<125 mEq per L), which can cause seizures and worsen neurologic status. The differential diagnosis is often between the syndrome of inappropriate secretion of antidiuretic hormone (SIADH) and the cerebral salt wasting (CSW) syndrome. Distinguishing between the two causes is important because the treatment of each condition is very different. In both, there is hyponatremia and inappropriately concentrated urine. SIADH is associated with increased extracellular fluid volume (ECF). In CSW syndrome, there is clinical evidence of a contracted ECF volume.

SYNDROME OF INAPPROPRIATE SECRETION OF ANTIDIURETIC HORMONE

This syndrome, although common in the pediatric critical care setting, is rarely the reason for admission to the pediatric intensive care unit (PICU). The expansion of the ECF volume in SIADH is due to a nonphysiologic or inappropriate secretion of the antidiuretic hormone (ADH), or due to the increased sensitivity of the kidneys to the effect of ADH. ADH acts on the distal collecting ducts and tubules resulting in increased permeability to water, increased fluid reabsorption and increased intravascular volume. In response to the latter, the glomerular filtration rate and renal plasma flow increase, and proximal sodium reabsorption decreases, thereby increasing the urine sodium levels and decreasing the serum sodium level. The increased ECF volume is accompanied by weight gain but is not associated with distended neck veins or edema because only one third of retained water is distributed in the ECF space.

With progressively decreasing levels of sodium, the patients gradually develop malaise, hypotonia, nausea, vomiting, anorexia, mental alterations, followed by convulsive crises, stupor, and coma. Other signs and symptoms include pseudobulbar paralysis, Babinski sign, and extrapyramidal symptoms. Patients with existing neurologic disorder will have neurologic symptoms at higher levels of sodium than those without such disorders.

SIADH is uncommon in children.[1] A summary of the different conditions associated with SIADH is given in

TABLE 11.1

CAUSES OF SYNDROME OF INAPPROPRIATE SECRETION OF ANTIDIURETIC HORMONE

Malignancies	Medications
Bronchogenic carcinoma	Vincristine
Thymoma	Carbamazepine
ALL	Cyclophosphamide (IV)
Lymphoma	SSRI antidepressants
Neuroblastoma	Opiates
Duodenal or pancreatic	Clofibrate
adenocarcinoma	Chlorpropamide
	Lamotrigine

Central Nervous System Disorders	Pulmonary Disorders
Infection: meningitis, encephalitis	Infection: pneumonia, tuberculosis
Neoplasms near the pituitary or hypothalamus	Asthma
Vascular anomalies, stroke	Pneumothorax
Trauma	Positive pressure ventilation
Hydrocephalus	
Pituitary surgery	
Hypoxia-ischemia	
Psychosis	

ALL, acute lymphoblastic leukemia; SSRI, selective serotonin reuptake inhibitors; IV, intravenous.

Table 11.1. The release of ADH can be stimulated by pain, stress, increased intracranial pressure, and hypovolemic states.[2] SIADH can also develop 1 week after transsphenoidal pituitary surgery in 35% of patients or as phase 2 in a triphasic phase following intrasellar surgery.[3] The retrograde neuronal degeneration with cell death and vasopressin release has been thought to be the mechanism behind this phenomenon.[4]

To confirm the diagnosis of SIADH, the following approximate measurements are used: hyponatremia ($Na^+ \leq 135$ mEq per L), serum hypo-osmolality (≥ 280 mOsm per L), decreased urine output to <1 mL/kg/hour with high urine osmolality (>600 mOsm per L), or an inappropriately high urine osmolality (with sodium excretion >20 to 25 mEq per L) in the presence of a low serum osmolality, and in the absence of clinically evident dehydration. Measurement of plasma hormones including ADH, natriuretic peptide, renin activity, and aldosterone are impractical because the results are not immediately available for use in making rapid clinical changes. In addition, the results may cause confusion because of the short half-life and mutual influence of the hormones on each other.

Treatment

Pediatric intensivists should anticipate the development of SIADH for prompt and effective therapy to be given. Mortality may be as high as 50% in acute hyponatremia

if untreated.[5] Treatment is based on the duration of the hyponatremia and the intensity of the neurologic disturbance such as seizure or altered mental status. There are two basic principles to be remembered when correcting hyponatremia: (i) the serum sodium level should be increased at a safe rate and (ii) the underlying disease should be treated. In general, the serum sodium should be corrected slowly at a rate not exceeding 1.3 mEq/L/hour with a total correction of no more than 10 mEq per L in the first 24 hours and <20 mEq per L over the first 48 hours.[6] If too rapid correction of serum sodium occurs, the patient may develop central pontine myelinolysis.[7] This is a disorder characterized by confusion, dysarthria, pseudobulbar palsy, and quadriplegia as a result of demyelination in the base of the pons.

In severe "acute" hyponatremia with neurologic symptoms, occurring within <48 hours, 3% saline solution, 3.0 to 5.0 mL per kg can be administered rapidly to increase the serum sodium faster at 1.5 to 2.0 mEq per L for 3 to 4 hours or until the neurologic symptoms resolve. The infusion rate may be calculated by multiplying the body weight in kilograms by the desired rate of increase in Na^+ level in mEq/L/hour. A loop diuretic such as furosemide 1.0 to 2.0 mL per kg may be added to increase water excretion.

SIADH, which is asymptomatic and therefore has likely developed over a longer period of time, is best treated with fluid restriction. This is usually sufficient to normalize the sodium level. In a young child, fluid intake may be restricted to the range of 30% to 75% of maintenance requirement or to 1,000 mL/m²/day.[8,9] If this fails to correct the hyponatremia, the addition of demeclocycline, may be indicated to allow for higher volume intake. Lithium may also be used for this purpose, but demeclocycline is superior in causing a nephrogenic diabetes insipidus (DI)-like state, thereby decreasing the renal concentrating ability and decreasing water reabsorption in the collecting ducts and tubules.[10] It may take several days before an optimal response is appreciated.

CEREBRAL SALT WASTING SYNDROME

CSW syndrome is not uncommon in a critically ill pediatric patient. CSW syndrome and SIADH have many similar clinical findings, that is, hyponatremia, high urine osmolality, and elevated urinary sodium concentration higher than 150 mEq per L. They can both be caused by the same intracerebral diseases. Vasopressin level is also elevated in CSW syndrome; however, it is an appropriate response to volume depletion. Unlike SIADH, in CSW syndrome, the urinary output is not low and the ECF volume is decreased due to primary natriuresis.[11] Clinical signs of dehydration are evident. Therefore, volume restriction is not effective in restoring normal serum sodium levels in CSW syndrome, and fluid restriction in a patient with CSW syndrome may cause further volume depletion, a decrease in brain perfusion and cerebral lesion, and an increase in mortality rate. On the other hand, large amounts of salt infusion required to restore normal sodium concentrations in CSW syndrome may prove detrimental in a patient with SIADH who is already volume expanded. The leading hypothesis in the pathophysiology of CSW syndrome is that brain natriuretic peptide (BNP), produced predominantly in the ventricles of the brain, is secreted in abnormal amounts. These natriuretic peptides, including atrial natriuretic peptide, C-type natriuretic peptide, and the recently discovered dendroaspis natriuretic peptide (DNP), exert their effect by antagonizing the renal effects of ADH, suppressing the renin–angiotensin–aldosterone axis, and centrally inhibiting salt appetite and thirst, causing diuresis and natriuresis.[12] Treatment of CSW syndrome consists of restoring normal intravascular volume with water and sodium chloride, as with the treatment of systemic dehydration. The underlying CNS disorder should be also treated, if possible.

DIABETES INSIPIDUS

DI is not uncommon and its occurrence should be anticipated in the pediatric intensive care setting. Central DI is likely if serum osmolality is >300 mOsm per kg with very dilute and high volume urine, exceeding 200 mL/m^2/hour. Children with an underlying neurologic disturbance are at highest risk. The most common situation is following suprasellar surgery. Here, the onset of DI is anticipated and intervention can be promptly initiated. DI should also be anticipated to occur in patients following accidental head trauma, infection, or massive brain ischemia. Because infants and children have a smaller body size and higher total body water content than adults, a small disturbance in volume homeostasis may cause significant acute fluid and electrolyte disturbance contributing to the course of the critical illness. Therefore, it is important to recognize, evaluate, and promptly treat DI when it occurs.

An intact thirst mechanism is an important regulator of volume homeostasis and serum osmolality, particularly in DI. Thirst is stimulated when the osmotic threshold for thirst is exceeded, commonly when the serum osmolality is 2% to 3% above the basal level. The initial perception of thirst is in direct proportion to the sodium level and osmolality. Patients with DI and an intact thirst mechanism will increase their fluid intake to maintain normal serum osmolality if antidiuretic therapy is inadequate, but they are allowed free access to water. The subset of DI patients with absent thirst mechanism (adipsia) are much more likely to present with severe dehydration and hypernatremia if their antidiuretic treatment is stopped or wears off too quickly, and are much more likely to require an admission to the PICU to correct the problem.

Acquired DI is more commonly seen than the congenital forms, although the latter should not be overlooked.

DI is a heterogeneous group of disorders, which can be divided into: (a) vasopressin-sensitive or (b) vasopressin resistant. The causes of vasopressin-sensitive DI (also called *hypothalamic, neurogenic,* or *central DI*) include trauma to the hypothalamic-neurohypophyseal system (either accidental or surgical), infiltrative disease including tumors or infection, destruction by the autoimmune process, genetic defects in vasopressin production, and congenital anomalies or defects of the hypothalamic or pituitary gland. The cause of central DI is unknown in 10% of pediatric cases.[13]

Vasopressin-resistant DI (also called *nephrogenic DI*) results from genetic or acquired causes. Genetic causes are more common in children than in adults and are more severe than the acquired form. Familial vasopressin-resistant DI is due to a defect in the vasopressin (V_2) receptor, inherited in an X-linked pattern. An autosomal dominant or recessive form of inheritance linked to a mutation in the aquaporin-2 water channel, with an intact V_2 receptor, has also been reported.[14] The acquired form of vasopressin-resistant DI is more common and less severe. It may be due to: disorders in the kidney and ureter, sickle cell disease; Sjögren syndrome, intake of drugs such as lithium, demeclocycline, and foscarnet (used to treat cytomegalovirus infection in immunosuppressed patients); electrolyte imbalance such as hypokalemia, osmotic diuresis due to glycosuria in diabetes mellitus; primary polydipsia; hypercalcemia; decreased protein or sodium intake; and washout from massive diuretic use.

THE TRIPHASIC RESPONSE

Injury to the supraopticohypophyseal tract causes bilateral neuron degeneration in the supraoptic neuron (SON) and the paraventricular neuron (PVN); when approximately 90% of the magnocellular neurons in the SON and PVN are lost, permanent diabetes insipidus ensues. Diabetes insipidus after surgery or trauma to the pituitary or hypothalamus may exhibit one of the three patterns: transient, permanent, or triphasic.[15] In the first phase of the triphasic pattern, total or partial DI begins on the first postoperative day and persists for 0.5 to 5 days. This phase is due to edema in the area interfering with normal ADH secretion. This is the most common pattern (50% to 60%) of postsurgical diabetes insipidus. The second phase is the SIADH phase. This is due to the unregulated release of arginine vasopressin (AVP) because of retrograde degeneration of the AVP secreting neurons. This may last for 5 to 10 days, during which the urine output falls abruptly. During the third phase, around the tenth postoperative day, a permanent form of DI appears. The last phase occurs if insufficient neurons survive to release an adequate amount of AVP. Usually, a marked degree of SIADH in the second phase is a preface to permanent DI. In patients with combined vasopressin and adrenocorticotropic hormone

(ACTH) deficiency, symptoms of DI may be masked because glucocorticoid deficiency impairs renal free water excretion. Treatment with glucocorticoid may unmask DI with sudden onset of polyuria leading to the diagnosis. In anticipation of this phenomenon, daily monitoring of urinary specific gravity, serum sodium, and review of fluid balance will provide adequate warning of the transition from one phase to another. Recording daily weight is also helpful in this regard. The risk for developing SIADH is greatest in the first and second postoperative weeks.

Diagnosis

Central DI is characterized by increased urinary flow (≥ 3 mL/kg/hour), low urine osmolality (<300 mOsm per L; in severe cases, <200 mOsm per L), urine specific gravity <1.010, and serum sodium >145 mEq per L or serum osmolality ≥ 300 mOsm per L, and polydipsia with craving for cold fluids, especially water. Loss of approximately 75% of the ADH-secreting neurons is required for polyuria to occur.

Differential diagnosis of polyuria includes: osmotic diuresis following infusion of mannitol, glycerol, or x-ray contrast agents; normal diuresis of fluids given during surgery; or nonoliguric renal failure. Diuresis following surgery is usually associated with normal serum osmolality, uncharacteristic of true DI. Review of the intraoperative report will help in distinguishing this from acute postsurgical central DI. Management involves limiting or equalizing intake and output.

Serum sodium, urine osmolality, and urine specific gravity almost always determine the diagnosis of central DI. In rare situations, it may be difficult to distinguish between central and nephrogenic DI, but the response to administration of desmopressin 1-deamino-8-D-arginine vasopressin (DDAVP) generally confirms the diagnosis.

Treatment

Newborns and young infants receive their nutrition primarily in the liquid form and have a high oral fluid requirement of approximately 3 L/m^2/day. DI occurring in these children is better managed with fluid therapy alone given by oral, G-tube (if in place), or intravenous routes. If combined with vasopressin treatment, this may cause dangerous hyponatremia and water intoxication.

Postoperative DI in young children can be managed with fluids alone; however, addition of antidiuretic therapy is preferred but must be used cautiously to minimize the occurrence of hyponatremia. Table 11.2 provides a summary of the different formulations of antidiuretic therapy. Also, antidiuretic therapy can mask the emergence of SIADH following a neurosurgical procedure or injury. If fluid alone is used, intravenous fluid given as 5% dextrose with 37 mEq of sodium per L (D5$\frac{1}{4}$ normal saline) is administered. The amount is calculated between

1 and 3 L/m^2/day (40 to 120 mL/m^2/hour); the initial amount is 40 mL/m^2/hour followed by matching hourly urine output volumes (only if >40 mL per m^2) up to 120 mL/m^2/hour. This limit is necessary to allow a mildly volume-contracted state to stimulate fluid reabsorption in the renal tubules eventually causing water/solute and osmolality to equilibrate. Otherwise, the kidneys will promptly excrete whatever fluid is given to the patient. This regimen will result in a serum sodium concentration in the 150 mEq/L range and allow one to determine whether the thirst mechanism is intact or whether SIADH is developing. Serum sodium levels measured every 4 hours are a sensitive indicator of the adequacy of replacement therapy. Serum and urine osmolalities (or urine specific gravity) are also determined at frequent intervals for monitoring. The infusion of dextrose may cause some patients to become hyperglycemic, especially if they are receiving glucocorticoid therapy. If there is concomitant hyperglycemia, only half-normal saline should be used until normal blood sugar level is restored. Correction of DI should occur within 48 to 72 hours.

If vasopressin therapy is added, it can be given in the form of synthetic aqueous vasopressin (Pitressin). Its effect is maximal within 2 hours of starting the infusion and the duration of action is 4 to 8 hours. The half-life is 10 to 20 minutes allowing convenient dosing as needed. The recommended initial dose is 2.5 to 10 units given IV every 6 to 12 hours. To prevent rapid decrease in sodium level, the smallest dose is started and gradually increased to achieve the desired effect. The therapeutic goals should include: urine output 2 to 3 mL/kg/hour, urine specific gravity of 1.010 to 1.020, and serum sodium of 140 to 145 mEq per L. Urine specific gravity and volume of urine output are the most sensitive parameters in assessing adequacy of treatment. Serum sodium level and serum osmolality do not correlate with the pitressin dose. Intravenous DDAVP should not be used in combination with fluid therapy in the management of acute central DI due to its long half-life (8 to 12 hours), which therefore increases the risk for dangerous hyponatremia. In addition, patients who are receiving fluid infusion and are not fully alert may not be able to regulate their own thirst, possibly leading to significant hyponatremia.

Continuous vasopressin infusion is another option for managing central DI. This is most helpful in two situations, (i) during the initial postoperative days in children in whom DI develops following CNS surgery and the child is not eating or drinking, and (ii) in patients with established central DI who require high fluid volume infusion and have high urine output during induction with cancer chemotherapy. Another useful application of continuous vasopressin infusion is intraoperative management of fluid in patients with known DI. Owing to its short half-life, continuous vasopressin infusion can be easily turned off with rapid return of diuresis. Continuous vasopressin infusion may also obviate the need for large volumes of

TABLE 11.2

SUMMARY OF THE DIFFERENT FORMULATIONS OF ANTIDIURETIC THERAPY

Product	Administration	Formulation	Half-life	Dosing	Duration	Indications
Vasopressin injection	IV	Synthetic aqueous solution	5–10 min	0.5–10 mU/kg/h	Max effect in 2 h	Acute central DI
Desmopressin solution	IV/SQ	4 μg/mL	8–12 h	0.2 to 1 μg b.i.d		Temporary central DI due to trauma or surgery; best if unable to use oral or nasal forms
Desmopressin intranasal	Intranasal spray or rhinal tube (for delivery of <0.1 mL)	10 μg per spray (0.1 mL)	75 min	0.1–0.4 mL (10 to 40 μg) per day divided b.i.d or t.i.d	8–15 h	Central DI due to trauma or surgery. May be difficult to give to infants or if nasal congestion exists
Desmopressin tablets	Oral, can be dissolved in water	0.1 mg, 0.2 mg	1.5 to 2.5 h	Start with 0.05 mg; increase to 0.1–0.4 mg b.i.d or t.i.d	8–12 h	Maintenance therapy for central DI
Lysine vasopressin	Intranasal spray	50 U/mL	2.5 to 14.5 min	Titrate to desired effect	2–8 h	If duration shorter than desmopressin is desired

DI, diabetes insipidus; SQ, subcutaneous; IV, intravenous.

fluid infusion and may avoid inducing osmotic diuresis from the dextrose. The recommended dose is 0.25 to 0.5 mU/kg/hour. It is started with the smallest dose and the amount is gradually increased by titrating with the urine output and serum sodium level. It will take 2 hours to establish an antidiuretic effect. Patients on this treatment regimen require careful monitoring of their intake and output. Placement of a urinary catheter is sometimes necessary for the accurate measurement of urine output. Sodium levels should be checked every 2 hours until it becomes stable, and then every 3 to 4 hours. Intake and output are reviewed every 3 hours and adjustments are made accordingly to achieve euvolemia, serum sodium of 135 to 145 mEq per L, and urine output of at least 2 to 3 mL/kg/hour.

Patients with established central DI on oral DDAVP, requiring high fluid infusion during cancer chemotherapy are best managed with continuous vasopressin infusion at 0.05 to 0.1 mU/kg/hour titrated according to urine output checked hourly and serum sodium level checked every 2 hours during the induction and infusion of the chemotherapeutic agent. Oral DDAVP should be discontinued 12 hours before the initiation of intravenous fluid and vasopressin infusion to maintain fluid homeostasis.

Intravenous, subcutaneous, or oral DDAVP should not be used initially in combination with fluid therapy in the management of acute central DI owing to its long half-life with associated higher risk for dangerous hyponatremia. DDAVP given intranasally or by the subcutaneous route is

not as safe. When oral intake is re-established, the patient can be transitioned to oral DDAVP for maintenance therapy. The initial dose should be 0.05 mg for infants and small children, 0.1 mg for older children, and 0.2 mg for adolescents repeated every 8 to 12 hours. Before the next dose of DDAVP, one should wait until the effect of the previous dose has worn off (when diuresis with dilute urine reappears) and the serum sodium is >135 mEq per L. This will prevent severe hyponatremia. After 1 to 3 days, it is usually possible to find a dose of oral DDAVP that controls urine output for close to 12 hours without causing hyponatremia, and the DDAVP can then be given on a fixed schedule.

REFERENCES

1. Sklar C, Fertig A, David R. Chronic syndrome of inappropriate secretion of antidiuretic hormone in childhood. *Am J Dis Child.* 1985;139(7):733–735.
2. Diringer MN. Sodium disturbances frequently encountered in a neurologic intensive care unit. *Neurol India.* 2001;49(Suppl 1):S19–S30.
3. Sane T, Rantakari K, Poranen A, et al. Hyponatremia after transsphenoidal surgery for pituitary tumors. *J Clin Endocrinol Metab.* 1994;79(5):1395–1398.
4. Hung SC, Wen YK, Ng YY, et al. Inappropriate antidiuresis associated with pituitary adenoma–mechanisms not involving inappropriate secretion of vasopressin. *Clin Nephrol.* 2000;54(2):157–160.
5. Baran D, Hutchinson TA. The outcome of hyponatremia in a general hospital population. *Clin Nephrol.* 1984;22(2):72–76.
6. Sterns RH. The treatment of hyponatremia: First, do no harm. *Am J Med.* 1990;88(6):557–560.
7. Schwartz WB, Bennett W, Curelop S, et al. A syndrome of renal sodium loss and hyponatremia probably resulting from

inappropriate secretion of antidiuretic hormone 1957. *J Am Soc Nephrol.* 2001;12(12):2860–2870.

8. King LS, Kozono D, Agre P. From structure to disease: The evolving tale of aquaporin biology. *Nat Rev Mol Cell Biol.* 2004; 5(9):687–698.

9. Casulari LA, Costa KN, Albuquerque RC, et al. Differential diagnosis and treatment of hyponatremia following pituitary surgery. *J Neurosurg Sci.* 2004;48(1):11–18.

10. Judd BA, Haycock GB, Dalton N, et al. Hyponatraemia in premature babies and following surgery in older children. *Acta Paediatr Scand.* 1987;76(3):385–393.

11. Olson BR, Rubino D, Gumowski J, et al. Isolated hyponatremia after transsphenoidal pituitary surgery. *J Clin Endocrinol Metab.* 1995;80(1):85–91.

12. Rabinstein AA, Wijdicks EF. Hyponatremia in critically ill neurological patients. *Neurologist.* 2003;9(6):290–300.

13. Wang LC, Cohen ME, Duffner PK. Etiologies of central diabetes insipidus in children. *Pediatr Neurol.* 1994;11(4):273–277.

14. Mulders SM, Bichet DG, Rijss JP, et al. An aquaporin-2 water channel mutant which causes autosomal dominant nephrogenic diabetes insipidus is retained in the Golgi complex. *J Clin Invest.* 1998;102(1):57–66.

15. Seckl JR, Dunger DB, Lightman SL. Neurohypophyseal peptide function during early postoperative diabetes insipidus. *Brain.* 1987;110(Pt 3):737–746.

Diabetic Ketoacidosis

Rajani Prabhakaran   Lynne L. Levitsky

Diabetic ketoacidosis (DKA) is caused by insufficiently circulating insulin or diminished insulin action. Insulin deficiency induces a profoundly catabolic state. Hyperglycemia is the result of the failure to store or utilize ingested carbohydrate, and the loss of suppression of glycogenolysis and gluconeogenesis. Without insulin, ingested glucose cannot be metabolized or stored in liver, muscle, or other tissues. The muscle and fat glucose transporter, GLUT-4 requires insulin for glucose transport into cells for metabolism and storage. Glycogen synthetase is activated by insulin in the liver to permit glucose storage as glycogen. Insulin deficiency and concomitant elevations in catecholamines and glucagon, deplete the glycogen in the liver and muscle. Insufficient insulin leads to increased substrate for gluconeogenesis from the gluconeogenic amino acids released during proteolysis and glycerol released during lipolysis.

Deficiency of insulin is associated with concomitant increases in counter-regulatory hormones including glucagon, cortisol, growth hormone (GH), and catecholamines. Glucagon is particularly important in the maintenance of ketoacidosis because of its role in ketogenesis. Individuals with glucagon deficiency (diabetes secondary to pancreatitis, or cystic fibrosis) rarely develop ketoacidosis. Excess of glucagon stimulates hepatic ketogenesis, and low levels of insulin prevent ketone body utilization by muscle and other tissues.

The kidneys can compensate to some extent for the catabolic state induced by insulin deficiency and counter-regulatory hormone excess. However, hyperglycemia induces a forced diuresis with renal losses of electrolyte. Insulin deficiency and glucagon excess enhances natriuresis. Dehydration and loss of electrolyte inhibit renal excretion of excess hydrogen ion and promote worsening acidosis. Death eventually results from severe dehydration, myocardial and central nervous system (CNS) energy depletion and electrolyte imbalance.

DIAGNOSIS

Presentation

Patients classically present with lethargy, hyperventilation with deep sighing breaths (Kussmaul breathing), and a fruity breath odor of ketones. Depression of the respiratory center, if the arterial pH is <7.0, may inhibit Kussmaul respirations in very severe DKA. General debility or cachexia may be noted if the illness is of a long duration. Abdominal or back pain, on occasion, can be severe enough to mimic a surgical emergency. Children may show signs of dehydration including dry mucous membranes, tachycardia, and poor capillary perfusion. A flushed face is common. Fever may be a symptom of an underlying precipitating infection, but hypothermia can be seen, and patients with underlying infection may not become febrile until treated for DKA. Patients with severe DKA can be stuporous with profound dehydration.

Clinical Evaluation

A prodrome of weight loss, polyuria, and polydipsia can usually be elicited. Although questioning about a family history of diabetes is important, more than half of the children with newly diagnosed diabetes mellitus do not have a relevant family history. Confusion of DKA with common viral vomiting illnesses and dehydration often leads to delayed diagnosis in very young children. Urination continues because of osmotic diuresis and cannot be used as a gauge of dehydration. A rapid respiratory rate secondary to metabolic acidosis might lead to initial confusion with pneumonia or asthma, particularly if the clinician does not detect an acetone odor. Other causes of metabolic acidosis including lactic acidosis, uremic acidosis, alcoholic acidosis, and metabolic acidosis secondary to drug ingestion (salicylates) must be considered in the differential diagnosis. In the first 1 to 2 years of life, some inborn errors of metabolism may present with ketoacidosis and variable elevations in blood glucose (BG) levels. Treatment with insulin and glucose is effective in reversing the catabolic state and improving the condition of these children, and so therapy for DKA, followed by a delayed diagnosis of an amino acid or metabolic acid disorder is not an inappropriate approach to diagnosis and therapy.

Physical Examination

Initial evaluation should include assessment of the level of consciousness, state of hydration, nutritional status, presence of acetone odor, stability of vital signs, presence of signs of infection, hepatomegaly, abdominal or back pain or tenderness, and examination of fundi for papilledema.

Laboratory Evaluation

The laboratory criteria for diagnosis of DKA are hyperglycemia with a BG level of at least 200 mg per dL, venous pH <7.3, and/or serum bicarbonate of <15 mmol per L. Occasionally, young or partially treated children or pregnant adolescents, may develop ketoacidosis with near normal glucose values. This has been termed *euglycemic* ketoacidosis. On the basis of the severity of the acidosis, DKA has been classified as mild (pH ≤7.3, serum bicarbonate ≤15), moderate (pH ≤7.2, HCO_3 ≤10), or severe (pH ≤7.1, HCO_3 ≤5).[1] The initial recommended laboratory studies are described under the section on "Treatment".

TREATMENT

Prognosis

DKA is the leading cause of death in children with insulin-dependent diabetes mellitus. Mortality rates are relatively constant in national population-based studies and in North America vary between 0.15% and 0.25%. One in 100 to one in 300 children with DKA develop cerebral edema. This accounts for more than 60% of all DKA deaths. Other causes of morbidity and mortality during treatment include electrolyte disturbances such as hypokalemia and hyperkalemia, hypoglycemia if BG is not carefully monitored, hypercoagulable state and CNS complications, hematomas, deep vein thrombosis, sepsis, infections including rhinocerebral mucormycosis, aspiration pneumonia, pulmonary edema, adult respiratory distress syndrome, subcutaneous emphysema, pneumomediastinum, malignant hyperthermia, and rhabdomyolysis. Although predictors for cerebral edema are recognized, no therapeutic regimen absolutely prevents the occurrence of cerebral edema. The other complications of DKA can be avoided entirely, reduced in frequency, or treated successfully if management is careful and attentive.[1,2]

Symptomatic cerebral edema is the most serious complication in the treatment of DKA in children. It is unclear why this complication almost never develops after adolescence. Brain swelling occurs in most children with DKA, even before treatment, but in a small number, it is significant enough to cause cerebral herniation and irreversible neurologic damage or death. Risk factors for the development of cerebral edema during therapy include younger age at onset and presentation with a new onset type 1 diabetes mellitus. In one study, children with low partial pressures of arterial carbon dioxide and high serum urea nitrogen at presentation, treated with bicarbonate were at increased risk (see Table 12.1).[3] Most studies show no correlation between the degree of hyperglycemia and the risk of cerebral edema. Although case–control studies have not convincingly demonstrated that the rapidity, volume, or osmolality of fluid rehydration correlates with the development of cerebral edema, it is generally conceded that overload with relatively hypotonic fluid could be a risk factor for this serious complication.

Children who develop symptomatic cerebral edema generally do so during recovery and are not very acidotic when they develop signs of acute intracranial pressure elevation. Symptoms usually develop between 6 and 24 hours after onset of therapy, but rarely can occur after 24 hours of therapy and have been reported at diagnosis. Initial symptoms and signs include reappearance of vomiting, worsening headache, and depressed sensorium. More ominous signs are slowing pulse rate, decreasing oxygen saturation, widening pulse pressure, and changes in the state of consciousness progressing to stupor, with incontinence and appearance of new neurologic deficits such as change in pupillary response and cranial nerve palsies.

An evidence-based protocol has been developed for use in the early diagnosis of cerebral edema in patients with DKA. Clinical diagnostic criteria include abnormal motor/verbal response to pain, decorticate or decerebrate posture, cranial nerve palsy (especially third, fourth, and sixth nerves), and abnormal neurogenic respiratory pattern (e.g., grunting, tachypnea, Cheyne-Stokes respiration, apneusis). The major criteria for impending cerebral edema

---

TABLE 12.1

RISK FACTORS FOR DEVELOPMENT OF CEREBRAL EDEMA

- Younger age at onset (younger than 5 y)
- Vigorous rehydration
- Administration of bicarbonate
- Presentation with a new onset T1DM
- Hypocapnia
- High serum urea nitrogen concentrations at presentation

T1DM, type 1 diabetes mellitus.

are altered mentation or fluctuating level of consciousness, sustained heart rate deceleration (decline of >20 bpm) not attributable to improved intravascular volume or sleep state, and age-inappropriate incontinence. The minor criteria are vomiting, headache, lethargy or difficulty in arousing from sleep, diastolic blood pressure (BP) >90 mm Hg, and age <5 years. One study showed that appearance during treatment of one diagnostic criterion or two major criteria, or one major and two minor criteria had a sensitivity of 92% with a false-positive specificity of 4% in the diagnosis of cerebral edema.[4] Further prospective validation of these criteria is needed.

Treatment should begin as soon as cerebral edema is suspected (discussed later in this chapter).

Management

The guidelines proposed in this chapter for the management of DKA are compatible with a recent international consensus statement on the treatment of DKA in children.[1] If there is frequent evaluation by health care providers experienced in diabetes management (by telephone or direct observation), mild cases of ketoacidosis without vomiting can be managed at home or in an outpatient care facility. Moderate to severe DKA should be treated in an intensive care or specialized pediatric setting. An experienced and trained nursing staff, availability of frequent on-site physician monitoring, clear written guidelines, and access to frequent laboratory evaluation are essential. Compromised circulation, depressed level of consciousness, risk factors

of cerebral edema such as younger age (<5 years) or new onset mandates treatment in an intensive care unit (ICU) setting where minute-to-minute monitoring is possible and neurosurgical consultation is readily available.

In a child appearing sick, documentation of a BG level >250 mg per dL on bedside testing and ketonuria documented on a urine ketone strip should be sufficient to begin treatment while waiting for the remaining lab results. Venous blood gas results are sufficient to guide management in most children with mild to moderate DKA, but in severe DKA, arterial blood gases might be more appropriate.

See Table 12.2 for a concise guide to management of DKA.

Monitoring

A tabular format for clinical monitoring is suggested in Figure 12.1.

Clinical Assessment

- Hourly monitoring of heart rate, respiratory rate, and BP.
- Strict fluid input and output, measured hourly, with bladder catheterization if necessary on the basis of the severity of illness and state of consciousness.
  - At least hourly monitoring of clinical condition for signs and symptoms of impending cerebral edema.
- An initial electrocardiogram (ECG) may be helpful in identifying EKG changes associated with hypo- or hyperkalemia. EKG can be repeated at 4-hour intervals if there is concern about cardiac status or hyperkalemia.

TABLE 12.2

CONCISE PLAN FOR MANAGEMENT OF DIABETIC KETOACIDOSIS

1. Administer bolus of 0.9% saline or Ringer lactate. Repeat bolus if necessary. Begin IV fluids calculated as fluid deficit (to be replaced over 36 h) and maintenance of fluid at a constant rate. Fluids should consist of 0.45% saline. Once the patient has voided, add 40 mEq/L of potassium salts (20 mEq of Kphos and 20 mEq of KCl or acetate) to the IVF. If the serum sodium begins to decrease or remains 132 mEq/L or less as glucose decreases, increase the saline concentration to 0.9% and re-evaluate the rate of rehydration
2. Once the BG level has decreased to 300 mg/dL, add 5% dextrose to the infusion. If acidosis persists, even after the BG level drops to 200 mg/dL or less, increase the dextrose infusion to 10%. Simultaneous administration of two bags (one with 5% dextrose and the other with 10% dextrose in salt solution) speeds IVF therapy changes
3. Give regular insulin intravenously at a rate of 0.1 U/kg/h (made up as 1 U/kg in 100 mL of 0.9% saline). The risk of hypoglycemia, if the IVF stops infusing accidentally, is reduced if the insulin is piggybacked into the IVF infusion. Do not decrease the insulin infusion rate while acidosis persists. Occasionally, higher rates of infusion (0.2 U/kg/h) may be needed to achieve the goal of reducing the level of BG by 75–100 mg/dL/h (4.2–5.6 mM), indicating resistance to insulin or a problem with dilution. The rate of insulin infusion can be reduced to 0.05 U/kg/h *after* acidosis has cleared (pH ≥7.3) and BG level is ≤300 mg/dL. Transition to subcutaneous insulin regimen should be considered only after the venous pH is >7.3, the patient is ready to eat, and the glucose is <300 mg/dL
4. Add potassium to the infusate after the patient voids; add 40 mEq/L of K salts, half as potassium phosphate (to replace phosphate losses) and the other half as KCl. If the patient is hyperchloremic, use potassium acetate instead of KCl. Persistently low (<3.6 mEq/L) or high (>5 mEq/L) potassium suggests the need for ECG monitoring to detect arrhythmias
5. Avoid bicarbonate administration, except if necessary for resuscitation
6. Monitor constantly the vital signs, fluid balance, neurologic state, hourly glucose levels, blood gases, and ketones with at least q2h electrolyte levels including HCO_3 levels while the patient is acidotic. Also monitor the calcium and phosphorus levels q4–6h. Measure urine output q4–6h once the patient has stabilized, more frequently in the first 6 h of treatment. Urinary catheterization may be needed depending upon neurologic status
7. Treat the underlying condition/precipitating illness, if possible

---

DKA, diabetic ketoacidosis; ECG, electrocardiogram; IVF, intravenous fluid; BG, blood glucose.

Hour	Heart rate	Blood pressure	Headache	Eyes	Emesis	Mental status	Fluid intake	Fluid output	Fluid balance	Blood glucose	pH	O₂ sat
1												
2												
3												
4												
5												
6												
7												
8												

Figure 12.1   Suggested clinical monitoring in diabetic ketoacidosis (DKA).

Laboratory Assessment

Initial laboratory studies should include a venous blood gas (arterial may be indicated in the most severely ill children), BG, electrolytes, bicarbonate level, phosphate, calcium, magnesium, blood urea nitrogen (BUN), creatinine, complete blood count and differential white blood cell count, and a urinalysis to document urine glucose and ketones. A serum osmolality is sometimes of interest and may be important in a child where there is concern about a complicated course.

- Other laboratory studies may be indicated on the basis of clinical findings, such as serum lactate if acidosis is disproportionate to ketonuria, serum lipase and amylase if abdominal pain is severe, or blood, urine or sputum culture if infection is a concern. If the laboratory can provide rapid β-hydroxybutyrate results or bedside monitoring capacity is available, measurement of serum β-hydroxybutyrate can be useful.
- BG should be obtained hourly. Hourly, bedside monitoring values using state-of-the-art calibrated meters are often adequate, but formal laboratory values should be obtained every 2 hours for confirmation.
- Blood gases and serum bicarbonate should be obtained at 2-hour intervals until the serum pH is clearly improving, and then every 4 hours until pH is normal.
- Potassium, phosphate, and calcium can be repeated every 4 hours until resolution of ketoacidosis and unless abnormal values prompt more frequent analysis.

Pitfalls in laboratory assessment include:

- Overinterpretation of a high white blood cell count with a shift to the left as a sign of infection. It usually represents the stress of DKA.
- Misinterpretation of a low serum sodium concentration as true hyponatremia. It usually represents a response to hyperglycemia because water is driven from cells into the extracellular fluid to balance osmolality, or may be factitious because of elevated triglycerides. The serum sodium concentration should be corrected for hyperglycemia by adding 1.6 mmol to the reported sodium level for every 5.6 mmol per L (100 mg per dL) increase in glucose >5.6 mmol per L.
- Overinterpretation of an elevated amylase level as pancreatitis. If the lipase is not concomitantly elevated, this represents release of salivary amylase.
- Factitiously elevated serum creatinine levels may create concern for renal failure if the laboratory uses an older nonenzymatic creatinine assay, which cross-reacts with acetoacetate.
- Rising levels of acetoacetate may be seen in the first 4 to 6 hours of treatment. Acetoacetate (measured as urine or serum ketones) and β-hydroxybutyrate are in equilibrium related to the redox state of the body. As acidosis and perfusion improves, the ratio of acetoacetate to β-hydroxybutyrate, which may be as high as 1:8 in the patient with severe acidosis, drops to 1:2 as β-hydroxybutyrate is converted to acetoacetate. The resulting transient increase in urine ketones should not be taken as a sign of worsening ketoacidosis.

Rehydration

General Guidelines to Fluid Management

Patients presenting with DKA are generally, moderately to severely (7% to 10%) volume depleted.[5] The high osmolality because of hyperglycemia is compounded by dehydration, and results in the shift of fluid from the intracellular compartment to the extracellular compartment.

In addition, patients have both intracellular and extracellular electrolyte deficits. Studies in adults have shown fluid deficits of up to 5 L and approximately 20% loss of total body sodium and potassium. The goal of the treatment is to restore circulatory volume, replace extracellular and intracellular fluid losses, replace the electrolyte deficits, and restore the glomerular filtration rate, while avoiding development of symptomatic cerebral edema or other serious complications of treatment. The following general management suggestions are assumed to decrease the risk of cerebral edema, although one retrospective case–control study did not confirm their validity:

- Fluid and electrolyte deficits should be replaced gradually over at least 36 hours.
- Treatment should cause a gradual decrease in BG levels, not exceeding 75 to 100 mg/dL/hour (4.2 to 5.6 mmol per hour).
- Rapid reductions in osmolality should be avoided by the use of rehydration solutions that are relatively isosmolar to serum.

Initial Fluid Bolus

Rehydration can begin with a 20 mL per kg bolus of isotonic fluid (normal saline or Ringer lactate). If circulation remains compromised, this bolus can be repeated if necessary. The initial fluid rehydration may lower blood and serum osmolality substantially because hyperglycemia and hyperosmolality is in part related to dehydration. If self-hydration with sugar-containing fluids had contributed to a markedly elevated blood sugar level at presentation (>500 mg per dL or 27.8 mmol), rehydration can cause a precipitous drop in serum glucose levels.

Rehydration Fluids

After the initial bolus, rehydration should be continued using at least 0.45% saline solution. Use of either colloid or more dilute solutions is likely to lead to rapid decreases in osmolality and movement of fluid into the intracellular compartment. The use of large amounts of 0.9% saline solution leads to hyperchloremic metabolic acidosis. Urinary loss leads to depletion of potassium, but serum potassium concentration may initially be normal or elevated because of shifts of potassium from the intracellular to the extracellular compartment. Because there is a small risk of prerenal failure early in the course of rehydration, potassium should be replaced only after the patient has voided and the serum potassium level is 5 mEq per L or less. We recommend beginning with 40 mEq per L of potassium salts in the form of 20 mEq per L potassium phosphate and 20 mEq per L potassium chloride. This replenishes phosphate losses to some extent and minimizes hyperchloremia while avoiding hypocalcemia as a result of larger quantities of infused phosphate. Alternatively, potassium acetate may be used to replace potassium losses without increasing hyperchloremia. Potassium supplementation can

be increased to 60 mEq per L if required. Serum phosphate levels are usually replaced from endogenous stores, but effects of phosphate depletion such as muscle weakness might be prevented by exogenous supplementation.

When the BG level has decreased to 300 mg per dL, 5% dextrose can be added to the intravenous infusion. If acidosis persists after the BG level drops to 200 mg per dL or less, the dextrose infusion should be increased to 10% to permit continued administration of insulin. Elevated blood glucose almost always improves more rapidly than acidosis. Simultaneous administration of two bags of intravenous fluid (IVF) (each with different dextrose concentrations whose rates can be titrated) decreases response time in making fluid therapy changes (Table 12.2).[6]

Insulin Therapy

Insulin should be given as soon as DKA is confirmed by documentation of hyperglycemia and urine ketones. Insulin is necessary for reversal of the catabolic state of DKA. It stimulates peripheral glucose uptake, suppresses glucose production, and inhibits lipolysis and ketogenesis. Regular human insulin should be administered by a continuous intravenous drip at a usual initial rate of 0.1 U/kg/hour. Insulin-resistant individuals may require 0.2 U/kg/hour or more, and babies who are very insulin sensitive may require a rate of 0.05 U/kg/hour. Lispro (Humalog) and insulin aspart (NovoLog), act faster when given subcutaneously because they do not form tight hexamers, and offer no advantage when given intravenously. There is no evidence that an initial insulin bolus improves the outcome or rapidity of recovery from DKA. The insulin preparation, usually diluted in saline for ease of infusion and flushed through the tubing to block insulin binding, should be piggybacked into the infusate to decrease the risk of hypoglycemia if there is a failure of the intravenous infusate. Adequacy of the insulin infusion is assessed by glycemic response and improvement in serum pH. If the BG level is not decreasing by 75 to 100 mg/dL/hour, the rate can be increased, and if it is decreasing more rapidly, glucose concentration in the infusate can be increased to prevent hypoglycemia while facilitating recovery from acidosis. The need for a higher dose of insulin in the first few hours augurs insulin resistance or a problem with the insulin or the insulin dilution. Acidosis is monitored by measuring pH with the goal being a venous pH >7.3. If the BG level falls <300 mg per dL before acidosis has resolved, as often happens, the glucose infusion rate should be increased by increasing the dextrose concentration. The rate of insulin infusion can be reduced to 0.05 U/kg/hour only after acidosis has cleared (pH ≥7.3) and BG is ≤300 mg per dL.

Treatment of Acidosis

Acidosis in DKA is associated with an increased anion gap.

$$Anion\ gap = [Na^+] - ([Cl^-] + [HCO_3^-])$$
$$\times\ Normal\ range\ is\ 12 \pm 2\ mmol\ per\ L$$

The contributing anions are primarily the ketoacids β-hydroxybutyrate and acetoacetate (see Chapter 2), and to a lesser extent (approximately 25%) lactic acid associated with poor tissue perfusion. Administration of IVFs to correct the dehydration helps in the correction of the lactic acidosis. Administration of insulin halts further generation of ketoacids. As renal perfusion improves, excretion of ketoacid increases. Metabolism of acetoacetate and β-hydroxybutyrate the acidosis.

Bicarbonate therapy in the treatment of DKA is controversial. There are several controlled trials in the pediatric and adult population that have been unable to show any advantage in using bicarbonate, and there are potential risks associated with bicarbonate therapy. Intracellular acidosis can be aggravated owing to the increased production of CO_2. Bicarbonate therapy may cause paradoxical CNS acidosis because of the delayed equilibration of bicarbonate ion compared to CO_2 across the blood–brain barrier. In addition, the rapid correction of the acidosis can cause intercompartmental movement of potassium leading to hypokalemia, putting the patient at a risk for cardiac arrhythmias. However, patients with life-threatening hyperkalemia, or decreased cardiac contractility and peripheral vasodilatation because of extreme acidosis (arterial pH <7) may on rare occasions benefit from rapid administration of bicarbonate. In such patients, bicarbonate should be administered to replace one third of the calculated deficit, solely as a resuscitative measure to treat or prevent impending circulatory collapse. Close laboratory follow-up is imperative.

Hyperosmolar Hyperglycemic State

Hyperosmolar hyperglycemic state (HHS) is a serious potentially life-threatening hyperglycemic complication in diabetes mellitus. It is characterized by hyperglycemia, hyperosmolality, and a mild metabolic acidosis. The diagnostic criteria for HHS are a BG level >33 mmol per L (>600 mg per dL) and a serum osmolality >320 mmol per kg (>320 mOsm per kg) in the absence of severe acidosis (pH >7.3) and ketosis. HHS is more common in patients with type 2 than with type 1 diabetes,[7] and is occasionally seen in pediatric patients who either have type 2 diabetes or who are developmentally disabled and not able to communicate their need for oral hydration to replace urinary losses.

The pathogenesis of HHS is not well understood; but the basic mechanism is a net reduction in the effect of circulating insulin coupled with the hyperglycemic action of counter-regulatory hormones. Insulin activity is insufficient to prevent glucose production or promote glucose utilization. Lower circulating levels of free fatty acids and/or higher portal vein insulin levels decrease ketogenesis. BG levels are often much higher than in DKA, and therefore associated with more pronounced osmotic diuresis, leading to more profound dehydration. HHS can take days or weeks to fully develop. Water loss is estimated as 15% to 20% rather than the 5% to 7% in DKA and hypertonic dehydration is pronounced. Patients frequently present in coma.

Treatment guidelines for HHS in pediatric patients have been developed by a consensus group under the auspices of the American Diabetes Association.[8] These guidelines are based on expert opinion but not confirmed by clinical studies. Because HHS can also be associated with the development of symptomatic cerebral edema, we recommend that it be managed in a manner similar to DKA, but with a recognition of the severity of the dehydration and hyperosmolality. Initial fluid replacement with boluses of 0.9% saline, followed by continued replacement with 0.7% to 0.9% saline with appropriate potassium supplementation provides a relatively hypo-osmolar replacement fluid. Sodium levels should be monitored and the percent of saline in the infusate reduced, if levels rise. Fluid replacement should be similar to that for DKA and based upon changes in glycemia and electrolytes. Insulin replacement should be initiated at 0.1 U/kg/hour but insulin infusion rates may need to be increased in obese, insulin-resistant young individuals.

Monitoring for cerebral edema should be similar to that in DKA. Rhabdomyolysis and multiorgan failure are some of the important complications of HHS. Creatine kinase levels, electrolyte levels, glucose levels, and osmolality should be monitored frequently. Despite intensive treatment, the mortality rate continues to be as high as 15%.

Treatment of Cerebral Edema

Cerebral edema in other disorders has been attributed to vasogenic edema (increases in extracellular volume) or cytotoxic edema (astrocytic brain cell swelling). The development of cerebral edema by vasogenic mechanisms has been attributed to cerebral ischemia/hypoxia and the generation of various inflammatory mediators, reperfusion injury, and disruption of cell membrane ion transport and aquaporin channels. Cytotoxic edema has been attributed to the generation of intracellular organic osmolytes (myoinositol, taurine, glycerylphosphoryl choline, betaine—previously known as *idiogenic* osmoles) and subsequent cellular osmotic imbalance and swelling. It is likely that both general mechanisms are important at different stages of the evolution of symptomatic cerebral edema.[9,10]

Therapy must be instituted as soon as cerebral edema is suspected. It should not be postponed for confirmation by radiologic studies. This delays treatment, and also places the patient at potential risk during transport or imaging because intensive monitoring and treatment might be less available in the event of brain herniation. The patient should be given intravenous mannitol at 0.25 to 1.0 g per kg over 20 minutes. If there is no initial response, the mannitol may be repeated in 1 to 2 hours. Hypertonic saline 5 to 10 mL per kg over 30 minutes can be used as an alternative to mannitol in controlling apparent intracranial hypertension.[11] The rate of fluid administration should usually be reduced. Intubation and mechanical ventilation may be necessary. The value of hyperventilation is questioned in cerebral edema, and there is at least one retrospective study that has shown an association of aggressive hyperventilation with adverse outcomes in DKA-related cerebral edema. Intracranial pressure monitoring and neurosurgical decompression are sometimes required.

Transition to a Subcutaneous Insulin Regimen

Once the venous pH has improved to >7.3, the BG level has fallen to <300 mg per dL, and the patient is ready to eat, plans should be made for transition to a subcutaneous insulin regimen. Intravenous insulin must be continued for half an hour after the administration of subcutaneous insulin to permit time for absorption. In children with known diabetes, restoration of the previous regimen is usually appropriate. There are many insulin management protocols. Two relatively simple approaches to management that are relatively easily implemented in children whose families have not yet become sophisticated in diabetes management are suggested. The initial daily dose for subcutaneous insulin is between 0.5 and 1.0 U per kg.

- NPH/short-acting insulin: Give two third of the dose in the morning and one third at dinnertime. Two thirds of the morning dose is given as NPH insulin and one third of the morning dose is given as short-acting insulin; the predinner dose is similarly split or can be given half the evening dose as NPH with the remaining half as short acting.

- Glargine (Lantus) and short-acting insulin (Humalog, or NovoLog): With this regimen, half of the total daily dose is given as glargine, and the rapidly acting insulin is given at mealtimes. Ideally, one must match insulin to carbohydrate with this regimen but at early stages, three equal short-acting insulin doses will be adequate.

REFERENCES

1. Dunger DB, Sperling MA, Acerin CLi, et al. ESPE/LWPES consensus statement on diabetic ketoacidosis in children and adolescents. *Arch Dis Child.* 2004;89:188–194.
2. Worly JM, Fortenberry JD, Hansen I, et al. Deep venous thrombosis in children with diabetic ketoacidosis and femoral central venous catheters. *Pediatrics.* 2004;113:e57–e60.
3. Glaser N, Barnett P, McCaslin I, et al. Risk factors for cerebral edema in children with diabetic ketoacidosis. *N Engl J Med.* 2001;344:264–269.
4. Muir AB, Quisling RG, Yang MCK, et al. Cerebral edema in childhood diabetic ketoacidosis. *Diabetes Care.* 2004;27:1541–1546.
5. Koves I, Neutze J, Donath S, et al. The accuracy of clinical assessment of dehydration during diabetic ketoacidosis in childhood. *Diabetes Care.* 2004;27:2485–2487.
6. Poirier MP, Greer D, Satin-Smith M. A prospective study of the "two-bag system" in diabetic ketoacidosis management. *Clin Pediatr.* 2004;43:809–813.
7. Morales AE, Rosenbloom AL. Death caused by hyperglycemic hyperosmolar state at the onset of type 2 diabetes. *J Pediatr.* 2004;144:270–273.
8. Position Paper, American Diabetes Association. Hyperglycemic crises in diabetes. *Diabetes Care.* 2004;27:S94–S102.
9. Glaser NS, Wootton-Gorges SL, Marcin JP, et al. Mechanism of cerebral edema in children with diabetic ketoacidosis. *J Pediatr.* 2000;145:164–171.
10. Levitsky LL. Symptomatic cerebral edema in diabetic ketoacidosis: The mechanism is clarified but still far from clear. *J Pediatr.* 2004;145:149–150.
11. Kamat P, Vats A, Gross M, et al. Use of hypertonic saline for the treatment of altered mental status associated with diabetic ketoacidosis. *Pediatr Crit Care Med.* 2003;4:239–242.

Thyroid Disorders

13

Audrey Austin

Alterations in thyroid functions are the most common metabolic changes that occur in critically ill patients. There may be overproduction of thyroid hormone causing hypermetabolic activity, or underproduction promoting a hypometabolic state. Either state might affect the healing process in a seriously ill child and negatively impact the outcome of the illness. This chapter discusses thyroid storm and the abnormalities associated with the use of iodine-containing products, and the sick euthyroid syndrome. Normal thyroid physiology and the regulation of thyroid function in critical illness have been discussed in Chapter 2. Diagnosis and management of the specific conditions are discussed in this chapter.

THYROID STORM

Hyperthyroidism is a state of increased production and sustained release of the thyroid hormones thyroxine (T_4) and tri-iodothyronine (T_3) into the circulation. A hypermetabolic state, thyrotoxicosis, develops when peripheral tissues are exposed to excessive thyroid hormones. By far, the most common cause is autoimmune-mediated Graves disease due to the production of antibodies, which bind to and stimulate the thyroid stimulating hormone (TSH) receptors in the thyroid gland. The clinical symptoms include tachycardia, hyperactivity, anxiety, and tremors. Weight loss is common and may be dramatic. A goiter is usually evident and exophthalmos may be present initially or develop later.

Thyroid storm is a life-threatening exacerbation of hyperthyroidism. The condition may be precipitated by the stress of surgery in children and adolescents with hyperthyroidism in the postoperative period after thyroidectomy, and by the use of certain drugs or by discontinuing antithyroid drug therapy. Early recognition and treatment are essential in reducing the morbidity and mortality associated with this condition.

Thyroid storm may also occur in the neonatal period, in infants born to mothers with Graves disease. Although this disease is rare in neonates, when it occurs it may present within hours of birth, but symptoms may be delayed up to 10 days postnatally if the mother was treated with thionamide drugs, and up to 6 weeks when the transplacental passage of maternal blocking antibodies occurs.[1] There are no specific laboratory tests that distinguish thyroid storm from hyperthyroidism; therefore the treating physician must always have a high degree of clinical suspicion to make the diagnosis.

Iodine-containing agents have been implicated in the development of thyroid storm. Specifically, amiodarone, useful in the management of cardiac arrhythmias, iodine-containing contrast medium, and topical iodine-containing antiseptic agents have been documented to trigger this condition, which is sometimes refractory to medical treatment.

Clinical Manifestations

The signs and symptoms of thyroid storm are an exaggerated replica of those in thyrotoxicosis and are characterized by hyperthermia, high output cardiac failure, gastrointestinal (GI) disturbances, and mental status changes.[2] (See Table 13.1). The precipitating causes of thyroid storm in children and adolescents are frequently different from those in adult patients (see Table 13.2), and most cases in the pediatric population are associated with a prior history of Graves disease. The thyroid is not always enlarged, but when a goiter is present it will help direct attention to the possibility of thyroid storm.

Laboratory Testing

The diagnosis of thyroid storm is made on the basis of clinical factors and this condition must be treated with the utmost urgency if morbidity is to be prevented. To document that a hyperthyroid state exists, one needs to

TABLE 13.1

SIGNS AND SYMPTOMS ASSOCIATED WITH THYROID STORM

Cardiac
Hypertension
Hypotension
Tachycardia
Shock
Congestive heart failure

Hyperthermia
Fever >102°F

CNS
Mental status changes
Seizures
Coma

GI
Nausea and vomiting
Diarrhea
Jaundice

Thyroidal
Goiter
Ophthalmopathy

General
Anorexia
Diaphoresis
Anxiety
Hyperactivity
Tremors

CNS, central nervous system; GI, gastrointestinal.

measure total or free thyroxine (FT$_4$), tri-iodothyronine (T$_3$), and TSH levels. FT$_4$ and T$_3$ levels are increased and TSH is suppressed to <0.1 μU per mL; however, the severity of the clinical condition does not correlate well with the degree of elevation of FT$_4$ and T$_3$.

TABLE 13.2

PRECIPITATING FACTORS OF THYROID STORM IN CHILDREN AND ADOLESCENTS

Graves disease
Thyroid surgery
Iodide therapy
Thyroid ingestion
Drug therapy (amiodarone)
Radioiodine therapy
Diabetic ketoacidosis
McCune-Albright syndrome

A complete blood count is important in determining whether an infectious process is implicated in the presenting condition. If jaundice is present, alanine aminotransferase (ALT), aspartate aminotransferase, alkaline phosphatase (ALK), and serum bilirubin levels are elevated.

Although no radiographic studies are required to make the diagnosis, a chest x-ray will be valuable to show whether cardiac enlargement or pulmonary edema are present. An electrocardiogram will identify the presence of atrial fibrillation, the most common arrhythmia associated with thyroid storm.[3]

Treatment

The cardiac status of the patient must receive immediate attention, especially if atrial fibrillation is present. Atrial fibrillation rates of 32% to 39% in elderly individuals have been reported,[4] but there is less information on how often this occurs in children and adolescents. The most important aspect of therapy is stability of the cardiac function, and the use of β-blocking agents is of primary importance. Esmolol given intravenously has been used successfully in the emergency treatment of thyroid storm because of its rapid onset and shorter duration of action than propranolol. It also has the benefit of blocking peripheral conversion of T$_4$ to T$_3$. The recommended dose for children (2 to 16 years) is 300 to 1,000 μg/kg/minute intravenously (IV) until the desired effect has been achieved. The β-blocking agent most frequently recommended for use in children is propranolol at an initial dose of 0.1 mg/kg/dose given intravenously, slowly over 5 minutes, followed by an oral dose of 10 to 20 mg at 6- or 8-hour intervals. Neonatal doses are 0.05 to 0.15 mg per kg IV given slowly over 5 minutes followed by oral doses of 0.2 to 0.5 mg per kg every 6 hours.[5]

The same thionamide antithyroid drugs used in the treatment of uncomplicated hyperthyroidism are effective in patients with thyroid storm. Propylthiouracil (PTU) can be given at 5 to 10 mg/kg/day in three divided doses and methimazole (MMI) is used at 0.5 to 1 mg/kg/day in two divided doses.[5] Because iodide in large doses will block thyroid hormone synthesis and release, a saturated solution of potassium iodide (SSKI) is an additional therapeutic agent used in the treatment of thyroid storm. The dose for children and adolescents is 0.3 to 0.5 mL orally at 6- to 8-hour intervals.

Lithium carbonate may be used as an alternative drug in patients with an allergy to iodine or with serious toxic reactions to the thionamides. However, this drug is also implicated in rare cases of thyroid storm because it decreases glomerular filtration and may therefore affect the clearance of thyroxine.

Fever should be controlled with an antipyretic agent, but not with salicylates, which competitively inhibit binding of thyroid hormones to serum proteins. Fluid losses due to fever and diaphoresis, nausea, and vomiting must be

TABLE 13.3					
THYROID FUNCTION CHANGES IN MODERATE AND SEVERE					
NONTHYROIDAL ILLNESS VERSUS PRIMARY HYPOTHYROIDISM					
	rT$_3$	T$_3$	T$_4$	FT$_4$	TSH
N-T illness (moderate)	↑	↓	NL/↑	NL	NL
N-T illness (severe)	↑	↓	↓	↓	NL/↓
HIV/AIDS	↓	↓	↑	NL/↓	NL/↑
Hypothyroidism	↓/NL	↓/NL	↓	↓	↑

N-T, nonthyroidal; NL, normal thyroid function; ↑, increased; ↓, decreased hormone levels compared to healthy subjects; HIV, human immunodeficiency virus; AIDS, acquired immunodeficiency syndrome; rT$_3$, reverse tri-iodothyronine; T$_3$, tri-iodothyronine; T$_4$, thyroxine; FT$_4$, free thyroxine; TSH, thyroid stimulating hormone.

replaced to prevent dehydration, vascular collapse, and to provide nutritional support.

Glucocorticoid therapy plays an important role in the management of those patients who seem to develop a relative adrenal insufficiency. This treatment also has the effect of reducing peripheral conversion of T$_4$ to T$_3$ and therefore aids in decreasing the hypermetabolic state. Hydrocortisone at a dose of 2 mg per kg IV at 8-hour intervals, is recommended.[5]

Additional treatment modalities that may be needed to correct other systemic dysfunction include oxygen, vasopressor agents, diuretics, and nutritional support.

SICK EUTHYROID SYNDROME

The complex of different patterns of thyroid abnormalities in critically ill patients have been studied in detail, and the degree of abnormality appears to correlate with the severity of the illness. Investigators have determined that the syndrome has been estimated to occur in approximately 50% of all patients in the medical intensive care[6] and is associated with a high mortality rate.[7] The syndrome has no clear etiology, and what is known about the pathophysiology associated with the syndrome has been discussed in Chapter 2.

Diagnosis

Thyroid function studies show abnormalities of tri-iodothyronine (T$_3$), thyroxine (T$_4$), and TSH levels (see Table 13.3).[8] Elevations of T$_4$ levels could be explained by thyroid hormone–binding abnormalities, but the considerable changes that occur in response to the stress of severe or chronic illnesses may make a correct diagnosis difficult. If there is a concern for hyperthyroidism in a patient with a low TSH, a serumfree T$_4$ must be obtained, preferably by an equilibrium dialysis method with minimum dilution of the serum, to prevent alteration of the equilibrium between free and bound T$_4$.[9] Elevated FT$_4$ in the presence of suppressed TSH (<0.1 μU per mL) is consistent with a hyperthyroid state. Greater difficulty exists in interpreting results with minimally decreased TSH (0.1 to 0.5 μU per mL) associated with low T$_4$ and T$_3$. In these cases, a serum reverse T$_3$ (rT$_3$) that is increased will aid in making a diagnosis of sick euthyroid syndrome. Serum T$_3$ and rT$_3$ are affected by fasting and they rapidly return to baseline within 24 to 36 hours of refeeding.[10] Similar abnormalities are observed in patients within a few hours after initiation of general anesthesia and surgery, and they return to normal in a few days if the postoperative course is uncomplicated.[10]

In most cases, serum TSH concentration is normal in patients with nonthyroidal illnesses. However, moderately elevated TSH level (>20 μU per mL) in the presence of low FT$_4$ is consistent with a primary hypothyroid state, and abnormally low TSH in the presence of low FT$_4$ concentration is consistent with a secondary hypothyroid state (TSH deficiency).

Treatment

Although it is important to make the diagnosis of sick euthyroid syndrome, the question of whether to use thyroid hormone replacement remains controversial. Brent and Hershman gave l-thyroxine at a dose of 1.5 μg/kg/day IV for 2 weeks to half of a group of 23 critically ill patients who had a serum T$_4$ level of <5, and found that although total and free T$_4$ increased as early as 3 days, there was no difference in mortality (approximately 75% in both groups). They suggested that the inhibition of TSH secretion by giving T$_4$ may suppress an important mechanism for the normalization of thyroid function during recovery.[11] This formulation is supported by Stathatos and Wartofsky in a recent review, in which, having discussed the components of the thyroid axis involved in the syndrome, they speculated that the low TSH levels are likely related in part to suppression by steroids, dopamine, and other medications used in critically ill patients.[12]

Patients with clearly determined hypothyroid states, primary or secondary, should be prescribed l-thyroxine in doses normally used in children (usually 50 to 100 μg per day according to age and size) and the dose should be titrated after at least a week to achieve an euthyroid state.

REFERENCES

1. Smith CM, Gavranich J, Cotterill A, et al. Congenital neonatal thyrotoxicosis and previous maternal radioiodine therapy. *BMJ* 2000;320:1260–1261.
2. Wartofsky L. Thyrotoxic storm. In: Braverman LE, Utiger RD, eds. *Werner and Ingbar's the thyroid: A fundamental and clinical text.* 8th ed. Philadelphia, PA: Lippincott Williams & Wilkins; 2000.
3. Klein I, Omajaa K. Thyroid hormone and the cardiovascular system. *N Engl J Med.* 2001;344:501–509.
4. Cobler JL, Williams ME, Greenland P. Thyrotoxicosis in institutionalized elderly patients with atrial fibrillation. *Arch Intern Med.* 1984;144:1758–1760.
5. Drugdex System. *Thompson Micromedex.* Healthcare Series, Vol. 125. Greenwood Village, CO; 2005.
6. Tuazon CU, Labriola AM. Infectious diseases and endocrinology. In: Becker KL, ed. *Principles and practice of endocrinology and metabolism.* Philadelphia, PA: JB Lippincott; 1990.
7. Kaptein E, Weiner JM, Robinson WS, et al. Relationship of altered thyroid hormone indices to survival in nonthyroidal illnesses. *J Endocrinol.* 1982;16:565–574.
8. Wartofsky L, Burman KD. Alterations in thyroid function in patients with systemic illness: The "euthyroid sick syndrome". *Endocr Rev.* 1982;3:164.
9. Hay ID, Bayer MF, Kaplan MM, et al. American Thyroid Association assessment of current free thyroid hormone and thyrotropin measurements and guidelines for future clinical assays. *Clin Chem.* 1991;37:2002.
10. Wiersinga WM. Nonthyroidal illness. In: Braverman LE, Utiger R, eds. *Werner and Ingbar's the thyroid: A fundamental and clinical text.* 8th ed. Philadelphia, PA: Lippincott Williams & Wilkins; 2000.
11. Brent GA, Hershman JM. Thyroxine therapy with severe nonthyroidal illnesses and low serum thyroxine concentration. *J Clin Endocrinol Metab.* 1986;63:1–8.
12. Stathatos N, Wartofsky L. The euthyroid sick syndrome: Is there a physiologic rationale for thyroid hormone treatment? *J Endocrinol Invest.* 2003;26:1174–1179.

Adrenal Disorders

14

Christiane O. Corriveau

The adrenal glands produce four classes of hormones: catecholamines, glucocorticoid, mineralocorticoid, and androgens (see Chapter 2). Catecholamine synthesis occurs in the adrenal medulla and requires cortisol and so it may be decreased in patients with hypothalamic–pituitary disease. The adrenal glands release cortisol under the control of the hypothalamic–pituitary axis, in response to stresses such as infection, surgery, and trauma. Aldosterone primarily responds to the renin–angiotensin system and potassium levels. Secretion of adrenal androgen is partly under the control of pituitary adrenocorticotropic hormone (ACTH), but other poorly understood factors regulate their production.[1] This chapter focuses on adrenal responsiveness to illness affecting production of glucocorticoids and mineralocorticoids.

SYNDROMES OF ADRENAL INSUFFICIENCY

Adrenal insufficiency is caused by a large variety of insults. It can be acute or chronic and may result from primary direct destruction of the adrenal glands (primary adrenal insufficiency) or from the loss of the hypothalamic–pituitary axis function (secondary adrenal insufficiency). The central pathophysiologic alteration secondary to adrenal insufficiency is cardiovascular—reduced cardiac output and decreased vascular tone with relative hypovolemia. Cardiac output is related to catecholamines and they have decreased inotropic and pressor effects in the absence of cortisol. Patients with catecholamine-resistant shock need to be evaluated for the presence of adrenal insufficiency. Relative hypovolemia is multifactorial. The response to hypovolemia is increased vasopressin secretion, leading to water retention, decreased plasma osmolality, and hyponatremia. Hyponatremia is exacerbated by aldosterone deficiency causing excessive urinary sodium loss,

which is usually accompanied by moderate to severe hyperkalemia. Therefore, hyperkalemia is often an important laboratory finding in aldosterone deficiency.

Primary Adrenal Insufficiency

Primary adrenal insufficiency is relatively rare. The primary causes are listed in Table 14.1. The adrenal glands have a large reserve but adrenal insufficiency develops in patients who have >90% destruction or replacement of the adrenal glands with inflammation, tumor, infection, or hemorrhage. In primary adrenal insufficiency, congenital or acquired lesions of the adrenal cortex prevent production of cortisol and often aldosterone. Autoimmune adrenal insufficiency spares the adrenal medulla. Depending on the pathologic lesion, symptoms may be severe or mild, and become manifest abruptly or insidiously. The most common pediatric causes are discussed subsequently.

Congenital Adrenal Hyperplasia

The most common cause of adrenocortical insufficiency in infancy is the salt-losing form of congenital adrenal hyperplasia (CAH). The most prevalent form of CAH (>90% of cases) is caused by the deficiency of the cytochrome P-450 enzyme, 21-hydroxylase, which in its severest form causes deficiency of both cortisol and aldosterone. In women, ambiguous genitalia without palpable testes provide a clue to the diagnosis.

Hemorrhage

Hemorrhage may occur during difficult labor, especially during breech presentation, or its cause may be unknown. An incidence of 3 per 100,000 live births has been reported. Postnatal adrenal hemorrhage occurs in patients being anticoagulated or those injured after blunt trauma, most notably nonaccidental trauma.

TABLE 14.1
ETIOLOGY OF ADRENAL INSUFFICIENCY

Cause	Occurrence
Primary Adrenal Insufficiency	
Autoimmune (polyendocrine deficiency syndrome)	70%
Tuberculosis	20%
Other	10%
Fungal infections	
Adrenal hemorrhage	
Congenital adrenal hypoplasia	
Sarcoidosis	
Amyloidosis	
Acquired immunodeficiency syndrome	
Adrenoleukodystrophy	
Adrenomyeloneuropathy	
Metastatic neoplasia	
Congenital unresponsiveness to corticotropin	
Secondary Adrenal Insufficiency	
After exogenous glucocorticoids or corticotropin	Very common
After the cure of Cushing syndrome (removal of endogenous glucocorticoids)	Common
Hypothalamic and pituitary lesions	Uncommon

Adapted with permission from Loriaux DL. Adrenocortical insufficiency. In: Becker KL, ed. *Principles and practice of endocrinology and metabolism.* 3rd ed. Philadelphia, PA: Lippincott Williams & Wilkins; 2001:739.

Autoimmune Adrenal Insufficiency (Addison Disease)

The most common cause of Addison disease is autoimmune destruction of the adrenal glands. In advanced disease, all adrenal cortical function is lost, but early in the clinical course, isolated cortisol deficiency may occur. Usually the adrenal medulla is not affected. Addison disease sometimes occurs as a part of two syndromes, each consisting of a constellation of autoimmune disorders. *Type 1 autoimmune polyendocrinopathy syndrome* (APS-1) is a recessive disorder also known as *autoimmune polyendocrinopathy/candidiasis/ectodermal dystrophy* (APECED) syndrome. The first disease manifestation is often chronic mucocutaneous candidiasis, commonly followed by hypoparathyroidism and then by Addison disease, which typically develops by adolescence. Adrenal failure may develop rapidly in APS-1. *Type 2 autoimmune polyendocrinopathy* (APS-2) consists of Addison disease with autoimmune thyroid disease or type 1 diabetes mellitus. Gonadal failure, vitiligo, alopecia, and chronic atrophic gastritis, with or without pernicious anemia may occur.

Infection

Infection and systemic inflammation are the most common causes of primary adrenal insufficiency in the critical care setting. Waterhouse-Friderichsen syndrome is adrenal failure caused by meningococcemia. Patients with HIV/AIDS may have a spectrum of clinical abnormalities associated with the hypothalamic–pituitary–adrenal (HPA) axis. Although adrenal insufficiency may result from direct invasion of the glands by the human immunodeficiency virus, more cases result from opportunistic infections (fungus, cytomegalovirus, tuberculosis).[1]

Drugs

Ketoconazole can cause adrenal insufficiency by directly inhibiting adrenal steroidogenic enzymes. Anticonvulsive drugs such as phenobarbitol and phenytoin may reduce the effectiveness and bioavailability of corticosteroid replacement therapy by inducing liver enzymes that are involved in steroid metabolism, leading to adrenal insufficiency.

Secondary Adrenal Insufficiency

Secondary adrenal insufficiency has three causes: adrenal suppression after exogenous glucocorticoid or ACTH administration, adrenal suppression after the correction of endogenous glucocorticoid hypersecretion, and abnormalities of the hypothalamus or pituitary gland leading to ACTH deficiency.

Adrenal suppression by exogenous glucocorticoids is the most common cause of secondary adrenal insufficiency.[2] Supraphysiologic doses of glucocorticoids suppress corticotropin-releasing hormone (CRH) production and the ability of the anterior pituitary gland to produce ACTH. The degree of adrenal suppression depends on three variables: dosage, schedule of administration, and duration of administration. Significant adrenal suppression is rarely seen with doses of hydrocortisone (or its equivalent) of <15 mg/m^2/day. Treatment periods of <14 days, rarely lead to significant suppression of adrenal function.

Secondary adrenal insufficiency can manifest shortly after the cessation of corticosteroid therapy or months later in a stressful situation such as surgery or injury. Full recovery of the HPA axis may take up to a year.[2] Patients with secondary adrenal insufficiency usually have intact mineralocorticoid function through the renin–angiotensin–aldosterone system, but require stress dose glucocorticoid supplementation when an acute disease develops or a stressful procedure is performed.

Functional Hypoadrenalism

Severe, acute stress leads to a strong activation of the HPA axis. Major stress can increase glucocorticoid production by 5- to 10-fold.[2] An insufficient response of the

TABLE 14.2

SIGNS AND SYMPTOMS OF ADRENAL INSUFFICIENCY IN PEDIATRIC PATIENTS

Symptoms	Findings on Clinical Examination
Generalized weakness and fatigue	Increased pigmentation
Anorexia, vomiting, nausea	Hypotension (postural)
±Weight loss	Tachycardia
Abdominal pain	Fever
Myalgia or arthralgia	Decreased body hair
Postural dizziness	Vitiligo
Craving for salt	Features of hypopituitarism
Headaches	Amenorrhea
Memory impairment	Intolerance of cold
Clinical Problems	**Laboratory Findings**
Hemodynamic instability	Hyponatremia
Hyperdynamic (common)	Hyperkalemia
Hypodynamic (rare)	Hypoglycemia
Ongoing inflammation with no obvious source	Eosinophilia
Multiorgan dysfunction	Elevated thyrotropin levels
Hypoglycemia	
Poor linear growth	

HPA axis in critical illness has been termed *functional hypoadrenalism* (also called *adrenocortical dysfunction, transient hypoadrenalism*, or *adrenal hyporesponsiveness*). During severe illness, many factors can impair the normal corticosteroid response.[3]

It is difficult to assess the adequacy of glucocorticoid secretion in critically ill adults and children; normal physiologic responses will vary on the basis of stimulus and insult. There is no agreement on the definition of an "insufficient" cortisol level during critical illness. Elevated plasma cortisol levels can be detrimental as well, contributing to the hyperglycemia, leukocytosis, immune suppression, and hypermetabolism seen in critical illness. Recent studies have focused on functional adrenal insufficiency in critically ill adults and neonates. The reported incidence varies with the criteria used to define the condition. Although there is lack of data of functional adrenal insufficiency in children, there is a belief that adrenal dysfunction is as common in children as it is in critically ill adults. Pediatric studies with limited numbers of subjects report an incidence close to that observed in adults, 52% in patients with septic shock[4] and 31% in critically ill pediatric patients.[5] In a recent prospective study in pediatric patients with septic shock, relative adrenal insufficiency ranged from 9% to 44% depending on the criteria used to classify adrenal function.[6]

Clinically, the signs and symptoms of adrenal insufficiency are nonspecific; therefore, all patients with sudden unexplained deterioration should be screened for adrenal insufficiency. Patients with coagulopathy, thromboembolic disease, chronic or recent glucocorticoid usage, hyponatremia, hyperkalemia, hypoglycemia, traumatic shock, and sepsis are more likely to have adrenal insufficiency (see Table 14.2).

DIAGNOSIS

The controversy about "relative" functional adrenal axis failure in acute stress conditions such as sepsis focuses on diagnosis. There is no consensus definition of corticosteroid insufficiency in critically ill adults, newborns, or children, and common diagnostic approaches are lacking.[7] Several of the more common methods are discussed subsequently.

Random Cortisol Levels

The highest levels of cortisol are found in patients with the severest of illness; however, both low and high cortisol levels are associated with increased mortality in critically ill adults.[8] Presumably, low cortisol levels indicate adrenal insufficiency, whereas high levels are associated with increased severity of illness and adequate stress responses; this is consistent with limited pediatric data.[9] Proposed "normal" levels of cortisol in adult critical illness have ranged from 10 to 34 μg per dL. Unfortunately, no absolute serum cortisol level exists that distinguishes an adequate from an insufficient adrenal response.[1] Several studies have identified <15 μg per dL as the threshold that best identifies the patient with clinical features of adrenal insufficiency or who would benefit from steroids.[3] Baseline random cortisol levels of <25 μg per dL were shown to be a better discriminator of adrenal insufficiency when compared to the standard or low-dose ACTH stimulation test (see subsequent text) in patients with septic shock.[10] On the basis of hemodynamic response to corticosteroids, adult studies have used a "random" cortisol of 25 μg per dL for the diagnosis of an adequate adrenal response to critical illness. In patients with vasopressor-dependent conditions treated with corticosteroids, a baseline serum cortisol of 20 μg per dL has been used to define steroid-responsive patients and 49 μg per dL to define nonresponders.[11] In catecholamine-resistant septic shock, adrenal insufficiency is assumed at random total cortisol concentrations ≤18 μg per dL. An increase in serum cortisol of ≤9 μg per dL, 30 or 60 minutes post-ACTH, also supports the diagnosis.[12]

There are no strict definitions of adrenal "sufficiency" for critically ill children. Children with adrenal insufficiency, defined as low serum cortisol concentrations after an ACTH stimulation test, required higher doses of vasopressors for a longer period than those with a normal HPA, but there was no difference in mortality.[4] An important problem in interpreting cortisol levels is that >90% of cortisol measured in the serum is protein bound (80% to cortisol-binding protein and 10% to albumin), whereas only 10%

is in the free biologically active form. During acute illness, there is a decrease in the corticosteroid-binding globulins and alterations in the concentrations of cortisol-binding protein, and this would be expected to affect the utility of the total plasma cortisol levels. Consistent with this data, baseline and ACTH-stimulated total serum cortisol concentrations were lower in critically ill patients with hypoproteinemia compared to those with higher albumin concentrations, and the response to ACTH correlated better with free cortisol changes than with the changes of the total cortisol levels.[13] Although the total plasma cortisol response to an ACTH challenge was low in some patients, the response of free bioactive cortisol was appropriate, suggesting that the HPA axis feedback was intact. This study indicates that initiating steroid replacement on the basis of absolute total cortisol levels may be in error most of the time. Currently, free plasma cortisol measurements are not widely available for clinical use.

Cortrosyn (Adrenocorticotropic Hormone) Stimulation Test

The best single test for the evaluation and diagnosis of primary adrenal insufficiency is the response to a challenge with synthetic ACTH 1 to 24 (250 μg of Cortrosyn) administered as a single intravenous bolus. Cortisol levels are measured at baseline, 30 and 60 minutes after ACTH stimulation. Normally, the plasma cortisol response should be >20 μg per dL. This test has clear limitations with hypoadrenalism. This test remains controversial in detecting functional adrenal insufficiency in critical illness because the "appropriate" response to ACTH stimulation has not been defined. Circulating ACTH concentrations during stress are in the range of 20 to 200 pg per mL, but levels reached after the administration of a 250 μg dose of Cortrosyn can be as high as 60,000 pg per mL. Therefore, a low-dose 1-μg Cortrosyn test has also been used which better approximates ACTH levels found in severe stress, with the suggestion that it might be more sensitive than the 250 μg test to assess adrenal competency.[14]

Recent pediatric recommendations define adrenal insufficiency in the face of catecholamine-resistant septic shock as a random total cortisol concentration <18 μg per dL or a post-ACTH increase in cortisol ≤9 μg per dL.[6,12] It is possible that the HPA axis (secondary adrenal insufficiency) may not be as serious a problem as primary adrenal insufficiency in children. In a recent prospective study in 57 pediatric patients with septic shock, relative adrenal insufficiency was observed in 26% of children; of this, 80% had catecholamine resistance and 20% had dopamine/dobutamine-responsive shock.[6] Although children with adrenal insufficiency had increased risk of catecholamine-resistant shock, this was not associated with higher mortality. In a smaller study, pediatric patients with septic shock likely had secondary adrenal insufficiency with baseline cortisol level <7 μg per dL and low–normal

ACTH levels. Cortisol levels increased after ACTH stimulation and all patients survived.[5] Hatherill et al. found that there was no difference in the mortality rates, or changes in the peak cortisol in response to ACTH stimulation in critically ill children with adrenal insufficiency and in those with normal adrenal function.[4] In the few pediatric studies published, none have demonstrated that responsiveness to cortrosyn or hydrocortisone replacement positively affected mortality.

Treatment

The overall significance of relative adrenal insufficiency in children is still unclear. Although glucocorticoid replacement will effectively treat patients with known or acquired absolute adrenal insufficiency, supplementation in patients with relative insufficiency or impaired-adrenergic receptors may also be beneficial. This positive effect is postulated to be a consequence of enhanced antiinflammatory activity, inhibition of deleterious proinflammatory activity, and/or diminution of nitric oxide-induced vasodilatation and hypotension. Although acute adrenal insufficiency is an emergency and immediate replacement of glucocorticoids, and fluids are essential, treatment of critical illness with glucocorticoids can potentially aggravate muscle wasting, and lead to immune suppression and metabolic derangements. The "Surviving Sepsis Campaign" recommends treatment with "low dose" hydrocortisone (adult dose: 200 to 300 mg per day for 7 days) in adults with inotrope-dependent shock.[12]

Recent pediatric recommendations for pediatric sepsis are that hydrocortisone therapy should be reserved for children with catecholamine-resistant hypotension and as well as suspected or proven adrenal insufficiency.[12] High-risk patients include those with severe septic shock and purpura, those who have previously received steroids, and children with pituitary or adrenal abnormalities. Dose recommendations for hydrocortisone vary from 1 to 2 mg per kg for stress coverage (based on a clinical diagnosis of adrenal insufficiency) to 50 to 100 mg/m^2/day for empirical therapy for shock followed by the same dose given as a 24-hour infusion. Two randomized controlled trials used very high doses of hydrocortisone (25 times higher than the stress dose) in children with dengue fever and shock, and had conflicting results.[12]

REFERENCES

1. Zaloga GP, Marik P. Endocrine and metabolic dysfunction syndromes in the critically ill. *Crit Care Clin.* 2001;17:1–20.
2. Loriaux DL. Adrenocortical insufficiency. In: Becker KL, ed. *Principles and practice of endocrinology and metabolism.* 3rd ed. Philadelphia, PA: Lippincott Williams &Wilkins; 2001:739–742.
3. Cooper MS, Stewart PM. Current concepts: Corticosteroid insufficiency in acutely ill patients. *N Engl J Med.* 2003;348:727–734.
4. Hatherill M, Tibby SM, Hilliard T, et al. Adrenal insufficiency in septic shock. *Arch Dis Child.* 199;80:51–55.
5. Menon K, Clarson C. Adrenal function in pediatric critical illness. *Pediatr Crit Care Med.* 2002;3:112–1166; Annane D. Time for a

consensus definition of corticosteroid insufficiency in critically ill patients. *Crit Care Med.* 2003;31:1868.

6. Pizarro CF, Troster EJ, Daiani D, et al. Absolute and relative adrenal insufficiency in children with septic shock. *Crit Care Med.* 2005;33:855–859.

7. Annane D. Time for a consensus definition of corticosteroid insufficiency in critically ill patients. *Crit Care Med.* 2003;31:1868.

8. Annane D, Sebile V, Troche G, et al. A three-level prognostic classification in septic shock based on cortisol levels and cortisol response to corticotrophin. *JAMA.* 2000;283(2):10448.

9. De Kleijn ED, Joosten KFM, Van Rijn B, et al. Low serum cortisol in combination with high adrenocorticotrophic hormone concentrations are associated with poor outcome in children with severe meningococcal disease. *Pediatr Infect Dis J.* 2002;21:330–336.

10. Marik PE, Zaloga GP. Adrenal insufficiency during septic shock. *Crit Care Med.* 2003;31:141–145.

11. Rivers EP, Gaspari M, Abi Saad H, et al. Adrenal insufficiency in high-risk surgical ICU patients. *Chest.* 2001;119:889–896.

12. Dellinger RP, Carlet JM, Masur H, et al. Surviving Sepsis Campaign guidelines for management of severe sepsis and septic shock. *Crit Care Med.* 2004;32:858–873.

13. Hamrahian AH, Oseni TS, Arafah BM. Measurements of serum free cortisol in critically ill patients. *N Engl J Med.* 2004;350:1629–1638.

14. Richards ML, Caplan RH, Wickus GC, et al. The rapid low-dose (1 microgram) cosyntropin test in the immediate postoperative period: Results in elderly subjects after major abdominal surgery. *Surgery.* 1999;125:431–440.

Disorders of Micronutrients

15

Angela A. Hsu   Cynthia L. Gibson

Electrolyte disturbances are very common in critically ill children. Early recognition and proper therapy for these disorders are vital. This chapter focuses on the etiologies, clinical manifestations, and therapies for these disorders, because the pathophysiology of these disorders has been discussed elsewhere (see Chapter 2 and Chapter 13). The micronutrients that are discussed in this chapter include sodium, potassium, calcium, phosphorus, and magnesium.

SODIUM

Serum sodium concentration is closely linked to water homeostasis and a disruption of this balance manifests as either hyponatremia or hypernatremia.

Hyponatremia

Etiologies

Hyponatremia is defined as a serum Na^+ of <135 mEq per L with severe hyponatremia characterized by a serum Na^+ <125 mEq per L. The etiologies of hyponatremia are extensive; however, they can be categorized on the basis of serum osmolality and urine Na^+ concentration. A diagnostic algorithm for hyponatremia is shown in Figure 15.1. Pseudohyponatremia occurs if a plasma substance draws water into the vascular space owing to the oncotic or osmolar forces. This can be caused by hyperlipidemia, hyperproteinemia, hyperglycemia, or mannitol use.

Hyponatremia may be classified into three categories on the basis of the total body water balance—hypovolemic, euvolemic, or hypervolemic. Hyponatremic dehydration can be caused by either extrarenal or renal losses (see Fig. 15.1).

Hypervolemic hyponatremia occurs from acute or chronic renal failure and edematous states such as those listed in Figure 15.1. There is an effective circulatory volume depletion and low urine Na^+ (<25 mEq per L).

With euvolemic hyponatremia, the serum osmolality is low, the urine osmolality is usually >100 mOsm per L, and the urine Na^+ is usually >25 mEq per L. After exclusion of hypothyroidism and glucocorticoid deficiency, the remainder fit into the category of secretion of antidiuretic hormone (SIADH). SIADH is one of the most common causes of hyponatremia and frequently leads to severe hyponatremia. Table 15.1 lists some common causes of SIADH.

Clinical Manifestations

Symptoms of hyponatremia vary greatly from mild (headache, nausea, vomiting, lethargy, weakness, and dizziness), to moderate (behavioral changes with agitation, mild confusion or psychosis, and encephalopathy), to severe (seizures, respiratory arrest, decorticate posturing, and coma). Symptoms may present acutely or be progressive.

Laboratory Data

Useful laboratory values in the evaluation of hyponatremia include BUN/Cr, serum Na^+, K^+, osmolality, glucose, urine Na^+, urine osmolality, and occasionally serum triglyceride and total protein levels.

Management

Symptomatic hyponatremia is a medical emergency. Treatment regimens should be instituted to restore serum Na^+ to 120 mEq per L or until symptoms are alleviated. Final correction to the normal range can then occur over the next 24 to 48 hours. Hypertonic saline solutions (including 3% and 11.5%) have been used to immediately treat severe hyponatremia. Infusion of these solutions would be adjusted to raise the Na^+ level by 1 mEq/L/hour. The amount of Na^+ necessary to achieve a desired Na^+ level can be calculated

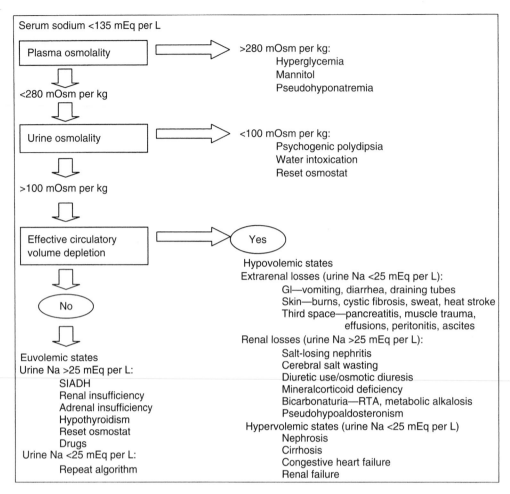

Serum sodium <135 mEq per L

Plasma osmolality → >280 mOsm per kg:
  Hyperglycemia
  Mannitol
  Pseudohyponatremia

<280 mOsm per kg

Urine osmolality → <100 mOsm per kg:
  Psychogenic polydipsia
  Water intoxication
  Reset osmostat

>100 mOsm per kg

Effective circulatory volume depletion → Yes

Hypovolemic states
Extrarenal losses (urine Na <25 mEq per L):
  GI—vomiting, diarrhea, draining tubes
  Skin—burns, cystic fibrosis, sweat, heat stroke
  Third space—pancreatitis, muscle trauma,
    effusions, peritonitis, ascites
Renal losses (urine Na >25 mEq per L):
  Salt-losing nephritis
  Cerebral salt wasting
  Diuretic use/osmotic diuresis
  Mineralcorticoid deficiency
  Bicarbonaturia—RTA, metabolic alkalosis
  Pseudohypoaldosteronism
Hypervolemic states (urine Na <25 mEq per L)
  Nephrosis
  Cirrhosis
  Congestive heart failure
  Renal failure

No

Euvolemic states
Urine Na >25 mEq per L:
  SIADH
  Renal insufficiency
  Adrenal insufficiency
  Hypothyroidism
  Reset osmostat
  Drugs
Urine Na <25 mEq per L:
  Repeat algorithm

Figure 15.1 Diagnostic approach to hyponatremia. SIADH, syndrome of inappropriate antidiuretic hormone; GI, gastrointestinal; RTA, renal tubular acidosis. (Adapted from Adrogue H. Primary care: Hypernatremia. *N Engl J Med.* 2000;342(20):1493–1499; Fouser L. Disorders of calcium, phosphorus, and magnesium. *Pediatr Ann.* 1995;24(1):38–46; Sperling M. *Pediatric endocrinology.* Philadelphia, PA: WB Saunders; 2002.)

by the formula:

$$\text{mEq Na}^+ \text{ required} = \text{Desired Na}^+ \text{ (mEq/L)} - \text{Present Na}^+ \times 0.6 \times \text{Weight (kg)}$$

As a guide, approximately 1 mL/kg/hour of 3% saline will normally raise the serum Na^+ by 1 mEq/L/hour.

Brain damage as a result of cerebral demyelination can develop if there is an excessive change in Na^+ levels. Central pontine myelinolysis is a rare complication of the treatment of hyponatremia. Patients may be asymptomatic or develop symptoms of confusion, quadriplegia, pseudobulbar palsy, and pseudocoma. These symptoms may present one to several days after the correction of hyponatremia. The rate of correction may have no relationship to the development of these demyelinating lesions, but rather the magnitude of the correction and the underlying diagnosis are the major contributing factors.

Mild hyponatremia with few or no symptoms can be treated in a conservative manner with isotonic saline to maintain the extracellular volume. If SIADH or an edematous state is present, a trial of water restriction is indicated. If the Na^+ is unresponsive to water restriction, treatment with demeclocycline could be used to inhibit antidiuretic hormone (ADH). All medications known to cause SIADH should be discontinued, as well as treatment of any underlying conditions.

Hypernatremia

Etiologies

Hypernatremia represents a deficit of water in relation to the body's Na^+ stores and can result from a net water loss or hypertonic Na^+ gain. Hypernatremia is usually multifactorial and a thorough history evaluating for gastrointestinal (GI) water losses, dermal water losses, medication history, sources of exogenous sodium intake, and decreased fluid intake may be helpful in the diagnosis. Table 15.2 lists the causes of hypernatremia. As in hyponatremia, children may be hypovolemic, euvolemic, or hypervolemic.

TABLE 15.1
CAUSES OF SYNDROME OF INAPPROPRIATE SECRETION OF ANTIDIURETIC HORMONE

Malignancies	Medications
Bronchogenic carcinoma	Vincristine
Thymoma	Carbamazepine
ALL	Cyclophosphamide (IV)
Lymphoma	SSRI antidepressants
Neuroblastoma	Opiates
Duodenal or pancreatic adenocarcinoma	NSAIDS

Central Nervous System Disorders	Pulmonary Disorders
Infection: meningitis, encephalitis	Infection: pneumonia, tuberculosis
Neoplasms	Asthma
Vascular anomalies, stroke	Pneumothorax
Trauma	Positive pressure ventilation
Hydrocephalus	
Pituitary surgery	
Hypoxia-ischemia	
Psychosis	

ALL, acute lymphoblastic leukemia; SSRI, selective serotonin reuptake inhibitors; NSAIDS, nonsteroidal anti-inflammatory drugs; IV, intravenous.

Hypovolemia (hypernatremic dehydration) and a low urine Na^+ (<20 mEq per L) implies extrarenal water losses, whereas a high urine Na^+ (>20 mEq per L) implies renal water losses. Children with euvolemia have variable urine Na^+ levels, whereas those with hypervolemia normally have increased urine Na^+ (as well as increased total body Na^+ in relation to total body water).

Clinical Manifestations
Children are often agitated and may manifest signs of hyperpnea, muscle weakness, lethargy, seizures, and coma. Infants may exhibit a high-pitched cry, but older children will normally exhibit increased thirst as a primary symptom.

Laboratory Data
As in hyponatremia, blood urea nitrogen (BUN), creatinine (Cr), serum Na^+, glucose, osmolality, urine Na^+, and urine osmolality must be measured.

Management
Treating the underlying condition, as well as correcting the serum Na^+ and circulatory volume is vital. Circulatory collapse should be treated first with normal saline, with subsequent correction of the Na^+ abnormality. The serum Na^+ should be reduced by 1 mEq/L/hour to a goal of 145 mEq per L. More rapid corrections of hypernatremia can lead to complications, including cerebral cell swelling, edema, and herniation in extreme cases. However, if hypernatremia has developed over a period of several hours, rapid correction improves the prognosis without

TABLE 15.2
CAUSES OF HYPERNATREMIA

Renal Water Loss	Decreased Fluid Intake
Central diabetes insipidus	Neurologic impairment
Nephrogenic diabetes insipidus	Hypothalamic disorder
Diuretics	Restricted access to fluids
Tubulopathy, renal dysplasia	Fluid restriction
Hyperglycemia	Ineffective breastfeeding

Insensible Water Loss	Excessive Sodium Intake
Fever	Hypertonic sodium chloride
Exercise	Sodium bicarbonate administration
Burns	Blood products
Respiratory illness	Sodium ingestion
Excessive sweating	↑ solute feed from improper formula mixing

Gastrointestinal Water Loss	
Gastroenteritis, vomiting	
Osmotic diarrhea	
Colostomy/ileostomy	
Malabsorption	

↑, increased.

increasing the risk of cerebral edema. Judicious use of hypotonic fluids will provide adequate free water to correct the sodium level. A simple method of determining the minimum amount of fluid necessary is by calculating the free water deficit:

$$\text{Free water deficit} = 4 \text{ mL} \times \text{Body weight (kg)} \times \text{Desired change in serum } Na^+$$

The calculated deficit does not account for insensible losses or those that are ongoing. Therefore, fluids required for maintenance should be continued. The rate of correction depends on the severity of symptoms. In severe hypernatremia (>170 mEq per L), serum Na^+ should not be corrected to below 150 mEq per L in the first 48 hours. In cases of excessive Na^+ intake, diuretics may be useful to facilitate Na^+ excretion.

POTASSIUM

Potassium plays an important role in a variety of cellular functions. Disturbances, if untreated, can be associated with high mortality and morbidity.

Hypokalemia

Etiologies
Hypokalemia is defined as a serum K^+ <3.5 mEq per L with severe hypokalemia being <2.5 mEq per L. Hypokalemia

can result from increased loss, transcellular shift, or decreased intake. Potassium is excreted through either the GI tract (diarrhea) or the kidney. Excessive renal losses of K^+ occur with diuretic use, and direct tubule damage by chronic interstitial nephritis, pyelonephritis, or nephrotoxic medications. The distal tubule may be a site for K^+ loss because of excess mineralocorticoid, increased Na^+ delivery to the distal tubule because of proximal renal tubular acidosis (RTA), Fanconi syndrome, diuretics, or hypercalcemia. Increased sweat loss and magnesium depletion can cause hypokalemia. Transcellular shifts of K^+ from metabolic alkalosis, medications (particularly, β_2 sympathomimetics, insulin, and phosphodiesterase inhibitors), and from syndromes (such as familial hypokalemic periodic paralysis) can cause decreased serum K^+ concentrations.

Clinical Manifestations

Mild hypokalemia is usually asymptomatic, although nonspecific changes in electrocardiograms (EKGs) can be observed. The manifestations of severe K^+ depletion are skeletal muscle weakness with hyporeflexia (ultimately culminating in rhabdomyolysis), smooth muscle dysfunction, and disorders of GI motility. Lethargy, confusion, and cardiac dysrhythmias (see Table 15.3 for EKG findings) are common manifestations of severe hypokalemia, and children with an underlying heart disease are at increased risk for the cardiovascular effects.

Laboratory Data

In addition to an EKG, other lab values to be obtained in the evaluation of hypokalemia include arterial blood gas (ABG), serum electrolytes with BUN, Cr, glucose, and urine electrolytes.

Management

Any concurrent conditions or medications that may result in K^+ shift should be treated and disorders of acid/base homeostasis should be addressed. K^+ replacement can be accomplished through oral or intravenous dosing. The acute K^+ deficit can be calculated by the following formula:

$$K^+ \text{ deficit} = [ICF\ K^+] \times 40\% \text{ of total fluid deficit}$$

Care must obviously be taken when infusing K^+ intravenously because rapid infusion can cause dysrhythmias or asystole, and extravasation of K^+ can cause severe local injury.

Hyperkalemia

Etiologies

Mild to moderate hyperkalemia is defined as a serum K^+ level between 6 to 7 mEq per L. Levels >7 mmol per L are considered severe hyperkalemia. Artifactual hyperkalemia can be caused by tight tourniquets or squeezing at the site of blood collection, hemolysis, thrombocytosis, or leukocytosis of the blood sample. True hyperkalemia is caused by increased K^+ intake, abnormal distribution, or decreased renal output. Increased intake can be iatrogenic owing to K^+ salts of medications or increased K^+ content of red cell products reaching their time of expiration. Abnormal distribution occurs with metabolic acidosis, tissue catabolism, hyperosmolarity due to hypernatremia or hyperglycemia, decreased insulin, and drug side effects (i.e., digitalis, β-blockers, or succinylcholine). Decreased renal output occurs with renal failure, hypoaldosteronism, or K^+-sparing diuretics.

Clinical Manifestations

Mild hyperkalemia is often asymptomatic. Severe hyperkalemia may present with generalized weakness, paralysis, paresthesias, and cardiac arrhythmias and represents a medical emergency. Typical EKG findings are listed in Table 15.3.

Laboratory Data

Serum electrolytes with BUN/Cr should be obtained, as well as an ABG, EKG, and urine electrolytes.

Management

Severe hyperkalemia with EKG changes should be treated emergently with intravenous (IV) calcium gluconate (100 mg/kg/dose), glucose (2 mL per kg of D_{25} W), and insulin (0.1 U per kg). The EKG should be continuously monitored. Sodium bicarbonate can be beneficial even in the absence of acidosis. Diuretics may be helpful to increase the K^+ excretion. These therapies may only be transient in

TABLE 15.3	
ELECTROLYTE ABNORMALITIES AND ELECTROCARDIOGRAM CHANGES	
Electrolyte Abnormalities	**Associated EKG and Cardiac Findings**
Hypokalemia	A prominent U wave with a flattened T wave
Hyperkalemia	
5.5–6.5 mmol/L	Tall peaked T waves (leads II, III, V2–V4)
6.5–7.5 mmol/L	Loss of P waves
7–8 mmol/L	Widening of QRS complexes
8–10 mmol/L	Sine wave, ventricular arrhythmias, asystole
Hypocalcemia	Prolonged QT interval
Hypercalcemia	Shortened QT interval
Hypomagnesemia	Ventricular arrhythmias (i.e., torsades de pointes)
Moderate	Widening QRS complex with peaked T waves
Severe	Prolonged PR interval, progressive widening of the QRS complex, diminution of T wave

the presence of renal failure, and in such cases, hemodialysis should be instituted. In mild hyperkalemia, sodium polystyrene resin (kayexelate) may be effective to increase excretion.

CALCIUM

Calcium exists in the serum in three forms: bound to protein (40% to 45%), complexed to inorganic anions (5% to 10%), and ionized (40% to 50%). The ionized fraction is the physiologically active form. Normal Ca^{2+} levels vary with age in the pediatric population. Normal neonatal values are between 9 to 10 mg per dL. This remains the average serum Ca^{2+} concentration until approximately 18 months of life. Serum Ca^{2+} levels between 8.5 to 10.5 mg per dL are considered to be normal in children and adolescents.

Hypocalcemia

Etiologies
Hypocalcemia is defined as a serum Ca^{2+} level <8.5 mg per dL in older children and <8.0 mg per dL in neonates. The total protein or albumin level is necessary to interpret the total Ca^{2+} level because of the considerable amount of serum Ca^{2+} that is protein bound. In recent years, accurate and immediate ionized calcium determination has improved. Therefore, ionized calcium concentrations <1.0 mg per dL can also be used to define hypocalcemia. The causes of hypocalcemia vary with age. Common etiologies in neonates include birth asphyxia, prematurity, toxemia in pregnancy, infants of diabetic mothers, intrauterine growth restriction, maternal hyperparathyroidism, and DiGeorge syndrome with congenital heart diseases. Other etiologies in childhood include hypoparathyroidism (primary or secondary), vitamin D deficiency, hyperphosphatemia, malabsorption states/malnutrition, pancreatitis, hypomagnesemia, and medications (i.e., anticonvulsants). Hypocalcemia is common after cardiac surgery because of induced hypocalcemia during preischemic cooling by using a Ca^{2+} free crystalloid priming solution and citrate in the pump prime. This has been found to provide myocardial preservation and reduce ischemic injury during the cooling phase of cardiopulmonary bypass.

Clinical Manifestations
Symptoms of hypocalcemia include tetany and its associated symptoms such as neuromuscular irritability, weakness, fatigue, paresthesias, cramping, altered mental status, seizures, laryngospasm, and cardiac arrhythmias. Infants with hypocalcemia may also demonstrate vomiting due to pylorospasm, wheezing from bronchospasm, and inspiratory stridor from laryngospasm. Many infants may also be asymptomatic. Trousseau and Chvostek signs are clinical signs of hypocalcemia. EKG changes are listed in Table 15.3.

Laboratory Data
Initial evaluation of suspected hypocalcemia in a child should include a serum total and ionized Ca^{2+}, phosphate, magnesium, alkaline phosphatase, 25-OH vitamin D, total protein, pH, BUN, Cr, parathyroid hormone (PTH), and an EKG. The albumin level should also be obtained because a decrease in serum albumin of 1.0 g per dL decreases serum Ca^{2+} by 0.8 mg per dL. Other tests to be obtained in the evaluation of hypocalcemia include urinary Ca^{2+}, phosphate, Cr, and radiographic tests to evaluate for evidence of rickets, the presence of a thymic shadow, and bone age.

Management
Treatment of hypocalcemia is best accomplished by treating the underlying cause or disease. However, in acute symptomatic patients, Ca^{2+} supplementation is best accomplished with IV forms of Ca^{2+} such as calcium gluconate, calcium chloride ($CaCl_2$), or calcium gluceptate. CaCl is three times as potent as calcium gluconate, and it should be infused through a central venous catheter to prevent tissue necrosis owing to extravasation. Oral Ca^{2+} supplements may be used in less acute situations. Refractory hypocalcemia may also be due to hypomagnesemia and so magnesium supplementation may be required before hypocalcemia can be corrected.

Hypercalcemia

Etiologies
Hypercalcemia is defined as a serum Ca^{2+} level >10.5 mg per dL or an elevated ionized Ca^{2+}. Hypercalcemia occurs rarely in children owing to the relatively low incidence of hyperparathyroidism and various malignancies common to adults (i.e., lung, breast, kidney, myeloma, etc.). Hypercalcemia in children with malignancies is usually a result of direct bony invasion, tumor metastasis, and tumor lysis. Other etiologies of hypercalcemia vary widely on the basis of the child's age and the differential diagnosis is listed in Table 15.4. Hypophosphatemia is associated with hypercalcemia as elevated levels of the PTH leads to decreased phosphate absorption. Hypercalcemia is also seen in William syndrome as a result of increased sensitivity to vitamin D.

Clinical Manifestations
Common symptoms of hypercalcemia include weakness, respiratory distress/apnea, headache, irritability, seizures, lethargy, abdominal pain, anorexia, nausea, vomiting, constipation, and bone pain. Other findings associated with hypercalcemia include polydipsia, polyuria, renal calculi, pancreatitis, abnormal deep tendon reflexes, and hypertension. A shortened QT interval is seen on EKG (Table 15.3). Dysmorphisms and hypercalcemia, such as elflike facies and hypertelorism, can be suggestive of William syndrome.

Laboratory Data
Initial laboratory evaluation of hypercalcemia should include serum total and ionized Ca^{2+}, phosphate, albumin,

TABLE 15.4
ETIOLOGIES OF HYPERCALCEMIA IN THE PEDIATRIC POPULATION

Hyperthyroidism	Granulomatous disease (i.e., sarcoidosis)
Primary hyperparathyroidism	Blue diaper syndrome
Secondary hyperparathyroidism	Adrenal insufficiency
Maternal hypocalcemia	Hypothyroidism
Renal disease/failure	Thyrotoxicosis including Grave disease
FHH	Vitamin D intoxication
MEN I and MEN IIa	Vitamin A intoxication
Milk-alkali syndrome	Excessive intake/iatrogenic causes (i.e., TPN)
Williams syndrome	Prolonged immobilization
Malignancy	Medications (i.e., thiazide diuretics, lithium, theophylline, tamoxifen, oral contraceptives)

FHH, familial hypocalciuric hypercalcemia; MEN, multiple endocrine neoplasia; TPN, triphosphopyridine nucleotide.

total protein, PTH, BUN, Cr, alkaline phosphatase, vitamin D levels, and an EKG. Additional laboratory tests may include thyroid function tests, complete blood count (CBC) with differential, urinary Ca^{2+}, phosphate and Cr levels, and radiography to evaluate for metastatic bone lesions and possible renal calculi as clinically indicated. Maternal Ca^{2+} and PTH levels may prove helpful in neonates with hypercalcemia.

Management

The treatment of hypercalcemia is based on an understanding of the etiology and its mechanism of action. In malignancy-associated hypercalcemia, which results from enhanced intestinal absorption, oral phosphorous therapy can be effective. Vitamin D intoxication or sarcoidosis can be treated with glucocorticoids, which suppress calcitriol effects and inhibit lymphokine secretions. Steroids may also be useful in the setting of malignancy to decrease vitamin D and Ca^{2+} absorption. However, irrespective of the underlying cause, (i) discontinuing or restricting further Ca^{2+} intake, (ii) correcting dehydration with saline infusion followed by furosemide, (iii) avoiding medications or supplements that will increase the serum Ca^{2+} concentration such as vitamin D, Ca^{2+} containing antacids, and thiazide diuretics, and (iv) administering phosphate can lead to decreases in serum Ca^{2+}. Severe or persistent hypercalcemia can be treated with calcitonin or bisphosphonate. It is important to note that correcting dehydration in the setting of hypercalcemia is crucial. The use of diuretics before rehydration can cause volume contraction and subsequently increase serum Ca^{2+}. Normal saline is the replacement fluid of choice because Na^+ blocks tubular Ca^{2+} reabsorption and enhances its excretion.

Accelerated bone resorption is an important factor in the pathogenesis of hypercalcemia in most patients with acute hypercalcemia. Bisphosphonates such as pamidronate is the treatment of choice for the inhibition of bone resorption. Other treatment modalities for hypercalcemia in extreme cases include dialysis and parathyroidectomy.

PHOSPHATE

Approximately 85% of our body phosphate stores are in our bones in the form of hydroxyapatite. The remaining 15% is in the interstitial fluid, serum, or within the cells. Normal serum phosphate concentrations are highest in infancy and early childhood (4 to 7 mg per dL) and decrease during midchildhood, and in adolescence the values range between 2.5 and 4.5 mg per dL.

Hypophosphatemia

Etiologies

Causes of hypophosphatemia include starvation, malnutrition, malabsorption syndromes, increased renal losses, vitamin D deficiency and vitamin D-resistant rickets, intracellular shifts associated with respiratory or metabolic alkalosis, treatment of diabetic ketoacidosis (DKA), and the administration of corticosteroids. Hypophosphatemia also occurs commonly in the very low birth weight (VLBW) neonates because their demands are usually greater than their intake.

Clinical Manifestations

Signs and symptoms of hypophosphatemia are only evident at very low levels (<1.0 mg per dL). At these levels, irritability, paresthesias, confusion, seizures, apnea in VLBW infants, and coma may be seen. Rare cases of cardiomyopathy have been reported. However, it is unclear if these symptoms are caused by the electrolyte disturbance or by the illness associated with hypophosphatemia.

Laboratory Data

The evaluation of hypophosphatemia should include serum phosphate, total and ionized Ca^{2+}, Na^+, K^+, magnesium, BUN, Cr, vitamin D, and PTH levels. Urinary studies such as urine Ca^{2+}, phosphate, Cr, and pH may prove helpful.

Management

Acute symptomatic hypophosphatemia should be treated with potassium phosphate or sodium phosphate as a slow infusion over 6 hours. Caution must be exercised in the administration of these solutions because an increase in serum K^+ or Na^+ can be anticipated.

Hyperphosphatemia

Etiologies

Hyperphosphatemia is relatively rare. Common etiologies include hypoparathyroidism, renal insufficiency with a reduction of glomerular filtration rate (GFR) of <25%, excessive intake/iatrogenic administration, and use of cytotoxic drugs to treat malignancies resulting in tumor lysis syndrome.

Clinical Manifestations

Signs and symptoms of hyperphosphatemia are generally the result of hypocalcemia caused by the effects of the PTH. As such, clinical symptoms include tetany and neuromuscular sequelae, altered mental status and seizures, and cardiac manifestations such as dysrhythmias and prolonged QT interval can be observed (Table 15.3).

Laboratory Data

Similar to children with hypocalcemia, laboratory analysis should begin with BUN, Cr, and serum phosphate, total and ionized Ca^{2+} levels. Vitamin D, PTH levels, and ABG may also be helpful. In cases of tumor lysis syndrome, a CBC should also be obtained along with urinary studies such as urinalysis and urine phosphate, calcium, and Cr levels.

Management

Treatment of hyperphosphatemia includes: (i) restricting further dietary phosphate intake, (ii) giving phosphate binders such as calcium carbonate and aluminum hydroxide (must be used with caution in patients with renal failure), (iii) hydrating with normal saline and IV mannitol in tumor lysis syndrome, and (iv) instituting dialysis if patient has poor renal function and hyperphosphatemia is refractory to above measures.

MAGNESIUM

Magnesium plays a critical role in metabolic processes and its deficiency is often associated with multiple biochemical abnormalities. Hypermagnesemia is much less common. Ionized magnesium is the physiologically active form; however, measurement of the ion is not yet available in most laboratories and so total magnesium is the monitored electrolyte.

Hypomagnesemia

Etiologies

Magnesium deficiency can occur from decreased intake or from increased losses (from the GI tract or kidney). GI losses may occur from intestinal malabsorption including cystic fibrosis, regional enteritis, ulcerative colitis, small bowel resection, and familial primary hypomagnesemia. Renal losses are generally a result of diuretic use, RTA, diffuse tubular disorders, hypercalciuria, and nephrotoxic medications. Other etiologies are DKA, hyperaldosteronism, and PTH disorders. Hypomagnesemia may also develop during cardiopulmonary bypass possibly owing to chelation by free fatty acids or citrate and enhanced cellular uptake induced by circulating catecholamines.

Clinical Manifestations

Low serum magnesium is manifested by anorexia, nausea, weakness, malaise, depression, and nonspecific psychiatric symptoms. Neurologic signs include clonus, tetany, hyperreflexia, and positive Chvostek and Trousseau signs. It can also be associated with hypokalemia, hypocalcemia, and metabolic acidosis, and arrhythmias may present as atrial or ventricular ectopy or torsades de pointes (Table 15.3).

Laboratory Data

Serum electrolytes including total and ionized magnesium (if available), Ca^{2+}, BUN/Cr, glucose, and urine electrolytes should be obtained.

Management

Replacement of magnesium with intravenous magnesium sulfate is the therapy for hypomagnesemia. Because a wide variety of clinical conditions can cause this electrolyte disturbance, an underlying condition should be determined and corrected promptly.

Hypermagnesemia

Etiologies

The most common cause of hypermagnesemia is acute or chronic renal failure. As with other electrolyte disturbances, excessive administration of magnesium (from enemas, cathartics, triphosphopyridine nucleotide (TPN), or in the treatment of preeclampsia/eclampsia) can also cause this disorder.

Clinical Manifestations

Increased magnesium can cause lethargy, hyporeflexia, confusion, hypotension, respiratory failure, and cardiac dysfunction.

Laboratory Data

Initial laboratory evaluation should include total magnesium, ionized magnesium (if available), Ca^{2+}, BUN and Cr.

Management

Stopping any supplemental magnesium is vital. Diuresis and calcium administration are beneficial in the treatment of hypermagnesemia. Hemodialysis may be necessary in renal failure or life-threatening cases.

CARDIAC EFFECTS OF ELECTROLYTE ABNORMALITIES

Abnormal serum electrolytes can have profound effects on cardiac conduction. These effects can be demonstrated as mild or dramatic changes on the EKG. Fluctuations in extracellular K^+, Ca^{2+}, and Mg^{2+} levels can change myocyte membrane potential gradients and alter the cardiac action potential. Characteristic EKG changes may provide diagnostic clues to these abnormalities. Table 15.3 is a summary of these changes and their associated electrolyte abnormality.

Increases in serum K^+ can have dramatic effects on the EKG and cardiac disorders should be suspected when the amplitude of the T wave is greater than or equal to the R wave in more than one lead.

Calcium affects the duration of the ST segment. Hypercalcemia shortens the ST segment thereby shortening the QT interval, and hypocalcemia has the reverse effects. At high Ca^{2+} concentrations, the duration of the T wave increases and the QT interval may become normal. These effects may be more pronounced in patients receiving digoxin therapy.

Magnesium regulates several cardiac ion channels, including Ca^{2+} channels and outward K^+ currents. Low Mg^{2+} increases these outward currents, shortening the action potential and increasing the susceptibility to arrhythmias.

RECOMMENDED READINGS

1. Adrogue H. Primary care: Hypernatremia. *N Engl J Med*. 2000; 342(20):1493–1499.
2. Agus Z. Hypomagnesemia. *J Am Soc Nephrol*. 1999;10:1616–1622.
3. Avner E. Clinical disorders of water metabolism: Hyponatremia and hypernatremia. *Pediatr Ann*. 1995;24(1):23–30.
4. Becker KL. *Principles and practice of endocrinology and metabolism.* Philadelphia, PA: Lippincott Williams & Wilkins; 2001.
5. Chang A. *Pediatric cardiac intensive care.* Philadelphia, PA: Lippincott Williams & Wilkins; 1998.
6. Fouser L. Disorders of calcium, phosphorus, and magnesium. *Pediatr Ann*. 1995;24(1):38–46.
7. Moritz M. Disorders of water metabolism in children: Hyponatremia and hypernatremia. *Pediatr Rev*. 2002;23(11):371–379.
8. Pescovitz OH, Eugster EA. *Pediatric endocrinology: Mechanisms, manifestations, and management.* Philadelphia, PA: Lippincott Williams & Wilkins; 2004.
9. Rastergar A. Hypokalemia and Hyperkalemia. *Postgrad Med*. 2001; 77:759–764.
10. Sperling M. *Pediatric endocrinology.* Philadelphia, PA: WB Saunders; 2002.
11. Yeates K. Salt and water: A simple approach to hyponatremia. *Can Med Assoc J*. 2004;170(3):365–369.

Inborn Errors of Metabolism

16

Dina J. Zand   Cynthia J. Tifft

Scientific and medical advances have challenged our initial approach to and understanding of inborn errors of metabolism (IEM). In 1908, when Sir Archibald Garrod first suggested the term, he believed that these diagnoses affected an individual throughout life and were essentially untreatable. Although most IEM are still life-long afflictions, advances in biochemistry, genetics, and pathophysiology have significantly altered our understanding of them. In general, IEM are disorders affecting the intermediary metabolism of protein, glucose, fat, and complex substrates. Some IEM, such as phenylketonuria (PKU), are treatable with consistent dietary intervention. Many, but not all IEM present during infancy or childhood. Our improved diagnostic abilities demonstrate that IEM are more common than initially believed. And, although consanguinity often increases the risk for diagnosis of IEM, most affected families are without known consanguinity.

The presenting symptomatology for IEM is often nonspecific. Within the first few weeks of birth, clinical findings may include lethargy, poor feeding, emesis, irritability, hypotonia, and seizures. However, loss of developmental skills, encephalopathy, and organ-specific abnormalities such as cardiomyopathy, hepatomegaly, and cataracts may present additional clues. IEM should be included in the differential diagnosis with any of these presentations.

A few general concepts are essential in understanding IEM. First, the pathophysiology most commonly results from a specific defect in metabolism. This may be a dysfunctional enzyme, a cofactor, or a transport protein. Second, this defect results in the accumulation of substrate and/or the deficiency of metabolic product. Either of these metabolic perturbations may give rise to clinical symptoms. Abnormally elevated levels of substrate may act as a toxin, affecting normal cellular mechanism

or organ pathophysiology. Similarly, decreased levels of product may force the cell to "overuse" other systems to compensate. Secondary affects from toxin buildup can also be observed. For example, elevations of plasma ammonia can be seen during illness with propionic aciduria (PA) and methylmalonic aciduria (MMA), although they are organic acidurias and not primary hyperammonemia disorders. In general, the pathophysiology of IEM is caused by a perturbation in normal cellular function, and clues to pinpointing the precise abnormality include a thorough history, repetitive clinical examinations, particularly during acute metabolic crisis, and prompt laboratory evaluation. Above all, clinical suspicion is paramount.

NEWBORN SCREENING

The public health paradigm for newborn screening (NBS) in the United States began when Dr. Robert Guthrie developed a test for PKU utilizing dried blood spots on filter paper. The analysis was rapid, inexpensive, and the prompt diagnosis led to the initiation of a specific therapy that could prevent the severe mental retardation characteristic of this disorder. Presently, NBS is conducted by state mandate. Each state determines those diagnoses that will be screened for, the methodology, and the subsequent follow-up for children identified. Some states require analysis of two serial blood samples because shortened hospital stays do not allow for adequate feeding of the newborn before sample collection. Initially, NBS tests involved individual enzyme analysis. Recently, a number of states have moved to tandem mass spectroscopy (MS/MS) to expand the number of IEM that can be identified on a single sample to include multiple aminoacidopathies, fatty acid oxidation disorders, and organic acidurias. The use of this technology allows for early identification of a greater number of presymptomatic newborns with disorders that would typically present with metabolic coma and neurologic decompensation. A negative screen, however, does not exclude a diagnosis of IEM because some disorders, such as nonketotic hyperglycinemia (NKH) or tyrosinemia remain difficult to diagnose using this technology. Clinical suspicion should always prevail.

ACUTE NEUROLOGIC DECOMPENSATION OR METABOLIC COMA

When a child presents with acute decompensation and encephalopathy, particularly in the newborn period, sepsis is the most common etiology. However, IEM should also be strongly considered. Because metabolic pathways often converge at common points, the clinical presentations of different IEM may, in fact, be quite similar. Fortunately, acute management is also similar to the goal of providing enough calories to reverse catabolism. The laboratory studies listed in Table 16.1 should be considered for any child with an unexplained acute encephalopathy. Specialized testing should be anticipated, and may require special tubes or sample handling (see Table 16.2). Intravenous fluids containing dextrose and electrolytes should be started immediately while laboratory results are pending. Testing performed at the bedside (dextrostick, I-STAT, and/or urine dipstick) may give quick clues toward changes in management. For example, hypoglycemia should be addressed immediately, with enough glucose to normalize levels promptly and provide the calories needed to reverse catabolism. For IEM, this may mean a continuous infusion of 8 to 10 mg/kg/minute or 10% dextrose at one-and-a-half-times the maintenance level (see Fig. 16.1). During these interventions, a complete and thorough history may help elucidate the etiology of the clinical symptoms. Specific information about changes in oral intake, illnesses, decrease in urine production, unusual odors (see Table 16.3), and family history inclusive of neonatal deaths and stillbirths should be elicited. A thorough and accurate clinical examination is essential. Any indication of increased intracranial pressure (pupillary reflexes, papilledema, increased reflexes, exaggerated startle, or clonus) should be evaluated quickly. If increased dextrose is required in the context of cerebral edema, a central line should be placed and the dextrose should be concentrated to limit further cerebral injury from excess intravenous fluid. An insulin drip may be needed to force dextrose into the cells, to further promote anabolism. Cataracts, cardiac arrhythmia, hepatosplenomegaly, poor growth, and dysmorphia are all important clues and should be documented while the patient is being stabilized. The results of initial laboratory studies for urine ketones, hypoglycemia, metabolic acidosis or alkalosis, and lactate may

preliminarily place a child into the IEM diagnostic category (see Table 16.4).

With the advent of MS/MS NBS, some patients may be referred for evaluation on the basis of the report of an abnormal newborn screen. Evaluation of these infants should be the same as for a child with an unknown presentation, with targeting of specialized testing on the basis of the screening result. NBS may also identify children who, although not acutely ill, may have biochemical evidence of a partial deficiency that under conditions of metabolic stress could/would produce clinical symptoms and neurologic compromise. Disorders of branched-chain amino acid (BCAA) metabolism, such as maple syrup urine disease (MSUD), PA, and MMA are some of the most common IEM in the pediatric population (see Fig. 16.2). PA and MMA are considered as organic acidurias because these enzyme deficiencies result in an abundance of organic acid metabolites found in plasma and urine. MSUD is located in the same pathway, and results in an elevation of the initial substrates—leucine, valine, and isoleucine. The initial presentation of all three conditions, as well as isovaleric acidemia (IVA) is similar with acidosis, ketone body formation, hypoglycemia, and possible encephalopathy.

Maple Syrup Urine Disease

The most common cause of this disorder is a decrease in the branched-chain α-keto dehydrogenase EI activity. Thiamin (vitamin B_1) is an important cofactor, and its administration may reduce the symptomatology in some cases. The characteristic sweet odor of maple syrup may be

---

TABLE 16.1

LABORATORY TESTS FOR INBORN ERRORS OF METABOLISM

Stat Initial Tests

Bilirubin (total and direct)
Blood gas
Blood glucose (D-stick and serum)
CBC with differential
Creatinine and BUN
Liver function tests (ALT and AST)
Plasma ammonia
Plasma lactate
Serum electrolytes to include calcium, magnesium, and phosphorus
Urine analysis: pH, ketones, glucose, protein, reducing substances

Additional Specialized Testing

Acylcarnitine profile
Carnitine level (total and free)
Plasma amino acids
Urine organic acids

CBC, complete blood count; BUN, blood urea nitrogen; ALT, alanine aminotransferase; AST, aspartate aminotransferase.

TABLE 16.2

SPECIALIZED TESTING FOR INBORN ERRORS OF METABOLISM

Test	Volume	Tube	Comments
PAA	1–3 mL	Green (Na heparin)	If cannot be processed immediately, spin down to separate and freeze plasma (not the entire sample)
Branched-chain amino acids	1–3 mL	Green (Na heparin)	Same as with PAA
Acylcarnitine profile	1–3 mL	Green (Na heparin)	Same as with PAA
Carnitine, total and free	1–3 mL, on ice	Green (Na heparin)	Same as with PAA
Biotinidase	1–3 mL	Green (Na heparin)	Same as with PAA
Homocysteine, total and free	3 mL, on ice	Green (Na heparin)	Same as with PAA
Lactate/pyruvate	1–2 mL, on ice	Grey (K oxalate and NaCl) or 8% perchloric acid	Collection container is institution dependent
Very long-chain fatty acids	3 mL	Lavender (EDTA)	
Karyotype	1–3 mL	Green (Na heparin)	DO NOT freeze or separate
Transferrin isoelectric focusing	5 mL	Yellow (acid citrate dextran)	
UOA	5–10 mL	Urine container	If it cannot be processed immediately, it may be frozen
Urine amino acids	5–10 mL	Urine container	Same as with UOA

PAA, plasma amino acids; EDTA, ethylenediaminetetraacetic acid; UOA, urine organic acids.

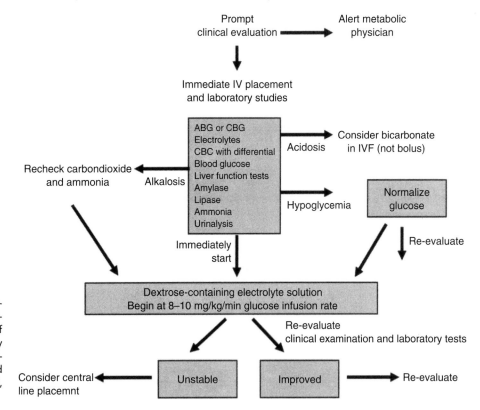

Figure 16.1 Suggested emergency treatment algorithm for individuals with known inborn errors of metabolism (IEM) with a tendency toward catabolism and encephalopathy during illness. ABG, arterial blood gas; CBG, capillary blood gas; IVF, intravenous fluid.

TABLE 16.3

UNUSUAL ODORS IN INBORN ERRORS OF METABOLISM

Disease	Odor
Maple syrup urine disease	Maple syrup, burned sugar
Isovaleric acidemia	Cheesy or sweaty feet
Multiple carboxylase deficiency	Cat's urine
Phenylketonuria	Musty
Hypermethioninemia	Rancid butter, rotten cabbage
Trimethylaminuria	Fishy

appreciated in either urine or cerumen, particularly during periods of acute illness, and allo-isoleucine detected by plasma amino acid analysis is diagnostic. Elevations of leucine-induced cerebral edema, and acute treatment with high dextrose-containing fluids are imperative. The leucine level returns to normal only by its incorporation into synthesized proteins; therefore, either formula or total parenteral nutrition (TPN) lacking BCAAs are also essential for therapy. Because valine and isoleucine levels fall more quickly, supplementation with these amino acids is usually needed to reduce plasma leucine to keep up with new protein synthesis. Repeat acute metabolic episodes of encephalopathy, as a result of routine childhood illness may result in cognitive impairment and dysmyelination.

Propionic Aciduria

Deficiency of propionyl-CoA carboxylase, a biotin-dependent enzyme, results in PA. The α subunit of the heteromeric enzyme binds biotin. However, as mutations are more commonly identified in the β subunit, most of the affected individuals do not respond to biotin supplementation. Elevations of free propionic acid in blood or urine may not be easily detectable, but organic acid by-products can be identified in urine (3-hydroxypropionate, methylcitrate, tiglylglycine, and unusual ketone bodies) by plasma acylcarnitine (propionylcarnitine) analysis. Elevations of organic acids may also be seen in multiple carboxylase deficiency owing to similar dependence on biotin as a cofactor.

Treatment begins during the acute metabolic crisis by arresting catabolism with intravenous dextrose (8 to 10 mg/kg/minute) and lipid (2 g/kg/day). Hypoglycemia, acidosis, vomiting, lethargy, and ketonuria are common initial features. A secondary effect of hyperammonemia owing to the toxin-mediated effects upon the urea cycle may be significant enough to warrant consideration of hemodialysis.

Parenteral administration of a formula that is deficient in the offending BCAAs is preferable once vomiting has resolved and the encephalopathy has improved. A secondary carnitine deficiency is common, and supplementation with l-carnitine (50 to 100 mg/kg/day) may aid in the removal of excess propionic acid and prevent the cardiomyopathy caused by carnitine depletion. Once the acidosis and urine ketones have resolved, the child should be maintained on a diet that is low in natural protein (0.5 to 1.5 g/kg/day) and a formula that is deficient in BCCAs to provide the remaining recommended daily protein allowance for that age. Because gut flora may contribute significantly to propionic acid production, some children have derived clinical benefit from metronidazole (10 mg/kg/day for 1 week twice per month) to decrease fecal propionate production.

Methylmalonic Aciduria

MMA is most often caused by mutations in the methylmalonyl-CoA mutase gene. Vitamin B_{12}, or cobalamin,

TABLE 16.4

INITIAL LABORATORY TESTS AND SUSPICION FOR METABOLIC DISEASE

Metabolic Category	Branched-Chain Amino Acids	Organic Acid Production	Urea Cycle (NH$_4$ Production)	Fatty Acid Oxidation	Energy Metabolism	Carbohydrate Utilization
Example diagnosis Test	MSUD	PA	OTC deficiency	MCAD deficiency	PDH deficiency	GSD type I
Blood pH	Acidotic	Acidotic	Alkalotic	Normal/++	Acidotic	Acidotic
Anion gap	++	++	Normal	Normal/++	++	++
Ammonia	Normal/++	Normal/++	++++	Normal/++	Normal/++	Normal
Glucose	Normal/−−	Normal/−−	Normal/−−	−−−−	Normal/−−	−−
Lactate	Normal	Normal/++	Normal	Normal/−−	++++	++
Urine ketones	Normal/++++	Normal/++++	Normal	Inappropriately/−−	Variable	Normal

MSUD, maple syrup urine disease; PA, propionic aciduria; OTC, ornithine transcarbamylase; MCAD, medium-chain acyl-CoA dehydrogenase; PDH, pyruvate dehydrogenase; GSD, glycogen storage disease.

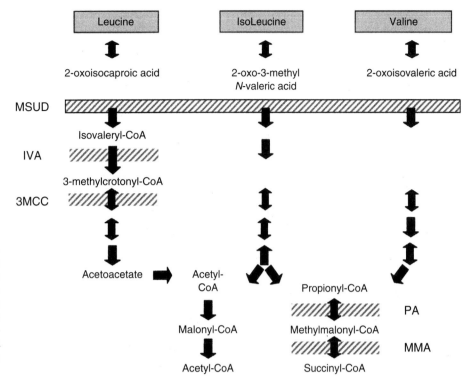

Figure 16.2 Inborn errors of metabolism within the branched-chain amino acid (BCAA) pathway. Both aminoacidopathies and organic acidurias can result from aberrations within the BCAA pathway. MSUD, maple syrup urine disease; IVA, isovaleric acidemia; MCC, 3-methylcrotonyl-CoA carboxylase; PA, propionic aciduria; MMA, methylmalonic aciduria.

is an essential cofactor, and less severe symptomatology may also arise with severe malabsorption or a strict vegan diet. Other derangements in cobalamin metabolism may also cause MMA (subtypes labeled cobalamin A through F). Cobalamin C has symptomatology of both MMA and homocystinuria, with a high risk of thromboembolism. As in PA, patients with severe MMA present with hypotonia, lethargy, hypoglycemia, ketonuria, and acidosis. Marked elevation of methylmalonate in urine is observed, as well as the presence of 3-hydroxypropionate and methylcitrate. The brain magnetic resonance imaging (MRI) may reflect basal ganglia, thalamic edema, and necrosis, and magnetic resonance (MR) spectroscopy can be helpful for identifying metabolites such as lactate. Additionally, vascular concerns may be present in MMA (cobalamin C and D), and ocular disease is common. Long-term renal disease caused by thrombotic microangiopathy and pancreatitis (also present in PA) are concerns. Formal diagnosis of the MMA subtype requires enzyme complementation analysis on cultured skin fibroblasts.

Acute management for MMA, similar to PA, involves aggressive therapy with intravenous dextrose and lipids to promote anabolism. Immediate dialysis may be needed if hyperammonemia and obtundation are present. Interim administration of high doses of vitamin B_{12} with both clinical and laboratory re-evaluation is important to rule out a rare but more easily treated form of MMA. The long-term management of MMA requires a protein-restricted diet, vitamin, and L-carnitine supplementation.

Urea Cycle Disorders

Hyperammonemia with hyperventilation and worsening encephalopathy in the newborn are hallmarks of urea cycle disorders (see Fig. 16.3); however, symptoms and age of onset vary considerably. In the most severe forms, newborns also develop lethargy, poor feeding habits, seizures, temperature instability, loss of reflexes, and intracranial hemorrhage due to coagulopathy. Infants and children with less severe disease may present with failure to thrive, feeding difficulty, vomiting, and chronic neurologic symptoms, or episodic ataxia, lethargy, and seizures. In addition to lethargy and recurrent encephalopathy, adolescents may show psychiatric or behavioral problems, or episodes of disorientation particularly during times of stress or in association with high protein intake. Patients with less severe or episodic symptoms may have partial enzyme deficiencies.

The diagnosis of urea cycle defect should be considered in any sick neonate. Plasma ammonia level should be drawn, placed on ice and run within 30 minutes. Improper sample handling can result in an ammonia level two to three times the normal level. The nonspecific signs of feeding intolerance and somnolence can rapidly progress to lethargy and coma if hyperammonemia goes unrecognized and therapy is delayed. Any infant with symptomatic hyperammonemia should be transported to a tertiary care center where hemodialysis and ammonia-scavenging drugs are available. Initial management should include stopping all protein feeds and infusing glucose and lipid to prevent catabolism. Patients may also be

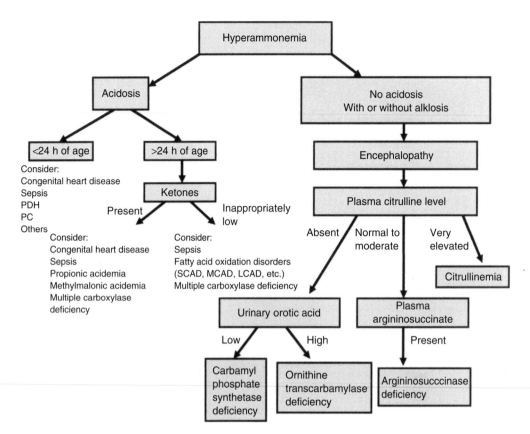

Figure 16.3 The differential diagnosis of hyperammonemia. PDH, pyruvate dehydrogenase; PC, pyruvate carboxylase; SCAD, short-chain acyl-CoA dehydrogenase; MCAD, medium-chain acyl-CoA dehydrogenase; LCAD, long-chain acyl-CoA dehydrogenase.

dehydrated. During hyperammonemic crisis, particularly in the newborn, plasma ammonia is usually >300 μm per L and may be much higher. Samples should be sent for PAA, plasma acylcarnitine profile, urine amino acids, urine organic acids, and urine orotic acid determinations in order to determine the etiology of the hyperammonemia (see Figs. 16.3 and 16.4).

Intravenous therapy with ammonia-scavenging drugs should be started in the child with suspected or documented urea cycle defect when ammonia elevation corresponds with central nervous system (CNS) symptomatology. It may be prudent to contact a metabolic specialist who has experience with these drugs because they are not without potentially toxic side effects. For acute neonatal hyperammonemic coma where the specific defect has not been documented, a 600 mg per kg loading dose of 10% L-arginine–HCl in 10% dextrose and 250 mg per kg loading dose each of sodium benzoate and sodium phenylacetate in 10% dextrose over a 2-hour period followed by a sustaining infusion of 250 mg per kg each of sodium benzoate and sodium phenylacetate over 24 hours are given. The arginine-sustaining dose varies according to the particular suspected or known enzyme deficiency. Arginine should ideally be given through a central catheter because extravasation into the peripheral tissues causes sclerosis.

Hemodialysis is the most rapid way to remove ammonia from the circulation. If hemodialysis is unavailable, then hemofiltration should be used. Peritoneal dialysis may be helpful but may not remove ammonia quickly enough to be clinically effective. Nitrogen-scavenging drugs should be continued during hemodialysis because they act synergistically and ammonia levels should be monitored frequently (every 2 to 4 hours initially, if the patient is obtunded).

After 48 hours, and following the acute phase of management, small amounts of protein (0.5 g/kg/day) should be added to the intravenous dextrose and lipids to prevent further catabolism. An experienced metabolic nutritionist should be involved in the care of the patient as oral feeding begins. Despite aggressive management, neonates with severe hyperammonemic coma may have significant residual neurologic deficits.

Other Inborn Errors with Acute Neurologic Presentation

There are many rare IEM that can produce acute neurologic decompensation in an infant or young child. Careful physical examination and laboratory testing may be

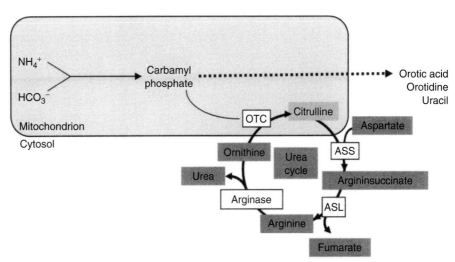

Figure 16.4 Urea cycle enzymes and cellular localization. Ornithine transcarbamylase (OTC) binds ornithine to carbamoylphosphate, to form citrulline. After citrulline is transported into the cytosol, aspartate is bound by argininosuccinate synthetase (ASS) to form argininosuccinate, which is then converted by argininosuccinate lyase (ASL) to arginine and fumarate. Arginase then converts arginine to urea and ornithine. Ornithine is then transported into the mitochondria by an ornithine transporter to complete the urea cycle.

suggestive of one of these disorders and a few of them are listed here.

Glutaric acidemia type 1 presents with macrocephaly and acute encephalopathic crisis with a dystonic–dyskinetic movement disorder typically between 6 and 18 months. The presence of glutaric acid and 3-hydroxyglutaric acid on urine organic acid analysis is diagnostic. Patients should be treated with carnitine 100 mg/kg/day and a lysine- and tryptophan-restricted diet. Glutaric acidemia type 2 or multiple acyl-CoA dehydrogenase deficiency presents with facial and cerebral malformations, metabolic acidosis, hypoglycemia, Reye syndrome, progressive encephalopathy, and epilepsy. Diagnostic testing shows elevated acylcarnitines (C4 to C18 species), and elevated organic acids (lactic, glutaric, ethylmalonic, and dicarboxylic acids). Treatment consist in the inclusion of a low-fat diet and avoidance of fasting.

Nonketotic hyperglycinemia presents acutely in the neonate or more transiently in early childhood with severe epileptic encephalopathy, hypotonia, and progressive neurologic symptoms. Diagnosis is based on elevations of glycine in the plasma and cerebrospinal fluid (CSF) with a CSF/plasma ratio >0.06 (normal <0.04). Valproate treatment may complicate interpretation of the CSF/plasma ratio. Treatment is experimental and suspected patients should be referred to a tertiary care center with experience in NKH. Sulfite oxidase and molybdenum cofactor deficiencies present in early infancy with intractable seizures, psychomotor retardation, microcephaly, and lens dislocation. Diagnosis is based on the presence of sulfites in fresh urine, measured at the bedside with diagnostic urine dipsticks (e.g., Merckoquant 10013, Merck Darmstadt, Germany), and a very low serum uric acid. The presence of S-sulfocysteine in plasma is diagnostic. Again, therapy is supportive and experimental.

Menkes disease presents in male infants with neonatal hypothermia, severe jaundice, epilepsy, a typical facial profile, "kinky" hair, and connective tissue and bone abnormalities. Decreased levels of serum copper and ceruloplasmin are diagnostic. Microscopic examination of the hair reveals characteristic "pili torti." Daily copper injections may be helpful if started early in the disease course.

Biotinidase deficiency is tested in some, but not in all neonatal screening programs, and is characterized by metabolic acidosis, hypotonia, seizures, psychomotor retardation, hair loss, a skin rash, and immune defects. Metabolic abnormalities such as elevations in serum lactate and ammonia and plasma alanine may be present, but deficient biotinidase activity is diagnostic. The condition is treatable with 5 to 10 mg per day of oral biotin. Infants identified by NBS often are asymptomatic and have only a partial deficiency.

INBORN ERRORS OF ENERGY METABOLISM

The generation of energy by oxidative phosphorylation takes place in most organ systems and involves mitochondrial and nuclear genes. Consequently, deficiencies in respiratory chain enzymes can give rise to any symptom, in any tissue, at any age, and by any inheritance pattern.

A respiratory chain deficiency should be considered in any infant or child who presents with progressive neuromuscular symptoms in association with symptoms in a seemingly unrelated organ system. Typically, an increasing number of organ systems are involved with advancing age, and worsening of symptoms often accompanies an intercurrent illness. These patients often experience a "stair steplike" downhill course that may be rapid or may progress over years. Clinical presentation can include progressive skeletal and cardiomyopathies, failure to thrive or poor growth accompanied by anorexia and poor feeding, proximal renal tubulopathy, hepatic failure, sensorineural hearing loss, diabetes, anemia, neutropenia, dermatologic changes, and facial dysmorphism. Leukodystrophy may be apparent on MRI. Progressive cardiomyopathy with recurrent apnea, dyspnea, cyanosis, or bronchitis in the newborn period may be the only finding in a severe presentation. Screening for respiratory chain deficiencies includes a plasma lactate and pyruvate. An elevated lactate to pyruvate ratio >20 is suggestive of a respiratory chain disorder. These samples are very sensitive to improper handling. For example, pyruvate degrades if the sample is not handled in a timely manner, and a difficult blood draw may artificially raise lactate levels—which may affect the ratio. An increase in plasma alanine and proline by quantitative amino acid analysis is also suggestive of the disorder, as is an elevation in CSF lactate or a lactate peak on MR spectroscopy.

Mitochondrial DNA mutation analysis on peripheral blood, if positive, is diagnostic; however, most genes encoding respiratory chain proteins are nuclear genes. Ragged-red fibers on muscle biopsy indicate mitochondrial disease and the diagnosis can be established by demonstrating reduced enzyme activity of one or more of the respiratory chain complexes or mitochondrial DNA mutations on snap frozen muscle. Treatment is symptomatic and includes avoidance of drugs that inhibit the respiratory chain (sodium valproate and barbiturates) or mitochondrial protein synthesis (tetracyclines and chloramphenicol), administration of additional respiratory chain cofactors (coenzyme Q_{10} 5 to 10 mg/kg/day, biotin 20 mg per day), and the use of L-carnitine (50 to 100 mg/kg/day) if a secondary carnitine deficiency is present. Acidosis can be corrected with sodium bicarbonate. Adequate caloric consumption should be ensured with a high-lipid, low-carbohydrate diet, and aggressive treating conditions with high-energy consumption (i.e., fevers and seizures) will minimize sequelae.

Pyruvate Dehydrogenase and Pyruvate Carboxylase Deficiency

The pyruvate dehydrogenase (PDH) complex is crucial for the oxidative metabolism of pyruvate catalyzing the production of acetyl-CoA, an important substrate for the Krebs cycle—the final common pathway for the oxidation of fatty acids, amino acids, and carbohydrates. Deficiency of PDH complex is the most common disorder producing lactic acidemia. The complex is composed of several subunits and deficiency of the E1 subunit, located on the X chromosome, is the most common. The spectrum of clinical manifestations reflects mutation severity, from overwhelming lactic acidemia and death in the newborn period, to moderate lactic acidemia and profound progressive psychomotor retardation and death in infancy, to carbohydrate-induced episodic ataxia and mild developmental delay seen only in women. Elevation of plasma and CSF lactate and pyruvate is suggestive of the diagnosis, but enzyme assay on cultured fibroblasts is confirmatory. Children with PDH deficiency benefit from a high-fat diet, and indeed the ketogenic diet has been

beneficial for seizure control for some patients. A high carbohydrate diet appears to worsen the lactic acidosis in these patients.

By contrast, pyruvate carboxylase (PC) is another enzyme important for the conversion of pyruvate to oxaloacetate, a substrate required at the end of the Krebs cycle for synthesis of citrate. These patients can also present with severe lactic acidosis at birth. Later presentations can involve failure to thrive, microcephaly, hepatomegaly developmental delay, and proximal renal tubular acidosis, and multiple carboxylase. Initial testing for PC is similar to that of testing for PDH deficiency. Skin biopsy with enzymatic analysis of PC activity is diagnostic. In contrast to PDH, treatment of PC with carbohydrates appears to be better tolerated.

PRIMARY INBORN ERRORS OF METABOLISM OF THE LIVER

The pathophysiology of many IEM are because of abnormal liver metabolism as a result of genetic mutations with predominant hepatic expression. The enzymes responsible for the IEM previously mentioned, such as aminoacidopathies (tyrosinemia type I, with concern for hepatocellular carcinoma), organic acidurias (MMA and PA), and the urea cycle are vital for routine hepatic processes. The IEM related to energy metabolism—glycogen synthesis, glycogenolysis, glycolysis, and gluconeogenesis—are also essential hepatic processes. Clinical presentation of these diagnoses can be somewhat varied and a thorough examination eliciting subtle clinical differences may be essential for diagnosis.

Aminoacidopathies

Aminoacidopathies with acute neurologic involvement, such as MSUD, PA, and MMA have been previously discussed. Of the aminoacidopathies which present acutely owing to primary hepatic symptoms, tyrosinemia type I hepatorenal tyrosinemia is the most common. The enzyme deficiency of fumarylacetoacetase results in the accumulation of fumarylacetoacetate and maleylacetoacetate believed to be responsible for hepatic damage. Tandem MS/MS newborn screening does not consistently identify infants at birth, and so clinical suspicion must be high if NBS is negative. The presence of succinylacetone in urine is pathognomonic for diagnosis. However, analysis in blood should be considered if levels in urine are only mildly elevated. The presentation of tyrosinemia type I during infancy can be severe, and may be accompanied by any combination of sepsis, vomiting, hypoglycemia, renal tubular acidosis, and signs of liver synthetic dysfunction (bleeding, edema, ascites, and jaundice). Dietary restriction of tyrosine and phenylalanine combined with treatment with nitisinone(NTBC) (1 to 2 mg/kg/day) helps limit the level of toxic metabolites. However, the risk for hepatocellular carcinoma is still present and must be screened for by imaging and frequent screening for elevations in α-fetoprotein. Ultimately, liver transplantation is necessary to eliminate the risk of hepatocellular carcinoma caused by tyrosinemia type I. The donor liver has normal enzyme function and therefore dietary restriction and NTBC are no longer required. However, the risk for renal failure remains.

Tyrosinemia type II, or oculocutaneous tyrosinemia, results from a deficiency in tyrosine aminotransferase, the first step in the metabolism of tyrosine, and is not generally seen in the critical care setting. It is characterized as painful corneal lesions, hyperkeratosis of the palms and soles, and mild mental retardation. Diagnosis is based on marked elevation of tyrosine in both plasma and CSF, and the presence of urine organic acids 4-hydroxyphenylpyruvate, 4-hydroxyphenyllactate, and 4-hydroxyphenylacetate. Treatment involves a phenylalanine- and tyrosine-restricted diet.

Disorders of Fatty Acid Oxidation

Metabolic pathways that utilize fat for energy production are vital during fasting. Fatty acids are the preferred source of fuel for cardiac muscle, and for skeletal muscle during sustained periods of exercise. There are four different metabolic pathways that combine to oxidize fatty acids to produce energy. These pathways can be identified as the following: (i) the carnitine cycle, which transfers fatty acids into the mitochondrial membrane for further utilization, (ii) the β-oxidation cycle, which facilitates the breakdown of long-chain fatty acids into shorter chains, coupled with (iii) the electron transport pathway; as a by-product of fatty acid oxidation (iv) the ketone synthesis pathway which is also utilized for energy.

The most common fatty acid oxidation disorder is a deficiency of the medium-chain acyl-CoA dehydrogenase (MCAD) enzyme. Children classically present in metabolic crisis in 8 to 12 hours after fasting, during an illness, or postsurgically with lethargy, nausea, vomiting, and subsequently seizures and coma. Affected individuals may have profound hypoglycemia with inappropriately low ketone formation. Acute management should focus on the evaluation of the neurologic status, and immediate correction of the hypoglycemia with intravenous dextrose. Intravenous lipids should be avoided because they are mostly derived from long-chain fats. Carnitine depletion may exacerbate an acute episode, and supplementation (50 to 100 mg/kg/day) may be beneficial. The initial presentation may occur during the first year of life, after nocturnal feedings have ceased; however, some children remain asymptomatic. Smaller children may be placed on a nighttime dose of uncooked cornstarch to provide carbohydrate during sleep.

The diagnosis of MCAD deficiency is established by an elevated C8:C10 ratio of acylcarnitines in plasma that is present even when the child is not ill. With avoidance of fasting, the prognosis is excellent; however, the first crisis can be fatal or it can produce residual neurologic damage. Children in some states of the United States are now identified by MS/MS NBS, and avoidance of fasting can be instituted before the child experiences an acute decompensation.

There are many other disorders of fatty acid oxidation which are less common. Additional diagnoses involving the β-oxidation pathway include short-chain acyl-CoA dehydrogenase (SCAD) deficiency that can present with failure to thrive and developmental delay, and children with long-chain 3-hydroxy acyl-CoA dehydrogenase (LCHAD) deficiency may present with myoglobinuria because of muscle breakdown. Maternal fatty liver of pregnancy has been associated with LCHAD deficiency and should be elicited when obtaining a family history.

The full spectrum of the disorders of fatty acid metabolism are beyond the scope of this chapter; however, the evaluation of a child presenting with hypoglycemia, especially after a period of fasting, should prompt the search for a fatty acid oxidation defect. Urine organic acids, total and free plasma carnitine levels, an acylcarnitine profile, and urinary ketone determinations are all essential for diagnosis.

Glycogen Storage Diseases

Glycogen stores predominate in the liver and muscle, and therefore, glycogen storage diseases (GSDs) most commonly and seriously affect these tissues. In the liver, the glycogen is responsible for glucose homeostasis and GSDs that preferentially affect the liver (types I, III, IV, VI, and IX) often present with hepatomegaly and hypoglycemia. In the muscle, the glycogen is the major substrate for the generation of ATP; therefore, in GSDs affecting primarily the muscle (types II, V, and VII), muscle cramps, exercise intolerance, susceptibility to fatigue, and progressive weakness are common features. With the exception of type IX, all of the GSDs are inherited as autosomal recessive disorders. Diagnosis is by DNA mutation analysis or enzyme assay that may require liver biopsy.

GSD Ia, or von Gierke disease, is the most common GSD and is caused by a deficiency of glucose-6-phosphatase in the liver, kidney, and intestinal mucosa. The clinical manifestations beginning in the first few months of life include growth retardation, hepatomegaly, severe hypoglycemia with fasting, lactic acidemia, hyperuricemia, and hyperlipidemia. Indeed hypoglycemic seizures can be the initial presentation of these infants when feeding intervals are increased. Type Ib, caused by impairment in the transport of glucose-6-phosphatase, has the additional features of neutropenia and poor neutrophil function resulting in recurrent bacterial infections. Acute management involves correction of the hypoglycemia with intravenous glucose, and long-term care involves frequent daytime feedings and nocturnal nasogastric infusions of glucose in the young child, and transitioning to orally administered uncooked cornstarch in the older child. This regimen effectively improves growth, reduces hepatomegaly, and corrects the lactic acidemia in these patients. Hyperuricemia can be effectively treated with allopurinol. Long-term complications include proteinuria, hepatic adenoma, and gout, and may be avoided or reduced with good metabolic control.

GSD II, also termed *acid maltase deficiency*, is caused by a deficiency of lysosomal enzyme acid α-glucosidase. In infantile, GSD II (Pompe disease) muscle involvement predominates with the typical presentation at 4 to 5 months of age. The infants come for clinical attention owing to respiratory distress, massive cardiomegaly, hypotonia, macroglossia, and hepatomegaly. Progressive hypertrophic cardiomyopathy leading to left ventricular outflow tract obstruction is also common. The characteristic electrocardiogram (EKG) shows a shortened pulse rate (PR) interval and large QRS complexes. The diagnosis can be made by enzyme assay on cultured fibroblasts. Clinical trials of treatment with weekly infusions of recombinant enzyme are currently ongoing, but show promise for treatment of this uniformly fatal disorder. These patients are clinically fragile and management in a tertiary care center that has experience in treating Pompe disease is recommended. The more chronic forms of GSD II feature progressive skeletal muscle weakness and are not typically seen in the intensive care setting until adolescence or adulthood when they present with respiratory compromise owing to progressive diaphragm weakness.

Galactosemia

Galactose, a major energy source for most infants, is present in milk and milk products as disaccharide lactose. Galactose is utilized by metabolism to glucose through a pathway involving three enzymes: galactokinase, galactose-1-phosphate uridyltransferase (GALT), and uridine diphosphate galactose 4'-epimerase. Specific disorders result from deficiencies in each of these enzymes; however, only classic galactosemia, or severe GALT deficiency, produces acute metabolic decompensation. Increasingly, states have added testing for galactosemia in the newborn metabolic screen.

Classic galactosemia most often presents in the first weeks of life with poor feeding habits and weight gain, vomiting, diarrhea, lethargy, and hypotonia. Physical examination often reveals jaundice, hepatomegaly, bruising, prolonged bleeding, and a full fontanelle. *Escherichia coli* sepsis is common, and galactosemia should be considered in any infant with *E. coli* sepsis. Laboratory evaluations typically show unconjugated or combined hyperbilirubinemia, elevated liver transaminases, elevated amino acids phenylalanine, tyrosine and methionine, and renal tubular disease including metabolic acidosis, galactosuria, glycosuria, albuminuria, and aminoaciduria. Hematologic abnormalities include hemolytic anemia and disordered clotting due to liver disease. Congenital or progressive

cataracts can be present and a comprehensive ophthalmologic evaluation including slit lamp examination should be preformed in any patient with suspected galactosemia. The initial presentation may be confusing if galactose feeding has been inconsistent because of formula changes or periods of intravenous fluid administration used to treat the nonspecific presenting features. Treatment of classic galactosemia, which is by the elimination of galactose from the diet, is straightforward and results in rapid resolution of the acute findings (see Table 16.5). Cataracts, if present, are not reversible. Long-term complications, despite early diagnosis and treatment, include speech delay and premature ovarian failure in women, as well as ataxic neurologic disease in a few patients.

Disorders of Fructose Metabolism

Fructose, an important source of dietary carbohydrates, is metabolized mainly in the liver, kidney, and small intestine. Two disorders of fructose metabolism produce acute decompensation and may be encountered in the intensive care setting. Hereditary fructose intolerance (HFI), an autosomal recessive disorder caused by a deficiency of fructaldolase B, is characterized by severe hypoglycemia and vomiting, shortly after the intake of fructose. Prolonged intake of fructose, such as fructose-containing infant formulas (Table 16.5), results in poor feeding, vomiting, hepatomegaly, jaundice, hemorrhage, proximal renal tubular syndrome, and eventual hepatic failure and death. Laboratory findings include hyperuricemia and hyperuricosuria, lactic acidemia, positive reducing substances (fructose and glucose), aminoaciduria, elevated

TABLE 16.5

INFANT FORMULAS CONTAINING LACTOSE, SUCROSE, OR FRUCTOSE

Lactose-Containing	Sucrose or Fructose-Containing
Similac Advance 20 and 24	Carnation Follow-up Soy
PM 60/40	Carnation Alsoy
Natural Care Human Milk Fortifier	Enfamil Lipil
Neosure	Next Step Soy
Special Care 24	Portagen
Calcilo XD	Isomil 20, 24, and DF (dietary fiber)
Enfamil Lipil 20, 24, and AR (added rice)	Alimentum
Premature 20 and 24	Wyeth store brands (except powders)
EnfaCare	
Carnation Good Start	
Carnation Follow-Up	
Wyeth store brands	
Human breast milk	

transaminases, hyperbilirubinemia, anemia, and thrombocytopenia. Treatment is by removal of fructose and sucrose from the diet and benefit is usually seen within days. If the child survives infancy without symptoms because of breast- or fructose-free infant formula feeding, or inadvertent dietary manipulation at the onset of nonspecific early symptoms, a more long-term course is observed as patients develop a strong aversion to offending foods. Diagnosis can be made by mutation analysis or by enzyme deficiency documented on liver biopsy.

Hereditary fructose 1,6-bisphosphatase deficiency, a severe disorder of gluconeogenesis, is characterized by life-threatening episodes of hyperventilation caused by profound acidosis. Irritability, somnolence or coma, apnea, dyspnea and tachycardia, hypotonia, and hepatomegaly may be seen. Laboratory studies reveal hypoglycemia, lactic acidemia, urinary ketosis, and elevated pyruvate. Symptoms respond to the administration of IV glucose and bicarbonate (but not glucagon) and the child may be asymptomatic for weeks to months before the next attack, often brought on by a febrile illness, again depleting the glycogen stores. In contrast to HFI, liver and renal tubular function are generally unaffected and children do not develop an aversion to sweet foods. Similar to HFI, treatment involves elimination of fructose and sucrose from the diet. Diagnosis is established by mutation analysis or enzyme deficiency on liver biopsy.

Lysosomal Storage Disorders

With a collective incidence of 1 in 5,000 live births the >40 lysosomal storage disorders (LSDs) represent an important cause of morbidity and mortality in children and adults. Most are autosomal recessive disorders resulting from a specific enzyme deficiency and have CNS involvement. Although they are not generally considered as disorders of acute onset, many of the complications of these disorders can develop acutely and produce critical illness. A detailed description of these disorders is beyond the scope of this chapter; however, some general principals for critical care management deserve mention.

With a few exceptions, children with LSDs generally appear healthy at birth and develop progressive disease over months to years. For each disorder, the age of onset and progression of disease reflect the amount of residual enzyme activity, which is determined by the specific genetic mutation(s). Whereas many of the disorders described in this chapter involve a metabolic imbalance of small molecules, the LSDs are characterized by the failure of degradation and subsequent storage of large molecules in subcellular compartments (lysosomes) predominantly in tissues where their rate of synthesis is the highest.

The eight subtypes of mucopolysaccharidoses (MPS) are enzyme deficiencies in the degradation of glycosaminoglycans dermatan, heparan and/or chondroitin sulfate. Major clinical features include hepatosplenomegaly, corneal clouding, dysostosis multiplex, and joint stiffness. Coarsening of the facial features and developmental delay or behavioral disturbances can be the presenting features. Storage is widespread. Airway complications such as stridor, obstructive sleep apnea, and respiratory distress particularly with intercurrent infections are common in progressive disease. Storage in cardiac tissues results in valvular insufficiency or cardiomyopathy. Children with CNS involvement are at risk for seizures and often show progressive feeding and swallowing difficulty, leading to aspiration and pneumonia.

Other LSDs involve the degradation of glycosphingolipids (Tay-Sachs and Sandhoff disease, and G_{M1} gangliosidosis), glycoproteins (α- and β-mannosidosis, fucosidosis, and sialidosis), and sphingomyelin (Niemann-Pick disease). These are autosomal recessive disorders that predominantly involve the CNS with progressive neurodegeneration. Seizures, loss of vision and hearing are common. Progressive difficulties with feeding and swallowing can also lead to aspiration, a frequent cause of death.

Even if the diagnosis of a progressive LSD has been made previously, an acute exacerbation in the critical care setting often raises questions about available therapies and interventions. It may be necessary to consider placement of a gastrostomy for the child who can no longer feed, or a tracheostomy for a child with acute airway compromise. These questions are best addressed in collaboration with the metabolic physician who regularly cares for the child and who may have a better understanding of the family dynamics, or be aware of new therapeutic modalities, many of which are currently in clinical trials.

UNEXPLAINED DEATH—THE METABOLIC AUTOPSY

The death of a child is devastating for parents and extended families. This is particularly true when the cause of death in unknown or when a metabolic disorder is suspected but not confirmed. Arriving at a diagnosis often hinges on timely peri- and postmortem sampling. Postmortem examinations on blood or tissue and a careful autopsy may be invaluable in determining the cause of death and may alter recurrence risks and genetic counseling for the immediate and extended family.

During the discussion with the family, before withdrawing life support or soon after the child dies, discuss with the parents the importance of an autopsy. If family members are resistant to a complete autopsy, then a limited study with exclusions, or permission to obtain tissue samples can also be very important in arriving at a diagnosis. Just before or immediately after death, re-examine the child with an eye to subtle dysmorphic features or malformations, abnormalities of the hair, digits, or genitalia. Many IEM have dysmorphic features or minor malformations. If possible, obtain photographs and request a genetics consultation.

Contact the hospital laboratory immediately to save any unused portions of blood specimens previously sent for routine tests.

When death is imminent and a metabolic workup has not been completed, with the family's permission, obtain blood samples for the tests listed in Table 16.2. Obtain an extra 5 mL of blood in a purple-top (ethylenediaminetetraacetic acid [EDTA]) tube for DNA isolation and 5 mL in a green-top (sodium or lithium heparin) tube and freeze the plasma for future studies. Obtain as much urine as possible and freeze immediately. If possible, obtain CSF, freeze on dry ice immediately, and store at $80°C$, if possible. Perform a skin biopsy by cleaning the inside of the forearm or anterior thigh with numerous alcohol swabs (povidone-iodine will impair cell growth) and use a 3- or 5-mm biopsy punch or scalpel to obtain a full thickness of skin. Place the biopsy in sterile culture medium (sometimes designated "viral culture medium") or, if unavailable, sterile saline. Store refrigerated or at room temperature, but *do not freeze*.

To reduce the possibility of artifact owing to cell lysis, obtain a liver biopsy as close to the time of death as possible, preferably within an hour of death. If a complete autopsy is not performed for several hours and the hospital pathologist concurs, an open wedge biopsy or percutaneous hepatic biopsy can be performed at the bedside. A pathologist, surgeon, or gastroenterologist, if available, may be more adept at obtaining the tissue. Hepatic tissue should be cut into 5-mm cubes and placed in a plastic cryotube and snap frozen in liquid nitrogen or dry ice. If an inborn error of energy metabolism is suspected, try to obtain a skeletal muscle biopsy shortly after death. A surgeon may be more experienced in obtaining a specimen. Three muscle fibers from the quadriceps muscle should be obtained using muscle clamps, if available, to prevent contraction. One specimen should be placed on a saline-soaked pad and refrigerated for light microscopy, a second placed in 1.5% glutaraldehyde in buffer (obtained from the pathology lab) for electron microscopy, and a third specimen, snap frozen in isopentane or liquid nitrogen for enzyme analysis.

It is important to stay in contact with the family. When the autopsy and any additional studies are complete, schedule a family conference. If not done previously, obtain a complete three-generation family history, paying particular attention to pregnancy losses or unexplained infant or childhood deaths and parental consanguinity. A genetic counselor may be helpful in this regard. Explain the results of the autopsy and any special testing that was performed. It is also often important to explain what did not lead to the child's death. With the help of a geneticist or genetic counselor, discuss the recurrence risks for future pregnancies and what types of tests could be used to monitor future pregnancies. If there are living siblings, determine whether they are at risk and whether they should undergo any additional testing. Provide the family and the primary care physician with the autopsy report, as well as a letter documenting the conference. This may be invaluable to them and to your physician colleagues in the future. Lastly, remain available to the family to answer additional questions as they grieve and come to accept the loss of their child.

RECOMMENDED READINGS

1. Clarke JTR. *A Clinical guide to inherited metabolic disease.* Cambridge, MA: Cambridge University Press; 1996.
2. Fernandes J, Saudubray JM, van den Berghe G. *Inborn metabolic diseases: Diagnosis and treatment.* 3rd ed. Berlin: Springer-Verlag; 2000.
3. Gunn VL, Nechyba C. *The Harriet Lane handbook.* 16th ed. Philadelphia, PA: Mosby; 2002.
4. Hoffmann GF, Nyhan WL, Zschocke J, et al. *Inherited metabolic diseases.* Philadelphia, PA: Lippincott Williams & Wilkins; 2002.
5. Scriver CR, Beaudet AL, Sly WS, et al. *The metabolic and molecular bases of inherited disease.* 8th ed. New York: McGraw-Hill; 2001.
6. The Urea Cycle Disorders Conference Group. Proceedings of a consensus conference for the management of patients with urea cycle disorders. *J Pediatr.* 2001;138(Suppl 1): S1–S72.
7. Zschocke J, Hoffmann GF. *Vademecum metabolicum: Manual of metabolic pediatrics.* 2nd ed. Friedrichsdorf, Germany: Milupa GmbH; 2004.
8. www.genereviews.org (This site provides comprehensive, updated reviews including diagnosis and management of specific genetic and metabolic disorders) 2005.

Disorders of Host Defense

Anthony D. Slonim

Immune Complications of Transplantation

17

Mark D. Sorrentino

Bone marrow transplantation (BMT) and solid organ transplantation (SOT) are widely used to treat a variety of pediatric disease states. Although these two medical interventions are different, they share a number of common problems, the major one of which is immunosuppression. The major barriers to a successful transplantation in both cases include infection, rejection, and graft versus host disease (GVHD). These problems often result in critical illness for the child who has undergone transplant and is treated in the pediatric intensive care unit (PICU). This chapter provides the intensivist with an understanding of the serious immune complications of BMT and SOT with an emphasis on infectious diseases.

COMPLICATIONS OF BONE MARROW TRANSPLANTATION

Children can receive a BMT for a variety of inherited and acquired disease states (see Table 17.1). The recipient can either receive their own marrow (autologous donation) or that of a human leukocyte antigen (HLA)–compatible donor (allogeneic donation). Recipients of an allogeneic BMT tend to have more serious complications and the issues about appropriate tissue matching become paramount. The induction phase of allograft BMT has the highest potential for serious complications. The goal of this phase is to ablate all cancerous cells, to create a space in the bone marrow for new elements, and to suppress any immunologically active host cells that would reject the transplant.[1] Post-BMT neutropenia usually lasts for 2 to 6 weeks while the transplanted marrow engrafts and is a time of heightened concern for infectious complications.

TABLE 17.1

PEDIATRIC DISEASES WHERE BONE MARROW TRANSPLANTATION IS UTILIZED

Leukemia
Solid organ tumors:
    Lymphoma
    Neuroblastoma
    Medulloblastoma
    Sarcoma
Aplastic anemia
Thalassemia major
Sickle cell disease
Severe combined immunodeficiency disease
Wiskott-Aldrich
Hurler syndrome
Fanconi anemia
Adrenoleukodystrophy
Metachromatic leukodystrophy
Osteopetrosis

INFECTIOUS COMPLICATIONS

Marrow ablation results in pancytopenia and creates an opportunity for serious infection. Opportunistic infections result from the neutropenia that occurs as a consequence of the preparative regimen. The immunosuppressed patient is unable to mount an effective response to a broad range of pathogens and therefore presents relatively late in the clinical course with an overwhelming infection.

The most common life-threatening infections occur during the neutropenic period and involve gram-negative and aerobic gram-positive bacteria often originating from organisms colonizing the child's skin, oral cavity, perineal area, and the gastrointestinal (GI) or respiratory tract.

Fungal Infections

Invasive fungal infections have become the leading infectious cause of mortality in those receiving a BMT.[2] These infections occur most frequently during periods of neutropenia or during steroid therapy for GVHD. *Candida* and *Aspergillus* species are the most common fungal pathogens. There has recently been an increase in the prevalence of non-*albicans Candida* and azole-resistant *Candida* spp. in the BMT population. The 1-year survival rate after a mold infection is approximately 32%, despite the use of aggressive antifungal prophylaxis and therapy. Although there are no large studies to document meaningful outcomes in pediatric patients, many transplant centers treat infected patients with multiple antifungal agents including voriconazole, caspofungin, and liposomal amphotericin.[3]

Cytomegalovirus Infection

Cytomegalovirus (CMV) continues to be an important pathogen in the BMT population. Most children, who develop CMV related-disease, do so as a reactivation of a previous primary infection. Reactivation tends to occur 3 weeks to 100 days post-transplantation, and is strongly associated with acute GVHD and pretransplant CMV seropositivity. Clinical features of CMV disease include severe pneumonitis, hepatitis, GI involvement, and colitis. Therapeutic approaches include the use of ganciclovir, valganciclovir, and CMV-specific intravenous immunoglobulin.[4]

Respiratory Syncytial Virus and Adenovirus Infection

Seasonal respiratory viruses including respiratory syncytial virus (RSV) and adenovirus are frequent causes of PICU admissions in the BMT population. There are few therapeutic options for the treatment of either severe adenovirus or RSV infection, and the mortality rates can be >50%. Aerosolized ribavirin has not been found to be particularly effective in either case. Recently, clinical improvement was demonstrated when cidofovir had been used in combination with intravenous ribavirin for disseminated adenovirus infection.[5] The goal to successful therapy appears to be early diagnosis and treatment.

Severe RSV disease is often manifested in the PICU as acute respiratory failure. Early aerosolized ribavirin can suppress viral replication, but has not been shown to impact the severity or duration of disease. Supportive therapy with supplemental oxygen and mechanical ventilation remain the hallmarks of therapy.

IMMUNE COMPLICATIONS OF SOLID ORGAN TRANSPLANTATION

Worldwide, there are approximately 40,000 solid organ transplantations performed each year. Immune system stimulation by foreign proteins (transplanted organs) results in the activation of both cell-mediated and humoral-mediated immune responses that result in cell destruction and tissue rejection. The greatest improvement in transplantation medicine has been the discovery of effective immunosuppressants, necessary to both prevent and treat organ rejection. The goal of these medications is to maintain a balance between adequate immunosuppression to protect the graft, while minimizing the patient's susceptibility to infection. Corticosteroids remain an important part of the immunosuppressive regimen, especially in the early post-transplant period. Unfortunately, they inhibit proinflammatory cytokine production, decrease the accumulation of polymorphonuclear leukocytes at sites of infection, inhibit arachidonic acid metabolites, block vascular permeability in inflammatory processes, and impede nitric oxide production. With immunologic defenses to infection and malignancy suppressed, the body's normal inflammatory responses become muted or absent. As a result, children with severe inflammatory diseases, including sepsis, may present with very few specific complaints or physical findings. The pediatric intensivist needs to be vigilant in caring for children on immunosuppressive regimens and always consider the possibility of overwhelming infection in the differential diagnosis for these children even when clinical signs may be minimal.

INFECTIOUS COMPLICATIONS

Infection remains the leading cause of death during the first year of post-transplantation. There is a well-described temporal relationship between the types of infection seen in the immunosuppressed solid organ transplantation patient. The basic timetable is the same for all patients with SOT, and can be divided into three periods: the first post-transplant month, 1 to 6 months post-transplant, and >6 months post-transplant (see Fig. 17.1). Up to 75% of transplantation patients will have evidence of microbial invasion during the first post-transplant year.

Infection in the First Post-transplant Month

The most serious infections that occur in the first month post-transplant are due to technical problems relating to the procedure itself, and to the management of perioperative devices including drains, vascular access devices, catheters, and endotracheal tubes. In addition, some infections may be conveyed with the allograft.

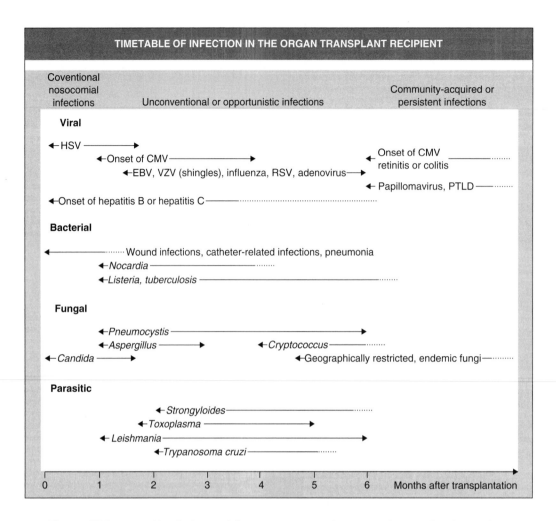

Figure 17.1   Timetable of infection following organ transplantation. Infections that deviate from this schema suggest a higher level of immunosuppression or a more intense environmental exposure. CMV, cytomegalovirus; EBV, Epstein-Barr virus; VZV, varicella-zoster virus; RSV, respiratory syncytial virus; PTLD, post-transplant lymphoproliferative disorder; HSV, herpes simplex virus. (From Rubin RH, Wolfson JS, Cosimi AB, et al. Infection in the renal transplant patient. *Am J Med.* 1981; 70:405–411, with permission.)

Infection 1 to 6 Months Post-transplant

In the period between 1 and 6 months post-transplantation, the highest incidence of clinical infections are secondary to the immunomodulating viruses such as CMV, Epstein-Barr virus (EBV), human herpes virus (HHV)-6, hepatitis B virus (HBV), hepatitis C virus (HCV), and human immunodeficiency virus (HIV). The incidence of CMV pretransplant seropositivity is approximately 30% in children >5 years old, and approximately 60% in adolescents. Therefore, the younger the child, the greater the potential for serious primary infection when a CMV-seropositive organ is transplanted. Ganciclovir remains the effective therapy for proven CMV infection in children. The pathogenesis of CMV includes four major mechanisms. First, the virus is reactivated. Second, the virus undergoes amplification and dissemination. Third,

major histocompatibility (MHC)–restricted, virus-specific, cytotoxic T cells become activated to attack virus-infected cells. Finally, cytokines, chemokines, and growth factors are produced in response to the replicating virus to further recruit immune cells to control the infection.[6]

This is also the time when opportunistic infections such as *Pneumocystis*, *Listeria*, and *Aspergillus* present. These infections arise from the combined effects of sustained immunosuppressive therapy and the immunomodulating effects of the viruses themselves. *Aspergillus* infection is a therapeutic emergency, especially in lung transplant recipients. The mortality rates have exceeded 50% despite treatment with amphotericin.[7] Finally, the respiratory viruses, RSV, and adenovirus, are of particular importance in the pediatric transplantation patient during this period of aggressive immunosuppressive therapy. These viruses are common in the pediatric community, especially during the winter months. Unfortunately, if the child develops a lower respiratory tract infection from these viruses, the mortality rates can exceed 70%. Therapeutic options are limited and are generally supportive.[8]

Infection >6 Months Post-transplant

Chronic infections with the hepatitis viruses, papillomavirus, HHV-8, or HIV are the most common during this time frame. In addition, children with poor allograft function, and acute or chronic rejection (CR) requiring increased levels of immunosuppressive therapy, remain at a high risk for opportunistic infections. Post-transplant lymphoproliferative disorder (PTLD) is a rare malignant disease that remains a major cause of serious morbidity and mortality when it arises in young children. PTLD is an EBV–CMV infection–related disease which should be actively pursued in the febrile transplantation patient presenting with lymphadenopathy, GI manifestations, seizures, or a mediastinal mass. Its manifestations are particularly aggressive in primary EBV infection, which is often the case in the usually EBV-seronegative pediatric population. PTLD treatment includes both a reduction in immunosuppression and aggressive chemotherapy with a combination of agents often including cyclophosphamide, doxorubicin, vincristine, and prednisone (CHOP protocol).[9,10]

REJECTION

Transplantation of any solid organ results in an initial cycle of heightened immune activation followed over time by a state of immune tolerance. This series of events can be attributed to the donor hematolymphoid cells that migrate from the allograft into the recipient's lymphoid tissues, concurrently with an influx of the recipient's cells into the allograft. Direct interaction between donor and recipient cells at these sites causes stimulation of both donor and recipient T cells. This results in T-cell blastogenesis, cytokine secretion, and mitogenesis in a process known as *direct allorecognition*. In addition, a direct allostimulation causes maturation of cytotoxic T cells, expansion of B cells, and recruitment of macrophages, eosinophils, neutrophils, and other effector cells which have the potential to damage the organ.[11] There is evidence that acute rejection (AR) is dominated by direct allorecognition.[12] Controlling the severity of this reaction is the goal of patient management during the first year post-transplantation. The hallmark histopathologic feature of severe AR, which is predictive of graft failure, is arterial inflammation or necrosis. This can be diagnosed with an allograft biopsy. Fortunately, the pathway of direct allostimulation is highly sensitive to increased immunosuppression, and is generally controllable.

CR usually begins within weeks to months after transplantation, often coinciding with multiple or persistent episodes of AR. The incidence of CR increases over time, and by 5 years post-transplant, it affects up to 80% of lung recipients, 30% to 40% of heart, kidney, and pancreas recipients, and 5% of liver recipients. The most common manifestation of CR is a progressive narrowing of the muscular arteries, or obliterative arteriopathy (OA). This damages the allograft by compromising the blood flow, and thereby predisposing to chronic ischemia and infarction. Other characteristics include patchy interstitial inflammation, fibrosis and parenchymal atrophy, and destruction of epithelial-lined conduits such as bronchioles in lung allografts (bronchiolitis obliterans syndrome), or bile ducts. Treatment of end-stage CR is impossible because the major structural damage is irreversible. Because CR appears to evolve directly from the damage incurred during AR episodes, the goal must be to control the frequency, severity, and duration of these events by adjusting immunosuppression and adding corticosteroids and additional agents as needed.

SUMMARY

Considerable progress has been made to control infection and contain rejection in the immunosuppressed transplantation patient. Early diagnosis and aggressive multidrug therapy is the key to reducing morbidity and mortality in patients with these complications.

REFERENCES

1. Gillis TA, Donovan ES. Rehabilitation following bone marrow transplantation. *Cancer.* 2001;92:998–1007.
2. Brown JMY. Fungal infections in bone marrow transplant patients. *Curr Opin Infect Dis.* 2004;17:347–352.
3. Mossad SB. Prevention and treatment of fungal infections in bone marrow transplantation. *Curr Hematol Rep.* 2003;2:302–309.
4. Ljungman P, Aschan J, Lewensohn-Fuchs I, et al. Results of different strategies for reducing cytomegalovirus-associated mortality in allogeneic stem cell transplant recipients. *Transplantation.* 1998;66:1330–1334.
5. Walls T, Shankar AG, Shingadia D. Adenovirus: An increasingly important pathogen in paediatric bone marrow transplant patients. *Lancet Infect Dis.* 2003;3:79–86.
6. Tolkoff-Rubin N, Rubin RH. Recent advances in the diagnosis and management of infection in the organ transplant recipient. *Semin Nephrol.* 2000;20:148–163.
7. Fishman JA, Rubin. Infection in organ transplant recipients. *N Engl J Med.* 1998;338:1741–1751.
8. Rubin R. Infection in the organ transplant recipient. In: Rubin RH, Young L, eds. *Clinical approach to infection in the compromised host.* New York: Plenum; 2002.
9. Cockfield S. Identifying the patient at risk for post-transplant lymphoproliferative disorder. *Transpl Infect Dis.* 2001;3(2):70–78.
10. Tanner J, Alfieri C. The Epstein-Barr virus and post-transplant lymphoproliferative disease: Interplay of immunosuppression, EBV, and the immune system in disease pathogenesis. *Transpl Infect Dis.* 2001;3(2):60–69.
11. Shirwan H. Chronic allograft rejection. *Transplantation.* 1999; 68(6):715–726.
12. Pattison JM, Krensky AM. New insights into mechanisms of allograft rejection. *Am J Med Sci.* 1997;313(5):257–263.

Immunosuppression Induced by Therapeutic Agents

18

William T. Tsai   John N. van den Anker

The use of immunosuppressive and immunomodulatory agents has changed the practice of pediatric medicine significantly and introduced an innovative set of therapeutics which hold not only exciting promises, but also significant challenges. These agents are primarily used in solid organ and hematologic transplantation, but are also used for treating rheumatologic and autoimmune diseases.

The current use of immunotherapeutics has focused not only on modulating the entire immune system cascade, but also on modulating specific immune cells using specific antibodies and cytokine receptor agonists and antagonists. Although the use of these agents has increased significantly in pediatric medicine, the numerous idiosyncrasies and side effects associated with their use have also become increasingly prominent. Table 18.1 provides a list of the common immunosuppressive medications, their mechanism of action, and their side effects.

The major classes of therapeutic agents used in immunosuppression include the calcineurin inhibitors, the glucocorticoids, the antimetabolites, and the biologic agents. Frequently, the approach to treatment with these agents is sequential, and multilayered, similar to that employed in the use of anticancer treatment. Combinations of these agents are used in the treatment of organ transplants to impact specific components of the immune cascade. This chapter discusses the common immunosuppressive and immunomodulatory agents used in the pediatric intensive care unit (PICU).

CLASSES OF IMMUNOSUPPRESSIVE AND IMMUNOMODULATORY AGENTS

Calcineurin Inhibitors

The introduction of the calcineurin inhibitor, cyclosporine A (CsA), to medicine has revolutionized transplantation medicine by improving early engraftment and by preventing acute graft rejection. Although earlier immunosuppressive regimens relied heavily on glucocorticoids and cytotoxic agents to produce a nonspecific suppression of the immune system, these immunomodulators are relatively specific, inhibiting T-cell transduction and T-cell activation.

Cyclosporine

CsA is the prototypical calcineurin inhibitor. It is a metabolite of the fungal species *Beauveria nivea*. CsA binds a cytoplasmic molecule, cyclophylin, which then binds calcineurin. Calcineurin is another cytoplasmic protein which, when complexed with activated cyclophylin, dephosphorylates NF-AT (nuclear factor of activated T), cells allowing the nuclear transcription of interleukin-2 (IL-2) mRNA and other lymphokines.

CsA is frequently used in solid organ transplantation and in autoimmune diseases such as rheumatoid arthritis. CsA is available both for injection and for oral administration. Oral bioavailability is poor, with wide inter- and intra-patient variability, narrow therapeutic index, and a large number of drug interactions (see Table 18.2). Close

TABLE 18.1

COMMON IMMUNOSUPPRESSIVE MEDICATIONS

Medication	Mechanism of Action	Side Effects
Corticosteroids	Upregulate IκB Decrease IL-1, tumor necrosis factor-α, IFN γ Anti-inflammatory	Cushing syndrome
Azathioprine	Antimetabolite	Marrow suppression GI, liver toxicity
Mycophenolate mofetil	Lymphocyte-specific Antimetabolite	Marrow suppression GI intolerance
Cyclosporine	Calcineurin inhibitor Down-regulates IL-2	Nephrotoxicity Neurologic symptoms
Tacrolimus (FK506)	Calcineurin inhibitor Down-regulates IL-2, IFN γ	Nephrotoxicity Neurotoxicity Diabetogenic
Sirolimus (rapamycin)	Blocks IL-2R signaling Also IL-4, IL-6; platelet-derived growth factor signaling	Impaired healing Hypertriglyceridemia
Antilymphocyte Globulin (antilymphocytic globulin, antithymocyte γ globulin, antithymocyte globulin)	Cytolytic antibody Blocks and depletes T cells	Leukopenia Thrombocytopenia "Serum sickness"
Ornithine-ketoacid transaminase-3 (OKT3)	Cytolytic antibody Blocks T-cell receptor Depletes T cells	Cytokine release Aseptic meningitis
Daclizumab (or basiliximab)	Blocks IL-2R Inhibits T-cell activation	Minimal

GI, gastrointestinal; IFN, interferon; IL, interleukin.
From Irwin RS, Rippe JM. *Intensive care medicine*. 5th ed. Philadelphia, PA: Lippincott Williams & Wilkins; 2003.

therapeutic drug monitoring (TDM) is therefore crucial in maximizing graft survival while minimizing toxicity. CsA is a substrate for intestinal P-glycoprotein, a drug efflux pump in the brush border on the luminal surface of the intestinal epithelium, as well as for intestinal and hepatic cytochrome P-450 3A. Marked interindividual and ethnic differences in the activity of these enzyme systems owing to genetic polymorphisms, account for reduced and variable oral absorption. Currently there are two oral formulations available: Sandimmune and Neoral. There are substantial differences in the bioavailability between these two formulations, and therefore, care must be taken when switching between formulations.

Although cyclosporine has little bone marrow suppression, its major limiting toxicity is nephrotoxicity. This effect is magnified when used in combination with other nephrotoxic agents, including tacrolimus. CsA causes afferent arteriolar vasoconstriction of the glomerulus by an unclear mechanism. Nephrotoxicity is managed by dosage reduction or by drug cessation. CsA, when used in combination with glucocorticoids, is diabetogenic. Bacterial, fungal, and viral infections occur commonly in patients treated with CsA.

TABLE 18.2

DRUGS THAT AFFECT CYCLOSPORINE A, TACROLIMUS, AND SIROLIMUS BLOOD LEVELS

Increased Levels	Decreased Levels
Grapefruit juice	Rifampin
Fluconazole, itraconazole, ketoconazole	Carbamazepine
Protease inhibitors	Barbiturates
Clarithromycin, erythromycin	Phenytoin
NSAIDs	Carvedilol
Glucocorticoids	St. John wort
Diltiazem, amlodipine, verapamil, nicardipine	Amiodarone
	Quinidine

NSAIDs, nonsteroidal anti-inflammatory drugs.

Tacrolimus

Tacrolimus is a macrolide antibiotic produced by *Streptomyces tsukubaensis*. It is a molecule that is structurally unrelated to CsA and binds to a cytoplasmic protein, FK- binding protein (FKBP). This complex then binds calcineurin and modulates the dephosphorylation action of NF-AT. As with CsA, this inhibits the production of IL-2 and other lymphokines responsible for T-cell activation.

Tacrolimus is indicated for the prophylaxis of solid organ transplant rejection or as rescue therapy in rejection episodes despite the use of CsA. Although graft survival rates comparing CsA and tacrolimus appear to be equivalent in children, tacrolimus has the ability to reverse established, ongoing rejection. CsA lacks this ability. Tacrolimus is available for injection and for oral use. Oral bioavailability is poor, with wide inter- and intra-patient variability, and a large number of drug interactions (see Table 18.1), but is higher in children than in adults. Tacrolimus is a substrate for intestinal P-glycoprotein, as well as for intestinal and hepatic cytochrome P-450 3A. Close TDM, for the same reasons as described for CsA, is crucial.

The renal effects of tacrolimus appear to be similar to CsA and concomitant use results in an additive nephrotoxic effect. Nephrotoxicity may require dosage adjustment or drug discontinuation. Neurotoxic effects include seizure, tremor, and headache and are more common than with CsA. The diabetogenic effect of tacrolimus is caused by its effect on pancreatic β cells and insulin homeostasis. Hypertension and gastrointestinal tract disturbances are present.

In children who are taking tacrolimus, the development of post-transplant lymphoproliferative disorder may occur in patients who develop primary Epstein-Barr virus infection. Discontinuation of tacrolimus may reverse the disorder.

Antimetabolites, Antiproliferative, and Alkylating Agents

Sirolimus (Target-of-Rapamycin Inhibitor)

Sirolimus is a macrocyclic lactone produced by *Streptomyces hygroscopicus*. Although structurally similar to tacrolimus, sirolimus is an antiproliferative agent that stops cell-cycle progression. It inhibits T-cell proliferation by binding to the FKBP. In contrast to tacrolimus, which functions by inhibiting cytokine gene transcription, the sirolimus-FKBP complex inhibits a serine–threonine kinase, mTOR, which blocks cell-cycle progression at the G1-S phase transition.

Sirolimus is indicated in the prophylaxis of solid organ transplant rejection in combination with other immunomodulatory agents. It is available as an oral formulation with poor bioavailability. It's toxicities include myelosuppression, fever, and gastrointestinal effects. Pulmonary interstitial fibrosis has been reported in adults. Sirolimus is a substrate for intestinal P-glycoprotein, as well as for intestinal and hepatic cytochrome P-450 3A. Close TDM, for the same reasons as described for CsA, is crucial. Importantly, it has been recommended that there be at least a 4-hour difference in timing of full-dose CsA and sirolimus administration because both share the same metabolic pathway. When using low doses of either CsA or tacrolimus, spacing of drug delivery is not important as long as TDM is used.

Azathioprine

Azathioprine is an imidazolyl derivative of 6 mercaptopurine (6MP), a purine antimetabolite. Azathioprine is then metabolized to 6MP, a false purine, which is incorporated into the DNA. This abnormal DNA results in abnormal gene replication, thereby inhibiting normal cellular function and cell division. Azathioprine is more potent in immunosuppression than 6MP.

Azathioprine has been used as an adjunct in the prophylaxis of solid organ transplant rejection and in the treatment of autoimmune diseases. Azathioprine is available for injection and for oral administration. Therapeutic activity and toxicity are related to tissue levels, which renders TDM ineffective. Approximately 1% of Whites are homozygous for an abnormal allele, causing deficiency of thiopurine methyltransferase (TPMT), a key enzyme in azathioprine metabolism. These individuals are at a high risk for developing drug-induced toxicity and can be potentially identified by TPMT genotyping. In general, dose-limiting myelosuppression occurs 1 to 2 weeks after the institution of therapy, and pancytopenia, thrombocytopenia, and megaloblastic anemia are the usual patterns. Hepatotoxicity and gastrointestinal tract disturbances are seen, and as with all immunosuppressives, there is an increased risk of serious infections and neoplasms. It should be used with caution when used in combination with other agents, which cause myelosuppression. Marked dose reductions are necessary with concomitant use with allopurinol and renal failure.

Mycophenolate Mofetil

Mycophenolate mofetil is a prodrug that is hydrolyzed to mycophenolic acid, a reversible inhibitor of inosine monophosphate dehydrogenase. This important enzyme is responsible for the synthesis of guanine nucleotides. B cells and T cells are dependent on this pathway for cell proliferation and function. Mycophenolate mofetil was developed to replace azathioprine for maintenance of immunosuppression and as rescue therapy for rejection episodes refractory to ornithine-ketoacid transaminase-3 (OKT3).

Mycophenolate mofetil is indicated for use in the prophylaxis of solid organ transplant rejection in combination with other immunomodulatory agents, and for reversal of acute rejection episodes. It is supplied both for injection and for oral administration. Concurrent administration of antacids, cholestyramine, or iron should be avoided because they will decrease its bioavailability. Levels of mycophenolic acid decrease when used in combination with CsA but not when used together with tacrolimus or sirolimus. Toxicity is dose-related, and leukopenia, diarrhea, and vomiting are seen commonly. Children have an increased incidence of severe side effects, necessitating cessation of therapy. The concomitant use of acyclovir or ganciclovir may raise serum concentrations of both the antivirals and mycophenolate mofetil. There is an increased incidence of serious infections.

Alkylating Agents

Cyclophosphamide and ifosfamide are prodrugs that require hepatic activation and they are used in the treatment of neoplastic disease and autoimmune disorders such as Wegener granulomatosis and refractory nephrotic syndrome. They are the progeny of the nitrogen mustard gas vesicants used in World War II and exert their effect by the nonspecific alkylation of tissue macromolecules. The alkylation of macromolecules such as DNA and RNA results in missense disruptions of nuclear transcription and inhibits cell division in tumor cells, and in the rapid division of normal tissues such as the bone marrow and gastrointestinal mucosa. This causes the therapeutic effect and toxicities seen with the use of these agents.

Cyclophosphamide is available for injection and oral administration. Oral bioavailability is good. It is eliminated by spontaneous hydrolysis and neither liver failure nor renal failure affects its half-life. Most patients experience nausea, vomiting, and hair loss. Many alkylating agents can cause pulmonary fibrosis and there is a predisposition to develop secondary hematologic malignancy. Urinary tract toxicity, which used to be limiting in the initial use of this agent, has been lessened with the use of mesna, a compound used to prevent hemorrhagic cystitis.

Methotrexate

Methotrexate is a dihydrofolate reductase inhibitor used not only for its antineoplastic effects but also for its ability to inhibit cell-mediated immunity. Methotrexate binds to dihydrofolate reductase and disrupts the carbon transfer necessary for purine nucleotide synthesis. In normal human tissues, this results in the disruption of DNA and RNA synthesis, leading to the death of rapidly growing tissues such as bone marrow and gastrointestinal mucosa.

Methotrexate is used in bone marrow and solid organ transplantation, in graft versus host disease, and in the treatment of autoimmune diseases such as juvenile rheumatoid arthritis. It is available for intravenous, intrathecal, and oral administration. Toxicities include myelosuppression, gastrointestinal symptoms, hepatic fibrosis, and hepatic cirrhosis. The myelosuppression presents an increased risk of life-threatening infections and spontaneous hemorrhage.

Corticosteroids

Corticosteroids are used extensively in the PICU for their anti-inflammatory effects. These agents are used in refractory septic shock, in respiratory distress syndrome, in neoplastic disorders, in asthma exacerbations and laryngotracheobronchitis, and in uncommon conditions such as systemic lupus erythematosus and juvenile idiopathic arthritis. Although its therapeutic uses are quite wide, this section focuses on its immunomodulatory effects.

The immunosuppressive effect of corticosteroids results in part from the suppression of T-cell activity by inhibiting cytokine production. Steroids bind intracellular molecules that affect the regulation of nuclear transcription elements responsible for cytokine production and programmed cell death (apoptosis). Steroids not only modulate cell-mediated effects by its action on T cells, but also have wide anti-inflammatory properties. Stabilization of lysosomal membranes, decreased capillary permeability, and inhibition of histamine release antagonize inflammatory mechanisms.

Glucocorticoids are used in combination with other immunomodulatory agents for prophylaxis against organ transplant rejection. High-dose steroids are used to reverse acute rejection episodes. Glucocorticoids are available for intravenous injection and oral administration. Prednisone is metabolized in the liver to prednisolone and the serum half-life is approximately 2 to 3 hours. Glucocorticoid toxicity causes significant morbidity. Growth retardation, poor wound healing, hyperglycemia, and hypertension are side effects seen in the PICU. In addition, serious infections are associated with steroid use and are well documented.

Polyclonal and Monoclonal Antibodies

Polyclonal and monoclonal antibodies play an important role in modulating the immune response in transplantation medicine and in the treatment of autoimmune diseases. These antibodies are directed at specific hematopoeitic cell surface molecules and lead to cell death and the blockade of important cell functions. These agents are most commonly used to prevent and reverse acute rejection episodes.

Antithymocyte Globulin

Antithymocyte globulin (ATG) is a polyclonal antibody purified from the sera of rabbits that have been injected with human thymocytes. These polyclonal antibodies bind to CD2, CD3, CD4, CD8, CD11a, CD18, CD25, CD44, CD45, and human leukocyte antigen (HLA) I and HLA II cell surface molecules of the T cell. T-cell depletion occurs by complement-mediated and cell-mediated destruction. Surviving T cells have decreased function owing to antibody-binding to cell surface molecules.

ATG is used in prophylaxis of solid organ transplant rejection and is used in reversing acute rejection episodes. It is available for intravenous use. Intradermal skin testing should be performed before the initial use. Its major toxicities include fever, chills, and hypotension which may be ameliorated by preadministration of steroids, acetaminophen, and antihistamines. Serum sickness and anaphylaxis can occur. An increased risk of serious infection and malignancy is present.

Ornithine-ketoacid transaminase-3—Anti CD3 Monoclonal Antibody

OKT3 is a monoclonal antibody that binds to the T-cell CD3 molecule. CD3 is part of the T-cell receptor complex and plays an important role in T-cell signal transduction. Binding of antibody to the CD3 receptor results in a rapid reduction of T cell numbers secondary to cell death resulting from both complement activation and activation-induced cell death. CD3 binding by this antibody also results in the reduced function of surviving T cells.

OKT3 is used for the prophylaxis of solid organ transplant rejection and for the reversal of established rejection episodes. It is available as an intravenous injection. Toxicity includes the cytokine release syndrome and manifests as nausea, vomiting, and myalgias that may occur approximately 30 minutes after infusion of OKT3. Symptoms are generally worse with the first dose of medication. The administration of steroids before the infusion lessens the severity of the response. Cytokine release syndrome occurs secondary to the release of IL-1, IL-2, tumor necrosis factor (TNF) α, and other lymphokines. Potentially fatal pulmonary edema, respiratory distress syndrome, arrhythmias, and cardiac arrest can develop. Use of this agent is associated with an increased risk of serious infections and secondary neoplasms.

Basiliximab/Daclizumab
(Anti-interleukin-2–Receptor Antibody)

Basiliximab is a chimeric (murine/human) monoclonal IL-2–receptor antibody. This IgG_1-receptor antibody binds to the α or Tac subunit of the IL-2 receptor and inhibits IL-2–mediated activation of lymphocytes. There is no decrement in circulating lymphocyte numbers, nor is there any significant change in lymphocyte cell phenotype.

Basiliximab is used in renal transplant recipients in combination with other immunosuppressive agents. It is administered intravenously and IL-2 receptors are fully saturated when serum concentrations exceed 0.2 μg per mL. Episodes of severe anaphylaxis have been reported on initial and repeat exposure to basiliximab. Patients should be re-exposed to a second course with extreme caution.

Daclizumab is a humanized monoclonal IL-2 receptor antibody that acts in a similar manner to basiliximab. It also binds to the α subunit of the IL-2 receptor and inhibits IL-2–mediated activation of lymphocytes. There is no decrement in circulating lymphocyte numbers, nor is there any significant change in lymphocyte cell phenotype.

Daclizumab is used in renal transplant recipients in combination with other immunosuppressives and has been investigated in pediatric bone marrow transplant and steroid-resistant graft versus host disease. It is available for intravenous use. When administered at the recommended dosage, daclizumab saturates IL-2 receptor for approximately 120 days. Toxicity includes severe hypersensitivity reactions on both initial exposure and re-exposure to the medication. Diarrhea, postoperative pain, fever, aggravated hypertension, pruritis, and infections of the upper respiratory and urinary tracts were reported more often in pediatric patients than adult transplant patients.

ACKNOWLEDGMENTS

Supported in part by grant 1 U10HD045993-02, National Institute of Child Health and Development, Bethesda, MD.

RECOMMENDED READINGS

1. Allison AC, Eugui EM. Mycophenolate mofetil and its mechanisms of action. *Immunopharmacology*. 2000;47:85–118.
2. Auphan N, DiDonato JA, Rosette C, et al. Immunosuppression by glucocorticoids: Inhibition of NF-Kappa B activity through induction of I Kappa B synthesis. *Science*. 1995;270:286–290.
3. Butani L, Palmer J, Baluarte HJ, et al. Adverse effects of mycophenolate mofetil in pediatric renal transplant recipients with presumed chronic rejection. *Transplantation*. 1999;68:83–86.
4. Ellis D. Clinical use of tacrolimus (FK-506) in infants and children with renal transplants. *Pediatr Nephrol*. 1995;9:487–494.
5. Ettenger RB. New immunosuppressive agents in pediatric renal transplantation. *Transplant Proc*. 1998;30:196–1958.
6. European FK506 Multicentre Liver Study Group. Randomised trial comparing tacrolimus (FK506) and cyclosporine in prevention of liver allograft rejection. *Lancet*. 1994;344:423–428.
7. Henry ML. Cyclosporine and tacrolimus (FK506): A comparison of efficacy and safety profiles. *Clin Transplant*. 1999;13:209–220.
8. Hooks MA, Wade CS, Millikan WJ. Muronanab CD-3: A review of its pharmacology, pharmacokinetics, and clinical use in transplantation. *Pharmacotherapy*. 1991;11:26–37.
9. Jungraithmayer T, Staskewitz A, Kirste G, et al. Pediatric renal transplantation with mycophenolate mofetil-based immunosuppression without induction: Results after three years. *Transplantation*. 2003;75:454–461.
10. Kahan BD. Cyclosporine. *N Engl J Med*. 1989;32:1725–1738.
11. Kahan BD. The potential role of rapamycin in pediatric transplantation as observed from adult studies. *Pediatr Transplant*. 1999;3:175–180.
12. Kuo CJ, Chung J, Fiorentino DF, et al. Rapamycin selectively inhibits interleukin-2 activation of p70 S6 kinase. *Nature*. 1992;358:70–73.
13. Mannick JA, Davis RC, Cooperband SR, et al. Clinical use of rabbit antihuman lymphocyte globulin in cadaver-kidney transplantation. *N Engl J Med*. 1971;284:1109–1115.
14. McAlister VC, Gao Z, Peltekian K, et al. Sirolimus-tacrolimus combination immunosuppression. *Lancet*. 2000;29:376–377.
15. Mihatch MJ, Kyo M, Morozumi K, et al. The side-effects of cyclosporine A and tacrolimus. *Clin Nephrol*. 1998;49:356–363.
16. Neu AM, Ho PL, Fine RN, et al. Tacrolimus vs. cyclosporine A as primary immunosuppression in pediatric renal transplantation: A NAPRTCS study. *Pediatr Transplant*. 2003;7:217–222.
17. Norman DJ, Leone MR. The role of OKT3 in clinical transplantation. *Pediatr Nephrol*. 1991;5:130–136.
18. Offner G, Broyer M, Niaudet P, et al. A multicenter, open-label, pharmacokinetic/pharmacodynamic safety, and tolerability study of basiliximab (simulect) in pediatric de novo renal transplant recipients. *Transplantation*. 2002;74:961–966.
19. Plosker GL, Foster RH. Tacrolimus: A further update of its pharmacology and therapeutic use in the management of organ transplantation. *Drugs*. 2000;59:323–389.
20. Ransahoff RM. Cellular responses to interferons and other cytokines: The JAK-STAT paradigm. *N Engl J Med*. 1998;338:616–618.
21. Shapiro R. Tacrolimus in pediatric renal transplantation: A review. *Pediatr Transplant*. 1998;2:270–276.
22. Venkataramanan R, Swaminathan A, Prasad T, et al. Clinical pharmacokinetics of tacrolimus. *Clin Pharmacokinet*. 1995;29:404–430.
23. Vicenti F, Kirkman R, Light S, et al. Interleukin-2-receptor blockade with daclizumab to prevent acute rejection in renal transplantation. Daclizumab Triple Therapy Study Group. *N Engl J Med*. 1998;338:161–165.

Allergic, Vasculitic, and Rheumatologic Illnesses

19

David C. Stockwell   *Aditi Sharangpani*

Allergic, vasculitic, and rheumatologic disorders are relatively unusual in the pediatric intensive care unit (PICU) population. These disorders can lead to PICU admission because of the underlying disease itself (e.g., hereditary angioedema), of a complication of the underlying disorder (e.g., pulmonary hypertension from scleroderma), or of a complication of the treatment (e.g., sepsis from immunosuppression). The focus of this chapter is on disease manifestations, treatments, and complications of these disorders that can cause or worsen critical illness in children.

ALLERGIC DISEASES

A range of allergic reactions, from skin rashes to life-threatening anaphylaxis, can occur in the PICU patient. Here, the focus is on the manifestations of allergic disease of interest to the PICU clinician.

Anaphylaxis

An *anaphylactic* reaction is an immediate (Type I) hypersensitivity reaction that occurs when antigen binds to specific immunoglobulin E (IgE) antibodies, and leads histamine release from mast cells or basophils. The most common allergens are drugs, foods, hymenoptera, and latex (see Table 19.1). Inflammation occurs and increases capillary permeability, mucosal edema, and smooth muscle spasm. When mast cell or basophil degranulation occurs from a non-IgE mechanism, the reaction is termed *anaphylactoid*, but the clinical manifestations and treatments are the same. Because they are clinically indistinguishable, anaphylaxis, and anaphylactoid reactions are discussed together.

Some patients have a predisposition to anaphylaxis with a hyper-IgE syndrome and may display crossover to allergens of other classes or subtypes. However, these predispositions are not easily recognizable or cannot be easily tested. Diagnostic IgE testing is available, but can only distinguish anaphylaxis from anaphylactoid reactions and is not an appropriate screening method by which high-risk individuals can be identified.

The clinical presentation of anaphylaxis is variable in its onset and duration. Common clinical features are due primarily to histamine release and include urticaria, flushing, stridor, wheezing, angioedema, congestion, sneezing, nausea, vomiting, and diarrhea, as well as constitutional symptoms such as fatigue. The more severe symptoms are airway obstruction associated with angioedema, hypotension, arrhythmias, shock, and cardiac arrest[1–3] (see Fig. 19.1).

Radiocontrast media causes represent an anaphylactoid reaction of importance to the intensivist and occur in approximately 3% of patients. Although the incidence of reaction has decreased owing to the use of lower osmolarity radiocontrast media, it is still reported to cause an estimated 900 deaths per year in the United States. The pretreatment with glucocorticoids and H_2 blockers can reduce the recurrence of an allergic reaction in patients with a known sensitivity. Shellfish or an "iodine allergy" is not a contraindication to the use of radiocontrast media and does not necessitate a pretreatment regimen.

Anaphylaxis Treatment

The mainstay of treatment of anaphylaxis is epinephrine, which can produce dramatic improvements within minutes. Epinephrine stimulates α-adrenoceptors, increases peripheral vascular resistance, improves blood pressure and coronary perfusion, reverses peripheral vasodilation, and decreases angioedema. Stimulation of β_1-adrenoceptors

TABLE 19.1

COMMON ALLERGENS AND TYPES OF ALLERGIES

Type of Allergy	Agents Commonly Responsible
Drug allergy 2%–3% of hospitalized patients Estimated anaphylaxis US death rates/year = penicillin 400, radiocontrast media = 900	Penicillin and its derivatives (Most common initiator of anaphylaxis worldwide) Sulfonamides Radiocontrast media Vincristine Asparaginase Aspirin and other NSAIDs Immune globulin Opiates Insulin (Bovine>Porcine>Human) Protamine Glucocorticoids
Food allergy 1%–2% of the general population 33%–50% of pediatric anaphylaxis Estimated anaphylaxis US death rates/year = 100	Peanuts Tree nuts Fish Shellfish Eggs Grains Milk
Hymenoptera allergy 0.5%–5% of the general population Estimated anaphylaxis US death rates/year = 40–100	Bees Wasps Ants Yellow jackets
Latex allergy 1%–6% of the general population Estimated anaphylaxis US death rates/year = 3	Gloves Catheters IV tubing Blood pressure cuffs Ventilator tubing

NSAIDs, nonsteroidal anti-inflammatory drugs; IV, intravenous.

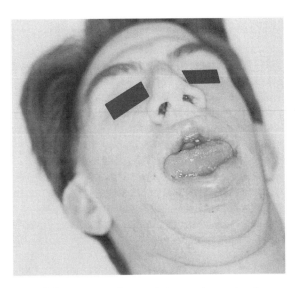

Figure 19.1 Facial swelling and airway obstruction from acute allergic reaction and anaphylaxis. (From Fleischer GR, Ludwig S, Baskin M. *Atlas of emergency medicine*. Philadelphia, PA: Lippincott Williams & Wilkins; 2004.) (See color Figure 19.1.)

Urticaria and Angioedema

Urticaria is a generalized manifestation of allergy that results from complement-mediated reactions, specific drug reactions, or it can be idiopathic. Urticaria lesions, known as *wheals or hives*, are pruritic, erythematous lesions with pale or dusky centers. These lesions can resolve rapidly or shift to new sites within hours. Urticarial reactions often occur in combination with angioedema, a deep mucocutaneous swelling, which if present in the airway can cause rapid, life-threatening airway compromise. Treatment options for urticaria and angioedema include glucocorticoids and histamine (H_1 and H_2) receptor antagonists depending on the severity of the reaction (Table 19.2).

Serum Sickness

Serum sickness is a non-IgE–mediated Type III hypersensitivity reaction that results from the injection of foreign protein, nonprotein drugs, or serum. This reaction is initiated by the formation of immune complexes resulting in vasculitis, specifically inflammation and necrosis of small vessels, and activation of compliment and granulocyte accumulation. Because the use of animal sera has decreased dramatically, drugs (especially antibiotics) and viral infections are the most common initiators.

The reaction typically occurs 1 to 3 weeks following administration of the inciting antigen, unless the patient has been previously sensitized. Cutaneous symptoms, fever, lymphadenopathy, arthritis, or arthralgias are the classic findings, but edema and involvement of the renal, cardiovascular, neurologic, and pulmonary systems have also been noted. Serum C3 and C4 complement levels are dramatically reduced.

has both positive inotropic and chronotropic cardiac effects. Stimulation of β_2-receptors causes bronchodilation, as well as increasing intracellular cyclic adenosine monophosphate (cAMP) production in mast cells and basophils, reducing release of inflammatory mediators. The subsequent administration of corticosteroids, intravenous fluids, and histamine (H_1 and H_2) receptor antagonists are required next (see Table 19.2). Glucagon can be given for refractory hypotension if a β-adrenergic blocker has been given because it increases intracellular cAMP levels by a mechanism that does not depend upon β-receptors.

Epinephrine for self-administration should be prescribed to individuals at risk for anaphylactic reactions. Prevention with monoclonal anti-IgE antibody may offer specific prophylaxis for individuals with a known hypersensitivity to certain antigens.[4]

TABLE 19.2

ALLERGIC REACTION TREATMENT GUIDE

Drug	Indication	Dose	Route	Frequency
Oxygen	Any patient with signs of allergic reaction	As needed to maintain oxygen saturations over 92%	Nasal cannula, face mask, or through endotracheal tube	Continuous until resolution of allergic reaction
Epinephrine	Any sign of moderate (stridor, wheezing, angioedema), or severe (airway obstruction associated with angioedema, hypotension, arrhythmias, shock, and cardiac arrest) allergic reaction	1:1,000 solution Pediatric: 0.01 mL/kg up to 0.3 mL Adult: 0.5 mL Use half of above doses if patient is taking tricyclic antidepressants or β-blockers	IM preferred, IV reserved for cases refractory to IM dosing	Every 5 min or sooner if needed; use of a continuous infusion is advised with refractory cases
Diphenhydramine	Mild to severe allergic reaction	1 mg/kg	IM/IV/PO	Every 4–6 h as needed
Ranitidine	Moderate to severe allergic reaction	1 mg/kg	IV/PO	Every 8 h as needed
Methylprednisolone	Moderate to severe allergic reaction	1 mg/kg	IV	Every 6 h as needed
Albuterol	Refractory bronchospasm	0.15 mg/kg	Nebulized	Continuous or every 4 h as needed for bronchospasm
Crystalloid	Continued hypotension	20 mL/kg	IV	Every 30 min or sooner if needed for refractory shock
Glucagon	Refractory shock in patients on β-blockers	0.02 mg/kg	IV/IM/SC	Every 5 min as needed

IM, intramuscular; IV, intravenous; SC, subcutaneous; PO, by mouth.

The initial treatment of serum sickness is discontinuation of the offending antigen. If the reaction requires further intervention, treatment is similar to that for allergic reactions: histamine (H_1 and H_2) receptor antagonists, glucocorticoids, and epinephrine if the patient develops airway compromise or shock (Table 19.2).

Adverse Drug Reactions

Adverse drug reactions are undesirable and unintended responses to a drug or a drug product. They are responsible for 5% of all hospital admissions and occur in 10% to 20% of hospitalized patients. These reactions fall into two broad categories. Type A reactions are approximately 80% of all adverse drug reactions, and are dose dependent and predictable events related to the pharmacologic actions of the substance. These reactions are easily treated by the discontinuation of the drug. Type B reactions are much less common, idiosyncratic, often immune mediated and less predictable. Drug hypersensitivity falls into this category.[5]

The intensivist will, at times, need to administer medications, despite a history of severe allergic reactions. For these patients, specific desensitization, which is the progressive administration of an allergenic substance, can help to blunt the allergic response. This procedure is typically used with agents that induce IgE-mediated reactions including penicillin, a number of non–β-lactam antibiotics, and insulin. The initial desensitization dose is usually 100 to 1,000 times lower than the concentration of the drug that produced the reaction. Dosage increases are administered at 15- to 30-minute intervals until therapeutic levels are achieved. Epinephrine, antihistamines, corticosteroids, and the appropriate equipment to treat anaphylaxis need to be immediately available in case of a reaction.

DERMATOLOGIC DISEASES (VASCULITIC DISEASES)

Erythema multiforme (EM), Stevens-Johnson syndrome (SJS), and toxic epidermal necrolysis (TEN) represent a spectrum of disease with manifestations that range from incidental rashes to mortality; they are presented in the order of their severity. Common causes of each of these diseases are presented in Table 19.3.

TABLE 19.3

COMMON CAUSES OF DERMATOLOGIC DISEASES (VASCULITIC DISEASES)

Reaction	Inciting Agents
Erythema Multiforme	Herpes simplex virus
Minor: zero to one mucosal surface involved	Epstein-Barr virus
Major: more than one mucosal surface involved	Enteroviral infections
Characteristic target-shaped lesions	Mycoplasmal although more commonly associated with SJS
Typically related to preceding viral or mycoplasma infection	Medications: sulfonamides, penicillins anticonvulsants, salicylates
Biopsy: inflammatory reaction with numerous T cells	Pregnancy
SJS	**Infections**
Typically medications are the inciting agent	Mycoplasma
25%–50% of cases no etiology is identified	**Medications**
5%–15% associated mortality	**Antibiotics**
<10% BSA involvement	Sulfonamides
Biopsy: necrotic changes without the large inflammatory reaction seen in EM.	Penicillin and its derivatives
Immunoreactivity for TNF-α	Quinolones
	Chloramphenicol
	Anticonvulsants
	Phenytoin and related antiepileptic drugs
	Carbamazepine
Toxic Epidermal Necrolysis	Lamotrigine
Represents SJS with larger involvement	Phenobarbital
>10% BSA involvement	Valproic acid
>40% associated mortality	**Other**
	Allopurinol
	Nevirapine
	NSAIDs, especially oxicams
	Carvedilol
	Vaccines
	Immune globulin
	Malignancies
	Lymphoma
	Bone marrow transplantation and acute graft versus host disease (TEN)

SJS, Stevens-Johnson syndrome; BSA, body surface area; EM, erythema multiforme; TNF, tumor necrosis factor; TEN, toxic epidermal necrolysis; NSAIDs, nonsteroidal anti-inflammatory drugs.

Erythema Multiforme

EM is frequently associated with infections. The lesions of EM usually consist of erythematous papules surrounded by a raised, erythematous ring, encircled by an additional outer erythematous ring on the extremities. The presence of these three zones distinguishes EM from urticaria, which has two zones. These target lesions also distinguish EM from SJS where target lesions are not typically seen.

These patients are typically not ill appearing, have an acute but self-limited course, and low morbidity. Although previously considered as a milder form of SJS, it is currently considered as its own entity. EM minor can be distinguished from EM major by the number of mucous membranes involved. Both forms are self-limited and have an excellent prognosis. Treatment is not typically needed.

Stevens-Johnson Syndrome and Toxic Epidermal Necrolysis

SJS differs in etiology from EM, and usually occurs as a drug hypersensitivity reaction. Sulfonamides are the most frequently implicated drugs (see Fig. 19.2). Both SJS and TEN represent mucocutaneous disorders with extensive necrosis and denuding of the epidermis. The initial skin lesions are ill-defined macules with darker purpuric centers. As the rash grows, it evolves into irregularly shaped bullous, purpuric lesions that often have overlying blisters or necrotic centers (see Fig. 19.3). These lesions occur on the face, trunk, and mucous membranes including the linings of the respiratory and gastrointestinal tracts. Classically, SJS involves <10% body surface area and TEN >30% body surface area. The area between 10% and 30% represents an overlap of the two disorders.

The pathophysiology is believed to be a cell-mediated cytotoxic reaction, which destroys keratinocytes that express a foreign antigen. Lesions contain a scarce infiltrate of T lymphocytes, mainly of CD8 phenotype, suggesting that apoptosis could be initiated by cytotoxic T lymphocytes. Tumor necrosis factor-α (TNF-α) overexpression in the epidermis may augment the epidermal destruction. TNF-α mediates this directly through apoptosis, indirectly through stimulating cytotoxic T cells, or through both. Finally this epidermal necrosis and apoptosis leads to the characteristic skin lesions.

Morbidity arises from the mucosal manifestations and can include mucosal scarring, strictures, and corneal ulcerations. Bronchiolitis obliterans and renal failure from acute tubular necrosis are complications of concern for the intensivist. The mortality rate for SJS is estimated at 5% to 15%, and for TEN it is approximately 40%. Typical criteria for PICU admission include the need for intensive nursing care for their burnlike wounds and monitoring of the airway because mucosal sloughing from the tracheobronchial tree may lead to respiratory failure.

Overall management is similar to that for burns. If the areas of involvement exceed 10% of the body surface area, transfer to a burn unit is suggested. Ophthalmology consultation is required to minimize corneal ulcerations, which is a major complication in these diseases. Adequate enteral or parenteral nutrition is an important aspect of care. Steroids are not recommended and may increase morbidity and mortality. Intravenous immunoglobulin (IVIg) therapy has been used to treat this disorder. A recent multicenter study noted a rapid cessation of skin and mucosal detachment in 90% of patients with TEN and survival in 88% with early infusion of IVIg at a total dose

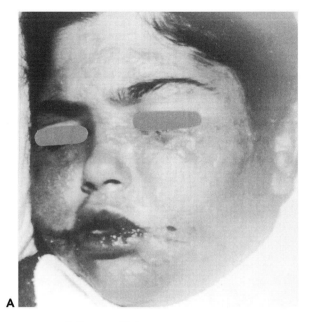
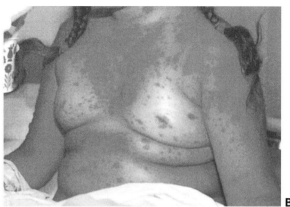

Figure 19.2 Stevens-Johnson syndrome. **A:** Adolescent with Stevens-Johnson syndrome secondary to sulfonamides. Note the involvement of the mucous membranes of the mouth. **B:** Same child. Note the distribution of lesions. (From Fleischer GR, Ludwig S, Baskin M. *Atlas of emergency medicine.* Philadelphia, PA: Lippincott Williams & Wilkins; 2004.) (See color Figure 19.2.)

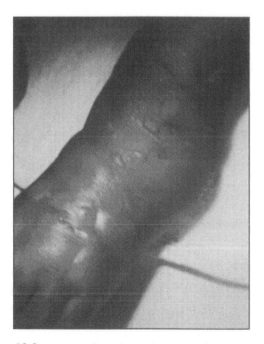

Figure 19.3 Toxic epidermal necrolysis (TEN) demonstrating the diffuse erythema and edema with overlying bullae. (From Anderson JA, Allergic drug reactions. In: Lieberman PL, Blaiss MS. *Atlas of allergic diseases.* Philadelphia, PA: Lippincott Williams & Wilkins and Current Medicine:2002:260.) (See color Figure 19.3.)

of 3 g per kg over 3 consecutive days (1 g/kg/day for 3 days). The use of cyclosporine with these disorders remains unproven. Withdrawal of the suspected cause is mandatory. Because sepsis is the most frequent cause

of death, close monitoring for secondary infections is critical, although prophylactic antibiotics are not indicated. Insensible fluid losses may be high and require large amounts of fluid replacement; in fact, some authors advocate rehydrating with the same fluid replacement formula as burns, depending on the total surface area of involvement. Surgical consultation and debridement are advised. Since sulfonamides are frequently an inciting agent, the use of silver sulfadiazine is contraindicated.[6]

VASCULITIC AND RHEUMATOLOGIC DISORDERS

The clinical manifestations and treatments associated with vasculitic and rheumatologic disorders of importance to the intensivist are presented here.

Henoch-Schönlein Purpura

Henoch-Schönlein purpura (HSP) is a small vessel vasculitis of childhood characterized by the deposition of IgA in arterioles, venules, and capillaries.[7] Its clinical presentation consists of a palpable purpuric rash, commonly over the lower extremities and buttocks, as well as arthritis, renal and gastrointestinal involvement (see Fig. 19.4). Renal involvement, which occurs in 20% to 80% of children, usually resolves, but can progress to renal failure in 3% to 18% of children.[8] The risk factors for renal failure are presented in Table 19.4. Severe HSP nephritis is treated with immunosuppressive therapy, including methylprednisolone and

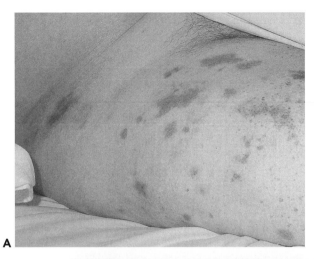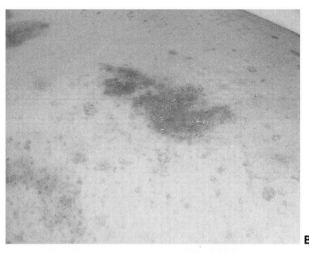

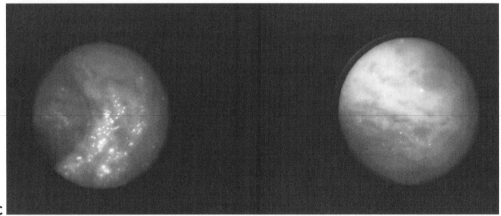

Figure 19.4 Vascular lesions of a patient with Henoch-Schönlein purpura. **A, B:** Veins of macular and papular pruritic lesions on the thigh. **C:** Endoscopic view of gastric mucosa demonstrates purpura. (From: Yamada T, Alpers DH, Kaplowitz N, et al. *Atlas of gastroenterology.* 3rd ed. Philadelphia, PA: Lippincott Williams & Wilkins; 2003.) (See color Figure 19.4.)

TABLE 19.4

RISK FACTORS FOR RENAL FAILURE IN CHILDREN WITH HENOCH-SCHÖNLEIN PURPURA

Nephrotic syndrome or proteinuria
Hypertension
Decreased factor XIII activity
Decreased renal function or renal failure at presentation
Nephritis at presentation
Crescenteric nephritis on biopsy

cyclophosphamide.[8] Gastrointestinal involvement ranges from diarrhea, which can be bloody, to intussusception and bowel necrosis.[9,10] Intussusception is managed by reduction, either by enema or surgery, and usually resolves completely; bowel perforation requires careful fluid management and close attention for the development of shock.

Finally, hemorrhagic complications are rare, but can be life threatening. Both pulmonary and cerebral hemorrhage have been reported.[11,12] The treatment of manifestations of HSP, other than renal insufficiency and intussusception, is supportive.

Systemic Lupus Erythematosus

Systemic lupus erythematosus (SLE) is a multisystem inflammatory illness in which dysregulation of both the innate and acquired immune systems allows the formation of autoantibodies. Between 10% and 20% of cases begin in childhood. Childhood onset is more common in Latino and African American children and is associated with a more severe disease at diagnosis and has a more aggressive course.[13] The diagnostic criteria for children are the same as for adults (see Table 19.5), but children are more likely to have neurologic and renal disease at diagnosis.[14]

Renal involvement is present in approximately 80% of children at the time of diagnosis, and 50% of children

TABLE 19.5

CRITERIA FOR DIAGNOSIS OF SYSTEMIC LUPUS ERYTHEMATOSUS

Constitutional

Failure to thrive, weight loss, anorexia, fatigue, fever

Skin

Discoid rash[a], malar rash[a], photosensitivity[a], aphthous ulcers[a]

Joints

Arthritis[a], arthralgias

Neurologic

Seizures[a] or psychosis[a] without other cause, stroke, pseudotumor cerebri, aseptic meningitis, cerebritis

Pulmonary

Pleuritis, pulmonary hemorrhage

Cardiologic

Pericarditis

Renal

Persistent proteinuria[a] or cellular casts[a], glomerulonephritis, nephrotic syndrome, ESRD

Hematologic

Hemolytic anemia[a], anemia of chronic disease, leukopenia[a], lymphopenia[a], thrombocytopenia[a]

Immunologic

Positive LE preparation[a], anti-DNA antibodies[a], anti-Smith antibodies[a], false-positive RPR[a], positive antinuclear antibody absent, administration of drugs known to cause lupus[a]

ESRD, end-stage renal disease; LE, lupus erythematosus; RPR, rapid plasma reagin.
[a]From Tan EM, Cohen AS, Fries JF, et al. The 1982 revised criteria for the classification of systemic lupus erythematosus. *Arthritis rheum.* 1982;25(11):1271–1277. Four of these strongly suggest the diagnosis of lupus.

diagnosed with lupus nephritis will progress to end-stage renal disease (ESRD) within 5 years, despite treatment.[15] Risk factors for ESRD include prolonged hypertension, anemia, abnormal urinalysis, increased creatinine levels, and diffuse proliferative glomerulonephritis on biopsy.[16] Following kidney transplant, both patient and allograft survival are shorter than in children who have undergone transplantation for SLE than other reasons.[15]

Cardiac manifestations include accelerated atherosclerosis leading to ischemia, even in asymptomatic children. Lupus anticoagulant and antiphospholipid antibodies can cause thromboembolic disease, necessitating long-term anticoagulation. Neuropsychiatric disease includes headache, cognitive and mood disorders, as well as seizures and cerebrovascular accidents,[14] and is associated with increased morbidity and mortality. Restrictive lung disease is commonly found on pulmonary function testing. Pulmonary hemorrhage, while rare, is also frequently fatal.

Nonsteroidal anti-inflammatory drugs (NSAIDs) and methotrexate may be used for serositis, skin, and joint symptoms, whereas corticosteroids remain the main treatment of active lupus and lupus flares. Lupus nephritis is often treated with cyclophosphamide, but azathioprine and mycophenolate may also have a role,[17] depending on biopsy and laboratory data. Other immune suppressive agents such as cyclosporine, thalidomide, and sex hormones may have a role in refractory lupus or severe organ disease. Treatment with exogenous antibodies against specific antigens (e.g., rituximab) is a more recent approach that holds promise. Finally, immune ablation, both with and without stem cell reconstitution has been used for severe or refractory lupus.[14,17]

Finally, critical illness can also arise from the complications of immunosuppressive agents, the most common of which are sepsis and malignancies. Children on long-term corticosteroid therapy may have related adrenal insufficiency. Although the overall mortality from lupus has significantly improved over the past few decades, long-term morbidity, most commonly from renal disease, and the complications of long-term immunosuppression, play a significant role in the care of these patients.[13]

Scleroderma

Although scleroderma is unusual in pediatrics, its associated gastrointestinal, cardiac, and pulmonary manifestations can necessitate PICU admission.[18] Scleroderma is associated with abnormal collagen deposition. Lung involvement, of interest to the intensivist, includes restrictive disease, pulmonary hypertension, and pulmonary fibrosis. Most children with scleroderma have abnormal lungs upon imaging and abnormal results of pulmonary function tests, with a restrictive pattern.[19] Pulmonary hypertension improves with the agent Bosentan,[18] but can be fatal despite maximal treatment. Gastrointestinal manifestations consist of altered esophageal motility causing acid reflux and potentially leading to stenosis, as well as altered intestinal motility.[20] Approximately 10% to 20% of patients with systemic sclerosis will develop "renal crisis" which is rapidly progressive renal failure associated with vasospasm and the release of large amounts of renin.[9]

Kawasaki Disease

Kawasaki disease (KD) is one of the most common acute vasculitides of childhood, and in the developed world, the most common cause of acquired heart disease.[21] It occurs most commonly in children aged 6 months to 5 years, with a peak at 9 to 11 months,[22] and is more common in boys and Asian children.[21] Risk factors for the development of coronary artery disease include male gender, atypical age or presentation, and the delayed administration of IVIg.

The pathogenesis of KD is unclear. One hypothesis is that a preceding infection results in exposure to an antigen

TABLE 19.6

CRITERIA FOR THE DIAGNOSIS OF KAWASAKI DISEASE

Fever and Four of the Physical Findings Must Be Present. (Atypical Kawasaki May Present with Fewer Findings But Will Still Have Evidence of Inflammation)

Fever $\geq$5 d

AND four of the following

Eyes: bilateral, nonpurulent conjunctivitis
Mouth: red lips, "strawberry tongue"
Skin: rash, most commonly maculopapular
Lymph nodes: lymphadenopathy, usually cervical
Hands/feet: red, edematous; desquamation in recovery phase

Associated Laboratory Derangements

Increase in acute-phase reactants
Erythrocyte sedimentation rate
C-reactive protein
Increased white blood cell count with leukocytosis
Anemia
Thrombocytosis (7–10 d after illness onset)
Hypoalbuminemia
Sterile pyuria
Negative evaluation for infection

TABLE 19.7

SYSTEM-SPECIFIC MANIFESTATIONS OF KAWASAKI DISEASE BY ORGAN/SYSTEM

Organ	Manifestations
Cardiovascular	Myocarditis, pericarditis, coronary artery aneurysm
Neurologic	Seizures; subdural collections; aseptic meningitis; stroke
Gastrointestinal	Hydrops of the gallbladder; increased transaminases; intestinal stenoses; acute abdomen
Renal	Sterile pyuria; nephrotic syndrome; renal failure
Pulmonary	Abnormal chest radiographs; pneumonia

or superantigen, thereby activating the immune system and causing systemic inflammation and panvasculitis.[21] Siblings or children of parents who had Kawasaki have an increased risk for the development of Kawasaki.

The diagnosis is based on clinical findings—diagnostic criteria and associated laboratory findings (see Table 19.6, Fig. 19.5). Children with an atypical presentation may have only three, rather than four of the additional criteria. An atypical presentation is more likely to lead to the development of coronary artery abnormalities.

The vasculitis of Kawasaki affects nearly every organ (see Table 19.7), but is usually self-limited, the coronary arteries being the notable exception. The most devastating complication of KD is the formation of coronary artery aneurysms. Echocardiography, to evaluate the formation of coronary artery aneurysm should be performed at diagnosis, particularly in children with prolonged fever. The treatment of KD with IVIg in the acute phase has decreased the incidence of coronary lesions from approximately 20% to 5%.[21] The coronary vessel wall may be permanently altered, which may account for some of the late mortality associated with Kawasaki. The acute phase of KD is associated with myocarditis and pericarditis, which usually resolve.

Neurologic effects of Kawasaki, which occur in approximately 1% of cases[23] include seizures, subdural collections, and stroke, which may be asymptomatic.[24] Both Kawasaki itself and the IVIg used to treat it are associated with aseptic meningitis.[25,26]

Gastrointestinal involvement includes hydrops of the gallbladder and increased transaminases, but more severe gastrointestinal tract disease, including intestinal stenoses requiring resection[27] and acute abdomen, has been reported. Of note, in a study of 10 children with Kawasaki who presented with acute abdomen, toxic shock syndrome requiring critical care occurred in four children, and coronary artery abnormalities occurred in five children, despite treatment with IVIg.[28]

Sterile pyuria is often observed in the acute phase of Kawasaki. Both acute renal failure and nephrotic syndrome have been reported. Pulmonary involvement, although uncommon, is suggestive of more aggressive vasculitis. Abnormal chest radiographs, found in 14.7% of all patients, are associated with more severe inflammation and increased incidence of pericardial effusion and coronary artery abnormalities.[29] Finally, in fatal acute KD, pathologic examination of the lungs reveals pneumonia most of the time.[30] The recent guidelines by the Committee on Rheumatic fever, Endocarditis, and Kawasaki Disease, Council on Cardiovascular Disease in the Young recommends that "all patients who are diagnosed with KD should be treated with IVIg," preferably in the first 7 to 10 days. Additional doses of IVIg or initial dose of IVIg after 10 days should be considered in the face of continuing inflammation.[21] Aspirin is usually given at a dose of 80 to 100 mg/kg/day initially, and continued at a dose of 3 to 5 mg/kg/day. Children with documented coronary artery aneurysms may also undergo systemic anticoagulation. The duration of aspirin therapy varies. Steroids may decrease the duration of clinical inflammation[31] but do not improve outcome. In patients with inflammation refractory to IVIg and aspirin, plasmapheresis, and immunosuppressive medication have been used, but data supporting these therapies are sparse.

In hospital, the mortality is only 0.17%. There is a mortality peak at 15 to 45 days following the onset of fever, a time of coronary vasculitis coupled with thrombocytosis

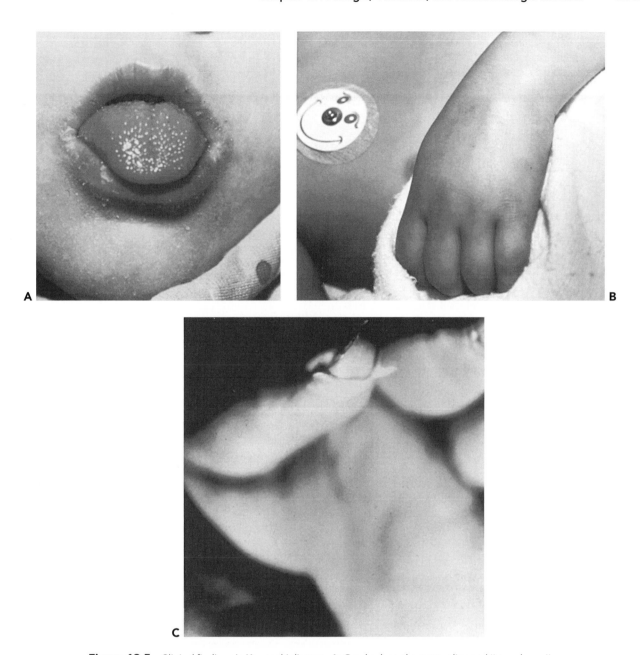

Figure 19.5   Clinical findings in Kawasaki disease. **A:** Cracked, erythematous lips and "strawberry" tongue. **B:** Brawny edema of the dorsum of the hand and small joint polyarthritis. **C:** Peeling of the skin on the thumbs. (From Fleischer GR, Ludwig S, Baskin M. *Atlas of emergency medicine.* Philadelphia, PA: Lippincott Williams & Wilkins; 2004.)

and a hypercoagulable state. Myocardial infarction and sudden death may occur many years after diagnosis both in patients who had unrecognized KD as children, and in those with a known history of Kawasaki and coronary lesions.[21] Recent evidence suggests a predisposition for an adverse lipid profile and increased arterial stiffness, years after the resolution of Kawasaki, even in children without coronary abnormalities in the acute phase.[32] Also, new coronary aneurysm, as well as worsening dilatation of known aneurysms have been reported to occur as late as 19 years after diagnosis.[33]

Juvenile Rheumatoid Arthritis

Juvenile rheumatoid arthritis (JRA) affects approximately 285,000 children in the United States. The disease is heterogeneous with four subtypes: rheumatoid factor positive, negative polyarticular, pauciarticular, and systemic onset. Although morbidity is high, critical illness and mortality are uncommon. Two complications of systemic JRA of interest to the PICU clinician are infections due to chronic immunosuppression and the rare, but life-threatening macrophage activation syndrome (MAS).[34]

In MAS, uncontrolled proliferation and activation of T lymphocytes and macrophages results in cytokine over-production, pancytopenia, coagulopathy, liver and neurologic pathology. Clinical features specific to MAS include hepatosplenomegaly, hyperferritinemia, and hypertriglyceridemia. The fever, lymphadenopathy, arthritis, rash, and increased erythrocyte sedimentation rate (ESR) that accompany MAS may initially suggest a flare up of the underlying rheumatic disease, and so an index of suspicion for MAS needs to be maintained. The treatment includes immunosuppression with steroids, cyclosporine A, or etanercept.[35]

Rheumatic Fever

Rheumatic fever is the most common cause of acquired heart disease in children in the underdeveloped world in which antibiotic treatment of pharyngitis may not be as readily available as in developed countries.[36] It is a multisystem inflammatory disorder that follows infection by certain serotypes of group A streptococcus (GAS)—hemolytic. These strains express a streptococcal surface protein that "mimics" the proteins of the brain and heart, resulting in antibodies cross-reacting with native antigens. In the brain, these result in Sydenham chorea, which includes both chorea and psychiatric symptoms, such as emotional lability and personality changes. Carditis, manifesting as a new murmur, pericardial friction rub or effusion, or overt congestive heart failure, is a result of antibodies reacting with cardiac antigens. Involvement of the joints, brain, and subcutaneous tissue is transient; the heart has the potential for permanent damage, and carditis can be fatal in the acute phase.[37] The diagnosis of rheumatic fever is made using the modified Jones criteria (see Table 19.8) and requires either one major and two minor, or two major signs or symptoms for diagnosis, as well as evidence of GAS infection. Recurrences of rheumatic fever require only one major or two minor criteria, as well as evidence of GAS infection. Not all criteria may be present at the time of clinical presentation. Signs and symptoms generally occur 1 to 3 weeks following GAS infection and during the last 6 to 14 weeks. The initial treatment includes the eradication of streptococci with benzathine penicillin G, treatment of carditis with steroids, treatment of arthritis with aspirin, and treatment of chorea with haloperidol or valproic acid.[38] Patients who have repeat infections with GAS are treated prophylactically with penicillin.

Wegener Granulomatosis

Wegener granulomatosis is an antineutrophil cytoplasmic antibody (ANCA)-positive necrotizing vasculitis of the small and medium vessels. Affected organs include the sinuses, nasopharynx, oropharynx, lungs, and kidneys. Necrotizing lesions can also form in the skin, central nervous system, or gastrointestinal tract.[7] Most children present with respiratory tract symptoms, both

TABLE 19.8

JONES CRITERIA FOR THE DIAGNOSIS OF ACUTE RHEUMATIC FEVER

Major Criteria	Comment
Carditis	
Polyarteritis	Usually migratory
Chorea	"Sydenham chorea," bilateral, purposeless movements; associated with emotional lability and irritability
Erythema marginatum	
Subcutaneous nodules	

Minor Criteria	Comment
Arthralgia	May not be used as a minor criterion if polyarteritis is being used as a major criterion
Fever	
Increase in acute-phase reactants	Erythrocyte sedimentation rate; C-reactive protein
Prolonged PR interval	

Evidence of GAS infection

Positive throat culture
Positive rapid streptococcal antigen test
Rising antistreptolysin O or anti-DNAse B titer

For initial presentation, evidence of GAS infection and two major, or one major and two minor criteria are required. For "relapses," evidence of GAS infection and only one major or two minor criteria are needed. GAS, group A streptococcus.
From Dajani AS, Ayoub E, Bierman FZ, et al. Special Report: Guidelines for the diagnosis of rheumatic fever. Jones Criteria, 1992 update. Special Writing Group of the Committee on Rheumatic Fever, Endocarditis, and Kawasaki Disease of the Council on Cardiovascular Disease in the Young of the American Heart Association. *Circulation.* 1993;87(1):302–307.

in the upper and lower respiratory tract. These symptoms include epistaxis, chronic cough, and dyspnea. Massive pulmonary bleeding, although rare, can be rapidly life threatening and has been successfully treated with extracorporeal life support. Compared to adults, children with Wegener granulomatosis are more likely to develop subglottic stenosis, a problem which can cause significant long-term morbidity, and which may require PICU admission for airway management. The development of renal disease is common, and can be asymptomatic until significant renal impairment has occurred. The treatment includes immunosuppression and trimethoprim--sulfamethoxazole, but patients are likely to experience at least one relapse.[39]

Takayasu Arteritis

Takayasu arteritis is an inflammatory disorder of the aorta and its main branches. Infiltration of the vessel wall causes thickening and narrowing of the lumen, whereas vessel walls proximal to the obstruction can undergo dilatation, aneurysm formation, and thrombosis. Patients can be asymptomatic, present with cardiovascular problems (such as aortic coarctation, congestive heart failure, or hypertension), or with neurologic problems (ranging from postural presyncope to stroke with permanent neurologic impairment).[40] The disease generally has a triphasic course. First, a prepulseless period with constitutional symptoms occurs. This is followed by a period of vessel inflammation. Finally, clinically significant fibrosis with bruits and ischemia result.[7] Arteritis can be diagnosed by magnetic resonance imaging (MRI) or conventional angiography. The long-term prognosis often depends on the control of cardiac complications such as congestive heart failure and dilated cardiomyopathy. The hallmark of treatment is immunosuppression.

Sarcoid

Sarcoidosis is characterized by the development of non-caseating granulomas that release inflammatory mediators. Signs and symptoms arise from organ dysfunction owing to the presence of granulomas or from the resultant inflammation,[41] and range from asymptomatic to multi-organ system failure and death.[42] Respiratory involvement is common and can result in significant obstruction to airflow. Cardiac sarcoidosis can cause rhythm disturbances, cardiomyopathy, or pericarditis. Despite its potentially serious consequences, it can go unrecognized and present as sudden death.[42] Finally, a metabolic consequence of sarcoid, of interest to the intensivist, is significant hypercalcemia due to unregulated production of Vitamin D by macrophages. The treatment is supportive.[41]

CONCLUSIONS

Allergic, vasculitic, and rheumatologic diseases can lead to PICU admission and require that the pediatric intensivist is familiar with the clinical manifestations, treatments, and complications of this group of diseases.

REFERENCES

1. Neugut AI, Ghatak AT, Miller RL. Anaphylaxis in the United States: An investigation into its epidemiology. *Arch Intern Med.* 2001;161(1):15–21.
2. Kay AB. Allergy and allergic diseases. Part I. *N Engl J Med.* 2001; 344:30–37.
3. Kay AB. Allergy and allergic diseases. Part II. *N Engl J Med.* 2001; 344:109–113.
4. Sampson HA. Anaphylaxis and emergency treatment. *Pediatrics.* 2003;111:1601–1608.
5. Roujeau JC, Stern RS. Medical progress: Severe adverse cutaneous reactions to drugs. *N Engl J Med.* 1994;331:1272–1285.
6. Prins C, Kerdel FA, Padilla RS, et al. Treatment of toxic epidermal necrolysis with high-dose intravenous immunoglobulins: Multicenter retrospective analysis of 48 consecutive cases. *Arch Dermatol.* 2003;139(1):26–32.
7. Ozen S. The spectrum of vasculitis in children. *Best Pract Res Clin Rheumatol.* 2002;16(3):411–425.
8. Kawasaki Y, Suzuki J, Suzuki H. Efficacy of methylprednisolone and urokinase pulse therapy combined with or without cyclophosphamide in severe Henoch-Schönlein nephritis: A clinical and histopathological study. *Nephrol Dial Transplant.* 2004; 19(4):858–864.
9. Cunard R, Kelly C. Immune-mediated renal disease. *J Allergy Clin Immunol.* 2003;111(2, part 3):S637–S644.
10. Langford C. Vasculitis. *J Allergy Clin Immunol.* 2003;111(2, part 3):S602–S612.
11. Nadrous HF, Yu AC, Specks U, et al. Pulmonary involvement in Henoch-Schönlein Purpura. *Mayo Clin Proc.* 2004;79(9): 1151–1157.
12. Ballinger S. Henoch-Schönlein purpura. *Curr Opin Rheumatol.* 2003;15(5):591–594.
13. Stichweh D, Arce E, Pascual V. Update on pediatric systemic lupus erythematosus. *Curr Opin Rheumatol.* 2004;16(5):577–587.
14. Carreno L, Lopez-Longo FJ, Monteagudo I, et al. Immunological and clinical differences between juvenile and adult onset of systemic lupus erythematosus. *Lupus.* 1999;8:287–292.
15. Gipson DS, Ferris ME, Dooley MA, et al. Renal transplantation in children with lupus nephritis. *Am J Kidney Dis.* 2003; 41(2):455–463.
16. McCurdy DK, Lehman TJ, Bernstein B, et al. Lupus nephritis: Prognostic factors in children. *Pediatrics.* 1992;89(2):240–246.
17. Ginzler EM, Moldovan I. Systemic lupus erythematosus trials: Successes and issues. *Curr Opin Rheumatol.* 2004;16(5):499–504.
18. Foeldvari I. Scleroderma in children. *Curr Opin Rheumatol.* 2002;14(6):699–703.
19. Murray KJ, Laxer RM. Scleroderma in children and adolescents. *Rheum Dis Clin North Am.* 2002;28(3):603–624.
20. Athreya BH. Juvenile scleroderma. *Curr Opin Rheumatol.* 2002;14(5):553–561.
21. Newburger JW, Takahashi M, Gerber MA, et al. Diagnosis, treatment, and long-term management of Kawasaki disease: A statement for health professionals from the Committee on Rheumatic Fever, Endocarditis and Kawasaki disease, Council on Cardiovascular Disease in the Young, American Heart Association. *Pediatrics.* 2004;114(6):1708–1733.
22. Tulloh R, Wood L. Coronary artery changes in patients with Kawasaki disease. *Acta Paediatr.* 2004;93(Suppl 446):75–79.
23. Terasawa K, Ichinose E, Matsuishi T, et al. Neurologic complications in Kawasaki disease. *Brain Dev.* 1983;5(4):371–374.
24. Fujiwara S, Yamano T, Hattori M, et al. Asymptomatic cerebral infarction in Kawasaki disease. *Pediatr Neurol.* 1992;8(3): 235–236.
25. Boyce TG, Spearman PM. Acute aseptic meningitis secondary to intravenous immunoglobulin in a patient with Kawasaki syndrome. *Pediatr Infect Dis J.* 1998;17(11):1054–1056.
26. Loh M, Janner D. Fever, aseptic meningitis and rash in a twenty-one-month-old male. *Pediatr Infect Dis J.* 1996;15(1):97, 100, 101.
27. Krohn C, Till H, Haraida S, et al. Multiple intestinal stenoses and peripheral gangrene: A combination of two rare surgical complications in a child with Kawasaki disease. *J Pediatr Surg.* 2001; 36(4):651–653.
28. Zulian F, Falcini F, Zancan L, et al. Acute surgical abdomen as presenting manifestation of Kawasaki disease. *J Pediatr.* 2003; 142(6):731–735.
29. Umezawa T, Saji T, Matsuo N, et al. Chest x-ray findings in the acute phase of Kawasaki disease. *Pediatr Radiol.* 1989;20(1–2):48–51.
30. Freeman AF, Crawford SE, Finn LS, et al. Inflammatory pulmonary nodules in Kawasaki disease. *Pediatr Pulmonol.* 2003; 36(2):102–106.
31. Sundel RP, Baker AL, Fulton DR, et al. Corticosteroids in the initial treatment of Kawasaki disease: Report of a randomized trial. *J Pediatr.* 2003;142(6):611–616.
32. Cheung Y-F, Yung TC, Tam SC, et al. Novel and traditional cardiovascular risk factors in children after Kawasaki disease. *J Am Coll Cardiol.* 2004;43(1):120–124.
33. Tsuda E, Kamiya T, Ono Y, et al. Dilated coronary artery lesions in the late period after Kawasaki disease. *Heart.* 2005;91(2):177–182.
34. Schneider R, Passo MH. Juvenile rheumatoid arthritis. *Rheum Dis Clin North Am.* 2002;28(3):503–530.

35. Ravelli A. Macrophage activation syndrome. *Curr Opin Rheumatol.* 2002;14(5):548–552.

36. McDonald M, Currie BJ, Carapetis JR. Acute rheumatic fever: A chink in the chain tat links the heart to the throat? *Lancet Infect Dis.* 2004;4(4):240–245.

37. Rullan E, Sigal LH. Rheumatic fever. *Curr Rheumatol Rep.* 2001; 3(5):445–452.

38. Hilario MOE, Terreri MTSLRA. Rheumatic fever and post-streptococcal arthritis. *Best Pract Res Clin Rheumatol.* 2002;16(3): 481–494.

39. Frosch M, Foell D. Wegener granulomatosis in childhood and adolescence. *Eur J Pediatr.* 2004;163(8):425–434.

40. Weyand CM, Goronzy JJ. Medium- and large-vessel vasculitis. *N Engl J Med.* 2003;349(2):160–169.

41. Leigh MW. Chapter 155-Sarcoidosis. In: Behrman RE, Kliegman RM, Jenson HB, eds. *Behrman: Nelson textbook of pediatrics.* 17th Ed. Philadelphia, PA: WB Saunders; 2004:822–823.

42. Newman LS, Rose CS, Maier LA. Sarcoidosis. *N Engl J Med.* 1997;336(17):1224–1234.

Immunodeficiency Syndromes in Children

20

Thomas J. Cholis III   Anthony D. Slonim

Immunodeficiency syndromes are an important component of pediatric critical care practice. Patients with primary immunodeficiencies may present with a spectrum of illnesses that ranges from pneumonia to respiratory failure to sepsis with shock. For children with repetitive or frequent infections, the pediatric intensivist needs to maintain vigilance and a keen index of suspicion to make the diagnosis of the underlying primary immunodeficiency syndrome. In part, the care that is provided in the pediatric intensive care unit (PICU) may contribute to relative immunologic compromise and resulting immunodeficiency. Examples of these so-called secondary immunodeficiencies include medications, surgery, and therapies such as continuous venovenous hemofiltration that affect the care and prognosis of these children. This chapter provides the necessary background on the primary and secondary immunodeficiency syndromes for the pediatric intensivist.

SUSPICION OF IMMUNODEFICIENCY

Primary immunodeficiency syndromes occur with a frequency between 1 in 10,000 and 1 in 100,000. Immunodeficiency syndromes should be considered when a child presents with infections that are unusual, longer in duration, or more severe than usual (see Table 20.1). For example, commonly considered criteria for an immunologic workup include patients who have been hospitalized with two or more pneumonias, or the occurrence of eight otitis media infections within a year.

The first step in diagnosing an immunodeficiency includes obtaining a thorough history and performing a physical examination. The history should focus on key elements of the past medical history of the child's illnesses,

TABLE 20.1

CRITERIA SUGGESTING THAT AN IMMUNODEFICIENCY WORKUP SHOULD BE PERFORMED

Unusual Pathogens (Examples)

Staphylococcal aureus
Burkholderia cepacia
Pneumocystis carinii
Nocardia sp.
Serratia marcescens
Aspergillus sp.

Increased Duration or Severity of Infections

Delayed umbilical cord separation
Poor dentition/delayed tooth loss/gingivitis
Poor wound healing
Recurrent meningitis
Recurrent sepsis with bacteremia
Failure to thrive

Other Criteria

Family history of recurrent infections
Consanguinity

a family history of repetitive infections, medication history, and immunization status. The physical examination may also provide insight into immunologic abnormalities. Skin lesions, abnormal facies, and poor development are all global indicators that may provide insight into an underlying immunodeficiency. A complete blood count, peripheral smear, and erythrocyte sedimentation rate should be performed next. Chronic granulomatous disease (CGD) may present with a personal or family history of repeated infections. DiGeorge syndrome presents with facial anomalies, and Wiskott-Aldrich and Chediak-Higashi syndromes are two conditions that can be diagnosed with simple blood tests. Wiskott-Aldrich syndrome presents with microcytic thrombocytopenia and Chediak-Higashi with characteristic-appearing granules in the neutrophils.

Beyond this simple approach, more specific diagnostic testing can be performed to refine the assessment of the immune disorder. Sorting immune cells into subsets has been useful as a diagnostic test for assessing immune function. The CD4/CD8 classification has become a standard for evaluating immune function in patients with human immunodeficiency virus. This technology can also be used to evaluate primary immunodeficiency syndromes involving neutrophils, lymphocytes, and monocytes. To evaluate the humoral arm of the immune system, immunoglobulin levels (IgA, IgM, and IgG) can be obtained. Isohemagglutins (ABO) are IgM antibodies that are directed against the group A and B antigens on red blood cells. They should be present by the third year of life. T-cell function can be tested with delayed hypersensitivity testing. This test is performed by administering antigens (e.g., Candida, tuberculin, and tetanus) in the skin and observing the localized reaction. The degree of wheal is evaluated within 24 to 48 hours and tests Type IV delayed hypersensitivity, which is a cell-mediated immune phenomenon. Recurrent *Neisseria* infections may be a marker for complement deficiency, and a CH50 will provide a quick assessment of total complement levels. If a child is experiencing recurrent infections to catalase-positive organisms, a nitroblue tetrazolium reduction test, which is an assay of superoxide or hydrogen peroxide production of the respiratory burst, could provide insight into the diagnosis of CGD.

PRIMARY IMMUNODEFICIENCY SYNDROMES

Primary immunodeficiency syndromes arise from genetic mutations that impair the functioning of the immune system (see Table 20.2). These conditions typically present in infancy up to early childhood, but some may not be diagnosed until adulthood. There have been more than 100 primary immunodeficiency disorders identified. These conditions have been traditionally classified by the component of the immune system that is most affected (Table 20.2). For example, T-cell immunodeficiency syndromes include DiGeorge and Wiskott-Aldrich syndromes. With an improved understanding of the genetic abnormalities that lead to these diseases, considerable overlap of these diseases between the different arms of the immune system has become more clearly understood.

B-Cell Disorders

B cells are a major component of humoral immunity. After being exposed to antigens, they become activated and evolve into plasma cells, which produce the various immunoglobulins described in more detail in Chapter 3.1. A deficiency can arise at many different steps of the process and produce a B-cell immunodeficiency. Maternal IgG antibodies typically cover these infants for the first few months of life. Children with B-cell immunodeficiencies usually present with symptoms after this period (i.e., 6 to 9 months).

In general, humoral deficiencies typically alter antibody production, causing the patient to be more susceptible to encapsulated organisms such as *Staphylococcal pneumoniae* and *Haemophilus influenzae*, and enteric gram-negative organisms (Table 20.2). Patients are also susceptible to enteroviral meningitis and *Giardia* gastroenteritis (Table 20.2). Recurrent infections and atypical organisms are the hallmarks of these diseases.

Congenital Hypogammaglobulinemia X-linked (Bruton)

This X-linked disorder provides an example of a classical B-cell immune disorder. The concentrations of immunoglobulins are low in all patients with this disorder and usually reach an important threshold as maternal antibody wanes at approximately 6 months of age (Table 20.2). As an X-linked disease, the condition presents in males. There is also a much less frequent autosomal recessive variant of hypogammaglobulinemia. The tonsils are very small, and these patients typically have no palpable lymph nodes (Table 20.2). They present with the classic recurrent bacterial infections affecting many different organ systems (e.g., sinusitis, otitis media, and conjunctivitis). Because the T-cell arm of acquired immunity is usually functional, fungal, viral, or opportunistic organisms (Toxoplasmosis, *Pneumocystis carinii*), are not usually a problem in these patients. The exception is that these patients are very susceptible to enteroviral meningitis. The diagnosis is made by quantitative serum immunoglobulin levels of <100 mg per dL of IgG and no IgM or IgA concentration (Table 20.2). These patients are typically treated with monthly intravenous immunoglobulin infusions.

Selective IgA Deficiency

Selective IgA deficiency is the most common antibody deficiency. The frequency in blood donors may be as high as 3 per 1,000 donors. Although the levels of other immunoglobulins are typically normal, the level of IgA is usually <10 mg per dL. Many of these patients are asymptomatic. Those more immunosuppressed may present with chronic sinopulmonary, gastrointestinal, or urogenital diseases with bacterial infections, resulting from the absence of IgA on mucosal surfaces. Some patients may have chronic diarrhea or severe malabsorption. Although there is no specific therapy for selective IgA deficiency, supportive care with antimicrobial therapy is important. These patients can have anaphylactic reactions against IgA in transfused blood products, so these products must be washed before transfusion.

TABLE 20.2

THE SYMPTOMS, DIAGNOSTIC EVALUATION, AND EXAMPLES OF PRIMARY IMMUNODEFICIENCY SYNDROMES

Symptoms	Evaluation of Immune System Needed	Diseases

Humoral immunity
  Recurrent pyogenic infections
  Lymphopenia
  Low globulin levels
  Hypoplastic tonsils
  Small lymph nodes
  >8 Otitis media infections in 1 y
  >2 Serious episodes of sinusitis,
  pneumonia, deep-seated infection
  Enteroviral meningitis
  Giardia
  Streptococcus pneumoniae, Haemophilus
    influenzae
	Serum immunoglobulins levels
	  IgG, IgM, IgA, IgE
	  IgG subclass
	Antibody function
	  Diphtheria or tetanus evaluate G1 and G3
	  Pneumococcal/meningococcal G2 and G4
	  Isohemagglutins ABO present at 1 y
	    of life
	  Lymphocytes in peripheral blood
		Bruton
		  Low IgG, No IgM, IgA
		Selective IgA deficiency
		  IgA <10
		Hyper IgM syndrome
		  IgM elevated, low IgG, IgA

Cell-mediated immunity
  Fungal (*Candida*)
  Protozoal (*Pneumocystis carinii*)
  Viral infections (EBV, HSV, CMV)
  Failure to thrive
  Chronic diarrhea
  GVHD to transfusion
	Total lymphocyte count
	Fluorescence-activated cell sorting
	  CD3, CD4, CD8
	DHT
	  Candida, tetanus, mumps, tuberculin
		DiGeorge
		  FISH for 22q11
		SCID
		  Hypogammaglobulinemia,
		    lymphopenia
		Wiskott-Aldrich
		  Thrombocytopenia, low IgM, IgA
		Ataxia-telangiectasia
		  Low IgA, CD3, CD4

Phagocytes
  Delayed separation of umbilical cord
  Catalase-positive organisms
  (*Staphylococcus aureus, Klebsiella*
    pneumoniae, Escherichia coli)
  Severe, recurrent skin infections
  Pneumatoceles
  Osteomyelitis
  Hepatosplenomegaly
  Granulocytosis
  Poor wound healing
  Gingivitis with periodontal disease
	Total neutrophil count
	Peripheral smear
	NBT reduction
	Fluorescence-activated cell sorting
		CGD
		  Catalase-positive organisms,
		    Absent NBT reduction
		Chediak-Higashi
		  Giant granules on smear

Complement
  Recurrent infection with Neisserial
    disease
	CH50
	  Total complement levels
	  Complement assay
		C5-9 deficiency
		  Low CH50

Ig, immunoglobulin; FISH, florescent *in situ* hybridization; SCID, severe combined immunodeficiency disorder; EBV, Epstein-Barr virus; HSV, herpes simplex virus; CMV, cytomegalovirus; DHT, delayed hypersensitivity skin test; GVHD, graft versus host disease; CGD, chronic granulomatous disease; NBT, nitroblue tetrazolium.

IgG Subclass Deficiency

Four subclasses of IgG exist, each having different biologic functions. IgG1 and IgG2 are responsible for the response to protein and polysaccharide antigens, respectively. The symptomatology of each subclass deficiency varies from asymptomatic to signs and symptoms of agammaglobulinemia manifested by recurrent pyogenic infections or *Giardia* infections. These deficiencies are identified by low laboratory levels of IgG subclasses (although the total level may be normal), and can be treated with intravenous immune globulin (IVIg).

Hyper IgM Syndrome

These patients have a clinical picture that is similar to X-linked agammaglobulinemia (Table 20.2). However, these patients also have an elevated IgM, low IgG, and no IgA. The genetic defect most commonly associated with this syndrome is on the CD40 ligand of the T cell. This ligand assists B cells in transitioning from IgM to IgG, IgA, and IgE. There are autosomal recessive and X-linked variants of this disorder. In addition to the usual presentation of recurrent pyogenic infections, these patients can present with opportunistic infections (*P. carinii*), and have a greater propensity toward the development of autoimmune disorders. One approach to therapy, described in a case report, consists of monthly IVIg and the aggressive treatment of bacterial infections. Some patients with neutropenia improved with granulocyte colony stimulating factor. This disease provides an example of the considerable crossover between the T- and B-cell lines and the resulting difficulty in classifying diseases into either B- or T-cell–specific immunodeficiencies.

T-Cell Disorders

T lymphocytes are primarily responsible for cell-mediated immunity and the recruitment of B cells in acquired immunity. These cells provide direct immune responses against viruses, fungi, and opportunistic infections such as *P. carinii*. These patients are also susceptible to graft versus host disease (GVHD) with nonirradiated blood transfusions. They can present with chronic diarrhea and failure to thrive (Table 20.2). Often, defects in T cells can cause damage to humoral immunity as well, causing combined immunodeficiency.

DiGeorge Syndrome

DiGeorge syndrome results from the abnormal development of the third and fourth branchial pouches, leading to thymic and parathyroid hypoplasia. These patients present with hypocalcemia (no parathyroid), congenital heart disease (conotruncal abnormalities, right-sided aortic arch, ventricular septal defects, atrial septal defects), esophageal atresia, hypothyroidism, and facial abnormalities (hypertelorism, low-set ears, and short philtrum) (see Fig. 20.1). Postcardiac surgery hypocalcemia can be recalcitrant to standard medical therapy. The lack of a thymus prevents the normal development of T cells, and makes these patients susceptible to fungi, viruses, opportunistic infections, and bacteria. The most common genetic defect is found on the 22q11, and diagnostically, a florescent *in situ* hybridization (FISH) assay for 22q11 is sent (Table 20.2). There are case reports of patients with complete DiGeorge being successfully treated with bone marrow transplantation (BMT). Fetal alcohol syndrome, velocardial syndrome, and retinoic acid exposure have similar clinical presentations.

Chronic Muco-cutaneous Candidiasis

This T-lymphocyte disorder presents with superficial candidal disorders in the mucosal areas and the skin. Patients may present early in life with candidal infections. This condition is associated with many other endocrinopathies including hypothyroidism or hypoparathyroidism. The tissues affected with candida can include the skin, nails, and oral mucosal membranes. Patients have a normal immune system except that they lack delayed hypersensitivity to *Candida* antigens. Chronic prophylaxis with antifungal agents is the therapy.

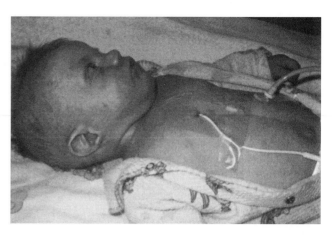

Figure 20.1 DiGeorge syndrome. A number of abnormalities that involve structures from the face to the thorax may be seen in this syndrome. Involvement of the thymus is variable. Patients with typical heart lesions and a microdeletion of 22q11 may have perfectly normal immune function. If the thymus is absent, the patient will have essentially no T cells and no response to mitogen stimulation of peripheral blood mononuclear cells. This situation is referred to as complete DiGeorge syndrome. This infant had complete DiGeorge syndrome and also a number of nonimmunologic and noncardiac problems. He demonstrates the small mandible and low-set, simple ears sometimes seen in those with the syndrome. He also has a severe swallowing disorder and gastroesophageal reflux that required fundoplication and feeding by the gastric tube shown. Swallowing difficulties, reflux, and aspiration are common among babies with DiGeorge syndrome. (From Williams LW, Roberts JL. Immunodeficiency disorders. In: Lieberman PL, Blaiss MS, eds. *Atlas of allergic diseases.* Philadelphia, PA: Lippincott Williams & Wilkins Current Medicine; 2002.) (See color Figure 20.1.)

X-linked Lymphoproliferative Disorder (Duncan Disease)

This disease affects a protein receptor on T cells causing them to hyperproliferate when exposed to the Epstein-Barr virus (EBV). Boys are healthy until the first exposure to EBV, which can have a fatality rate of 50%. This defect on T cells allows the T cells and the natural killer (NK) cells to self promote without negative feedback. If patients survive the first EBV infection, they have cellular immune defects, lymphomas, anaplastic anemia, and hypogammaglobulinemia. There is 70% mortality by age 10 for these children. There is a case series that reported a 50% success rate for these patients using BMT.

Combined B- and T-Cell Disorders

Severe Combined Immunodeficiency Disorders

Severe combined immunodeficiency disorders (SCIDs) encompass a wide range of genetic abnormalities where both the humoral and cell-mediated arms of immunity are affected (Table 20.2). Infants can be diagnosed with lymphopenia at birth, but typically present with failure to thrive, diarrhea, and symptoms of a more classical T-cell deficiency. These patients also have little to no antibody production. Infants present with opportunistic organisms, have a higher risk of mortality from viruses, and are at risk of GVHD from the transfusion of nonirradiated products. Usually, the lymph nodes, thymus, tonsils, and adenoidal tissue are all hypoplastic. There are many genetic abnormalities that can cause SCID, and one of the most common is the deficiency of adenosine deaminase, on 20q13. This deficiency creates a metabolite that causes premature apoptosis of thymocytes and lymphocytes. These patients have a much lower absolute lymphopenia than other variants of SCID. The definitive treatment includes BMT within the first year. Treatment with IVIg and gene therapy is ineffective.

Wiskott-Aldrich

This X-linked disease presents with the classic triad of microcytic thrombocytopenia, eczema, and immunodeficiency. These patients can present at birth with bleeding symptoms and are susceptible to recurrent infections with encapsulated bacteria. Patients with Wiskott-Aldrich have a poor antibody response to antigen exposure, and have low IgM, low IgG, and elevated IgA and IgE. T-cell counts are also diminished. In later life, these patients present with deficiencies related to cell-mediated immunity that present as opportunistic infections; some also have autoimmune disease. Death occurs from bleeding due to thrombocytopenia and bacterial infections. Some patients are treated with splenectomy or bone marrow transplant.

Ataxia-Telangiectasia

Ataxia-telangiectasia is an autosomal recessive disorder, which has been mapped to the long arm of chromosome 11. These patients present with progressive cerebellar ataxia within the first 6 years of life. Oculo-cutaneous telangiectasias develop at approximately 3 years of age. Most patients have a component of antibody deficiency, with some reported cases of T-cell deficiency as well. The immunodeficiency and presentation are variable and depend on the components of the immune system that are affected, but the typical presentation involves recurrent bacterial sinopulmonary disease. Other neurologic sequelae, such as mental retardation, speech, and gait disturbances, are also present. Currently, there is no known therapy.

Phagocytic Disorders

Phagocytic defects typically present with a susceptibility to nonpathogenic organisms or more severe presentations with pathogenic organisms (Table 20.2). Recurrent infections and abscesses in the skin, lungs, liver, and bone are common. Infections with catalase-positive microorganisms (*Staphylococcal aureus*) and fungi (*Aspergillus*) provide a clue that the patient may have a defect in the phagocyte function. These diseases may not respond to typical antibiotic or antifungal therapy, which should further raise clinical suspicion.

Chronic Granulomatous Disease

Patients with CGD experience recurrent infections with catalase-positive organisms (*S. aureus*, *Burkholderia cepacia*,

Aspergillus, *Nocardia*, and *Serratia marcescens*) and atypical mycobacteria of the skin, soft tissues, and the liver. The most common genetic defect in CGD is a mutation in the phagocyte oxidase glycoprotein, and is X linked, accounting for its higher frequency in boys. However, there are also variants that are autosomal recessive. The granulocytes of these patients have defects in the generation of hydrogen peroxide for the oxidative burst in killing these organisms. These patients can have gingivitis and acne, but do not have the dental disease seen with other defects in phagocytosis. CGD is diagnosed by the nitroblue tetrazolium (NBT) test. If untreated, these patients will succumb to systemic infections. Therapy includes prophylactic trimethoprim–sulfamethoxazole and itraconazole, which decreases the number of infections. Interferon γ has also been a useful therapy for this disease.

Chediak-Higashi Syndrome

This autosomal recessive disorder on chromosome 1 creates a susceptibility to recurrent *S. aureus* and β-hemolytic streptococcal infections. The genetic defect affects cytoplasmic proteins and causes giant lysosomal granules, which in turn, causes peripheral neuropathy, mild mental retardation, and platelet dysfunction. Normal granules in neutrophils have peroxidase, esterase, and acid phosphatase, providing oxidative burst for killing bacteria. However, these giant granules are unable to bind with phagosomes decreasing this capability. Patients have normal immunoglobulins with mild neutropenia. However, T cells are also delayed in this disease. The treatment is bone marrow transplant.

Leukocyte Adhesion Disorders

This condition arises from an impairment of the neutrophil binding to the endothelium and an inability to migrate to the site of inflammation. There are several genetic components to these syndromes varying with the severity of the disease. These patients usually present with a delay of umbilical cord separation, impaired wound healing, and recurrent infections of the teeth, mucosa skin, and respiratory tract (see Fig. 20.2). Patients are susceptible to a variety of pathogens including *S. aureus*, gram-negative bacteria, *Candida*, and *Aspergillus*. In Type I leukocyte adhesion disorders (LAD), the defect is at CD18. The amount of CD18 affects the severity of the disease. These patients lack the B_2 integrin adhesion molecule. This prevents neutrophil aggregation in response to infection. These impaired leukocytes do not adequately bind to the endothelial adhesion molecules, thereby preventing transport to sites of infection. No therapy is currently recognized.

Hyper IgE Syndrome (Job Syndrome)

This autosomal recessive syndrome is recognized from the patient's extraordinarily high levels of IgE. Patients present with recurrent *S. aureus* skin and pulmonary infections that are unresponsive to therapy. Eosinophilia, elevated IgE levels, and decreased chemotaxis, eczematoid rash, and

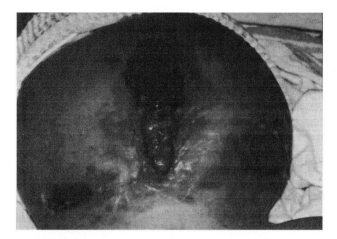

Figure 20.2 Leukocyte adhesion deficiency (LAD). In LAD, there is severe impairment of the migration of leukocytes to areas of inflammation or infection. If the CD11/18 complex is totally (or nearly) absent from leukocytes, circulating leukocytes are unable to firmly adhere to the capillary endothelium and pass into tissues. With such severe deficiency of CD11/18, infection may begin in the first weeks of life. Omphalitis extending to peritonitis may occur and is likely to be severe or fatal. The umbilical cord is slow to separate, but the features most suggestive of LAD are omphalitis and extreme elevation of the absolute neutrophil count, often >50,000 per mm³. This picture demonstrates necrotic, nonhealing surgical incisions and colostomy in a 2-year-old boy. Before it was known that he had LAD, he had an abdominal exploration for surgical abdomen that was actually peritonitis. Several subsequent procedures were attempted because of poor healing. The lesions improved with granulocyte transfusions. (From Williams LW, Roberts JL. Immunodeficiency disorders. In: Lieberman PL, Blaiss MS, eds. *Atlas of allergic diseases.* Philadelphia, PA: Lippincott Williams & Wilkins Current Medicine; 2002.) (See color Figure 20.2.)

coarse facies are the hallmarks of this condition. No current therapy exists for these patients.

Complement Disorders

Complement proteins are an integral part of the innate immune system. They provide a wide range of activities including lysis of bacteria, immunologic memory, and clearance of infected cells and complement complexes. Activation of the complement system activates C5 through C9, which provides for the lysis of bacteria. Lack of these complement components typically presents as recurrent Neisseria infections. C3 binds to the bacterial surface and promotes phagocytosis of the organism. Therefore, the lack of this binding protein presents with recurrent bacterial infections. Low CH50 levels are diagnostic for complement disorders. Deficiencies of the early complement components are characterized as autoimmune disorders.

SECONDARY IMMUNODEFICIENCY

Secondary immunodeficiencies are a class of conditions that create a situation of increased risk of infection for the host. These disorders are more common than primary

TABLE 20.3
A CLASSIFICATION SYSTEM FOR SECONDARY IMMUNODEFICIENCY SYNDROMES
Immune Dysfunction Related to Physiologic Changes
Age
Splenic abnormalities
Hypothermia
Malnutrition
Immune Dysfunction Related to Traumatic Disorders
Trauma
Burns
Immune Dysfunction Related to Medical Interventions
Surgery
Bone marrow transplant
Radiation therapy
Medications
Immune Dysfunction Related to Acquired Nonimmunologic Diseases
Sickle cell disease
Uremia
Nephrotic syndrome
Diabetes mellitus

immunodeficiency syndromes and can affect any component of the immune system. Table 20.3 presents a simple classification schema for these conditions. Secondary immunodeficiency states can vary in severity from asymptomatic to life threatening.

Immune Dysfunction Related to Physiologic Changes

Age

Age is an important determinant of immune function. In the newborn, the immune system is immature and unable to respond effectively to infection. This immaturity is exaggerated in the preterm infant below 34 weeks of gestation and affects all the components of the immune system including phagocytes, complement, splenic function, T cells, and antibody responses. Newborn infants have high levels of IgG, but these levels arise from transplacental maternal immunoglobulin transfer, and not from endogenous production. These underdeveloped components of the immune system provide a risk for bacteremia and mortality in the newborn.

Splenic Abnormalities

The spleen is responsible for a variety of immune-related activities including the phagocystosis of microorganisms, the removal of antibody-coated cells, and the production of cytokines and antibodies. Although splenectomy after trauma is an important component of this immunodeficiency, functional splenectomy, as it occurs in congenital asplenia or with certain diseases (e.g., sickle cell disease), is clinically important as well. Asplenia should be suspected in patients with heterotaxy and congenital heart disease. Important clinical clues include the presence of Howell-Jolly bodies and erythrocyte inclusions on a peripheral blood smear. *S. pneumoniae, Neisseria meningitidis, S. aureus, Salmonella* spp., and *E. coli* account for most postsplenectomy bacterial infections. Those who are at increased risk of postsplenectomy complications include infants and those patients within 2 years of their splenectomy. The focus of therapy is in assuring appropriate prophylaxis encapsulated organisms either through vaccination or through the use of suppressive antibiotics.

Hypothermia

Hypothermia in postcardiac surgery has been proved to cause increased risk of infection. Interest in active cooling for traumatic brain injury or postcardiac arrest is increasing, although earlier studies had shown increased risk of infection. The potential source of immune dysfunction is that cold damages normal neutrophil chemotaxis and adhesion, phagocytosis, and oxygen burst.

Malnutrition

Malnutrition is a major cause of immunodeficiency in children. Protein calorie malnutrition causes T-cell and NK-cell immunodeficiency, as well as deficiencies in complement. The lack of nutrients can cause thymic atrophy and a decreased cytokine response to infection. However, immunoglobulin levels are usually increased. These defects can result from malnutrition of any etiology and are associated with poor wound healing and higher mortality. For example, patients with cystic fibrosis, liver disease, or inflammatory bowel disease may experience a wasting syndrome with malnutrition that results in a secondary immunodeficiency and an increased susceptibility to infections. Improvement of the patient's immunodeficiency can be corrected by appropriate attention to nutrition and an adequate supply of protein and calories.

Immune Dysfunction Related to Traumatic Disorders

Trauma

Trauma and other stress-related syndromes provide an example of the intimate interactions between the immune and endocrine systems. Patients with multiple trauma often demonstrate a diffuse inflammatory response. The origin behind this immune dysfunction is not entirely understood, although it appears that T-cell function and cytokine production are compromised after traumatic insults. Patients with acute trauma in the PICU also have a number of interventions that compromise their immunity. They

are catabolic, have multiple invasive catheters and drains, which intrude on the mechanical barriers to infection, and are at considerable risk for aspiration.

Burns

Patients with burns are at a significantly higher risk for infection owing to the impairment of the physical barrier of the skin. Sepsis is a major cause of morbidity and mortality in these patients. The most common immune dysfunction after burns is T-cell deficiencies and dysfunction. In addition, because of the impaired cytokine response, the function of neutrophils including phagocytosis, opsonization, and chemotaxis is also impaired after a burn wound. Currently, the treatment is supportive and includes adequate nutrition and the prevention of complications. Prophylactic antibiotics are not indicated for this immune dysfunction.

Immune Dysfunction Related to Medical Interventions

Surgery

Anesthesia and major surgery can cause immune dysfunction by affecting both lymphocyte and neutrophil function. Lymphopenia can occur after anesthesia, but the return to normal levels occurs several days after surgery. Inhaled anesthetics can cause reduced ciliary clearance within the lungs and also impair the oxidative killing of neutrophils, thereby increasing the risk of pulmonary infections.

Bone Marrow Transplantation

The preparatory regimen for BMT requires chemotherapy to kill tumor cells and prepare the marrow for the graft. These patients experience pancytopenia for a period of 2 to 4 weeks, but can experience B- and T-cell depression for more than a year. These patients are at a high risk for infections of many etiologies including bacterial, viral, protozoal, fungal, and opportunistic. These infections occur at different times during the post-transplant period and are associated with considerable mortality. However, effective prophylactic regimens are available as a part of the supportive post-BMT transplant regimen (see Chapter 29). Irradiated and cytomegalovirus (CMV)-negative blood products should be provided to these patients to prevent the transmission of infection.

Radiation Therapy

Patients receiving radiation therapy have a higher risk of infection owing to the impaired cell-mediated immunity. This therapy can also cause lymphopenia and decreased lymphocyte reactivity to antigens. There is a dose response to radiotherapy with a higher degree of immunosuppression occurring with increasing doses of radiotherapy.

Medications

A number of medications cause immunodeficiency. For some of these medications, immunosuppression is the intended therapeutic effect, but for other medications, the resulting immunosuppression is an unintended adverse drug event. For example, corticosteroids are often used for their immunosuppressive effects. They can induce deficiencies in T-cell number and function, inhibit phospholipase A2 conversion to eicosanoids, and inhibit neutrophil and complement function. Alternatively, anticonvulsant medications, although primarily intended for their beneficial effects against seizures, can cause selective IgA deficiency, IgG subclass deficiency, and transient hypogammaglobulinemia.

Immune Dysfunction Related to Acquired Nonimmunologic Diseases

Sickle Cell Disease
Patients with sickle cell disease have a high risk of death from bacterial infections particularly those caused by encapsulated bacteria, including *S. pneumoniae* and *Mycoplasma pneumoniae*. In part, the immune dysfunction arises from functional asplenia related to repeated sickle cell crises. Prophylactic penicillin is started for patients below 5 years.

Uremia
Renal failure produces elevated levels of urea. Uremia inhibits phagocytosis, chemotaxis, and bacterial killing by neutrophils. It also inhibits T-cell production and function. Humoral immunity is mildly affected, but immunoglobulin levels are typically normal. *S. aureus* is a common pathogen for these patients and is often associated with the presence of vascular access devices for dialysis.

Nephrotic Syndrome
Patients with nephrotic syndrome experience protein loss in the urine and through the gastrointestinal tract that leads to low serum IgG and IgM. Immunodeficiencies result from the loss of these immunoglobulins and lead to a higher risk for pneumococcal, *S. aureus*, and *Streptococcus pyogenes* infections. These pathogens can cause bacteremia, cellulitis, and peritonitis. There are also defects in cell-mediated and complement function in these patients. Prophylaxis with penicillin and vaccination are important in protecting the patients.

Diabetes
Type 1 diabetes is caused by autoimmune destruction of pancreatic islet cells. The immunosuppressions in these patients are influenced by the metabolic derangements, vasculopathy, and denervation, which are inherent in long-standing diabetes. The immunologic deficiencies involve impaired neutrophil function including chemotaxis, phagocytosis, and killing activities. NK-cell cytotoxicity, complement, and T-cell defects can also occur. Fungal and bacterial infections, especially *S. aureus* infections, can occur and affect the skin and urinary tract.

CONCLUSION

Immunodeficiency syndromes, either primary or secondary, are important conditions for the pediatric intensivist. The outcome for primary immunodeficiencies depends in part on their appropriate assessment and prophylaxis. Secondary immunodeficiencies are commonplace in the PICU and often require aggressive physiologic support while antimicrobial therapies are being administered.

ACKNOWLEDGMENTS

Supported in part by grant KO-8 HS14009-01, Agency for Healthcare Research and Quality, Rockville, MD.

RECOMMENDED READINGS

1. Buckley RH, Primary immunodeficiency disease due to defects in lymphocytes. *N Engl J Med.* 2000;343:1313–1324.
2. Walport MJ. Advances in immunology: Complement (first of two parts). *N Engl J Med.* 2001;344:1058–1066.
3. Walport MJ. Advances in immunology: Complement (second of two parts). *N Engl J Med.* 2001;344:1140–1144.
4. Lekstrom-Himes JA, Gallin JI. Advances in immunology: Immunodeficiency diseases. Caused by defects in phagocytes. *N Engl J Med.* 2000;343:1703–1714.
5. Ballow M. Stress-related immunodeficiencies: TRAUMA, surgery, anesthesia, burns, exercise, and splenic deficiencies. In: Stiehm ER, Ochs HD, Winkelstein JA, eds. *Immunologic disorders in infants and children.* Philadelphia, PA: Elsevier; 2004.
6. Cunningham-Rundles S, McNeely DF, Ananworanich J. Immune responses in malnutrition. In: Stiehm ER, Ochs HD, Winkelstein JA, eds. *Immunologic disorders in infants and children.* Philadelphia, PA: Elsevier; 2004.
7. Ananworanich J, Shearer WT. Immune deficiency in metabolic diseases. In: Stiehm ER, Ochs HD, Winkelstein JA, eds. *Immunologic disorders in infants and children.* Philadelphia, PA: Elsevier; 2004.
8. Buckley RH. Primary immunodeficiency diseases. In: Paul WE, ed. *Fundamental immunology.* Philadelphia, PA: Lippincott Williams & Wilkins; 2003.
9. Tanginsmankong N, Bahna SL, Good RA. The immunologic workup of the child suspected of immunodeficiency. *Ann Allergy Astham Immunol.* 2001;87:362–370.
10. Williams LW, Roberts JL. Immunodeficiency disorders. In: Lieberman PL, Blaiss MS, eds. *Atlas of allergic diseases.* Philadelphia, PA: Lippincott Williams & Wilkins; 2002.

Pediatric Acquired Immunodeficiency Syndrome in the Pediatric Intensive Care Unit

21

Sophia R. Smith   *Hans M. L. Spiegel*

The worldwide dissemination of human immunodeficiency virus (HIV) over the past four decades is one of the most catastrophic examples of the emergence, transmission, and propagation of a microbial agent. In industrialized countries, only 15% to 20% of untreated children die before the age of 4 years. Since the introduction of modern therapies, the average survival of perinatally infected children in the United States has currently increased to 14.8 years. During 2004, <100 children died in the United States owing to the complications of HIV infection. Contrast these improved results to sub-Saharan Africa where in 2004, 460,000 HIV-positive children <15 years of age died.

There are limited data available on the epidemiology of pediatric intensive care unit (PICU) admission patterns, as well as the outcome for children and youth with HIV infection who require PICU admission, since the development of highly active antiretroviral therapy (HAART). Recent retrospective studies from Europe, which span the period before and after the start of HAART, still reveal the predominance of PICU admissions early in life for symptomatic infants with HIV infection. In these studies, the age at admission ranged between 2 months and 11 years.[1] Respiratory failure due to *Pneumocystis carinii* (*jiroveci*) pneumonia (PCP) is consistently recognized as the most common cause for intensive care unit (ICU) admission among children with HIV disease. One third of the other admissions to the ICU for respiratory failure were due to different respiratory pathogens including *Mycobacterium tuberculosis* pneumonia, fungal pneumonias such as those due to *Cryptococcus neoformans*, *Histoplasma capsulatum*, *Coccidioides immitis*, and *Aspergillus fumigatus*, cytomegalovirus (CMV) pneumonia, and *Toxoplasma gondii* pneumonitis.

ICU mortality in the United Kingdom over the last 10 years was 38% and more than 80% of their survivors were being treated with HAART.[1] Recently, the incidence of PICU patients with acquired immunodeficiency syndrome (AIDS) has been declining, which can be attributed to HAART therapy. Although the outcome of HAART in the studied adult populations has been variable, once started on HAART, post-ICU survival has considerably improved.[2]

PATHOGENESIS

HIV has a predilection for the activated HIV-specific CD4+ cells, although other cells are also susceptible to the virus (i.e., macrophages). This tropism for particular cells is determined mainly by cellular receptors to which HIV attaches in order to enter the cells. HIV seems to function as a "master regulator" of cellular gene expression. Recent studies suggest that HIV infection can influence the expression of many host genes, and some of these may have critical roles in the HIV replication cycle.

HIV disease progression is characterized by the development of functional abnormalities and numeric depletion of CD4$^+$ T cells. Uninfected infants have higher CD4$^+$ T-cell counts during the first 2 years of life, which reach adult levels by approximately 6 years of age.[3] Both CD4$^+$ T-cell counts and viral load are predictors of HIV disease progression and mortality in children.[4] According to the current guidelines from the Centers for Disease Control (CDC), CD4$^+$ T-cell counts <15% constitute severe immune suppression and an increased risk for AIDS-defining opportunistic infections, recurrent severe invasive bacterial infections, and malignancies. Other immune defects include B-cell deficiencies, phagocytic abnormalities due to impairments in neutrophil number and function, dysfunction of macrophages and monocytes, and occasional complement defects.

Ninety percent of today's HIV-positive children contracted the virus from their infected mothers (vertical transmission) during or near the time of birth with most of the infection occurring in the intrapartum period. In the United States, vertical transmission has decreased to <2% among infants born to HIV-positive mothers due, in part, to the introduction of universal prenatal HIV counseling and testing, maternal and infant perinatal antiretroviral prophylaxis, and elective cesarean section delivery of HIV-infected pregnant woman.

Other routes of infection include sexual abuse, blood, and blood products. With the introduction of HIV antibody screening of blood in 1985, the risk of HIV infection through transfusion has considerably diminished. A minimal residual risk remains because of donors who are in the window period of their infection when HIV serum antibodies are not yet present.

DIAGNOSIS

Adults and children develop serum antibodies to HIV by 6 to 12 weeks after infection. In this group, the diagnosis of HIV infection depends on the detection of virus or viral nucleic acid, which is achieved by polymerase chain reaction (PCR) assay of DNA. By 1 month of age, almost all infected infants are HIV DNA PCR–positive. HIV-uninfected infants may carry their mother's antibodies until 18 months of age. The use of plasma HIV RNA is only licensed currently in the United States as a quantitative test but has diagnostic relevance when positive. In children older than 18 months of age, the HIV enzyme immunoassay (EIA) is the initial diagnostic test. Western blot analysis remains the gold standard for diagnostic confirmation.

CLINICAL PRESENTATION OF HIV INFECTION IN PEDIATRICS

Most infected infants do not have abnormal findings on clinical examination at birth. The initial manifestations of the disease are mild and nonspecific. These may include generalized lymphadenopathy, chronic or recurrent diarrhea, failure to thrive, oral thrush, or developmental delay. HIV disease progresses more rapidly in children and has a shorter latency period as compared to adults.[5] The disease progression in children at the time of diagnosis of AIDS is 8 to 17 months compared to 8 to 11 years in adults, owing to an immature immune system. The clinical manifestations of pediatric HIV infection are varied and differ from those in adults. Clinical manifestations in children are mostly dependent on the level of immune compromise present, host factors, as well as exposure to potential opportunistic pathogens (see Tables 21.1 and 21.2). As an example, lymphocytic interstitial pneumonitis (LIP), chronic parotid swelling, and HIV encephalopathy are encountered more frequently in children than in adults.

On the basis of age of presentation, patterns that have been described include manifestations in the form of opportunistic infections and neurologic manifestations seen within the first few months of life. These children are considered "rapid progressors." Other children may show a more gradual development of manifestations that tend to materialize after 1 year of age and usually present as failure to thrive, recurrent bacterial infections, or lymphoid interstitial pneumonitis. Finally, there is a third smaller group of children who present later in childhood or during the adolescent years with minor or more severe manifestations.

COMPLICATIONS OF ACQUIRED IMMUNODEFICIENCY SYNDROME OF INTEREST TO THE INTENSIVE CARE PHYSICIAN

In studies of critical care medicine and HIV-infected patients, acute respiratory failure is the most common diagnosis at the time of admission and accounts for approximately 40% to 50% of ICU admissions. The need for mechanical ventilation after failure of initial therapy is a key marker for poor prognosis in HIV-infected patients, especially those with PCP. Although the overall mortality rate for HIV-positive patients with PCP was 30%, patients with ventilation-related risk factors have a higher mortality. Other factors associated with a poor prognosis include nosocomial infections, pneumothorax, and prolonged mechanical ventilation.

Other frequently reported causes of ICU admissions include central nervous system (CNS) dysfunction, gastrointestinal bleeding, and cardiovascular disease. HIV-infected patients are also admitted to the ICU for reasons unrelated to their immunodeficiency. Patients may be admitted for associated conditions including postoperative care, infections secondary to indwelling catheters, noninfectious pulmonary diseases including asthma and chronic obstructive pulmonary disease, renal failure, metabolic disturbances such as lactic acidosis, and drug overdoses.

TABLE 21.1

1994 REVISED HUMAN IMMUNODEFICIENCY VIRUS PEDIATRIC CLASSIFICATION SYSTEM: CLINICAL CATEGORIES

Category N: Not Symptomatic

Children who have no signs or symptoms considered to be the result of HIV infection, or who have only one of the conditions listed in category A

Category A: Mildly Symptomatic

Children with two or more of the following conditions but none of the conditions listed in categories B and C
- Lymphadenopathy ($\geq$0.5 cm at more than two sites; bilateral = one site)
- Hepatomegaly
- Splenomegaly
- Dermatitis
- Parotitis
- Recurrent or persistent under respiratory tract infection, sinusitis, or otitis media

Category B: Moderately Symptomatic

Children who have symptomatic conditions other than those listed for category A or category C that are attributed to HIV infection. Examples of conditions in clinical category B include but are not limited to the following:
- Anemia (<8 g/dL), neutropenia (<1,000/mm^3), or thrombocytopenia (<100,000/mm^3)
- Bacterial meningitis, pneumonia, or sepsis (single episode)
- Candidiasis, oropharyngeal (i.e., thrush) persisting for >2 mo in children older than 6 mo
- Cardiomyopathy
- Cytomegalovirus infection with onset before age 1 mo
- Diarrhea, recurrent or chronic
- Hepatitis
- HSV stomatitis, recurrent (i.e., more than two episodes within 1 y)
- HSV bronchitis, pneumonitis, or esophagitis with onset before age 1 mo
- Herpes zoster (i.e., shingles) involving at least two distinct episodes or more than one dermatome
- Leiomyosarcoma
- LIP or pulmonary lymphoid hyperplasia complex
- Nephropathy
- Nocardiosis
- Fever lasting >1 mo
- Toxoplasmosis with onset before age 1 mo
- Varicella, disseminated (i.e., complicated chicken pox)

Category C: Severely Symptomatic

Children who have any condition listed in the 1987 surveillance case definition for acquired immunodeficiency syndrome, with the exception of LIP (which is a category B condition)

HIV, human immunodeficiency virus; HSV, herpes simplex virus; LIP, lymphoid interstitial pneumonia.
From Centers for Disease Control and Prevention. 1994 revised classification system for human immunodeficiency virus infection in children less than 13 years of age. *MMWR Morb Mortal Wkly Rep.* 1994;43:1–10, with permission.

Adverse effects of antiretroviral therapy include pancreatitis and severe immune reconstitution inflammatory syndrome (IRIS), which is the result of an exuberant inflammatory response toward previously diagnosed or incubating opportunistic pathogens, as well as responses toward other, as yet, undefined antigens.

Complications of pediatric HIV infection can be grouped into organ-specific sequelae including generalized lymphadenopathy, hepatosplenomegaly, recurrent diarrhea (idiopathic or infectious), parotitis, cardiomyopathy, hematologic abnormalities, pancreatitis, nephropathy, endocrine dysfunction, LIP, and CNS disease, including cerebral vascular complications. Malignancies are of low incidence. Kaposi sarcoma, which occurs more commonly among children with HIV infection in areas where the tumor is highly endemic, is rare in children within the United States.

Infectious complications of HIV remain the major cause of respiratory failure or sepsis in the ICU. Included among

TABLE 21.2

PEDIATRIC HUMAN IMMUNODEFICIENCY VIRUS CLASSIFICATION FOR CHILDREN YOUNGER THAN 13 YEARS

	Clinical Category			
Immune Category	(N) No Symptoms	(A) Mild Symptoms	(B)[a] Moderate Symptoms	(C)[a] Severe Symptoms
1. No suppression	N1	A1	B1	C1
2. Moderate suppression	N2	A2	B2	C2
3. Severe suppression	N3	A3	B3	C3

Using this system, children are classified according to three parameters: infection status, clinical status, and immunologic status. The categories are mutually exclusive. Once classified in a more severe category, a child is not reclassified in a less severe category even if the clinical or immunologic status improves. Children whose human immunodeficiency virus infection status is not confirmed are classified by using this grid with a letter *E* (for vertically exposed) placed before the appropriate classification code (e.g., EN2).
[a]Both category C and lymphoid interstitial pneumonitis in category B are reportable to state and local health departments as acquired immunodeficiency syndrome.
From Centers for Disease Control and Prevention. Revised classification system for human immunodeficiency virus infection in children less than 13 years of age. *MMWR Morb Mortal Wkly Rep.* 1994;43(RR-12):1–12, with permission.

the other infectious complications are candida infection, ranging from oral candidiasis, local or disseminated CMV infection, herpes simplex and varicella zoster virus infections, PCP, *Mycobacterium* avium complex (MAC) infection, chronic enteritis caused by *Cryptosporidium* species, *Isospora* species, or *Microsporidium, T. gondii* infections, and cryptococcal meningitis.

PCP is the most common cause for ICU admissions. The appearance of the chest radiograph is highly variable (see Fig. 21.1). Perinatal PCP may occur as early as 4 weeks of age, but the incidence attains a peak between 3 and 6 months of age. Hospital survival for adults with PCP and respiratory failure was 40% in a retrospective study from 1995 to 1997.[6] In the post-HAART era, survival rates have improved significantly. HAART initiation was an independent predictor for improved survival of patients with severe PCP.[7] The preferred therapy for PCP is intravenous trimethoprim–sulfamethoxazole (TMP–SMX). Corticosteroids significantly improve survival in both adults and children with moderate to severe PCP.[8]

Sepsis is common, especially as the disease progresses, and worsening immune dysfunction occurs. The overall incidence of gram-negative bacteremia was 10.6%. Pathogens isolated in the order of frequency were *Pseudomonas aeruginosa*, nontyphoidal *Salmonella, Escherichia coli*, and *Haemophilus influenzae*.[9] In a recent retrospective study of children with HIV infection, the case-fatality rate due to gram-negative bacteremia was 54.2% in infants and 43.0% in children older than 12 months. Antibiotic drug resistance of bacterial isolates is common and must be anticipated. Initial broad-spectrum empiric therapy is essential.

ORGAN-SPECIFIC ADVERSE REACTIONS TO ANTIRETROVIRAL THERAPY

Neutropenia

Neutropenia is a dose-limiting toxicity of antiretroviral drugs. While it occurs, in particular with azidothymidine (AZT), it also occurs with medications used for long-term prophylaxis against opportunistic infections such as TMP– SMX and ganciclovir. Use of recombinant granulocyte colony-stimulating factor (rG-CSF) leads to an increase in neutrophil number and improvement of microbicidal activity of neutrophils. Reversal of

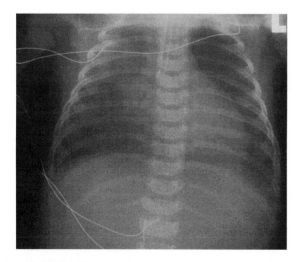

Figure 21.1 *Pneumocystis carinii* pneumonia. This infant with congenital human immunodeficiency virus presented with pneumonia and respiratory failure caused by *P. carinii*. (From Fleisher GR, Ludwig S, and Baskin M. *Atlas of emergency medicine.* Philadelphia, PA: Lippincott Williams & Wilkins, 2004:211.)

HIV-associated neutropenia in studies in adults with HIV infection was significantly correlated with decreased morbidity and mortality due to bacterial infections.[10]

Thrombocytopenia

Thrombocytopenia in children with HIV infection can result from a direct effect of the HIV infection, overwhelming sepsis from opportunistic infections, autoimmune platelet destruction, as a side effect of antiretroviral medications, or splenic sequestration. Preferentially, intravenous immunoglobulin and Rho (D) immune globulin are used for therapy. Rarely will plasmapheresis or splenectomy be necessary.

Coagulopathies

Among the coagulopathies reported in children with HIV infection, there can be decreased activity of natural anticoagulants such as protein S, presence of antiphospholipid–anticardiolipin antibodies, which is known to increase the activated partial thromboplastin time, and increase platelet activation.

Cardiovascular Abnormalities

Cardiovascular abnormalities in children with HIV infection include dilated cardiomyopathy evidenced as decreased left ventricular function.[11] Other vascular lesions included are those within the CNS that manifest as cranial artery aneurysms and acute stroke. Protease inhibitors are known to cause lipid profile disturbances that may impact the onset of cardiovascular disease.

Hepatic Abnormalities

Elevations in the levels of hepatic transaminases can be due to coinfections with hepatitis B or C, acute or reactivated CMV, Epstein-Barr virus (EBV) infection, or disseminated *Mycobacterium* intracellulare complex (MAC) infection. Drug-induced hepatotoxicity is seen with commonly used drugs such as antifungal azoles, macrolides, and rifamycins. The nucleoside reverse transcriptase inhibitor (NRTI) component of the HAART regimen can be the cause of acute and chronic pancreatitis or hepatic steatosis in children with HIV infection. ICU management focuses on parenteral nutrition, pain management, and compartmental fluid balance.

Nephropathy

HIV-associated nephropathy is characterized clinically by proteinuria, azotemia, and enlarged kidneys.[12] In perinatally infected children, the prevalence of nephropathy in the pre-HAART era ranged, depending on ethnicity, from 0.5% to 16%,[13] and was observed in the post-HAART era in up to 12% of patients.[14] Renal complications due to HAART or prophylactic drugs include acute interstitial nephritis, renal tubular damage, crystalluria, and tubular obstruction. In patients with HIV, commonly used antimicrobial agents such as amphotericin B, aminoglycoside antibiotics, and pentamidine are all potentially nephrotoxic and must be adjusted for renal failure.

Hyponatremia, Hypokalemia, and Lactic Acidosis

Hyponatremia is the most common electrolyte abnormality in HIV-infected patients and is often due to fluid losses and less commonly due to inappropriate secretion of antidiuretic hormone (SIADH) or adrenal insufficiency. Hypokalemia may occur as a side effect of drugs such as pentamidine and amphotericin. Lactic acidosis is also a well-documented side effect of the NRTI component of HAART, which results in a high anion-gap metabolic acidosis.

TREATMENT

The goals of therapy are to prevent replication of the virus, which will control the mutagenesis of the HIV virus and prevent drug resistance, and to prevent the progression of immunodeficiency and restore immunologic function delaying the onset of AIDS. Initiation of antiretroviral therapy depends on virologic, immunologic, and clinical criteria. Combination antiretroviral therapy is more effective than monotherapy. Clinical trials demonstrate antiretroviral therapy including a protease inhibitor or a non-NRTI to be the most effective therapeutic means for long-term viral suppression, when >90% adherence with the regimen can be maintained. Except for AZT, no parenteral preparations of antiretrovirals are available. Reduced enteral absorption in patients with circulatory compromise, as well as abrupt discontinuation of antiretroviral combinations with markedly different serum half-life can lead to the development of HIV antiretroviral drug resistance. Both protease inhibitors and non-NRTIs can interfere with the metabolism of drugs, involved with the cytochrome P-450 isoenzyme.

SPECIAL CONSIDERATIONS

Prophylaxis Against Opportunistic Infections

For infants younger than 12 months of age with possible or proven HIV infection, PCP prophylaxis should be started at 4 to 6 weeks of age and continued for the first year of life unless HIV infection is excluded. The need for PCP prophylaxis for HIV-infected children 1 year of age and older is determined by age-specific CD4+ T-lymphocyte counts. Guidelines for the prevention and treatment of opportunistic infection (OIs) in children, adolescents, including PCP, MAC, CMV, and toxoplasmosis prophylaxis are available online (www.aidsinfo.nih.gov).

REFERENCES

1. Cooper S, Lyall H, Walters S, et al. Children with human immunodeficiency virus admitted to a pediatric intensive care unit in the United Kingdom over a 10-year period. *Intensive Care Med.* 2004;30:113–118.
2. Casalino E, Wolff M, Ravaud P, et al. Impact of HAART advent on admission patterns and survival in HIV-infected patients admitted to an intensive care unit. *AIDS.* 2004;18:1429–1433.
3. The European Collaborative Study. Age-related standards for T lymphocyte subsets based on uninfected children born to human immunodeficiency virus 1-infected women. *Pediatr Infect Dis J.* 1992;11(12):1018–1026.
4. Palumbo PE, Raskino C, Fiscus S, et al. Predictive value of quantitative plasma HIV RNA and CD4+ lymphocyte count in HIV-infected infants and children. *JAMA.* 1998;279(10):756–761.
5. Frederick T, Mascola L, Eller A, et al. Progression of human immunodeficiency virus disease among infants and children infected perinatally with human immunodeficiency virus or through neonatal blood transfusion. Los Angeles County Pediatric AIDS Consortium and the Los Angeles County-University of Southern California Medical Center and the University of Southern California School of Medicine. *Pediatr Infect Dis J.* 1994;13(12):1091–1097.
6. Randall Curtis J, Yarnold PR, Schwartz DN, et al. Improvements in outcomes of acute respiratory failure for patients with human immunodeficiency virus-related Pneumocystis carinii pneumonia. *Am J Respir Crit Care Med.* 2000;162:393–398.
7. Morris A, Wachter RM, Luce J, et al. Improved survival with highly active antiretroviral therapy in HIV-infected patients with severe Pneumocystis carinii pneumonia. *AIDS.* 2003;17:73–80.
8. Gatell JM, Marrades R, el-Ebiary M, et al. Severe pulmonary infections in AIDS patients. *Semin Respir Infect.* 1996;11:119–128.
9. Rongkavilit C, Rodriguez ZM, Gomez-Marin O, et al. Gram-negative bacillary bacteremia in human immunodeficiency virus type 1-infected children. *Pediatr Infect Dis J.* 2000;19(2):122–128.
10. Kuritzkes DR. Neutropenia, neutrophil dysfunction, and bacterial infection in patients with human immunodeficiency virus disease: The role of granulocyte colony-stimulating factor. *Clin Infect Dis.* 2000;30(2):256–260.
11. Harmon WG, Dadlani GH, Fisher SD, et al. Myocardial and pericardial disease in HIV. *Curr Treat Options Cardiovasc Med.* 2002; 4(6):497–509.
12. Kimmel PL, Bosch JP, Vassalotti JA. Treatment of human immunodeficiency virus (HIV)-associated nephropathy. *Semin Nephrol.* 1998;18(4):446–458.
13. Zilleruelo G, Strauss J. HIV nephropathy in children. *Pediatr Clin North Am.* 1995;42(6):1469–1485.
14. Garcia I, Merchan A, Chaparro PE, et al. Overview of the HIV/tuberculosis coinfection in Bogota, Colombia, 2001. *Biomedica.* 2004;24(suppl. 1):132–137.

RECOMMENDED READINGS

1. Hilbert G, Gruson D, Vargas F, et al. Non-invasive ventilation in immunosuppressed patients. *Rev Mal Respir.* 2003;20:68–76.
2. Huault G. Development of intensive care for pediatric infectious diseases over the last 20 years. *Arch Pediatr.* 2001; 8(suppl. 4):665s–672s.
3. Leifeld L, Rockstroh J, Skaide S, et al. Indication, outcome and follow up of intensive care in patients with HIV-infection. *Eur J Med Res.* 2000;5:199–202.
4. Notterman DA. Pediatric AIDS and critical care. *Crit Care Med.* 1993;21:S319–S321.
5. Richard N, Stamm D, Floret D. Pneumocystis carinii infections in a pediatric intensive care unit: A retrospective study 1980–2002. *Arch Pediatr.* 2003;10(suppl. 5):539s–544s.
6. Rosenberg AL, Seneff MG, Atiyeh L, et al. The importance of bacterial sepsis in intensive care unit patients with acquired immunodeficiency syndrome: Implications for future care in the age of increasing antiretroviral resistance. *Crit Care Med.* 2001;29: 548–556.
7. Vincent B, Timsit JF, Auburtin M, et al. Characteristics and outcomes of HIV-infected patients in the ICU: Impact of the highly active antiretroviral treatment era. *Intensive Care Med.* 2004;30: 859–866.

Health Care–Associated Infections

Jennifer Hurst   Nalini Singh

Health care–associated infections (HAIs) are important for the pediatric intensivist because they are common occurrences associated with a high overall (11%) and age-adjusted mortality. The risk factors for the transmission of pathogens in critically ill children are well known and are greater because of the increased need for physical contact between the patients and the providers. Most importantly, many of these infections are preventable with an approach that includes management of risk factors, prevention of infection, and attention to patient safety. This section, outlines the epidemiology of major HAI surveillance, prevention, and control practices.

EPIDEMIOLOGY

The epidemiology of HAI among hospitalized children in pediatric intensive care units (PICUs) has been described by the Centers for Disease Control and Prevention-National Nosocomial Infection Surveillance (CDC-NNIS) system and the point prevalence study of PICU patients of the Pediatric Prevention Network (PPNs). Primary blood stream infections (28%), followed by pneumonia (21%), and urinary tract infections (15%) are the most frequent HAIs in PICU patients.[1] The remaining HAIs include lower respiratory tract infections other than pneumonia (tracheitis), surgical site, eye, ear, nose, or throat, gastrointestinal, skin, and soft tissue, and cardiovascular infections. More than 70% of HAI occur in children <5 years of age. Of these, most (39%) infections occur in infants <2 months of age. According to multicenter studies, the frequency of HAI in individual PICUs varies from 11% to 27%.[2]

The CDC-NNIS reports blood stream, urinary tract infection, and pneumonia rates of 6.6 (0.9 to 11.2), 2.9 (0 to 8.1), and 4 (0 to 8.1) per 1,000 device days, respectively.[3] The cost per incident bloodstream infection (BSI) in the PICU is estimated at approximately $46,000.[4] Coagulase-negative staphylococci (38%) and gram-negative rods (25%) are the most common pathogens causing BSI. *Pseudomonas aeruginosa* (22%) followed by *Staphylococcus aureus* (17%) and viral pathogens, such as respiratory syncytial virus, were the most common pathogens causing pneumonia. Gram-negative rods followed by fungi mostly caused urinary tract infections. Of these, *Escherichia coli* (19%) and *Candida albicans* (14%) were the most common pathogens.

Surgical site infections cause approximately 6% to 10% of HAI in the PICU. The most common surgical procedures included cardiovascular surgery (41%), gastrointestinal surgery (24%), neurosurgery (13%), transplant surgery (8%), orthopedic surgery (5%), vascular surgery (3%), and head and neck surgery (3%). *S. aureus* (34%), *P. aeruginosa* (16%), and coagulase-negative staphylococci (23%) were the most common pathogens associated with surgical site infections after cardiovascular, gastrointestinal, and neurosurgical procedures.[1]

Multidrug-resistant organisms, such as methicillin-resistant *Staphylococcus aureus* (MRSA), vancomycin-resistant *Enterococcus* (VRE), and resistance to third-generation cephalosporins, such as resistant *Enterobacteriaceae* extended-spectrum β-lactamase (ESBL)-producing gram-negative rods, have emerged as major causes of HAI. According to the CDC-NNIS, in the United States, the incidence of multidrug-resistant organisms continues to increase in the intensive care units (ICUs).[3] As of 2004, approximately 60% of *S. aureus* isolates were MRSA and 89% of coagulase-negative staphylococci were resistant to methicillin, 28.5% of enterococcal isolates were VRE and 20% of *Klebsiella pneumoniae* were resistant to third-generation cephalosporins. This increase continues despite the implementation of standard infection control measures. Limited data exist for specific resistance rates for children admitted to the PICU.[5]

In a national point prevalence survey performed by the PPN, approximately 20% of gram-negative bacteria were resistant to third-generation cephalosporins. The clinical manifestations of HAI with multidrug-resistant organisms are indistinguishable from susceptible organisms, thereby making diagnosis and treatment a challenge. Identifying children at risk of developing HAI can be complex, and risk models have attempted to provide objective criteria to identify children with the highest risk of acquiring HAI. Models to predict a future event such as the risk of developing an HAI incorporated intrinsic and extrinsic risk factors for interhospital comparison.[6,7] The best predictors for HAI infections were device utilization ratio, antimicrobial therapy, and length of stay. Many of the difficulties in comparing interhospital rates can be decreased using standardized surveillance methodologies.

SURVEILLANCE

Surveillance is a tool that provides for the regular, ongoing collection and analysis of data to establish baselines and identify trends. Surveillance data are important for infection prevention and control activities, and heightens PICU staff awareness of such efforts. Specifically in the PICU, surveillance should be conducted to detect risk factors for HAIs, including the presence of invasive devices, indwelling catheters, and the compliance with infection control policies, such as the implementation of the correct isolation precautions. The number of total patient and device days is used as the denominator for calculating device-associated infection rates. Utilizing appropriate denominator data, site-specific infection rates such as catheter-associated BSI, ventilator-associated pneumonia, and urinary tract infection rates can be calculated. In the United States, the CDC-NNIS is the primary data source on the epidemiology of HAIs. Member institutions voluntarily submit their infection data, and benchmarks are established that allow these institutions to comparatively analyze infection rates. Reports published by the CDC-NNIS provide information on site-specific device-associated infection rates and can be used as external benchmarks. These infection rates are reported as 10th to 90th percentiles including pooled mean and device utilization ratios. The device utilization of a PICU is a measure of the unit's invasive practice and is an external risk factor for HAI. Device utilization can also serve as a marker for severity of illness for PICU patients. If the infection rates are below the 10th or above the 90th percentile, this may indicate either under-reporting or high rates of HAI.

PREVENTION AND CONTROL EFFORTS

Hand Hygiene

Good hand hygiene is the cornerstone of an effective infection control program in the PICU. However, health care providers often fail to recognize its primary role in the reduction of morbidity and mortality. Adequate hand hygiene is used <50% of the total opportunities, and one study done in the PICU showed the overall compliance among nurses, respiratory therapists, and physicians to be 34%. Reasons for this poor compliance have included complaints of skin dryness and irritation from hand hygiene products, lack of supplies, poor placement of sinks, and insufficient time. Alcohol-based hand gels have provided an effective strategy to avert many of these reasons for ineffective hand hygiene. In the absence of visible blood or body fluids, these gels are even more efficacious in decreasing the infectious pathogens on hands than traditional soap and water. These gels are easily mounted in convenient locations, require less time for application, and cause less skin irritation. Therefore, intensive care providers should take advantage of these products.[3]

Early and Accurate Isolation Precautions

Standard and transmission-based precautions are effective strategies to prevent the transmission of infectious organisms from health care workers (HCW) to patients and vice versa. Standard precautions are used in caring for all patients when there is the potential to come into contact with blood, body fluids, secretions, excretions, mucous membranes, and nonintact skin either when directly caring for the patient or when the provider may get in contact with used equipment or soiled linen. In addition to good hand hygiene, it includes the use of barrier devices such as gloves, gowns, masks, and goggles to prevent cross-contamination. Contaminated linen, waste, equipment, and sharp instruments should be disposed of in separate biohazardous waste containers, as per the recommendations of the Occupational Safety and Health Administration (OSHA).

On the basis of clinical syndromes or diagnoses, patients may be placed on transmission-based precautions (see Tables 22.1 and 22.2). Transmission-based precautions are used because there is a potential for contracting or passing infectious organisms or illnesses by one of three modes—contact, droplet, or airborne. Contact transmission is the most frequent route of transmission. It can occur by either direct or indirect contact with infective substances and/or equipment. Using a private room, cohorting patients, wearing a gown and gloves for all patient contact, and appropriate hand hygiene can prevent contact transmission. Droplet transmission occurs when droplets containing microorganisms are transmitted over a short distance (usually defined as ≤3 feet) and come in contact with the mucous membranes of a potential host. Droplet precautions require the use of a private room, cohorting of affected patients, and using a mask for direct patient care. Airborne transmission occurs with small particles (usually defined as <5 μm in size) that contain microorganisms that can be propelled over large distances and that which circulate in the environment for extended periods (up to 1 hour).

TABLE 22.1

CLINICAL SYNDROMES OR CONDITIONS WARRANTING ADDITIONAL EMPIRIC PRECAUTIONS TO PREVENT TRANSMISSION OF EPIDEMIOLOGICALLY IMPORTANT PATHOGENS PENDING CONFIRMATION OF DIAGNOSIS

Clinical Syndrome or Condition	Potential Pathogens	Empiric Precautions
Diarrhea		
Acute diarrhea with a likely infectious cause in an incontinent or diapered patient	Enteric pathogens	Standard plus contact
Meningitis		
	Neisseria meningitidis	Droplet for first 24 h of antimicrobial therapy; mask and face protection for intubation
	Enteroviruses	Contact for infants and children
Rash or Exanthems, Generalized, Etiology Unknown		
Petechial/ecchymotic with fever	*N. meningitidis*	Droplet for first 24 h of antimicrobial therapy
Vesicular	Varicella, smallpox, or vaccinia virus	Airborne infection isolation plus contact; contact if vaccinia
Maculopapular with cough, coryza, and fever	Rubeola (measles) virus	Airborne infection isolation
Respiratory Infections		
Respiratory infections, particularly bronchiolitis and pneumonia, in infants and young children	Respiratory syncytial, parainfluenza, adeno, influenza viruses	Contract plus droplet; droplet may be discontinued when adenovirus and influenza have been ruled out
Cough/fever/upper lobe pulmonary infiltrate in an HIV-negative patient or a patient at low risk for human immunodeficiency virus (HIV) infection	*Mycobacterium tuberculosis*; severe acute respiratory syndrome virus (SARS-CoV)	Airborne infection isolation; add contact plus eye protection if history of SARS exposure, travel
Cough/fever/pulmonary infiltrate in any lung location in an HIV-infected patient or a patient at high risk for HIV infection	*M. tuberculosis*	Airborne infection isolation

Adapted from Richards MJ, Edwards JR, Culver DH, et al. Nosocomial infections in pediatric intensive care units in the United States. National nosocomial infections surveillance system. *Pediatrics.* 1999;103:e39.

In caring for these patients, a private room with negative air pressure, and the National Institute for Occupational Safety and Health (NIOSH)–approved N-95 or higher respirators should be worn.[8] Table 22.2 provides a list of specific diagnoses that require transmission-based precautions.

Aseptic Technique

Central venous access devices, which are commonly used in critically ill patients, have a substantially higher rate of infection than peripheral intravenous catheters. Aseptic technique refers to the use of maximal barrier precautions when inserting, manipulating, and maintaining these devices. It has been shown that during insertion of intravenous catheters, the use of a large sterile drape, sterile gown, sterile gloves, and mask decreases the incidence of

BSIs compared to the use of only sterile gloves and smaller sterile drapes.[9]

Skin antisepsis is the preparation of the skin before an invasive procedure and is warranted any time this first line of defense against infection is bypassed. Until 2000, the most common antiseptics were 70% alcohol and 10% povidone-iodine. The newest approved product, 0.5% chlorhexidine gluconate has been shown to be effective in both immediate disinfection and residual skin decolonization. A range of skin preparations may be selected depending on the extent of the intrusion. Alcohol-based products can be used to eliminate skin flora for simple procedures such as peripheral IV insertion. The skin should be cleansed with the alcohol solution for at least 30 seconds before the procedure. Povidone-iodine inactivates skin flora upon drying and is appropriate for the aseptic technique with invasive and surgical procedures. Commonly referred to as Betadine,

TABLE 22.2

DESCRIPTION OF ROUTINE PRECAUTION TYPES AND EXAMPLES OF SPECIFIC CONDITIONS REQUIRING THESE PRECAUTIONS

	Standard Precautions	Contact Precautions	Droplet Precautions	Airborne Precautions

Description	■ Hand hygiene
	■ PPE when anticipated contact with blood or body fluids
	  • Gloves
	  • Gowns
	  • Face masks
	  • Eye shields
	■ Minimal contact with soiled linen
	■ Proper disinfection of patient care equipment
		Standard precautions +
		■ Gown/glove with all patient care
		■ Private room if available
		■ May cohort patients with same infectious disease diagnoses e.g., respiratory syncytial virus
			Standard precautions +
			■ Mask with all patient care within 3 feet of patient
			■ Private room
				Standard precautions +
				■ N-95 respirator or higher face mask; powered air purifying respirator for bearded men or those who are not protected by N-95 (failed fit testing)
				■ Private room with negative airflow and HEPA filtration

Examples of specific disease/conditions requiring isolation	■ Applies to all patients	■ Multidrug resistant bacteria (e.g., ESBLs producing gram-negative rods, VRE, MRSA) ■ *Clostridium difficile* colitis ■ Hemorrhagic colitis due to *Escherichia coli* 0157:H7 or *Shigella* ■ Abscess or draining wound ■ Croup/parainfluenza virus ■ Bronchiolitis/respiratory syncytial virus	■ Influenza ■ *Neisseria meningitidis* ■ Parvovirus B-19 ■ Pertussis ■ Serious invasive Streptococcal disease	■ *Mycobacterium tuberculosis* ■ Measles virus ■ Varicella-zoster virus ■ Severe acute respiratory syndrome (in combination with contact precautions)

PPE, personal protective patient; HEPA, high efficiency particulate air; ESBL, Enterobacteriaceae-extended spectrum β-lactamase; VRE, vancomycin-resistant enterococcus; MRSA, methicillin resistant *Staphylococcus aureus*.

this antiseptic should be applied in concentric circles outward from the procedure or incision site for maximal effectiveness and allowed to completely dry. Chlorhexidine can be used any time if skin asepsis is warranted except in the premature neonate (<36 weeks). Chlorhexidine need not be applied in concentric circles, but the entire surface of the skin should be cleansed for at least 30 seconds.

Process of Care

Establishment and adherence to evidence-based care practices are of benefit in the prevention of HAI. In a study conducted by Yogaraj et al., it was suggested that risk factors for developing BSIs in the PICU were more directly related to the process of care than the severity of illness (see Fig. 22.1). These factors included the frequent manipulation of multiple central venous catheters, use of arterial

catheters, performance of procedures at the bedside, and movement of the patient out of the PICU.[10]

Perhaps one of the best predictors for the development of catheter-associated infections (CAI) is the duration of catheterization. Timely discontinuation of invasive devices is of central importance to decreasing the risk of HAI. For example, it has been shown that for each day that an arterial catheter remains in place, the risk of CAI increases 3% to 5%, and by 21 days, the risk of infection is as high as 60%. In addition, the risk of contamination of the IV ports increases with the length of catheterization and frequency. Intravenous tubing should be changed in accordance with recommendations from CDC, and ports of entry should be cleansed with alcohol for at least 10 seconds before access.[11] The use of tubing with three-way stopcocks and intermittent flush systems which can be opened to the air should also be avoided because they could contribute to

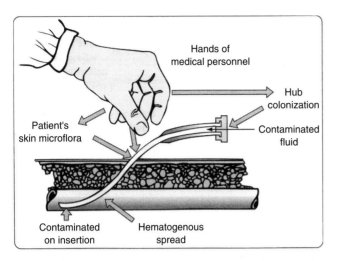

Figure 22.1 Potential sources for contamination of intravascular devices. Intravascular catheters can become colonized or infected with a variety of organisms from various sites, including the normal flora of the skin, pathogens introduced on the hands of health care workers, and—less likely—contaminated devices and infusates. (From Bone RC, Campbell GD, Payne DK. *Bone's atlas of pulmonary and critical care medicine*. Philadelphia, PA: Lippincott Williams & Wilkins; 2001:168.)

colonization of the tubing and subsequent infection in the patient. Instead, a system that employs a continuous flush system should be utilized.

In a study conducted by Elward et al. it was suggested that the risk factors for developing ventilator-associated pneumonias in the PICU were also more directly related to the process of care than the severity of illness. These factors included the diagnosis of a genetic syndrome, reintubation, and transfer out of the PICU.[12] Basic hygiene and positioning measures can help to reduce the rate of ventilator-associated pneumonias. These measures include an oral hygiene regimen with subglottic suctioning as frequently as every 2 hours and the prone or the semirecumbent position (45 degree angle).[12] Table 22.3 provides the recommended practice principles for the prevention of ventilator-associated pneumonia and CAI.

The institution of appropriate antimicrobial prophylaxis before surgery is an important component of patient care in the PICU. Optimal prophylaxis ensures that an adequate concentration of an appropriate antimicrobial agent is present in the blood, tissue, and wound during the entire time the incision is open and while there is a risk of bacterial contamination. The appropriate antimicrobial should be administered approximately 60 minutes before the surgical incision. For cardiothoracic, orthopedic, or vascular surgeries the recommended antimicrobial prophylaxis is cefazolin or cefuroxime. In the presence of a β-lactam allergy or sensitivity, vancomycin or clindamycin are the suggested alternatives. The duration of treatment following surgery is generally 24 to 72 hours. However, the most recent guidelines propose that <24 hours of therapy is sufficient.[13]

Implementing a system that ensures that antibiotics with appropriate sensitivities are used against pathogens and the institution uses antimicrobial agents judiciously is important. A multidisciplinary committee to review the antimicrobial utilization patterns and compare them with resistance patterns is useful for minimizing selective pressures, and may be part of a hospital program to prevent and control multidrug-resistant organisms.[8]

Education

The OSHA requires that the education of health care workers occur on the principles of infection control, at least annually. This education is generally performed by the Infection Control Program and should provide the health care provider with the knowledge and skills necessary to protect themselves and their patients from contracting or passing communicable illnesses. In addition to the basic infection control information, the feedback of targeted infection rates to unit staff is a positive motivator for the reduction of infection rates.

Environmental Control

Microorganisms can live for extended periods on surfaces and if they are able to gain entry into a host they can create disease. The purpose of cleaning, disinfection, and sterilization is to reduce the risk of this environmental transmission. Policies on the appropriate methods of cleaning should be established for environmental surfaces and equipment in the hospital. Equipment that will come into contact with the mucous membranes such as endoscopes and intubation equipment require a high-level of disinfection. Instruments that enter sterile body cavities must be sterilized. Defective bronchoscopes and improper disinfection or sterilization of equipment has led to poor outcomes in patients.[14,15] After utilizing reusable patient care items, they should be sent to the sterile processing department of the health care facility for processing before reuse. Many facilities now practice event-related sterilization rather than dated expiration. This means that sterile items do not have expiration dates printed on them and are considered sterile unless the integrity of the packaging is compromised. This is an effective and efficient model of practice. However, in this model, the responsibility for assuring package integrity is placed upon the practitioner. It is important that the nurse, physician, or patient care technician inspect all sterile item packaging before using it for patient procedures. If damaged, dusty, wet, or otherwise compromised, the item should not be used and should be returned to the sterile processing area for resterilization.

TABLE 22.3

RECOMMENDED PRACTICE PRINCIPLES FOR THE PREVENTION OF VENTILATOR-ASSOCIATED PNEUMONIA AND CATHETER-ASSOCIATED INFECTIONS

Prevention of Catheter-Associated Bloodstream Infections	Prevention of Ventilator-Associated Pneumonia	When to Call an Infection Control Practitioner
■ Wash hands before insertion or manipulation ■ Use maximal sterile precautions during insertion procedure ■ Disinfect all access ports with alcohol for 10 s prior to use ■ Place a line with the least amount of access ports as is possible ■ Change IV administration sets every 72 h ■ Do not touch sterile IV tubing connections or allow them to come into contact with nonsterile surfaces ■ Take out all devices as soon as clinically prudent	■ Position patient to decrease potential for aspiration of oropharyngeal secretions in either the prone or semirecumbent position ■ Practice subglottic suctioning with a sterile catheter every 2 h and as needed ■ Practice good oral hygiene, including the use of antiseptic mouthwash at least every 4 h ■ Wash hands and use clean gloves before all procedures ■ Follow hospital policy for the maintenance and routine care of respiratory equipment	■ When a patient is diagnosed or suspected of having a reportable communicable illness[a] ■ When there has been a staff or patient exposure to a communicable disease, including blood borne pathogens, tuberculosis, chicken pox, pertussis, scabies, or other concerning illness ■ When there is a concern for suspected nosocomial spread of a communicable illness or pathogen ■ Clarification on hospital infection control policy

[a]The CDC yearly publishes the list of reportable illnesses which should be available in the Epidemiology/Infection Control Program policy and on the CDC Website. These illnesses are reported to the local department of health for national tracking.

Collaboration of the Health Care Team and Administrative Support

The education of HCW will provide the basic foundation for good infection control knowledge. Clinical implementation of standard and transmission-based precautions will promote environmental safety. However, frequent communication and interdisciplinary collaboration yields the greatest benefit. The involvement of providers in infection-control decision making is imperative for the success of infection control preventative interventions.[16] In addition, this approach provides the ability to push evidence-based best practices to the patient–provider interface and improve the organization's culture. Collaboration between the intensive care providers and the infection control professionals is essential to combating hospital-acquired infections.

REFERENCES

1. Richards MJ, Edwards JR, Culver DH, et al. Nosocomial infections in pediatric intensive care units in the United States. National Nosocomial Infections Surveillance System. *Pediatrics.* 1999;103:e39
2. Grohskopf LA, Sinkowitz-Cochran RL, Garrett DO, et al. A national point-prevalence survey of pediatric intensive care unit-acquired infections in the United States. *J Pediatr.* 2002;140: 432–438.
3. Healthcare Infection Control Practices Advisory Committee and Hand-Hygiene Task Force; Society for Healthcare Epidemiology of America; Association for Professionals in Infection Control and Epidemiology; Infection Diseases Society of America. Guideline for hand hygiene in healthcare settings. *J Am Coll Surg.* 2004;198:121–127.
4. Slonim AD, Kurtines HC, Sprague BM, et al. The costs associated with nosocomial bloodstream infections in the pediatric intensive care unit. *Pediatr Crit Care Med.* 2001;2:170–174.
5. Siegel JDK, Karen K, Levine G, et al. Prevalence of antimicrobial resistant bacteria in Pediatric Prevention Network (PPN) Intensive Care Units (ICUs). *Abstracts of the IDSA 39th Annual Meeting,* 2001:311.
6. Singh-Naz N, Sprague BM, Patel KM, et al. Risk assessment and standardized nosocomial infection rate in critically ill children. *Crit Care Med.* 2000;28:2069–2075.
7. Arantes A, Carvalho Eda S, Medeiros EA, et al. Pediatric risk of mortality and hospital infection. *Infect Control Hosp Epidemiol.* 2004;25:783–785.
8. Pirwitz S. HICPAC guidelines for isolation precautions: Hospital infection control practices advisory committee. *Am J Infect Control Practices Advisory Committee.* 1997; 25:287–888. Guideline for isolation precautions: Preventing transmission of infectious agents in healthcare settings. 2004.
9. Raad II, Hohn DC, Gilbreath BJ, et al. Prevention of central venous catheter-related infections by using maximal sterile barrier precautions during insertion. *Infect Control Hosp Epidemiol.* 1994; 15:231–238.
10. Yogaraj JS, Elward AM, Fraser VJ. Rate, risk factors, and outcomes of nosocomial primary bloodstream infection in pediatric intensive care unit patients. *Pediatrics.* 2002;110:481–485.
11. O'Grady NP, Alexander M, Dellinger EP, et al. Guidelines for the prevention of intravascular catheter-related infections. *Infect Control Hosp Epidemiol.* 2002;23:759–769.
12. Elward AM. Pediatric ventilator-associated pneumonia. *Pediatr Infect Dis J.* 2003;22:445–446.
13. Bratzler DW, Houck PM. Antimicrobial prophylaxis for surgery: An advisory statement from the National Surgical Infection Prevention Project. *Clin Infect Dis.* 2004;38:1706–1715.
14. Alvarado CJ, Reichelderfer M. APIC guideline for infection prevention and control in flexible endoscopy. Association for Professionals in Infection Control. *Am J Infect Control.* 2000;28:138–155.
15. Singh N, Belen O, Leger MM, et al. Cluster of trichosporon mucoids in children associated with a faulty bronchoscope. *Pediatr Infect Dis J.* 2003;22:609–612.
16. Coombs M, Ersser SJ. Medical hegemony in decision-making–a barrier to interdisciplinary working in intensive care? *J Adv Nurs.* 2004;46:245–252.

Systemic Inflammatory Response Syndrome

23

M. Nilufer Yalindag-Ozturk   **Oral Alpan**

The term *Systemic inflammatory response syndrome* (SIRS) describes the generalized reaction of a host to a nonspecific insult, which can be due to an infectious etiology, or due to noninfectious causes such as trauma, pancreatitis, and burns. This reaction is characterized by a cascade of events, which may lead to severe endothelial damage, and to microvascular and hemodynamic disturbances (see Fig. 23.1). When SIRS presents as a result of an infection, it is called sepsis. Irrespective of the etiology, SIRS can progress to multiple organ dysfunction syndrome (MODS) and death. This terminology was introduced in 1991 at a consensus conference of the American College of Chest Physicians and Society of Critical Care because of the apparent need for a uniform language to report and compare interventions and to establish inclusion criteria for clinical trials in sepsis.[1]

EPIDEMIOLOGY

The incidence of SIRS/sepsis has been difficult to assess owing to inconsistencies in definitions. It is estimated that approximately 750,000 American adults are affected every year with severe sepsis, with a mortality rate that ranges from 28% to 60%. The most comprehensive epidemiologic study in children reported an incidence of 0.56 cases per 1,000 population per year, with infants being particularly at risk.[2] The in-hospital mortality rate was 10%. Half of the patients who died had an underlying disease. The death rate increased progressively with the number of failed organ systems (7% with single organ failure to 53.1% with four or more failing organs). The mean length of stay and cost were 31 days and $40,600, respectively. Estimated annual total costs were $1.97 billion nationally.

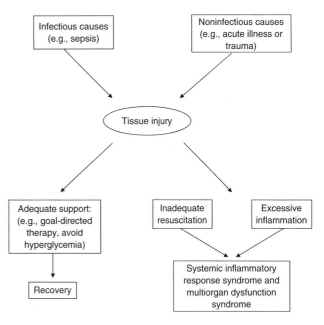

Figure 23.1 The relationships between the causes of systemic inflammatory response, their effect on tissues, and how interventions may affect the outcome.

PATHOGENESIS

Although many different mechanisms for SIRS have been proposed, none of them have explained the exact immune characteristics of the response. Why should both an infectious and noninfectious insult create a seemingly similar response, and what kind of systemic response is seen in SIRS?

The Danger model of the immune system seems to explain some of the features of SIRS. It suggests that the immune system is more associated with damage than with foreignness, and is called into action by alarm signals from the injured tissues (infectious or noninfectious), rather than by the recognition of nonself.[3] Cells dying by the normal programmed processes are usually scavenged before they disintegrate, whereas cells that die by necrosis release their contents, and any released intracellular product could potentially be a danger signal. The important feature is that danger or alarm signals should not be sent by healthy cells or by cells undergoing normal physiologic deaths. Resting antigen-presenting cells can be activated by one of the following four processes:

1. Toll-like receptors (TLRs) which bind a wide range of biologic molecules;
2. Tissue injury resulting in the release of endogenous, nonforeign alarm signals, including mammalian DNA, RNA, heat shock proteins, interferon-α (an inducible protein often made by virus-infected cells), interleukin-1, CD40-L (a surface molecule on activated platelets and T cells), and breakdown products of hyaluron (made when vessels are damaged);
3. Nucleotide-binding oligomerization domain (NOD) receptors, which respond to both injury or pathogen-related signals and normal physiologic signals involved with apoptosis;
4. And finally, any hydrophobic portion (Hyppo) of a given molecule, which is buried in the depths of that molecule, but could act as an alarm signal if exposed.

Recently, there has been a major influx of information related to the inflammatory response at the cellular and molecular level. Interactions between the metabolic, neural, endocrine, and immune systems seem to play important roles in the inflammatory responses. Measurements of single mediators and their inhibitors do not seem to reflect the overall picture because they can exhibit different actions in different physical settings or toward different cell types. The natural tendency is to think in linear terms about a response, but the extensive feedback and cross-regulatory activities of the body can yield very nonlinear, even chaotic system behavior. Complex systems often display all or none of the responses; the consequence is that small differences in both the nature of inputs (insult) and the state of an individual host's immune system can lead to very different outcomes.

The most popular theory for SIRS is that inflammation causes additional harm to the host by creating endothelial damage, microvascular derangements, tissue hypoxia, and possibly by causing MODS while fighting off the initial insult. Immunologically, this can be explained by an immune response of the wrong class. This is commonly seen in autoimmune disorders, where an inappropriate immune response to a pathogen (e.g., a T_H1 response in the intestinal tract or the eye) can lead to tissue destruction. SIRS may result from an inappropriate systemic response. For example, experimental animal data showed that high tumor necrosis factor (TNF) levels in the blood correlated with the severity of sepsis. Blocking the mediator resulted in a decreased mortality. In human trials, blockage of the proinflammatory mediators was uniformly unsuccessful. One likely reason was that patients with sepsis are a heterogeneous group of patients that present at very different stages of their illness. The targets for these trials were the early sepsis mediators, but the administration and the timing of therapy could simply have been wrong, given the lead-time of the patient's disease. Alternatively, there is current interest in late mediators of sepsis like the high mobility group box 1 (HMGB1) protein, and animal studies show that its inhibition reverses lethality, suggesting a potentially therapeutic role for sepsis during a wider clinically relevant treatment window.

Anti-inflammatory therapies may also fail with sepsis/SIRS because there could be a change toward the anti-inflammatory state over time. This phase is called compensatory anti-inflammatory response syndrome (CARS) and it deserves special attention because definitive evidence for a dominant systemic inflammatory response has been difficult to obtain. Although numerous studies have suggested major proinflammatory forces at local sites of infection or injury, it has not been possible to demonstrate their dominance in the circulation or distant tissues. According to a different view by Munford and Pugin, the body's systemic anti-inflammatory responses to stress may not be simply compensatory, but they dominate outside the affected local site. Stresses such as strenuous exercise, cold exposure, or a major injury trigger have many of the same adaptations. Normal responses to injury usually prevent systemic inflammation and can sometimes be immunosuppressive, allowing survival and the further multiplication of microorganisms that enter the host through disrupted epithelia.[4] Other findings suggestive of systemic anti-inflammatory states in SIRS/sepsis are the loss of delayed type hypersensitivity, an inability to clear infection, or a predisposition to nosocomial infections. Autopsy studies performed in children with sepsis and MODS show an 80% incidence of persistent or unrecognized infection.[5] Adult autopsy series demonstrate less severe damage than expected for the clinical condition, show a profound apoptosis-induced loss of cells of the adaptive immune system.[6] Depending on the pathogen, apoptosis of host cells may be beneficial or detrimental to host survival. Whether or when apoptosis can be targeted is an area that deserves further exploration.

DIAGNOSIS

SIRS is defined by the presence of at least two abnormalities of temperature, respiratory rate, heart rate, and white blood cell count. Although very sensitive, the SIRS criteria are nonspecific, and have been revised twice in international

TABLE 23.1

DEFINITIONS OF SYSTEMIC INFLAMMATORY RESPONSE SYNDROME, SEPSIS, SEVERE SEPSIS, AND SEPTIC SHOCK

SIRS	Minimum two criteria required, *one of which must be* either abnormal temperature or leukocyte count
	■ Core temperature of >38.5°C or <36°C
	■ Unexplained tachycardia (mean HR>2SD), or bradycardia <1 y
	■ Tachypnea (mean RR>2SD) or mechanical ventilation for an acute process
	■ Leukopenia or 10% immature neutrophils
Sepsis	SIRS in the presence or the result of suspected or proven infection
Severe sepsis	Sepsis plus one of the following:
	■ Cardiovascular dysfunction
	■ Acute respiratory distress syndrome,
	■ Two or more organ dysfunctions (see Table 23.2)
Septic shock	Sepsis and cardiovascular organ dysfunction

HR, heart rate; RR, respiratory rate; SIRS, systemic inflammatory response syndrome; SD, standard deviation.
Modified from Carcillo JA, Fields AI. Clinical practical parameters for hemodynamic support of pediatric and neonatal patients with septic shock. American College of Critical Care Medicine Task Force Committee Members. *Crit Care Med.* 2002;30:1365–1378.

expert meetings, resulting in some additions, but not in major definition changes because of the lack of evidence to support a change. The recently proposed pediatric-specific SIRS-sepsis and organ dysfunction criteria were developed in 2002 and are summarized in Tables 23.1 and 23.2.[7]

Although useful for identifying the population at risk, SIRS criteria do not allow precise staging or prognostication of the host's response. Therefore, a hypothetical model, called PIRO, is being evaluated, which may characterize the syndrome on the basis of predisposing factors and premorbid conditions (P), the nature and extent of the insult (I), the nature and magnitude of host responses (R), and the degree of the resultant organ dysfunction (O). The objective of this model would be to develop interventions on the basis of the nature of the response, to evaluate baseline risk factors on the basis of premorbid condition and genetic predisposition, and to quantify organ dysfunction. This model has the potential to differentiate morbidity arising from an insult versus morbidity arising from the response to the insult.

The definition of sepsis does not require a proven infection; the diagnosis can be made by a high clinical suspicion. Microorganisms are only isolated in half of the patients with SIRS and MODS, despite a clinical picture that resembles sepsis. Potential biomarkers for differentiating infectious from noninfectious causes of SIRS lack adequate specificity, although procalcitonin (PCT) and C-reactive protein (CRP) appear to hold the most promise. PCT is a propeptide of calcitonin, and the levels are low in healthy individuals (<0.1 ng per mL). Various conditions such as major surgery, tissue trauma, and prolonged circulatory failure may induce PCT elevation, although the rise of PCT under those conditions is not as high as in sepsis. Levels exceeding 10 ng per mL are almost

exclusively seen in severe sepsis. CRP is an acute-phase protein, which is released by the liver after the onset of inflammation or tissue damage. During infections, CRP has both proinflammatory and anti-inflammatory effects, but the levels do not adequately reflect the severity and the kinetics are slower.

TREATMENT

The treatment of SIRS remains supportive. The timely recognition and early supportive interventions are key factors. Early and adequate fluid resuscitation is of fundamental importance, and it reduces mortality. Goal-directed therapy predefines the resuscitation end points for clinicians. Recent studies based on the task force guidelines of the American College of Critical Care Medicine[8] reported mortality ranging from 5% to 10%. The choice of vasoactive and inotropic agents depends on clinical findings (warm vs. cold shock) and invasive hemodynamic data.[8] Therapeutic goals include improving end-organ perfusion, and are measured by the surrogates of capillary refill, a good pulse strength without a differential between the central and peripheral pulses, warm extremities, adequate urine output, normal mental status, decreased lactate, normalization of base deficit, and goal-mixed venous oxygen saturation (>70%). Evidence is accumulating that fluid balance correlates with the outcome, and fluid overload predicts survival in MODS in critically ill patients.[9] MODS is associated with high mortality in children, ranging from 35% to 54%. Renal replacement therapies are used frequently in this setting, although some small underpowered randomized controlled trials (RCTs) failed to demonstrate any significant change in the outcome. Retrospective pediatric studies

TABLE 23.2

ORGAN DYSFUNCTION CRITERIA

Cardiovascular dysfunction	Despite fluid bolus ≥40 mL/kg in 1 h,
	■ Hypotension, *or*
	■ Need for vasoactive drug to maintain BP in normal range, *or*
	■ Two of the following:
	  Unexplained metabolic acidosis (base deficit >5 mEq/L)
	  Increased arterial lactate > two times upper limit of normal
	  Oliguria: Urine output <0.5 mL/kg/h
	  Prolonged capillary refill >5 s
	  Core to peripheral temperature gap >3°C

Respiratory dysfunction	Any of the below: ■ Pao_2/Fio_2 <300 in absence of cyanotic heart disease or preexisting lung disease, ■ $Paco_2$ >65 mm Hg or 20 mm Hg over baseline ■ Proven need or >50% Fio_2 to maintain Sao_2 ≥92 Need for nonelective, invasive, or noninvasive mechanical ventilation.
Neurologic dysfunction	GCS ≤11 or change in GCS ≥3 points
Hematologic dysfunction	Platelet count <80,000 per mm^3 or a decline of 50% or INR >2
Renal dysfunction	Serum creatinine ≥ two times the upper normal limit or twofold increase in baseline
Hepatic dysfunction	Total bilirubin ≥4 mg/dL (except newborn) or ALT two times the upper normal limit

BP, blood pressure; GCS, Glasgow coma score; INR, international normalized ratio; ALT, alanine transaminase.
Modified from Carcillo JA, Fields AI. Clinical practical parameters for hemodynamic support of pediatric and neonatal patients with septic shock. American College of Critical Care Medicine Task Force Committee Members. *Crit Care Med.* 2002;30:1365–1378.

show that early initiation of continuous renal replacement therapies, as identified by less fluid accumulation, appear to affect the outcome.

There are four major interventions associated with decreased mortality in adults: (i) administration of early goal-oriented therapy (as described earlier), (ii) use of recombinant human-activated protein C, (iii) use of low-dose steroids, and (iv) strict regulation of blood glucose levels in patients with severe sepsis/septic shock. Whether supportive evidence for all of these interventions will be found in the pediatric population remains to be seen.

Recombinant Human-Activated Protein C

Recombinant human-activated protein C (rAPC), an anticoagulant, is the first biologic agent shown to be effective in reducing the mortality of patients with severe sepsis. The efficacy of an anticoagulant has been attributed to the feedback between the coagulation system and the inflammatory cascade (see Chapter 3.2). The question arises as to why the other recently tested anticoagulant therapies such as antithrombin-III (AT-III) and tissue factor pathway inhibitor (TFPI) failed. Inhibition of thrombin has an indirect anti-inflammatory action, which is not specific for rAPC if anti-inflammatory properties made a difference in

the outcome. Whether rAPC has direct anti-inflammatory or antiapoptotic actions *in vivo* needs to be shown. Serious bleeding is the major complication. The incidence of bleeding in a pediatric safety study during infusion and during the entire study period was 2.4% and 4.8%, respectively. A large, phase 3 RCT is currently under way to formally assess the safety and efficacy of APC in children.

Low-Dose Steroids

The failure of adrenocorticotropic hormone (ACTH) to appropriately augment the plasma cortisol levels appears to be a poor prognostic finding in vasopressor-dependent sepsis, and may indicate "relative adrenal insufficiency (RAI)." A recent RCT showed that the use of replacement steroid therapy for more than 7 days was beneficial in individuals in whom ACTH failed to respond.[10] ACTH responders, on the other hand, showed a trend to lower survival with steroid therapy. Unfortunately, a consensus about the reference values for baseline and stimulated cortisol levels are missing. An ongoing European multicenter RCT (Corticus study) will hopefully provide additional information on the more precise definition of RAI and the role of steroids in sepsis. In addition, the acute respiratory distress syndrome (ARDS) network study evaluating the use of steroids will also be available soon. Currently, there is no consensus about the role of steroids or the best dose of steroids suitable for children with septic shock. Their use should be reserved to children with catecholamine resistance and with suspected or proven adrenal insufficiency.[8]

Glycemic Control

Strict control of blood glucose levels by insulin therapy decreases mortality and morbidity in critically ill adults. The metabolic control rather than insulin is thought to be related to the benefits. Current evidence draws attention to hyperglycemia, emphasizes maneuvers to prevent its occurrence such as early enteral feeding, and efforts to avoid factors and medications known to induce hyperglycemia. If preventative measures fail, in view of the risks for hypoglycemia, normoglycemic control should only be done with frequent glucose monitoring.

CONCLUSION

The nature and extent of the host response in SIRS is variable and likely to be affected by the genetic background, environmental factors, type of initial insult, any significant premorbid condition, and the treatment strategy applied. It is not likely that there will be a single target in the treatment of SIRS. Emphasis still needs to be on timely recognition and avoidance of delays in initial supportive therapy. With the help of further research, future strategies will screen the immune, genetic, and neuroendocrine profile of the host and create a custom-made treatment.

REFERENCES

1. Bone RC. American College of Chest Physicians/Society of Critical Care Consensus Conference: Definitions for sepsis and organ failure and guidelines for the use of innovative therapies in sepsis. *Crit Care Med.* 1992;20:724–726.
2. Watson RS, Carcillo JA, Linde-Zwirble WT, et al. The epidemiology of severe sepsis in children in the United States. *Am J Respir Crit Care Med.* 2003;167(5):695–701.
3. Matzinger P. The Danger Model: A renewed sense of self. *Science.* 2002;296:301–305.
4. Munford RS, Pugin J. Normal responses to injury prevent systemic inflammation and can be immunosuppressive. *Am J Respir Crit Care Med.* 2001;163:316–321.
5. Carcillo JA. Pediatric septic shock and multiple organ failure. *Crit Care Clin.* 2003;19:413–446.
6. Hotchkiss RS, Karl IE. Medical progress: The pathophysiology and treatment of sepsis. *N Engl J Med.* 2003;348:138–150.
7. Goldstein B, Giroir B, Randolph A, et al. International pediatric sepsis consensus conference: Definitions for sepsis and organ dysfunction in pediatrics. *Pediatr Crit Care Med.* 2005;6:2–8.
8. Carcillo JA, Fields AI. Clinical practical parameters for hemodynamic support of pediatric and neonatal patients with septic shock. American College of Critical Care Medicine Task Force Committee Members. *Crit Care Med.* 2002;30:1365–1378.
9. Bunchman T. Fluid overload in multiple organ dysfunction syndrome: A prediction of survival. *Crit Care Med.* 2004;32:1805–1806.
10. Annane D, Sebille V, Charpentier C, et al. Effect of treatment with low doses of hydrocortisone and fludrocortisone on mortality in patients with septic shock. *JAMA.* 2002;288:862–871.

Hematologic and Oncologic Disorders

Naomi L. C. Luban   *Edward C. Wong*

Sickle Cell Disease

24

Karen E. King

Sickle cell disease is a hemoglobinopathy characterized by the presence of hemoglobin S, a variant form of hemoglobin. It results from the substitution of a valine for a glutamate at the sixth residue from the amino terminus of the β chain of hemoglobin A. As a consequence of this single base substitution, molecules of hemoglobin S aggregate and polymerize in the deoxygenated state, ultimately leading to the characteristic sickle-shaped red cell which is rigid and lacks deformability.[1] These changes in cellular morphology, increased blood viscosity, and increased adherence to vascular endothelium lead to vascular sludging, microcirculatory occlusion, inadequate oxygenation, and multiorgan failure.

It is estimated that 8% of African Americans are heterozygous for the *hemoglobin S gene*. Sickle cell anemia, in which patients are homozygous for the *hemoglobin S gene*, affects approximately 1 in 600 African Americans.[2] Sickle cell disease also includes compound heterozygous states, such as hemoglobin SC disease and hemoglobin S β-thalassemia. Individuals of African, Mediterranean, Indian, Middle Eastern, and Hispanic descent can be affected.

Clinically, sickle cell anemia is characterized by a chronic hemolytic anemia and the occurrence of frequent vaso-occlusive crises (VOC), which result in tissue hypoxia and end-organ damage. Although extraordinarily painful, many patients with VOC can be managed as outpatients; other life-threatening complications, such as acute chest syndrome (ACS) and stroke, require hospitalization and critical care for their management.

INFECTION

In children with sickle cell anemia, infection is the most common cause of death. In a recent report of 711 children with sickle cell disease, 25 patients died with a mean age of 5.6 years at death.[3] Fifteen of the deaths were attributable to sickle cell disease, including five deaths due to sepsis. The organisms most commonly seen were *Streptococcus pneumoniae*, *Haemophilus influenzae*, *Staphylococcus aureus*, *Streptococcus viridans*, *Escherichia coli*, and *Salmonella* species.

The most common cause of bacteremia in children with sickle cell disease is *S. pneumoniae*. This life-threatening infection may be associated with an aplastic crisis, disseminated intravascular coagulopathy, and meningitis. *H. influenzae* is the second most common cause of bacteremia and meningitis, and is often seen in older children. Osteomyelitis, occurring because of infection involving an infarcted bone, is often attributable to the *Salmonella* species or *E. coli* and must be differentiated from vaso-occlusive bony pain. Pneumonia, clinically presenting as ACS, may be caused by community-acquired organisms, such as *Mycoplasma pneumoniae* and *Chlamydia pneumoniae*.

The risk of life-threatening infection in these patients is predominantly due to impaired splenic function, which is evident early in life. During the first year of life, patients with sickle cell anemia will have red cells with Howell-Jolly bodies and irregular pitted surfaces. These morphologic findings are indicative of splenic dysfunction with decreased clearance of particles from the intravascular space. Ultimately, patients with sickle cell anemia will experience repeated splenic infarcts, resulting in fibrosis and calcification. As a consequence, these patients should be considered asplenic.

Infants with sickle cell disease should receive both a pneumococcal vaccine and the *H. influenzae* vaccine. By 8 weeks of age, a regimen of prophylactic penicillin should be initiated and continued until the age of 5 to 6, at which time penicillin should be kept readily available. Despite this preventive regimen, a high index of suspicion for a life-threatening bacterial infection must be maintained. Patients with a septic presentation should have cultures drawn and antibiotics started immediately.

ACUTE SPLENIC SEQUESTRATION CRISES

Acute splenic sequestration is the sudden pooling of blood in the spleen resulting in anemia, which may be life threatening. This type of crisis occurs most often in young children between 10 and 27 months of age in whom autoinfarction of the spleens has not yet happened. It occurs less frequently, but at older ages, in patients with hemoglobin SC disease and hemoglobin S β-thalassemia. The cause of this syndrome is unclear; it may be seen in the setting of concurrent bacterial or viral infection. The diagnostic criteria for acute splenic sequestration include an acutely enlarging spleen, a decrease in hemoglobin level of at least 2 g per dL below baseline, thrombocytopenia often with a platelet count <100,000 per mm,[3] leukopenia, and evidence of bone marrow compensation with reticulocytosis. In its most severe form, acute splenic sequestration results in life-threatening anemia, hypovolemia, and shock. Decreases in the levels of hemoglobin <4 g per dL are associated with 35% mortality rates. It is estimated that as much as 50% of the patient's red cells can be sequestered in the spleen. Approximately 50% of patients who survive an episode of acute splenic sequestration will experience a recurrence.[4]

Emergency management is aimed at restoring circulatory blood volume and hemodynamic stability. Although therapy may begin with crystalloid resuscitation, red blood cell transfusions must be given promptly. Repeated small volume transfusions (2 mL/kg/transfusion) or normovolemic exchange transfusions may be required. Aggressive transfusion (5 to 10 mL per kg) may result in high hematocrits and should be avoided. This approach can lead to the suppression of endogenous erythropoiesis, and more critically, an "overshoot" phenomenon can be seen in which the hematocrit rises out of proportion to transfusion. This phenomenon is attributed to contraction of the enlarged spleen with the release of the sequestered red blood cells.

Long-term management is complicated because there is a high rate of recurrence of either acute or subacute sequestration. Splenectomy has been advocated when recurrent episodes occur. Short-term chronic transfusion programs have also been advocated.

Acute hepatic sequestration is a similar phenomenon in which red cells are acutely sequestered within the liver (see Fig. 24.1). Hepatic sequestration occurs less frequently and is more often seen in older children and adults who present with acute anemia and pain due to the enlargement of the liver. Differential diagnosis includes acute cholecystitis.

APLASTIC CRISES

Because sickle cell anemia is a congenital hemolytic anemia, there is ongoing red cell destruction, which must be supported by endogenous erythropoiesis manifest as reticulocytosis. Any concurrent illness that suppresses endogenous erythropoiesis will result in reticulocytopenia and a decrease in hemoglobin level and hematocrit. Acute aplastic crises are characterized by a decrease in the level of hemoglobin of >3.0 g per dL in the setting of reticulocytopenia. These crises often occur in association with an infection that leads to transient bone marrow suppression; human parvovirus B19, the etiologic agent of erythema infectiosum (fifth disease), is notorious for causing this complication.

Patients should be given supportive red cell transfusions when they have hemodynamic instability, which may present with tachycardia, tachypnea, postural hypotension, and unstable blood pressure. Symptomatic anemia, indicative of the need for transfusion, includes dyspnea, dizziness, excessive fatigue, and difficulty in concentrating. Clinical management depends on the degree of anemia and cardiovascular compromise. Aggressive transfusions should be avoided, because transfusion to levels much above the

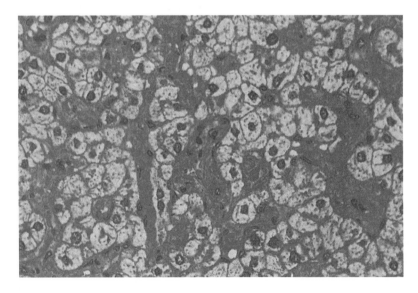

Figure 24.1 Clumps of sickled red blood cells packed in the sinusoidal spaces. (H&E stain; original magnification × 200.) (From Yamada T, Alpers DH, Laine L, et al. *Atlas of gastroenterology*, 3rd ed. Philadelphia, PA: Lippincott Williams & Wilkins; 2003:938.) (see color Figure 24.1.)

patient's baseline hematocrit may suppress endogenous erythropoiesis further.

ACUTE CEREBROVASCULAR ACCIDENTS

Cerebrovascular accidents (CVAs) are one of the most devastating sequelae of sickle cell anemia. The Cooperative Study of Sickle Cell Disease evaluated data from more than 4,000 patients enrolled from 1978 to 1988: CVAs were most common in sickle cell anemia (homozygous hemoglobin S disease) with a prevalence of 4.0% and an incidence of 0.61 per 100 patient-years. In smaller cohort studies, approximately 7% of children develop a CVA with the highest rates in children between 5 and 10 years. In untreated patients, the mortality is 20% with a 70% recurrence rate within 3 years. Infarctive, nonhemorrhagic CVAs are most common (70% to 80%) and most often occur in children between the ages of 2 and 5 (see Fig. 24.2),[5] whereas hemorrhagic stroke is less frequent (10%) occurring in adolescents and young adults who often have a history of a transient ischemic attack.

Typical findings on magnetic resonance imaging (MRI) within 2 to 4 hours of an infarctive event include major vessel obstruction (distal internal carotid and proximal middle cerebral artery) or distal obstruction of smaller vessels leading to infarction in the border zone between the anterior and middle cerebral arteries. Presentation ranges from acute neurologic signs with visual changes, focal seizure, weakness, and hemiparesis, to transient loss of consciousness, to frank tonic clonic seizures. In adolescents, intracranial hemorrhage, either subarachnoid or intracranial is the more usual central nervous system (CNS) event. This presents with headache, vertigo, syncope, and meningismus, and these symptoms are likely the results of aneurysmal bleeding. The aneurysms have arisen from intimal damage occurring from multiple VOC during childhood. Rupture of some of the multiple aneurysms with collateral vessel development, as is seen in moyamoya disease, may be the cause of many of these hemorrhagic CVAs.

Transfusion therapy is initiated at presentation with partial or full exchange transfusion aimed at reducing the hemoglobin S percentage to 30% while maintaining the hematocrit at 30%. Manual partial or automated exchange can be performed. The timing of initiation of the exchange has not been studied. Simple repetitive transfusions should be avoided because they may cause an increase in whole blood viscosity if the hemoglobin level exceeds 11 to

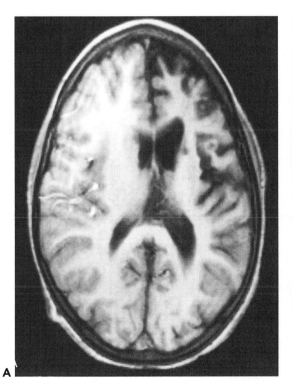
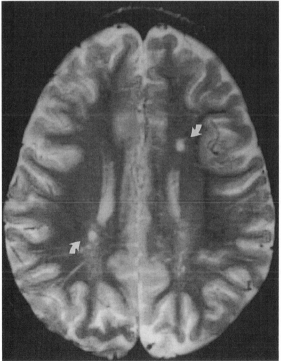

A   B

Figure 24.2   Vaso-occlusive effects in central nervous system. **A:** T1-weighted magnetic resonance imaging in a 6-year-old with HB SS and a history of stroke. There is extensive atrophy involving the distributions of the left anterior and middle cerebral arteries with compensatory enlargement of the left lateral ventricle. **B:** T2-weighted sagittal magnetic resonance imaging in a 4-year-old boy with silent infarcts. Small areas of leukomalacia are seen in deep white matter in frontal and parietal areas. (From Lee G, Foerster J, Lukens J, et al. *Wintrobe's clinical hematology*, 10th ed. Philadelphia, PA: Lippincott Williams & Wilkins; 1998:1360.)

12 g per dL. Therapy with a long-term transfusion program by simple transfusion often follows the initial event because of the high rate of recurrence(s) ranging from 40% to 90%.[6] The optimal duration in years of chronic transfusion therapy has not been well studied. In one study, stopping transfusion after 5 to 12 years resulted in a 50% recurrence rate within 1 year, whereas in another study, recurrence was after 3 to 18 years. Transfusional hemochromatosis, one of the major complications of chronic transfusion, can be obviated with programs designed to reduce the rate of iron accumulation. Modified simple transfusion programs using higher hemoglobin S percentage and erythrocytopheresis may lead to reduction in iron overload while providing the benefit of hemoglobin S reduction;[7] many modifications of such programs are in clinical trials. The landmark Stroke Prevention Trial in Sickle Cell Disease was the first study to confirm that children with elevated transcranial Doppler (TCD) measurements could be protected from subsequent strokes by a transfusion regimen. Current randomized studies will evaluate whether those who have subtle neurocognitive defects and may have had silent strokes can benefit from pre-emptive transfusion to avoid CVAs.

ACUTE CHEST SYNDROME

ACS is a leading cause of mortality and morbidity. ACS presents with fever, cough, and chest pain accompanied by leukocytosis and infiltrates as shown by chest x-rays of patients with hypoxemia. In children, the infiltrates are often middle or upper lobe, whereas in older children and adults, they are in lower lobes and are accompanied by pleural effusions. The infiltrates may progress to multilobular disease, which is indistinguishable from acute respiratory distress syndrome. The etiology of ACS is unknown and likely multifactorial; potential causes include infection, pulmonary vasculature vaso-occlusion with pulmonary infarction, pulmonary embolism, and fat embolism.[8] Release of plasma phospholipase A2 and free fatty acids from fat embolism may result in bronchoconstriction, increased pulmonary vascular permeability, and leukocyte chemotaxis. Patients with fat emboli as the cause of ACS often have bone pain, neurologic symptoms, and decrease in platelet count. In children, acute infection is implicated most often, and asthma and airway hyperreactivity may also contribute to a ventilation perfusion mismatch with hypoxia and acidosis. Other risk factors associated with the development of ACS include younger age, lower Hgb F concentration, higher steady state hemoglobin concentration, and higher steady state white blood cell (WBC) count. Half of the patients who have an episode of ACS will experience recurrence.[9] Repeated episodes of ACS and pulmonary infarction contribute to the poor prognosis of ACS which results in pulmonary fibrosis, pulmonary hypertension, and cor pulmonale. This chronic pulmonary disease results in mortality rates of 4.3% in adults and

1.8% in children. In one study reporting 538 patients with 671 episodes of ACS, 13% of patients required mechanical ventilation and 3% of patients died.[8] Seventy-six percent of these patients experienced their first episode of ACS below the age of 20. In a report by the Cooperative Study of Sickle Cell Disease, the highest incidence of ACS was seen in children 2 to 4 years of age with a gradual decrease in incidence with increasing age.[10]

Conventional management includes empiric antibiotics for the possibility of infection and supportive care for potential infarction, including oxygen, pain medication, incentive spirometry, and transfusion. Transfusion has proven to be useful in the treatment of ACS; partial or full volume red cell exchange is indicated in the more severe episodes. Several new therapies have been advocated. These include inhaled nitric oxide and L-arginine, both being advocated in clinical trials. Bone marrow and hematopoietic stem cell transplantation may also prove beneficial, especially in those children with recurrent ACS without evidence of end-organ failure. The following criteria have been used to determine the need for red cell exchange transfusion: high hematocrit, worsening pulmonary infiltrates, marked infiltrates involving more than one lobe, moderate to severe hypoxemia which does not improve with oxygen therapy, and clinical respiratory compromise. Persistent hypoxia (pO_2 of <75 mm Hg or decrease of 25% from baseline) is an indication for simple transfusion. Analgesia should be used with extreme caution because hypoventilation, which further exacerbates hypoxia, may occur.

MULTIORGAN FAILURE SYNDROME

Multiorgan failure syndrome (MFS) is a rare and life-threatening complication which often follows a severe vaso-occlusive crisis and is characterized by the simultaneous failure of several organ systems. Diagnostic criteria require that two of the following three organs be affected: lung, liver, or kidney.[11] Characteristic findings include hypoxia, pulmonary infiltrates, hepatic transaminitis, hyperbilirubinemia, renal impairment, encephalopathy, rhabdomyolysis, and coagulopathy. MFS has been attributed to widespread microvascular occlusion and, of interest, is reported most often in patients with a mild clinical course and relatively normal hemoglobin concentrates. Pulmonary dysfunction may require supplemental oxygen, and possibly intubation with ventilatory support. Patients often have a nonfocal encephalopathy which may progress to coma and resembles thrombotic thrombocytopenic purpura (TTP). Bone marrow dysfunction, as evidenced by severe anemia and thrombocytopenia, can be confirmed by bone marrow biopsy where extensive marrow necrosis may be seen. Fever and pancreatic dysfunction may also occur.

MFS is a life-threatening complication, requiring intensive supportive care. Treatment includes aggressive transfusion therapy, which should begin with an urgent red cell exchange. Red cell exchange is recommended because this syndrome is felt to result from a global lack of adequate oxygenation, possibly aggravated by hyperviscosity. Red cell exchange can rapidly lower hemoglobin S levels to 20% to 30%, improving whole blood viscosity. For patients with severe anemia, it may be preferable to give multiple red cell transfusions as opposed to performing a red cell exchange. Subsequent transfusion support should be given to maintain a hemoglobin S level of 20% to 30%, with a hematocrit not higher than 30%. When transfusion therapy is initiated quickly, patients may dramatically respond with rapid clinical improvement and resolution of organ dysfunction.

PERIOPERATIVE MANAGEMENT

Patients with sickle cell disease who undergo surgery have an increased risk of morbidity and mortality as compared to patients who do not have sickle cell disease. Some of the complications of anesthesia, such as hypoxia, hypotension, and hypothermia, may lead to intravascular sickling and subsequent vaso-occlusion.

In the past, many have advocated routine preoperative transfusion or, if emergent, red cell exchange to decrease the perioperative morbidity and mortality. More recently, a prospective, randomized, multicenter trial has shown that red cell exchange to achieve a hemoglobin S <30% with a hemoglobin level of 10 g per dL has no clinical advantage over simple transfusion to a preoperative hemoglobin level of 10 g per dL. As compared with the patients receiving simple transfusion, the patients undergoing exchange transfusion had twice the number of transfusion-related complications, including red cell alloimmunization.[12] As a consequence, patients undergoing surgery with general anesthesia should be transfused to a preoperative hemoglobin level of 10 g per dL.

Patients with hemoglobin SC disease typically have a higher baseline level of hemoglobin and hematocrit. If the patient presents with a hemoglobin level of 10 g per dL or greater, it is not feasible to give simple transfusions. These patients may benefit from preoperative red cell exchange to decrease whole blood viscosity and the amount of hemoglobin S.[13]

TRANSFUSION MANAGEMENT

Transfusion therapy has a major role in the treatment of sickle cell disease, both in the critical care setting and in the long-term management of specific complications (see Table 24.1). Transfusion therapy achieves many beneficial effects including improved oxygen-carrying capacity and better oxygen delivery to the tissues. Patients with sickle cell disease should not be transfused above a hematocrit of 30% to avoid hyperviscosity. Red cell exchanges have the

TABLE 24.1
INDICATIONS FOR RED CELL TRANSFUSION IN SICKLE CELL DISEASE

Episodic or Acute Transfusion
Acute exacerbating of anemia
Acute hepatic/splenic sequestration
Aplastic crisis
Symptomatic anemia
Acute chest syndrome
CVA or other acute neurologic event
Acute multiorgan failure
Preparation for major surgery

Chronic Transfusion
CVA—primary prevention (abnormal TCD) or secondary prevention (recurrent stroke)
Silent infarct (abnormal MRI) with abnormal neurocognitive testing
Recurrent acute chest syndrome
Chronic heart failure
Symptomatic anemia associated with chronic renal failure
Pulmonary hypertension with chronic hypoxia

Controversial
Acute
Priapism
Acute pain crisis
Before administration of radiographic contrast
Chronic
Pregnancy
Normal MRI with abnormal neurocognitive testing
Chronic leg ulcers
Early renal disease
Early retinopathy

CVA, cerebrovascular accident; TCD, transcranial Doppler; MRI, magnetic resonance imaging.

additional benefit of reducing whole blood viscosity, by decreasing the patient's percent hemoglobin S. Patients must be monitored for the potential adverse effects of transfusion, including febrile and allergic transfusion reactions, hemolytic transfusion reactions that can be more complex in patients with sickle cell disease, transfusion transmitted disease, and long-term complications such as transfusional hemosiderosis or iron overload.

Although automated erythrocytopheresis is generally the preferred method of performing red cell exchange, there are circumstances in which a manual exchange may be indicated. Automated erythrocytopheresis has the advantage of being accomplished within 60 to 90 minutes; however, a double lumen catheter is required. Manual exchange may be preferable when it is logistically difficult to place a double lumen catheter, when the patient is very young with a low weight and low total blood volume, or when the patient is critically ill and may not tolerate the automated procedure.

A manual red cell exchange or double red cell exchange, is performed as follows:

1. Insert two catheters, either two venous catheters (one large bore) or one venous and one arterial catheter.
2. Send baseline laboratory samples for complete blood count, and percent Hgb S. Send sample for ABO, Rh, antibody screening, and cross match of appropriate red cells.
3. Calculate volume of red cells to exchange:

$$2 \times EBV \times Patient's\ Hct \div Hct\ of\ transfused\ unit$$
(usually 60% to 80%)

EBV is the estimated blood volume.

4. Transfuse for more than 4 to 6 hours, while withdrawing blood at 10- to 15-minute intervals from the large bore venous catheter or arterial line. Larger volume exchanges may require up to 12 hours to accomplish. Balance should be maintained within 5% to 10% of blood volume. The patient should never be >15% below the baseline blood volume.
5. Monitor vital signs continuously. Hct should be checked every 2 hours and at completion. Percent Hgb S should be checked at completion of the procedure.
6. The goal of the procedure is to achieve a percent Hgb S of 30% to 40% with a Hct of 30%.

Leuko- reduced red cells are preferable because of their decreased risk of nonhemolytic febrile transfusion reactions and human leukocyte antigen (HLA) alloimmunization. It is preferable to transfuse hemoglobin S-negative red cells because hemoglobin A can provide a means to quantify the effect of transfused red cells and their survival. When performing red cell exchange, hemoglobin S-negative red cells should always be used, because one of the goals of the procedure is to reduce the percentage of hemoglobin S-red cells in circulation. More specialized manipulation such as washed red cells or frozen deglycerolized red cells are only indicated in specific clinical situations.

Patients with sickle cell disease have rates of alloimmunization against red cell antigens ranging from 8% to 35%. These high rates of alloimmunization place them at a risk for delayed hemolytic transfusion reactions, which can have serious adverse clinical outcomes such as life-threatening anemia, hemolysis, and renal dysfunction. Many have advocated the prophylactic use of antigen-matched red cells to decrease alloimmunization. Recommendations range from extensive phenotypic matching for up to 17 antigens to limited matching for only Rh antigens and Kell. In the critical care setting, it may be difficult or impossible to obtain antigen-matched red cells within the needed time constraints, especially if the patient's red cell phenotype is not previously known and are not on file. Urgent red cell exchange or simple transfusion should not be delayed in an effort to provide prophylactic matching. Routine pre-transfusion testing should be performed and the sample can be retained so that when time permits, phenotyping can be performed.

REFERENCES

1. Bunn HF. Pathogenesis and treatment of sickle cell disease. *N Engl J Med.* 1997;33:762–769.
2. Steinberg MH. Management of sickle cell disease. *N Engl J Med.* 1999;340:1021–1030.
3. Quinn CT, Rogers ZR, Buchanan GR. Survival in children with sickle cell disease. *Blood.* 2004;103:4023–4027.
4. Emond AM, Collis R, Darvill D, et al. Acute splenic sequestration in homozygous sickle cell disease: Natural history and management. *J Pediatr.* 1985;107:201–206.
5. Ohene-Frempong K, Weiner SJ, Sleeper LA, et al. Cerebrovascular accidents in sickle cell disease: Rates and risk factors. The cooperative study of sickle cell disease. *Blood.* 1998;91:288–294.
6. Danielson CF. The role of red blood cell exchange transfusion in the treatment and prevention of complications of sickle cell disease. *Ther Apher.* 2002;6:24–31.
7. Cohen AR, Martin MB, Silber JH, et al. A modified transfusion program for prevention of stroke in sickle cell disease. *Blood.* 1992; 79:1657–1661.
8. Vichinsky EP, Neumayr LD, Earles AN, et al. Causes and outcomes of the acute chest syndrome in sickle cell disease. The National Acute Chest Syndrome Study Group. *N Engl J Med.* 2000;342: 1855–1865.
9. Vichinsky EP. Current issues in blood transfusion in sickle cell disease. *Semin Hematol.* 2001;38:14–22.
10. Castro O, Brambilla DJ, Thorington B, et al. The acute chest syndrome in sickle cell disease: Incidence and risk factors. The cooperative study of sickle cell disease. *Blood.* 1994;84:643–649.
11. Hassell KL, Eckman JR, Lane PA. Acute multiorgan failure syndrome: A potentially catastrophic complication of severe sickle cell pain episodes. *Am J Med.* 1994;96:155–162.
12. Vichinsky EP, Haberkern CM, Neumayr L, et al. A comparison of conservative and aggressive transfusion regimens in the perioperative management of sickle cell disease. The Preoperative Transfusion in Sickle Cell Disease Study Group. *N Engl J Med.* 1995;333: 206–213.
13. Ohene-Frempong K. Indications for red cell transfusion in sickle cell disease. *Semin Hematol.* 2001;38:5–13.

Thrombotic and Fibrinolytic Disorders

25

Guy Young

Thromboembolism (TE) in children has been increasing significantly, largely owing to the technologic advances in the care of critically ill children with most TE occurring in intensive care units.[1] The increased incidence has led to substantial gains in the understanding of the epidemiology and etiology of pediatric thrombosis; however, management is still based on data extrapolated from adult studies and uncontrolled pediatric studies. To date, there are no randomized controlled trials evaluating various modes of therapy, and therefore, therapy is largely based on the experience of the treating physician (most often pediatric hematologists with a specific interest in coagulation disorders). The near future holds promise for collaborative trials exploring the important questions of which patient to treat, with what methods/agents, and for what length of time.

The etiology of childhood TE differs considerably from that of adults. The most common conditions leading to thrombosis in children are the placement of central venous catheters (CVC) and congenital heart disease (CHD). Other risk factors include infections, inflammatory disorders, surgery, trauma, immobilization, renal disease, and congenital prothrombotic disorders (thrombophilia). In most cases, there are several risk factors in place at the time of presentation. For most patients admitted to the intensive care unit, several of the factors mentioned earlier may be in place even upon admission, and additional risk factors may accumulate during the admission. Therefore, it is incumbent upon the intensive care unit team to be vigilant for the symptoms and signs of thrombosis and to institute laboratory and imaging investigations as soon as a thrombotic event is suspected. Consultation with the experts in pediatric thrombosis belonging to a particular institution is also suggested.

DIAGNOSIS

Clinical Manifestations

The clinical presentation (and subsequent management) depends on the type of thrombosis (arterial or venous) and the location (central, peripheral, or central nervous system). Arterial thrombosis occurs most often in children with CHD, and may involve femoral artery thrombosis status post cardiac catheterization or atrial and rarely ventricular thrombi. It could also occur in patients with artificial heart valves and grafts. Arterial thrombosis could also occur in acquired vasculitic disorders such as Kawasaki disease, vasculitis of large vessels, for example, Takayasu arteritis, and stroke in sickle cell anemia. Idiopathic arterial thrombosis in children is rarely seen.

Typically, arterial TE leads to signs of decreased perfusion to the area distal to the thrombus. For peripheral arteries, one would expect to see changes in the color and temperature of the affected extremity. Initially, one sees mottling of the skin and a subtle coolness of the overlying skin. This will be followed by pallor and a more pronounced reduction in temperature when compared to that of the contralateral limb. Once perfusion is drastically affected, a blue–purple discoloration with a cold feel to the skin will occur. Eventually, skin necrosis with a black color will occur (see Fig. 25.1). In addition, peripheral pulses will be affected, evolving from decreased palpable

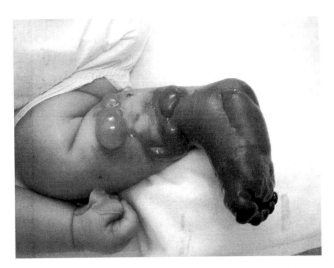

Figure 25.1 Physical findings of a child with a popliteal artery thrombosis. Note the discoloration and line of demarcation, which are late findings. (See color Figure 25.1.)

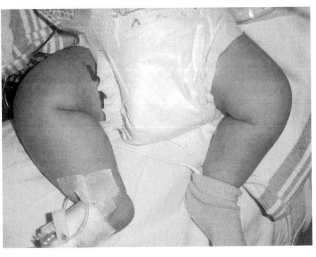

Figure 25.2 Physical findings of a child with a femoral vein thrombosis. Note the asymmetry in the size of the two extremities which is the key finding on examination of an extremity DVT. (See color Figure 25.2.)

pulses to the complete absence of a pulse. In the later stages, a line of demarcation is often noted. The early identification of an arterial thrombosis is crucial in order to prevent irreversible damage that can result in amputation of the digits or limbs. Central arterial thrombosis is harder to diagnose. Most often it is found incidentally on echocardiography or ultrasonography. If there is a significant occlusion leading to decreased perfusion of one or two extremities, the signs mentioned earlier may be noted. If there is decreased perfusion to the affected organs such as the liver or kidney, then one may note elevated levels of transaminases (a sign of hepatic necrosis) or systemic hypertension or decreased urine output, and signs of decreased perfusion to one or both kidneys. Aortic thrombosis may lead to widely differing blood pressures in the upper and lower extremities. Finally, one must consider the potential for stroke to be caused by a thromboembolic event. Children with stroke may present with subtle neurologic signs or more obvious abnormalities such as hemiparesis, cranial nerve palsies, or seizures. Because diagnostic imaging of the brain will generally be undertaken in such patients, it is likely that the diagnosis will be made then.

Venous thrombosis has an altogether different presentation. Deep vein thrombosis (DVT) is usually associated with CVC, especially in patients in the intensive care unit. Other patient populations for whom venous thrombosis may occur without the presence of a CVC include patients with infection (particularly head and neck), malignancy, autoimmune disorders, renal disease (especially nephrotic syndrome), orthopedic disease especially following surgery, and in trauma patients, particularly with head trauma. Although idiopathic extremity DVT does occur in children, it rarely requires admission to an intensive care unit.

The typical signs of venous thrombosis are related to decreased venous drainage of the area distal to the thrombus. Thrombosis affecting the limbs (usually as a result of CVC) will initially result in swelling and pain of the affected extremity (see Fig. 25.2). Discoloration and reduced temperature of the overlying skin are late signs and are caused by reduced perfusion to the skin because of increased pressure in the subcutaneous space. In general, venous thrombosis should be diagnosed before it reaches this stage. Occlusion of the central veins can result in both dramatic physical signs such as in superior vena cava syndrome (see Fig. 25.3) or the signs may be subtler such as ascites or splenomegaly. However, the same physiologic principle applies, which is decreased venous

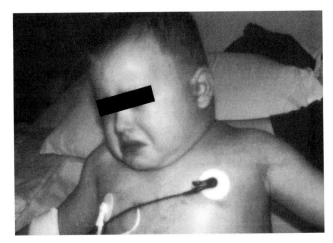

Figure 25.3 Physical findings of a child with superior vena cava syndrome. Note the severe swelling of the head and neck including periorbital and perioral edema. (See color Figure 25.3.)

drainage of an affected organ or location. In superior vena cava syndrome, the onset of symptoms is fairly acute, with an often dramatic swelling of the head and neck associated with notable headache and discomfort. The presence of engorged superficial veins may be noted early on. Thrombosis affecting particular organs will often result in nonspecific signs and symptoms such as ascites (portal vein), splenomegaly and/or hypersplenism (splenic vein), hematuria (renal vein), abdominal pain (mesenteric vein), or hepatomegaly and hyperbilirubinemia (hepatic vein). Visceral thrombosis should be considered in the differential diagnosis for any of these signs in the absence of a clear cause. Another manifestation of venous thrombosis is cerebral sinus thrombosis. It most often presents in neonates and infants with dehydration or older children and adolescents with severe sinusitis. It can also present idiopathically. The symptoms again are related to decreased venous drainage with the brain being the affected organ. Symptoms are often nonspecific and include signs of raised intracranial pressure such as headache, vomiting, and visual disturbances. In addition, seizures may occur (usually in infants), and occasionally, focal neurologic signs may be noted if venous infarcts have occurred. Early diagnosis of the thrombosis, as well as diagnosing its underlying cause (dehydration, sinusitis) is important for the treatment to be effective in preventing permanent neurologic sequelae. Lastly, pulmonary embolism (PE) is an important and often undiagnosed event in children. The symptoms are usually subtle owing to the inherent ability of children to compensate for hypoxemia. Furthermore, the symptoms, when they do occur, are nonspecific and include tachypnea, cough, chest pain, and rarely respiratory distress. Hypoxemia is not always present. Owing to the numerous conditions that can lead to these symptoms, and the relative rarity of PE in children, it is likely that the diagnosis is made in few children. It is also believed (although certainly not proven) that children often recover from PE without long-term sequelae. Nevertheless, PE should be in the differential diagnosis for any child with a known thrombus and with the symptoms mentioned earlier, or for any child with unusual or unexpected pulmonary symptoms when alternative diagnoses have been eliminated.

Diagnostic Studies

Laboratory Studies

Once the diagnosis for thrombosis is made, there are laboratory tests that can assist in delineating the likelihood for a thrombus. The most readily available test is the D-dimer. The D-dimer is formed when cross-linked fibrin is lysed by plasmin. This only occurs in patients with thrombosis or disseminated intravascular coagulation. Studies in adults have demonstrated both a very high positive and negative predictive value (approximately 95% to 99%) when there is an *a priori* high level of suspicion for a thrombotic event. Therefore, an elevated D-dimer in a patient with physical signs of thrombosis is highly suggestive, while negative results should lead to the evaluation of alternative diagnoses. Other laboratory tests including prothrombin fragment 1.2 and thrombin–antithrombin complexes have demonstrated a high level of sensitivity and specificity; however, these tests are less available and less studied than the D-dimer. A discussion of the evaluation of thrombophilia is discussed in the subsequent text.

Diagnostic Imaging Studies

Once a thrombus is suspected, the appropriate diagnostic imaging study to confirm the clinical suspicion should be performed. Arterial thrombosis can be diagnosed by the following modalities: color Doppler ultrasonography, magnetic resonance imaging (MRI) and/or magnetic resonance angiography (MRA), echocardiography (atrial, ventricular, aortic root, and coronary thrombi), or computerized tomography (CT) and/or CT angiography. A stroke can be diagnosed by MRI/MRA, or less effectively by CT scan. Transcranial Doppler ultrasonography can also be performed and has been validated as an effective tool for the prediction of thrombosis in sickle cell anemia. If there is a high clinical suspicion, and these studies do not identify a thrombosis, standard angiography may be required. The "gold" standard for venous thrombosis is venography. Despite its high sensitivity and specificity, it is not utilized frequently because of the need for the placement of a peripheral intravenous line, the availability and relative ease of Doppler ultrasonography, and the reluctance of many radiologists to perform the test. It is nonetheless the most reliable study. For the lower venous system, compression Doppler ultrasonography has a reasonably high sensitivity (80% to 90%) and is therefore the first option. If the study is negative and yet the clinical suspicion persists, venography should be performed. For the upper venous system, ultrasonography has very poor sensitivity (approximately 30%) for the veins proximal to the distal subclavian owing to the presence of the clavicle overlying the subclavian vein, the inability to compress the veins, and the depth of the veins in the chest. Venography is therefore required to properly assess the upper venous system; however, venography is not sensitive for thrombosis in the internal jugular veins because the injected dye will not flow in a retrograde fashion. Therefore, both ultrasonography and venography are required for a complete assessment of the upper venous system. Of note, venography involves injection of the dye into the peripheral veins (generally in the antecubital fossa) because injection of the dye into a CVC will not allow for the assessment of the portions of the venous system proximal to the tip of the catheter.

Evaluation of the central abdominal and visceral veins is usually accomplished by color Doppler ultrasonography. Alternatively, MRI and magnetic resonance venography (MRV), or CT scan and CT venography can be performed, although data on sensitivity and specificity are lacking. Superior vena cava syndrome is best evaluated with bilateral upper venography, although it may be noted by MR or CT venography. Ultrasound, as mentioned previously, is a poor technique for evaluating the superior vena cava, innominate, and subclavian veins. Cerebral sinus thrombosis is most effectively diagnosed using the MRI/MRV of the brain. Although a CT scan will often reveal the abnormality, a normal study does not exclude the diagnosis. As mentioned in the preceding text, it is difficult to diagnose PE in children and there are no validated diagnostic methods. Although ventilation/perfusion (V/Q) scanning can be performed, the sensitivity and specificity are not known. This, combined with the nonspecific symptoms make the interpretation of results difficult. Studies on adults have demonstrated the utility of spiral CT angiography as an effective method with a greater degree of sensitivity and specificity; however, this method has not been formally evaluated in children. Currently, the diagnosis can be made when either V/Q scanning or CT angiography are suggestive and the clinical suspicion is high.

Laboratory Evaluation for Prothrombotic Disorders

The need for a detailed laboratory evaluation for thrombophilia depends on the clinical situation. Because this is an area that has not been studied systematically, the need and extent for such a laboratory evaluation will differ depending on physician preference and experience. Although it is reasonable not to further evaluate a child with a catheter-related thrombus and one or more additional risk factors (surgery, bacteremia, immobilization), an effort can be made to evaluate all such children. Despite risk factors being present, most children will *not* develop a thrombus, suggesting additional unseen risk factors. Therefore until further studies are done, the need and extent of a laboratory evaluation for such patients will depend on physician preference. For the child with an idiopathic thrombus or for a child with an unusual, unexpected, or recurrent thrombosis, a thorough laboratory investigation is warranted.

Although the extent of the laboratory investigation is controversial, in general, the following first-line tests should be included: genetic analysis for factor V_{Leiden} and the prothrombin G20210A mutation, assays for fibrinogen, proteins C and S and antithrombin, homocysteine level, factor VIII activity, lipoprotein (a) level, and evaluation for antiphospholipid antibodies including lupus anticoagulant, anticardiolipin, and anti–β_2-glycoprotein I antibodies. Additional conditions and the tests to assess them, which are not usually part of the first-line of tests include: factor XII deficiency (activated partial thromboplastin time [aPTT]), dysfibrinogenemia (thrombin time, reptilase time, functional fibrinogen), and disorders of fibrinolysis (euglobulin clot lysis time). Other conditions for which the link with thrombosis remains unclear include: elevated factors VII, IX, and XI, methylene tetrahydrofolate reductase (MTHFR) polymorphisms with normal homocysteine levels, plasminogen deficiency, plasminogen-activator inhibitor-1 4G/5G polymorphism,

and heparin cofactor II deficiency. New genetic abnormalities associated with an increased risk for thrombosis are being identified on a regular basis. Some of the emerging candidates include protein Z deficiency, tissue factor pathway inhibitor deficiency, factor XIII Val34Leu polymorphism, and others. It is recommended that before any laboratory investigation is undertaken, consultation with an expert in childhood thrombosis be sought in order to assist in this investigation. Finally, it should be noted that children and particularly infants have different normal ranges for many of the above mentioned tests than adults and that tests performed during the acute phase may be abnormal simply because of the consumption of proteins. Therefore, laboratory results should be interpreted with these caveats.

TREATMENT

Currently, there are no randomized clinical trials that have addressed any aspect of the management of thrombosis in children. Treatment is largely based on guidelines put together by expert panels and derived from adult studies and the personal experience of these experts. References 2 and 3 are suggested.[2,3] It is again recommended that the guidance of the institutional expert in childhood thrombosis be sought to assist in the management of such patients. Furthermore, it is best to involve the physicians likely to care for these patients upon discharge from the intensive care unit, early in the diagnostic and treatment process.

There are several general principles that guide the choice of therapy in children with thrombosis. First, it should be noted that children with limb thrombosis are at high likelihood of developing post-thrombotic syndrome, a condition of chronic venous insufficiency, which can be debilitating. Second, children will likely survive for many decades following the thrombotic event necessitating management, which will reduce the likelihood of long-term sequelae (post-thrombotic syndrome, amputations, neurologic damage). Third, it is possible, if not likely, that during the diagnostic process children will be found to have risk factors that may be long term or even permanent. Finally, children have fewer bleeding complications from thrombolytic and anticoagulant therapy allowing for more aggressive therapy than especially elderly patients.

Arterial Thrombosis

Arterial thrombosis is a medical emergency. Early identification and aggressive management are warranted in order to prevent severe sequelae and death. For acute limb-threatening thrombosis, the treatment of choice is thrombolysis with systemic tissue-type plasminogen activator (tPA). It should be administered as soon as possible after the thrombus is identified. tPA is given by continuous infusion with a standard dose of 0.1 to 0.5 mg/kg/hour.

A recent study suggests that smaller doses may be as effective,[4] but given the rapidity of vascular compromise, starting at a dose that will prove ineffective may result in amputation or death. Some guidelines recommend an infusion of low-dose heparin (10 U/kg/hour) to be given with the tPA, but this has not been studied and is not universally adopted. tPA should be infused for only as long as is necessary, so as to minimize the risk of bleeding. The affected artery should be re-evaluated by imaging frequently (at least daily), and the duration of the infusion should continue until perfusion is restored or until further treatment is deemed ineffective by follow-up imaging, so as long as clinically significant bleeding does not occur. Once the tPA is discontinued, therapeutic anticoagulation with heparin or low-molecular-weight heparin (LMWH) should begin immediately (see subsequent text for details). Arterial thrombosis in central arteries or the left atrium should be treated the same way. Patients should be monitored with the aPTT, fibrinogen, and D-dimer. The aPTT should increase, the fibrinogen should decrease, and there should be a sharp rise in the D-dimer, indicating effective thrombolysis. If these do not occur and there is no symptomatic improvement, the options are to increase the dose and/or to give fresh frozen plasma to replenish plasminogen. Treatment of stroke in children is unclear with the exception of patients with sickle cell anemia.[5] Although dosing tPA using adult guidelines is reasonable,[6] it is rare that children are diagnosed early enough for this to be feasible. Furthermore, while most adult stroke is the result of atherothrombosis, the etiology of childhood stroke is diverse, and not necessarily thrombotic in nature. In the subacute phase a variety of options exist including anticoagulation (see subsequent text), antiplatelet therapy with aspirin or other agents or no therapy. The decision on which therapy to choose should be guided by the likelihood of recurrence based on the underlying cause of the stroke and the risk for bleeding from the above therapies. These decisions should be made with the assistance of an expert in pediatric stroke.

Venous Thrombosis

The management of venous thrombosis in children is less straightforward than arterial thrombosis. The options range from aggressive thrombolysis as in arterial thrombosis to no therapy. Consideration for tPA should be given to patients with severe, life-threatening acute thrombosis such as superior vena cava syndrome or clinically significant PE and visceral vein thrombosis. Alternatively, less severe forms of these symptoms can be treated just with anticoagulation as can typical cases of limb DVT and cerebral sinus thrombosis. In situations in which acute and easily reversible causes for the thrombotic event are evident, it is possible that simply correcting the underlying cause can resolve the thrombus and no anticoagulation is needed. For example,

the infant with severe dehydration who develops cerebral sinus thrombosis may have complete resolution with appropriate rehydration and does not necessarily need anticoagulation. Similarly, the patient with an acute catheter-related thrombosis may respond simply to the removal of the catheter. It should be noted, however, that if the catheter is still required to treat the underlying disease, it may be best to leave the catheter in place and begin anticoagulation. It is suggested that the decision not to treat be done in consultation with an expert in pediatric thrombosis.

The choice of agents, dosing regimen, and the duration of therapy are all controversial because there are no pediatric trials which adequately address these issues. Nevertheless, the following principles apply. For patients with a temporary risk factor (catheter, immobilization, etc.), the duration of therapy should continue until that risk factor is no longer present and the thrombus has resolved or at least recanalized. This could be as little as several days to several weeks. For patients with chronic risk factors, be they acquired (antiphospholipid syndrome, nephrotic syndrome, etc.) or congenital (factor V_{Leiden}, protein C deficiency, etc.), treatment should continue for at least 3 months and perhaps much longer. The duration of long-term therapy will rarely need to be decided in the intensive care unit. For patients with ongoing risk factors who have had a recurrence, indefinite anticoagulation is necessary. It is important to emphasize that these are merely guidelines and that specific therapy for each patient will depend upon their individual circumstances.

As to which agent to use and to what intensity, it is again important to note that no pediatric clinical trials exist on which to base these recommendations. In the acute setting, the current choices are unfractionated heparin and LMWH. There are pros and cons to each and details can be found in Reference 7.[7] Unfractionated heparin is administered with a bolus of 50 to 75 U per kg followed by a continuous infusion of 20 to 28 U/kg/hour with younger patients requiring higher doses. Dosing is usually adjusted on the basis of the aPTT with a goal of 1.5 to 3 times baseline. It should be noted, however, that the aPTT is not as accurate in assessing the degree of anticoagulation as the antifactor Xa assay. Although it is indeed more accurate to guide therapy with the antifactor Xa assay (goal of 0.35 to 0.70 U per mL), many institutions do not have the test available onsite leading to a long turnaround time for results. Even in those institutions where the test is available, it is often run only once a day. Therefore until the widespread availability of the antifactor Xa assay is achieved, it is reasonable to dose unfractionated heparin on the basis of the aPTT.

For LMWH, most of the available data on dosing is with enoxaparin, although some data exist for dalteparin as well. LMWH can be used in the acute setting; however, because of its long half-life and requirement for twice-daily dosing and dosing adjustment based on antifactor Xa levels (LMWH does not affect the aPTT), it is not generally recommended for acutely ill patients who may require invasive procedures. In addition, LMWH is not easily reversible (protamine is only partially effective). Subcutaneous twice-daily administration is more of an advantage for outpatients than for critically ill patients. If it is used, the dosing is 1.5 mg/kg/dose every 12 hours for children younger than a year and 1 mg/kg/dose every 12 hours for children older than 1 year. Intravenous LMWH has been reported but has been associated with severe bleeding and is not recommended. Several novel anticoagulants have become available and are undergoing clinical trials in children. These agents for now are being used in patients for whom heparin is contraindicated such as those with heparin-induced thrombocytopenia. These agents have been recently reviewed and compared to unfractionated heparin and LMWH.[7] Long-term anticoagulation with oral vitamin K antagonists is not generally done in the intensive care unit although patients on these agents such as those with CHD may be admitted to intensive care units. A detailed discussion of this agent is beyond the scope of this chapter but can be found in the following reference.[8]

REFERENCES

1. Hoppe C, Matsunaga A. Pediatric thrombosis. *Pediatr Clin North Am.* 2002;49:1257–1283.
2. Hirsh J, Guyatt G, Albers GW, et al. The seventh ACCP conference on antithrombotic and thrombolytic therapy: Evidence-based guidelines. *Chest.* 2004;126(suppl. 3):172S–173S.
3. Andrew M, Michelson AD, Bovill E, et al. Guidelines for antithrombotic therapy in pediatric patients. *J Pediatr.* 1998;132:575–588.
4. Wang M, Hays T, Balasa V, et al. Pediatric coagulation consortium. Low-dose tissue plasminogen activator thrombolysis in children. *J Pediatr Hematol Oncol.* 2003;25:379–386.
5. Adams RJ, McKie VC, Hsu L, et al. Prevention of a first stroke by transfusions in children with sickle cell anemia and abnormal results on transcranial Doppler ultrasonography. *N Engl J Med.* 1998;339:5–11.
6. Albers GW, Amarenco P, Easton JD, et al. Antithrombotic and thrombolytic therapy for ischemic stroke: The seventh ACCP conference on antithrombotic and thrombolytic therapy. *Chest.* 2004;126(suppl. 3): 483S–512S.
7. Young G. Current and future antithrombotic agents in children. *Expert Rev Cardiovasc Ther.* 2004;2:523–534.
8. Streif W, Andrew M, Marzinotto V, et al. Analysis of warfarin therapy in pediatric patients: A prospective cohort study of 319 patients. *Blood.* 1999;94:3007–3014.

Coagulation Disorders

26

W. Tait Stevens

EVALUATION

Coagulopathic bleeding is common in the pediatric intensive care unit. Fortunately, there are a limited number of common causes of coagulopathic bleeding, and the relatively rapid turnaround in modern laboratories can help guide treatment. This chapter discusses initial evaluation, specific disease entities, and treatment modalities targeted to achieve hemostasis in the pediatric acute care setting.

Patients with pathologic bleeding should have emergent coagulopathy screening, even if there are obvious explanations for the bleeding. The basic laboratory screening panel for neonates includes a complete blood count (CBC) (for platelet count and hemoglobin levels), prothrombin time (PT), activated partial thromboplastin time (aPTT), thrombin time (TT), plasma fibrinogen, and a chemistry panel. In older children, fibrinogen degradation products (FDP) or D-dimer levels are also indicated. Most tests are based on physiologic assumptions and may be invalid in certain circumstances. For example, the amount of citrate in sodium citrate tubes (light-blue-top tubes) is based on a particular amount of plasma expected in the tube. Excessive anticoagulation can occur when insufficient plasma is added to the tube, as may occur if the tube is incompletely filled or if the blood has a very high hematocrit. Heparin contamination may be avoided by carefully flushing the catheter or by drawing samples from a fresh phlebotomy site. Particular care should be paid to avoid hemolysis when drawing the samples. Samples should be gently mixed by inversion immediately after being drawn, to avoid clotting.

Any bleeding in neonates should be evaluated. A detailed bleeding history should include onset, duration, rate, amount, location, and frequency of bleeding. Other history should take into account medications including herbals and over-the-counter drugs, clinical events, previous surgical challenges, comorbid conditions, laboratory trends, and administration of blood products. A family history of bleeding can be particularly helpful in identifying and diagnosing inherited coagulopathy, particularly X-linked disorders.

The physical examination should attempt to identify the sources of bleeding. A complete physical examination may identify abnormalities associated with hemostatic defects such as neurologic changes, lymphadenopathy, absent radii and organomegaly. Imaging tests may be needed to confirm organomegaly or hemorrhage into viscera or surrounding areas.

Test Interpretation

Disseminated intravascular coagulation (DIC) may present with essentially any combination of abnormal tests. Scoring systems have been established to diagnose DIC, most of which rely on a combination of decreased platelet counts, decreased fibrinogen level, aPTT prolongation, and elevated markers of fibrinolysis (FDP or D-dimer).

Thrombocytopenia is classically due to platelet consumption (as in active clot formation, necrotizing enterocolitis, sepsis, immune thrombocytopenia, or DIC), sequestration (splenomegaly), dilution (massive transfusion), or production failure (aplastic anemia). Thrombocytopenic bleeding is rarely spontaneous. Other factors contributing to bleeding should be identifiable unless the thrombocytopenia is profound.

A prolonged aPTT may indicate heparin contamination or coagulopathy. A correction of TT after treatment with protamine sulfate confirms heparin effect, whereas correction of the aPTT on a mixing study, or by use of a heparin absorption test, rules it out. A prolonged aPTT and normal PT suggests hemophilia A or B, von Willebrand disease (vWD), the presence of lupus anticoagulant, or, possibly, contact-factor deficiencies. If the PT is prolonged, vitamin K deficiency, liver disease, or, possibly, hereditary deficiency of factors II, V, VII, or X should be considered. If the aPTT, PT, and TT are all prolonged in the presence of a normal platelet count, hypofibrinogenemia, afibrinogenemia, early liver disease, vitamin K deficiency, or a common pathway inhibitor should be in the differential diagnoses.

An isolated PT prolongation suggests hereditary factor VII deficiency, liver disease, mild vitamin K deficiency, or rarely, the presence of a factor VII inhibitor.

Low fibrinogen levels suggest consumption (such as trauma or DIC), dilution (massive transfusion), or congenital hypofibrinogenemia. Dysfibrinogenemia may present with a prolonged thrombin or reptilase time.

Suspected fibrinolytic disorders may be evaluated with assays for α_2-antiplasmin (α_2-AP) deficiency or plasminogen activator inhibitor-1 (PAI-1) deficiency.

Increased levels of FDP and D-dimer are classic in DIC and hyperfibrinolytic syndromes and may be elevated in thrombotic states (e.g., following surgery, in the presence of marked inflammation, or following a deep vein thrombosis or pulmonary embolus). FDP includes fibrin and fibrinogen breakdown products; D-dimer is a specific FDP resulting from plasmin-mediated fibrinolysis (see Chapter 4).

Normal screening tests may reinforce an impression of postsurgical bleeding or relate to hematologic defects, such as mild hemophilia A or B, vWD, an inherited or acquired platelet function defect, or, more rarely, factor XIII deficiency. Additional testing to narrow down the etiology may include specific factor function assays and platelet function tests.

ACQUIRED DISORDERS

Disseminated Intravascular Coagulation

DIC is a state of widespread activation of the coagulation and fibrinolytic systems, generally initiated by coagulation with accompanying compensatory fibrinolysis and secondary consumption of platelets and clotting factors. DIC may range in severity from very mild with transient lowering of factors to profound coagulopathy with RBC fragmentation and generalized hemorrhage, and is an independent predictor of mortality in sepsis and severe trauma. Newborns have lower levels of coagulation inhibitors (protein C, protein S, and antithrombin) and lower fibrinolytic function, making them more susceptible to DIC than older children.

The common causes of DIC are listed in Table 26.1. Intravascular coagulation may be initiated by a large number of agonists including tissue factor, endotoxins, amniotic fluid, and foreign material (e.g., collagen). If coagulation does not sequester the initiating substance, activation continues and thrombin and fibrin continue to be produced.

In DIC, plasmin-mediated fibrinolysis fails to keep up with disseminated fibrin production. Elevated levels of circulating fibrin may lead to microvascular thrombosis and organ failure. There is a simultaneous bleeding tendency;

TABLE 26.1
COMMON CAUSES OF DISSEMINATED INTRAVASCULAR COAGULATION

Sepsis/severe infection
Trauma
Malignancy
Solid tumors
Acute leukemia
Neonatal issues
Amniotic fluid embolism
Dead twin
Vascular malformations
Severe allergic or other toxic reactions
Severe immunologic reactions (e.g., transfusion reaction)
Heat stroke

Modified from Handin RI, Lux SE, Stossel TP, eds. *Blood: Principles and practice of hematology.* 2nd ed. Philadelphia, PA: Lippincott Williams & Wilkins; 2003.

ongoing activation of coagulation consumes clotting factors (e.g., fibrinogen, platelets, and factors V and VIII), leading to more severe coagulopathy.

Thrombosis may be present in varying locations and amounts. Mild microangiopathic hemolytic anemia is present in many cases and is more severe when associated with widespread malignancy. Systemic thrombosis may occur when fibrinolysis is inadequate (more common in the presence of antifibrinolytics, sepsis, or inadequate levels of protein C in the neonate); sites of thrombosis may result in renal insufficiency, skin infarction, and respiratory failure.

In addition to coagulopathy with thrombosis, the classic findings of DIC are elevated markers of fibrinolysis; with prolonged fibrinolysis, FDP accumulate. At high plasma concentrations, FDP themselves may have an anticoagulant effect.

Monitoring

The classic laboratory findings of DIC are not always present; low platelet count, low fibrinogen levels, and increased D-dimer, PT, aPTT, TT, and fragmented RBCs on the peripheral blood smear. In premature infants, D-dimer levels >500 ng per mL are more indicative than coagulation tests for diagnosing DIC.

Treatment and resolution of DIC can be tracked by following fibrinogen levels. Changes in the platelet count can also be used as an indicator of ongoing thrombogenesis; they will decrease or be extremely low during active DIC because of intravascular aggregation. If there are no other causes for thrombocytopenia, the platelet count will stabilize or rise following resolution of DIC. The PT is often used to measure response of sepsis-related DIC to treatment; aPTT may correlate well. Alternatively, protein

C levels may indicate severity of DIC and may predict the outcome.

Treatment Guidelines

DIC is best treated by aggressive treatment of the underlying disorder to remove the procoagulant stimulus. The decision to replace consumed factors can be challenging and must balance "feeding the fire" with controlling hemorrhage. With persistent bleeding, consumed factors may be replaced as necessary with fresh frozen plasma (FFP) or cryoprecipitate to increase the fibrinogen to >100 mg per dL and platelet transfusions to ≥50,000 per μL. Factor assays may be useful when necessary to guide replacement therapy and to help treat comorbid coagulopathies.

In chronic DIC or DIC complicated by thrombosis, low to moderate doses of heparin (5 to 8 U/kg/hour) have been successful in inhibiting the activation of coagulation, but this approach may be contraindicated in liver disease. Increased platelet and clotting factor support may be indicated since heparin can increase the risk of bleeding in DIC.

In adults, rare cases of DIC associated with malignancy have exhibited marked hyperfibrinolysis. In these cases, antifibrinolytics have been helpful in resolving bleeding.

Procedure-Related Coagulopathy

Bleeding following major procedures has three major causes: inadequate surgical hemostasis, dilutional coagulopathy, and heparin effect. Because all of these conditions may be present simultaneously, a coagulation workup should be performed even when surgical bleeding is suspected.

Cardiopulmonary Bypass and Extracorporeal Membrane-Oxygenation

Platelets are consumed during cardiopulmonary bypass surgery (CPB); additionally, they may partially degranulate, reducing platelet function. Hypothermia may also contribute to suppression of platelet function. Infants normally have lower levels of coagulation factors than adults, and patients with heart disease and decreased hepatic synthetic function may also exhibit lower than normal concentrations of plasma coagulation factor. Coagulopathy due to constitutively low factors is exacerbated by dilution during bypass and heparinization. Factor levels improve spontaneously a few hours after CPB surgery. Since anticoagulant factors are also reduced and the procedure itself may be procoagulant, FFP is recommended only when coagulopathy is problematic or prolonged.

Causes of coagulopathy in patients on extracorporeal membrane-oxygenation (ECMO) are similar to those in CPB. Since ECMO may continue for days or weeks, the overall incidence of bleeding is higher (intracranial hemorrhage will occur in 25% to 50% of newborns on ECMO). Prophylactic FFP and cryoprecipitate transfusions are recommended to correct deficiencies to normal ranges. Platelet transfusions are recommended to keep counts above 80,000 to 100,000 per μL or higher for additional invasive procedures.

Massive Transfusion

Coagulopathy following massive transfusion is not uncommon and is associated with dilution of both procoagulant and anticoagulant factors as well as with decreased body temperature. General considerations in bleeding following massive transfusion include maintaining an adequate hematocrit to ensure adequate oxygen delivery, restoring platelets to ≥50,000 per μL (100,000 per μL in neurosurgical patients), correcting gross PT and aPTT elevations with FFP, and correcting hypofibrinogenemia with cryoprecipitate. Uncontrollable bleeding has been successfully treated with recombinant factor VIIa, but it should be used cautiously in hypercoagulable states. Anticoagulants such as protein C, protein S, and antithrombin are also diluted in massive transfusion, so full correction of procoagulant factors may lead to a net hypercoagulable state. DIC should also be considered following prolonged operative procedures, particularly if blood-salvage techniques have been employed.

RBCs, platelets, and FFP are anticoagulated by citrate, which works by binding ionized calcium. In massive transfusion, enough citrate may be infused to cause symptoms of hypocalcemia and hypotension. This effect is exacerbated in infants and neonates because of their limited hepatic clearance function. Bolus intravenous calcium based on laboratory tests of ionized calcium can rapidly correct the symptoms and the hemostatic defect.

Rapid infusion of multiple units of cold RBCs may induce hypothermia. A body temperature of <35°C contributes to coagulopathy by reducing platelet function, impairing secondary clot formation (through the coagulation cascade), and limiting citrate metabolism.

The effects of massive transfusion are body-size dependent, manifesting more quickly in neonates and infants than in older children.

Thrombocytopenia

Approximately one in eight neonates admitted to a neonatal intensive care unit (NICU) will develop thrombocytopenia of <100,000 per μL. Nonalloimmune neonatal thrombocytopenia presents by day 2 of life, is maximal by day 4, and then recovers over the next week. Prophylactic platelet transfusions in nonbleeding patients are not recommended unless thrombocytopenia is profound or platelet function defects are suspected. If coexisting risk factors suggest an increased likelihood of bleeding, transfusion may be considered in a nonbleeding patient at platelet counts of 20,000 per μL or less. For patients with active bleeding, and in the absence of platelet function defects, a platelet count of 50,000 per μL is sufficient for hemostasis; this target is usually raised to 80,000 or 100,000 per μL when bleeding may be of profound clinical significance, such as in the central nervous system (CNS) and retinal bleeding.

Neonatal Alloimmune Thrombocytopenia

Neonatal alloimmune thrombocytopenia (NAIT) occurs when fetal platelets express an antibody that the mother is lacking and to which the mother produces an antibody. NAIT presents with unexpected moderate or severe thrombocytopenia in approximately 1 in 2,000 live births. NAIT may be diagnosed by identifying maternal antibody to infant (or paternal) platelets. The most common inciting antigen (HPA-1a) is absent in 2% of the population. Treatment consists of transfusing platelets collected from an antigen-negative donor; washed, irradiated, maternally derived platelets are used most frequently.

Idiopathic Thrombocytopenic Purpura

In idiopathic thrombocytopenic purpura (ITP), a common hemorrhagic disorder with thrombocytopenia, there is autoantibody-mediated destruction of platelets. New cases occur in 4 in 100,000 children per year, typically following a viral infection. Neonates may experience an ITP-like syndrome secondary to maternal ITP. Most cases of ITP are relatively mild and may not need treatment.

Platelet-associated antibodies are of limited diagnostic benefit due to poor specificity; an increase in reticulated platelets has a better positive predictive value, although this test is not widely available. The PT and aPTT are usually normal. Platelet counts of <20,000 per μL are not uncommon.

In children, acute ITP with bleeding may be treated by corticosteroids, anti-D immune globulin, intravenous immunoglobulin, local interventions, or careful observation. Because of the etiology of ITP, platelet transfusions should be reserved for life-threatening bleeding. Splenectomy may be considered in refractory cases.

Platelet Function Defects

Acquired platelet function defects may be multifactorial and are frequently difficult to diagnose. The most common causes of acquired platelet function defects are uremia, liver failure, dysproteinemias, myeloproliferative disorders, and drug effect (see in the subsequent text). Platelet function disorders may be challenging to diagnose, as PT, aPTT, TT, and CBC can be normal. Platelet function may be tested in the laboratory by measuring platelet response to agonists such as collagen or epinephrine. The most common sites of bleeding are skin and mucous membrane; petechiae and ecchymosis, nosebleeds, bleeding from venipuncture sites, and gastrointestinal bleeding are common.

Drug-Related Platelet Dysfunction

Drug-related platelet dysfunction is likely underdiagnosed. Drugs known to interfere with platelet function include aspirin and other conventional nonsteroidal anti-inflammatory drugs, ω-3 fatty acids, sulfinpyrazone, ticlopidine, clopidogrel, propofol, and many antimicrobial drugs (including early generation penicillins and cephalosporins). Platelet inhibition by antimicrobial agents may not occur for days to weeks. Drug-induced platelet dysfunction can be tested with platelet function tests. The suspected agent should be changed or discontinued if possible; transfusions may be helpful in controlling problematic bleeding. 1-Deamino-8-D-arginine vasopressin (DDAVP; desmopressin) may also be useful.

Uremia

Bleeding associated with renal failure has reduced with the use of dialysis and erythropoietin, but it still occurs. Retroperitoneal bleeding may follow femoral catheterization. Subdural hematomas occur in approximately 10% of adult patients on hemodialysis and may be life threatening.

The first-line treatment for uremic bleeding is the correction of anemia to a hematocrit of 30% with recombinant erythropoietin or with RBC transfusions; this promotes margination of platelets to the vessel wall. RBC transfusions are preferred because of their speed in correcting anemia. One or two doses of DDAVP at 0.3 μg per kg may help stop active bleeding, although tachyphylaxis may occur if doses are given more frequently than at 24-hour intervals. Cryoprecipitate may be helpful for up to 36 hours in some cases. Conjugated estrogens at 0.6 mg/kg/day for 4 to 5 days may improve bleeding times within a few hours and remain effective for up to 2 weeks.

Myeloproliferative Disorders

Myeloproliferative disorders include polycythemia vera, chronic myelogenous leukemia, essential thrombocytosis, and myeloid metaplasia. Bleeding in myeloproliferative disorders may be related to increased numbers of dysfunctional platelets or secondary thrombocytopenia. Platelet transfusions may be effective in reducing bleeding. Diagnosis and control of the myeloproliferative disorder are critical to long-term hemostasis.

Liver Disease

Coagulopathy in patients with liver disease is caused by low clotting factor levels, anemia (with low endogenous erythropoietin), and low platelet counts. Treatment of coagulopathy of liver disease includes correction of anemia with erythropoietin or RBC transfusions, correction of factor deficiencies with FFP or cryoprecipitate, and improvement of thrombocytopenia with transfusions. Low-dose recombinant factor VIIa has also been used successfully in cases of refractory bleeding due to liver disease.

Vitamin K Deficiency

Vitamin K is necessary for proper, fully formed function of prothrombin, factor VII, factor IX, and factor X, as well as proteins C and S. The classic presentation of neonatal vitamin K deficiency is hemorrhagic disease of the newborn, with gastrointestinal bleeding, ecchymosis, bleeding from puncture sites, or even intracranial hemorrhage between days 2 and 5 of life. However, vitamin K–deficient bleeding may present within the first 24 hours, particularly if the mother was on medications that affect vitamin K storage or function, such as oral anticoagulants, anticonvulsants, rifampin, and isoniazid. Alternatively, vitamin K deficiency may show up weeks to months later in children with liver disease or other morbidities.

Vitamin K deficiency may be suspected on history, clinical presentation, or isolated deficiencies of vitamin K–dependent factors. Vitamin K levels can be measured directly, as can decarboxylated forms of the vitamin K–dependent factors. In bleeding patients, FFP may be given to partially correct vitamin K–dependent factor deficiency; 10 to 20 mL per kg is usually adequate to achieve hemostasis. However, time is required to thaw FFP, and the volume may be excessive. Vitamin K deficiency may be corrected by subcutaneous, intramuscular, or intravenous administration of 0.5 to 1 mg of the vitamin. If immediate control of bleeding is necessary, as in intracranial hemorrhage, prothrombin complexes, or even relatively low-dose recombinant factor VIIa are suggested.

Hypofibrinogenemia

Clot formation is dependent on adequate levels of functional fibrinogen. Acquired hypofibrinogenemia may be due to increased consumption of clotting factors (e.g., DIC), dilution (due to massive transfusion), or decreased production (e.g., liver disease or insult). Management involves transfusion of fibrinogen-containing products such as cryoprecipitate or FFP. (See also section on "Hypofibrinogenemia and Dysfibrinogenemia.")

INHERITED DISORDERS

Inherited coagulation disorders can be very complex and should be managed in conjunction with an experienced hematologist whenever possible.

Hemophilia A

Hemophilia A, an X-linked recessive bleeding disorder with decreased factor VIII concentration or function, is found in approximately 1 in 5,000 males. A variety of molecular etiologies lead to clinical diseases of varying severity. Bleeds present as spontaneous musculoskeletal bleeding, CNS bleeding, and disproportionate bleeding following minor trauma.

Definitive treatment of an acute bleed is rapid restoration of factor VIII function, ideally with recombinant factor VIII concentrates. If factor VIII is unavailable, either recombinant or human concentrate, or if there are other factor deficiencies, cryoprecipitate may also be acceptable. DDAVP causes release of von Willebrand factor (vWF) and factor VIII from endothelium and may be adequate therapy in mild or moderate disease. Antifibrinolytic therapy may help stabilize and maintain a clot and has been a useful adjunct in treating mucosal bleeds.

Patients with hemophilia may develop inhibitors to transfused factors and can be particularly challenging to manage.

Hemophilia B

Hemophilia B is an X-linked recessive bleeding disorder with a deficiency of factor IX level or function, found in approximately 1 in 30,000 males. Clinically, it is very similar to hemophilia A. There are several hundred variants of hemophilia B, manifesting clinically with a wide range of severity. Other reported causes of low factor IX levels include liver disease, vitamin K deficiency, warfarin therapy, and nephrotic syndrome.

Acute bleeds may be treated with recombinant or, when unavailable, human-derived factor IX concentrate.

von Willebrand Disease

vWD, an autosomal dominant bleeding disorder, with a defect of vWF level or function, is found in approximately 1% of the general population. Most have a mild functional defect with mildly prolonged bleeding; 5% have more severe disease with clinically significant bleeding. Laboratory findings vary with specific disease types. Treatment varies with disease type and severity of the bleeding episode: DDAVP is the first-line treatment of type 1 vWD in most settings. Since patient response varies, a trial may be indicated before use in surgery. Human plasma–derived antihemophilic factor/vWF containing factor VIII and vWF (Humate P) is the first-line treatment of patients with type 1 vWD undergoing major surgery and the second line-treatment for type 1 vWD in other settings. Factor replacement is the first-line therapy in types 2 and 3. DDAVP may be helpful in some type 2 vWD, but is usually contraindicated in type 2b. DDAVP is not useful in type 3 vWD.

Platelet Defects

A variety of inherited platelet function defects result from reduced platelet adhesion, aggregation, or secretion. The inherited platelet function defects share a final common pathway; even in the presence of normal platelet counts, they produce bleeding consistent with thrombocytopenia: petechiae, ecchymosis, epistaxis, gastrointestinal hemorrhage, menorrhagia, and excessive bleeding following trauma or surgery. Acute bleeding in patients with most forms of acquired platelet function defects can be ameliorated with platelet transfusions or DDAVP.

One exception is Glanzmann thrombasthenia, an autosomal recessive absence of IIb/IIIa receptors or receptor function that is not responsive to DDAVP. Bleeding in Glanzmann thrombasthenia may be profound and generally requires platelet transfusion, although some have reported success using recombinant factor VIIa for surgical bleeding and epistaxis.

Platelet-type pseudo-vWD occurs when a defective platelet vWF receptor (glycoprotein Ib) spontaneously binds to plasma vWF, leading to increased clearance of vWF and platelets. Platelet-type pseudo-vWD may be effectively treated with platelet transfusions; vWF-enriched concentrates are rarely needed.

Fibrinolysis

α_2-AP (also known as α_2-plasmin inhibitor, or α_2-PI) normally down-regulates plasmin-mediated breakdown of fibrin. PAI-1 indirectly downregulates fibrinolysis by inhibiting tissue plasminogen activator (tPA). Absent or nonfunctional α_2-AP or PAI-1 leads to unopposed plasmin-mediated fibrinolysis, causing a profound bleeding tendency. Family history is particularly important in diagnosis. Since α_2-AP and PAI-1 disorders are rare, testing may require a referral to a specialized coagulation reference laboratory. Bleeding due to hyperfibrinolysis in α_2-AP and PAI-1 disorders has been effectively treated with lysine-analog antifibrinolytics (e.g., Amicar or tranexamic acid).

Hypofibrinogenemia and Dysfibrinogenemia

Congenital hypofibrinogenemia and dysfibrinogenemia are rare. Treatment of bleeding is directed at achieving hemostatic levels of functional fibrinogen (approximately 100 mg per dL) by cryoprecipitate transfusion. Prophylactic transfusions are usually avoided because patients with congenital afibrinogenemia may form antibodies to fibrinogen.

Other Factor Deficiencies

Coagulopathy may also be associated with defects in a number of other factors. Deficiencies of factors II, V, VII, X, and XI are rare; factor-specific assays can detect reduced factor function. They can be treated with factor concentrates or with FFP, and response to treatment can be measured directly.

THERAPIES

Perfect hemostasis may not always be safely achievable. Since all treatments have drawbacks, clinical judgment is important to determine whether nonhematologic control of bleeding is preferable to the drawbacks of aggressive treatment.

TABLE 26.2

CONTENT AND *IN VIVO* HALF-LIFE OF THE MAJOR COAGULATION FACTORS IN A UNIT OR BAG (10 TO 20 ML) OF CRYOPRECIPITATE

Coagulation Factor	Per Bag	Half-life (h)
Fibrinogen	150–250 mg	100–150
Factor VIII	80–150 U	12
Factor XIII	50–75 U	150–300
von Willebrand factor	100–150 U	24

Modified from Mintz PD, ed. *Transfusion therapy: Clinical principles and practice.* 2nd ed. Bethesda, MD: AABB Press; 2005.

Calculations

Clotting factors are measured in "units," (U), with 1 U being the amount of activity in 1 mL of normal plasma. Since laboratory measurements of factor levels are reported as percentages of normal function, it is relatively straightforward to calculate the dose needed to correct a known deficiency. Physicians must also know the activity in the product to be administered. For example, cryoprecipitate is expected to have approximately 100 U of factor VIII per bag (see Table 26.2).

Fresh Frozen Plasma

FFP is prepared by freezing plasma from the collection of a unit of whole blood. Because the plasma is frozen within a few hours of collection, even labile clotting factors remain (see Table 26.3). FFP is particularly useful for correcting multiple simultaneous factor deficiencies, such as massive transfusion, or for factor deficiencies when

TABLE 26.3

CONCENTRATION AND *IN VIVO* HALF-LIFE OF COAGULATION FACTORS IN FRESH FROZEN PLASMA

Coagulation Factor	Concentration	Half-life (h)
Fibrinogen	2–4.5 mg/dL	100–150
Prothrombin (factor II)	~1 U/mL	50–80
Factor V	~1 U/mL	12–24
Factor VII	~1 U/mL	6
Factor VIII	~1 U/mL	12
Factor IX	~1 U/mL	24
Factor X	~1 U/mL	30–60
Factor XI	~1 U/mL	40–80
Factor XIII	~1 U/mL	150–300
von Willebrand factor	~1 U/mL	24

Modified from Mintz PD, ed. *Transfusion therapy: Clinical principles and practice.* 2nd ed. Bethesda, MD: AABB Press; 2005, with permission.

appropriate concentrates are not available. FFP may be indicated when the PT or aPTT are >1.5 times normal. Transfusion of 10 to 20 mL per kg should increase coagulation protein levels by 20% to 30%. A unit of FFP ranges from approximately 250 to 300 mL. In practice, smaller volumes are transfusable from pediatric packs (70 to 80 mL) or from aliquots taken from a full unit. Risks associated with FFP transfusion include volume overload, transfusion-transmitted diseases, and transfusion-related acute lung injury (TRALI). TRALI is a serious pulmonary complication of transfusion with pulmonary injury thought to be due to neutrophil activation, with a 5% to 10% fatality rate. FFP is also indicated for urgent reversal of Coumadin toxicity and in active bleeding with a history or clinical course suggesting inherited or acquired coagulopathy.

Cryoprecipitate

Cryoprecipitate is prepared by slowly thawing FFP at 1°C to 6°C and collecting the precipitated proteins. This product contains most of the factor VIII, vWF, fibrinogen, and some of the factor XIII in the original unit of plasma (Table 26.2). Transfusion-transmitted viruses can be transmitted despite freezing. Cryoprecipitate is the first-line therapy for treating factor XIII deficiency and hypofibrinogenemia (1 U per 7 kg of body weight may raise fibrinogen levels to 100 mg per dL). Cryoprecipitate may also be a useful adjunct therapy when DDAVP or conjugated estrogens fail to control uremic bleeding. Cryoprecipitate is not virally inactivated; the risk of transfusion-transmitted viruses is similar to that of FFP and whole blood.

Platelets

Platelet concentrates are collected by centrifugation of whole blood or by apheresis. Platelet transfusions should be administered to raise counts to 50,000 per μL for most invasive procedures and 100,000 per μL for procedures in which related bleeding may be particularly problematic. In the acute setting, the risk of procedure-induced bleeding may be less than the risk of delaying a procedure for platelet transfusion. A platelet dose of 5 mL per kg will ideally raise the count by 100,000 per μL, but response to platelets is usually much less. Increments may be decreased in the presence of active bleeding, DIC, sepsis, fever, splenomegaly, human leukocyte antigen alloimmunization, and immune thrombocytopenic purpura. Platelet concentrates are stored in plasma that includes nonlabile clotting factors. Risks of platelet transfusion include febrile and allergic reactions, TRALI, transfusion-transmitted diseases (including bacterial contamination), and volume overload. Neonates and other immunosuppressed patients are at particular risk for transfusion-associated-graft versus host disease (TA-GVHD), due to transfused passenger lymphocytes. This can be eliminated by irradiation; some facilities irradiate all cellular products.

Red Blood Cells

RBCs are collected by centrifugation of whole blood or by apheresis and stored at 1°C to 6°C. Hemostasis may be improved by transfusing to a target hematocrit of 30% to 35%. Risks of RBC transfusion include alloimmunization and acute and delayed hemolytic transfusion reactions, transfusion-transmitted diseases, and volume overload. Patients requiring cytomegalovirus- (CMV-) attenuated blood products should receive either CMV seronegative or third-generation leukodepleted blood products that are considered to be equivalent to CMV seronegative products. As in the case of platelets, irradiation is necessary to preclude TA-GVHD by red blood cell transfusions.

Specific Clotting Factors

The readily available factor concentrates vary widely by hospital formulary, but generally include recombinant preparations of factors VIII and IX and Humate P for vWD.

Activated recombinant factor VII (rVIIa) is a powerful procoagulant that has been formally approved by the U.S. Food and Drug Administration (FDA) for treatment of bleeding in factor VIII and factor IX–deficient hemophiliacs (hemophilia A and B) with inhibitors at a recommended dose of 90 μg per kg every 2 hours until cessation of bleeding. It is also used to control bleeding in patients with factor VII deficiency. Anecdotal reports suggest rVIIa may help control refractory bleeding in patients without hemophilia, particularly in post-traumatic or postoperative bleeding and in vitamin K deficiency. A lower dose may be effective in these settings; however, it should not be used when there is active clotting present (DIC, thromboembolic disease/deep venous thrombosis). Its use with procoagulant drugs, such as antifibrinolytics, has not been well studied.

The goal of factor VIII or IX replacement therapy is to reach a target plasma factor level, selected on the basis of the severity of bleed (see Table 26.4). In an intensive care setting, a loading dose bolus followed by continuous intravenous drip provides efficacy with the lowest drug use. Pharmacokinetics varies by age, blood volume, blood group, and from individual to individual, so response to factor VIII or IX administration must be monitored and dosing titrated appropriately. Inhibitory antibodies to factor VIII develop in up to 20% of severe factor VIII cases and in approximately 3% of factor IX cases. There are limited treatment options for patients who are bleeding and have inhibitory antibodies to factor VIII or IX; in particular, recombinant factor VIIa has been approved by the FDA for use in this setting.

1-Deamino-8-D-Arginine Vasopressin; Desmopressin

DDAVP (0.3 μg per kg parenterally) causes release of stored vWF and factor VIII from stores in endothelial cells. The effect on coagulopathy begins in about an hour and lasts 4 to 12 hours. The response to DDAVP administration

TABLE 26.4
FACTOR VIII AND IX DOSING GUIDE

Type of Bleeding	Factor Correction	Duration	Comments
Head trauma	100% for all head trauma in severe hemophilia	30%–50% correction every 12 h for 1–2 doses	Always treat before diagnostic imaging, even without bleeding or neurologic symptoms
Tongue or neck swelling	100%	As necessary for hemostasis	Patients should be evaluated to rule out airway obstruction
Compartment syndrome	70%–100% correction	30%–50% correction every 12 h	
Flank or abdominal pain	70%–100% correction	Duration dependent on nature of bleeding	Obtain CT scan of abdomen/pelvis to evaluate bleeding
Hemarthrosis (minor or early)	50%–70% correction	30% in 12 h, repeat at 24 or 36 h	Splint joint
Hemarthrosis (chronic, late, or target joint)	70% correction	30% correction at 12 and 24 h	Patients with factor IX should receive second dose at 4–8 h and third at 24 h
Muscle bleeding	30% correction	Follow-up at 12–24 h	Immobilize area
Thigh/iliopsoas bleeding	70% correction	Maintain factor above 30% for 2–6 d	Monitor Hb for blood loss; bed rest recommended
Fractures	70% correction	Maintain above 30% for 5–7 d	
Sutures	70% correction	30% correction during removal	Attempt steri-strips if possible

CT, computed tomography.
Modified from Herman JH, Manno CS, eds. *Pediatric transfusion therapy*. Bethesda, MD: AABB Press; 2002.

progressively diminishes as stores are depleted. Endothelial synthesis will partially restore levels in approximately 24 hours.

Antifibrinolytics

ε-Aminocaproic acid (EACA) and tranexamic acid (aminomethylcyclohexane carboxylic acid; AMCA) are lysine-analog antifibrinolytics. They help ensure clot stability by blocking fibrinolysis through competitive inhibition of plasmin and tPA at lysine binding sites. EACA and AMCA are used systemically as definitive treatment of congenital and procedure-related hyperfibrinolytic states and have been shown to reduce blood loss in cardiac surgery. They also may be used locally (e.g., to control oral or uterine bleeding) with a decreased risk of systemic effects. Attempted use in urologic bleeding has been associated with ureteral obstruction, but antifibrinolytics may be helpful with bladder irrigation to control bleeding localized to the bladder. Antifibrinolytics are contraindicated in DIC and should be used only after careful consideration in fibrinolytic conditions or in prothrombotic states (e.g., within 12 hours of prothrombin concentrate administration). Prolonged use of EACA may lead to myonecrosis. Another antifibrinolytic, aprotinin, inhibits a variety of proteases and has been shown to reduce blood loss, need for re-exploration, and mortality in open-heart surgery in adults. Aprotinin is more expensive than lysine analogs. It is a bovine-derived protein, and it may cause anaphylactic shock or even death.

RECOMMENDED READINGS

1. Handin RI, Lux SE, Stossel TP, eds. *Blood: Principles and practice of hematology*. 2nd ed. Philadelphia, PA: Lippincott Williams & Wilkins; 2003.
2. Hathaway WE, Goodnight SH, eds. *Disorders of hemostasis and thrombosis: A clinical guide*. 2nd ed. New York: McGraw-Hill; 1993.
3. Herman JH, Manno CS, eds. *Pediatric transfusion therapy*. Bethesda, MD: AABB Press; 2002.
4. Hillyer CD, Silberstein LE, Ness PM, et al. eds. *Blood banking and transfusion medicine: Basic principles and practice*. Philadelphia, PA: Churchill Livingstone; 2003.
5. Hoffman RH, Benz EJ, Shattil SJ, et al. eds. *Hematology: Basic principles and practice*. Philadelphia, PA: Churchill Livingstone; 2005.
6. Huang WY, Kruskall MS, Bauer KA. The use of recombinant activated factor VII in three patients with central nervous system hemorrhages associated with factor VII deficiency. *Transfusion*. 2004;44:1562–1566.
7. Kitchens CS, Alving BM, Kessler CM, eds. *Consultative hemostasis and thrombosis*. Philadelphia, PA: WB Saunders; 2002.
8. Loscalzo J, Schafer AI, eds. *Thrombosis and hemorrhage*. 3rd ed. Philadelphia, PA: Lippincott Williams & Wilkins; 2003.
9. Mintz PD, ed. *Transfusion therapy: Clinical principles and practice*. 2nd ed. Bethesda, MD: AABB Press; 2005.
10. Simon TL, Dzik WH, Snyder EL, et al. eds. *Rossi's principles of transfusion medicine*. 3rd ed. Philadelphia, PA: Lippincott Williams & Wilkins; 2002.

Oncologic Emergencies

Edward C. Wong   Anne L. Angiolillo

The pediatric oncology patient poses special problems for the pediatric intensive care specialist. Oncologic emergencies largely arise because of the underlying disease and the sequelae of intensive chemotherapy. Treatment can cause profound immunosuppression and impaired hematopoiesis, as well as marked organ system and metabolic perturbations. In this chapter, we review the assessment and management of various oncologic emergencies in children. Table 27.1 summarizes the various emergencies according to the organ system. The reader is referred to excellent reviews of this topic for further details.[1,2]

CARDIOTHORACIC EMERGENCIES

Cardiothoracic emergencies in pediatric oncology patients range from superior vena cava syndrome (SVCS), which may be characterized only by respiratory distress, to entities such as the retinoic acid syndrome, which involves pulmonary damage by interstitial infiltration of maturing leukocytes. In general, these cardiothoracic emergencies may be classified by their anatomic location. In the anterior mediastinum, conditions such as the SVCS and superior mediastinal syndrome (SMS) predominate, whereas cardiac tamponade, myopathy/myocarditis, and intracardiac masses are the primary concerns in the middle mediastinum. In the posterior thoracic region, cord compression can result from mass lesions, and within the lung parenchyma, a number of diseases can threaten normal physiologic gas exchange.

Superior Vena Cava Syndrome and Superior Mediastinal Syndrome

SVCS and SMS arise from compression, obstruction, or thrombosis of the superior vena cava (SVC) (see Fig. 27.1).

TABLE 27.1

TYPE OF PEDIATRIC ONCOLOGIC EMERGENCY ACCORDING TO THE ORGAN SYSTEM

Organ System	Type
Cardiothoracic	Superior vena cava syndrome/superior mediastinal syndrome
	Pleural and pericardial effusions
	Cardiac tamponade
	Massive hemoptysis
	Pneumothorax/pneumomediastinum
	Retinoic acid syndrome
Abdominal	Gastrointestinal hemorrhage
	Gastrointestinal obstruction
	Gastrointestinal perforation
	Gastrointestinal infection/inflammation
	Acute massive hepatomegaly in neuroblastoma
	Hemorrhagic pancreatitis
Genitourinary	Oliguria/anuria
	Hypertension
	Hemorrhagic cystitis
Neurologic	Cerebrovascular accident
	Seizure
	Intrathecal chemotherapy overdose/error
	Spinal cord compression
	Hyperleukocytosis
Metabolic	Tumor lysis syndrome
	Malignant hypercalcemia
	Hyponatremia (SIADH)

SIADH, syndrome of inappropriate secretion of antidiuretic hormone.

When tracheal compression occurs, SMS results. Because both syndromes are often present, both terms are used synonymously. In children with malignancies, the most common symptoms of SMS and SVCS include facial swelling, cough, dyspnea, dysphagia, orthopnea, wheezing,

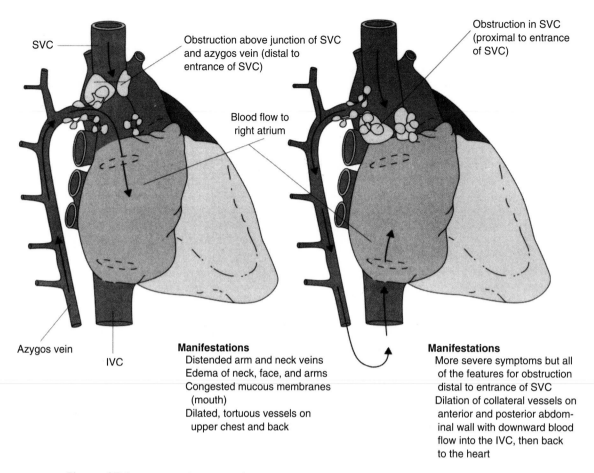

SVC

Obstruction above junction of SVC and azygos vein (distal to entrance of SVC)

Obstruction in SVC (proximal to entrance of SVC)

Blood flow to right atrium

Azygos vein

IVC

Manifestations
Distended arm and neck veins
Edema of neck, face, and arms
Congested mucous membranes (mouth)
Dilated, tortuous vessels on upper chest and back

Manifestations
More severe symptoms but all of the features for obstruction distal to entrance of SVC
Dilation of collateral vessels on anterior and posterior abdominal wall with downward blood flow into the IVC, then back to the heart

Figure 27.1 Anatomic locations of superior vena cava (SVC) obstruction leading to the SVC syndrome. IVC, inferior vena cava. (From Skarin AT, ed. *Atlas of diagnostic oncology.* 2nd ed. St Louis, MO: Mosby; 1996.)

and hoarseness. These symptoms can be aggravated when the patient is in the supine position or when placed in the fetal position for a lumbar puncture. Symptoms will typically worsen rapidly over several days. Diagnostic imaging studies are necessary for the diagnosis. Clues to the presence of SMS or SVCS include the presence of mediastinal widening, pleural effusions, and tracheal deviation in the chest radiograph. Computerized tomography (CT) may be helpful in delineating the anatomic distortions. However, because the symptoms just described are also commonly observed in other pathologic processes, echocardiography and pulmonary function tests may help in ascertaining a pericardial effusion or thromboembolism. It is often useful to obtain a tissue specimen to confirm that the tumor is the cause of the SMS or SVCS. This is best obtained by direct biopsy; however, examination of the peripheral blood smear and bone marrow aspirate or cytologic examination of fluid obtained by pleurocentesis or pericardiocentesis may also provide evidence of tumor involvement. Patients who require anesthesia should have an evaluation by an anesthesiologist because of known intolerance to anesthesia and occasional difficulty in intubating these patients. A

suggested algorithm for assessment and treatment of SMS or SVCS is seen in Figure 27.2.

Emergent therapy for SVCS or SMS can be problematic if a tissue diagnosis is not possible. Presently, there are no established recommendations for therapy; however, if there is strong suspicion that the patient has a tumor type that is radiosensitive, radiotherapy may be effective. For instance, in non-Hodgkin lymphoma, radiotherapy can effectively produce symptomatic relief within 12 hours. Although radiotherapy is also preferred in the presence of renal failure in order to avoid tumor lysis syndrome (TLS), this can render postradiation tissue diagnosis difficult. Radiotherapy is not without its problems, and in fact, significant tracheal swelling can occur, with further respiratory deterioration. This latter problem is partially addressed by using focused radiation portals to the tracheal region or using small, bilateral opposing fields that include the trachea, subclavicular region, and proximal right auricle. Timing and dosage of radiotherapy will depend on the presumed radiosensitivity of the tumor. In contrast, the use of chemotherapy (generally indicated in acute lymphoblastic leukemia [ALL] with high white blood cell [WBC] counts in the presence of a

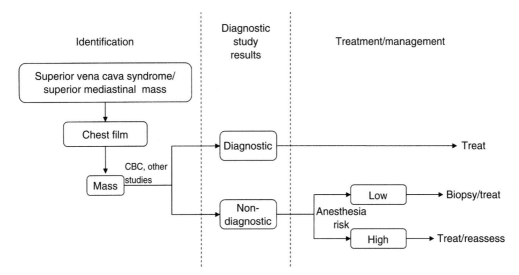

Figure 27.2 Suggested algorithm for assessment and management of symptomatic superior vena cava syndrome or superior mediastinal mass with a known anterior mediastinal mass. If radiographic and laboratory studies are nondiagnostic, anesthesia risk versus the need to obtain tissue must be weighed. If the risk is low, a biopsy for diagnostic studies is recommended. On the other hand, if anesthesia risk is high and there is marked clinical urgency, treatment should be initiated after consultation with a pediatric hematology/oncology specialist. If, after reassessment, anesthesia risk is low, then obtaining tissue sample may be feasible to confirm the diagnosis; otherwise continued empirical treatment may be necessary. CBC, complete blood count.

mediastinal mass) including steroids (to prevent worsening of radiation-induced tracheal swelling) may also confound the pathologic diagnosis. Signs or symptoms of SVCS present in a patient with a central venous line should always prompt a workup for an extensive thromboembolus as chemotherapy or radiotherapy may not be always appropriate. Thrombolytic therapy (see Chapter 25) can be initiated if there are no contraindications. In general, systemic heparin therapy should be initiated after thrombolytic therapy at a loading dose of 75 U per kg, with a maintenance dose of 20 U per kg for children older than 1 year, maintaining activated partial thromboplastin time (aPTT) between 60 and 85 seconds.[3] This should correspond to an anti-Xa activity between 0.35 and 0.70 U per mL. Anticoagulation should be continued for 3 to 6 months using coumadin or low-molecular-weight heparin (LMWH). Recommended guidelines can be seen in Reference 4.

Life-Threatening Effusions

Life-threatening effusions can be caused by either a primary malignancy or an infection (exudative effusion), or from fluid overload, heart failure, hypoproteinemia, or a reactive response to tumor presence in the chest or the abdomen (transudative effusion). Overall, symptoms may include dyspnea, orthopnea, cough, and chest pain. Chylous effusions can also result from thoracic duct obstruction. In patients with untreated cancer and respiratory distress, a single thoracentesis is often adequate as little reaccumulation of fluid occurs during treatment. In contrast, patients with advanced disease often require repeated thoracenteses with the use of a percutaneous catheter for drainage. In these cases, the use of a sclerosing agent such as tetracycline or talc may be helpful. Although surgical pleurectomy or pericardiectomy may be necessary if sclerosis is not effective, this procedure is associated with considerably increased morbidity and mortality.

Large pericardial effusions resulting in cardiac tamponade may necessitate emergent thoracentesis or pericardiocentesis for rapid cardiopulmonary relief. Cardiac tamponade may occur as a result of pericardial inflammation or infection, leukemic infiltration, postradiation fibrosis, or occlusion by tumors situated within the cardiac muscle or endocardium. Infectious pericarditis or myocarditis is usually the most common cause of tamponade in immunocompromised children with cancer. Marantic vegetations or clots within the heart can also cause tamponade. Symptoms of impending tamponade resemble congestive heart failure and include dyspnea, chest pain, cough, hiccups, and abdominal pain. Typical signs include tachycardia, hypotension, cyanosis, and a pulsus paradoxus of >10 mm Hg. Cardiac tamponade must be distinguished from congestive heart failure, infectious pericarditis or myocarditis, and therapy-induced cardiomyopathy. Radiographic studies may be informative. In the anteroposterior view of the chest film, a "waterbag" cardiac shadow may be evident. In the lateral view, there may be an abnormal space between the pericardial fat and pericardium. Echocardiography of the posterior wall often displays two echoes, one from the cardiac muscle and one from the pericardium. Thickening of the pericardium consistent with pericarditis or tumor can also be noted by echocardiography. Electrocardiogram (EKG) findings may include low-voltage QRS complexes, flattened or inverted T waves, and electrical atrial and ventricular alternans. If pericardiocentesis is performed, diagnostic studies of the fluid should, at a minimum, include evaluation for protein, glucose, cell counts and differential, culture, Gram stain, and cytology.

Therapy for malignant pericardial effusions and constrictive pericarditis is largely supportive and consists of hydration, oxygenation, and optimizing of patient position to maximize cardiac output. Diuretics are contraindicated. Definitive treatment is the immediate removal of fluid under echocardiographic guidance. More invasive procedures such as subxiphoid pericardiotomy or pericardial window are associated with a high success rate, with low morbidity and mortality. For palliation, sclerosing agents can be used in recurrent or refractory tumors. If a Wilms' tumor thrombus is found to extend into the right side of the heart and if the thrombus does not occlude the chambers, therapy with dactinomycin and vincristine has been found to reduce the size of the thrombus within a week.

Massive Hemoptysis

Massive hemoptysis can lead to asphyxiation as a result of thrombus formation in the bronchial tree and infrequently, exsanguination. Mild hemoptysis in a patient with cancer usually results from aspiration of blood from epistaxis whereas massive hemoptysis usually results from invasive pulmonary aspergillosis. The incidence of pulmonary hemoptysis from pulmonary aspergillosis ranges from 2% to 26%. Although a chest x-ray can reveal nodular or cavitary lesions or peripheral wedge-shaped or disseminated infiltrates, CT scans can better delineate the extent of fungal disease. Differential diagnoses include all invasive fungi, bacterial pneumonia, and consolidation with invasive organisms such as *Staphylococcus aureus*, *Klebsiella*, and *Pseudomonas* sp. It is important to assess for any coagulation abnormality (by review of complete blood count [CBC], prothrombin time, partial thromboplastin time, fibrinogen and fibrin degradation product levels) and transfuse appropriately, in order to minimize hemoptysis and maintain adequate oxygenation (see Chapter 26). Therapy is largely directed at the prevention of asphyxiation, localizing and stopping the site of bleeding. Although transcatheter embolization or occlusion with a balloon catheter can be successful in massive hemoptysis, these measures are largely unsuccessful in patients with invasive pulmonary aspergillosis. Shapiro et al.[5] described the successful use of a no. 12 French Ring-McLean sump catheter to aspirate the aspergillus cavity and instill a solution containing *N*-acetylcysteine and amphotericin B. In most cases of mild hemoptysis, bleeding eventually stops; however, in patients with fungal disease, the lesion often requires excision to treat the hemoptysis. If the underlying malignancy is the cause of the hemoptysis, surgical resection may be necessary; however, initiation of chemotherapy or irradiation may also improve symptoms rapidly. Therefore, consultation with a hematology/oncology specialist is advised in these situations.

Pneumothorax/Pneumomediastinum

Pneumothorax or pneumomediastinum may be a rare presentation of an undiagnosed malignancy but is more often due to infection, chemotherapy-related emesis, perforation of the esophagus, recurrent or metastatic disease, pulmonary fibrosis secondary to radiation or bleomycin, pulmonary histiocytosis, or idiopathic causes. Treatment of tension pneumothorax or pneumomediastinum includes placement of 100% oxygen, needle thoracentesis (or subxiphoid incision for tension pneumomediastinum), and chest tube for long-term evacuation. Recurrent pneumothoraces can be treated by pleurodesis with mechanical abrasion or a chemical agent. Treatment of the underlying problem should be initiated as soon as the patient is stable.

Retinoic Acid Syndrome

Retinoic acid syndrome is seen in patients with acute promyelocytic leukemia (APML) who are treated with all-trans-retinoic acid. This syndrome occurs in up to 26% of patients within days to weeks of starting the treatment. Overall mortality is significant, ranging from 5% to 13%. Signs and symptoms include respiratory distress, fever, hypotension, weight gain, fluid retention, pleural and pericardial effusions, and renal failure. This syndrome occurs in APML patients during induction chemotherapy. Chest x-ray may demonstrate pulmonary edema or infiltrates and a pleural or pericardial effusion. Retinoic acid syndrome can occur during the development of hyperleukocytosis or during low WBC counts. Treatment consists of 10 mg of dexamethasone given intravenously every 12 hours in adults or 0.5 to 1.0 mg per kg every 12 hours in children. Chemotherapy can be withheld if the symptoms are life-threatening.

GASTROINTESTINAL EMERGENCIES

Abdominal pediatric oncologic emergencies occur because of predisposition to hemorrhage, mechanical obstruction, perforation, or inflammation. Coagulopathy, thrombocytopenia, mucosal ulceration, or abnormal tumor vessel formation predisposes a child with cancer to gastrointestinal hemorrhage. Compression of the gastrointestinal lumen by tumor or abscess or therapy-induced ileus can result in obstruction. Similarly, unresolved obstruction, ulceration, and segmental necrosis can result in perforation. Abdominal processes that are localized in healthy children may be generalized in the child with cancer. Inflammation in response to chemotherapy, tumor, or infection is abnormal because of leukopenia and poor wound healing. In addition, fever does not always accompany infection in these patients. Although pain is the principal symptom of an acute abdominal process, it is essential that a physical examination be performed by a pediatric surgeon and hematology/oncology specialist to ascertain potential causes of an acute abdomen. In addition, the hematology/ oncology specialist following up the individual should be consulted for appropriate laboratory and diagnostic testing.

Gastrointestinal Hemorrhage

Gastrointestinal hemorrhage can result from either bleeding esophageal varices or upper (nonesophageal) and lower gastrointestinal hemorrhage. Patients with Langerhans cell histiocytosis, with refractory abdominal tumors compressing the portal vein, or with chronic viral hepatitis have a predilection to develop esophageal varices. Initial management consists of head elevation by 30 to 45 degrees, and volume expansion with crystalloid solution, and transfusion of packed red blood cells (RBCs) to correct anemia. Broad-spectrum antibiotics should be given to febrile patients with bleeding esophageal varices as this may be an indication of sepsis in patients with cirrhosis. To monitor the rate of bleeding, a nasogastric tube should be inserted with frequent normal saline lavage. Emergent management is needed if bright red blood persists in the lavage fluid. Intravenous infusion of vasopressin may be attempted and followed by endoscopic variceal ligation or sclerotherapy, if necessary. Balloon tamponade under direct observation may be necessary to control refractory bleeding but is associated with considerable morbidity and mortality. Splenorenal shunts should only be used as a last resort if bleeding cannot be controlled and all other interventions have failed.

Upper gastrointestinal bleeding can also result from swallowed blood either from epistaxis or oropharyngeal mucositis. Extensive bleeding may come from Mallory-Weiss tears that can be caused by chemotherapy-related emesis. Other sources of bleeding include stress ulcers that are especially common in children with cancer and those children taking high-dose corticosteroids. In addition, those children with cancer who have undergone high-dose irradiation are also at risk for stress ulcer. In contrast, lower gastrointestinal bleeding can be associated with typhlitis, a necrotizing colitis, localized to the cecum. This is usually associated with *Clostridium difficile*, cryptosporidium, and fungal infections. Intussusception can cause intermittent bleeding or "currant jelly" stools. However, the etiology is often multifactorial in a patient with cancer. Although bleeding from hemorrhoid and anal fissures occurs occasionally, rarely is this a clinically significant source of lower gastrointestinal bleeding.

Gastrointestinal Obstruction

Gastrointestinal obstruction can occur in the child with cancer as a result of adjuvant therapy or previous abdominal surgery. Differential diagnosis includes obstipation or paralytic ileus caused by many factors, including medications such as vinca alkaloids, narcotics or tricyclic antidepressants, adhesions or strictures, and intussusception. Burkitt lymphoma of the ileum can present initially as bowel obstruction. Gastrointestinal obstruction can also be seen in patients with refractory sarcomas, particularly desmoplastic small-cell sarcoma, or colon, or ovarian stromal cell cancer. Furthermore, presacral teratomas and pelvic sarcomas may occlude the rectum also, causing obstruction. Small bowel obstruction is managed initially by making the patient NPO and placing a nasogastric tube. Rectal obstruction can be managed by the use of a stool softener and placement of a small rectal tube in severe cases until cytotoxic therapy reduces the tumor mass.

Gastrointestinal perforation is usually the outcome of unresolved obstruction, ulcers, or gastritis unresponsive to medical therapy, infections, or erosion by the primary tumor.

In the case of abdominal Burkitt lymphoma, perforation may occur at various points during diagnosis and treatment including at presentation, during steroid therapy, or after clinical resolution in association with the treatment of penetrating metastasis. Abdominal radiographs may demonstrate the presence of air under the diaphragm with concomitant tracking of air into or along the flank of the liver. Gastrointestinal perforation is a surgical emergency and must be managed either by resection of the affected area and secondary closure or by primary reanastomosis. Massively disseminated abdominal Burkitt tumor may require cytotoxic therapy, in order to reduce tumor burden prior to surgery.

Gastrointestinal Infection and Inflammation

Gastrointestinal infection and inflammation are often seen in children with cancer. One of the most common problems in pediatric oncologic patients is fungal and viral esophagitis. Often neutropenic enterocolitis, typhlitis, and appendicitis have similar presentations in this population, a small percentage of which will develop appendicitis. In a study at St. Jude's Children's Research Hospital, 0.5% of children with cancer were diagnosed with appendicitis that required either ultrasound or CT scan in addition to physical examination.[6,7] Typhlitis is often a concern in the neutropenic child with cancer and often confounds the diagnosis of appendicitis. Typhlitis can occur after the initiation of cytotoxic chemotherapy. Up to a third of patients with acute myelogenous leukemia (AML) can have typhlitis during induction therapy.[8] The pathophysiology often involves bacterial or fungal invasion of the cecal mucosa, with progression to full-thickness infarction and possible perforation. Major fungal organisms include *Candida* and *Aspergillus* sp., whereas bacteria that are involved include *Pseudomonas* sp., *Escherichia coli* and other gram-negative organisms, *S. aureus*, α-hemolytic streptococci and *Clostridium* sp. Mortality rates for typhlitis range from 20% to 100% with either surgical or medical treatment. On the basis of the criteria for surgical intervention given by Shamberger et al.[8] that include: (a) persistent gastrointestinal bleeding despite resolution of thrombocytopenia and correction of clotting abnormalities, (b) evidence of free air, (c) need for vasopressor support or large volumes of fluid, suggesting uncontrolled sepsis from intestinal infarction, and (d) development of symptoms of an intra-abdominal process that would normally require an operation, approximately 70% to 80% cases of typhlitis can be managed medically with broad-spectrum antibiotics that include clindamycin or metronidazole for gastrointestinal anaerobes. Patients who have signs and symptoms of enterocolitis and do not have typhlitis, may have transverse colitis, intussusception, or antibiotic-related pseudomembranous or clostridial enterocolitis.

Acute Massive Hepatomegaly and Hemorrhagic Pancreatitis

Acute massive hepatomegaly is often a complication of stage IV-S neuroblastoma in the neonate and can result in fatal respiratory compromise. Chemotherapy, irradiation, or rarely surgical enlargement of the abdominal wall using a Silastic pouch may be necessary. Another gastrointestinal emergency is hemorrhagic pancreatitis, which has a 2% incidence in standard risk patients with ALL. This should be considered when there is vomiting and abdominal pain in a child receiving L-asparaginase or steroids. Ultrasound or CT scan should be performed and serum chemistries including lipase and amylase should be obtained in order to confirm the diagnosis. Appropriate consultation with hematology/oncology and surgical specialists is often necessary for management.

GENITOURINARY EMERGENCIES

Genitourinary pediatric oncologic emergencies result from tumor related complications or complications related to therapy. Prerenal causes of anuria or oliguria require an evaluation for septic shock, the most common prerenal cause of reduced output in the child receiving chemotherapy. In addition, any cause of intravascular volume depletion (chemotherapy-induced emesis, infectious diarrhea, decreased oral intake, and/or metabolic abnormalities) should be considered. Postrenal causes of oliguria include the presence of bulky abdominal or pelvic tumor causing ureteral or bladder obstruction. Mass effect must be differentiated from TLS (discussed later), as both can present with similar serum chemistry laboratory findings, including elevated uric acid, potassium, and phosphorus. Often blood urea nitrogen (BUN) and creatinine are helpful in discerning between TLS and postrenal obstruction as very high levels of both favor postrenal failure secondary to

obstruction. The effect of medications such as narcotics, vincristine, or phenothiazines on urinary retention and even the presence of herpes zoster, which affects the sacral nerves resulting in urinary retention, should be considered in the differential for oliguria.

Hypertension

Hypertension in the patient with cancer is often due to compression of the renal artery or the renal parenchyma, which results in increased renin production. Symptoms may include headache, lethargy, irritability, mental status changes, and ultimately seizures and coma. This commonly occurs in Wilms tumor, neuroblastoma, ganglioneuroblastoma, abdominal lymphomas, and pheochromocytomas. Renin can also be ectopically produced by Wilms tumor and neuroblastoma, contributing to hypertension. The presence of hypertension in association with other signs or symptoms may be indicative of specific disease entities. For example, the presence of elevated arterial systolic blood pressure in association with hematuria may be an indication of renal vein thrombosis. Furthermore, hypertension in conjunction with bradycardia and respiratory depression (Cushing triad) may indicate increased intracranial pressure in a patient with central nervous system (CNS) leukemia or infection or brain tumor. Hypertension can also result from medications commonly given to pediatric oncology patients. These include medications such as steroids, cyclosporine A, and amphotericin B. Pain, a common symptom experienced by patients with cancer, can also cause hypertension that is often associated with tachycardia. Therefore, evaluation requires review of current medications, frequent monitoring of blood pressure, CT scan of the head for any increased intracranial pressure, urine and plasma catecholamine levels and plasma renin levels to evaluate for paraneoplastic causes of hypertension, abdominal CT scan to evaluate for a mass effect, and Doppler ultrasonography to evaluate renal blood flow. Medical management is often preferred in patients with normal renal function. However, furosemide can be used in patients with fluid overload. If hypertension is caused by increased intracranial pressure, dexamethasone or mannitol can be used to decrease cerebral edema, which, in turn, will decrease blood pressure. Cytotoxic therapy or surgical resection may be necessary if the tumor is the cause of the hypertension.

Hemorrhagic Cystitis

Hemorrhagic cystitis often results from bladder inflammation and bleeding. In the immunosuppressed patient with cancer, adenovirus, cytomegalovirus, and polyomavirus BK are frequent causes of this disease that often occurs in patients who have received cytoxan or ifosfamide. This toxicity results from a metabolite, acrolein, which becomes toxic when it precipitates in the bladder. Hemorrhagic cystitis involves gross hematuria with passage of painful clots. Preventive treatment consists of hydration and diuresis to reduce acrolein accumulation in the bladder. If prevention fails, then therapy consists of further hydration, correction of any coagulation or platelet abnormalities, maintenance of hemoglobin/hematocrit with red cell transfusion, and continuous bladder irrigation. Oxybutynin chloride, baclofen, belladonna, or opioids may be necessary to control painful bladder spasms. Any concurrent bladder irradiation or chemotherapy with radiomimetic agents should be held. For continued bleeding, endoscopy with electrocauterization, installation of formalin, alum, or prostaglandin E_2 (PGE_2) may be useful. However, in patients with reflux, formalin is contraindicated. The mildest treatment consists of PGE_2 instillation that has been shown to resolve hematuria within 5 days of starting infusions, without any systemic effects.

NEUROLOGIC EMERGENCIES

Neurologic pediatric oncologic emergencies result from the direct mass effect of the tumor, which often leads to increased intracranial pressure or from cancer-related therapy. Any altered mental status, seizure activity, and cerebrovascular accidents (CVAs) and other neurologic findings should be evaluated by a prompt, careful, detailed neurologic examination, in order to localize the deficit and thereby avoid potentially harmful investigations that can further delay diagnosis and increase morbidity and mortality.

Acute Alterations in Consciousness

Acute alterations in consciousness in the child with cancer range from lethargy to coma and are associated with a number of etiologies. Evaluation begins with evaluation of airways, breathing, and circulation and emergent stabilization as needed, followed by a focused, yet thorough, history and formal neurologic examination. CBC, serum glucose, electrolytes and ammonia level, hepatic and renal function tests, blood cultures, and a coagulation profile should be obtained. Signs and symptoms of increased intracranial pressure should be managed with intravenous dexamethasone and possibly mannitol. Emergent CT scan or magnetic resonance imaging (MRI) with osmotic contrast agents should be performed only if they are not contraindicated. Broad-spectrum antibiotics should be initiated prior to imaging in patients with signs and symptoms of increased intracranial pressure because of suspected sepsis or meningitis. Neurosurgical intervention is indicated for mass lesions or hydrocephalus unresponsive to medical management. Lumbar puncture should not be performed until a mass lesion has been ruled out and after and/or thrombocytopenia and coagulopathy has been corrected.

Chemotherapy-Related Neurotoxicity

Chemotherapy-associated neurologic alterations should prompt decreased dosing or discontinuation of the medication. Specific antidotes include methylene blue for ifosfamide encephalopathy and leucovorin or carboxypeptidase for elevated methotrexate levels. Errors in the administration of intrathecal chemotherapy have been reported and summarized by Dropcho.[9] These include overdoses of intrathecal methotrexate with symptoms ranging from none to headache for doses of <100 mg and seizure and coma within hours for overdoses in excess of 500 mg. Doses <100 mg require minimal intervention (cerebrospinal fluid [CSF] drainage with systemic leucovorin), whereas doses >500 mg are usually fatal. However, if the overdose is recognized within 2 hours and the dosage is >100 mg, immediate action should involve removal of as much CSF as possible, as 30% to 50% of the original dose may be recovered. Alternatively, CSF can be exchanged with saline or Ringer lactate if more time has elapsed. Ventricular catheter placement should be considered if the patient's clinical condition continues to deteriorate or if the overdose is severe. Recently, the use of carboxypeptidase G_2 (CPG_2) for the management of methotrexate doses >100 mg has been evaluated. In this study, CSF was drained by gravity for 5 minutes followed by the instillation of 2,000 units of $CPDG_2$. High-dose systemic leucovorin (100 mg every 6 hours for 24 hours) and intravenous dexamethasone (0.5 mg per kg) every 6 hours for 24 to 72 hours was recommended to decrease the severity of the chemically induced meningitis symptoms.[10] Another much less frequently reported error is accidental administration of intrathecal vincristine. Unfortunately, only one of the eight reported cases has survived, with the survival likely related to rapid identification of the error and prompt treatment. Although the use of systemic corticosteroids is felt to decrease meningeal inflammation, the current data is insufficient to evaluate efficacy in medication errors. The use of intrathecal corticosteroids cannot be used because of the need to drain and exchange the CSF immediately.

Cerebrovascular Accidents

CVAs in the child with cancer are associated with cerebral arterial or venous thrombosis, intracerebral hemorrhage, tumor enlargement, chemotherapy, CNS infections, or hematologic abnormalities. Embolic phenomenon is rarely associated with CVAs. Early in the disease process, CVAs are associated with coagulation abnormalities, whereas chemotherapy- or infection-related etiologies predominate during treatment. In contrast, disseminated intravascular coagulation (DIC), CNS infection, sepsis, and tumor progression account for most etiologies at the end of the disease. Strokes can occur months to years after therapy has been completed and are likely related to radiation-related vasculopathy.

Patients with AML, especially APML, with hyperleukocytosis are at high risk for strokes, particularly at diagnosis or early in treatment. Leukemic promyelocytes enhance thrombin activation, as well as production of plasmin (by expression of annexin II), resulting in an often-striking DIC picture. The use of L-asparaginase is associated with an increased risk of venous thrombosis, especially near the end of induction therapy in ALL patients with most of the thromboemboli localized to the CNS. The etiology of this is felt to be related to acquired deficiencies of antithrombin III, proteins C and S, and plasminogen, which increase the risk of thromboembolism. Radiation therapy (which can be potentiated by concomitant chemotherapy such as methotrexate and cytosine arabinoside) can cause delayed large- and small-vessel occlusions months to years after treatment. Hemorrhagic CVA can occur in patients with neuroblastoma metastatic to the dura or torcula and those with platelet-refractory thrombocytopenia. Lateral and transverse sinus thrombosis can also be a feature of metastatic neuroblastoma.

Evaluation of a presumed CVA in a child with cancer requires understanding of the type, extent, and status of the cancer, chemotherapy treatment, and any associated medical conditions. CVAs will usually present as acute impairment of motor function or speech, often with associated seizures. If the symptoms do not clear within 24 hours, there must be an evaluation for a structural CNS lesion. Obtundation, which must be differentiated from lethargy or coma, can result from a sagittal sinus thrombosis or brain stem stroke. Once stable, an emergent CT scan or MRI should be performed with and without contrast. Magnetic resonance angiography can help confirm a specific diagnosis such as postradiation vasculopathy, but is rarely needed initially. In particular, the torcular region of the calvarium and dura in patients with neuroblastoma should be evaluated for a possible sinus thrombosis. Absence of a mass lesion on CT scan or MRI will allow the performance of a lumbar puncture that can provide useful information such as opening pressure and enable obtainment of CSF samples for protein and glucose levels, cell count, cytology and bacterial, viral, and fungal cultures.

Therapy is primarily supportive and can include platelets and fresh frozen plasma in the case of DIC. It is suggested that platelets be kept >75,000 per μL for hemorrhagic CVA. The use of antithrombin III has been found to improve survival in patients with DIC secondary to sepsis, who have low antithrombin III levels.[11] However, the use of fresh frozen plasma (as a source of antithrombin III) does not affect the acquired antithrombin III deficiency seen in L-asparaginase-related CVA.[12] Although all-trans-retinoic acid can often resolve the associated coagulopathy/DIC in APML within 5 to 7 days, many CVAs occur at diagnosis and early in the course of treatment. Patients with neuroblastoma metastatic to the torcular region, may benefit from emergency irradiation which can rapidly resolve symptoms. Treatment of nonmetastatic sagittal sinus thrombosis in patients without

hypernatremia requires corticosteroids and hyperosmolar agents to decrease the intracranial pressure. Although surgery may be life-saving in cases of intracerebral hemorrhage, such intervention may be unwarranted in patients with uncontrolled coagulopathy and in end-stage disease.

Seizures

Seizures reflect an underlying pathologic process and account for >50% of neurologic consultations on pediatric oncology services.[13] Seizures usually result from the underlying malignancy, which include primary and metastatic CNS tumors, meningeal leukemia, and chemotherapy. Medications such as intrathecal cytarabine, intrathecal methotrexate, and high-dose intravenous methotrexate can cause seizures, especially in children who have received cranial irradiation. Vincristine can also be associated with seizures but it is unclear if this association is related to the syndrome of inappropriate secretion of antidiuretic hormone (SIADH). Radiation-related small-vessel disease, cerebral necrosis, and leukoencephalopathy can also increase the risk of seizures. CVAs of any etiology, CNS infections, coagulopathy, and metabolic derangements can also cause seizures. Evaluation is similar to that previously described for CVAs. Most seizures are self-limited; however, a prolonged seizure requires emergency management. Initial management consists of adequate provision of ventilation and circulation and correction of any metabolic abnormality, followed by initiation of anticonvulsants. Valproic acid and carbamazepine should be avoided owing to their potential marrow suppression. Those patients without markedly abnormal electroencephalograms and normal CNS imaging studies usually can discontinue therapy without a recurrence; however, prolonged or repetitive seizures generally require prolonged therapy with anticonvulsants. Antibiotics are indicated in at-risk patients who are febrile and neutropenic, patients with meningeal signs or symptoms and other at-risk patients.

Spinal Cord Compression

Spinal cord compression is a common presenting finding at diagnosis. This occurs in 3% to 5% of children with cancer. Another 5% to 10% present with back pain that must be differentiated form spinal cord compression. Although spinal cord compression can occur with any tumor type, metastatic spread from sarcomas account for most cases, with neuroblastoma, germ cell tumors, lymphoma, and metastatic primary CNS tumors accounting largely for the remainder. In the evaluation of children with cancer and back pain, spinal cord compression should be considered until proven otherwise. Although pain can be present weeks to months before diagnosis, once neurologic abnormalities become apparent, paraplegia and quadriplegia can occur rapidly and may be irreversible. Clearly a detailed neurologic examination is necessary. History and physical examination can rule out vincristine as the cause of back pain. It should be noted that the absence of weakness or sensory abnormalities does not exclude spinal cord compression. Radiographic studies should include craniospinal T_1- and T_2-weighted MRI; this will allow demonstration of epidural disease, intraparenchymal tumor spread and identification of lesions compressing the nerve roots in the cauda equina. CSF studies are necessary for the evaluation of subarachnoid disease, meningeal leukemia, or carcinomatosis. Patients with complete spinal cord block have elevated CSF protein concentration; but it should be noted that in patients with partial obstruction, CSF protein concentrations are often normal. Therefore, treatment strategy is dependent on clinical and physical findings. Dexamethasone (bolus 1.0 to 2.0 mg per kg) followed by MRI is recommended in the child with rapidly progressive spinal cord dysfunction. However, if spinal cord compression is possible in a child with cancer and back pain, but in whom symptoms are not apparent, dexamethasone at a lower dose (0.25 to 0.50 mg per kg orally every 6 hours) is usually sufficient. If, however, there is an epidural mass compressing the spinal cord, the cord must be decompressed immediately using local radiotherapy, surgical decompression, or chemotherapy. The clearest indication for surgery is the patient who has spinal cord compression with an unknown primary tumor. Surgery offers the benefit of decompression in addition to obtaining tissue for diagnosis. Surgery often involves laminectomy and posterior decompression because the frequent route of the tumor through the intervertebral foramina. Vertebral body metastasis or radioresistant tumor that results in spinal cord compression may also require surgery. Surgery is also indicated if there is radiotherapy failure. If the diagnosis is known and the tumor is known to be radiosensitive, then radiotherapy is the treatment of choice. Chemotherapy is an appropriate alternative especially in patients with spinal cord compression due to lymphoma, leukemia, and neuroblastoma. The use of high-dose dexamethasone and systemic chemotherapy can result in prompt improvement in symptoms associated with a reduction in tumor size. Although prognosis in patients with spinal cord compression is dependent on the neurologic findings at presentation, a study by Lewis et al.[14] found that approximately one-half of children who could not walk at the beginning of treatment regained the ability to do so after emergency treatment.

Hyperleukocytosis

Hyperleukocytosis is defined by a peripheral leukocyte count >100,000 per μL. However, clinically significant hyperleukocytosis often occurs with WBC counts >200,000 per μL in patients with AML and >300,000 per μL in ALL or chronic myelogenous leukemia (CML). Hyperleukocytosis occurs in 9% to 13% of children with ALL and 5% to 22% of children with AML and almost all children with CML in the chronic phase. Mortality related to hyperleukocytosis usually occurs as a result of CNS hemorrhage or thrombosis,

pulmonary leukostasis or tumor lysis. In a study by Bunin et al.[15] pulmonary leukostasis and CNS hemorrhage were the primary causes of death in AML patients with hyperleukocytosis (23% of patients during early induction), whereas metabolic derangements from tumor lysis were the principle causes of death (5%) in similar patients with ALL. In preparation for tumor lysis by chemotherapy, intravenous hydration at two to four times the maintenance volume, alkalinization with sodium bicarbonate and allopurinol should be started. Platelet counts should be maintained above 10,000 per μL. However, because red cell transfusion can significantly increase whole blood viscosity, red cell transfusions should not be given to patients to raise the hemoglobin to over 10 g per dL. Exchange transfusion and leukapheresis can lower the WBC count and improve coagulopathy that is often present. However, both modalities are only temporizing. WBC count can be decreased by 52% to 66% with exchange transfusion and 48% to 62% with leukapheresis resulting in improved neurologic abnormalities, respiratory distress, and priaprism, if present.

METABOLIC EMERGENCIES

Tumor Lysis Syndrome

TLS is a commonly encountered entity in the child with cancer. This syndrome results from the release of intracellular contents of lysed or dying cells. This can occur before any cytotoxic therapy or within hours to days of the start of therapy. Patients who have tumors with high growth fraction, that are widely disseminated or large in volume and that are sensitive to cytotoxic therapy, are particularly prone to TLS. These include patients with Burkitt lymphoma, lymphoblastic lymphoma, and ALL, especially T-cell ALL patients with hyperleukocytosis and extensive extramedullary disease. In contrast, TLS is rarely seen in AML or CML, despite high WBC counts. The classic metabolic triad includes hyperuricemia, hyperkalemia, and hyperphosphatemia. These metabolic derangements can be accentuated in the presence of poor urine output or low glomerular filtration rate. Increases in serum potassium can be rapid enough to cause cardiac arrest in minutes or hours if left unchecked. Because urine is concentrated in the collecting ducts of the renal tubules, this can be a site of uric acid crystal precipitation if hyperuricemia is present. Elevated serum phosphate levels are especially seen in lymphoblast lysis as these cells contain four times as much phosphate as normal lymphocytes. Metabolic acidosis can also contribute to hyperphosphatemia as a shift of intracellular phosphate into the extracellular space occurs under this condition. Secondary hypocalcemia can occur when the solubility product is exceeded causing calcium phosphate precipitation in the microvasculature. Furthermore, precipitation of uric acid crystals and calcium phosphate within the renal tubules may also lead to acute renal failure.

Symptoms of TLS may include abdominal pain, fullness, back pain, nausea, vomiting, diarrhea, dehydration, anorexia, cramps, spasms, tetany, seizure, and altered consciousness. Studies should include CBC, electrolytes, BUN, creatinine, calcium, phosphorus, and urinalysis. Evaluation of low serum calcium requires evaluation of ionized calcium and serum albumin levels. Typical EKG findings of hypocalcemia include prolonged QTc intervals. In contrast, if hyperkalemia is present, the EKG may demonstrate QRS widening and peaked T waves. Patients who demonstrate EKG findings should be placed on a cardiac monitor. As mentioned previously, obstructive causes of acute renal failure often present with similar metabolic derangements as in TLS and must be ruled out because the treatment strategy is very different. For example, hydration, an essential part of treatment in the prevention and treatment of TLS, can exacerbate obstructive renal failure. Early and aggressive intervention is necessary to reduce the morbidity associated with TLS. Patients with newly diagnosed leukemia or non-Hodgkin lymphoma should receive hydration, alkalinization, and allopurinol. This regimen is sufficient for most patients to prevent clinically significant tumor lysis and renal failure.

Hydration is the most critical factor in treatment. Patients should receive two to four times maintenance fluid as 5% dextrose in 0.25% normal saline, with 40 to 80 mEq of sodium bicarbonate per L, to maintain a urine pH between 7.0 and 7.5. Urine output should be maintained at >100 dL/m^2/hour with a specific gravity <1.010. Potassium and calcium should not be added to these fluids unless the patient is symptomatic. Diuretics and mannitol may be indicated in patients with poor urine output because of accumulation of infused fluid in the third space. If urine output falls below 60 mL/m^2/hour, mannitol can be given at 0.5 mg per kg over 15 minutes, followed by furosemide (0.5 to 1.0 mg per kg).

Allopurinol inhibits the formation of uric acid by blocking the enzyme xanthine oxidase, which converts hypoxanthine and xanthine to uric acid. Uricase can also be used for elevated uric acid levels as it converts uric acid to allantoin. It has a particular advantage in that alkalinization is not necessary. Although alkalinization helps to solubilize uric acid, sodium bicarbonate should be discontinued when serum levels of uric acid normalize and cytotoxic therapy begins. Over alkalinization may result in xanthine and hypoxanthine stones and calcium phosphate may crystallize in the kidneys at pH ≥ 8. Metabolic studies should be repeated at least four times daily until the electrolyte and metabolic disturbances have subsided. The use of aluminum hydroxide (administered per nasogastric tube) can be used to increase the excretion of phosphate. Calcium gluconate (100 to 200 mg/kg/dose) can shift potassium from the extracellular to the intracellular space and stabilize myocardial conduction. An alternative is rapid-acting insulin (0.1 units per kg) in 2 mL per kg of 25% glucose in water, which can promote intracellular influx of potassium. Caution should be taken

while correcting hypocalcemia as the infusion of calcium gluconate can increase the calcium phosphate solubility product and result in the increased risk of calcium phosphate deposition with resultant renal failure. If medical intervention cannot correct the electrolyte disturbances or if oliguria persists, dialysis may be necessary. Hemodialysis is preferred to peritoneal dialysis for several reasons; these include more rapid correction of electrolyte abnormalities and the contraindication of peritoneal dialysis in patients with abdominal or pelvic tumors. Both leukapheresis and exchange transfusion have been used to reduce tumor load; however, this use has not been subject to a randomized controlled trial and current use is limited to patients with leukemia and hyperleukocytosis who have evidence of neurologic deterioration because of hyperviscosity. Overall, careful management of these patients requires constant consultation with the pediatric hematology/oncology and nephrology specialists who follow up these patients.

Hypercalcemia

Hypercalcemia is a serum calcium that exceeds 12 mg per dL. Levels >20 mg per dL can be fatal. Hypercalcemia is more common in adults with cancer (5% to 20%) than in children with cancer (0.4%).[16] Although a variety of tumors may cause hypercalcemia, in a 29-year study at St. Jude's Children's Hospital, a large proportion of patients (10 out of 29) who were diagnosed with ALL, and four out of 29 patients who had rhabdomyosarcoma, developed hypercalcemia.[17] Children with acute leukemia are more likely to have treatment-responsive hypercalcemia at presentation, compared to children with solid tumors or lymphomas; the latter of which were more likely to develop therapy-resistant hypercalcemia later in the course of their disease. This resistance to treatment of hypercalcemia is likely related to the cause of the malignant hypercalcemia. Malignant hypercalcemia can be classified into three categories: humoral, osteolytic, and calcitriol-mediated. A variety of growth factors such as PTH-related peptide in patients with rhabdomyosarcoma, osteoclast-activating factor in Burkitt lymphoma, and calcitriol in Hodgkin disease and non-Hodgkin lymphoma have been implicated in hypercalcemia.

Hypercalcemia typically has nonspecific symptoms including nausea, constipation, and polyuria, which can be followed by profound muscle weakness, renal insufficiency, bradyarrhythmias, and coma if left unchecked. Patients will typically develop dehydration related to anorexia, vomiting, and polyuria, which worsen the dehydration. Early symptoms can mimic TLS and metabolic derangements can be similar. Several medications can exacerbate malignant hypercalcemia including thiazide diuretics, oral contraceptives, antacids with calcium carbonate and lithium. Other diseases and conditions such as hypervitaminosis A or D, granulomatous and renal disease, adrenal insufficiency, fractures and immobilization may also contribute.

Any calcium level exceeding 12 mg per dL requires immediate correction. Principles of treatment include hydration, enhancement of renal excretion, decreasing calcium mobilization from bone, and treating the underlying malignancy. For a serum calcium of <14 mg per dL, hydration coupled with furosemide-mediated diuresis may be sufficient. At higher levels, forced diuresis with normal saline repletion at two to three times maintenance volume is recommended, followed by furosemide (2 to 3 mg per kg every 2 hours) once good urine output is obtained. Furosemide blocks calcium resorption by the kidney and can decrease serum calcium by 3 mg per dL in 48 hours. Prednisone can reduce serum calcium level if the mechanism of hypercalcemia is mediated by osteoclast-activating factor, PGE_2 or calcitriol. Salmon calcitonin and mithramycin have also been used to lower serum calcium; however, with salmon calcitonin, the effect may only last for days; longer, if used with steroids. Mithramycin can lower calcium levels within days but is too cytotoxic for prolonged use. Bisphosphonates can inhibit osteoclast-mediated resorption of bone and reduce osteoclast viability. Although studies in adults have demonstrated that this agent is highly effective and has a long duration of action, reports in children are limited. A medication being increasingly used is intravenous pamidronate that can result in normalization of calcium levels within 3 to 7 days.[18]

Hyponatremia

Hyponatremia, as it relates to the SIADH, can be life-threatening depending on the magnitude or rate of decrease. In general a fall to <120 mmol per L within 24 hours or a gradual decrease in serum sodium to <115 mmol per L requires immediate correction. Hyponatremia found with SIADH is associated with the use of vincristine, vinblastine, cyclophosphamide, ifosfamide, cisplatin, and melphalan. The mechanism of action of cyclophosphamide and ifosfamide is thought to be related to reduced free-water clearance that is independent of antidiuretic hormone (ADH); the resultant hyponatremia may be aggravated by aggressive hydration, which is used to prevent cystitis caused by cyclophosphamide and ifosfamide. SIADH can occur in a number of clinical settings including CNS injury or disease, pulmonary infection and inflammation, stress, pain, surgery, or positive-pressure ventilation, and is often seen with tumors such as small-cell lung carcinoma, lymphoma, or gastrointestinal carcinoma. Early symptoms include fatigue, anorexia, and nausea, whereas later symptoms typically include lethargy, confusion, seizures, and coma. The most common cause of mild hyponatremia is iatrogenic over hydration with a hypotonic solution. Hyponatremia can also be caused by failure to administer stress doses of glucocorticoid in a patient who has recently discontinued systemic steroids. Diabetes insipidus in patients with Langerhans cell histiocytosis or with suprasellar tumors can be associated with hyponatremia if the patient

has had losses replaced with water or other hypotonic solutions. In patients with CNS tumors and renal damage, SIADH may need to be differentiated from cerebral salt wasting.[19] Diagnosis of SIADH is made if the serum osmolality (usually <280 mmol per L) is lower than the urine osmolality (often >500 mmol per L). Fluid restriction is the mainstay of treatment of mild hyponatremia. In cases of severe neurologic involvement (seizures, coma), boluses of 3% hypertonic saline to replace sodium losses should be started followed by furosemide diuresis. Sodium correction should not be >2 mmol/L/hour in order to avoid cerebral edema, which can further exacerbate neurologic deterioration and death. Urine output should be monitored closely, and frequent monitoring of serum electrolytes is essential.

SUMMARY

In summary, pediatric oncology emergencies largely result from either direct tumor invasion or mass effect, consequences of altered hemostasis and immunity, and/or from the side effects of chemotherapy and supportive medications. Pediatric oncology patients should be cared for by the pediatric intensivist in close collaboration with the pediatric hematology/oncology specialist in order to provide optimal care.

REFERENCES

1. Rheingold SR, Lange BJ. Oncologic emergencies. In: Pizzo PA, Polack DG, eds. *Principles and practice of pediatric oncology.* 4th ed. Philadelphia, PA: Lippincott Williams & Wilkins; 2004: 1177–1203.
2. Kelly KM, Lange B. Oncologic emergencies. *Pediatr Clin North Am.* 1997;44:809–830.
3. Andrew M, Michelson AD, Bovill E, et al. Guidelines for antithrombotic therapy in pediatric patients. *J Pediatr.* 1998;132:575–588.
4. Monagle P, Chan A, Massicotte P, et al. Antithrombotic therapy in children: The Seventh ACCP Conference on Antithrombotic and Thrombolytic Therapy. *Chest.* 2004;126(Suppl 3):645S–687S.
5. Shapiro MJ, Albelda SM, Mayock RL, et al. Severe hemoptysis associated with pulmonary aspergilloma. *Chest.* 1988;94:1225–1231.
6. Kaste SC, Rodriguez-Galindo C, Furman WL. Imaging pediatric oncologic emergencies of the abdomen. *AJR Am J Roentgenol.* 1999;173:729–736.
7. Wade DS, Marrow SE, Balsara ZN, et al. Accuracy of ultrasound in the diagnosis of acute appendicitis compared with the surgeon's clinical impression. *Arch Surg.* 1993;128:1039–1044.
8. Shamberger RC, Weinstein HJ, Delorey M, et al. The medical and surgical management of typhlitis in children with acute nonlymphocytic (myelogenous) leukemia. *Cancer.* 1986;57:603–609.
9. Dropcho EJ. Neurotoxicity of cancer chemotherapy. *Semin Neurol.* 2004;24:419–426.
10. O'Marcaigh AS, Johnson CM, Smithson WA, et al. Successful treatment of intrathecal methotrexate overdose in using ventriculolumbar perfusion and intrathecal instillation of carboxypeptidase G2. *Mayo Clin Proc.* 1996;71:161–165.
11. Levi M, Ten Cate H. Disseminated intravascular coagulation. *N Engl J Med.* 1999;341:586–592.
12. Mitchell L, Hoogendoorn H, Giles AR, et al. Increased endogenous thrombin generation in children with acute lymphoblastic leukemia: Risk of thrombotic complications in L-asparaginase-induced antithrombin III deficiency. *Blood.* 1994;83:386–391.
13. DiMario FJ, Packer RJ. Acute mental status changes in children with systemic cancer. *Pediatrics.* 1990;85:353–360.

14. Lewis DW, Packer RJ, Raney B, et al. Incidence, presentation and outcome of spinal cord disease in child with systemic cancer. *Pediatrics*. 1986;78:438–443.

15. Bunin NJ, Pui CH. Differing complications of hyperleukocytosis in children with acute lymphoblastic or acute nonlymphoblastic leukemia. *J Clin Oncol*. 1985;3:1590–1595.

16. Mundy GR, Ibbotson KJ, D'souza SM, et al. The hypercalcemia of cancer. *N Engl J Med*. 1984;310:1718–1727.

17. McKay C, Furman WL. Hypercalcemia complicating childhood malignancies. *Cancer*. 1993;72:256–260.

18. Young G, Shende A. Use of pamidronate in the management of acute cancer-related hypercalcemia in children. *Med Pediatr Oncol*. 1998;30:117–121.

19. Diringer M, Ladenson PW, Borel CB, et al. Sodium and water regulation in a patient with cerebral salt wasting. *Arch Neurol*. 1989;46:928–930.

Therapeutic Apheresis

28

Anne F. Eder

Therapeutic apheresis describes blood-processing techniques that selectively remove pathogenic substances or abnormal cells from the bloodstream while simultaneously replacing the needed blood components. Erythrocytapheresis is also known as *red cell exchange* because the patient's defective red cells are replaced with red cells collected from healthy, volunteer blood donors. Leukapheresis and plateletpheresis (thrombocytapheresis) remove excessive or malignant white blood cells (WBCs) and platelets, respectively. Plasmapheresis, or plasma exchange, efficiently reduces the plasma concentration of pathogenic autoantibodies, immune complexes, plasma proteins, cytokines, lipoproteins, protein-bound drugs, or metabolic toxins. During all therapeutic apheresis procedures, replacement fluids such as albumin, crystalloid, or blood components are administered in order to treat the underlying disease as well as to maintain intravascular volume, red cell mass, or hemostasis.

Because therapeutic apheresis targets specific blood elements or plasma, these procedures are often used as initial treatment or adjunctive therapy for a wide variety of disorders and diseases. In a collaborative effort, the American Society for Apheresis and the AABB have evaluated the clinical indications for therapeutic apheresis on the basis of available published evidence and clinical experience.[1] In the pediatric critical care setting, indications that are considered standard and acceptable as primary or first-line adjunct therapy include erythrocytapheresis for infarctive crises in sickle cell patients, leukapheresis or thrombocytapheresis for symptomatic hyperleukocytosis or thrombocytosis, respectively, and plasmapheresis for atypical hemolytic uremic syndrome (HUS)/thrombotic thrombocytopenic purpura (TTP)[2,3] (see Table 28.1). The emerging interest in therapeutic apheresis for other critical care indications in pediatrics is also briefly reviewed in this chapter.

In order to safely and effectively treat affected children, standard procedures developed for adults must be modified to ensure adequate vascular access, intravascular fluid support, and red cell balance throughout the procedure.[4,5] In addition, the clinical team must promptly recognize and appropriately manage adverse reactions that occur in young patients who may not be able to cooperate fully or communicate effectively during a procedure.

TECHNICAL CONSIDERATIONS

Vascular Access

Therapeutic apheresis devices separate whole blood into its component parts by centrifugation and selectively remove plasma or cellular fractions while returning the remaining components and additional replacement fluids to the patient. Adequate vascular access is a key to a successful procedure and the peripheral veins of young children usually will not accommodate the necessary catheters or needles required for the blood draw and flow rates for the procedure. Children requiring multiple or sequential apheresis procedures usually require a temporary percutaneous central line or a surgically implanted tunneled central venous catheter to allow for a longer course of treatment.[4,5] Hemodialysis catheters such as the MedComp catheter (MedComp, Inc., Harleysville, PA) are frequently used in pediatrics because of their large bore, double lumen, and rigid walls that support the requisite blood flow rates during apheresis procedures. The size of the catheter must be appropriate for the patient and is often guided by the patient's weight (see Table 28.2).[5] Hickman catheters, Infuse-a-Port, or peripherally inserted central venous catheters (PICC lines) cannot be used for the draw line, but can be used for returning replacement fluids during apheresis procedures. The expected benefit of therapeutic apheresis should justify the risks associated with intravascular catheters, which include vessel damage, bleeding, infection, and thrombosis.

TABLE 28.1
THERAPEUTIC APHERESIS IN THE PEDIATRIC CRITICAL CARE SETTING

Erythrocytapheresis

Sickle cell disease	I
■ Acute crises	
Stroke	
Acute chest syndrome	
Retinal infarction	
Life- or organ-threatening ischemia	
Hyperparasitemia	III
■ Malaria or babesiosis	
Polycythemia/erythrocytosis	II
■ Polycythemia vera	
■ Congenital heart disease, cyanotic	

Leukapheresis

Leukemia with symptomatic leukocytosis, in order of likelihood of occurrence	I
■ AML	
■ CML, blast crisis, accelerated phase	
■ ALL (uncommon)	
■ CML, chronic phase with high percentages of immature myelocytes (uncommon)	

Plateletpheresis

Symptomatic thrombocytosis, associated with	I
■ Essential thrombocythemia	
■ Polycythemia vera	
■ CML	
■ Myeloproliferative disorder	

Plasmapheresis

■ Renal and metabolic disease: thrombotic thrombocytopenic purpura	I
■ Glomerular basement membrane antibody disease	I
■ HUS	III
■ Acute hepatic failure	III
■ Recurrent focal segmental glomerulonephritis	III
Neurologic disorders	
■ Acute/chronic inflammatory demyelinating polyradiculoneuropathy	I
■ Myasthenia gravis	I
■ PANDAS	II
Solid organ transplant	
■ Presensitization to donor organ	III
■ Transplantation across ABO barrier	III
■ Humoral rejection—cardiac transplant	III
■ Renal allograft rejection (cellular)	IV
■ Acute hepatic failure	III
Sepsis and multiple organ failure	NR

Category definitions: I, standard acceptable therapy; II, sufficient evidence to suggest efficacy usually as adjunctive therapy; III, inconclusive evidence on efficacy or uncertain risk/benefit ratio; IV, lack of efficacy in controlled trials; NR, not rated.
AML, acute myeloid leukemia; CML, chronic myelogenous leukemia; ALL, acute lymphoblastic leukemia; HUS, hemolytic uremic syndrome; PANDAS, pediatric autoimmune neuropsychiatric disorders associated with streptococcal infection.

TABLE 28.2
PEDIATRIC THERAPEUTIC APHERESIS GUIDELINE FOR CENTRAL VENOUS CATHETERS

Patient Weight (kg)	MedComp[a]
<10	7 Fr
10–20	8 Fr
20–50	9 Fr
>50	9 or 11.5 Fr

[a]MedComp Inc., Harleysville, PA. Other catheters of comparable size and rigidity may also be utilized.

Intravascular Fluid and Red Cell Balance

At the beginning of a standard apheresis procedure, blood is drawn from the patient into the extracorporeal circuit and must fill the centrifuge before the continuous exchange process begins. The blood remaining in the tubing at the end of the procedure is given back to the patient in the "rinseback" phase. The net result is an intravascular volume and red cell deficit during the procedure followed by return of most of the red cells along with a net fluid gain at the end of the procedure. These volume shifts are usually inconsequential for an adult, but account for proportionately more of a smaller patient's total blood volume and may not be well tolerated by a young child. The standard procedure must be modified so that intravascular volume shifts are limited to <15% of the patient's total blood volume.[5] Therapeutic apheresis procedures must be carefully planned to appropriately manage intravenous fluid shifts, and additional fluid should be administered as needed from the start of the procedure.

In addition, the extracorporeal circuit or the return line may be filled or "primed" with donor red cells before starting the procedure, so that red cells are given as soon as the blood draw begins and the patient's hematocrit remains constant during the procedure. Red cell priming is generally indicated when (i) drawing whole blood into the extracorporeal circuit will result in depletion of >30% of the patient's original circulating red cell volume or (ii) any degree of impairment of oxygen-carrying capacity poses a risk to the patient because of concomitant illness.[5] As a general rule, children weighing <20 kg or below the age of 6 usually require red cell priming, as well as older children with anemia or underlying cardiopulmonary disease, hemodynamic instability, or tissue ischemia. If a red cell prime is given at the beginning of the procedure, the final rinseback phase is often omitted to avoid volume overload. Alternatively, a partial rinseback of up to 15% of the patient's total blood volume may be given, if the therapeutic goal is to further increase the patient's hematocrit and the patient can tolerate the additional volume.

Adverse Reactions

Apheresis personnel must recognize the early signs of adverse reactions and effectively manage these complications. Despite the critical nature of the diseases being treated, clinically significant adverse reactions occur in only approximately 5% of therapeutic apheresis procedures, according to a survey of 18 institutions.[6] The incidence of reactions was not reported with respect to the age of the patient, and it is likely that most of the patients in the survey were adults. Irrespective of this finding, the most frequently encountered adverse effects in both pediatric and adult patient populations are reactions to citrate, blood components, volume shifts, or vasovagal responses. Citrate, which chelates calcium to prevent clotting, is rapidly metabolized by the liver, but may cause transient, symptomatic hypocalcemia. Adults are likely to experience perioral tingling, chills, numbness, or parasthesias as the first indication of citrate-induced hypocalcemia. In contrast, children rarely experience or report these classic signs and symptoms of hypocalcemia, but they may experience acute onset of abdominal pain, nausea, and/or vomiting, agitation, pallor, and sweating accompanied by tachycardia and hypotension. Severe hypocalcemia may be associated with frank tetany, electrocardiogram abnormalities, and dysrhythmias. The administered citrate dose and the rate of infusion during a procedure are primary factors that affect the probability of citrate reactions. Patients undergoing leukapheresis are at the greatest risk because of the large blood volumes processed, followed by patients receiving fresh frozen plasma (FFP) replacement during plasmapheresis. Patient-related factors also increase sensitivity to the effects of citrate, such as liver disease, serum pH, and electrolyte imbalances. Citrate reactions often may be avoided or mitigated by careful monitoring of symptoms, blood pressure, and serum ionized calcium concentration during the procedure, and effectively managed by reducing the flow rate, and/or providing calcium supplementation. Alternatively, anticoagulation regimens for leukapheresis procedures have used heparin, either alone or in combination with citrate, to reduce the risk of citrate toxicity. Heparin, however, will result in systemic anticoagulation lasting 4 to 6 hours after completion of the procedure.

Hypotension during apheresis may be caused by citrate, vasovagal reactions, or hypovolemia. A vasovagal reaction can be distinguished from a hypovolemic reaction by the effect on the pulse rate—bradycardia occurs in vasovagal reactions and tachycardia with the loss of intravascular volume and hypovolemia. Vasovagal reactions are treated by pausing the procedure and placing the patient in the Trendelenberg position (i.e., supine with head lower than legs). Hypovolemic reactions are treated with the administration of additional replacement fluids or a saline bolus.

Adverse reactions during therapeutic apheresis procedures may also be due to blood component administration which can cause hemolytic, allergic, febrile, or septic reactions. The signs and symptoms of transfusion reactions may suggest a specific reaction, such as hives and urticaria in allergic responses, or back pain and disseminated intravascular coagulation in hemolytic reactions. Often, however, signs and symptoms are nonspecific, and the differential diagnosis of fever, chills, tachycardia, or hypotension must include hemolytic, febrile, and septic transfusion reactions. When a reaction occurs, the transfusion should be discontinued, and supportive treatment should be directed at the underlying or suspected cause. An immediate investigation should be conducted to rule out acute hemolysis and bacterial contamination of blood components. In planning subsequent procedures, pretreatment with acetaminophen and administration of leukocyte-reduced cellular blood components may prevent recurrent febrile reactions; pretreatment with antihistamines or washing red cell units to remove residual plasma may prevent recurrent allergic reactions.

CLINICAL INDICATIONS

Erythrocytapheresis

Acute Emergencies in Sickle Cell Disease

Sickle cell disease is characterized by acute and chronic complications of anemia, vascular occlusion and thrombosis that result from the predominance of hemoglobin S (HbS), chronic hemolysis, and the propensity of the sickled red cells to impede blood flow and increase blood viscosity. Red cell transfusion is indicated to alleviate or prevent acute life- or organ-threatening ischemic complications of sickle cell disease, such as stroke, acute chest syndrome, retinal infarction, and acute hepatic crisis. Although acute painful crises are usually managed without transfusion, red cell exchange may be used to treat chronic, debilitating pain and multiorgan failure syndrome associated with severe painful crises. Exchange transfusion for priapism is controversial because of its association with neurologic complications, but chronic red cell exchange transfusion may prevent recurrent priapism.[7] Also controversial is the role of exchange transfusion in pregnant women with sickle cell disease, but transfusion may be appropriate for obstetric emergencies such as preeclampsia, septicemia, and possibly for general anesthesia and surgery.[2]

Both simple transfusion and exchange transfusion abrogate the sickling process and increase the oxygen-carrying capacity. However, exchange transfusion offers several important advantages over simple transfusion, especially in the setting of acute sickle complications. Simple transfusion increases blood viscosity, which may further increase the risk of vascular occlusion in previously untransfused patients with sickle cell disease or in those with high baseline HbS concentration. In contrast, red cell exchange transfusion simultaneously decreases HbS while replacing sickled red cells with donor red cells, thereby avoiding the unfavorable condition of having a high HbS and a high hematocrit. Simple transfusion also carries a risk of circulatory overload and cardiac compromise in patients with sickle cell disease with chronic, compensated anemia; in contrast, exchange transfusions enable careful control of intravascular fluid balance and avoid volume overload.

In acute emergencies, the therapeutic goal of exchange transfusion is to decrease the patients' HbS levels to approximately 30% or less of the total hemoglobin and increase their hematocrit at the end of the procedure to 30% or greater, but not >36%. If the patient has not been transfused within the previous 3 months, the HbS level should be assumed to be 100% in order to calculate the amount of donor red cells needed for the procedure. An exchange transfusion of a volume equal to the total red cell volume of the patient is predicted to decrease HbS to approximately 35% and produce an HbA level of approximately 65%. For example, a single blood volume exchange transfusion in a 10-year-old child weighing 27 kg (total blood volume, 1,890 mL) with a 25% hematocrit will require approximately 3 units of red cells (300 mL per unit with 60% hematocrit) [calculation: $(1,890 \text{ mL})(0.25) = (\text{number of units needed})(300 \text{ mL})(0.60)$].

Alternatively, the volume that must be exchanged to achieve the desired goal, which is expressed as the FCR (fraction of the patient's cells remaining in circulation after the exchange transfusion), can be automatically calculated by the apheresis device on the basis of the patient's weight, height, initial hematocrit, and the desired end hematocrit. On completing the procedure, hemoglobin electrophoresis should be performed and hematocrit determined to evaluate the efficiency of the exchange transfusion.

Patients who have experienced a stroke should be started on a schedule of periodic transfusion after recovery from the acute event, to prevent recurrent stroke. Long-term transfusion therapy is also recommended to prevent the first occurrence of stroke in patients at risk as determined by abnormal results on transcranial Doppler ultrasonography.[8,9] The treatment goal of long-term transfusion therapy is to maintain the patients' HbS levels between 30% and 50% of the total hemoglobin. The incidence of stroke in patients with sickle cell disease is decreased by 90% with long-term transfusion therapy, and a recent study suggests that transfusions cannot be safely discontinued in patients at risk.[9] Consequently, long-term transfusion therapy for stroke prevention is an extended commitment, and exchange transfusion prevents or markedly reduces iron accumulation and obviates the need for iron chelating therapy in some patients undergoing long-term transfusion.[10]

In addition to iron overload, complications of long-term transfusion therapy include red cell alloimmunization, delayed hemolytic transfusion reactions, and viral transmission. The risks of infectious diseases associated with blood have been significantly decreased with the use of nucleic acid testing (NAT) for HIV and hepatitis C. The risk of red cell alloimmunization is reduced by selecting donor red cell units for crossmatch that are matched to those of the patient for blood group antigens at ABO,

Rhesus (D, C, E), Kell (K1), and other loci.[11] The red cell units intended for patients with sickle cell disease should also be HbS-negative, to avoid interference in laboratory evaluation of HbS after the exchange transfusion, as well as to avoid the potential risks associated with sickle-trait units. Leukocyte reduction of cellular components is indicated for sickle cell transfusion recipients, primarily for prevention of recurrent febrile nonhemolytic transfusion reactions. Irradiation of units selected for transfusion to patients with sickle cell disease is not required, unless there is a coexistent medical condition that places them at risk of transfusion-associated graft versus host disease, such as bone marrow transplantation.

Erythrocytapheresis in Other Medical Emergencies

Red cell exchange has been used to treat patients with protozoal infection, poisoning, and incompatible transfusion.[2] In case reports of malaria or babesia infection, red cell exchange combined with pharmacotherapy has led to a rapid reduction in peripheral parasite load and clinical improvement.[2] Consequently, red cell exchange may be indicated in cases of babesiosis and malaria if parasitemia exceeds 5% to 10%, or for lesser degrees of parasitemia in immunocompromised or critically ill patients or those with renal failure or cerebral malaria.

Erythrocytapheresis may be performed instead of manual phlebotomy to alleviate symptoms attributable to increased red cell mass in polycythemia vera or secondary polycythemia resulting from cyanotic congenital heart disease, and to reduce iron stores in hemochromatosis.[2] The primary advantage of erythrocytapheresis in this clinical setting is the ability to maintain constant intravascular volume during the procedure in hemodynamically unstable patients.

Plasmapheresis

Plasmapheresis effectively reduces the plasma concentration of pathogenic antibodies, immune complexes, plasma proteins, cytokines, lipoproteins, protein-bound drugs, or metabolic toxins. Indications for plasmapheresis are less commonly encountered in young children than in adults; nevertheless, the same treatment strategy with plasmapheresis is often used (Table 28.1). Plasmapheresis has a well-established role in treating thrombotic thrombocytopenia purpura, and its use has been extended to clinical overlap syndromes with atypical hemolytic uremic syndrome in children. In addition, plasmapheresis is emerging as a potentially beneficial intervention for treating sepsis and for preventing rejection of incompatible solid organ transplants.

Atypical Hemolytic Uremic Syndrome/Thrombotic Thrombocytopenic Purpura

Classic HUS is characterized by the acute onset of thrombocytopenia, microangiopathic hemolytic anemia, and renal dysfunction and accounts for approximately 90% of childhood HUS cases. Symptoms usually develop following a diarrheal illness most often caused by enterotoxigenic bacteria, such as *Escherichia coli* O157:H7. Most children with classic HUS recover fully with supportive treatment and dialysis, do not require plasmapheresis, and do not experience relapses or recurrences. The remaining 10% of cases of childhood HUS have been referred to as atypical, nondiarrhea-associated, or sporadic HUS and are either idiopathic or secondary to drugs, malignancy, bone marrow transplantation, or systemic infections.[3] Clinically, atypical HUS in children resembles TTP in adults, and neurologic features may dominate the clinical picture, reflecting the clinical overlap between TTP and HUS. TTP is typically characterized by thrombocytopenia and microangiopathic hemolytic anemia, with varying degrees of renal failure, neurologic dysfunction, and fever. Acquired idiopathic TTP is caused by autoantibodies that inhibit the function of the enzyme, ADAMTS-13, a metalloprotease that cleaves unusually large von Willebrand factor (vWF) and renders it less thrombogenic. Enzyme activity may be decreased in HUS, but it is usually severely decreased or undetectable in TTP.[12] Chronic relapsing TTP in children is a rare disease caused by a congenital deficiency of ADAMTS-13.[12]

Laboratory tests for ADAMTS-13 activity have not yet proven useful in distinguishing HUS from TTP in acute emergencies. Because of this difficulty and the extremely poor prognosis, plasma exchange should be promptly initiated if there is doubt about the cause.[2,12] If neurologic symptoms are present, most practitioners would also promptly initiate plasma exchange. In cases of TTP, plasma exchange effectively removes offending inhibitors of ADAMTS-13 activity and replenishes functional enzyme, but its mechanism of benefit in cases of atypical HUS/TTP is not clearly defined.

Treatment of TTP requires daily plasma exchange and replacement of 1 to 1.5 plasma volumes with FFP or plasma depleted of cryoprecipitate (cryosupernatant or cryoprecipitate-poor plasma). Exchange of 1.5 plasma volumes is predicted to remove 85% of circulating immunoglobulin G (IgG); however, redistribution of IgG between the intravascular and extravascular space occurs in the hours following the procedure so that the efficiency of removal is less than for an ideal solute (e.g., fibrinogen) that is restricted to the intravascular space. Daily treatment is required until the patients' lactate dehydrogenase (LDH) normalizes and their platelet count increases to >100 to 150×10^9 per L for 2 to 3 consecutive days.[2] Periodic measurement of fibrinogen should be performed to avoid deficiency, especially if cryoprecipitate-poor plasma is used as replacement. The duration of treatment necessary to affect a response among adults with TTP varies widely, but many patients demonstrate improvement in symptoms or laboratory parameters within 10 to 14 days. Laboratory tests of ADAMTS-13 activity and the presence of inhibitors

may be useful to guide therapeutic decisions and monitor the efficacy of plasma exchange.[12] If a patient experiences an acute exacerbation of TTP following withdrawal of treatment or a recurrence of the disease several weeks after treatment, plasmapheresis must be emergently resumed. In contrast to acquired TTP, congenital TTP is treated with plasma infusions alone; plasma exchange is not needed because inhibitors are not present.

Sepsis-Associated Thrombotic Microangiopathy

Unlike TTP, the role of plasmapheresis has not been clearly defined for other conditions associated with thrombotic microangiopathy such as sepsis, disseminated intravascular coagulopathy, and multiple organ failure.[13,14] Plasmapheresis is an intuitively attractive treatment option because cytokines, inflammatory mediators, and other plasma factor deficiencies have been implicated in the pathogenesis of these disorders; however, data on its efficacy from animal models and clinical studies have been conflicting. Plasma exchange was effective in correcting plasma deficiencies of vWF-cleaving protease activity and plasminogen-activator inhibitor (PAI-1) activity in children with thrombocytopenia-associated multiple organ failure (platelet count $<100 \times 10^9$ per L), which may improve clearance of microvascular thrombosis.[14] Children who were treated with plasma exchange also demonstrated a reduction in the severity of multiple organ failure, whereas children who were not treated with plasma exchange showed progressive worsening of organ dysfunction at 14 days.[14]

Busund et al. randomized 106 adults with sepsis to plasma exchange or standard supportive care, and reported a trend toward improved outcomes among patients who received plasma exchange.[15] Although these data suggest benefit from plasmapheresis in sepsis and thrombocytopenia-associated multiple organ failure, the available evidence is not sufficient to support a recommendation for routine practice. Further study is needed to determine if plasma exchange reduces mortality associated with sepsis and thrombotic microangiopathy and to define which patient groups are most likely to benefit.

Transplantation

The use of plasma exchange in the setting of solid organ transplantation has been explored most recently as part of an immunomodulatory preparative regimen to facilitate incompatible organ transplantation or to treat humoral rejection.[3,16] In renal transplantation, plasmapheresis to remove anti-HLA antibodies to prevent rejection has enabled transplantation in sensitized individuals with circulating donor-specific anti-HLA antibodies.[3] More recently, plasmapheresis has also been used as part of a conditioning regimen to allow successful ABO-incompatible renal transplantation.[16] Another indication for plasmapheresis is adjunctive therapy to prevent recurrent focal segmental glomerulosclerosis following renal transplantation, which may remove a circulating factor that alters glomerular permeability.[17] The use of plasma exchange to treat rejection mediated by donor-specific anti-HLA antibodies is controversial in renal transplantation. Similarly, plasma exchange for liver allograft rejection does not improve graft survival but may be effective in preventing life-threatening bleeding because coagulation status can be improved without volume overload.[18]

In contrast, histologic diagnosis of antibody-mediated rejection of cardiac transplants is often treated with plasmapheresis as part of the immunosuppressive regimen. If a patient is on extracorporeal membrane-oxygenation (ECMO) because of cardiac graft failure or other critical illness, plasmapheresis can be performed in tandem with the ECMO circuit.[19] Cardiac transplantation across ABO groups has been successful in infants and young children below 14 months. During the first year of life, the titer of anti-A and anti-B antibodies is low and the complement system is not fully mature at birth, which significantly decreases the risk of hyperacute rejection of ABO-incompatible heart transplants. Exchange transfusion is performed through the cardiopulmonary bypass circuit to further lower the titer of isohemagglutinins as part of the immunosuppressive regimen.[20]

Leukapheresis

Symptomatic Hyperleukocytosis

Leukapheresis is the emergent treatment to alleviate symptoms of hyperleukocytosis and vascular stasis in patients with leukemia with a preponderance of circulating blasts. Clinical manifestations resulting from leukostasis and impaired blood flow include tachypnea, dyspnea, pulmonary insufficiency, blurred vision, diplopia, dizziness, slurred speech, and coma. Pulmonary and cerebral hemorrhage or thrombosis are dire complications of hyperleukocytosis. The physical properties of the leukemic cells, as well as their number, influence their tendency to cause symptoms.[21] Although peripheral WBC counts may be extremely high in acute lymphoblastic leukemia (ALL), the blasts are smaller and less likely to adhere to peripheral vasculature than myeloid blasts. The risk of symptomatic leukocytosis is greatest for acute myeloid leukemia (AML), followed by the accelerated or blast crisis of chronic myelogenous leukemia (CML), and ALL. Complications from leukostasis are uncommon in chronic phase CML and are rare in chronic lymphocytic leukemia (CLL). Leukapheresis has also been used as an adjunct to chemotherapy to prevent metabolic complications associated with blast cell lysis in ALL and as a means to control leukocytosis in

CML when cytotoxic therapy is contraindicated, as in early pregnancy.[2]

The decision to initiate leukapheresis must be individualized and should not be based on an arbitrary white blood cell threshold. Peripheral WBC counts may be extremely high in ALL, but are often not accompanied by symptomatic leukocytosis, whereas a lesser degree of leukocytosis may occur in AML with pronounced leukostasis and clinical symptoms. As a general guideline, patients with peripheral WBC counts $>100 \times 10^9$ per L, with a high percentage of blasts and promyelocytes and neurologic or pulmonary manifestations of leukostasis are candidates for leukocyte depletion.[2] Different laboratory thresholds have been used to guide therapy, such as a fractional volume of leukocytes (leukocrit) above 10%, or circulating blasts above 50×10^9 per L, and additional clinical criteria may have to be taken into account, such as the rate at which the WBC or blast count is rising or the patient's coagulation status and general medical condition.[2]

Leukapheresis is a temporizing measure, and a definitive treatment of the underlying disease should be coordinated soon after the procedure(s) is (are) completed. Daily leukapheresis procedures may be performed for symptomatic improvement, or until the leukocyte count is substantially reduced and chemotherapy is under way. The treatment goal must also be individualized. The efficacy of the cytoreduction is variable and reflects total-body tumor burden, proliferative rate of the leukemic cells, and the response to concomitant chemotherapy. On average, a >50% reduction in circulating WBCs is achieved with each procedure that processes at least two blood volumes. Therefore, large volumes must be processed, corresponding to approximately 10 L for a 70-kg adult or approximately 5 L for a 35-kg child. Calculation of expected volume shifts before initiating the procedure is extremely important to avoid hypovolemia, dehydration, and acid–base imbalance, especially in small children.[5]

Patients with hyperleukocytosis are often severely anemic, but red cell transfusion should be given only after a degree of cytoreduction is achieved during the procedure or after the procedure, if clinically possible. Caution is warranted to avoid the risk of further increasing blood viscosity with red cell transfusion and aggravating existent vascular stasis and tissue ischemia. Citrate toxicity is a greater problem with leukapheresis than with exchange procedures because of the large volumes of blood processed and high doses of citrate administered. Patients should be closely monitored for citrate toxicity, and intravenous calcium supplementation will be required if citrate alone is used as an anticoagulant. Heparin may be used in combination with citrate to decrease the dose of citrate and the attendant risk of citrate toxicity. Contraindications to heparin use in this setting include significant coagulopathy or hemorrhage.

Peripheral Blood Stem Cell Collection

Leukapheresis to collect peripheral blood progenitor cells (PBPCs) is technically an autologous donation and not a therapeutic intervention, but pediatric patients with refractory or relapsed cancers often have significant underlying health problems that necessitate careful monitoring, often in the intensive care unit, and may require medical intervention during the procedure. PBPC transplantation has surpassed bone marrow transplantation as the preferred method to restore hematopoiesis in patients who have received myeloablative chemotherapy. Pediatric transplantation candidates typically have stage IV, high-risk neuroblastoma or malignant central nervous system (CNS) tumors. PBPC transplantation, in practice, achieves faster engraftment than bone marrow transplantation, shortening the duration of neutropenia and thrombocytopenia and reducing the attendant risks of infection and bleeding during recovery from myeloablation. Procedures to mobilize PBPCs into the circulation include a dose of a chemotherapeutic agent 10 to 14 days before apheresis with daily administration of granulocyte colony-stimulating factor (G-CSF, filgrastim) or granulocyte-macrophage colony-stimulating factor (GM-CSF, sargramostim). Typically, one to three daily leukapheresis procedures are sufficient for an adequate collection yield for transplantation, which corresponds to at least 2×10^6 to 5×10^6 CD34$^+$ mononuclear cells/kg/transplant. Leukapheresis procedures in pediatric transplantation candidates usually require red cell priming to maintain an adequate patient hematocrit during the collection. Platelet transfusion may also be needed before, during, or after the procedure, to maintain adequate platelet counts. Patients with brain tumors may be at increased risk of CNS bleeding, and therefore the platelet counts should be above 100×10^9 per L in susceptible patients.

Patients who have had extensive prior chemotherapy may require more procedures to collect adequate numbers of PBPCs and may have significant underlying morbidity necessitating additional precautions during apheresis procedures. Leukapheresis procedures require high blood flow rates to process large blood volumes (e.g., 5 to 10 L); consequently, citrate toxicity must be closely monitored especially if the patient's liver and renal functions are impaired. In addition to hypocalcemia, citrate could result in metabolic alkalosis and hypokalemia, as well as other electrolyte imbalances. Use of prophylactic intravenous calcium, alone or with magnesium, during full-dose citrate anticoagulation was shown to be effective and safe for children undergoing large-volume leukapheresis.[22] Alternatively, anticoagulation regimens using heparin, either alone or combined with citrate, reduce the risk of citrate toxicity.[5,23] Large-volume leukapheresis using a heparin–citrate strategy was associated with an overall risk of mild reactions of 16% and with no medically significant adverse reactions in a series of 72 pediatric patients with neuroblastoma,

weighing <20 kg.[24] Pediatric patients with brain tumors may be at increased risk for citrate toxicity and seizures.

Plateletpheresis (Thrombocytapheresis)

Symptomatic Thrombocytosis

Both malignant thrombocythemia, as is seen with myeloproliferative disorders such as essential thrombocythemia, and reactive thrombocytosis, as occurs following splenectomy, may result in platelet counts exceeding $1,000 \times 10^9$ per L; however, reactive thrombocytosis in children is transient, asymptomatic, and rarely requires treatment. In contrast, thrombocythemia associated with myeloproliferative disorders is unremitting and may require treatment to prevent bleeding or thrombosis. Bleeding may involve mucocutaneous (i.e., epistaxis), gastrointestinal, genitourinary, or cerebrovascular sites. Hemorrhagic and thrombotic complications are variable in severity and cannot be predicted on the basis of laboratory tests of coagulation or the platelet count.

Treatment of thrombocytosis is directed at controlling the underlying disease and managing patients with bleeding, thrombosis, or both complications. Pharmacologic options include single-agent chemotherapy with hydroxyurea, interferon, busulfan, or anegrilide. Aspirin and/or dipyridamole and antiplatelet agents may also be given for thrombotic complications; however, these agents and other anticoagulants are contraindicated if there are coexistent hemorrhagic complications. Because of the lag between initiation of pharmacologic agents and their clinical effect, plateletpheresis may be performed to immediately lower the platelet count as a temporizing measure. There is poor correlation between the platelet count and the risk of significant clinical problems. Plateletpheresis is generally recommended as an adjunct to chemotherapy for patients with platelet counts $>1,000 \times 10^9$ per L and for patients with markedly elevated platelet counts and manifestations of thrombosis or bleeding, irrespective of the platelet concentration.[2] In general, processing 1 to 1.5 blood volumes is expected to remove about 50% of circulating platelets, but the efficiency of removal demonstrates considerable variability and the reduction in platelet count may range from 30% to 80% with each procedure. As with leukapheresis procedures, red cell mass and intravascular fluid balance must be monitored carefully, with appropriate blood component therapy or fluid replacement during or after the procedure.

REFERENCES

1. Smith JW, Weinstein R, Hillyer KL. Therapeutic apheresis: A summary of current indication categories endorsed by the AABB and the American Society for Apheresis. *Transfusion.* 2003;43: 820–822.

2. Grima KM. Therapeutic apheresis in hematological and oncological diseases. *J Clin Apheresis*. 2000;15:28–52.

3. Winters JL, Pineda AA, McLeod BC, et al. Therapeutic apheresis in renal and metabolic diseases. *J Clin Apheresis*. 2000;15:53–73.

4. Eder AF, Kim HC. Pediatric therapeutic apheresis. In: Herman JH, Manno CS, eds. *Pediatric transfusion therapy*. Bethesda, MD: AABB Press; 2000.

5. Kim HC. Therapeutic pediatric apheresis. *J Clin Apheresis*. 2000; 15:129–157.

6. McLeod BC, Sniecinski I, Ciavarella D, et al. Frequency of immediate adverse effects associated with therapeutic apheresis. *Transfusion*. 1999;39:282–288.

7. Siegel JF, Rich MA, Brock WA. Association of sickle cell disease, priapism, exchange transfusion and neurological events: ASPEN syndrome. *J Urol*. 1993;150:1480–1482.

8. Adams RJ, McKie VC, Hsu L, et al. Prevention of a first stroke by transfusions in children with sickle cell anemia and abnormal results on transcranial doppler ultrasonography. *N Engl J Med*. 1998;339:5–11.

9. Clinical Alert from the National Heart, Lung and Blood Institute. December 5, 2004, http://www.nhlbi.nih.gov/health/prof/blood/sickle/clinical-alert-scd.htm.

10. Kim HC, Dugan NP, Silber JH, et al. Erythrocytapheresis therapy to reduce iron overload in chronically transfused patients with sickle cell disease. *Blood*. 1994;83:1136–1142.

11. Vichinsky EP, Luban NLC, Wright E. et al. Prospective RBC phenotype matching in a stroke-prevention trial in sickle cell anemia: A multicenter transfusion trial. *Transfusion*. 2001;41:1086–1092.

12. Sadler JE, Moake JL, Miyata T, et al. Recent advances in thrombotic thrombocytopenic purpura, Hematology (Am Soc Hematol Educ Program). 2004;407–423.

13. McMaster P, Shann F. The use of extracorporeal techniques to remove humoral factors in sepsis. *Pediatr Crit Care Med*. 2003; 4:2–7.

14. Nguyen T, Hall M, Han Y, et al. Microvascular thrombosis in pediatric multiple organ failure: Is it a therapeutic target? *Pediatr Crit Care Med*. 2001;2:187–196.

15. Busund R, Koukline V, Utrobin U, et al. Plasmapheresis in severe sepsis and septic shock: A prospective, randomised, controlled trial. *Intensive Care Med*. 2002;28:1434–1439.

16. Winters JL, Gloor JM, Pineda AA, et al. Plasma exchange conditioning for ABO-incompatible renal transplantation. *J Clin Apheresis*. 2004;19:79–85.

17. Savin VJ, Sharma R, Sharma M, et al. Circulating factor associated with increased glomerular permeability to albumin in recurrent focal segmental glomerulosclerosis. *N Engl J Med*. 1996;334: 878–883.

18. Singer AL, Olthoff KM, Kim H, et al. Role of plasmapheresis in the management of acute hepatic failure in children. *Ann Surg*. 2001;243:418–424.

19. Hernandez ME, Lovrekovic G, Schears G, et al. Acute onset of Wegener's granulomatosis and diffuse alveolar hemorrhage treated successfully by extracorporeal membrane oxygenation. *Pediatr Crit Care Med*. 2002;3:63–66.

20. West LJ, Pollock-Barziv SM, Dipchand AI, et al. ABO-incompatible heart transplantation in infants. *N Engl J Med*. 2001;344:793–800.

21. Lichtman MA, Rowe JM. Hyperleukocytic leukemias: Rheological, clinical and therapeutic considerations. *Blood*. 1982;60:279–283.

22. Bolan CD, Yau YY, Cullis HC, et al. Pediatric large-volume leukapheresis: A single institution experience with heparin versus citrate-based anticoagulant regimens. *Transfusion*. 2004;44: 229–238.

23. Gorlin JB, Humphreys D, Kent P, et al. Pediatric large volume peripheral blood progenitor cell collections from patients under 25 kg: A primer. *J Clin Apheresis*. 1996;11:195–203.

24. Pierson GR, Kim H, Dugan N, et al. Hematopoietic progenitor cell collection by apheresis in small children with high risk neuroblastoma. *Cytotherapy*. 2003;5:450.

Bone Marrow Transplantation

Edward C. Wong   *Evelio D. Perez-Albuerne*   *Naynesh R. Kamani*

Patients who have undergone hematopoietic stem cell transplantation (HSCT) often pose special problems for the pediatric intensive care unit (PICU) specialist. These patients often have profound immunosuppression, impaired hematopoiesis, and immunologic problems such as graft versus host disease (GVHD). Jacobe et al. found that[1] patients with HSCT admitted to the PICU have poor outcomes with an overall mortality rate of 44%. Several factors including the conditioning regimen, the source of the hematopoietic stem cells, and the immunosuppressive regimen are important in determining the host's susceptibility to complications in the post-transplantation period.

OVERVIEW

Depending on the patient's disease and condition, a conditioning regimen of high-dose chemotherapy and/or irradiation may be selected to destroy any remaining cancer, prepare the marrow for engraftment by donor hematopoietic stem cells, and prevent graft rejection. This regimen is usually administered 4 to 8 days before transplantation. Additionally, a source of hematopoietic stem cells is chosen. Often, these decisions are made as a part of an institutional research protocol. Complications will vary depending on the type of transplantation and time of occurrence (see Table 29.1).

There is an increasing trend toward using combined high-dose chemotherapeutic regimens with repeated infusion of autologous peripheral blood stem cells (PBSC). This approach rescues the patient from hematologic toxicity, which is the dose-limiting toxicity for many chemotherapeutic agents. The rescue also allows either the use of higher doses of chemotherapy in a single infusion or the repetition of chemotherapy cycles at shorter intervals. The goal is to completely eradicate the patient's tumor cells, as there is little, if any, graft versus tumor effect in an autologous transplant. These patients may be admitted to the PICU for a variety of reasons including the need for stem cell infusions and the use of automated cell separators in young children (often <2 years). Automated cell separators can harvest potentially more stem cells from peripheral blood with less contaminating tumor cells than can be obtained from bone marrow harvest. However, PICU issues include citrate toxicity, sedation, and an increased seizure risk during PBSC collection. These complications related to PBSC harvest are described in more detail in Chapter 28.

In contrast, the hematopoietic stem cells for allogeneic stem cell transplantation originate from the PBSC, bone marrow, and cord blood. In adult stem cell transplantation, PBSC are the primary source of hematopoietic cells. However, in pediatrics, cord blood is an attractive alternative because of the reduced stem cell dose and the availability of underrepresented ethnic groups in cord blood registries. Furthermore, cord blood has other features that make it unique as a source of hematopoietic stem cells. These include a reduced incidence of GVHD, the reduced need for strict human leukocyte antigen (HLA) matching, and the reduced cell dose needed for engraftment. However, there is an increased risk of graft failure and prolongation of hematopoietic recovery (particularly platelet recovery) after transplantation.[2,3]

Recipients of allogeneic transplants experience important complications that often lead to PICU admission. These include respiratory and infectious complications, cardiac toxicity, veno-occlusive disease (VOD), GVHD, renal dysfunction, neurologic complications, and graft failure. These complications may also be seen to a lesser extent in patients undergoing autologous transplantation. Complications related to the specific underlying diseases for which

TABLE 29.1

POTENTIAL COMPLICATIONS DURING THE COURSE OF TRANSPLANTATION[a]

	Before Transplantation	At Transplantation	First 100 d After Transplantation	After 100 d of Transplantation
Hematologic	Bleeding		Bleeding	
Infectious			Fungal infections, especially Candida and Aspergillus spp., Pneumocystis carinii	Fungal infections, especially Aspergillus spp. and Pneumocystis carinii
			Bacterial infections, especially gram-negative organisms	Bacterial infections, especially encapsulated organisms
			Parasitic infections	Parasitic infections
			Viral infections, especially CMV	Viral infections
Pulmonary		Pulmonary emboli[b]	Idiopathic pulmonary syndrome; diffuse alveolar hemorrhage	
Immunologic			Cytokine release/engraftment syndrome	
		Anaphylaxis[b]	Acute GVHD	Chronic GVHD
			Hemolytic anemia with ABO mismatch	
Metabolic	SIADH		Idiopathic hyperammonemia	
Genitourinary	Hemorrhagic cystitis		Hemorrhagic cystitis	
Hepatic			Veno-occlusive disease	
Renal			Acute renal failure	HSCT-associated TTP
Cardiovascular			Hemorrhagic cardiomyopathy	

[a]Occurrence is dependent on conditioning regimen, type of transplant, source of hematopoietic stem cells, disease status, post-transplantation GVHD treatment. Complications are indicated for the usual time of occurrence and may vary. See text for more details.
[b]Secondary to stem cell infusion.
CMV, cytomegalovirus; SIADH, syndrome of inappropriate antidiuretic hormone; GVHD, graft versus host disease; HSCT, hematopoietic stem cell transplantation; TTP, thrombotic thrombocytopenic purpura.

transplantation is being performed are beyond the scope of this chapter. The reader is referred to excellent reviews on this subject.[4] Diseases that have been treated with autologous and allogeneic stem cell transplantation are described in Table 29.2.

COMPLICATIONS

Infectious Complications

Infectious complications can occur from profound immunosuppression, impaired hematopoiesis, and pulmonary toxicity from the conditioning regimen, particularly with myeloablative conditioning regimens that include alkylating agents, podophyllotoxins, antimetabolites, or total body irradiation. In addition, rapidly dividing mucosal stem cells are damaged resulting in severe mucosal injury and a susceptibility to microorganisms. In contrast, the use of reduced-intensity conditioning regimens (nonmyeloablative or "mini" transplants) using purine analogs, anti-T-cell antibodies, or low-dose total body irradiation

have significantly less myelosuppression and little mucosal injury resulting in fewer infectious complications in the immediate post-transplantation period.

After bone marrow infusion, the patient remains aplastic for approximately 2 to 4 weeks; a slow recovery follows. In the case of PBSC transplant, hematopoietic recovery is achieved in approximately 8 to 12 days. Infection in this period of aplasia is commonly associated with a high degree of morbidity and mortality and is influenced by the duration of neutropenia, presence of GVHD, source of hematopoietic stem cells, patient age, underlying hematologic malignancy, relapsed disease status, extensive antibiotic use, higher radiation dose, and colonization with organisms before or soon after transplantation. Several studies describe that the return of functional immunity takes between 6 months to 2 years and, in many allogeneic transplant patients, may never return completely, often requiring reimmunization for childhood illnesses. Many patients, especially those with chronic GVHD and recipients of T-cell-depleted grafts, will continue to have impaired cellular and humoral immunity years after transplantation.

TABLE 29.2

MALIGNANT AND NONMALIGNANT DISEASES IN PEDIATRIC PATIENTS TREATED WITH HEMATOPOIETIC STEM CELL TRANSPLANTATION

Malignant Disorders	Nonmalignant Disorders
Acute lymphocytic leukemia	DiGeorge syndrome
Acute nonlymphocytic leukemia	Glycoprotein disorders
Preleukemia	Hematologic/immunologic disorders
Hairy cell leukemia	Aplastic anemia
Chronic myelogenous leukemia	Amegakaryocytic thrombocytopenia
Chronic lymphocytic leukemia	Chédiak-Higashi syndrome
Germ cell tumors (including CNS)	Chronic granulomatous disease
Hodgkin and non-Hodgkin lymphoma	Cyclic neutropenia
Juvenile myelomonocytic leukemia	Diamond-Blackfan anemia
Ovarian cancer	Fanconi syndrome
Primary brain tumors	Gaucher disease
Gliomas	IPEX syndrome
Medulloblastoma	Kostmann syndrome
Other primitive neuroectodermal tumors outside posterior fossa	Myelofibrosis
Brain stem tumors	Severe combined immunodeficiency disorder
Ependymoma	Sickle Hemoglobinopathy
Myelodysplastic syndromes	Shwachman-Diamond syndrome
Multiple myeloma	Thalassemia
Sarcoma	Wiskott-Aldrich syndrome
Solid tumors	X-linked agammaglobulinemia
Breast cancer	X-linked lymphoproliferative disorder
Melanoma	Juvenile dermatomyositis (severe)
Neuroblastoma	LDL receptor deficiency
	Lysosomal and Peroxisomal storage diseases
	Leukodystrophies
	Mucopolysaccharidoses
	Glycoprotein disorders
	Other lysosomal disorders
	Osteopetrosis

CNS, central nervous system; IPEX, immunodysregulation, polyendocrinopathy, enteropathy, X-linked; LDL, low density lipoprotein.

Pre-Engraftment Phase (<30 Days)

In the allogeneic transplant recipient, infectious complications in the pre-engraftment period are influenced by the presence of neutropenia, mucositis, and acute GVHD. Fever is the major manifestation of infection in this period; however, other signs and symptoms of infection are often attenuated because of neutropenia. Therefore, any cutaneous, mucosal, sinus, respiratory, or genitourinary symptoms require a thorough investigation. Physical examination should include special attention to the oropharynx, lungs, skin, and indwelling catheter sites. Any respiratory symptoms should prompt obtaining a chest radiograph or computed tomography (CT) scan. Likewise, urinalysis and culture should be obtained in a patient with urinary symptoms. The prompt evaluation for possible infection and early antibiotic treatment is imperative to reduce the risk of morbidity and mortality from infection in this period.

Common pathogens (>10% of patients) for infections include gram-negative bacilli, *Staphylococcus epidermidis*, streptococcal species of gastrointestinal origin, *Candida*, and *Aspergillus* species. Respiratory complications include both infectious and noninfectious pneumonitis and bacterial and fungal sinus infections. Signs and symptoms of fungal and bacterial pneumonia include dyspnea, cough, sputum production, fever, and intermittent or progressively worsening hypoxia. Chest radiographic findings typically consist of patchy or diffuse lower-lobe infiltrates. Atypical presentations of bacterial pneumonia are common, particularly in the presence of neutropenia.

Fungal pneumonia presents similarly but may have additional signs and symptoms including pleuritic chest pain, a pleural friction rub, hemoptysis, and tachycardia. On CT scans, fungal pneumonia appears as a wedge-shaped area of consolidation or as cavitary pulmonary nodules. Unfortunately, the diagnostic yield of bronchoscopy for fungal pneumonia is often poor. In future, use of galactomannan assays for suspected invasive aspergillosis may be helpful.[5,6] The evaluation of these assays in pediatric stem cell transplant patients is currently under way.

The most common viral infection in this period is herpes simplex infection, which usually manifests as ulcerative stomatitis. Patients who are seropositive before transplant are especially prone to developing this infection. In addition to herpes simplex virus, respiratory and enteric viral infections are seen in this and other posttransplantation periods and may be seasonal in occurrence.

Postengraftment Phase (30 to 100 Days)

In the postengraftment phase, impaired cellular immunity and acute or chronic GVHD predominate and contribute to a high incidence (>10%) of infections from *Staphylococcus epidermidis*, and streptococcal species of gastrointestinal origin. However, because the patient in this period is no longer neutropenic, gram-negative bacillus infections are rare. Epstein-Barr virus–mediated lymphoproliferative disease and *Toxoplasma gondii* and *Strongyloides stercoralis* infections occur in a small percentage of patients. Patients receiving corticosteroids, T cell–depleted grafts, or with GVHD are especially prone to invasive fungal infections such as *Pneumocystis carinii*, *Candida*, and *Aspergillus* species in this period. Furthermore, the risk of hemorrhagic cystitis by BK polyoma virus is increased by the development of acute GVHD.

The incidence of cytomegalovirus (CMV) infection is high in this period especially if the patient was seropositive before transplantation. Signs and symptoms of CMV interstitial pneumonia include dyspnea, low-grade fever, nonproductive cough, and diffuse bibasilar crackles. Initial chest radiographic findings include localized infiltrates, which can progress to diffuse bilateral interstitial infiltrates. Bronchoscopy with bronchoalveolar lavage or transbronchial biopsy may be useful in identifying actual CMV virus or early CMV antigen using shell vial culture, immunofluorescence, or polymerase chain reaction (PCR) techniques. Weekly surveillance of blood samples for CMV antigen or PCR should be performed from engraftment to day 100, as viremia typically occurs before the onset of symptoms. Other presentations of CMV infection such as enterocolitis, and rarely chorioretinitis, hepatitis, leptomeningitis, or encephalitis are possible. CMV, especially in allogeneic transplant patients can be life threatening. Patients who are CMV seronegative pretransplantation should receive CMV seronegative or CMV "reduced risk" (leukoreduced) products during hematopoietic recovery.

Postengraftment Phase (> 100 Days)

After 100 days of transplantation, the type of infection is influenced by impaired humoral (new) and cellular immunity, and chronic GVHD. This accounts for the high incidence of infection to CMV and varicella-zoster virus, encapsulated bacteria (especially *Streptococcus pneumoniae*, *Haemophilus influenzae*, and *Neisseria meningitidis*), *Aspergillus* species and *Pneumocystis carinii* and the continued low incidence among transplant recipients of *Toxoplasma gondii* infection and Epstein-Barr lymphoproliferative disease. Many medications including acyclovir, cidofovir, ganciclovir, and intravenous γ-globulin preparations with high titers to these infectious agents have been used to prevent or treat these infections. Foscarnet is used against CMV infections known to be refractory to ganciclovir and intravenous immunoglobulin.

Other viral infections can be problematic during bone marrow transplantation (BMT). These include adenovirus and human herpes virus-6 (HHV-6). Adenovirus infection can occur at a rate as high as 44%, which may lead to viremia in roughly one-third of cases.[7] HHV-6 is often detected during the immediate post-transplantation period using PCR techniques. HHV-6 antigenemia is often associated with fever, rash, and delayed engraftment. In rare cases, HHV-6 reactivation can lead to encephalitis. This reactivation can be detected using reverse transcriptase polymerase chain reaction (RT-PCR) techniques on the patient's cerebrospinal fluid to detect actively replicating virus. Although PCR of the HHV-6 genome can detect the presence of the virus, this technique has the disadvantage of not distinguishing between latent HHV-6 and actively replicating virus.[8]

Given the number of potential infectious complications and the time-dependent changes in cellular and humoral immunity, acute or chronic-GVHD in pediatric transplant patients, optimal management requires close consultation with a hematopoietic stem cell transplantation physician. For further details on management, the reader is referred to an excellent review by Wingard and Anaissie.[9]

Pulmonary Complications

Pulmonary complications are commonly seen in the allogeneic hematopoietic stem cell recipient. In a 5-year retrospective study of 363 pediatric patients undergoing BMT from 1995 to 1999, 90 (25%) developed new or persistent pulmonary infiltrates on chest imaging or pulmonary symptoms including hypoxemia or hemoptysis.[10] A major clinical challenge in the post-transplantation period is determining whether a pulmonary complication is infectious. However, despite the identification of a pathogen in 46% of patients using bronchoscopy and bronchoalveolar lavage, overall mortality was not decreased in one study.[10]

A major noninfectious pulmonary complication is idiopathic pneumonia syndrome, which results from cytokine-induced and alloreactive T cell–mediated lung injury. The widespread interstitial inflammation and alveolar damage can progress to pulmonary fibrosis. Although there is an association with GVHD, no definitive link has been established. The clinical presentation is characterized by a dramatic presentation of dyspnea, fever, and hypoxemia. Presentation can either be early with a median onset during the second to third week post-transplantation with an incidence of 6% to 8%. Chest radiographs demonstrate a diffuse process, and pulmonary function tests demonstrate a restrictive pattern with decreased diffusion capacity. Approximately 70% of patients require ventilatory support, with 50% requiring support within 2 days of presentation. High-dose methylprednisolone (2 to 10 mg/kg/day) may be beneficial. Antifungal prophylaxis is recommended because postmortem studies demonstrate that approximately 28% of patients with idiopathic pneumonia syndrome have a fungal etiology. The mortality can be as high as 70% with an almost 100% mortality if mechanical ventilation is required.[11] Recently, the use of etanercept (Enbrel), a soluble, dimeric tumor necrosis factor-α (TNF-α)–binding protein, has shown promise in the treatment of this disease.[12]

Another noninfectious pulmonary complication of allogeneic HSCT in children is diffuse alveolar hemorrhage (DAH). The pathogenesis of DAH is poorly understood. Several theories exist including the conditioning regimen, injury to alveolar capillary endothelial cells, inflammatory cytokine storm causing endothelial damage, and acute GVHD. Clinical signs and symptoms include diffuse infiltrates on chest radiograph, fever, dyspnea, cough, hemoptysis, and hypoxemia. The diagnosis is often established by bronchoscopy with repeated bronchoalveolar lavage demonstrating increasing hemorrhage and absence of microorganisms. DAH is a rarely described complication in children undergoing allogeneic HSCT. In a retrospective study[13] in pediatric allogeneic BMT, 6 of 138 (4.3%) patients (ages 3 to 120 months) developed DAH. Despite mechanical ventilation and optimization of any coagulopathy, mortality was seen in five out of six patients. The mean time to occurrence of DAH in these patients was 27 days with a range of 1 to 37 days post-transplantation. The treatment of this complication is largely supportive, with maintenance of platelet counts >50,000 per μL and correction of any thrombocytopathy or coagulopathy. Several studies have suggested that the administration of high-dose corticosteroids may be used to improve patient outcome;[14] however, the attendant risks of worsening unidentified fungal infections (especially pulmonary aspergillosis) causing increased morbidity and mortality and the lack of efficacy were noted in some studies.[13]

Veno-occlusive Disease

VOD of the liver is a clinical syndrome that occurs early after HSCT as a result of liver damage by the conditioning regimen. The incidence ranges from 22% to 28% among pediatric patients undergoing transplantation and is associated with a mortality rate of up to 47%. In a retrospective review of 142 pediatric patients who underwent hematopoietic stem cell transplantation, the mortality within 100 days of transplant was 4.97 times higher in the presence of VOD versus the absence of VOD.[15] Criteria for the diagnosis include hyperbilirubinemia, hepatomegaly, abdominal pain, and fluid retention. Initially, weight gain begins 6 to 8 days after transplantation with potentially severe liver dysfunction occurring by the second to third week after transplantation. Severe VOD can progress to multiorgan failure, which is associated with poor survival.

Risk factors for VOD include older age (older than 15 years), transplantation for diseases other than acute lymphoblastic leukemia, a preexisting history of liver disease or hepatic toxicity, use of HLA-matched unrelated donor stem cells, total parenteral nutrition, positive recipient CMV serology, and total body irradiation.[15] Chemotherapeutic agents such as azathioprine, cytosine arabinoside, and dacarbazine at conventional doses and cyclophosphamide, carmustine, busulfan, and mitomycin C at higher doses can cause VOD. Other new investigational medications may also increase the risk of VOD.

The overall treatment of VOD is largely supportive, consisting of maintenance of intravascular volume and renal perfusion. The goal of treatment is to prevent or minimize extravascular volume expansion and the consequences of hepatic dysfunction. The use of heparin or other agents (such as tissue plasminogen activator) used to prevent VOD is controversial, and there are currently no consensus guidelines regarding prophylactic therapy.[16] Studies of defibrotide, a polydeoxyribonucleotide, have been reportedly effective, but have not undergone controlled randomized

clinical trials.[17] Consultation with a pediatric hematopoietic stem cell transplantation physician is necessary to recognize and optimize treatment of this complication of BMT.

Acute and Chronic Renal Failure

Although renal dysfunction has been commonly reported in adult BMT patients, there are only a limited number of studies of renal dysfunction in pediatric patients. The incidence of acute renal failure occurring immediately after transplantation is 25% to 50%, with 5% to 10% requiring dialysis.[18] Although the causes of acute renal failure are multifactorial, sepsis, drug toxicity, and hepatorenal syndrome are most relevant. In a study by Patzer et al.[18] the risk factors for acute renal failure included allogeneic stem cell transplantation, sepsis, conditioning regimens consisting of cyclophosphamide and etoposide, VOD, and a hyperbilirubinemia >2 mg per dL. Although reported chronic renal failure rates have ranged from 0% to 28%, no end-stage renal failure has been reported. Treatment of acute renal failure is largely preventive, including adequate hydration, avoidance or minimization of exposure to nephrotoxic agents, and use of amifostine to minimize toxicity with high-dose chemotherapy, especially regimens containing *cis*-platinum. Once dialysis is initiated, mortality is markedly increased.[18]

Bone Marrow Transplantation–Associated Thrombotic Thrombocytopenic Purpura

An entity referred to as "BMT nephropathy" or BMT-associated thrombotic thrombocytopenic purpura (TTP) is also seen commonly. This syndrome occurs >100 days after transplantation and is characterized by hypertension, renal failure, negative direct antiglobin test (DAT) hemolytic anemia, and thrombocytopenia. This syndrome, unlike idiopathic TTP, often has a poor response to plasmapheresis. The basis for this poor response to plasmapheresis is related to lack of a functional decrease of a disintegrin and metalloproteinase with thrombospondin motifs (ADAMTS-13) secondary to an autoantibody response to ADAMTS-13 (see Chapter 28). As many as 54% of pediatric patients undergoing BMT may experience a variant of this disorder. The several contributing factors include previous total body irradiation, GVHD, CMV infection, mitomycin C, cyclosporin A, and an allogeneic source of stem cells. The pathogenesis of BMT nephropathy is secondary to endothelial cell damage from one of the above factors. The treatment is largely supportive. Platelet transfusions should be avoided in order to avoid worsening the ongoing thrombotic microangiopathy and should be given only in the case of life-threatening hemorrhage.

Central and Peripheral Nervous System Complications

Central and peripheral nervous system complications often result from radiotherapy and chemotherapy and medications such as cyclosporin A and corticosteroids; however, GVHD, changes in drug metabolism, thrombocytopenia, or relapsing disease also influence the clinical presentation. Central and peripheral nervous system complications present as neuropathies, somnolence, confusion or disorientation, seizures, encephalopathy, or coma. In a large retrospective study of 272 patients from 1985 to 2001, Faraci et al.[19] found that severe neurologic complications had an incidence rate of 14%, causing 8.5% of transplant-related mortality. The main risk factors for these complications included unrelated allogeneic transplantation, development of severe GVHD, and the use of total body irradiation in the preparative regimen. In this study, the median days of occurrence for cyclosporin A–mediated neurotoxicity ($n = 21$), total body irradiation- or chemotherapy-related leukoencephalopathy ($n = 7$), central nervous system (CNS) infections ($n = 7$), and cerebrovascular accident ($n = 3$) ranged from 82 to 95 days after transplantation depending on the type of neurologic complication. Rare immune-mediated complications were noted in one patient that led to Guillain-Barré syndrome that was refractory to plasmapheresis and high-dose intravenous immunoglobulins, and complications associated with diffuse subcortical and cortical involvement, responsive to etoposide and azathioprine, in a second patient with right-sided hemiparesis. These immune-mediated complications, however, occurred months to years after transplantation and were not seen in the immediate posttransplantation period. In this study, the most frequent CNS infections included viral infections, followed by (in decreased frequency) infection with *Toxoplasma* and *Aspergillus* species. Treatment largely consists of withholding or reducing the dose of the implicated medication (especially in the case of cyclosporin A–mediated toxicity), provision of anticonvulsant treatment, and treatment of the underlying infection, as necessary. The development of encephalopathy is associated with an extremely poor prognosis. In a study of 405 patients over a 10-year period in which 26 patients developed encephalopathy, 65% died of either progressive encephalopathy or relapse of primary disease or toxicity.[20] Consultations with specialists in neurology, hematopoietic stem cell transplantation, and infectious diseases are necessary to provide optimal management for these patients.

Hemorrhage

Because of the profound bone marrow suppression, thrombocytopenia and anemia are common complications of BMT. Thrombocytopathy, breakdown of mucosal barriers, and coagulopathy secondary to sepsis and disseminated intravascular coagulation (DIC) are commonly observed in these patients. Common sites of hemorrhage include the gastrointestinal tract and intracranial or pulmonary hemorrhage. Platelet counts should be maintained at >50,000 per μL and ideally at >100,000 per μL, particularly, in the case of intracranial hemorrhage. Monitoring

and correcting any coagulopathy or thrombocytopathy is critical to the control of life-threatening hemorrhage. Often patients are refractory to platelet transfusions that develop from anti-HLA antibodies, which occurs in previously pregnant women or patients who have had numerous red blood cell (RBC) or platelet transfusions. Many nonimmune causes for platelet refractoriness such as DIC, fever, infection, drugs (such as amphotericin), and hemorrhage exist and should be ruled out before consideration of HLA-matched or cross-matched compatible platelets.[21] The use of antifibrinolytic agents such as ε-aminocaproic acid or tranexamic acid may be considered (see Chapter 26). The use of activated factor VIIa as a hemostatic agent in patients with hematopoietic stem cell transplant is not yet validated by controlled clinical trials.[22]

Graft Versus Host Disease

GVHD is caused by the recognition of recipient tissue as foreign by the newly engrafted immune system. Donor T cells principally mediate this disease. Antigen-presenting cells present recipient antigens to donor T cells resulting in the activation and expansion of GVHD effector populations, ultimately leading to the development of cytotoxic T cells. This occurs in either an acute (<100 days after transplantation) or chronic (>100 days) form in a high percentage (40% to 50%) of patients with allogeneic bone marrow transplants and to a much smaller extent (5% to 10%) in patients with autologous BMT. The source of hematopoietic stem cells has an important influence in the development of chronic GVHD in patients who undergo allogeneic peripheral blood stem cell transplantation.[23]

Acute GVHD is an inflammatory disease that primarily affects the skin, liver, and gastrointestinal tract. The gastrointestinal tract and liver are commonly involved along with skin changes (see Figs. 29.1 and 29.2). Skin GVHD usually presents as a maculopapular rash that can be evanescent, often involving the palms and soles. Gastrointestinal GVHD can present with crampy abdominal pain and diarrhea that is watery, highly voluminous, and occasionally bloody with large amounts of mucus. Diagnosis can be made through rectal biopsies demonstrating lymphocytic infiltrates in the crypts, and necrosis and loss of crypt cells. Acute liver GVHD presents as unconjugated hyperbilirubinemia with mild to moderate increases in hepatic transaminases and alkaline phosphatase. Pathologically, acute liver GVHD demonstrates lymphocytic infiltrates in the interlobular and marginal bile ducts similar in appearance to cholestasis. Other conditions including drug toxicity, viral disease, and VOD, the last of which is associated with endothelial damage and clinical signs of ascites, hepatomegaly, and abdominal pain need to be considered. CT scan can reveal multiple, diffuse, fluid-filled bowel loops and an enhancement of bowel wall mucosae. A subset of acute GVHD known as *hyperacute GVHD* typically occurs

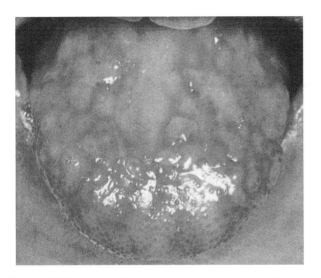

Figure 29.1 Ulcerated tongue in a patient with graft versus host disease following BMT. This phenomenon, where mature donor lymphocytes attack the recipient's tissues, consists of a tetrad of painful oral mucositis, enteritis, dermatitis, and hepatic dysfunction. (From Yamada T, Alpers DH, Laine L, et al. *Atlas of gastroenterology.* Philadelphia, PA: Lippincott Williams & Wilkins; 2003.) (See color Figure 29.1.)

in recipients of HLA-mismatched hematopoietic stem cells and is related to the massive release of interleukin-2 (IL-2), TNF, and interferon-γ (IFN-γ) immediately after transplantation. Hyperacute GVHD is characterized by a much stronger inflammatory response than that seen in acute GVHD and usually occurs within 72 hours of transplantation. Clinical signs and symptoms include fever, skin changes, diarrhea, hyperbilirubinemia, and occasionally lung collapse.

Steroids are the mainstay of treatment of acute and hyperacute GVHD and need to be used until the GVHD has resolved. Steroids have many side effects including infection (especially fungal and viral), osteoporosis, diabetes, hypertension, and cataracts. The medication dosage needs to be tapered slowly to minimize the symptoms. Other medications such as daclizumab (an antibody against the α-chain of the IL-2 receptor), mycophenolate mofetil,

rapamycin, tresperimus, basiliximab, denileukin diftitox, anti-CD40L, and CTLA-4-Ig are currently under investigation as adjunctive medications to steroids.

Chronic GVHD occurs >100 days after transplantation, and pathologically resembles an autoimmune vasculitis. Epithelial cell damage, mononuclear cell inflammation, fibrosis, and hypocellularity and atrophy of the lymphoid system eventually result and can lead to significant morbidity and even fatal disease. A major complication resulting from chronic GVHD is life-threatening viral infections, especially CMV. Treatment includes steroids with cyclosporin A, thalidomide, mycophenolate, or other similar agents. Supportive therapy is an important component of chronic GVHD and may include bronchodilator treatment, immunoglobulin replacement (containing e.g., high antibody titers to CMV), and lung transplantation for pulmonary involvement; prophylactic antibiotic prevention of infection and physical therapy for development of muscle weakness, contractures, and fasciitis due to epithelial cell damage and fibrosis. The use of extracorporeal photophoresis using methoxypsoralen as a possible useful adjunctive therapy is currently under investigation[24,25] and awaits randomized, controlled clinical trials.

Graft Failure or Rejection

Less than 5% of BMTs and only rare peripheral blood stem cell transplants experience graft failure or rejection. Graft failure is more likely to occur in patients with aplastic anemia and those with unrelated donor transplants (particularly patient mismatched at the HLA D locus). In a study by Woodard et al.[26] of 309 consecutive patients undergoing allogeneic BMT between 1989 and 1999, other potential etiologic factors for graft failure included lower total nucleated cell dose, transplantation for nonmalignant diseases, and conditioning regimens that did not include total body irradiation. Often a failing graft may be stimulated with growth factors and steroids; however, if this fails, then a second infusion of marrow stem cells or PBSC from the original donor may be necessary. Autologous back-up marrow infusion may be an appropriate alternative in certain patients.[27]

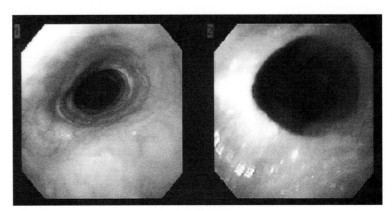

Figure 29.2 Graft versus host disease. Multiple fine mucosal webs are present in the esophagus. (From Yamada T, Alpers DH, Laine L, et al. *Atlas of gastroenterology.* Philadelphia, PA: Lippincott Williams & Wilkins; 2003:216.) (See color Figure 29.2.)

Otherwise, retransplantation is necessary requiring an aggressive conditioning regimen. In those patients requiring repeat transplantation, there is a significantly increased risk of VOD and GVHD with attendant complications.

Cardiac Toxicity

Cardiac toxicity arises from the cumulative toxicity related to anthracycline use, high-dose cyclophosphamide, chest, or total body irradiation. Mitral valve disease and cardiac ejection fraction <50%, although less commonly seen in pediatric patients, may also contribute to cardiac toxicity. Hemorrhagic cardiomyopathy secondary to high-dose cyclophosphamide can occur 1 to 10 days after administration of the preparative regimen. Signs and symptoms include cardiomegaly, pulmonary edema, poor peripheral perfusion, and systemic edema. The electrocardiogram often demonstrates low voltage readings. Resultant hemorrhagic myocarditis may lead to cardiac tamponade and death, if left unnoticed. Treatment includes fluid management and use of diuretics and inotropes (see Chapter 27).

Metabolic Complications

Cyclophosphamide commonly causes the syndrome of inappropriate antidiuretic hormone (SIADH). Patient intake and output and daily serum sodium levels must be closely monitored with frequent checks of urine electrolytes for evidence of SIADH. If SIADH occurs, fluid restriction or increasing the sodium content of the infusion until the drug is finished may be necessary. Other electrolyte abnormalities such as hypomagnesemia secondary to urinary losses following cyclosporine or tacrolimus and hypokalemia secondary to furosemide use are commonly seen and require replacement (see Chapter 27).

Cytokine Release/Engraftment Syndrome

Cytokine release syndrome is a shocklike syndrome that occurs primarily among patients undergoing matched unrelated donor BMT. This is felt to occur because of the tremendous cytokine release that occurs in patients who experience early hematopoietic recovery. In an adult study by Miller et al.[28] there was an associated mortality rate of 44% despite aggressive therapy with an incidence of 4% among patients undergoing allogeneic BMT. The median occurrence was 11 days after transplantation. Clinical symptoms are similar to toxic shock syndrome including refractory hypotension, fever, renal insufficiency, and hepatic failure, although additional symptoms include encephalopathy, hypoxia, pulmonary infiltrates, weight gain, and erythroderma. The treatment of this syndrome is largely supportive. Usually blood cultures are negative in these patients, but sepsis has a similar presentation and must be ruled out.

Engraftment syndrome occurs in recipients of autologous stem cell transplantation and has a very similar clinical presentation. Patients typically present with skin rash involving a significant portion of body surface (>27% in one series), fever, hypoxia, pulmonary infiltrates, hepatic dysfunction, renal insufficiency, weight gain, and occasional transient encephalopathy. In a study by Madero et al.[29] of patients with engraftment syndrome, overall transplant-related mortality was approximately 23% and significantly higher than in patients without engraftment syndrome. Greater associated morbidity (increased transfusion requirements, parenteral nutrition, and hospital stay) was also seen in these patients than in patients without engraftment syndrome.[29] In a follow-up study from the same group, using a multivariate analysis, high CD34+ stem cell dose, transplantation for solid tumors, early disease status, and use of conditioning regimens other than busulfan were associated with engraftment syndrome.[29] As with cytokine release syndrome, treatment of engraftment syndrome is also largely supportive.

Complications Related to Infusion of Hematopoietic Stem Cell Infusion

Complications from the infusion of hematopoietic stem cells also occur. Depending on the source and processing of the hematopoietic stem cells, these complications may include allergic and anaphylactic reactions, fluid overload, fat, or bone emboli. The symptoms of these reactions may include hyper- or hypotension, cardiac arrhythmias, urticaria, pruritus, dyspnea, wheezing, anaphylaxis, flanks pain, back pain, chills, and fever. PBSC can also elicit symptoms such as headache, nausea, vomiting, diarrhea, abdominal cramps, chills, tachycardia, tachypnea, and malaise. These symptoms are felt to be secondary to the large volume of PBSC and the high percentage of dimethyl sulfoxide (DMSO) in PBSC. The infusion of marrow results in exposure to toxic cell products and free hemoglobin, which, in combination with a nephrotoxic conditioning regimen, may result in acute renal failure. Some institutions require that a physician remains at the bedside during infusion or for a specified time after infusion, whereas others perform electrocardiograph monitoring, frequent vital signs, or a combination of both.[30]

FACTORS PREDICTING PEDIATRIC INTENSIVE CARE UNIT ADMISSION

Table 29.3 describes factors predicting PICU admission by recipients of hematopoietic stem cell transplants based on a study by Diaz et al.[31] In this study, the probability of complications requiring admission to the PICU was approximately 21%. For recipients of autologous and allogeneic transplants, the probability of complications requiring admission to the intensive care unit (ICU) was 10% and 34%, respectively. On the basis of a univariate analysis, underlying disease, status at transplantation (advance stage), multiorgan dysfunction, respiratory failure

TABLE 29.3

CLINICAL FACTORS PREDICTING INTENSIVE CARE UNIT ADMISSION IN PATIENTS UNDERGOING HEMATOPOIETIC STEM CELL TRANSPLANTATION

Allogeneic HSCT
Disease status[a]
Underlying disease[a]
GVHD [a,b]
Multiorgan dysfunction[a]
Autologous HSCT
Disease status[a]
Underlying disease[a,b]
Engraftment syndrome[a,b]
Multiorgan dysfunction during neutropenic period[a]

[a]Univariate analysis
[b]Multivariate analysis
HSCT, hematopoietic stem cell transplantation; GVHD, graft versus host disease.
Adapted from Diaz MA, Vicent MG, Prudencio M, et al. Predicting factors for admission to an intensive care unit and clinical outcome in pediatric patients receiving hematopoietic stem cell transplantation. *Haematologica*. 2002;87:292–298.

alone, and GVHD were significantly associated with PICU admission in patients undergoing allogeneic transplantation. Similar findings were seen in recipients undergoing autologous transplantation. However, upon multivariate analysis, only severe GVHD (grade III to IV) was independently associated with admission to the ICU among patients undergoing allogeneic transplantation. In contrast, advanced stage of disease and engraftment syndrome were associated with ICU admission among pediatric patients undergoing autologous transplantation using a similar analysis.

SUMMARY

The recipient of hematopoietic stem cells poses unique challenges to the PICU specialist. This is largely the result of the conditioning regimen, the underlying disease, transplant type (autologous or allogeneic), post-transplantation immunosuppression and hematopoietic stem cell source. Dynamic changes in cellular and humoral immunity along with early impaired hematopoiesis and the need to establish a graft versus tumor effect (which is often associated with GVHD) contribute to the many potential complications seen by the transplant recipient. Optimal management of these patients requires close consultation with many pediatric specialists, especially the pediatric hematopoietic stem cell transplant physician.

REFERENCES

1. Jacobe SJ, Hassan A, Veys P, et al. Outcome of children requiring admission to an intensive care unit after bone marrow transplantation. *Crit Care Med*. 2003;31:1299–1305.
2. Broxmeyer HE, ed. *Cord blood: Biology, immunology, banking, and clinical transplantation*. Bethesda, MD: AABB Press; 2004.
3. Ballen KK. New trends in umbilical cord blood transplantation. *Blood*. 2005;105:3786–3792.
4. Mehta P, ed. *Pediatric stem cell transplantation*. Sudbury, MA: Jones and Bartlett Publishers; 2004.
5. Musher B, Fredricks D, Leisenring W, et al. Aspergillus galactomannan enzyme immunoassay and quantitative PCR for diagnosis of invasive aspergillosis with bronchoalveolar lavage fluid. *J Clin Microbiol*. 2004;42:5517–5522.
6. Maertens J, Verhaegen J, Lagrou K, et al. Screening for circulating galactomannan as a noninvasive diagnostic tool for invasive aspergillosis in prolonged neutropenic patients and stem cell transplantation recipients: A prospective validation. *Blood*. 2001;97:1604–1610.
7. Heemskerk B, Lankester AC, van Vreeswijk T, et al. Immune reconstitution and clearance of human adenovirus viremia in pediatric stem-cell recipients. *J Infect Dis*. 2005;191:520–530.
8. Savolainen H, Lautenschlager I, Piiparinen H, et al. Human herpes-6 and -7 in pediatric stem cell transplantation. *Pediatr Blood Cancer*. 2005;45:820–825.
9. Wingard JR, Anaissie E. Infectious complications after hematopoietic cell transplantation. In: Mehta P, ed. *Pediatric stem cell transplantation*. Sudbury, MA: Jones and Bartlett Publishers; 2004:389–400.
10. Eikenberry M, Bartakova H, Defor T, et al. Natural history of pulmonary complications in children after bone marrow transplantation. *Biol Blood Marrow Transplant*. 2005;11:56–64.
11. Kantrow SP, Hackman RC, Boeckh M, et al. Idiopathic pneumonia syndrome: Changing spectrum of lung injury after marrow transplantation. *Transplantation*. 1997;63:1079–1086.
12. Yanik G, Hellerstedt B, Custer J, et al. Etanercept (Enbrel) administration for idiopathic pneumonia syndrome after allogeneic hematopoietic stem cell transplantation. *Biol Blood Marrow Transplant*. 2002;8:395–400.
13. Ben-Abraham R, Paret G, Cohen R, et al. Diffuse alveolar hemorrhage following allogeneic bone marrow transplantation in children. *Chest*. 2003;124:660–664.
14. Haselton DJ, Klekamp JG, Christman BW, et al. Use of high-dose corticosteroids and high-frequency oscillatory ventilation for treatment of a child with diffuse alveolar hemorrhage after bone marrow transplantation: Case report and review of the literature. *Crit Care Med*. 2000;28:245–248.
15. Barker CC, Butzner JD, Anderson RA, et al. Incidence, survival, and risk factors for the development of veno-occlusive disease in pediatric hematopoietic stem cell transplant recipients. *Bone Marrow Transplant*. 2003;32:79–87.
16. Reiss U, Cowan M, McMillan A, et al. Hepatic venoocclusive disease in blood and bone marrow transplantation in children and young adults: Incidence, risk factors and outcome in a cohort of 241 patients. *J Pediatr Hematol Oncol*. 2002;42:746–750.
17. Corbacioglu S, Greil J, Peters C, et al. Defibrotide in the treatment of children with veno-occlusive disease (VOD): A retrospective multicentre study demonstrates therapeutic efficacy upon early intervention. *Bone Marrow Transplant*. 2004;33:189–195.
18. Patzer L, Kentouche K, Ringelmann F, et al. Renal function following hematological stem cell transplantation in childhood. *Pediatr Nephrol*. 2003;18:623–635.
19. Faraci M, Lanino E, Dini G, et al. Severe neurologic complications after hematopoietic stem cell transplantation in children. *Neurology*. 2002;59:1895–1904.
20. Woodard P, Helton K, McDaniel H, et al. Encephalopathy in pediatric patients after allogeneic hematopoietic stem cell transplantation is associated with a poor prognosis. *Bone Marrow Transplant*. 2004;33:1151–1157.
21. Slichter SJ, Davis K, Enright H, et al. Factors affecting posttransfusion platelet increments, platelet refractoriness, and platelet transfusion intervals in thrombocytopenic patients. *Blood*. 2005;105:4106–4114.
22. Bacigalupo A. Haemopoietic stem cell transplants: The impact of haemorrhagic complications. *Blood Rev*. 2003;17(Suppl 1):S6–S10.
23. Remberger M, Beelen DW, Fauser A, et al. Increased risk of extensive chronic graft-versus-host disease after allogeneic

peripheral blood stem cell transplantation using unrelated donors. *Blood.* 2005;105:548–551.

24. Dall'Amico R, Messina C. Extracorporeal photochemotherapy for the treatment of graft-versus-host disease. *Ther Apher.* 2002; 6:296–304.

25. Halle P, Paillard C, D'Incan M, et al. Successful extracorporeal phototherapy for chronic graft-versus-host disease in pediatric patients. *J Hematother Stem Cell Res.* 2002;11:501–512.

26. Woodard P, Tong X, Richardson S, et al. Etiology and outcome of graft failure in pediatric hematopoietic stem cell transplant recipients. *J Pediatr Hematol Oncol.* 2003;25:955–959.

27. Mehta J, Powles R, Singhal S, et al. Outcome of autologous rescue after failed engraftment of allogeneic marrow. *Bone Marrow Transplant.* 1996;17:213–217.

28. Miller CB, Hayashi RT, Vogelsang GB, et al. Cytokine release syndrome after bone marrow transplantation (BMT). *Blood.* 1994;76:487.

29. Madero L, Vicent MG, Sevilla J, et al. Engraftment syndrome in children undergoing autologous peripheral blood progenitor cell transplantation. *Bone Marrow Transplant.* 2002;30:355–358.

30. Gorlin JB. Transfusion reactions associated with hematopoietic progenitor cell reinfusion. In: Popovsky MA, ed. *Transfusion reactions.* 2nd ed. Bethesda, MD: AABB Press; 2001:235–253.

31. Diaz MA, Vicent MG, Prudencio M, et al. Predicting factors for admission to an intensive care unit and clinical outcome in pediatric patients receiving hematopoietic stem cell transplantation. *Haematologica.* 2002;87:292–298.

Cardiac Diseases

John T. Berger III   *Richard A. Jonas*

Principles of Postoperative Care

30

Melvin C. Almodovar

Advances in diagnosis, surgical management, and perioperative care over the last 25 years have led to impressive survival rates in children with *all* types of congenital heart disease (CHD). Current operative management strategies are designed not only to optimize patient survival but also to achieve the best possible long-term functional outcomes, with emphasis on cardiac function, neurodevelopment, and quality of life.[1] Optimal care of the postoperative pediatric cardiac surgical patient (or adult patient with CHD) requires the orchestrated and collaborative efforts of a multidisciplinary care team with expertise in pediatric cardiac surgery, pediatric cardiology, pediatric and adult medicine, critical care medicine, neonatology, nursing, and cardiac anesthesiology.

PATIENT POPULATION AND PREOPERATIVE CONSIDERATIONS

Early primary repair is now advocated in most cases to prevent the secondary consequences of abnormal physiology associated with CHD. Even in premature infants, early surgical correction has demonstrated better survival as compared to the strategy of prolonged medical management.[2] Neonates often present specific challenges because of prematurity and low–birth-weight status, immature organ systems, a transitional circulation, coexisting malformations, and a propensity for multiorgan injury (i.e., intracranial hemorrhage, and necrotizing enterocolitis), all of which affect the timing of surgery, the surgical approach, and overall outcomes. Preoperative clinical status of the newborn with CHD has a significant impact on postoperative course; therefore, it is extremely important to establish a complete cardiac diagnosis and to provide necessary

interventions to optimize myocardial and other organ functions before surgery. Following the initial diagnosis, many neonates with CHD require specific interventions such as prostaglandin E_1 (PGE_1) infusion or balloon atrial septostomy to prevent end-organ dysfunction or injury preoperatively. Diffuse systemic inflammation, myocardial dysfunction, end-organ hypoperfusion, acquired lung disease, and endocrine dysfunction may all adversely affect recovery in neonates despite a technically successful operation.

Older children and adults with CHD may present for surgical intervention with new cardiac problems or, after years of deranged hemodynamics, with varying degrees of secondary end-organ dysfunction. An increasing number of symptomatic adult patients are referred to pediatric centers for surgical treatment of deteriorating hemodynamics due to valvar disease, residual intracardiac shunts, or complex arrhythmias following previous intervention. Despite good surgical outcomes in older patients, the cumulative effects of chronic cyanosis, systemic hypoperfusion, lifestyle choices, and other medical conditions lead to limited organ reserve and a potentially challenging course following surgery. Consequently, this patient population benefits greatly from advanced planning and collaboration among pediatric and adult specialists to identify and address coexisting medical and psychosocial issues.

Patient care systems designed to evaluate and provide timely intervention are extremely important for the successful care of patients with CHD of all sizes and ages. A detailed approach forms the basis for selecting the optimal timing of surgery and anticipating major problems and choosing the best management strategies following intervention. In all aspects, perioperative care should be *anticipatory* with regard to the individual patient's anatomic response to surgery and *proactive* with respect to evaluation and intervention of expected and unexpected events to optimize the chances for success.

ROUTINE POSTOPERATIVE MANAGEMENT

Critical care management of patients after cardiac surgery typically emphasizes the cardiovascular system and the state of the surgical repair; however, organ system interactions, limited organ reserve, and the tendency for rapid changes in hemodynamics must be addressed systematically by the critical care team. A major goal is to balance systemic oxygen (O_2) delivery and consumption while minimizing the potential for complications during the recovery period.

Postoperative Evaluation, Hemodynamic Monitoring, and Assessment of Vital Organ Perfusion

Standard Initial Evaluation and Monitoring

Standard initial evaluation of the patient should include a review of the preoperative and postoperative anatomy, the surgical procedure and operative course, a complete physical examination, and a survey of surgically inserted devices (e.g., drains, transthoracic catheters, and temporary pacing wires). Periodic blood sampling to evaluate acid–base status, gas exchange, O_2 content (co-oximetry), electrolyte concentrations, endocrine function, and indices of hepatic and renal function is performed regularly. Serologic markers of perfusion or organ injury may also be useful in tailoring treatment strategies and predicting postoperative outcome.

Invasive Monitoring

Continuous invasive monitoring is achieved by the use of percutaneous or transthoracic intracardiac catheters, which allow direct, simultaneous measurement of central venous or right atrial pressure, left atrial pressure, and pulmonary artery pressure. The hemodynamic consequences of various rhythm disturbances, responses to blood volume loss or repletion, responses to manipulation of inotropes or pacing maneuvers, and the evaluation of potential cardiac anatomic or functional lesions are all facilitated by monitoring intracardiac pressures and associated waveforms (see Tables 30.1 and 30.2) with little risk to the patient.[3] Co-oximetric analysis of blood sampled from select intracardiac monitoring lines allows for measurement of mixed venous O_2 saturation as a means of estimating cardiac index (Fick principle) or determining the presence of significant anatomic left-to-right shunting at the atrial or ventricular levels. Information obtained by invasive monitoring may identify the need for further anatomic

TABLE 30.1

ATRIAL AND PULMONARY ARTERY PRESSURES IN RELATION TO RESIDUAL ANATOMIC LESIONS, MYOCARDIAL FUNCTION, POSTOPERATIVE RHYTHM, AND VASCULAR VOLUME STATES

	Right Atrial Pressure	Left Atrial Pressure	Pulmonary Arterial Pressure
Left heart lesions			
MR, MS	nl, ↑[a]	↑, ↑↑, ↑↑↑	nl, ↑, ↑↑
LV dysfunction	nl, ↑[a]	nl, ↑, ↑↑	nl, ↑
LVVO	nl, ↑[a]	↑, ↑↑	nl, ↑
LV hypoplasia	nl, ↑[a]	↑, ↑↑	nl, ↑, ↑↑
LVOTO	nl, ↑[a]	nl, ↑, ↑↑	nl, ↑
Right heart lesions			
TR, TS	↑, ↑↑	nl	nl
RV dysfunction	nl, ↑, ↑↑	nl, ↑	nl, ↑
RVVO	↑, ↑↑	nl, ↑	nl
RV hypoplasia	↑, ↑↑	nl	nl
RVOTO	nl, ↑, ↑↑	nl, ↑	nl
PAH	nl, ↑, ↑↑	nl, ↓, ↑	↑, ↑↑, ↑↑↑
Loss of AV synchrony	↑	↑	nl
Cardiac tamponade	↑↑	↑↑	nl, ↑
Hypovolemia	↓	↓	↓
Hypervolemia	↑	↑	↑

[a]Right atrial pressure may be increased if left heart failure is associated with PAH.
↑, mildly increased; ↑↑, moderately increased; ↑↑↑, severely increased; ↓, decreased; nl, normal; MR, mitral regurgitation; MS, mitral stenosis; LV, left ventricle; LVVO, left ventricular volume overload; LVOTO, left ventricular outflow tract obstruction; TR, tricuspid regurgitation; TS, tricuspid stenosis; RV, right ventricle; RVVO, right ventricular volume overload; RVOTO, right ventricular outflow tract obstruction; PAH, pulmonary artery hypertension; AV, atrioventricular.

investigation by echocardiography, cardiac catheterization, or both.

Serologic Markers of Perfusion and Organ Injury

Monitoring the patient's metabolic status by careful analysis of arterial blood gas data, serum electrolyte profile, and indices of end-organ function also contribute to the information about the adequacy of the circulation or possible vital organ injury. Elevated blood lactate concentration may reflect tissue hypoxia or injury due to circulatory insufficiency or impaired function of the organs that are active in lactate metabolism. Measurement of serum lactate concentrations during cardiopulmonary bypass (CPB) or after admission to the intensive care unit (ICU) may be predictive of outcome, including the development of multiple organ failure, need for mechanical circulatory support, or death.[4] In addition to lactate, serum concentrations of neuron-specific enolase, S100 β protein, and various inflammatory-related adhesion molecules may serve as potential markers of early postoperative brain injury after CPB.[5] Cardiomyocyte

TABLE 30.2

ABNORMAL ATRIAL WAVEFORMS

Right or Left Atrial Wave	Physiology	Disease Example
Cannon A wave	Atrial contraction against an obstructed atrioventricular valve or resistance to ventricular filling	Tricuspid or mitral stenosis, complete heart block, ventricular hypertrophy
Absent A wave	Ineffective atrial contraction	Atrial fibrillation
Giant V wave	Transmission of ventricular pressure to the atria	Mitral or tricuspid regurgitation

injury resulting from atrial and ventricular incisions, cardioplegia with myocardial ischemia followed by reperfusion, aortic cross-clamping, and hypothermia during CPB leads to increased serum cardiac troponin I levels. Elevated cardiac troponin I levels, along with increased serum concentrations of the cardiac-specific creatine kinase, may predict the development of impaired myocardial performance and complicated postoperative course.[6]

Specialized Noninvasive Evaluation and Monitoring

Noninvasive techniques are available to evaluate and monitor cardiac function or to assess the adequacy of vital organ perfusion in critically ill patients with cardiac disorders. Monitoring of cerebral blood flow may be performed in the ICU using transcranial Doppler (TCD) ultrasonography to evaluate deep cerebral artery blood flow velocities and flow patterns or using cerebral near infrared spectroscopy (NIRS), a noninvasive oximetric technique that measures cerebral venous O_2 content, thereby allowing assessment of cerebral perfusion. NIRS has been used to continuously monitor brain perfusion during and following CPB in pediatric patients undergoing cardiac surgery.[7] On the basis of the same principle, NIRS has also been used to assess and monitor splanchnic and renal perfusion after coarctation repair in a pediatric population.[8] In ventilated patients, continuous monitoring of end-tidal carbon dioxide (CO_2) and volumetric CO_2 elimination (i.e., volume of CO_2 eliminated per minute) are useful not only to assess the adequacy of lung ventilation but also to potentially detect rapid changes in pulmonary blood flow (PBF) in patients whose PBF is provided through systemic-to-pulmonary artery or cavopulmonary shunts. Capnography can also be used to noninvasively measure cardiac output using partial CO_2 rebreathing measurements and the differential Fick equation.[9]

Cardiac Imaging and Intervention

When a patient fails to progress as anticipated or deteriorates unexpectedly, prompt evaluation using echocardiography and a review of invasive monitoring data should be performed. Echocardiography allows for accurate assessment of myocardial systolic and diastolic function, residual or previously unidentified anatomic lesions, intracardiac thrombi, or significant pericardial fluid collections. Postoperative cardiac catheterization may supplement findings by echocardiography and clinical data and may dictate the need for catheter-based or subsequent surgical reintervention.

Mechanical Ventilation

Following a successful operation, many infants and older children can wean from full mechanical ventilation and extubate within 12 to 24 hours. For those who require prolonged intubation, disease-specific cardiopulmonary interactions dictate a tailored ventilator strategy to optimize gas exchange while minimizing the negative effects of positive-pressure ventilation on the right side of the heart. Lung overdistension and, conversely, atelectasis, should be avoided while maintaining the lowest possible mean airway pressure to reduce pulmonary vascular resistance (PVR) in patients with right ventricular dysfunction. A weaning or maintenance strategy encouraging spontaneous respiration utilizing assist-control ventilation and decreasing the frequency of mandatory ventilator breaths (pressure or volume control modes) appears to work well in patients of all sizes and ages, including neonates. This approach seeks to minimize sedation and pain-control needs, optimize the lung volume–PVR relationship, minimize the mechanical effects of positive-pressure ventilation on right ventricle (RV) afterload, and enhance left ventricle (LV) function, and it allows for the assessment of circulatory function under conditions of increased metabolic demands and systemic O_2 consumption. A patient who fails to wean or extubate should be evaluated for residual cardiac lesions and myocardial dysfunction (see Table 30.3). Other etiologies of respiratory failure seen in patients after cardiac surgery include airway compression by enlarged or abnormally positioned cardiovascular structures, vocal cord paralysis, diaphragmatic paresis or paralysis, muscular weakness, and poor nutritional state.

Hemostasis and Coagulation Disturbance

Postoperative bleeding may occur after achieving hemostasis in the operating room and typically results from coagulation disturbance due to CPB-induced platelet dysfunction, thrombocytopenia, coagulation factor depletion or consumption, hypothermia, hepatic dysfunction, and profound metabolic disturbance. Patients with a history of previous cardiac surgery, newborns, and patients with

TABLE 30.3

ETIOLOGIES OF EXTUBATION FAILURE IN PATIENTS AFTER CARDIAC SURGERY

Cardiac	Residual surgical lesions
	Left (systemic) ventricle dysfunction
Neurologic	Phrenic nerve dysfunction
	Recurrent laryngeal nerve dysfunction
	Depressed respiratory center output (due to medications)
Respiratory	Hyperinflation
	Airway compression by enlarged or abnormally positioned cardiac structures
	Chronic lung disease of infancy (BPD)
	Atelectasis
	Pneumonia
	Pleural effusion or chylothorax
Metabolic	Malnutrition
	Hypomagnesemia
	Hypophosphatemia
	Hypocalcemia
	Hypokalemia

BPD, bronchopulmonary dysplasia.

chronic cyanosis are among those at highest risk for postoperative bleeding.[10]

Coagulation profile measurements, including activated prothrombin time, partial thromboplastin time, serum fibrinogen concentration, and fibrin split products, as well as the complete blood count, should be monitored regularly in patients experiencing bleeding immediately after surgery. Packed red blood cell transfusions should be provided to maintain a hematocrit of >40% to 45% in patients with cyanosis who have borderline cardiac output and ongoing bleeding. Abnormal coagulation profile with associated bleeding should be aggressively treated with fresh frozen plasma or cryoprecipitate transfusions to achieve hemostasis. Platelet transfusion, despite the relatively normal platelet count, may also be useful, given the common occurrence of platelet dysfunction following CPB. The use of protamine to neutralize the effects of residual heparin, ε-aminocaproic acid infusion to inhibit plasminogen activation, or aprotinin or tranexamic acid to inhibit fibrinolysis may all be effective in controlling life-threatening bleeding. Recently, recombinant, activated factor VIIa has been used with promising results in pediatric patients experiencing bleeding after cardiac surgery.[11] The use of these agents, however, must be balanced against the risk of inducing intravascular thrombosis in patients whose intracardiac and vascular anatomy may predispose to thromboembolism (e.g., patients with shunt-dependent circulations). In the event of persistent chest bleeding, it is important that mediastinal and pleural tubes remain patent to avoid the development of pericardial tamponade or lung compression. In cases of inadequate drainage and

the presence of tamponade physiology, pericardiocentesis, chest reopening, and/or thoracocentesis are necessary to avoid cardiorespiratory collapse.

Fluids, Electrolytes, and Nutrition

Fluid retention is common after cardiac surgery and can significantly impact outcome. Systemic inflammation and alterations in plasma oncotic pressure related to CPB result in tissue edema and intravascular depletion with diminished renal perfusion. In addition, increased antidiuretic hormone production and the need for blood product transfusion or volume resuscitation contribute to a rapid increase in total body water content, with secondary adverse effects on pulmonary, myocardial, gastrointestinal, and potentially, brain function. Postoperative decrease in cardiac output contributes to prerenal hypoperfusion, which, if sustained, predisposes to renal tubular necrosis and renal failure.

Fluid management, therefore, typically involves restricting intake to approximately 50% of the calculated maintenance water needs during the initial postoperative period. Additional volume expansion is given as needed to maintain adequate preload and support cardiac output. Diuretic therapy is typically started within 24 to 48 hours and serves to facilitate total body water removal, allowing for improved myocardial and pulmonary function. Once a consistent diuresis is established, maintained by adequate circulatory function, patients generally tolerate increased fluid and caloric intake by either enteral or parenteral routes and demonstrate increasing hemodynamic reserve, thereby facilitating the process of weaning from ventilator and inotropic support.

Diuretic use may lead to electrolyte depletion or metabolic alkalosis, resulting in symptomatic hypokalemia, hypocalcemia, hyponatremia, and hypomagnesemia, manifesting as arrhythmias, decreased vascular tone, and decreased myocardial contractility. Careful monitoring and routine repletion of electrolytes is critical during recovery after cardiac surgery. Alternative methods to facilitate fluid removal and solute clearance, in cases of renal dysfunction, include passive peritoneal drainage or peritoneal dialysis with ultrafiltration, continuous venovenous hemofiltration, and intermittent hemodialysis with ultrafiltration.

Early establishment of enteral feeding is preferred in most patients, especially neonates and those with preoperative malnourishment. Persistent chylothorax may develop (particularly in neonates), complicating nutritional management and, in some cases, resulting in the need for recurrent chest drainage procedures, mechanical ventilation, immunoglobulin and coagulation factor replacement, and treatment of secondarily acquired infections. Therapeutic options for persistent chylothorax include conversion to enteral formulas that are low in long-chain triglyceride content, a trial of total parenteral nutrition, trial of medication (e.g., octreotide, somatostatin), and surgical intervention including thoracic duct ligation and/or pleurodesis.[12] All of these options have been met with variable success in this generally self-limited, but problematic, postoperative condition.

SPECIFIC POSTOPERATIVE PROBLEMS

Recovery after congenital heart disease will be hindered by the development of complications related to low cardiac output states, pulmonary artery hypertension (PAH), and nosocomial infection, among others. Although most postoperative patients are at some risk of experiencing these complications, morbidity and mortality should be optimized by strategies to attenuate or prevent them altogether.

Postoperative Low Cardiac Output Syndrome

Low cardiac output states may develop after cardiac surgery because of structural lesions, myocardial dysfunction, elevated systemic or pulmonary afterload, arrhythmias, and pericardial tamponade (see Table 30.4). Myocardial dysfunction is frequent after CPB because of the production of inflammatory cytokines, ischemia-reperfusion injury, and direct myocardial trauma. Wernovsky et al. reported that 25% of neonates undergoing arterial switch for transposition of the great arteries had a decrease in cardiac index to <2 L/minute/m^2 during the first postoperative

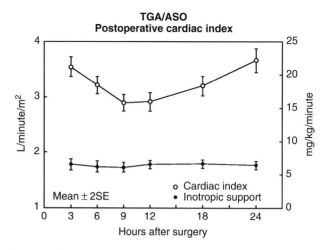

Figure 30.1 Decline in cardiac index in neonates following the arterial switch operation for transposition of the great arteries. TGA, transposition of the great arteries; ASO, arterial switch operation; SE, standard error. (From Wessel DL. Managing low cardiac output syndrome after congenital heart surgery *Crit Care Med.* 2001;29:S220–S230.)

night.[13] The time course and typical decline in cardiac output in this population is demonstrated in Figure 30.1. Although diminished myocardial function and preload are common causes of low cardiac index, other etiologies should be rigorously considered and treated, if found.

Residual structural defects leading to reduced systemic O_2 delivery or conditions resulting in increased myocardial O_2 consumption can complicate recovery after cardiac surgery. Residual defects are typically identified by physical examination, data provided by invasive monitoring, echocardiography, or catheterization, the significance of which is highly dependent on the cardiac lesion and repair. For example, outflow obstruction is well tolerated after repair of tetralogy of Fallot but not after surgery for hypoplastic left heart syndrome. Loss of atrioventricular synchrony almost invariably leads to decreased ventricular filling and cardiac output, the cause of which should be sought and restoration of sequential atrioventricular contraction promptly established. Patients with functional single ventricle anatomy and pulmonary and systemic circulations in parallel may require maneuvers to manipulate the ratio of pulmonary-to-systemic flow (Q_p/Q_s), modulate systemic vascular resistance, and augment total cardiac output as a means of optimizing systemic blood flow (Q_s) and end-organ (including myocardial) perfusion.

Appropriate anticipation of and early intervention in low cardiac output syndrome is required to decrease morbidity or the need for mechanical circulatory support. Select patients with right ventricular (RV) dysfunction benefit from creation or retention of an atrial-level right-to-left shunt. In such cases, the right-to-left shunt preserves left ventricular preload and systemic cardiac output, albeit at the expense of systemic cyanosis. Pharmacologic strategies designed to enhance myocardial contractility and reduce

TABLE 30.4

CAUSES OF LOW CARDIAC OUTPUT SYNDROME AFTER CONGENITAL HEART SURGERY

Structural lesions	a. Intracardiac shunts
	b. Valve stenosis or insufficiency
	c. Systemic or pulmonary outflow obstruction
Myocardial dysfunction	a. Systolic and/or diastolic
	b. Right ventricle and/or left ventricle
Arrhythmias	a. Loss of atrioventricular synchrony (e.g., JET, AV block)
	b. Atrial or ventricular tachyarrhythmias
	c. Sinus node dysfunction
Tamponade	a. Localized clot or uniform fluid collection
	b. Myocardial edema
	c. Tension pneumothorax or pneumopericardium
Elevated PVR	a. Fixed or reactive
	b. Anatomic or physiologic

JET, junctional ectopic tachycardia; AV, atrioventricular block; PVR, pulmonary vascular resistance.

systemic afterload, without adversely affecting myocardial O_2 demand, are important in supporting cardiac output during the immediate postoperative period. Extracorporeal membrane oxygenation or the use of ventricular assist devices, providing mechanical circulatory support, should be considered in patients with refractory ventricular dysfunction or low cardiac output states.

Postoperative Pulmonary Artery Hypertension

Elevated PVR, or rapid increases in PVR leading to acute PAH, may complicate the postoperative course after repair of CHD. Lesions associated with PAH are listed in Table 30.5. Other factors, including patient age, associated genetic abnormalities, the presence of preoperative elevation in PVR, and intraoperative factors, including the duration of CPB, are known to be associated with postoperative pulmonary vascular reactivity in at-risk patients. CPB promotes PAH by a variety of mechanisms, which include ischemic injury to the pulmonary vascular endothelium, pulmonary microemboli, local production of cytokines, endothelin release, and hypoxic pulmonary vasoconstriction. Patients at risk for PAH may demonstrate pulmonary vascular reactivity (lowering of PVR) on preoperative vasodilator testing with O_2, nitric oxide (NO), or other

agents. Consequently, it is important to assess reactivity before surgery in high-risk patients not only to determine operability but also to anticipate strategies of treatment should PAH develop postoperatively. In cases of postoperative PAH, anatomic causes of elevated pulmonary or RV pressures should be considered (peripheral pulmonary artery stenosis or RV outflow obstruction) because attempts to decrease PVR may not only be unsuccessful but may also even exacerbate the patient's clinical condition, as in the case of residual left-to-right shunt.

Patients with impaired RV function due to CPB, myocardial ischemia-reperfusion injury, and myocardial incision may experience profound reductions in cardiac output in the face of sudden or sustained increases in RV afterload. The overall management of postoperative PAH should involve consideration of the following: (i) review of preoperative risk and reactivity, (ii) anatomic investigation to rule out a fixed cause of increased RV afterload, (iii) mechanical ventilation strategy that avoids excessive tidal volume and high intrathoracic pressure, (iv) pulmonary vasodilator therapy, (v) aggressive treatment of metabolic acidosis, (vi) targeted RV support (pharmacologic or mechanical), (vii) sedation/anesthesia, and (viii) creation of small $R \rightarrow L$ atrial shunt. Pulmonary vasodilator therapy, an active area of clinical investigation, currently involves the use of supplemental O_2, NO, phosphodiesterase inhibitors (e.g., milrinone, sildenafil), prostacyclin analogs (PGI_2), endothelin receptor blockers, and calcium channel blockers. These agents may be used in the acute care setting, as well as in the long-term treatment of postoperative PAH.

Postoperative Infection

Superficial and deep surgical site infections, sepsis, and other nosocomial infections are uncommon after congenital heart surgery; however, the potential for prolonged ICU stay and secondary complications, including death, is substantial in cases of nosocomial infection.[14] Because skin and nasopharyngeal colonization with *Staphylococcus epidermidis* and *S. aureus* is common, most surgical programs have adopted a protocol of prophylactic antibiotic therapy using a first- or second-generation cephalosporin for a total duration of 24 hours, postoperatively. Patients requiring delayed sternal closure generally receive prophylactic antibiotics until chest closure or until thoracostomy tubes are removed. Broadening of antibiotic coverage should be considered in patients requiring repeated chest exploration or for those at risk for developing nosocomial infections due to common or resistant gram-negative organisms, in which case gentamicin and/or ceftazidime are reasonable additions.

Some patients with CHD present with innate immune system deficiency (DiGeorge syndrome) and are known to be colonized with antibiotic-resistant organisms; others may develop immune system deficiency during their postoperative course. The latter may occur in critically ill

TABLE 30.5

CAUSES OF PULMONARY ARTERY HYPERTENSION IN CONGENITAL HEART DISEASE

Anatomic or Physiologic Lesion	Examples
Chronic left-to-right shunt (increased PBF and PA pressures)	VSD, PDA, AP window, CAVC defect
Increased pulmonary venous pressure	MS, TAPVR, pulmonary vein stenosis, pulmonary veno-occlusive disease, LV failure
Cyanotic heart diseases	d-TGA with VSD, truncus arteriosus, TOF with PA, single ventricle lesions
Anomalies of pulmonary arteries or veins[a]	Isolation of RPA or LPA from the aorta, Scimitar syndrome
Systemic-to-pulmonary artery shunts (surgical)	Systemic-to-pulmonary central shunt, surgical AP window, Blalock-Taussig shunt

[a]With associated lung maldevelopment and abnormal microvasculature.
PBF, pulmonary blood flow; PA, pulmonary artery; VSD, ventricular septal defect; PDA, patent ductus arteriosus; AP, aortopulmonary; CAVC, complete atrioventricular canal; MS, mitral stenosis; TAPVR, total anomalous pulmonary venous return; LV, left ventricle; d-TGA, dextro-transposition of the great arteries; TOF, tetralogy of Fallot; RPA, right pulmonary artery; LPA, left pulmonary artery.

patients with poor hemodynamics requiring prolonged intubation and indwelling central vascular catheters or in those who are poorly nourished because of inadequate caloric intake and persistent catabolism. Patients experiencing large amounts of third-space fluids losses (drainage of chylous pleural effusions and/or ascites) for a prolonged period may develop lymphopenia and significant loss of serum immunoglobulins and other plasma proteins important in the defense against infection. Basic infection control practices are highly effective in reducing the likelihood of postoperative infection, particularly in the care of neonates, patients with open sternum, and sick patients with the need for prolonged vascular catheter access.

CONCLUSION

An anticipatory approach to the care of the postoperative patient with CHD is essential. Optimal postoperative care begins before the operation with careful review of the cardiac anatomy and physiology, comprehensive surgical planning, and medical stabilization, if required. In the postoperative period, the physiologic stress of surgery and CPB frequently produce organ disturbances. The distinction between expected and abnormal recovery is essential because aggressive investigation and intervention is required in cases of failed progress or unexpected clinical deterioration. A multidisciplinary approach to cardiovascular care is essential, as evidenced by reduced mortality and morbidity in children undergoing surgical treatment of CHD in the current era.

REFERENCES

1. Bellinger DC, Wypij D, duDuplessis AJ, et al. Neurodevelopmental status at eight years in children with dextro-transposition of the great arteries: The Boston Circulatory Arrest Trial. *J Thorac Cardiovasc Surg.* 2003;126(5):1385–1396.
2. Reddy VM, McElhinney DB, Sagrado T, et al. Results of 102 cases of complete repair of congenital heart defects in patients weighing 700 to 2500 grams. *J Thorac Cardiovasc Surg.* 1999;117(2):324–331.
3. Gold JP, Jonas RA, Lang P, et al. Transthoracic intracardiac monitoring lines in pediatric surgical patients: A ten-year experience. *Ann Thorac Surg.* 1986;42(2):185–191.
4. Munoz R, Laussen PC, Palacio G, et al. Changes in whole blood lactate levels during cardiopulmonary bypass for surgery for congenital cardiac disease: An early indicator of morbidity and mortality. *J Thorac Cardiovasc Surg.* 2000;119(1):155–162.
5. Arrowsmith JE, Grocott HP, Reves JG, et al. Central nervous system complications of cardiac surgery. *Br J Anaesth.* 2000;84(3):378–393.
6. Hammer S, Loeff M, Reichenspurner H, et al. Effect of cardiopulmonary bypass on myocardial function, damage and inflammation after cardiac surgery in newborns and children. *Thorac Cardiovasc Surg.* 2001;49(6):349–354.
7. Andropoulos DB, Stayer SA, Diaz LK, et al. Neurological monitoring for congenital heart surgery. *Anesth Analg.* 2004;99(5):1365–1375.
8. Berens RJ, Hoffman GM, Robertson FA. Near infrared oximetry (NIRS) allows noninvasive assessment of regional oxygenation during pediatric coarctation repair. *Anesthesiology.* 2003;99:A136.
9. Binder JC, Parkin WG. Non-invasive cardiac output determination: Comparison of a new partial-rebreathing technique with thermodilution. *Anaesth Intensive Care.* 2001;29(1):19–23.
10. Tempe DK, Virmani S. Coagulation abnormalities in patients with cyanotic congenital heart disease. *J Cardiothorac Vasc Anesth.* 2002;16(6):752–765.
11. Tobias JD, Simsic JM, Weinstein S, et al. Recombinant factor VIIa to control excessive bleeding following surgery for congenital heart disease in pediatric patients. *J Intensive Care Med.* 2004;19(5):270–273.
12. Suddaby EC, Schiller S. Management of chylothorax in children. *Pediatr Nurs.* 2004;30(4):290–295.
13. Wernovsky G, Wypij D, Jonas RA, et al. Postoperative course and hemodynamic profile after the arterial switch operation in neonates and infants. A comparison of low-flow cardiopulmonary bypass and circulatory arrest. *Circulation.* 1995;92(8):2226–2235.
14. Mehta PA, Cunningham CK, Colella CB, et al. Risk factors for sternal wound and other infections in pediatric cardiac surgery patients. *Pediatr Infect Dis J.* 2000;19(10):1000–1004.

Congenital Heart Disease: Single Ventricle Physiology

31

John T. Berger III   *Steven M. Schwartz*   *David P. Nelson*

Various categorical frameworks have been used to classify congenital heart defects, including anatomic features and presenting symptoms. Although careful delineation of the complex and numerous anatomic structures is essential for surgical treatment of a specific lesion, the management of a patient in the intensive care unit (ICU) is primarily dictated by the type of circulation and corresponding physiology. Children with congenital heart disease can be categorized into one of a distinct number of physiologic presentations (see Table 31.1).

UNIVENTRICLE, PARALLEL CIRCULATION (NEONATE WITH A SINGLE VENTRICLE)

The term "functional single ventricle" includes a variety of congenital cardiac anomalies where there is only one ventricle pumping blood to the systemic and pulmonary circulations (see Table 31.2). Physiology in this arrangement is a considerable clinical challenge because patients with single ventricle physiology often respond differently to common interventions, such as supplemental oxygen, mechanical ventilation, and vasoactive drugs, than patients with normal cardiac anatomy. The most important anatomic issues affecting planned interventions and ICU management are the connections of the single ventricle to the pulmonary and systemic circulations. The newborn may have either pulmonary or aortic obstruction, or bilaterally unobstructed outflows. Additionally, either the systemic or the pulmonary venous return may also be abnormally connected or obstructed in the newborn with a single ventricle circulation.

Obstruction of Systemic Outflow

Systemic obstruction is present in multiple anatomic variations, including hypoplastic left heart syndrome, tricuspid atresia with discordant ventriculo-arterial connections, and variants of double inlet left ventricle. The physiology encountered with systemic obstruction also applies to newborns with critical aortic stenosis, critical coarctation of the aorta, or interruption of the aortic arch where systemic blood flow is dependant on a patent ductus arteriosus. Important physiology of these lesions includes complete mixing of the systemic and pulmonary venous returns, with the ventricular outflow being directed primarily to the lungs. When systemic obstruction is severe, systemic blood flow is dependent on right-to-left ductal shunting. When the ductus arteriosus closes, the infant develops cardiovascular collapse. With a nonrestrictive duct, systemic blood flow itself is dependent upon the overall output from the functional single ventricle, the relative resistances of the pulmonary and systemic vascular beds, and the degree of intra-atrial communication. For example, infants with low pulmonary vascular resistance (PVR) and no atrial restriction will develop excessive pulmonary blood flow and show signs of congestive heart failure and shock, whereas infants with a very restrictive atrial septum will present with severe cyanosis and shock.

Obstruction of Pulmonary Outflow

Obstruction to the flow of blood to the lungs occurs in lesions such as tricuspid atresia, pulmonary atresia, and severe Ebstein's malformation of the tricuspid valve. Salient physiology includes complete mixing of systemic and pulmonary venous returns, with the ventricular outflow

TABLE 31.1

PHYSIOLOGIC PRESENTATIONS OF CONGENITAL HEART DISEASE

Physiologic Presentation	Anatomic Examples
Obstruction of Systemic Blood Flow	
■ Pressure overload of systemic ventricle	Aortic stenosis, severe coarctation of aorta
■ Ductal-dependant systemic blood flow[a]	Interrupted aortic arch, critical coarctation of aorta
Obstruction of Pulmonary Blood Flow	
■ Right-to-left shunt with diminished pulmonary flow[a]	Tetralogy of Fallot
■ Ductal-dependant pulmonary blood flow[a]	Pulmonary atresia/VSD
■ Pressure overload of pulmonary ventricle without intracardiac shunt	Pulmonary valve stenosis
Ventricular Volume Overload	
■ Left-to-right shunt with excessive pulmonary flow	ASD, VSD, PDA
Transposition Physiology[a]	D-TGA
Mixing Lesions[a]	
■ two ventricle	Truncus arteriosus, TAPVD
■ Functional single ventricle	HLHS, tricuspid atresia
• Neonatal single ventricle physiology	
• Bidirectional Glenn physiology	
• Fontan physiology	
Acute Myocardial Dysfunction	
■ *Left ventricular* dysfunction (systolic and/or diastolic)	Anomalous left coronary artery from pulmonary artery
■ *Right ventricular* dysfunction (systolic and/or diastolic)	

[a]Physiologic presentations associated with cyanosis.
VSD, ventricular septal defect; ASD, atrial septal defect; PDA, patent ductus arteriosus; D-TGA, dextrotransposition of the great arteries; TAPVD, total anomalous pulmonary venous drainage; HLHS, hypoplastic left heart syndrome.

directed predominantly to the aorta. The restricted flow of blood to the lungs imposes an obligatory intracardiac right-to-left shunt, generally at the atrial level, and results in deoxygenated blood reaching the systemic circulation. The clinical finding is one of cyanosis. Clinical consequences of obstructed blood flow to the lungs are variable, and depend on the severity of the lesion. Mild obstruction may permit excessive amounts of the total cardiac output to go to the pulmonary circulation, sometimes at the expense of the systemic cardiac output. Infants with this type of anatomy are only minimally cyanotic, and often develop signs and symptoms of congestive heart failure. Treatment in this group of patients is directed at limiting, rather than increasing the pulmonary flow. At the other end of the spectrum are those with severe obstruction, or even atresia of the pulmonary pathway. These patients are profoundly cyanotic unless an alternate source of flow to the lungs is quickly established. These lesions often require continued ductal patency to maintain pulmonary blood flow, and are therefore referred to as duct-dependent malformations.

The Atrial Septum

In the functional single ventricle, unobstructed pulmonary or systemic venous return often requires a nonrestrictive intra-atrial communication. When an atrioventricular valve is severely stenotic or atretic, as it occurs in hypoplastic left heart syndrome, tricuspid atresia, or pulmonary atresia with intact ventricular septum, a large atrial septal defect is necessary to decompress the atrium that exits through the inadequate atrioventricular valve. Restricted systemic venous return causes increased central venous pressures, interstitial edema, and limited cardiac output. Although patency of the oval foramen usually allows right-to-left shunting of blood across the atrial septum, it is occasionally inadequate to permit unobstructed flow of all systemic venous return to the systemic ventricle.

Obstructed flow from the pulmonary venous atrium causes pulmonary edema, elevated pulmonary venous pressure, and secondary pulmonary artery hypertension. Although elevated PVR can be helpful in the immediate newborn period to limit flow of blood to the lungs, and enhance systemic blood flow, the atrial septum must be opened at the time of the first palliative operation to avoid the long-term consequences of elevated PVR. A severely restrictive or intact atrial septum with pulmonary venous hypertension requires creation of a shunt at atrial level as an emergency to alleviate the profound cyanosis. These procedures carry a high risk of morbidity,

TABLE 31.2

ANATOMIC FEATURES COMMONLY ASSOCIATED WITH SINGLE VENTRICLE HEARTS IN THE NEWBORN

Physiology	Anatomy
Systemic outflow obstruction	Hypoplastic left heart syndrome Critical aortic stenosis Critical coarctation of the aorta Interrupted aortic arch Tricuspid atresia with discordant ventriculo-arterial connections. Double inlet left ventricle Double outlet right ventricle (some variations)
Pulmonary outflow obstruction	Tricuspid atresia with concordant ventriculo-arterial connections Pulmonary atresia with intact ventricular septum Critical pulmonary stenosis Severe Ebstein malformation of the tricuspid valve Double outlet right ventricle (some variations)

and may imply a worse prognosis for further palliative surgery.

Myocardial Function

Low total cardiac output in the single ventricle physiology manifests as cyanosis as well as signs of poor tissue perfusion. A single ventricle circulation places the newborn at an increased risk of ventricular contractile dysfunction because the single ventricle is volume loaded compared to a normal heart and may have a vulnerable myocardial oxygen supply. Two key factors reduce myocardial oxygen supply: (i) low systemic flows, particularly with low diastolic blood pressure as seen in the newborn with a large aortopulmonary shunt or patent arterial duct; and (ii) high end-diastolic ventricular pressure as occurs in a volume-loaded heart. Limited coronary perfusion can compromise systolic ventricular function, further raising end-diastolic pressure and lowering systemic arterial pressure. If not rapidly corrected, this type of situation can result in profound hemodynamic decompensation.

Postoperative Anatomy

The goal of all initial palliative procedures for the newborn with single ventricle anatomy is to establish unobstructed pulmonary and systemic venous return, unobstructed systemic outflow, and to deliver a limited amount of blood to the lungs at normal pulmonary arterial pressures. This is typically accomplished through the Norwood procedure, construction of a modified aortopulmonary shunt (e.g.,

Blalock-Taussig shunt), or banding of the pulmonary trunk. Although variations on these palliative procedures exist, they represent the spectrum of postoperative anatomy encountered in cardiac intensive care. Because each anatomic arrangement establishes similar physiology, the important differences are the means by which each operation accomplishes the ultimate goal defined in the preceding text. The Norwood procedure requires cardiopulmonary bypass, cardioplegia, and a period of deep hypothermic circulatory arrest, although newer techniques can limit the period of circulatory arrest. This operation subjects the tissues to ischemia-reperfusion injury which is often followed by transient postoperative cardiac dysfunction. An aortopulmonary shunt, either alone or as part of the first stage Norwood procedure, can lower diastolic arterial pressure, which may compromise coronary arterial perfusion. Unlike an aortopulmonary shunt, a band on the pulmonary trunk is not associated with diastolic run-off to the lungs and better preserves coronary perfusion. Pulmonary artery banding may increase the risk of subaortic obstruction and ventricular hypertrophy, although this has been disputed. The shunting and banding procedures both carry the risk of distorting the pulmonary arteries, or producing unilateral pulmonary arterial obstruction, which can contribute to cyanosis after either of these procedures.

Monitoring Systemic Oxygen Delivery in Neonates with Single Ventricle Physiology

Monitoring the adequacy of systemic oxygen delivery, especially in the immediate postoperative period, has proven difficult. Irrespective of the underlying anatomy, single ventricle physiology entails mixing of systemic and pulmonary venous return, and partitioning the total cardiac output to pulmonary and systemic flows on the basis of the amount of anatomic obstruction and the vascular resistance to flow in the respective circulations. Variables that are used to monitor adequacy of systemic oxygen delivery include arterial saturation, venous saturation, calculated pulmonary blood flow to systemic blood flow ratio (Qp:Qs ratio), and lactate levels.

Traditionally, the arterial oxygen saturation has been used as a surrogate of the Qp:Qs ratio and systemic oxygen delivery on the basis of a simplification of the Fick principle. Assuming that systemic oxygen consumption and pulmonary uptake are equal and knowing that aortic and pulmonary artery saturations are identical, the Qp:Qs ratio equals

$$(Sao_2 - Smvo_2)/(Spvo_2 - Sao_2)$$

where $Smvo_2$ is the oxygen saturation of mixed venous blood, Sao_2 is the oxygen saturation of arterial blood, and $Spvo_2$ is the oxygen saturation of pulmonary venous blood.

Because the lungs in most infants with congenital cardiac malformations are relatively healthy, one can assume that the saturation of oxygen in the pulmonary venous blood is normal, 95% in room air. Furthermore, if one also assumes that the difference between the systemic arterial and venous oxygen saturation is normal, at approximately 25%, the simplified equation for the ratio of pulmonary to systemic blood flow becomes

$$25/(95 - SaO_2)$$

This simplified version of the Fick equation allows the estimation of the pulmonary to systemic blood flow ratio based on systemic oxygen saturation alone. Theoretically, this allows one to assess the effects of interventions designed to alter flows by observing changes in arterial oxygen saturation. The importance of accurately estimating the ratio of pulmonary to systemic flow is depicted in Figure 31.1, which demonstrates the relationships between the ratio of flows, systemic oxygen delivery, and total cardiac output.[1,2] Because the total cardiac output of the functionally single ventricle is the combined flows, unless total cardiac output increases, an increase in pulmonary flow is accompanied by a decrease in systemic flow, and vice versa. The maximum oxygen delivery occurs at a Qp:Qs ratio between 0.5 and 1, depending upon total cardiac output. Further the relationship of Qp:Qs and systemic oxygen delivery is very steep at maximum delivery, suggesting that small changes in the ratio of flows are associated with large changes in oxygen delivery. The most important hemodynamic issue demonstrated in Figure 31.1, however, is that systemic oxygen delivery is increased much more effectively by augmenting total cardiac output than by altering the ratio of flows.

Estimation of the ratio of pulmonary to systemic blood flow is based on several assumptions about oxygen saturation of mixed venous and pulmonary venous blood. First, the assumption about the difference in systemic arterial–venous oxygen saturation is only accurate if systemic perfusion is normal. In low output states, which are common in neonates with single ventricle physiology, the SvO_2 can be quite low, so that arteriovenous oxygen saturation differences will be substantially >25%. If the decrease in systemic flow and mixed venous oxygen saturation is offset by an increase in the amount of well-saturated blood returning from the lungs, the arterial oxygen saturation may remain unchanged, or even increase. Second, although the saturation of oxygen in pulmonary venous blood is likely to be normal in the absence of pulmonary parenchymal disease, there are conditions under which this assumption is incorrect. Using catheters placed in the left lower pulmonary vein in infants undergoing Norwood palliation, Taeed et al. found that unexpected pulmonary venous desaturation is common early after Norwood palliation, particularly with fractional inspired oxygen levels <0.3.[3] Failure to account for pulmonary venous desaturation results in a falsely low estimate of the Qp:Qs ratio using equation 39-2. Even errors as small as 5% result in gross inaccuracy (25% to 60% error) in the estimated Qp:Qs ratio.[3] The clinical relevance is that maneuvers that decrease pulmonary venous oxygen

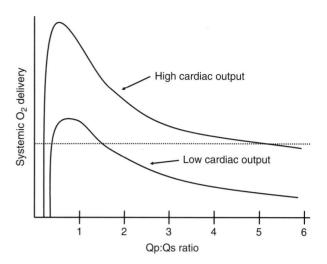

Figure 31.1 Systemic oxygen delivery versus ratio of pulmonary to systemic blood flow (Qp:Qs). The graph shows that systemic oxygen delivery varies as a function of cardiac output and Qp:Qs ratio. Maximal oxygen delivery occurs at a ratio between 0.5 to 1. The relationship between delivery and flow ratio is very steep at the maximal point. The *dashed line* indicates the anaerobic threshold, where delivery no longer meets demand. (Adapted from Barnea O, Santamore WP, Rossi A, et al. Estimation of oxygen delivery in newborns with a univentricular circulation. *Circulation.* 1998;98:1407–1413; Barnea O, Austin EH, Richman B, et al. Balancing the circulation: Theoretic optimization of pulmonary/systemic flow ratio in hypoplastic left heart syndrome. *J Am Coll Cardiol.* 1994;24:1376–1381.)

saturation rather than alter the Qp:Qs ratio of flows result in lower arterial oxygen saturation but not in increased systemic blood flow, and therefore not in increased systemic oxygen delivery.

Because very small changes in arterial saturation are associated with large changes in systemic oxygen delivery, other measures have been examined. Clinical data suggest that the oxygen saturation of mixed venous blood varies considerably in patients with single ventricle physiology. Many centers have begun to monitor this value routinely, following Norwood palliation for hypoplastic left heart syndrome, using a sample from the superior vena cava (SVC) as representative of mixed venous blood, because there is no true site of systemic mixed venous blood in the single ventricle circulation.[4,5] Even intermittent SVC sampling has proven more useful than arterial sampling in monitoring a patient's cardiovascular status. In a study of 18 patients with hypoplastic left heart syndrome, SVC saturation was significantly lower at admission and 6 hours after Norwood procedure in patients requiring extracorporeal membrane oxygenation (ECMO) although SaO_2 did not differ between the two groups.[6]

Optimizing Systemic Oxygen Delivery in Neonates with Single Ventricle Physiology

The goal of management in this setting is not to maximize the systemic arterial saturation, but to ensure adequate delivery of oxygen to all tissues. Optimization of systemic oxygen delivery requires maintenance of cardiac output while balancing systemic and pulmonary flows. Systemic oxygen delivery may be better in an infant with moderate cyanosis as compared to a well-saturated infant with poor perfusion. Although systemic delivery of oxygen is best augmented by optimizing total cardiac output, inherent interrelationships between the various hemodynamic variables can make this task challenging in the patient with a single ventricle. Although management of this situation in neonates has traditionally focused on manipulation of flows by changes in PVR, newer data suggest that management of total cardiac output and systemic vascular resistance (SVR) may be more effective. In all instances, maintenance of oxygen-carrying capacity by keeping hemoglobin in the range of 13 to 16 mg per dL is beneficial. In patients with intracardiac shunting, an increased concentration of hemoglobin increases mixed venous and arterial oxygen saturations, and decreases the ratio of pulmonary to systemic flow, by increasing the ratio of pulmonary to systemic resistances.[7]

Optimizing Systemic Oxygen Delivery by Manipulation of Pulmonary Vascular Resistance

Differential manipulation of the resistances in patients with single ventricle physiology has traditionally emphasized the use of oxygen, carbon dioxide, and acid–base status (see Table 31.3). In infants with unrestricted pulmonary flow, subatmospheric levels of oxygen, or induction of respiratory acidosis, can effectively raise pulmonary resistance and decrease systemic resistance, and thereby decrease the ratio between them.[8] Subatmospheric oxygen should be used with caution because it may cause pulmonary venous desaturation and reduce rather than increase systemic oxygen delivery, especially in the postoperative patient.[3] Further, prolonged exposure may result in increased PVR after surgical repair and cardiopulmonary bypass. Respiratory acidosis can be induced either through alveolar hypoventilation, or by altering inspired concentrations of carbon dioxide in patients who are paralyzed and are on ventilator support. Recent data from both pre- and postoperative newborns with hypoplastic left heart syndrome suggest that inhaled carbon dioxide may be more effective than subatmospheric oxygen in increasing cerebral and/or systemic perfusion in patients on ventilator assistance, although these studies did not differentiate whether inspired carbon dioxide improves systemic or cerebral delivery of oxygen, or both.[8-10] Although both inspired carbon dioxide and subatmospheric oxygen are often used to balance the ratio of flows in spontaneously breathing patients, data in this group are lacking.

In infants with low PVR and anatomically restricted pulmonary blood flow, it is even less clear that the manipulation of pulmonary resistance is useful to alter the ratio of flows. Because all palliative procedures are aimed to restrict blood flow to the lungs by mechanical obstruction,

TABLE 31.3

EFFECTS OF RESPIRATORY MANEUVERS ON PULMONARY AND SYSTEMIC VASCULAR RESISTANCE

Treatment	PVR	SVR	Q_p/Q_s
Decrease F_{IO_2}	Increase	Decrease	Decrease
Increase CO_2	Increase	Decrease	Decrease
Decrease pH	Increase	Decrease	Decrease
Increase PEEP	Increase	Decrease	Decrease

Note: PVR, pulmonary vascular resistance; SVR, systemic vascular resistance; F_{IO_2}, fraction of inspired oxygen; PEEP, positive end-expiratory pressure, Qp:Qs, ratio of pulmonary to systemic blood flow.

it is likely that pulmonary flow is primarily limited by the size of the systemic-to-pulmonary arterial shunt or the tightness of the pulmonary arterial band, so that further decreases in downstream resistance are of minimal consequence. Subatmospheric oxygen following Norwood palliation does not induce significant change in the Qp:Qs ratio of flows.[3] Although the arterial–venous difference in oxygen measured in the SVC increased with inspired carbon dioxide in postoperative Norwood patients, these alterations could result from effects of carbon dioxide and pH on SVR or cerebral circulation.[10]

Not all patients with single ventricle physiology demonstrate pulmonary overcirculation. Elevated pulmonary resistance can easily persist in the newborn with such physiology, and can cause severe cyanosis. When pulmonary flow is very low, it can effectively increase the pulmonary dead space and impair alveolar ventilation. The occurrence of respiratory acidosis in this setting is of grave concern, because this will further increase PVR, limiting the ability to hyperventilate or alkalinize the patient. Treatment of high pulmonary resistance in such patients is much the same as in any other population. Strategies of alveolar recruitment are appropriate when there is atelectasis or pulmonary disease, but airway pressures should be limited to the minimum necessary to maintain functional residual capacity. High-frequency oscillatory or jet ventilation may be effective to attain hyperventilation at low mean airway pressure. Use of supplemental inspired oxygen, hyperventilation, and alkalosis may be beneficial. Inhaled nitric oxide and infusion of prostaglandin have also been used in these patients to selectively lower PVR. Raising systemic blood pressure by vasoconstriction may increase pulmonary flow, and thereby increase systemic arterial oxygen saturation.

Optimizing Systemic Oxygen Delivery by Manipulation of Systemic Vascular Resistance

Another approach to differential regulation of the vascular resistances is pharmacologic manipulation of SVR.

Although intravenous vasodilators tend to have similar effects on the pulmonary and systemic vasculature, in the setting of poor systemic perfusion with high systemic and low pulmonary resistance, they will have a greater relative effect on the systemic vasculature. Systemic vasodilation may be particularly valuable after operations such as the Norwood operation that require deep hypothermic circulatory arrest. Systemic vasoconstriction in this setting as a response to low systemic output is a maladaptive response. Inappropriate increases in SVR increase pulmonary flow at the expense of systemic flow while maintaining blood pressure and systemic arterial saturation, therefore masking potential warning signs of low systemic output. Nitroprusside, phenoxybenzamine, inamrinone, and milrinone have been advocated to reduce systemic afterload, and to block the α-adrenergic–receptor mediated vasoconstriction that occurs with drugs such as epinephrine. Phenoxybenzamine lowers systemic resistance, decreases the ratio of pulmonary to systemic flow, and improves systemic delivery of oxygen after the Norwood operation, although it is associated with reductions in systemic blood pressure.[11] Beneficial effects reported with use of phenoxybenzamine may also result from increased use of inotropic agents in these patients. β-Adrenergic stimulation of the myocardium, in conjunction with vasodilating agents, can increase total cardiac output without associated vasoconstriction. Other vasodilating agents can be used to accomplish this same goal, although they involve different receptor mechanisms and cellular pathways. Data supporting manipulation of SVR to balance flows in neonates with a functional single ventricle is limited to postoperative patients. The utility of manipulating systemic resistance in newborns with unrestricted pulmonary flow has not been studied.

Optimizing Total Cardiac Output

Increasing total cardiac output is among the most effective ways to optimize systemic oxygen delivery, which may also increase systemic arterial saturation simply by increasing the mixed venous saturation. Inotropic agents can augment stroke volume for a given preload, but may be accompanied by undesired systemic vasoconstriction. Consequently, even if total cardiac output is increased, systemic oxygen delivery may not increase. In a porcine model of single ventricle physiology, Riordan et al. studied the effects of epinephrine, dobutamine, and dopamine on pulmonary and systemic blood flows.[12] They showed that although all three medications increased total cardiac output, only epinephrine increased systemic oxygen delivery. Although it is likely that these observations are not fully applicable to the clinical situation because human neonates are more likely to show systemic vasoconstriction to epinephrine or high-dose dopamine, these data illustrate the importance of using vasodilator drugs to accompany inotropic agents with prominent vasoconstrictor properties. Furthermore, because the neonatal heart is particularly sensitive to elevated afterload, vasodilator drugs may also augment

total cardiac output through afterload reduction. When systemic vasodilators are used in patients with single ventricle physiology, cardiac output and systemic arterial pressure are particularly sensitive to a reduction in preload, and so the clinician must be certain that adequate preload is maintained. Figure 31.1 demonstrates the importance of combining inotropic and vasodilator agents in patients with single ventricle physiology. Systemic oxygen delivery can be improved dramatically by increasing total cardiac output, and further optimized by adjusting the ratio flows; thereby the combination of inotropic support and decreasing systemic resistance is often the optimal strategy to maximize systemic oxygen delivery.

Optimizing Pulmonary Recruitment to Avoid Pulmonary Venous Desaturation

Clinical data suggest that postoperative Norwood patients may have abnormalities in pulmonary gas exchange resulting from cardiopulmonary bypass, circulatory arrest, and the extensive surgical procedure.[3] Ventilatory maneuvers used to manipulate PVR in these patients, such as controlled hypoventilation, or inhalation of low concentrations of oxygen, may also predispose patients to microatelectasis and ventilation–perfusion mismatch. The presence of unrecognized pulmonary venous desaturation will compromise systemic oxygen delivery by lowering the systemic arterial oxygen saturation. In each of the patients studied by Taeed et al. pulmonary venous desaturation normalized with higher inspired oxygen or increased positive end-expiratory pressure, which suggests that judicious use of inspired oxygen and/or positive end-expiratory pressure may be beneficial in select patients early after Norwood palliation.[3] These data suggest that optimal alveolar recruitment may be the best way to preserve pulmonary gas exchange and prevent pulmonary venous desaturation in the patient with a functional single ventricle.

BIDIRECTIONAL CAVOPULMONARY ANASTOMOSIS: BIDIRECTIONAL GLENN PHYSIOLOGY

Anatomy

The second stage of single ventricle palliation is the creation of a bidirectional cavopulmonary anastomosis (BCPA) in which the SVC is connected directly to the pulmonary artery and other sources of pulmonary blood flow are either eliminated or severely restricted (see Fig. 31.2). Surgical variations include the bidirectional Glenn and the hemi-Fontan. The BCPA has been remarkable for the relatively low level of associated morbidity and mortality. Single center reports suggest an overall perioperative mortality of 3% to 5% or less.[13]

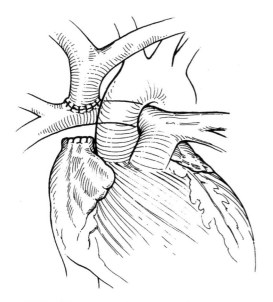

Figure 31.2 Bidirectional Glenn cavopulmonary anastomosis. The superior vena cava (SVC) is transected just above the right atrium, the cardiac end is oversewn, and the proximal end is anastomosed into the right pulmonary artery. (From Chang AC, Hanley FL, Wernovsky G, et al., ed. *Pediatric cardiac intensive care.* Philadelphia, PA: Lippincott Williams & Wilkins; 1998:278.)

Physiology

There are three significant aspects that separate the physiology of the BCPA from that of a normal circulation and/or neonatal single ventricle physiology. First, the driving force for pulmonary blood flow is SVC pressure. Second, pulmonary blood flow must pass through two separate and highly regulated vascular beds, the cerebral vasculature and the pulmonary vasculature, without an intervening pumping chamber. Finally, compared to neonatal single ventricle physiology, the BCPA removes a left-to-right shunt and

thereby the volume load from the single ventricle. The clinical physiology of the BCPA therefore centers on issues about the central venous–pulmonary artery pressure, pulmonary and cerebral vascular resistance, and alterations in ventricular loading and geometry.

Because pulmonary blood flow is supplied by upper body systemic venous return, one consequence of conversion to a BCPA is an acute rise in SVC pressure. Selection of patients with low PVR as candidates for the BCPA minimizes the risk of clinical complications arising from elevated SVC pressure, but SVC syndrome can occur nonetheless. Failure to maintain low SVC pressure following the BCPA can also lead to problems maintaining an adequate SaO_2. Small venovenous collateral vessels (such as a persistent left SVC or vein of Marshall) may enlarge in size following a BCPA and allow a "pop-off" for desaturated blood in the SVC to bypass the lungs and thereby contribute to arterial desaturation. Other causes of cyanosis after BCPA are listed in Table 31.4.

Another unique aspect of the physiology of the BCPA is that pulmonary blood flow is largely dependent on the resistance of two highly but differentially regulated vascular beds. The cerebral and pulmonary vasculatures have opposite responses to changes in carbon dioxide, acid–base status, and oxygen. This can make treatment of patients with excessive cyanosis particularly challenging. Hyperventilation and alkalosis, for example, have limited utility. Because pulmonary blood flow is dependent on venous return by the SVC (largely made up of cerebral blood flow), hyperventilation and alkalosis, by limiting cerebral blood flow, actually decrease pulmonary blood flow and exacerbate hypoxemia although these maneuvers reduce PVR.[14,15] In fact, hypoventilation improves cerebral blood flow, pulmonary flow, and arterial saturation after BCPA.[16] Other frequently used techniques for decreasing PVR such

TABLE 31.4
CAUSES OF HYPOXEMIA AFTER PARTIAL CAVOPULMONARY SHUNT

Etiology	Evaluation	Therapy
Obstruction of SVC-PA anastomosis	■ SVCp–PAp gradient >2 mm Hg ■ Echo	■ Removal of clot ■ Surgical revision
Increased PVR	■ Elevated SVC/PAp >18 mm Hg ■ Transpulmonary gradient >7–10 mm Hg	■ PVR therapy ■ Early extubation vs. negative pressure ventilator
Decreased ventricular function	■ SVC/PAp >18 mm Hg ■ LAp >12–15 mm Hg	■ Vasodilators and inotropes
AV valve regurgitation	■ Echo	■ AV valve repair
Anomalous venous connection	■ Contrast echo ■ Venography	■ Surgical or catheter-based therapy

SVC-PA, superior vena cava-pulmonary artery; SVCp, pressure in the SVC (preanastomosis); PAp, pulmonary artery pressure, PVR, pulmonary vascular resistance; AV, atrioventricular; LAp, left (or systemic) ventricular pressure.

as deep sedation/anesthesia may also reduce cerebral blood flow and therefore fail to increase pulmonary blood flow even if they successfully reduce PVR. In the patient with healthy lungs, early extubation is often beneficial, because negative-pressure ventilation is associated with increased pulmonary blood flow in this type of circulation. If mechanical ventilation is required, excessive mean airway pressures and tidal volume as well as atelectasis should be avoided to minimize PVR. Aprotinin and modified ultrafiltration have also been associated with decreased transpulmonary pressure gradient, less pleural drainage and improved SaO_2. Inhaled nitric oxide, which acts selectively on the pulmonary vasculature, has been reported to be effective in reducing the transpulmonary pressure gradient for patients after the BCPA and may therefore be the best treatment of high PVR and low SaO_2. When the degree of cyanosis is not prohibitive, expectant management with good hemodynamic support and maintenance of hemoglobin will often suffice. This is because SaO_2 tends to slowly improve in the first few days following surgery and again at the time of extubation as long as there are no intervening airway or pulmonary issues.

The major hemodynamic advantage of the BCPA compared to shunted or banded single ventricle physiology is in the reduction of the volume load on the ventricle. This occurs because the ventricle now only pumps systemic blood flow, not pulmonary and systemic flow. In addition, owing to the decreased volume load, the ventricle dimension decreases with improved atrioventricular valve function. Coronary blood flow decreases, probably in response to the lower metabolic demand of the myocardium, but coronary perfusion pressure is higher with the elimination of diastolic run-off into the pulmonary circulation with shunt ligation.

When a significant left-to-right shunt persists following BCPA because of aortopulmonary collateral blood vessels, persistent pleural effusions, high central venous pressures, and low cardiac output may result. It is also important to recognize that the changes in ventricular geometry that occur with volume reduction place infants with certain types of anatomy at risk for systemic outflow obstruction. Specifically, when systemic outflow is dependent on flow through a ventricular septal defect or bulboventricular foramen, acute decreases in ventricular volume may precipitate subaortic stenosis as the pathway for systemic outflow narrows. The appearance of an ejection murmur in a patient with susceptible anatomy following BCPA should prompt a complete assessment.

TOTAL CAVOPULMONARY ANASTOMOSIS: FONTAN PHYSIOLOGY

Anatomy

The complete Fontan operation or total cavopulmonary anastomosis (TCPA) has several commonly used anatomic variants, all designed to completely separate systemic and pulmonary blood flows. Although one may still encounter older individuals with direct right atrial to pulmonary artery connections, the current approaches are the creation of either an intracardiac lateral tunnel or extracardiac conduit to baffle the IVC blood flow into the pulmonary arteries. The lateral tunnel involves placement of a semicircular tube along the lateral wall of the right atrium from the inferior vena cava to the SVC. The extracardiac conduit uses a complete circular tube of Gore-tex or pericardium to connect the inferior vena cava to the pulmonary artery. The conduit is placed along the outer surface of the right atrium and therefore creates a connection incapable of dilating over time, unlike the classic Fontan. Either surgical variation can be fenestrated by leaving a hole of known size in the baffle in order to maintain cardiac output during periods of elevated PVR albeit with increased cyanosis.

Physiology

Fontan physiology is a hybrid of BCPA and normal cardiovascular physiology. Like the BCPA, the driving pressure for pulmonary blood flow is mean systemic pressure, but the entire systemic venous return enters the pulmonary circulation. If the Fontan baffle is fenestrated, there may still be a right-to-left shunt causing some mild systemic arterial desaturation, but the systemic and pulmonary circulation are largely separated, as with a normal heart. Potential hemodynamic problems in the postoperative period include systemic venous hypertension, low cardiac output and excessive cyanosis.

Elevated systemic venous pressure results either from elevated PVR, anatomical pulmonary artery obstruction or when myocardial dysfunction raises pulmonary venous pressure, and results in peripheral edema, pleural effusions, and/or ascites. Numerous studies demonstrate that elevated central venous pressure (15 mm Hg) is associated with poor outcome in Fontan patients.[17,18] Pleural effusions and ascites often worsen pulmonary function necessitating the increase of positive-pressure ventilation which further raises PVR and mean systemic pressure. In general, the Fontan fenestration can lower the risk of some of these complications by providing a source of systemic blood flow that is not dependent on passing through the pulmonary circulation. Fenestration can also decrease pulmonary artery pressure enough to reduce third-space losses of fluid and shorten the duration of postoperative pleural effusions. When an individual with Fontan physiology is in a low cardiac output state, it is essential to determine and treat the underlying cause (see Table 31.5). Low cardiac output with high left atrial and central venous pressures indicates myocardial dysfunction in the patient with Fontan physiology. Myocardial dysfunction can occur from ischemia-reperfusion injury during surgery or may be related to poor preoperative myocardial function. Several

TABLE 31.5

CAUSES OF LOW CARDIAC OUTPUT SYNDROME OR HYPOXEMIA AFTER FONTAN PROCEDURE

Etiology	Evaluation	Therapy
Hypovolemia	■ Low CVP/PAp and low LAp	■ Volume expansion
Obstruction of PA anastomosis (surgical or clot)	■ CVP–PAp gradient >2 mm Hg present ■ High CVP/PAp and low LAp	■ Remove clot ■ Surgical revision
Increased PVR	■ Transpulmonary gradient >15 mm Hg ■ High CVP/PAp and low LAp	■ PVR therapy ■ Early extubation or negative pressure vent ■ Drain pleural effusions
Ventricular dysfunction	■ Elevated CVP/PAp and elevated LAp	■ Vasoactive agents
AV valve regurgitation		■ Valve repair or replacement
Ventricular outflow obstruction	■ Elevated CVP/PAp and elevated LAp	■ Surgical repair

CVP, central venous pressure; PAp, pulmonary artery pressure; LAp, left (or systemic) ventricular pressure; PA, pulmonary artery; PVR, pulmonary vascular resistance; AV, atrioventricular.

studies demonstrate better outcome for the Fontan operation when performed in patients younger than 4 years, or when a BCPA has been performed as the second stage in single ventricle heart palliation, suggesting that long-standing ventricular volume overload is detrimental to myocardial function.[19,20] The only effective long-term therapy for low cardiac output with ventricular dysfunction following a Fontan operation is to improve the cardiac output and reduce the left atrial pressure. The use of inotropic agents that do not increase ventricular afterload, such as milrinone, dobutamine, and low-dose epinephrine (≤ 0.05 μg/kg/minute) may be helpful. If systemic blood pressure will tolerate it, aggressive afterload reduction with vasodilating agents may also lower left atrial pressure significantly. If there is good reason to believe that the insult to ventricular function is reversible, mechanical circulatory support can also be effective therapy. Persistent aortopulmonary collateral vessels which place a volume load on the systemic ventricle can exacerbate ventricular dysfunction. Aggressive assessment and embolization of these vessels may be useful in this situation.

Obstruction to pulmonary blood flow should be considered as the cause of low output when left atrial pressure is low and central venous pressure is high. If central venous pressure is not monitored, large third-space fluid losses with a low or normal left atrial pressure should raise the suspicion of this diagnosis. Even with a fenestrated baffle, the capability of the fenestration to preserve cardiac output in the face of anatomic or physiologic obstruction to pulmonary blood flow is limited. Therefore, limited pulmonary blood flow can result in low cardiac output and, when a fenestration is present, in significant cyanosis. Cyanosis can also result from intrapulmonary arteriovenous malformations or ventilation–perfusion mismatch

related to low cardiac output. If high PVR is responsible for the elevation of systemic venous pressure, institution of the standard ventilatory maneuvers of supplemental oxygen, hyperventilation, and alkalosis is indicated. As with the patient with BCPA, the use of high positive pressures to achieve these ends may be counterproductive. Negative-pressure ventilation can augment stroke volume and cardiac output and high-frequency jet ventilation may lower $Paco_2$ at low mean airway pressures. Intravenous vasodilators such as prostacyclin or prostaglandin E (PGE) should be used with caution because of the risk of systemic vasodilation with limited cardiac output. Inhaled nitric oxide has been reported to be effective in lowering the transpulmonary pressure gradient.

REFERENCES

1. Barnea O, Santamore WP, Rossi A, et al. Estimation of oxygen delivery in newborns with a univentricular circulation. *Circulation.* 1998;98:1407–1413.
2. Barnea O, Austin EH, Richman B, et al. Balancing the circulation: Theoretic optimization of pulmonary/systemic flow ratio in hypoplastic left heart syndrome. *J Am Coll Cardiol.* 1994;24:1376–1381.
3. Taeed R, Schwartz SM, Pearl JM, et al. Unrecognized pulmonary venous desaturation early after Norwood palliation confounds Qp:Qs assessment and compromises oxygen delivery. *Circulation.* 2001;103:2699–2704.
4. Hoffman GM, Ghanayem NS, Kampine JM, et al. Venous saturation and the anaerobic threshold in neonates after the Norwood procedure for hypoplastic left heart syndrome. *Ann Thorac Surg.* 2000;70:1515–1520.
5. Tweddell JS, Hoffman GM, Fedderly RT, et al. Patients at risk for low systemic oxygen delivery after the Norwood procedure. *Ann Thorac Surg.* 2000;69(6):1893–1899.
6. Charpie JR, Dekeon MK, Goldberg CS, et al. Postoperative hemodynamics after Norwood palliation for hypoplastic left heart syndrome. *Am J Cardiol.* 2001;87:198–202.

7. Beekman RH, Tuuri DT. Acute hemodynamic effects of increasing hemoglobin concentration in children with a right to left ventricular shunt and relative anemia. *J Am Coll Cardiol.* 1985;5: 357–362.

8. Tabbutt S, Ramamoorthy C, Montenegro LM, et al. Impact of inspired gas mixtures on preoperative infants with hypoplastic left heart syndrome during controlled ventilation. *Circulation.* 2001;104:I159–I164.

9. Ramamoorthy C, Tabbutt S, Kurth CD, et al. Effects of inspired hypoxic and hypercapnic gas mixtures on cerebral oxygen saturation in neonates with univentricular heart defects. *Anesthesiology.* 2002;96:283–288.

10. Bradley SM, Simsic JM, Atz AM. Hemodynamic effects of inspired carbon dioxide after the Norwood procedure. *Ann Thorac Surg.* 2001;72:2088–2093.

11. Tweddell JS, Hoffman GM, Fedderly RT, et al. Phenoxybenzamine improves systemic oxygen delivery after the Norwood procedure. *Ann Thorac Surg.* 1999;67:161–167.

12. Riordan CJ, Randsbaek F, Storey JH, et al. Inotropes in the hypoplastic left heart syndrome: Effects in an animal model. *Ann Thorac Surg.* 1996;62:83–90.

13. Reddy VM, McElhinney DB, Moore P, et al. Outcomes after bidirectional cavopulmonary shunt in infants less than 6 months old. *J Am Coll Cardiol.* 1997;29:1365–1370.

14. Fogel MA, Durning S, Wernovsky G, et al. Brain versus lung: Hierarchy of feedback loops in single-ventricle patients with superior cavopulmonary connection. *Circulation.* 2004;110(Suppl II):II–147–II–152.

15. Hoskote A, Li J, Hickey C, et al. The effects of carbon dioxide on oxygenation and systemic, cerebral, and pulmonary vascular hemodynamics after the bi-directional superior cavopulmonary anastomosis. *J Am Coll Cardiol.* 2004;44:1501–1509.

16. Bradley SM, Simsic JM, Mulvihill DM. Hyperventilation impairs oxygenation after bidirectional superior cavopulmonary connection. *Circulation.* 1998;98:II372–II376.

17. Kaulitz R, Luhmer I, Bergmann F, et al. Sequelae after modified Fontan operation: Postoperative haemodynamic data and organ function. *Heart.* 1997;78:154–159.

18. Gentles TL, Mayer JE Jr, Gauvreau K, et al. Fontan operation in five hundred consecutive patients: Factors influencing early and late outcome. *J Thorac Cardiovasc Surg.* 1997;114:376–391.

19. Masuda M, Kado H, Shiokawa Y, et al. Clinical results of the staged Fontan procedure in high-risk patients. *Ann Thorac Surg.* 1998;65:1721–1725.

20. Uemura H, Yagihara T, Kawashima Y, et al. What factors affect ventricular performance after a Fontan-type operation? *J Thorac Cardiovasc Surg.* 1995;110:405–415.

Myocardial Disease

32

Christopher F. Spurney

Cardiomyopathies (CMPs) are diseases of the myocardium associated with decreased cardiac function. There are four forms of CMP: dilated, hypertrophic, restrictive, and arrhythmogenic right ventricular dysplasia. The overall incidence of primary CMP in children is approximately 1.13 per 100,000, with a significantly higher incidence in children younger than 1 year (8.34) compared to those between 1 and 18 years (0.70).[1] Dilated CMPs account for the largest proportion (51%) and are characterized by an increase in ventricular size and reduced function. Hypertrophic CMP accounts for 42% of the cases and is characterized by a thickened ventricle without dilation. Restrictive CMP affects diastolic function, producing abnormal ventricular filling without ventricular hypertrophy. Arrhythmogenic right ventricular dysplasia is characterized by progressive replacement of the right ventricular myocardium with fatty tissue, leading to decreased function, ventricular arrhythmias, and sudden death.

DILATED CARDIOMYOPATHY

Dilated CMP is the most common form of CMP and while a number of secondary causes have been identified (see Table 32.1), most of these cases are idiopathic. Genetic mutation may account for 20% to 50%[2] of these idiopathic cases, and a significant number of the remaining cases are likely related to previous viral injections.

Presentation

Patients present to the intensive care unit with acute or chronic symptoms secondary to low cardiac output or congestive heart failure (CHF). The symptoms include poor feeding and growth failure in infants and exercise intolerance in older children. Superimposed infections may cause acute decompensation, which leads to cardiogenic

---

TABLE 32.1
CAUSES OF DILATED CARDIOMYOPATHY

Structural heart disease: mitral insufficiency, aortic stenosis or insufficiency, left ventricle noncompaction
Ischemia: Kawasaki disease, anomalous origin of the left coronary artery, atherosclerosis
Drug-induced: anthracyclines, ethanol, cocaine
Infections:
  Bacterial: *Streptococcus, Staphylococcus, Pneumococcus, Mycobacterium, Haemophilus, Meningococcus, Mycoplasma, Corynebacterium, Bordetella, Clostridium, Gonococcus, Brucella, Vibrio cholerae*
  Viral: coxsackie, adenovirus, echovirus, influenza, parainfluenza, parvovirus, human immunodeficiency virus, Epstein-Barr virus, cytomegalovirus, respiratory syncytial, varicella, rubella, measles, mumps
  Fungal: *Candida, Aspergillus, Histoplasma, Crytococcus, Coccidioides, Actinomyces, Nocardia, Sporothrix*
  Protozoal: *Trypanosoma cruzi, Plasmodium, Toxoplasma, Leishmania*
  Parasitic: *Ascaris, Schistosoma, Trichinella*
  Spirochetal: *Chlamydia, Borrelia*
  Rickettsial: *Rickettsia*
Autoimmune disorders: systemic lupus erythematosus, acute rheumatic carditis, rheumatoid arthritis, drug hypersensitivity, sarcoidosis, polymyositis, polyarteritis nodosa
Endocrine disorders: hypoparathyroidism, hypo/hyperthyroidism
Metabolic disorders: glycogen storage disease (often hypertrophic), carnitine deficiency, medium-chain acyl-CoA dehydrogenase deficiency, mitochondrial disorders
Hereditary disorders: autosomal dominant, autosomal recessive, X-linked
Muscular dystrophies: Duchenne muscular dystrophy, Becker muscular dystrophy, Friedreich ataxia, myotonic dystrophy
Nutritional disorders: deficiencies of vitamin B_1, vitamin D, selenium, malnutrition
Arrhythmia: supraventricular, ectopic, and ventricular tachyarrhythmias
Toxins: lead, copper, iron
Idiopathic

shock. Patients with cardiogenic shock have tachycardia, hypotension, and a narrow pulse pressure. The patient has cool extremities and poor capillary refill as a result of increased systemic vascular resistance. Signs of heart failure include jugular venous distension, pulmonary wheezes or crackles, hepatomegaly, and peripheral edema. Cardiac auscultation often reveals a gallop rhythm and regurgitant murmurs of mitral or tricuspid insufficiency.

Diagnostic Studies

In newly diagnosed patients, an investigation for secondary causes of dilated CMP is warranted, with an emphasis on causes requiring specific treatment (Table 32.1). Evidence of structural heart disease, infection, systemic inflammation, autoimmunity, and endocrine disorders should be ruled out. A metabolic or genetic evaluation may also be required. Skeletal muscle biopsies may be required in patients in whom the suspicion for metabolic disease is high.

The assessment of myocardial and other organ damage is important to the intensivist. Troponin I, a protein bound in the myocardial contractile apparatus, provides the most specific evidence of ongoing myocardial damage. B-type natriuretic peptide (BNP) is secreted from the left ventricle in response to volume overload and ventricular stretch. BNP levels are increased in patients with dilated CMP. Adult studies demonstrate that BNP is a useful diagnostic and prognostic marker for heart failure. In general, a declining BNP level correlates with a favorable outcome, whereas a rising BNP level may indicate that more intensive treatment is necessary.

An electrocardiogram usually demonstrates ventricular hypertrophy, and ST-segment and T-wave changes. Any evidence for arrhythmias including a prolonged QT interval should be sought. The chest x-ray usually demonstrates cardiomegaly and pulmonary venous congestion.

Cardiac Imaging Studies

Echocardiography is essential in the evaluation of cardiomyopathy, and characteristic findings include left ventricular dilation, left atrial enlargement, and decreased systolic function assessed by shortening fraction or ejection fraction (see Fig. 32.1). The ventricular dilation can lead to mitral or tricuspid valve insufficiency. Coronary anatomy must be delineated, ruling out anomalous coronary artery origins as an etiology. In very poorly functioning hearts, there is a risk for the development of mural thrombi in the atria and ventricles.

Cardiac catheterization can be performed after stabilization of the patient if the diagnosis remains unclear. During catheterization, hemodynamic information, coronary angiography, and a myocardial biopsy may be performed to differentiate CMP from myocarditis or intrinsic muscle disease.

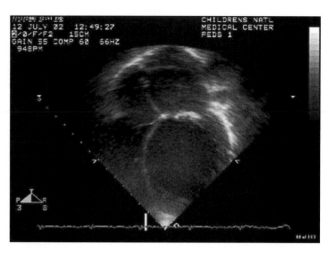

Figure 32.1 Apical four-chamber view of dilated cardiomyopathy. There is severe left ventricular and left atrial enlargement.

Treatment

Management of Acute Cardiac Failure

The management of acute cardiac failure is aimed at restoring end-organ perfusion, maintaining oxygen delivery, restoring fluid balance, and preventing cardiorespiratory arrest and death. These goals can be addressed while the underlying causes of the CMP are being investigated and more specific treatments are being considered.

Diuretics

Diuretics are widely used to reduce fluid retention secondary to cardiac failure. These drugs help decrease ventricular filling pressures and return the patient to a euvolemic state. Loop diuretics, such as furosemide, are most commonly used. However, overaggressive diuresis can result in reduced cardiac output secondary to reduced preload.

Nesiritide

Nesiritide is recombinant human BNP that reduces preload and afterload. By enhancing sodium excretion and diuresis, inhibiting the renin–angiotensin–aldosterone system, and decreasing the sympathetic nervous system activity, this drug addresses the mechanisms underlying the pathophysiology of heart failure. In adults with decompensated heart failure, nesiritide therapy improves the global clinical status including the symptoms of dyspnea and fatigue.[3]

Levosimendan

Levosimendan is a new calcium-sensitizing agent that increases myocardial contractility without significantly increasing myocardial oxygen demand, improves myocardial relaxation, and causes vasodilatation. In an adult study of low cardiac output heart failure, levosimendan was associated with improved hemodynamics and lower mortality when compared to dobutamine therapy.[4]

Nitrates and Nitroprusside

Nitroglycerin dilates systemic veins to reduce venous return and decreases filling pressures of the ventricles. It is used for patients with pulmonary congestion and elevated pulmonary capillary wedge pressures. Nitrates also dilate coronary arteries and relieve coronary vasospasm. Sodium nitroprusside is a rapid-onset afterload-reducing agent that acts to dilate arteriolar and venous vascular beds. It is useful for acute low ventricular output states with stable blood pressures, often seen with cardiac failure after heart surgery and myocardial infarction.

Inotropes

Intravenous inotropic infusions are associated with an increased risk of tachyarrhythmias and increased myocardial oxygen demand and are reserved for patients in cardiogenic shock. The phosphodiesterase inhibitors, milrinone and amrinone, decrease afterload, increase preload, and have putative benefits on myocardial relaxation. Sympathomimetics include dobutamine, dopamine, norepinephrine, and epinephrine. Norepinephrine and epinephrine both have potent inotropic and vasoconstrictor properties.

Mechanical Ventilation

Cardiopulmonary interactions have significant implications for patients with acute heart failure. Mechanical ventilation not only reduces oxygen consumption by decreasing the work of breathing but also favorably affects left ventricular afterload. Noninvasive positive-pressure ventilation is beneficial in acute and chronic failure.

Mechanical Support

In refractory cardiac failure, circulatory support with ventricular assist devices or extracorporal membrane oxygenation (ECMO) may be used as a bridge toward transplantation or for a limited period of myocardial rescue.[5]

Management of Chronic Cardiac Failure

Medications

The goals of treatment of chronic cardiac failure are to modulate the neurohormonal responses, thereby slowing the progression of myocardial injury and increasing survival. Other goals include symptomatic relief, arrhythmia control, and the prevention of sudden cardiac death. Most clinical studies in chronic heart failure were performed on adults, with pediatric guidelines being extrapolated from these results.[6] The mainstay of treatment include angiotensin-converting enzyme inhibitors, β-adrenergic blocking agents, and aldosterone antagonists, which modulate the rennin–angiotensin or sympathetic nervous systems. All three drug classes decrease hospitalizations and mortality.[7–9] Diuretics control congestion but require careful monitoring of electrolyte imbalance to prevent arrhythmias. Digoxin does not improve survival in adults and should not be used in asymptomatic patients.[10] It

may have a role, at low doses, in patients with significant symptoms.

Pacemakers and Automated Defibrillators

Patients with severe heart failure may require permanent pacemakers or intracardiac defibrillators. Biventricular pacing synchronizes the activation of the intraventricular septum and left ventricular free wall and improves left ventricular function. The Multi-site Stimulation in Cardiomyopathy (MUSTIC) trial in adult patients with severe heart failure and a widened QRS complex showed that biventricular pacing improved exercise tolerance and decreased hospitalizations by 66%.[11] In the three-arm Comparison of Medical Therapy, Pacing, and Defibrillation in Heart Failure (COMPANION) trial comparing optimal medical therapy to medical therapy plus biventricular pacing or medical therapy plus pacing and automated internal defibrillator, the risk of death was reduced by 36% in the automatic implantable cardioverter-defibrillator (AICD)/pacemaker group and by 24% in the pacemaker alone group as compared to optimal medical management.[12]

Transplantation

CMP remains the leading cause of cardiac transplantation in children older than 1 year. The rate of transplantation for primary dilated CMP was 12.7% in the first 2 years after diagnosis.[1]

Prognosis

Idiopathic dilated CMP has a progressive course that is difficult to predict on the basis of any single clinical or imaging parameter. Death usually occurs from either progressive cardiac failure or sudden death. Survival has been improved using maximal medical therapies, but the 5-year mortality rate still varies from 20% to 60%.

HYPERTROPHIC CARDIOMYOPATHY

Hypertrophic CMP is a primary disorder of the cardiac muscle, causing an asymmetric enlargement of the ventricular septum without dilation of the ventricular chamber. The myocardium shows poorly organized myocytes. A family history is found in half the cases; most of these are related to β-myosin heavy chain, myosin-binding protein C, and troponin T. Other causes and associated conditions are listed in Table 32.2. Hypertrophic CMP is the most common cause of sudden death in adolescents, including competitive athletes.[13]

Diagnosis

Symptoms usually begin in adolescence. In some cases, the first presentation itself may be an episode of sudden death. Other symptoms include chest pain, palpitations, presyncope, or syncope related to increased left ventricular

TABLE 32.2
CAUSES AND CONDITIONS RELATED TO HYPERTROPHIC CARDIOMYOPATHY

Genetic Mutations	Metabolic Disorders
Autosomal dominant	Glycogen storage diseases (Pompe)
Sporadic	Mucopolysaccharidoses (Hunters/Hurlers)
	Lysosomal storage disorders (Fabry)
	Infant of a mother with diabetes
Genetic Disorders	**Mitochondrial Disorders**
Noonan syndrome	Friedreich ataxia
Turner syndrome	
Amyloidosis	
Neuroectodermal Disorders	**Endocrine Disorders**
Multiple lentigines syndrome	Hyperparathyroidism/ hyperthyroidism
Tuberous sclerosis	Pheochromocytoma

outflow obstruction. In severe phenotypes, patients present with symptoms of CHF. The physical examination finding includes a systolic ejection murmur related to subaortic stenosis. The electrocardiogram shows left ventricular hypertrophy and a strain pattern with T-wave inversions and ST-segment depressions. Chest x-ray may show cardiomegaly, but the overall heart contour may not be enlarged at the time of diagnosis. Echocardiography shows the characteristic asymmetric septal hypertrophy (see Fig. 32.2). Measurement of the left ventricular outflow gradient is essential and can have prognostic implications.

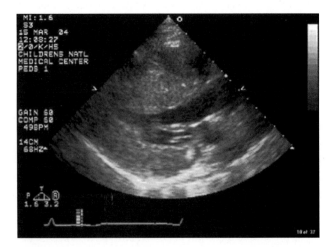

Figure 32.2 Parasternal long axis view of hypertrophic cardiomyopathy. Note the severe enlargement of the interventricular septum and left ventricular free wall.

Deceased left ventricular diastolic function is related to the hypertrophic myocardium.

Treatment

In patients with hypertrophic CMP, hemodynamic instability may develop when a patient is volume-depleted and treated with inotropes, both of which can increase the left ventricular outflow gradient. Peripheral vasoconstrictors, such as phenylephrine, and volume are used to support low blood pressures. Symptomatic patients with a significant outflow obstruction are treated with β-blockers. This treatment reduces the left ventricular outflow gradient and minimizes myocardial oxygen demand. Slower heart rates also enhance ventricular diastolic filling. Calcium channel blockers improve diastolic relaxation and reduce the outflow gradient. Diuretics can decrease ventricular filling pressures and improve symptoms but must be used cautiously. If a significant left ventricular outflow gradient is present after stabilization, additional interventions including dual chamber pacing, catheter-based alcohol septal ablation, and surgical myotomy–myectomy may be required.

Ventricular arrhythmias are the substrate for sudden death. These patients are difficult to stratify for their risk of sudden death, but risk factors include a history of cardiac arrest, documented sustained ventricular tachycardia, or sudden death in the family. These arrhythmias require treatment with medications such as sotalol and amiodarone or with implantable cardiac defibrillators.

Prognosis

The overall mortality for patients with hypertrophic CMP is approximately 1%.[13] Many patients with hypertrophic CMP remain asymptomatic throughout life. It is difficult to predict as to which patients are at risk for sudden death or progressive heart failure, and it is not clear at this time whether genetic testing will improve this ability.

RESTRICTIVE CARDIOMYOPATHY

Restrictive CMP is characterized by normal ventricular chamber size and function, with deceased diastolic function secondary to decreased ventricular compliance and filling. The differential diagnosis includes primary and secondary myocardial disorders and constrictive pericardial disease. Causes of restrictive cardiomyopathy include endomyocardial fibroelastosis, Loeffler hypereosinophilic syndrome, amyloidosis, sarcoidosis, hemochromatosis, glycogen storage diseases, and idiopathic fibrosis.

Diagnosis

Patients with restrictive CMP present with shortness of breath, decreased exercise tolerance, and peripheral edema. Physical examination findings include jugular venous

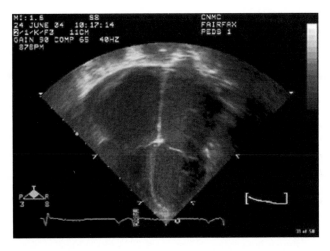

Figure 32.3 Apical four-chamber view of restrictive cardiomyopathy. Note the normal-sized ventricles and the severely enlarged atria.

distension, pulmonary rales, hepatomegaly, a gallop rhythm, and peripheral edema. Chest x-ray demonstrates a normal or enlarged cardiac silhouette with pulmonary venous congestion. An electrocardiogram often reveals biatrial enlargement. Echocardiogram also demonstrates biatrial enlargement with normal ventricular size and wall thickness (see Fig. 32.3). Doppler evaluation of atrioventricular valve inflow patterns can assist in making the diagnosis. Cardiac catheterization shows an increase in left ventricle end diastolic pressures, a characteristic "square-root" sign diastolic tracing, and possible pulmonary hypertension. Endocardial biopsy may be diagnostic, demonstrating interstitial fibrosis and endocardial sclerosis.

Treatment

This type of CMP is a clinical syndrome of heart failure due to isolated diastolic dysfunction. The treatment options are limited. Diuretics are an important therapy to reduce pulmonary congestion. However, these patients are preload-dependent, and excessive diuresis can easily lead to decreased cardiac output. β-Blockers and calcium channel blockers may improve ventricular relaxation and filling. Anticoagulation may be required for severe atrial enlargement to decrease the potential for thrombus formation. Antiarrhythmic therapy may be necessary to maintain atrioventricular synchrony. Patients often remain symptomatic even on maximal medical therapy. Patients refractory to treatment should be considered for heart transplantation.

ARRHYTHMOGENIC RIGHT VENTRICLE DYSPLASIA

This type of CMP predominately affects the right ventricle, where fibrofatty tissue progressively replaces normal ventricular myocardium. Even with treatment, the disease can progress to right ventricular and then biventricular failure. Arrhythmogenic right ventricle dysplasia (ARVD) is a cause of sudden death in athletes and young adults.

Diagnosis

Initial symptoms, which often occur with exertion, include palpitations, dizziness, light-headedness, and syncope. These are related to right ventricular arrhythmias. Diagnostic testing includes an electrocardiogram that may show ventricular ectopy with left bundle branch morphology. In older adolescents and adults, T wave inversions in the right precordial leads (V_1 to V_3) are important markers for ARVD. Echocardiography can demonstrate right ventricular dilation, decreased systolic function, and regional wall motion abnormalities. However, a normal echocardiogram does not rule out the diagnosis. Magnetic resonance imaging (MRI) is increasingly being used to evaluate patients with suspected ARVD. With the improved soft tissue contrast, MRI can detect the gross fatty changes in the right ventricular myocardium found in histopathologic specimens (see Fig. 32.4).

Treatment

Treatment includes suppressing ventricular arrhythmias with β-blockers. Other antiarrhythmics such as amiodarone or sotalol may also be considered. Pacemakers or implantable defibrillators may be required for the prevention of sudden death. If the patient experiences progressive CHF, medications or transplantation may be required.

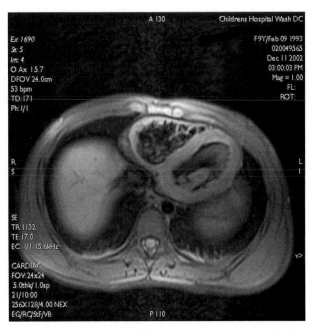

Figure 32.4 Magnetic resonance image of arrhythmogenic right ventricular dysplasia. Note the increased signal intensity of the right ventricular free wall, indicating fatty infiltration.

This chapter covers the major classification schema for cardiomyopathy in the critically ill child, with consideration of the major clinical, diagnostic, and treatment criteria of importance to the pediatric intensivist.

REFERENCES

1. Lipshultz SE, Sleeper LA, Towbin JA, et al. The incidence of pediatric cardiomyopathy in two regions of the United States. *N Engl J Med.* 2003;348:1647–1655.
2. Burkett EL, Hershberger RE. Clinical and genetic issues in familial dilated cardiomyopathy. *J Am Coll Cardiol.* 2005;45:969–981.
3. Colucci WS, Elkayam Y, Horton DP, et al. Intravenous nesiritide, a natriuretic peptide, in the treatment of decompensated congestive heart failure. *N Engl J Med.* 2000;343(4):246–253.
4. Follath F, Cleland JGF, Just H, et al. Efficacy and safety of intravenous levosimendan compared with dobutamine in severe low-output heart failure (the LIDO study): A randomized double-blind trial. *Lancet.* 2002;360:196–202.
5. Rosenthal D, Chrisant M, Edens E, et al. International society for heart and lung transplantation: Practice guidelines for management of heart failure in children. *J Heart Lung Transplant.* 2004;23:1313–1333.
6. The SOLVD investigators. Effect of enalapril on survival in patients with reduced left ventricular ejection fractions and congestive heart failure. *N Engl J Med.* 1991;325(5):293–302.
7. Pitt B, Zannad F, Remme WJ, et al. The effect of spironolactone on morbidity and mortality in patients with severe heart failure. *N Engl J Med.* 1999;341(10):709–717.
8. Packer M, Coats AJS, Fowler AB, et al. Effect of carvedilol on survival in severe chronic heart failure. *N Engl J Med.* 2001;344(22):1651–1658.
9. Garg R, Gorlin R, Smith T, et al. The effect of digoxin on mortality and morbidity in patients with heart failure. *N Engl J Med.* 1997;336(8):525–533.
10. Cazeau S, Leclerco C, Lavergne T, et al. Effects of multisite biventricular pacing in patients with heart failure and intraventricular conduction delay. *N Engl J Med.* 2001;344(12):873–880.
11. Bristow MR, Saxon LA, Boehmer J, et al. Cardiac-resynchronization therapy with or without an implantable defibrillator in advanced chronic heart failure. *N Engl J Med.* 2004;350:2150.
12. Duncan BW, Bohn DJ, Atz AM, et al. Mechanical circulatory support for the treatment of children with acute fulminant myocarditis. *J Thorac Cardiovasc Surg.* 2001;122:48.
13. Maron BJ. Hypertrophic cardiomyopathy: A systematic review. *JAMA.* 2002;287(10):1308–1320.

Pericardial and Endocardial Disease

33

George Ofori-Amanfo

INFECTIVE ENDOCARDITIS

Infective endocarditis is an inflammatory disease affecting the native endocardium, heart valves, or related structures. It can involve the prosthetic valves, aortopulmonary shunts, surgical patches, or indwelling central venous catheters. The inflammatory process occurs in the setting of a previous injury to these structures by surgical manipulation, trauma, or disease. The infecting organism can be bacterial, fungal, viral, chlamydial, or rickettsial.

Infective endocarditis has been reported to account for 1 in 1,280 pediatric admissions per year,[1] although the incidence continues to grow owing to improved survival among children with congenital heart disease (CHD). In 8% to 10% of pediatric cases, it develops without structural heart disease or other identifiable risk factors.[2] These cases are usually fulminant, affecting the aortic or mitral valve and are secondary to *Staphylococcus aureus* bacteremia.[3]

Three important factors play a significant pathogenetic role in the development of endocarditis (see Fig. 33.1):

a. The presence of structural abnormalities in the heart or great vessels with resultant pressure gradient or turbulent blood flow.
b. Endothelial damage and platelet–fibrin aggregation.
c. Bacteremia.

Most patients who develop infective endocarditis have a history of congenital or acquired heart disease. With the exception of secundum atrial septal defects, most cardiac defects, including bicuspid aortic valve and mitral valve prolapse with regurgitation, can predispose to infective endocarditis. In intravenous (IV) drug users, the disease may develop without antecedent cardiac defects. Although bacteremia can result from any localized infection such

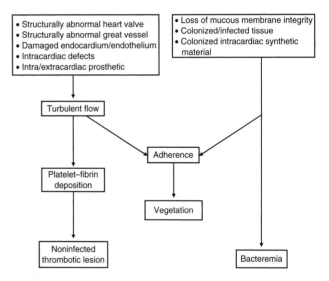

Figure 33.1 The development of endocarditis.

as cellulitis or osteomyelitis, it most commonly follows dental procedures.

The vegetation of infective endocarditis often develops on the low-pressure side of the defect; therefore, vegetations of mitral valve endocarditis will form on the atrial side of the valve or in the aorta in the case of aortic valve endocarditis. The common organisms that cause pediatric infective endocarditis are gram-positive cocci, including viridans group (α-hemolytic) streptococci, staphylococci, and enterococci. Other less frequent causative organisms are the HACEK group (*Haemophilus parainfluenzae*, *Actinobacillus*, *Cardiobacterium hominis*, *Eikenella* species, and *Kingella kingae*), group B *streptococci*, *Streptococcus pneumoniae*, *Pseudomonas aeruginosa*, *Serratia marcescens*, and *Candida* species.[4]

Clinical Manifestations

Although most patients have a past history of heart disease, infective endocarditis can present even in the absence of underlying cardiac defects. A recent history of dental disease or procedure is often present. The disease is rare in infants; when it occurs in this age-group, it usually follows open-heart surgery. In neonates without CHD, infective endocarditis has been associated with the long-term use of indwelling central venous catheters. The onset of symptoms (fever, anorexia, malaise, arthralgia, fatigue) is often insidious, although some patients may present with acute circulatory collapse secondary to severe valvar dysfunction.

Fever occurs in 80% to 90% of patients and splenomegaly occurs often less. Presence of a heart murmur is a universal finding, although in most patients the murmur is specific to their underlying cardiac disease. A new or changing murmur occurs in only 25% of pediatric patients. In IV drug users, the tricuspid valve is the most affected valve resulting in a murmur of tricuspid regurgitation, gallop rhythm, and pulsatile liver. These patients often have pulmonary complications including infarction, abscess formation, and signs and symptoms of pleural effusions. The typical cutaneous manifestations of the disease occur less often in children and are probably secondary to microemboli. These include Osler nodes (red, tender nodes on the finger and toe pads, sides of the fingers, and thenar and hypothenar eminences), Janeway lesions (hemorrhagic, painless lesions on the palms and soles), and splinter hemorrhages (linear streaks on the nail beds). Embolic phenomena to other organs may be seen in infective endocarditis and include Roth spots (oval retinal hemorrhages with pale centers), renal failure and hematuria, and seizures and stroke.

Presentation with a neurologic event occurs in approximately 25% of patients.[5] Acute hemiplegia, ataxia, focal neurologic defects, or seizures may be the presenting features. Therefore, infective endocarditis should be suspected in children with CHD who present with such findings.

A small group of patients may present in acute circulatory collapse because of the inability to maintain adequate cardiac output. This may result from (a) profound mitral or aortic valve insufficiency secondary to valve leaflet erosion or papillary muscle necrosis (mitral valve), (b) obstruction of mitral valve inflow by a large vegetation, or (c) abscesses or aneurysms around the aortic valve. Severe mitral insufficiency or obstruction of mitral valve inflow will result in increased left atrial pressure and result in rapidly progressive pulmonary edema. Such patients present an acute surgical emergency.

Diagnosis

Blood cultures are indicated in all patients. Because bacteremia is continuous, the yield of blood culture exceeds 90%. Bacteremia may also be low grade and therefore the yield is improved by obtaining multiple cultures. Failure to culture the organism may be because of inadequate microbiologic techniques, infections with highly fastidious bacteria or nonbacterial microorganisms, or prior antimicrobial therapy.

The most common hematologic abnormality is normochromic, normocytic anemia of chronic disease, reflecting chronic inflammation. Leukocytosis is common but variable. Erythrocyte sedimentation rate (ESR) and C-reactive protein (CRP) are always elevated at presentation. Hematuria results from embolization in renal arteries. Serum globulins are increased and the rheumatoid factor is elevated in 20% of patients.

Echocardiography should focus on identifying vegetations, intracardiac or para-valvar abscesses, new prosthetic valve dehiscence, or new valvar insufficiency. Transthoracic echocardiography (TTE) is noninvasive, rapid to obtain and has a specificity of 98% for vegetations but has an overall sensitivity <66%. Vegetations larger than 2 mm in size, especially those on right-sided valves, are readily seen by TTE.[6] Transesophageal echocardiography (TEE) should be considered in patients with limited echocardiographic windows. TEE also has a vital place in the management of infective endocarditis because it is more sensitive in identifying or ruling out important complications such as periannular abscess, valve leaflet perforation, or fistulae; it also offers a better visualization of prosthetic valves. False-negative echocardiographic findings may result from vegetations smaller than the limits of resolution, prior embolization of the vegetation, or from inadequate echocardiographic windows.

Clinical diagnosis is based on the Duke criteria (see Table 33.1). A definite diagnosis can be made by pathologic criteria, including the presence of microorganisms by culture or histology of a vegetation or intracardiac abscess, or by pathologic lesions including histologically confirmed intracardiac abscess. A diagnosis based on clinical criteria

TABLE 33.1

DUKE CRITERIA

Major Criteria	Minor Criteria

1. Positive blood culture for IE
  • Typical microorganisms consistent with IE on two separate blood cultures
  • Persistently positive blood cultures
2. Evidence of endocardial involvement
  • Positive echocardiogram
  • New valvar regurgitation
	1. Predisposition: previous cardiac disease
	2. Fever: temperature $\geq 38°C$
	3. Vascular phenomena (e.g., emboli)
	4. Immunologic phenomena
	5. Positive blood culture but does not meet major criterion
	6. Positive echocardiographic finding but does not meet major criterion

IE, Infective endocarditis.

can be made with two major criteria or one major criterion, and three minor or five minor criteria.

Management

Patients admitted to the pediatric intensive care unit (PICU) often have hemodynamic compromise or severe neurologic complication, and therefore need to be stratified according to the risk of progression of symptoms and the need for urgent intervention. Patients with the inability to maintain cardiac output (without evidence of stroke) present a surgical emergency for valve repair or replacement and need prompt hemodynamic stabilization. Such support can include fluid resuscitation, pharmacologic afterload reduction, and early intubation and mechanical ventilation to improve pulmonary edema and to decrease left ventricular (LV) afterload. Placement of a pulmonary artery catheter is highly recommended in this patient population, particularly for the assessment of the effects of interventions and for an objective guide to management. If medical management fails to maintain a stable hemodynamic status, urgent surgical intervention must be considered.

For patients presenting with acute stroke, the indication and timing of surgery are controversial.[7,8] In one large series, the surgical indication was recurrent cerebral embolisms and the outcome of surgery was most favorable if performed approximately 72 hours after a stroke.[7] Computed tomography (CT) scan of the head is mandatory, immediately before surgery to define the extent of cerebral infarction and identify early reperfusion hemorrhages. In patients with reperfusion hemorrhages, cardiac surgery must be postponed because of the high risk of severe cerebral bleeding during perioperative anticoagulation. The timing of surgery should be decided in consultation with the neurosurgeon. Patients with ruptured mycotic aneurysms may need to have them clipped before cardiac surgery.

Empiric antibiotic therapy must be initiated, pending sensitivities. Appropriate long-term antibiotic therapy and prophylaxis may be chosen after consulting infectious diseases.

PERICARDIAL EFFUSIONS

Pericardial effusion is the presence of fluid in the pericardial space in excess of the physiologic amount of 15 to 50 mL. An increase in intrapericardial pressure (as in pericardial effusion) or restriction of pericardial cavity (as in constrictive pericarditis) causes changes in ventricular interdependence and ventricular filling with resulting decrease in cardiac output and cardiac tamponade. The severity of symptoms and signs of pericardial effusion is determined by the rate of pericardial fluid accumulation and myocardial compliance. Rapid accumulation of even a small amount of fluid may be accompanied by cardiac tamponade and

TABLE 33.2	
CAUSES OF PERICARDIAL EFFUSION	
Pathologic Process	**Disease**
Cardiac	Heart failure, cardiac allograft rejection, postinfarction pericarditis, postpericardiotomy syndrome, postsurgical chylous effusion, postsurgical hematoma
Neoplastic	Mediastinal lymphomas, metastatic neoplasia (e.g., acute leukemia)
Infectious	Viral, bacterial, fungal, mycobacterial, atypical bacterial, parasitic diseases
Immune/inflammatory	Rheumatoid arthritis, systemic lupus erythematosus, systemic sclerosis, vasculitides
Miscellaneous	Uremia, trauma, central line erosion, radiation, drugs (hydralazine, procainamide)

circulatory embarrassment. Cardiac tamponade results in compensatory mechanisms and these include an increase in pulmonary and systemic vascular tone to improve diastolic filling, an increase in systemic vascular resistance to improve blood pressure, and tachycardia to enhance cardiac output. Pericardial effusion can be acute or chronic, and is the manifestation of local or systemic disorders. Table 33.2 outlines the causes of pericardial effusion. In addition to a pericardial fluid collection, a localized clot or myocardial edema can cause cardiac tamponade. Diagnosis depends on the presence of an underlying disease and on the results of pericardial fluid analyses.

Treatment of pericardial effusion is directed at removal of the fluid and treatment of the underlying cause. Fluid removal can be achieved by pericardiocentesis at the bedside or in the cardiac catheterization laboratory. Surgical options reserved for recurrent effusions include pericardial window or pericardial sclerosis. Before any invasive intervention, supportive treatment in the intensive care unit (ICU) is of paramount importance and should focus on intravascular volume expansion with crystalloid or colloid to sustain adequate systemic arterial pressures, optimizing cardiac output with inotropic agents such as dobutamine, and considering discontinuation of any β-blocker agents because these may blunt compensatory tachycardic responses. Application of positive pressure ventilation must be carefully done because increased intrathoracic pressure can lead to significant decrease in ventricular preload and cardiac output.

The indications for pericardiocentesis include hemodynamic or impending hemodynamic compromise (cardiac tamponade), an infectious etiology, or an unknown etiology.

ACUTE PERICARDITIS

Inflammation of the pericardium is largely idiopathic but may result from one of many processes: infective, vasculitic/autoimmune, metabolic, neoplastic, traumatic, postmyocardial infarction, or following cardiac surgery or radiation therapy. The pathophysiology of the disease originates from the mechanical constraint that the inflamed pericardium places on the heart.

Acute pericarditis presents with progressive, sharp, pleuritic chest pain that is generally worse in the supine position and relieved by upright sitting. This may be accompanied by fever. If moderate to severe cardiac tamponade is present, pulsus paradoxus may be appreciated on physical examination. Pericardial friction rub is pathognomonic for pericarditis, but is frequently not present. It is best heard at end-expiration with the patient leaning forward. A developing pericardial effusion may lower the intensity of the rub.

Electrocardiogram (ECG) typically shows low voltage QRS complexes caused by pericardial effusion and ST-segment elevation particularly in leads I, II, V_5, V_6. PR segment depression may accompany or precede the ST segment changes (see Fig. 33.2). The ECG changes may evolve through four phases: Stage I is marked with ST elevation with upright T waves. Stage II is marked by resolution of ST elevations. Stage III is characterized by T-wave inversion, and Stage IV is complete normalization of the ECG. These ECG changes evolve over 2 to 4 weeks.

Echocardiogram is most useful in establishing the diagnosis of pericardial effusion, usually seen both anteriorly and posteriorly. Evidence of cardiac tamponade is shown as right atrial collapse in late diastole and collapse or indentation of the right ventricle free wall.

Patients who present in stable hemodynamic status should be monitored closely because they may be at risk of acute decompensation. The compressed heart is preload-dependent and therefore optimum fluid repletion is required to maintain adequate cardiac output. Pericardiocentesis or surgical drainage of the effusion is mandatory for the establishment of diagnosis.

Urgent decompression by pericardiocentesis or surgical drainage is indicated for cardiac tamponade. While preparing for the procedure, the patient should be fluid resuscitated to increase central venous pressure, leading to cardiac filling. Urgent surgical drainage of the pericardium is indicated when purulent pericarditis is suspected and this must be followed by 4 to 6 weeks of intravenous antibiotic regimen.

Medical management of pericarditis is directed at the primary disease process (e.g., uremia, malignancy, etc.). Salicylate is used to treat precordial pain, rheumatic pericarditis, or postpericardiotomy syndrome (PPS). Corticosteroid may be indicated in patients with severe rheumatic carditis or PPS.

POSTPERICARDIOTOMY SYNDROME

PPS is believed to be an autoimmune response to damaged myocardium or pericardium and develops after a surgery involving pericardiotomy. It occurs in approximately 25% to 30% of patients after pericardiotomy and presents after a median time of 4 weeks postcardiac surgery. The nonsurgical correlate of PPS is Dressler syndrome following myocardial infarction.

PPS is characterized by fever and chest pain caused by both pericarditis and pleuritis. Tachycardia, tachypnea, rising venous pressure, decreased arterial pulse, and pulsus paradoxus may be present if the disorder is associated with cardiac tamponade. The chest radiograph shows enlarged cardiac silhouette, and ECG demonstrates ST-segment

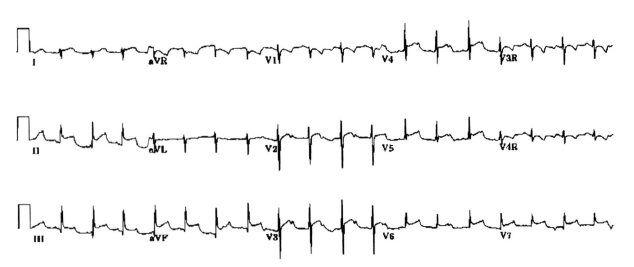

Figure 33.2 Electrocardiogram (ECG) of a 3-year-old with bacterial pericarditis. ECG shows diffuse ST segment elevation, most prominent in leads I, II, III, aVF, and V_4 to V_6. Reciprocal changes, ST depression, are present in lead aVR.

elevation and flattened or inverted T waves in the limb leads and left precordial leads. Echocardiogram confirms the presence and size of effusion. Laboratory data shows leukocytosis with a left shift and elevated ESR.

A nonsteroidal anti-inflammatory agent such as indomethacin or ibuprofen for 4 to 6 weeks is adequate treatment in most cases. Steroids are recommended for patients with more severe cases of PPS and large pericardial effusions. Emergency pericardiocentesis may be required if signs of cardiac tamponade are present. Diuretics may be used for pleural effusions. Although the prognosis is good, patients with recurrences may need pericardiectomy.

REFERENCES

1. Van Hare GF, Ben-Shachar G, Liebman J, et al. Infective endocarditis in infants and children during the past 10 years: A decade of change. *Am Heart J.* 1984;107(6):1235–1240.

2. Stockheim JA, Chadwick EG, Kessler S, et al. Are the Duke criteria superior to the Beth Israel criteria for the diagnosis of infective endocarditis in children? *Clin Infect Dis.* 1998;27(6):1451–1456.

3. Saiman L, Prince A, Gersony WM, et al. Pediatric infective endocarditis in the modern era. *J Pediatr.* 1993;122(6):847–853.

4. Ferrieri P, Gewitz MH, Gerber MA, et al. Unique features of infective endocarditis in childhood. *Circulation.* 2002;105(17):2115–2126.

5. Heiro M, Nikoskelainen J, Engblom E, et al. Neurologic manifestations of infective endocarditis: A 17-year experience in a teaching hospital in Finland. *Arch Intern Med.* 2000;160(18):2781–2787.

6. Bayer AS, Bolger AF, Taubert KA, et al. Diagnosis and management of infective endocarditis and its complications. *Circulation.* 1998;98(25):2936–2948.

7. Piper C, Wiemer M, Schulte HD, et al. Stroke is not a contraindication for urgent valve replacement in acute infective endocarditis. *J Heart Valve Dis.* 2001;10(6):703–711.

8. Filsoufi, F, Adams DH. *Surgical treatment of mitral valve endocarditis.* New York: McGraw-Hill; 2003.

Dysrhythmias

34

Jeffrey P. Moak

Disorders of cardiac rhythm are frequently observed in the pediatric intensive care unit (PICU), thereby making it imperative for the intensivist to be familiar with the techniques of diagnosis and treatment of the more common arrhythmias observed in this setting because consultation with a cardiologist or cardiac electrophysiologist may not be readily available.

Once an arrhythmia is recognized, it is important to obtain a 15-lead electrocardiogram (ECG). Analysis of cardiac rhythm disorders, solely from a bedside rhythm strip, is limited and will frequently result in the misclassification of the arrhythmia. Simultaneously, a careful assessment of the patient's hemodynamic state will determine the urgency and type of therapy. Therapy may be required because the cardiac arrhythmia actively impairs the hemodynamic state of the patient or, despite being hemodynamically stable, the arrhythmia may pose some future risk for an adverse cardiac event.

From the 15-lead ECG, the physician needs to evaluate several key features (see Figs. 34.1 and 34.2). First, the clinician should determine the atrial rate, P wave morphology, and regularity. If P waves are difficult to determine on the 15-lead ECG, a number of maneuvers are useful. The Lewis lead is a special bipolar chest lead that amplifies P wave activity. It is recorded by placing the right arm electrode in the second intercostal space to the right of the sternum, and the left arm electrode in the fourth intercostal space to the right of the sternum. The P wave will then be evident on ECG lead I. Additionally, a transesophageal recording catheter may be placed to record atrial activity. An estimate of the depth of insertion is made by externally measuring the distance from the external nares to the xiphisternum. Once inserted to the estimated depth, a bipolar electrogram is recorded, using the right and left arm electrodes from the electrocardiographic recorder. The esophageal atrial electrogram will be best observed on ECG lead I, but can as well be visualized on all the frontal plane leads (see Fig. 34.3).

A final technique is to administer adenosine to induce transient atrioventricular (AV) block to view atrial electrical activity in the absence of ventricular activity (see Fig. 34.4.).

Second, the ventricular rate, regularity and QRS morphology, and duration must be assessed. If a wide QRS with bundle branch block is present, then whether it is a right or a left bundle branch block should be determined. Third, the relationship between atrial and ventricular activity should be evaluated. Abnormalities such as interventricular conduction block (bundle branch block) may make it more difficult to derive the correct diagnosis solely from the ECG.

BRADYARRHYTHMIAS

Sinus Node Dysfunction

Bradycardia is the most common arrhythmia seen in the PICU, and results from either sinus node dysfunction or AV block. Manifestations of sinus node dysfunction include sinus bradycardia, severe sinus arrhythmia, sinus pauses, sinus arrest, slow escape rhythms, and sinoatrial exit block. Disorders of sinus node automaticity or conduction may be primary or secondary to autonomic nervous system imbalance or drug effects (see Table 34.1). Sinus node dysfunction may result in hemodynamic compromise. In most patients, a subsidiary pacemaker will take control of the cardiac rhythm (low atrial, junctional, or ventricular focus), preventing the development of overt symptoms. Other manifestations of sinus node dysfunction include a secondary tachycardia in the atrium (e.g., tachycardia-bradycardia syndrome) or other arrhythmias such as supraventricular tachycardia (SVT), atrial flutter, or atrial fibrillation. Atrial bradycardia may also result in excessive prolongation of the QT interval, premature ventricular contractions (PVCs), and ventricular tachycardia (VT) or fibrillation.

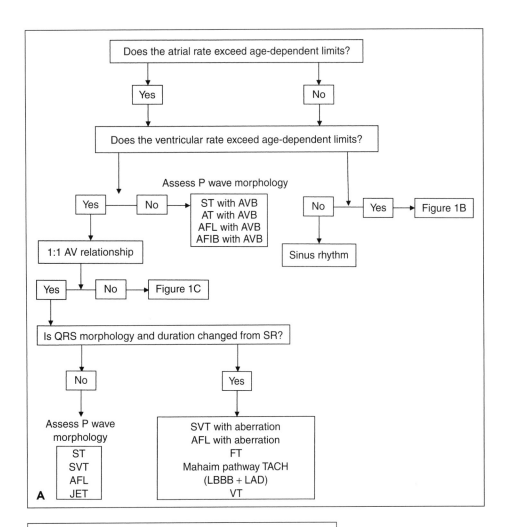

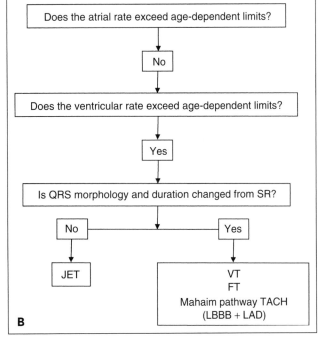

Figure 34.1 Algorithm for diagnosis of tachyarrhythmias. AFIB, atrial fibrillation; AFL, atrial flutter; AT, atrial tachycardia; AV, atrial to ventricular relationship; AVB, atrioventricular block; FT, fascicular tachycardia; JET, junctional ectopic tachycardia; LBBB + LAD, left bundle branch block and left axis deviation; SR, sinus rhythm; SVT, supraventricular tachycardia; TACH, tachycardia; VT, ventricular tachycardia; w, with; ST, sinus tachycardia.

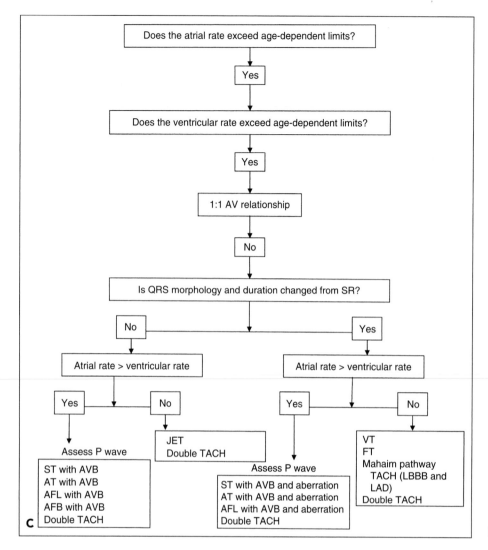

Figure 34.1   (*continued*)

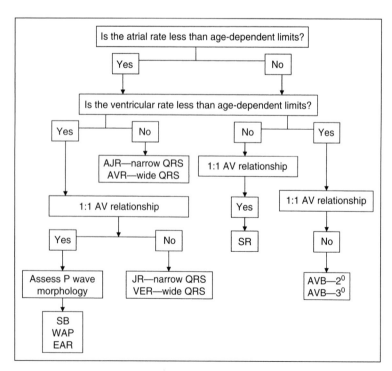

Figure 34.2 Algorithm for diagnosis of bradyarrhythmias. AJR, accelerated junctional rhythm; AVR, accelerated ventricular rhythm; AV, atrial to ventricular relationship; AVB, atrioventricular block; EAR, ectopic atrial rhythm; JR, junctional rhythm; SB, sinus bradycardia; SR, sinus rhythm; VER, ventricular escape rhythm; WAP, wandering atrial pacemaker.

Treatment is directed at the underlying precipitant, particularly if the patient is asymptomatic. If no acutely reversible cause is identified and the patient is unstable, acute emergency medical treatment includes intravenous atropine (0.01 to 0.04 mg per kg) or isoproterenol (0.01 to 0.1 mg/kg/minute). Placement of a temporary transvenous or transesophageal pacemaker is indicated in the symptomatic patient who does not respond to medical treatment.

Atrioventricular Block

AV block is defined as a block or prolongation in the time interval for an electrical impulse originating in the atrium (sinus node) to reach the ventricle, and result in ventricular depolarization. AV block can occur within the atrium,

AV node, bundle of His, or a combination of sites and is classified as first, second, and third degree. Major causes of AV block are listed in Table 34.2. First-degree AV block is defined as a prolongation of the AV conduction time of all impulses being conducted to the ventricles. It usually does not result in hemodynamic impairment or symptoms, nor does it require specific therapy. In the setting of an evolving disease such as Lyme carditis, patients with first-degree AV block warrant monitoring for development of more advanced block. First-degree AV block may result in decreased cardiac output in the patient with severe left ventricular dysfunction.

Second-degree AV block is defined as the failure of some, but not all, impulses to be conducted from the atrium to the ventricles. It is subdivided into Mobitz type I and II. The number of atrial beats that are conducted

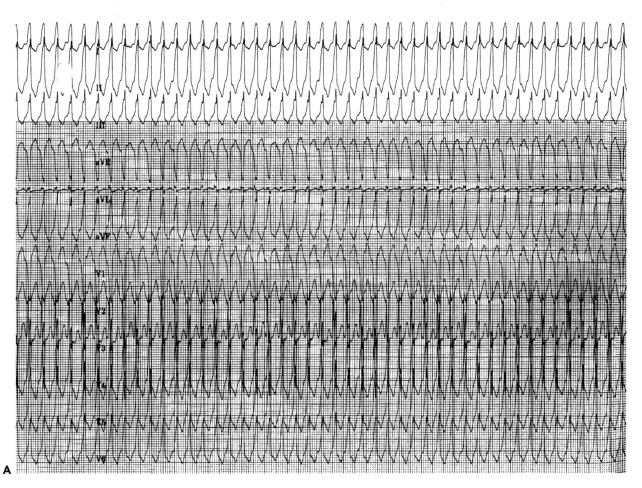

Figure 34.3 Utility of esophageal atrial electrogram to assist in arrhythmia diagnosis. **A:** Twelve-lead electrocardiogram (ECG) revealed wide complex tachycardia for age (left bundle branch block [LBBB] and normal axis, with ventricular rate = 250 per minute). Atrial activity was difficult to discern on the surface ECG. **B:** After placement of an esophageal catheter, atrial activity was easily observed (*arrows*). The atrial rate = 160 per minute, which was higher than normal for age. The ventricular rate = 250 per minute, also greater than normal for age. Atrial to ventricular relationship was not 1:1. QRS morphology differed from sinus rhythm (prolonged QRS duration in patient with normal heart). Ventricular rate exceeded atrial rate, therefore diagnosis was most consistent with double tachycardia = ventricular tachycardia and sinus tachycardia.

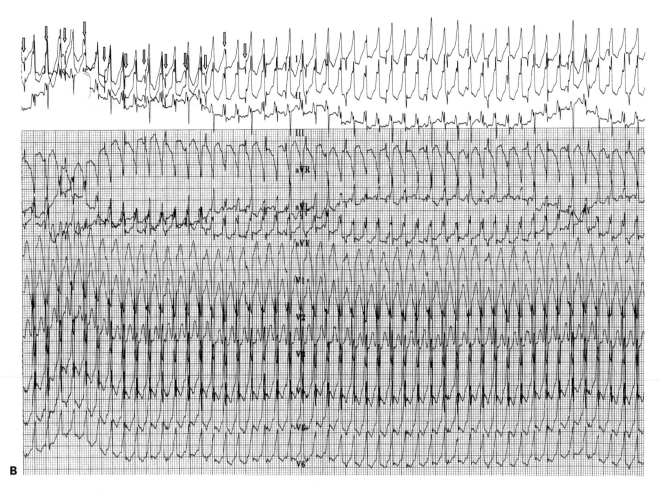

Figure 34.3   *(continued)*

to the ventricles is expressed as the AV conduction ratio. In Mobitz type I, second-degree AV block, also referred to as Wenckebach block, there is a progressive prolongation of the PR interval before a nonconducted P wave. Typical Wenckebach periodicity has the following characteristics: (i) the maximum increase in the PR interval occurs between the first and second conducted beats in a series, (ii) each successive PR interval lengthens, (iii) successive RR intervals shorten, and (iv) the pause created by the blocked P wave is less than twice the preceding RR interval. However, most Mobitz type I, second-degree blocks are atypical. Mobitz type I, second-degree block is associated with diseases affecting the AV node. Increased parasympathetic tone and medications are the most frequent causes. In Mobitz type II, second-degree AV block, the PR interval is constant. Mobitz type II, second-degree AV block is associated with diseases of the bundle of His and bundle branches and frequently progresses to complete heart block. In patients with 2:1 block, differentiating type I from type II is not possible. Type II block should be suspected in patients with a wide QRS complex, syncope, or structural heart disease.

Third-degree AV block is complete lack of transmission of atrial impulses to the ventricles. Long rhythm strips must be examined to be certain that atrial impulses do not conduct to the ventricle. If even occasional atrial impulses conduct, this is classified as advanced second-degree AV block (see Fig. 34.5). Third-degree or complete AV block is associated with either a junctional or ventricular escape rhythm. Patients who do not demonstrate an escape rhythm are dependent on a pacemaker.

The management of heart block is influenced by the patient's age, hemodynamic status, and whether the block is congenital or acquired. Treatment should be directed at the underlying cause. Acute medical treatment should be attempted with intravenous atropine (0.01 to 0.04 mg per kg) or isoproterenol (0.01 to 0.1 mg/kg/minute) for symptomatic patients. If the patient does not respond to medical therapy or has continuing hemodynamic compromise, temporary ventricular pacing should be instituted. Permanent pacing for complete heart block is indicated for a blocks that persist for more than 10 to 14 days after cardiac surgery, in patients with symptoms or an inadequate ventricular escape rate.

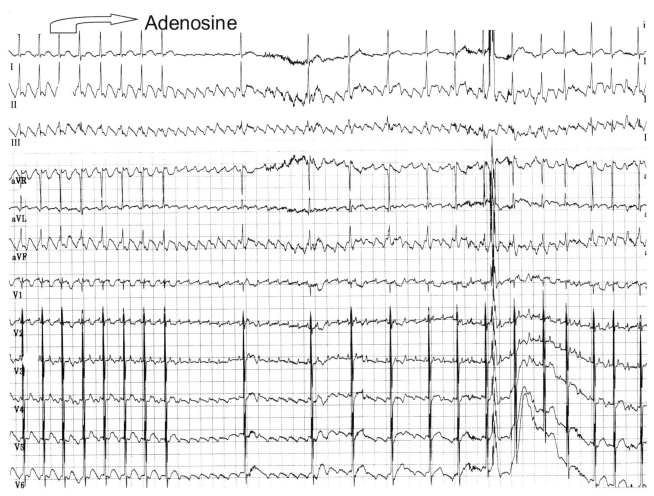

Figure 34.4 Utility of adenosine to assist in arrhythmia diagnosis. Transient complete atrioventricular (AV) block follows intravenous bolus administration of adenosine, allowing visualization of atrial activity without superimposed ventricular complexes. The atrial rate = 350 per minute, which was higher than normal for age. The ventricular rate = 165 per minute, also greater than normal for age. Atrial to ventricular relationship was not 1:1. QRS morphology was normal. Since atrial rate exceeds ventricular rate and characteristic sawtooth pattern of P wave morphology was evident on the surface electrocardiogram (ECG), the diagnosis was consistent with atrial flutter and second-degree AV block.

TACHYARRHYTHMIAS

Sinus Tachycardia

Sinus tachycardia is an arrhythmia that originates from the sinus node complex. The P wave morphology during sinus tachycardia has the same mean vector and a similar but not necessarily identical morphology to the P wave during normal sinus rhythm. In general, the heart rate during sinus tachycardia should be <220 beats per minute in an infant, and <180 beats per minute in a child. Major causes of sinus tachycardia include fever, hypovolemia, myocardial dysfunction, thyrotoxicosis, anemia, and pain. Persistent sinus tachycardia in the setting of dilated cardiomyopathy needs to be distinguished from an incessant ectopic atrial

tachycardia from the right atrial appendage. In ectopic atrial tachycardia, the P wave morphology in ECG lead V_1 is completely negative.[1] Treatment should be directed at the underlying cause. Very rarely, β-blockers (intravenous propranolol or esmolol) or a calcium channel blocker (intravenous diltiazem) can be administered to slow the heart rate.

Supraventricular Tachycardia

Re-entrant Supraventricular Tachycardia

SVT is any rapid regular tachyarrhythmia resulting from an abnormal mechanism originating above the bifurcation of the bundle of His. Re-entry and automaticity are the two underlying electrophysiologic mechanisms that

TABLE 34.1
CAUSES OF SINUS NODE DYSFUNCTION

Secondary Causes (Most Common in the PICU Setting)

Metabolic

Hypoxemia
Hypothyroidism
Hypothermia
Hypercalcemia
Hyperkalemia
Hypovolemia
Congenital homocystinuria

Hypervagotonia

Idiopathic
Nasopharyngeal stimulation/gastroesophageal reflux
Endurance athletes
Coughing/swallowing/vomiting/endotracheal tube stimulation
Breath holding/apnea
Increased intracranial pressure
Sleep
Baroreflex: increased blood pressure
Abdominal distention

Medications

Parasympathomimetic effects and side effects
Antiarrhythmic agents

Miscellaneous

Obstructive jaundice
Myocardial ischemia

Primary causes

Nonsurgical

Idiopathic/congenital
Familial: SCN5A defect in the sodium channel
Congenital heart disease: sinus venous ASD
Neuromuscular disease
　Emery-Dreifuss muscular dystrophy
　Guillain-Barré
　Friedreich ataxia
Inflammatory disorders of the heart: myocarditis/pericarditis
Long QT syndrome

Surgical

Congenital heart disease: postoperative atrial surgery (sinus venous ASD, bidirectional Glenn procedure, Mustard/Senning procedure)

PICU, pediatric intensive care unit; ASD, atrial septal defect.

TABLE 34.2
CAUSES OF ATRIOVENTRICULAR BLOCK

Acute Causes

Metabolic

Hypoxemia
Hypothermia
Hypercalcemia/hypocalcemia
Hyperkalemia/hypokalemia
Hypoglycemia

Hypervagotonia

Idiopathic
Nasopharyngeal stimulation/gastroesophageal reflux
Endurance athletes
Coughing/swallowing/vomiting/endotracheal tube stimulation
Breath holding/apnea
Increased intracranial pressure
Sleep
Baroreflex: increased blood pressure
Abdominal distention

Medications

Parasympathomimetic effects and side effects
Antiarrhythmic agents

Inflammatory/Infectious Disorders of the Heart

Myocarditis/endocarditis
Rheumatic fever, Lyme disease

Miscellaneous

Myocardial ischemia

Chronic Causes

Congenital: neonatal lupus syndrome
Familial inherited conduction system disease
Acquired/genetic: SCN5A defect in the sodium channel
Congenital heart disease: ASD, L-TGA
Neuromuscular disease
　Emery-Dreifuss muscular dystrophy
　Duchenne muscular dystrophy
　Myotonic dystrophy
Long QT syndrome
Postoperative after repair of congenital heart disease, especially any procedure involving VSD closure
Cardiomyopathy
Myocardial infarction
Inflammatory/infectious disorders of the heart, connective tissue disease, sarcoidosis
Tumors: mesothelioma, rhabdomyoma
Radiation

ASD, atrial septal defect; L-TGA, L-transposition of the great arteries; VSD, ventricular septal defect.

result in SVT in children (see Tables 34.3 and 34.4). SVT is the most common tachyarrhythmia in children, with an estimated incidence between 1 in 250 and 1 in 1,000 children.[2] Atrioventricular re-entry tachycardia (AVRT) or atrioventricular nodal re-entry tachycardia (AVNRT) can have its onset at any age during childhood, with 40% to 60% presenting by the age of 4 months. Most children with SVT have a structurally normal heart, but 20% to 30% have congenital heart disease. Congestive heart failure (CHF) at the time of presentation is observed in 20% to 25% of patients. If SVT persists untreated for at least 36 hours, CHF will develop in approximately 20% of patients, and if allowed to continue for more than 48 hours, 50% develop heart

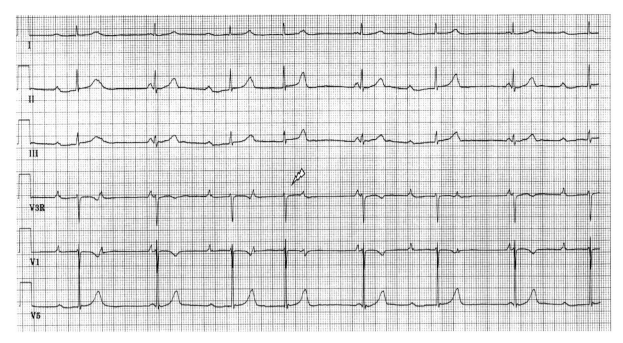

Figure 34.5 Advanced second-degree atrioventricular (AV) block. At first glance, the rhythm strip might be interpreted as third-degree AV block without a consistent relationship between the P waves and QRS complexes. However, the fourth QRS complex (*lightening bolt*) appears significantly earlier than would be anticipated if there was complete AV dissociation. The rhythm strip demonstrates advanced second-degree AV block.

failure. CHF rarely develops in the first 24 hours. Other symptoms include palpitations and lightheadedness. If an accessory pathway can conduct impulses antegrade during sinus rhythm, the ECG will show a δ (i.e., pre-excitation) wave. If a δ wave is not seen, the pathway is concealed.

TABLE 34.3
MECHANISM OF SUPRAVENTRICULAR TACHYCARDIA IN CHILDREN

Re-entry with Bypass Tract

Wolff-Parkinson-White syndrome
Mahaim "atriofascicular" accessory pathway
Concealed retrograde only conducting accessory pathway
Permanent form of junctional reciprocating tachycardia

Re-entry without Bypass Tract

Sinus node re-entry
AV node re-entry
Atrial muscle re-entry (micro–re-entry)
His bundle re-entry

Automatic Ectopic Focus

Atrial
Chaotic atrial tachycardia
Junctional
Fascicular

AV, atrioventricular.

Sinus rhythm can be restored using nonpharmacologic techniques or intravenous drug therapy. If the episode of SVT has resulted in hemodynamic compromise or shock, immediate termination using synchronized direct current (DC) electrical cardioversion should be performed (0.25 to 1.0 J per kg). Nonpharmacologic techniques for treatment of SVT include: (i) elicitation of the diving reflex by either facial immersion in cold water (5°C to 15°C) or the brief application of an ice bag (<15 seconds); (ii) vagal maneuvers including carotid sinus massage, gagging, coughing, or the Valsalva maneuver; (iii) esophageal or atrial overdrive pacing; or (iv) synchronized DC electrical cardioversion. Acute pharmacologic termination of SVT is directed at slowing or blocking conduction in the AV node using adenosine, propranolol, verapamil, diltiazem, or amiodarone. Calcium channel blockers should be avoided in children below 6 months of age. Intravenous therapy aimed at slowing atrial, ventricular, or accessory pathway conduction may be attempted using procainamide or amiodarone.

Atrial Ectopic Tachycardia

Atrial ectopic tachycardia (AET) is a SVT caused by an autonomic focus. The ECG shows a regular narrow complex tachycardia with a P wave morphology significantly different from sinus rhythm. Most patients have structurally normal hearts. Patients may present with CHF and secondary cardiomyopathy, which resolves with control of the arrhythmia. AET is often resistant to medical management.

TABLE 34.4

DETERMINATION OF SUPRAVENTRICULAR TACHYCARDIA MECHANISM FROM SURFACE ELECTROCARDIOGRAM

	P Wave					PR/RR		
	Not Visible	NL Axis 1:1	NL Axis and AV Dissociation	Inverted	Left Atrium	<0.50	0.51–0.79	>0.8
Re-entrant Tachycardias								
SNRT		+					+	
AMRT		+	+	+	+	+	+	
AVNRT	+							+
WPW		+		+	+			+
Concealed AP		+		+	+			+
Automatic Focus Tachycardias								
AET		+	+	+	+	+	+	
JET	+		+	+				
PJRT				+		+		

1:1, 1:1 AV conduction; +, suggestive of diagnosis; AET, atrial ectopic tachycardia; AMRT, atrial muscle re-entry tachycardia; AP, accessory pathway; AVNRT, atrioventricular nodal re-entry tachycardia; JET, junctional ectopic tachycardia; PJRT, permanent form of junctional reciprocating tachycardia; SNRT, sinus node re-entry tachycardia; WPW, Wolff-Parkinson-White.

Treatment with digoxin or β-blockers is often ineffective but may improve hemodynamics by decreasing the ventricular rate. Amiodarone, sotalol, or flecainide may be required for long-term management. Neither cardioversion, adenosine, nor overdrive pacing terminate this arrhythmia.

Atrial Flutter

Atrial flutter, sometimes referred to as an intra-atrial re-entrant tachycardia (IART), is a macro–re-entrant arrhythmia circuit that is usually confined to the right atrium, but may occur alone in the left atrium or incorporate both the right and left atria. The differentiation of IART from a micro–re-entrant tachycardia (atrial muscle re-entrant tachycardia) and other SVTs can be achieved using intravenous adenosine. Adenosine results in transient high-degree AV block revealing flutter waves, the rate of which is unaffected (Fig. 34.4). Atrial flutter can present in one of four typical situations (i) hydropic newborn with intrauterine tachycardia, (ii) infant with an otherwise normal heart, (iii) older child with pre- or postoperative congenital heart disease or dilated cardiomyopathy, and (iv) as a manifestation of cardiac rejection in the post-transplantation patient. The rate of IART can range from 280 to 450 per minute. Long-term antiarrhythmic medication may markedly slow atrial conduction enough to result in IART rates as slow as 120 to 200 beats per minute, making it difficult to differentiate this arrhythmia from sinus tachycardia or SVT.

The classic electrocardiographic pattern of atrial flutter is a sawtooth or picket fence appearance, most prominently observed in ECG leads II, III, aVF, and V_1 (initial negative P waves in the inferior leads). Other ECG patterns reflect alternative atrial activation patterns that may result from scar-related arrhythmias from previous cardiac surgery, or atrial remodeling due to volume or pressure overload. AV conduction in atrial flutter is frequently variable (Mobitz type I, second-degree AV block), and therefore results in an irregular ventricular rate. The most common AV conduction ratio is 2:1. The second flutter wave is often concealed by the QRS complex leading to the conclusion that the rhythm is sinus tachycardia, making this the most misdiagnosed arrhythmia.

Atrial flutter may be terminated using nonpharmacologic techniques or intravenous drug therapy. Treatment based on nonpharmacologic techniques include atrial overdrive pacing or synchronized DC electrical cardioversion (0.5 to 1.0 J per kg). If atrial flutter is associated with a rapid ventricular rate because of 1:1 AV conduction, slowing of the ventricular rate immediately may be desirable and can be achieved using intravenous pharmacologic agents that reduce AV node conduction such as calcium channel blockers, β-blockers, amiodarone, and digoxin. Intravenous therapy aimed at terminating atrial flutter by prolonging atrial refractoriness may be attempted using ibutilide or procainamide. If atrial flutter has persisted for more than 48 hours in a patient with heart disease, a transesophageal echocardiogram needs to be performed to document the absence of atrial thrombi (right or left atrium). If atrial clots are documented, cardioversion of the arrhythmia should be deferred until after 3 to 4 weeks of adequate anticoagulation. Postcardioversion, adequate anticoagulation should be given for at least 1 month depending on the clinical setting.

Atrial Fibrillation

Atrial fibrillation presents as a spectrum of rapid arrhythmia disorders that vary in the pattern of disorganization and regularity. Atrial rates vary typically from 400 to 700 per minute. Atrial fibrillation seems to result from multiple simultaneous wave fronts traveling in a chaotic and random manner. However, more sophisticated mathematical analyses can demonstrate a dominant frequency of electrical activation during atrial fibrillation. The surface ECG shows high-frequency "fibrillatory" waves without a true isoelectric baseline, and irregular and highly variable QRS to QRS intervals. Recent experience demonstrates that an ectopic pacemaker cell, firing irregularly from the pulmonary veins is the most common etiology underlying atrial fibrillation. Rarely atrial fibrillation may originate from the right atrium or atrial septum. Atrial fibrillation is rare in pediatric patients, and occurs in one of the following four clinical settings: (i) the older child or adolescent with Wolff-Parkinson-White syndrome, (ii) late adolescent or young adult with complex structural heart disease and residual hemodynamic abnormalities, (iii) the late adolescent or young adult with dilated cardiomyopathy, and (iv) the late adolescent or young adult with a structurally normal heart with "lone" paroxysmal atrial fibrillation.

Acute treatment is similar to atrial flutter. Nonpharmacologic techniques for treatment of atrial fibrillation are restricted to synchronized DC electrical cardioversion (1.5 to 4 J per kg). The careful placement of electrode patches or paddles, particularly in the anteroposterior position can improve success rates for cardioversion. If atrial fibrillation is associated with a rapid ventricular rate, immediate slowing of the ventricular rate may be desirable and can be achieved using intravenous agents that reduce AV node conduction such as calcium channel blockers, β-blockers, amiodarone, or digoxin. Intravenous therapy aimed at prolonging atrial refractoriness may be attempted using ibutilide or procainamide to convert the arrhythmia. Deliberate attention to anticoagulation is mandatory because of the high risk of left atrial thrombi and cerebral embolic events in patients with atrial fibrillation. Anticoagulation with heparin should be started immediately. Before attempting electrical or pharmacologic cardioversion, careful consideration needs to be given to the duration of the arrhythmia. If atrial fibrillation has persisted for more than 48 hours, a transesophageal echocardiogram needs to be performed to document absence of atrial thrombi. If atrial clots are documented, cardioversion of the arrhythmia should be delayed until after 3 to 4 weeks of adequate anticoagulation has been administered. Postcardioversion, adequate anticoagulation needs to be prescribed to all patients for a 1- to 6-month period.

Junctional Ectopic Tachycardia

Junctional ectopic tachycardia (JET) is another subtype of SVT that results from an ectopic focus in the AV node–His bundle region. JET occurs typically either in infants with a congenital (familial) form, which may be related to neonatal lupus syndrome or in the immediate postoperative period following intracardiac repair of congenital heart disease. The rhythm is an incessant tachycardia characterized by a narrow complex QRS or one that is unchanged from baseline. JET may occur in association with 1:1 ventricular–atrial (VA) conduction, retrograde Wenckebach VA conduction or VA dissociation (see Fig. 34.6).

Postoperative JET is associated with slower patient recovery and increased intensive care unit (ICU) length of stay. The rhythm usually resolves spontaneously (48 to 96 hours) and does not require long-term therapy. The protracted periods of very high heart rates and the loss of AV synchrony result in decreased ventricular filling and low cardiac output. JET occurs most frequently after the repair of tetralogy of Fallot (22%), and less commonly after the surgical repair of AV septal defect (10%) and ventricular septal defect (4%).[3] Resection of muscle bundles, higher bypass temperatures, and a transatrial approach for the relief of right ventricular outflow tract obstruction, each one by themselves, predicted postoperative JET. Other factors include operative procedures involving ventricular septal defect closure or younger age.

Postoperative JET is resistant to cardioversion and frequently refractory to most antiarrhythmic agents. In hemocompromised patients, treatment is largely supportive and is aimed at slowing the heart rate and restoring AV synchrony with temporary pacing. General support measures include: (i) adequate sedation to decrease stress-induced catecholamine release, (ii) correction of metabolic and electrolyte abnormalities, (iii) avoidance and prompt correction of hyperthermia, and (iv) limitation of the administration of positive inotropic agents. If these measures are inadequate, the heart is slowed using moderate hypothermia (rectal temperature between 33°C and 35°C) and/or administration of intravenous amiodarone or procainamide. In our experience, intravenous procainamide has been associated with greater morbidity than amiodarone. The treatment goal is to achieve a stable decrease in the ventricular rate below 140 to 150 per minute, allowing the possibility of atrial pacing to restore AV synchrony and improvement of cardiac output. Extracorporeal-membrane oxygenation (ECMO) or catheter ablation of the His bundle is rarely necessary.

VENTRICULAR ARRHYTHMIAS

Ventricular Tachycardia

VT is defined as a series of three or more repetitive ventricular complexes at a rate >120 beats per minute.

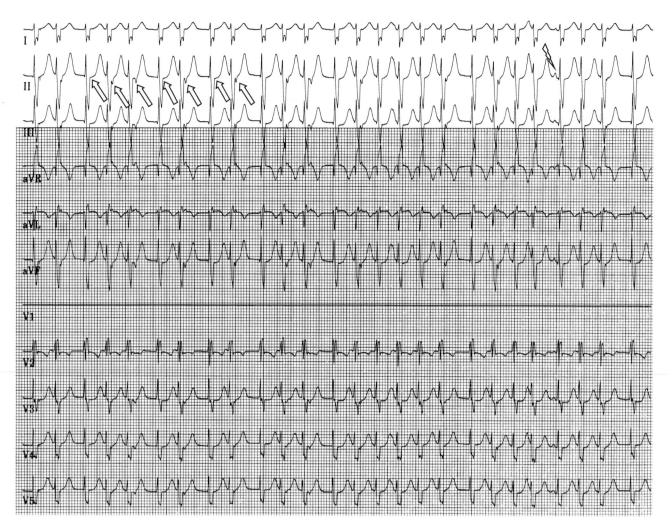

Figure 34.6 Junctional ectopic tachycardia associated with periods of retrograde decremental ventricular to atrial conduction (lengthening conduction time between ventricle and atrium; *arrows*) and AV dissociation with sinus capture beats (*lightening bolt*).

Because the origin of the ventricular complexes differs from sinus rhythm, the QRS is prolonged or "wide" for age (>90 millisecond up to age 4 years and >100 millisecond from 4 to 16 years). The following ECG features aid in the diagnosis of ventricular tachycardias (i) AV dissociation; (ii) intermittent sinus capture or fusion beats; and (iii) the similarity of the morphology of VT with that of single PVCs (see Fig. 34.7). The differential diagnosis of wide complex tachycardia includes VT and SVT in a patient with known bundle branch block, or SVT with aberration. In one series of 124 children presenting with SVT, only 2.4% of patients exhibited *de novo* aberrant ventricular conduction, and right bundle branch block was more common than left bundle branch block. Because SVT with aberration is so rare in children, VT should be strongly suspected unless there is a known bundle branch block. Acute and chronic conditions responsible for causing VT are listed

in Table 34.5. VT in children most often develops in association with metabolic disturbances, medications, and myocardial injury (myocarditis).

If the episode of VT has resulted in hemodynamic compromise, immediate termination using synchronized DC electrical cardioversion should be employed (0.5 to 1.0 J per kg). If the patient's hemodynamic status is stable, intravenous termination can be attempted using lidocaine, amiodarone, or procainamide. It is not recommended that amiodarone and procainamide be used simultaneously, because both may prolong the QT interval.

Torsade-de-Pointes Ventricular Tachycardia

Torsade-de-pointes VT is a multiform VT that develops in the setting of prolonged QT interval, whether congenital or acquired. The polarity of QRS complexes changes

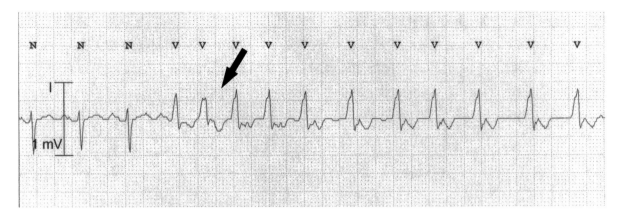

Figure 34.7 Ventricular tachycardia (VT). Atrioventricular dissociation is evident during the first two beats of VT (*arrow*).

TABLE 34.5
CAUSES OF VENTRICULAR TACHYCARDIA

Acute

Hypoxemia
Acidemia
Hypoglycemia
Hyperkalemia/hypokalemia
Myocarditis/endocarditis
Myocardial damage: immediate following cardiac surgery, chest
  trauma
Myocardial ischemia
Decompensated congestive heart failure
Intracardiac catheters
Medications
  Anesthetic agents
  Sympathomimetics: decongestants, cocaine
  Antiarrhythmic agents
  Tricyclic antidepressant overdose
  Digitalis toxicity

Chronic

Normal heart

Right ventricular outflow tachycardia
Left ventricular outflow tachycardia
Left posterior and anterior fascicular tachycardia
Prolonged QT syndrome
Short QT syndrome
Brugada syndrome
Catecholamine sensitive polymorphic ventricular tachycardia
Neuromuscular disorders

Heart disease

Ventricular tumors
Mitral valve prolapse
Postoperative congenital heart disease
Arrhythmogenic right ventricular cardiomyopathy
Hypertrophic cardiomyopathy
Dilated cardiomyopathy
"Tinman" syndrome
Postmyocardial infarction
Bundle branch re-entry ventricular tachycardia

from one morphology to another. *Torsade-de-pointes* tends to recur and may resolve spontaneously. Infrequently, *torsade-de-pointes* degenerates into ventricular fibrillation (VF). Prompt cardioversion is performed in patients with poor hemodynamics or when the rhythm degenerates into VF. Medical therapy includes correction of electrolyte abnormalities, discontinuation of drugs that prolong the QT interval, intravenous magnesium to suppress early after-depolarizations, and maneuvers to shorten the QT duration. The QT duration may be shortened with lidocaine, increasing the serum potassium level to 4 to 4.5 mEq per L or increasing the ventricular rate with pacing or isoproterenol.

Ventricular Fibrillation

VF is a relatively rare arrhythmia in the pediatric patient. The ECG presentation reveals a series of low-amplitude, chaotic, and irregular depolarizations without any identifiable QRS complexes. At the onset of VF, the pattern observed on the surface ECG is referred to as "coarse" VF. Several minutes later, a "fine" fibrillatory pattern can be recognized on the ECG, sometimes being confused with the patterns observed during cardiac asystole; therefore multiple ECG leads need to be checked before excluding VF. VF must also be differentiated from loss of ECG electrode contact. Most children with VF have a structurally abnormal heart, myocardial disease, or a prolonged QT interval. Isoproterenol, cardiac pacing, or magnesium may be indicated as outlined in the subsequent text (see Long QT syndrome). Prompt defibrillation (2 to 4 J per kg) is the definitive treatment of an episode of VF. If after three defibrillation attempts, sinus rhythm is not restored, consideration should be given to giving epinephrine along with amiodarone. Cardiopulmonary resuscitation may aid in facilitating successful defibrillation of the heart, particularly if VF has persisted for several minutes.

SPECIAL CLINICAL SITUATIONS

On occasion, the intensivist will be involved in the initial evaluation and stabilization of a child or adolescent who has had a recent cardiac arrest episode. *Sudden cardiac death* is usually defined as the abrupt *unexpected* death from a cardiovascular cause within 6 to 12 hours of the onset of symptoms. Sudden death may happen after exercise, at rest, or during sleep. The evaluation as to a possible precipitant of the event should center on a careful history (personal and family), physical examination, ECG, echocardiogram, and 24-hour Holter. Specialized testing may be required, depending on the finding of these previously mentioned studies. Known predisposing disorders are listed in Table 34.6.[4,5]

Syncope is the sudden temporary loss of consciousness associated with the loss of postural tone. Recovery is

TABLE 34.6
CAUSES OF SUDDEN CARDIAC ARREST

Heart disease

Cardiomyopathy

Hypertrophic cardiomyopathy
Arrhythmogenic right ventricular cardiomyopathy
Dilated cardiomyopathy

Coronary artery disease

Structural coronary artery abnormalities
Myocardial infarction

Structural heart disease

Congenital heart disease
Mitral valve prolapse
Valvular heart disease
Aortic dissection

Ion channelopathies and conduction anomalies

Long QT syndrome
Conduction system disease
Brugada syndrome
Catecholamine sensitive polymorphic ventricular tachycardia
Idiopathic ventricular fibrillation
Wolff-Parkinson-White syndrome

Miscellaneous

Myocarditis
Commotio cordis

Medications

Sympathomimetics: cocaine
Antiarrhythmic agents
Tricyclic antidepressant overdose
Digitalis toxicity

Noncardiac disease

Cerebral aneurysm
Cerebral embolus
Pulmonary embolus

TABLE 34.7
CAUSES OF SYNCOPE

Cardiovascular disease

Arrhythmia

Bradyarrhythmias: sinus node dysfunction, AV block
Tachycardias: supraventricular tachycardia, atrial flutter/fibrillation with rapid AV conduction, ventricular tachycardia

Structural heart disease

Cardiomyopathy
  Hypertrophic cardiomyopathy
  Dilated cardiomyopathy
Congenital heart disease: aortic stenosis, tetralogy of Fallot
Myocardial ischemia/infarction
Cardiac tamponade
Subclavian artery steal
Atrial myxoma
Dissecting/ruptured aortic aneurysm

Paroxysmal reflex activation

Neurally mediated cardiac syncope
Micturition syncope
Deglutition syncope
Defecation syncope
Postprandial syncope
Post-tussive syncope
Hair grooming syncope
Breath holding spells

Orthostatic hypotension

Dopamine β-hydroxylase deficiency
Monoamine oxidase deficiency
Medication-induced

Neurologic disorders

Migraine
Seizure
Cerebral vascular accident
Hyperventilation
Dysautonomia
Primary autonomic failure
Autonomic neuropathy: diabetes mellitus, phorphyria, Guillain-Barré syndrome, Lisker syndrome

Others

Psychogenic
Drug-induced
Hypoglycemia
Hypoxemia
Hypoadrenalism
Hypo/hyperkalemia
Hypo/hypercalcemia
Hypo/hypermagnesemia
Pulmonary embolus
Pulmonary artery hypertension
Systemic mastocytosis
Pheocytochroma

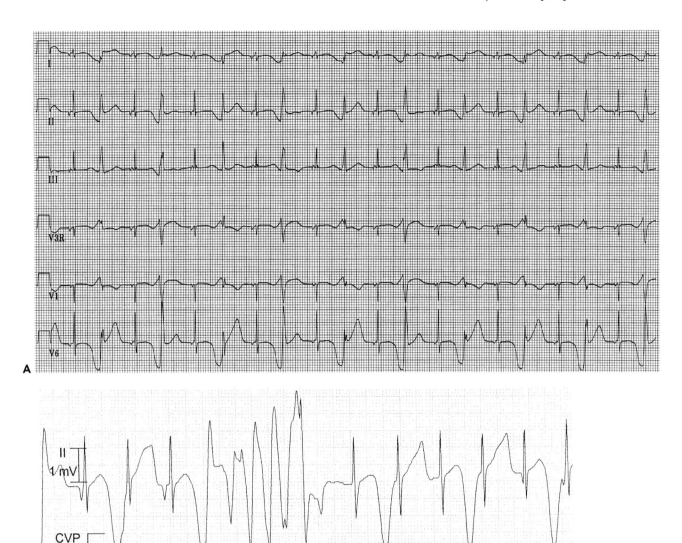

Figure 34.8 Long QT syndrome. **A:** Electrocardiogram (ECG) demonstrating marked QT prolongation with abnormal shaped T waves, and ventricular bigeminy. **B:** Same patient exhibiting periods of T wave alternans, and an episode of *torsade-de-pointes* ventricular tachycardia.

spontaneous and does not require electrical or chemical cardioversion. Syncope is a fairly common symptom, and is often recurrent. Because syncope may be a precursor to cardiac arrest, the evaluation of a patient with syncope must be considered seriously, although many of the causes of syncope have a benign prognosis. The evaluation as to a possible cause should focus on a careful history, physical examination, ECG, and echocardiogram (see Table 34.7).[6]

The long QT syndromes are a constellation of congenital ion channelopathies that result in prolongation of cardiac ventricular repolarization and a predisposition to *torsade-de-pointes* VT. The diagnosis of the congenital form of long QT syndrome is difficult because of borderline ECG findings (see Fig. 34.8). A scoring system has been developed to aid in diagnosis. Long QT syndrome should be considered in patients presenting with syncope, unexplained drowning, or sudden cardiac death. The intensivist is more likely to be faced with caring for children with acquired prolongation of the QT interval, which is also associated with increased risk of *torsade-de-pointes* (see Table 34.8).[7] Acute treatment consists of hemodynamic and electrocardiographic monitoring, discontinuing all QT-prolonging drugs, suppressing of early after-depolarizations with intravenous magnesium (30 mg per kg over 2 minutes, maximum dose is 2 g, then a continuous IV infusion 0.1 mg/kg/minute), and shortening QT duration. The QT duration may be shortened either through the administration of lidocaine, the elevation of serum potassium (4 to 4.5 mEq per L), increasing the ventricular rate by administering isoproterenol or by pacing to a heart rate of 100 to 140 per minute.

TABLE 34.8

LONG QT SYNDROMES

Genetic forms: LQT1-LQT7

Acquired forms:

Medications

Antiarrhythmic: quinidine, procainamide, disopyramide, ibutilide, amiodarone, azimilde, dofetilide, sotalol, propafenone

Antimicrobial/antifungal: erythromycin, clarithromycin, grepafloxacin, amoxifloxacin, levofloxacin, pentamidine, amantadine, chloroquine, trimethoprim–sulfamethoxazole, ketoconazole, itraconazole, halofantrine

Psychotropics: haloperidol, tricyclic antidepressants, risperidone, quetiapine, pimozide, lithium

Others: tacrolimus, droperidol, methadone

Electrolyte imbalance: hypokalemia, hypomagnesemia, hypocalcemia

Toxins: arsenic, organophosphorus compounds

Severe bradycardia: sinus node dysfunction, AV block

Neurologic: subarachnoid hemorrhage, stroke, autonomic neuropathy

Others: HIV, protein sparing diet, hypothermia, hypothyroidism

HIV, human immunodeficiency virus; AV, atrioventricular.

REFERENCES

1. Gelb BD, Garson A. Noninvasive discrimination of right atrial ectopic tachycardia from sinus tachycardia in "dilated cardiomyopathy". *Am Heart J*. 1990;120:886–891.
2. Garson A, Gillette PC, McNamara DG. Supraventricular tachycardia in children: Clinical features, response to treatment, and long-term follow-up in 217 patients. *J Pediatr*. 1981;98:875–882.
3. Dodge-Khatami A, Miller OI, Anderson RH, et al. Surgical substrates of postoperative junctional ectopic tachycardia in congenital heart defects. *J Thorac Cardiovasc Surg*. 2002;123:624–630.
4. Eckart RE, Scoville SL, Campbell CL, et al. Sudden death in young adults: A 25-year review of autopsies in military recruits. *Ann Int Med*. 2004;141:829–834.
5. Estes NAM, Saleem DN, Wang PJ, eds. *Sudden cardiac death in the athlete*. Armonk, New York: Futura Publishing; 1998.
6. Grubb BP, Olshansky B, eds. *Syncope: Mechanisms and management*. Armonk, New York: Futura Publishing; 1998.
7. Chiang CE. Congenital and acquired long QT syndrome. Current concepts and management. *Cardiol Rev*. 2004;12:222–234.

Pacemakers

35

Russell R. Cross   Jeffrey P. Moak

Pacemakers are increasingly common in the pediatric critical care setting in both the permanent and temporary forms. It is important to understand the principles of pacemaker function to efficiently program and use pacemakers for emergency indications, as well as to recognize when a pacemaker does not function properly.

INDICATIONS FOR PACING

The indications for temporary cardiac pacing follow from the indications for permanent pacemakers.[1] Pacemakers are generally indicated in patients who have or who are at risk of hemodynamic compromise from sinus node dysfunction, atrioventricular (AV) conduction abnormalities, or certain tachyarrhythmias, for which overdrive pacing can be beneficial (see Table 35.1). Patients who have undergone cardiac surgery or catheterization are at risk for various conduction disturbances resulting from direct myocardial tissue destruction or temporary injury, electrolyte

abnormalities, or increased adrenergic tone. Other pediatric conditions that can result in the need for pacing include endocarditis, myocarditis, cardiomyopathies, drug intoxications, and rarely, myocardial infarctions. Temporary pacing to achieve optimal hemodynamics and/or stability may be needed in cardiac trauma, overwhelming sepsis, other systemic illnesses, certain electrolyte abnormalities (hyperkalemia), or drug toxicities (digoxin, tricyclic antidepressants). Patients with certain tachyarrhythmias may benefit from overdrive (suppression) pacing of the atrium at a rate that is slightly faster than that of the tachyarrhythmia. Suppression pacing may also be useful in certain forms of ventricular tachycardia, *torsades de pointes*, and prolonged QT syndrome to prevent extra ventricular systoles, which can have negative hemodynamic effects.

PACEMAKER TYPES AND TECHNIQUES

Pacemaker systems are composed of the pacemaker generator and lead systems. The generator produces pacing pulses at the desired rate and output and has the capacity to sense intrinsic cardiac activity. The lead system conveys the energy to and from the heart. Permanent pacemakers are implanted subcutaneously. Leads are connected to the generator and they reach the heart either intravascularly for endocardial attachment or subcutaneously for epicardial attachment. The generator has an internal power supply that will typically last for 4 to 7 years. Programming and evaluation of the device is performed using a telemetry wand connected to a programmer, which is capable of emitting and receiving radiofrequency pulses.

With temporary pacemakers, the generator device is located outside the body, and various means are used to deliver the electrical impulse to the heart. The most readily available device for emergency use is the transcutaneous pacemaker, which uses large electrode pads attached directly to the chest wall. The pads are typically placed in an

TABLE 35.1
INDICATIONS FOR TEMPORARY PACING

Indications for Temporary Pacing

Sinus node dysfunction	Asystole Symptomatic sinus bradycardia
Atrioventricular conduction abnormalities	Advanced second-degree heart block Third-degree (complete) heart block Bifascicular block
Tachyarrhythmias	Atrial fibrillation or flutter Re-entrant supraventricular tachycardia Junctional ectopic tachycardia Certain ventricular tachycardias

Note that most indications are also based on evidence for hemodynamic compromise.

anteroposterior position with one pad in the midchest to the left of the sternum and the other on the left back below the scapula. An alternative anterolateral positioning may be used with the anterior pad positioned below the right clavicle and the other placed on the left lateral wall of the thorax. After the pads are adhered to the skin and attached to the pacemaker generator, the user selects the appropriate pacing rate and adjusts the output strength to the point at which electrical capture occurs. The general pacemaker setup and evaluation, described later in this chapter, should be followed. Transcutaneous pacing is currently being used as an emergency life-saving technique until more definitive pacing techniques can be established; patients often require sedation because it is so uncomfortable.

An alternative means of providing temporary pacing is through the esophagus. An esophageal pacing lead is passed into the esophagus to a position posterior to the heart for atrial pacing, or into the fundus of the stomach for ventricular pacing. The lead connected to the generator pacing at the desired rate is passed into the esophagus, and the surface electrocardiogram is observed for evidence of atrial or ventricular capture. If no capture is observed, the pacemaker output should be increased and the esophageal lead repositioned until pacing is successful. The general pacemaker setup and evaluation principles described later should be applied. Transesophageal pacing tends to be unstable and is not recommended for pacing that is long-term, unless the patient is intubated and sedated. Transesophageal pacing is also uncomfortable and usually requires sedation.

A more stable form of temporary pacing is the transvenous approach in which a lead is inserted into the venous system through a vascular sheath and advanced to the appropriate chamber for pacing. Various venous approaches for lead placement are used, with the femoral, jugular, or subclavian vein being the most common. The leads may be placed under fluoroscopic or echocardiographic guidance, and an electrocardiographic tracing from the lead tip or observation of cardiac capture on surface electrocardiogram monitoring is used to confirm positioning. Once the lead is in place, it should be well secured at the skin to maintain stability and sterility. Patients may require sedation to maintain lead placement. Newer technologies allow for temporary transvenous pacing leads to be "screwed" into the myocardial tissue, thereby providing enhanced stability, and patient ambulation.

The most common scenario of temporary pacing found in the intensive care unit (ICU) is the transcutaneous epicardial route that is frequently used in patients following cardiac surgery. The cardiac surgeon attaches one or multiple electrodes to the epicardial surface of the heart (atrium, ventricle, or both) and tunnels the wire subcutaneously to the outer chest wall where the pacemaker generator can be connected. The leads can be ultimately removed by gentle traction on the external wires when they are no longer needed or have stopped functioning.

PACING MODES

Pacemakers, both permanent and temporary, can function in a variety of configurations. To simplify pacemaker description, a code was established to describe how a pacemaker is configured. The first position in the code indicates the chamber(s) being paced, the second position indicates the chamber(s) being sensed, and the third position indicates the response of the pacemaker to sensing. The first two positions use the following code: A, atrium; V, ventricle; D, dual-chamber; and O, none. The third position is held by the code "T" to indicate that the pacemaker *triggers* pacing in response to a sensing event, "I" to indicate the pacemaker *inhibits* in response to sensing intrinsic activity, "D" to indicate *dual* response (inhibit and trigger), or "O" to indicate asynchronous response. A fourth and fifth position can indicate that the pacemaker is rate-responsive or has antitachycardia capabilities, such as overdrive pacing or defibrillation.

On the basis of the capabilities of the pacemaker, it can be set in an asynchronous mode (AOO, VOO, DOO) to pace at a preset rate irrespective of intrinsic activity, or in an inhibited mode (AAI, VVI) to pace at a preset rate, but inhibit if intrinsic activity is sensed. However, the most common mode of pacing is dual-pacing, dual-sensing, dual-mode (DDD), in which both the atrium and ventricle can be paced and sensed, and the pacemaker can be both inhibited and triggered on the basis of the intrinsic activity of the heart.

PACEMAKER TERMINOLOGY

Modern pacemakers have multiple parameters that can be set by the user, including mode of pacing, lower pacing rate limit, sensitivity to intrinsic activity, stimulation output, AV delay timing, upper rate limit, and refractory periods. Before establishing parameters for any particular pacemaker, it is important to understand some key concepts of pacing terminology. Capture indicates that there is myocardial contraction in response to energy applied by the pacemaker. The capture threshold is the minimum amount of energy that results in capture. Sensing threshold establishes the level of intrinsic myocardial activity the pacemaker can sense. The value of sensitivity selected on the device indicates the amplitude of the signal above which the pacemaker can detect intrinsic activity; therefore, decreasing the programmed pacemaker sensitivity value results in increased sensitivity. If the sensitivity is set too low (high number), the pacemaker may fail to detect intrinsic myocardial activity that it should be sensing, and if it is set too high (low number), the pacemaker may mistake artifact or noise for intrinsic myocardial activity. Improper sensing frequently results in the pacemaker failing to work properly and may create a proarrhythmic situation resulting in atrial

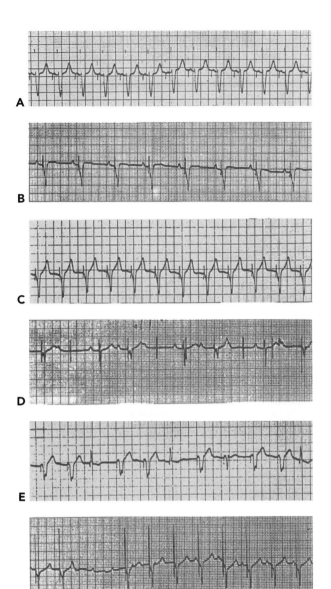

Figure 35.1 **A:** An electrocardiogram shows a pacemaker that paces the atrium and after 150 milliseconds paces the ventricle. Note the pacemaker stimulus artifact before the P wave and QRS complex. **B:** An electrocardiogram shows a pacemaker that senses the atrium and paces the ventricle after a 150-millisecond delay. Note that pacemaker stimulus artifact only precedes the QRS complex. **C:** An electrocardiogram shows ventricular pacing at 100 beats per minute with normal capture. Note the pacemaker stimulus artifact preceding the QRS. **D:** An electrocardiogram shows ventricular pacing at 85 beats per minute with intermittent failure of capture. Note that several pacemaker stimulus artifacts are not followed by a QRS complex, indicating failure of capture. **E:** An electrocardiogram shows ventricular pacing at 90 beats per minute, with normal sensing of the patient's intrinsic rhythm. **F:** An electrocardiogram shows ventricular pacing at 100 beats per minute, with inappropriate sensing and failure to stimulate the heart secondary to a wire fracture. (From Fleisher GR, Baskin M. *Atlas of emergency medicine.* Philadelphia, PA: Lippincott Williams & Wilkins;2004:62.)

tachyarrhythmias, ventricular tachycardia, or fibrillation (see Fig. 35.1).

Dual-chamber pacemakers have additional parameters that the operator should be familiar with to determine whether a pacemaker is functioning properly. The upper rate limit may be set to either allow the patient with complete AV block to track the atrium allowing 1:1 AV association or prevent undesirable tracking of a tachyarrhythmia (atrial flutter or atrial fibrillation). When the pacemaker is tracking the atrial rate and reaches the upper rate limit, it will begin to drop ventricular-paced beats so as not to surpass the upper rate limit (electronic Wenckebach behavior). To an observer unfamiliar with this function, it may appear that the pacemaker is transiently losing capture during this period. Another feature commonly used on dual-chamber pacemakers is the postventricular atrial refractory period (PVARP). In some circumstances, the atrial lead of a DDD pacemaker can oversense the QRS of a ventricular beat and misinterpret the signal as a P wave. If this happens, the pacemaker will wait for the appropriate AV delay and then trigger another ventricular-paced beat, resulting in a form of pacemaker-mediated tachycardia. This may be overcome by adjusting the atrial sensitivity, but if that is not possible, PVARP may be used to establish a time period after a paced or sensed ventricular activity during which the pacemaker ignores any sensed atrial activity. Finally, when dealing with implanted permanent pacemakers, one should realize that placing a magnet over the generator causes the device to default to a preset rate in asynchronous mode.

TEMPORARY PACEMAKER SETUP AND EVALUATION

Most temporary pacemakers default to nominal adult "safety" settings when first turned on. They also typically have an "emergency" button that can be used to set the pacemaker at maximum output in asynchronous dual-chamber pacing mode at a preset rate. These settings

TABLE 35.2
TEMPORARY PACEMAKER PARAMETERS

Parameters to Set When Using Temporary Pacemakers

All Pacemakers	Dual-Chamber Pacemakers
Mode (asynchronous/ synchronous)	AV delay
Lower pacing rate	Upper rate limit
Atrial and/or ventricular output (use capture threshold to determine)	Postventricular atrial refractory period
Sensing threshold	

usually are inadequate for pediatric patients. After leads are attached and the pacemaker is turned on, the user must set the pacing mode and other parameters appropriately (see Table 35.2). The pacemaker should be set at an appropriate lower rate limit, AV delay, upper rate limit, and PVARP setting appropriate for age.

The pacemaker capture and sensitivity thresholds in both the atrium and the ventricle should be tested when initiating pacing and as and when needed. To determine the capture threshold, the pacing rate must first be set higher than the intrinsic atrial or ventricular rate and the output must be set high enough to ensure capture. Capture is confirmed by visualizing a P wave or a QRS complex in response to a pacing spike on the monitor that correlates with the patient's pulse. The capture threshold is then determined by slowly decreasing the pacemaker output (usually measured in terms of milliamperes) to the point that a response to the pacing stimulus is no longer evident. This is the capture threshold. The pacemaker output should then be set with an adequate safety margin, typically twice the capture threshold. For example, if the ventricular capture threshold is 3 mA, the ventricular output of the pacemaker should be programmed to 6 mA.

Atrial and ventricular sensitivity is determined after determining the capture threshold and setting the pacemaker output. The pacemaker should first be set at a rate slightly below the intrinsic atrial or ventricular rate and at a high sensitivity value such that all intrinsic activity is sensed and no cardiac pacing is being performed. The device is then incrementally made less sensitive by increasing the value on the sensitivity dial (millivolts) to the point where the pacemaker begins to pace. The millivolt level that allows complete sensing and no pacing defines the sensing threshold. A sensing indicator light usually indicates sensing by the pacemaker. The sensitivity is then set at an acceptable safety margin, typically one-half the sensing threshold. For example

TABLE 35.3

EVALUATION OF COMMON PACEMAKER PROBLEMS

Problem	Diagnosis	Potential Causes	Troubleshooting
Loss of capture	Pacemaker spikes present No myocardial response (no P wave or QRS)	Tissue or metabolic changes that increase the stimulus threshold Drug effects Lead failure or disconnection Lead or patch dislodgement	Evaluate patient for change in condition Check lead position Reverse polarity of the connection: switch the + and − leads Increase pacemaker output or pulse width to obtain capture Check cables for loose or broken wires Change battery
Loss of pacing	No pacemaker spike No myocardial response	Lead failure or disconnection Battery/power failure Pacemaker oversensing Lead or patch dislodgement	Evaluate patient for change in condition Confirm that pacemaker is not being suppressed by intrinsic activity; increase EKG size on monitor Ensure that the pacemaker is not oversensing Consider changing to asynchronous mode Check lead position and cables for loose or broken wires Change battery
Oversensing	Random pacemaker response May inappropriately trigger or suppress pacing	T-wave sensing Far field sensing (sensing of P or R waves) Muscle sensing Lead problems Electrical noise	Decrease sensitivity of appropriate lead Decrease A or V output Increase PVARP if atrial oversensing Confirm cable connections Consider asynchronous mode
Undersensing	Random pacemaker spikes over intrinsic activity	Sensitivity too low Poor connection Lead failure or dislodgement	Increase sensitivity of appropriate lead Check lead position and cables for loose or broken wires Reverse polarity of the connection: switch the + and − leads

EKG, electrocardiogram; PVARP, postventricular atrial refractory period.

if the R wave (ventricle) sensing threshold is 8 mV, the ventricular sensing threshold should be programmed to 4 mV.

Because the sensing and capture thresholds and other settings are dynamic and can change because of multiple variables, it is imperative that the parameters are set with a safety margin and checked and adjusted regularly. Atrial, as well as, ventricular capture and sensing thresholds should be determined daily, or more frequently if pacemaker malfunction is noticed. The temporary pacemaker battery should also be changed every 24 to 48 hours. When any patient is being temporarily paced, caregivers must be familiar with the pacemaker settings and must be able to determine that the pacemaker is functioning as desired (see Table 35.3).

OVERDRIVE RAPID ATRIAL PACING

Overdrive rapid atrial pacing can terminate some forms of atrial flutter or re-entrant supraventricular tachycardias. The technique requires the use of transcutaneous pacing wires attached to the atrium, transesophageal, or transvenous pacing leads. The pacemaker generator may require a select setting for rapid atrial pacing, or a device dedicated for the technique may be used. In either case, the atrium is paced at a rate slightly faster than the rate of the tachyarrhythmia, usually 10 to 50 beats per minute faster. Rapid atrial pacing occurs at rates of 200 or more beats per minute. The energy is applied in a short burst of rapid pacing lasting several seconds (on the order of 3 to 5 seconds). If the tachyarrhythmia is not terminated at the end of the pacing burst, the rate and burst duration can be gradually increased until the arrhythmia is terminated. This form of intervention is frequently useful following cardiac surgery or when pharmacologic intervention is undesirable.

REFERENCE

1. Gregoratos G, Abrams J, Epstein AE, et al. ACC/AHA/NASPE 2002 Guideline Update for Implantation of Cardiac Pacemakers and Antiarrhythmia Devices: Summary Article: A Report of the American College of Cardiology/American Heart Association Task Force on Practice Guidelines (ACC/AHA/NASPE Committee to Update the 1998 Pacemaker Guidelines). *Circulation.* 2002;106:2145–2161.

Vasoactive Agents

36

Ronald A. Bronicki   *Paul A. Checchia*

Hemodynamic instability is a common problem in pediatric intensive care units (PICUs). There are a variety of strategies available to support the cardiovascular system, including fluid administration, positive pressure ventilation, provision of mechanical circulatory assistance, and utilization of vasoactive agents. The proper choice of vasoactive agent(s) requires an understanding of the hemodynamic disturbance and the pharmacology of the drug(s) utilized. This chapter will focus on the use of vasoactive agents in modifying circulatory dynamics.

CATECHOLAMINES

The available catecholamines are dopamine, dobutamine, epinephrine, norepinephrine, and isoproterenol (see Table 36.1). The hemodynamic effects of catecholamines are dose dependent, and are mediated by a variety of adrenergic receptors that use the cyclic adenosine monophosphate (cAMP)-dependent signaling cascade. Increased intracellular cAMP alters intracellular calcium metabolism and cellular function. Activation of endothelial β_2-receptors decreases cytosolic calcium levels resulting in vascular smooth muscle relaxation and vasodilation. Conversely, activation of endothelial α_1-receptors increases cytosolic calcium levels resulting in vasoconstriction. Activation of cardiomyocyte β_1-receptors increases cytosolic calcium levels resulting in enhanced contractility and, to a lesser extent, increased heart rate. Over time, β-adrenergic receptors become desensitized, a process by which β_1- and β_2-receptors generate an attenuated physiologic response to an agonist. This occurs with prolonged exposure to elevated levels of either endogenous or exogenous catecholamines. Catecholamines are primarily metabolized by two enzyme systems: catechol O-methyltransferase and monoamine oxidase. All catecholamines have a very short half-life, allowing for easy titration (see Table 36.2).

Catecholamines have similar side-effect profiles. All catecholamines increase myocardial oxygen demands as a result of their chronotropic and inotropic effects. If myocardial oxygen delivery does not increase to the same extent as demand, myocardial ischemia may ensue. Unfavorable changes in myocardial energetics are a particular concern with epinephrine and isoproterenol. Tachyarrhythmias result from stimulation of β_1-adrenergic receptors. The agents most commonly associated with induction of arrhythmias are isoproterenol and epinephrine. Finally, catecholamines with α-agonist activity, such as epinephrine, norepinephrine, and dopamine, should be administered through a central venous line to avoid the risk of extravasation and resulting tissue necrosis.

Dopamine is the immediate precursor of norepinephrine in the endogenous catecholamine biosynthetic pathway. In addition to its hemodynamic and renal effects, dopamine serves as a neurotransmitter in the central and peripheral nervous system. Dopamine directly stimulates α-, β-, and dopaminergic receptors. Approximately half of the dopamine-induced inotropic responses result from dopamine-induced release of norepinephrine from sympathetic nerve terminals. Dopamine is primarily used in the treatment of oliguria, septic shock, and ventricular dysfunction. Dopamine in low doses (<3 to 5 μg/kg/minute) stimulates renal vascular dopaminergic receptors, increasing renal blood flow and the glomerular filtration rate (GFR), although this has not been shown to prevent the acute renal failure or need for dialysis.[1] Moderate doses (<10 μg/kg/minute) have chronotropic and inotropic effects. In adults with congestive heart failure (CHF), dopamine significantly increases cardiac output (CO) by increasing stroke volume and, to a lesser extent, heart rate. Left ventricular filling pressures either remain unchanged or are increased; this results from venoconstriction and reduced venous capacitance. At higher doses (>10 μg/kg/minute), α-adrenergic effects predominate and systemic vascular resistance (SVR) begins to increase. The effects of dopamine on pulmonary vascular resistance (PVR) and pulmonary artery pressure are conflicting.

TABLE 36.1

CATECHOLAMINES

Agent	Receptors	Dose	Effect
Dopamine	Dopa-1, β_1, α_1	<5 μg/kg/min >10 μg/kg/min	↑Renal blood flow, ↑HR, ↑CO ↑HR, ↑CO, ↑SVR
Dobutamine	β_1	2–20 μg/kg/min	↑HR, ↑CO, ↓SVR
Epinephrine	β_1, β_2 β_1, α_1	0.01–0.1 μg/kg/min >0.1 μg/kg/min	↑HR, ↑CO, ↓SVR/PVR ↑HR, ↑CO, ↑SVR
Norepinephrine	α_1, β_1	0.01–1.0 μg/kg/min	↑SVR
Isoproterenol	β_1, β_2	0.01–1.0 μg/kg/min	↑HR, ↑CO, ↓SVR/PVR

HR, heart rate; CO, cardiac output; SVR, systemic vascular resistance; PVR, pulmonary vascular resistance.
↑, ↓ indicate increase or decrease, respectively.

Dobutamine is a synthetic catecholamine that provides inotropic support. In adults with ventricular dysfunction, dobutamine significantly improves CO and, in contrast to dopamine, consistently reduces ventricular filling pressures by increasing stroke volume and, to a lesser extent, by increasing heart rate and reducing SVR. The reduction in SVR has been attributed to β_2-stimulation, as well as a compensatory withdrawal of endogenous α_1-activation due to increased CO.

Epinephrine is an endogenous catecholamine formed from norepinephrine through N-methylation. It is largely produced by the adrenal medulla in response to stress. Epinephrine produces widespread metabolic and hemodynamic effects and is used frequently in the management of severe septic and cardiogenic shock and during cardiopulmonary resuscitation. In low doses (<0.1 μg/kg/minute), epinephrine provides significant inotropic and chronotropic support. Additionally, it stimulates β_2-receptors causing a reduction in SVR, PVR, and diastolic blood pressure. Unloading of baroreceptors contributes to its direct chronotropic effects. At higher doses, activation of α_1-receptors leads to progressive increases in SVR, which may compromise renal and mesenteric blood flow. Finally, because epinephrine significantly increases contractility, heart rate, and afterload, myocardial oxygen demands may increase more than myocardial oxygen delivery, worsening myocardial oxygen balance.

Norepinephrine is the neurotransmitter of the sympathetic nervous system. It is released from terminal nerve endings and acts locally. Norepinephrine primarily increases SVR by activating α_1-receptors, while providing minor inotropic support. The primary use of norepinephrine is to restore an adequate perfusion pressure in the setting of vasodilatory shock. As with epinephrine, significant increases in SVR may compromise renal and mesenteric blood flow.

Isoproterenol is a synthetic catecholamine. It is a potent, nonspecific β-agonist that provides significant inotropic and chronotropic support, as well as reductions in SVR and PVR. The primary indication for isoproterenol is symptomatic bradycardia. Isoproterenol is associated with significant tachycardia and the propensity to develop

TABLE 36.2

PHARMACOKINETIC PARAMETERS OF INTRAVENOUS INOTROPIC AGENTS

Drug	Clearance (mL/min/kg)	Half-life (min)	Adjustments		
			Children	Renal Failure	Hepatic Failure
Dopamine	50	2–20	CL increased	CL decreased	CL decreased
Dobutamine	60–120	2–3	CL variable	Unchanged	Unchanged
Epinephrine	16–80	3	—	—	—
Isoproterenol	33–50	2	—	—	—
Norepinephrine	24–40	2	Unchanged	Unchanged	Unchanged
Milrinone	2.0–2.5	120	CL and V_d increased	Half-life increased	Unchanged
Levosimendan	3.0–3.7	60	Unknown	Unchanged	Unchanged

CL, clearance; V_d, volume of distribution.

arrhythmias. Isoproterenol has a higher potential to compromise coronary perfusion because it shortens diastole and decreases diastolic blood pressure.

MILRINONE

Milrinone, like its predecessor amrinone, does not act through adrenergic receptors, but rather through selective inhibition of phosphodiesterase III, a member of a family of intracellular enzymes that degrade cyclic nucleotides such as cAMP and cyclic guanosine monophosphate (cGMP). Phosphodiesterase III inhibition leads to a reduction of cAMP degradation. The increases in cAMP result in enhanced myocardial contractility and relaxation of vascular smooth muscle (see Table 36.3). Milrinone also appears to improve diastolic function either by improving myocardial energetics or by having a direct effect on the myocardium. Half-life is age-dependent and ranges from <1 hour in children to >3 hours in infants and is much longer than most vasoactive agents used in the intensive care unit (ICU).[2] Milrinone is predominantly cleared by renal excretion; therefore dosing must be altered in patients with renal insufficiency (Table 36.2). In patients undergoing hemofiltration, the half-life is prolonged even further; that is, up to 20 hours.[3]

In children with acute ventricular dysfunction, the combined inotropic and afterload-reducing effects of milrinone produce a significant increase in CO and reduce ventricular filling pressures. Milrinone also increases venous capacitance, decreases PVR, and has minimal effect on heart rate. Hoffman et al. demonstrated the efficacy and safety of milrinone in children, following cardiac surgery.[2] They demonstrated a 64% relative risk reduction in the development of low-CO syndrome with the prophylactic use of high-dose milrinone (0.75 μg/kg/minute). Additionally, there was no significant difference in the incidence of adverse events (e.g., hypotension or arrhythmia) when compared to placebo.

Milrinone therapy in adult patients with decompensated heart failure has not been shown to improve outcome. One study found increased mortality in an adult population treated with an oral preparation of the drug.[4] In contrast, other randomized studies have demonstrated that milrinone is more efficacious than afterload reduction with nitroglycerin (NTG).[5] These studies highlight the potential difficulties in data interpretation between subpopulations of patients; that is, chronic versus acute heart failure, adult versus pediatric patients.

VASOPRESSIN

Vasopressin is a hormone that is essential for osmotic and cardiovascular homeostasis (see Chapter 2). In addition to its antidiuretic effect, physiologic levels of vasopressin are required for normal vascular tone. Vasopressin interacts with membrane-bound G protein–coupled vasopressin-specific receptors, V_1 and V_2. The V_1 receptors are located on vascular smooth muscle cells, whereas V_2 receptors are located on renal tubular epithelium. Vasopressin constricts systemic arterial and venous capacitance vessels in a dose-dependent fashion (Table 36.3). Vasopressin is more potent in skin, skeletal muscle, adipose tissue, and pancreas than in mesenteric, coronary, and cerebral circulations. On a molar basis, vasopressin is a more potent vasoconstrictor than angiotensin II or norepinephrine. On the basis of these properties, vasopressin has been used in the treatment of cardiac arrest and vasodilatory shock.

The resuscitation guidelines of the American Heart Association and the European Resuscitation Council currently recommend vasopressin as an alternative to epinephrine for the treatment of cardiac arrest and refractory ventricular fibrillation.[6] This recommendation is based on trials that demonstrated improved coronary perfusion pressure, myocardial blood flow, and a higher rate of successful resuscitation and survival in patients treated with vasopressin versus epinephrine. However, it should be noted that a recent meta-analysis failed to demonstrate a clear advantage of vasopressin over epinephrine in the treatment of cardiac arrest.[7]

TABLE 36.3

ADDITIONAL VASOACTIVE AGENTS

| | Hemodynamic Effects | | | | | | |
	Venous Capacitance	Inotropic Properties	Lusitropic Properties	SVR and PVR	LVFP	Mechanism of Action	Dose
Milrinone	Increased	Yes	Yes	Decreased	Decreased	PDE III inhibition	0.25–0.75 μg/kg/min
Vasopressin	Decreased	No	No	Increased	Increased	Vasopressin receptors	0.0003–0.002 U/kg/min
Nesiritide	Increased	No	Yes	Decreased	Decreased	Natriuretic receptors	0.01–0.03 μg/kg/min
Nitroprusside	Increased	No	Yes	Decreased	Decreased	Nitric oxide mediated	0.5–5.0 μg/kg/min
Nitroglycerin	Increased	No	Yes	Decreased	Decreased	Nitric oxide mediated	0.5–5.0 μg/kg/min

SVR, systemic vascular resistance; PVR, pulmonary vascular resistance; LVFP, left ventricular filling pressure; PDE, phosphodiesterase inhibitor.

Three unique attributes of vasopressin support its potential use in the management of vasodilatory shock: (i) there often exists a relative deficiency of vasopressin, (ii) the sensitivity of the systemic circulation to vasopressin is increased, and (iii) it potentiates the vasoconstrictive effects of catecholamines. Vasopressin has been demonstrated to significantly increase blood pressure, allowing for the reduction of catecholamine therapy in children with vasodilatory shock.[8] Although these studies demonstrated that CO and oxygen delivery remained unchanged, stroke volume increased significantly despite increases in afterload. It is controversial whether vasopressin provides inotropic support because of its effect on preload, heart rate, and most importantly, coronary perfusion. Despite available experimental data and increased enthusiasm for vasopressin in the management of vasodilatory shock, there are no clinical data to suggest any superiority over conventional vasopressor agents in reducing mortality, and vasopressin is not currently recommended as a replacement for norepinephrine or dopamine as a first-line agent. Potential side effects of vasopressin include excessive vasoconstriction and potential regional ischemia, hyponatremia, and fluid retention.

NESIRITIDE

The natriuretic peptide family consists of atrial natriuretic peptide (ANP), brain natriuretic peptide (BNP), and C-type natriuretic peptides, which modulate vascular tone and fluid homeostasis. They are an integral part of a cardiac–endothelium feedback mechanism, acting as counter-regulatory hormones to endothelin 1, norepinephrine, and the renin–angiotensin–aldosterone system (RAAS). The tissue-specific distribution and regulation of each peptide and their affinity for natriuretic peptide receptors differ between peptides. ANP is produced primarily by atrial myocytes, whereas BNP, first identified in the extracts of porcine brain, is predominantly synthesized and secreted by ventricular myocytes. The natriuretic peptides interact with receptors linked to the cGMP-dependent signaling cascade. ANP and BNP are secreted in response to an increase in myocardial wall stress (i.e., volume load or pressure load) and have very similar cardiovascular and renal effects. Nesiritide is the human recombinant form of BNP. It produces dose-dependent dilation of arterial resistance and venous capacitance vessels in the pulmonary and systemic circulations (Table 36.3). Nesiritide also affects vasomotor tone by inhibiting both the RAAS and the release of endothelin-1. Nesiritide causes dose-dependent natriuresis and diuresis by reducing sodium reabsorption in the proximal and distal tubules and by inhibiting adrenal cortical production of aldosterone. Nesiritide also increases the GFR by modulating renal hemodynamics. Nesiritide has a half-life of 15 minutes.

The primary indication for nesiritide is in the acute management of decompensated CHF. Because nesiritide decreases afterload and increases venous capacitance, CO is increased while ventricular filling pressures are reduced. The evaluation of nesiritide in pediatric patients has been limited to small, retrospective analysis. There is, however, limited data in children on the hemodynamic effects of infused ANP. Following the Fontan procedure, infused ANP reduced PVR and SVR, and increased CO without a significant effect on blood pressure.[9] In a subset of patients with pulmonary hypertension following congenital heart surgery, infused ANP significantly reduced PVR.[10] In contrast to other vasodilators, the use of nesiritide is not associated with reflex stimulation of adrenergic activity. Finally, nesiritide also appears to improve diastolic function because of increased intracellular cGMP.

Adverse events include dose-related hypotension and the risk of worsening renal function.[11]

NITROGLYCERIN

NTG undergoes biotransformation to yield nitric oxide, which diffuses across smooth muscle cell membranes activating the soluble form of guanylate cyclase resulting in increased cGMP synthesis. NTG produces dose-dependent dilation of systemic and pulmonary arterial and venous capacitance vessels (Table 36.3). NTG is hydrolyzed by hepatic glutathione-organic nitrate reductase into inorganic nitrite and denitrated metabolites. Tachyphylaxis develops rapidly to NTG, and may result from impaired biotransformation.

Intravenous NTG is primarily used in the acute management of CHF. In low to moderate doses ($<3\ \mu g/kg/minute$), NTG mainly increases venous capacitance; therefore ventricular filling pressures are reduced without significant changes in CO. In higher doses, NTG reduces SVR and PVR, and CO increases. Finally, as with other therapies that increase myocardial cGMP levels, NTG improves diastolic function.

Adverse events with intravenous NTG are similar to other vasoactive agents. Hypotension results from inadequate ventricular filling pressures. In addition, pulmonary vasodilation may worsen oxygenation by overcoming hypoxic pulmonary vasoconstriction and increasing ventilation–perfusion mismatch.

NITROPRUSSIDE

Nitroprusside (NTP) spontaneously releases nitric oxide which activates the soluble form of guanylate cyclase, producing increased levels of cGMP. NTP causes dose-dependent dilation of systemic and pulmonary arterial resistance and venous capacitance vessels (Table 36.3). NTP decomposes nonenzymatically in the blood, releasing cyanide, which undergoes transsulfuration to form thiocyanite. Thiocyanite is excreted by the kidneys and has a half-life of 3 days in patients with normal renal function. Although thiocyanite is not vasoactive, it does accumulate in the setting of renal failure and may cause neurotoxicity. When thiosulfate stores are depleted, cyanide toxicity ensues. NTP has a half-life of 2 minutes, allowing for easy titration and, in contrast to NTG, does not develop tolerance.

NTP is used in a variety of clinical settings where afterload reduction is desired. NTP is highly effective in the treatment of malignant hypertension. NTP is also effective in improving the hemodynamics of patients with valvular diseases including aortic stenosis (AS), aortic regurgitation (AR), and mitral regurgitation (MR).[12] Afterload reduction has long been considered contraindicated in patients with severe AS. It is thought that the stroke volume is fixed, and decreasing SVR will precipitate severe hypotension. However, because resistances in a series are additive, decreasing SVR reduces the effective afterload of the left ventricle. This is particularly beneficial for the failing ventricle, which is sensitive to afterload. In adult patients with severe decompensated heart failure due to severe AS (baseline mean cardiac index of 1.62 L/minute/m^2 and mean ejection fraction of 21%), NTP decreased SVR and significantly increased cardiac index, while reducing left ventricular filling pressures.[12]

In MR, NTP consistently increases CO by increasing the forward stroke volume and decreasing the regurgitant volume, while reducing ventricular volumes and pressure; the ejection fraction is unchanged. It therefore appears that the increase in CO results primarily from reduced ventricular volume, which leads to a decrease in the regurgitant orifice area and regurgitant volume. In AR, NTP consistently increases the ejection fraction, whereas ventricular volumes and pressure are decreased. Changes in regurgitant volume and forward stroke volume are less consistent. Therefore, NTP primarily improves the hemodynamics in AR by decreasing myocardial wall stress and improving ventricular emptying despite reductions in ventricular preload.

NTP is effective in the acute management of CHF. Because NTP decreases afterload and increases venous capacitance, CO is increased while ventricular filling pressures are reduced. In infants with low CO following intracardiac repair, NTP significantly increased CO while reducing pulmonary arterial and ventricular pressures.[13] Finally, as with other therapies that increase myocardial cGMP levels, NTP appears to improve diastolic function.

The primary adverse event resulting from the use of NTP is hypotension. One advantage of NTP is its short half-life, allowing for easy titration. And as with all vasoactive agents that increase venous capacitance, an adequate ventricular filling pressure is necessary to maintain stroke volume. By causing pulmonary vasodilation, NTP may worsen oxygenation by releasing hypoxic pulmonary vasoconstriction and increasing ventilation–perfusion mismatch. Finally, as mentioned, thiocyanite and cyanide toxicities may occur in the setting of renal failure or prolonged use. Cyanide toxicity is rare, however, when low-dose infusion rates (<3 μg/kg/minute) are used for a short period of time (<3 days).

LEVOSIMENDAN

Levosimendan represents the first of an entirely new class of agents, calcium sensitizers, that enhance the sensitivity of the myofilament to calcium without an increase in cytosolic calcium levels. Contraction of cardiac myofilaments is triggered when a calcium ion binds to troponin C. Levosimendan stabilizes calcium-induced changes in troponin C and inhibits troponin I, prolonging the troponin-mediated activation of the actin–myosin interaction. This results in a marked positive inotropic effect. Because cytosolic calcium level is not increased, levosimendan does not disturb myocardial energy balance unlike most other inotropic agents. Additionally, levosimendan activates adenosine triphosphate (ATP)-dependent potassium channels leading to pulmonary, coronary, and systemic vasodilation (Table 36.3). Its terminal elimination half-life after intravenous administration is about 1 hour (Table 36.2). Levosimendan undergoes significant metabolism by conjugation and results in the formation of active metabolites. These metabolites have a half-life as long as 80 hours, which enhances the hemodynamic effects of the parent drug, resulting in prolonged inotropic, chronotropic, and vasodilatory actions.[14]

Intravenously administered levosimendan significantly increases CO without appreciable changes in myocardial oxygen consumption, thereby improving myocardial energetics. Heart rate is unchanged and ventricular filling pressures are significantly reduced. Several trials have evaluated the safety and efficacy of levosimendan in adult patients. When compared to dobutamine, levosimendan significantly increased CO and reduced left ventricular filling pressures in adults with decompensated heart failure.[15,16] In addition, both the Randomized Study on Safety and Effectiveness of Levosimendan in Patients with Left Ventricular Failure After an Acute Myocardial Infarct (RUSSLAN) and Levosimendan Infusion versus Dobutamine (LIDO) studies demonstrated reduced mortality with levosimendan when compared to placebo and dobutamine, respectively.[15,17] Finally, the safety profile of levosimendan is good. The RUSSLAN study demonstrated no difference in the incidence of clinically significant hypotension when compared to placebo.[17] Pediatric data are limited, but it appears to have a similar safety and efficacy pattern.[18] Levosimendan has been approved for use in Europe, with ongoing pediatric and adult trials in the United States.

CONCLUSION

The cardiovascular system is commonly affected, either directly or indirectly, by a myriad of disease processes, often resulting in hemodynamic instability. By manipulating the determinants of CO, vasoactive agents play an integral role in restoring adequate cardiovascular function. Which of these agents is used depends on the baseline hemodynamic profile as well as the underlying pathophysiologic process.

REFERENCES

1. Kellum JA, Decker JM. Use of dopamine in acute renal failure: A meta-analysis. *Crit Care Med.* 2001;29:1526–1531.
2. Hoffman TM, Wernovsky G, Atz AM, et al. Efficacy and safety of milrinone in preventing low cardiac output syndrome in infants and children after corrective surgery for congenital heart disease. *Circulation.* 2003;107(7):996–1002.
3. Lehtonen LA, Antila S, Pentikainen PJ. Pharmacokinetics and pharmacodynamics of intravenous inotropic agents. *Clin Pharmacokinet.* 2004;43(3):187–203.
4. Packer M, Carver JR, Rodeheffer RJ, et al. Effect of oral milrinone on mortality in severe chronic heart failure. The PROMISE Study Research Group. *N Engl J Med.* 1991;325(21):1468–1475.
5. Loh E, Elkayam U, Cody R, et al. A randomized multicenter study comparing the efficacy and safety of intravenous milrinone and intravenous nitroglycerin in patients with advanced heart failure. *J Card Fail.* 2001;7(2):114–121.
6. Anonymous. Guidelines 2000 for Cardiopulmonary Resuscitation and Emergency Cardiovascular Care. Part 6: Advanced cardiovascular life support; Section 6: Pharmacology II: Agents to optimize cardiac output and blood pressure. The American Heart Association in collaboration with the International Liaison Committee on Resuscitation. *Circulation.* 2000;102(Suppl 8):I129–I135.
7. Aung K, Htay T. Vasopressin for cardiac arrest: A systematic review and meta-analysis. *Arch Intern Med.* 2005;165(1):17–24.
8. Rosenzweig EB, Starc TJ, Chen JM, et al. Intravenous arginine-vasopressin in children with vasodilatory shock after cardiac surgery. *Circulation.* 1999;100(Suppl 19):II182–II186.
9. Hiramatsu T, Imai Y, Takanashi Y, et al. Hemodynamic effects of human atrial natriuretic peptide after modified Fontan procedure. *Ann Thorac Surg.* 1998;65(3):761–764.
10. Ivy DD, Kinsella JP, Wolfe RR, et al. Atrial natriuretic peptide and nitric oxide in children with pulmonary hypertension after surgical repair of congenital heart disease. *Am J Cardiol.* 1996;77(1):102–105.
11. Sackner-Bernstein JD, Skopicki HA, Aaronson KD. Risk of worsening renal function with nesiritide in patients with acutely decompensated heart failure. *Circulation.* 2005;111:1487–1491.
12. Khot UN, Novaro GM, Popovic ZB, et al. Nitroprusside in critically ill patients with left ventricular dysfunction and aortic stenosis. *N Engl J Med.* 2003;348(18):1756–1763.
13. Appelbaum A, Blackstone EH, Kouchoukos NT, et al. Afterload reduction and cardiac output in infants early after intracardiac surgery. *Am J Cardiol.* 1977;39(3):445–451.
14. Kivikko M, Lehtonen L, Colucci WS. Sustained hemodynamic effects of intravenous levosimendan. *Circulation.* 2003;107(1):81–86.
15. Follath F, Cleland JG, Just H, et al. Efficacy and safety of intravenous levosimendan compared with dobutamine in severe low-output heart failure (the LIDO study): A randomised double-blind trial. *Lancet.* 2002;360(9328):196–202.
16. Nieminen MS, Akkila J, Hasenfuss G, et al. Hemodynamic and neurohumoral effects of continuous infusion of levosimendan in patients with congestive heart failure. *J Am Coll Cardiol.* 2000;36(6):1903–1912.
17. Moiseyev VS, Poder P, Andrejevs N, et al. Safety and efficacy of a novel calcium sensitizer, levosimendan, in patients with left ventricular failure due to an acute myocardial infarction. A randomized, placebo-controlled, double-blind study (RUSSLAN). *Eur Heart J.* 2002;23(18):1422–1432.
18. Turanlahti M, Boldt T, Palkama T, et al. Pharmacokinetics of levosimendan in pediatric patients evaluated for cardiac surgery. *Pediatr Crit Care Med.* 2004;5(5):457–462.

Respiratory Disorders

Heidi J. Dalton   *Mark J. Heulitt*

Pulmonary Diagnostic Procedures

37

Parthak Prodhan   Natan Noviski

IMAGING MODALITIES

A wide range of imaging options is now available to the physician in the intensive care unit (ICU). Collaboration between the patient care team and the radiologist helps maximize the diagnostic and therapeutic yield of procedures while minimizing costs.

Conventional Radiographs

Chest radiographs, obtained at the bedside (portable radiographs), are the most common imaging studies performed in the ICU. Recently, these images are being obtained using a photostimulable phosphor imaging plate, instead of film, which are scanned, read, and processed by the computer. The software allows image visualization from distant sites or through web-based systems.

The bedside radiograph for acutely ill patients is commonly obtained as an anteroposterior (AP) view. This view magnifies the mediastinum, and, therefore, caution is required while interpreting the size of these structures. In the supine position, air rises anteriorly and fluid collections layer posteriorly. Lateral decubitus views are often useful in determining whether the pleural abnormalities represent the freely flowing fluid, whereas apical lordotic views can often allow the visualization of the disease at the lung apices better than that in the standard AP view.

Studies of the glottic, subglottic, and large airways should be performed dynamically under airway fluoroscopy. This allows visualization of dynamic changes in the airway caliber (i.e., compression, exaggerated dilatation, and airway instability) and air movement within the lungs. Fluoroscopy is helpful in identifying diaphragmatic dysfunction and is also performed in contrast studies of the esophagus and the bronchi. A barium esophagogram may

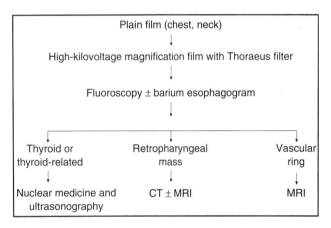

Figure 37.1 Recommended sequence for imaging the pediatric airway. CT, computed tomography; MRI, magnetic resonance imaging.

sometimes assist with the workup of a child with stridor, wheezing, or chronic cough. A recommended sequence for imaging the pediatric airway is illustrated in Figure 37.1.

Ultrasound

Ultrasound examination at the bedside in the ICU is relatively inexpensive and does not utilize ionizing radiation. Because ultrasound energy is rapidly dissipated in air, ultrasound imaging is not very useful for the evaluation of the pulmonary parenchyma. However, it can be effectively utilized to evaluate and localize pleural fluid collections, to determine whether such collections are free or loculated, and as a guide for placement of appropriate needle or tube during thoracentesis. It is also useful to estimate the diaphragm motion and detect pneumothoraces. In addition, Doppler ultrasonography can be used to evaluate the patency of blood vessels (e.g., in case of deep vein thrombosis and anomalous pulmonary blood vessels).

Computed Tomography

Computed tomography (CT) scan is clearly the superior method for assessing hilar and mediastinal disease, in identifying and characterizing disease adjacent to the chest wall or spine (including pleural disease), and in identifying areas of fat density or calcification in pulmonary lesions. With the additional use of contrast material, CT scan identifies normal or abnormal vascular structures. The demonstration of cross-sectional anatomy by CT scan, the density discrimination of which is ten times greater than that of the conventional radiographs, makes it an excellent method for evaluating solid masses, differentiating empyemas from lung abscesses, and selecting an approach for biopsy.

Recent advances in CT scan technology include high-resolution CT scan, multidetector CT scan, helical CT scan, CT scan angiography, and portable CT scan. High-resolution CT scan allows evaluation of slice thickness of 1.5 mm, rather than the usual 7 to 10 mm, enhancing the ability to recognize subtle parenchymal and airway disease. The limits of bronchial and blood vessel visibility on high-resolution CT scan are illustrated in Figure 37.2. Helical and multidetector CT scanning allows for a rapid scanning during a shorter time interval. These devices produce accurate images even in patients with tachypnea or in uncooperative pediatric patients. Recent advances in computer data processing as a result of helical CT scanning allow for images to be presented in three-dimensional reconstructions (virtual bronchoscopy) that mimic those seen by direct visualization of the airways. Helical CT scanning can also be combined with intravenous contrast (CT scan angiography) to detect pulmonary emboli in segmental and larger pulmonary arteries. Reconstructive techniques from thin-slice and helical CT scan can recreate images in coronal, sagittal, and axial planes with minute detail.

The main disadvantages of CT scan technology include cost, radiation exposure, and adverse reactions to intravascular radiocontrast media. The risks and benefits associated with the transportation of the critically ill patient to the radiology suite should always be considered.

Magnetic Resonance Imaging

When the nuclei of atoms having an odd number of neutrons and protons are placed in a magnetic field, they attempt to align to the magnetic field. Each nucleus rotates (precess) in the magnetic field at a specific frequency. These precessing nuclei absorb energy if they are exposed to a radio wave of the same frequency (resonance). After exposure to a radio-wave pulse, the nuclei release energy as they return to their resting state (relaxation). Longitudinal (T_1) and transverse (T_2) relaxation times can be measured on the basis of the amount of energy released. These energy pulses are recorded and transformed into images. This forms the basis of the magnetic resonance imaging (MRI) technology. Hydrogen nuclei are both magnetic and abundantly present in living tissues and are the nuclei that are commonly involved in imaging by most present-day devices.

MRI is well suited for imaging abnormalities near the lung apex, chest wall, spine, mediastinum, and the thoracoabdominal junction. It is the method of choice for evaluating posterior mediastinal neurogenic tumors that may involve the spinal canal. In addition, MRI can be used to evaluate vascular pathology within the thorax and to distinguish vascular from nonvascular structures. Flowing blood does not produce a signal on MRI, so vessels appear as hollow tubular structures. This feature is useful in defining the vascular origin of abnormal hilar or mediastinal densities. Intravascular contrast agents like gadolinium can enhance the imaging of vascular structures. MRI of the aorta is an excellent method to evaluate acquired diseases (aneurysms and dissections), as well as congenital lesions (vascular rings and coarctations). Recently, velocity-encoded cine MRI has been used to measure pulmonary blood flow and pressure and to identify the abnormal

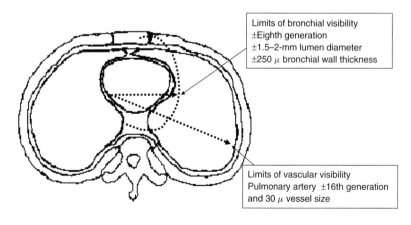

Limits of bronchial visibility
±Eighth generation
±1.5–2-mm lumen diameter
±250 μ bronchial wall thickness

Limits of vascular visibility
Pulmonary artery ±16th generation
and 30 μ vessel size

Figure 37.2 Schematic cross-sectional image of the chest illustrating the limits of visibility on high-resolution computed tomography (CT).

vessels in the chest. The signal from moving blood can be adjusted without the addition of contrast material. This advantage makes velocity-encoded cine MRI an alternative to CT scan in patients who are allergic to contrast.

Unlike CT scan, MRI does not expose the patient to ionizing radiation. However, in many cases, MRI is not feasible in critically ill patients because of the interference caused by ferromagnetic monitoring devices, the presence of implanted metallic devices (e.g., wire sutures, pacemakers, or surgical staples), the difficulty of adequately ventilating and monitoring patients within the narrow MRI gantry, and the long scan times.

SCINTIGRAPHIC IMAGING

Radioactive isotopes, administered either by intravenous or by inhaled routes, allow the lungs to be imaged with a gamma camera. This forms the basis of ventilation/perfusion (V/Q) lung scanning. The most common indication of such imaging is the evaluation for pulmonary embolism. The V/Q scan is a two-step process. First, a perfusion study is performed, in which technetium 99m (^{99m}Tc)-macroaggregated albumin is injected intravenously and becomes trapped within the pulmonary circulation. The distribution of the trapped radioisotope follows the distribution of blood flow. The diagnosis of pulmonary thromboembolism on the V/Q scan is based on documenting perfusion defects in an area of normal ventilation—a mismatched defect. The ventilation portion of the examination is performed with the patient inhaling xenon 133, krypton 81, or an aerosolized solution of ^{99m}Tc diethylenetriaminepentaacetic acid (DTPA). The aerosol is deposited deep into the lungs in proportion to the alveolar ventilation. Ventilation abnormalities are shown by failure of areas to fill during the wash-in phase or by the delayed clearance of the inhaled xenon from areas during the washout phase. In some centers, the property of the injectable form of xenon 133 allows both these steps to be carried out together.

PULMONARY ANGIOGRAPHY

Pulmonary angiography demonstrates either a defect in the lumen of a vessel (a "filling defect") or an abrupt termination ("cutoff") of the vessel. Occasionally, therapeutic transcatheter embolization can be accomplished for the treatment of pulmonary atrioventricular (AV) fistulas during angiography. Recently, with advances in CT scanning, traditional pulmonary angiography is increasingly being replaced by CT scan angiography. Although complications are uncommon, urticaria, bronchospasm, renal failure, hematoma, or respiratory distress may occur because of the contrast medium or the manipulation of the pulmonary vasculature. Death occurs in 0.5% of instances.

DIAGNOSTIC PROCEDURES

Clinicians have at their disposal several procedures for the diagnosis of pulmonary disease. They range from the essentially noninvasive analysis of expectorated sputum to the significantly invasive open lung biopsy through thoracotomy.

Sputum Examination

Sputum consists mainly of secretions from the tracheobronchial tree. The presence of squamous epithelial cells in a "sputum" sample indicates contamination by secretions from the upper airways. The sputum specimen can be subjected to various staining, culture, and immunologic tests. Lipid-laden vacuoles in alveolar macrophages can be seen in patients with aspiration pneumonia. The presence of large numbers of eosinophils (>20% to 30%) suggests atopic or parasitic disease. Patients with asthma may have sputum characterized by the presence of Charcot-Leyden crystals (formed by the crystallization of eosinophil lysophospholipase), Curschmann spirals (bronchiolar casts), or Creola bodies (formed of exfoliated epithelial cells). As for pneumonia, staining and culture for mycobacteria or fungi, culture for viruses, and staining for *Pneumocystis carinii* may be diagnostic. Immunologic techniques and molecular biologic methods (e.g., antigen detection tests, polymerase chain reaction amplification, and DNA probes) are used to diagnose pertussis, tuberculosis, respiratory syncytial virus, and influenza.

Thoracentesis

Thoracentesis is usually performed for diagnostic or therapeutic purposes in the case of a large effusion. The collected fluid allows biochemical, microbiologic, and cytologic studies to be performed. Table 37.1 provides the criteria to differentiate between the two major types of effusions: transudates and exudates. On occasion, these criteria misidentify transudates as exudates. If a pleural

---

TABLE 37.1

DIFFERENTIATION BETWEEN EXUDATES AND TRANSUDATES

Exudates fulfill at least one of the following criteria, whereas transudates meet none
1. Pleural fluid protein/serum protein level >0.5
2. Pleural fluid LDH/serum LDH level >0.6
3. Pleural fluid LDH level above two third the upper limit of the normal serum LDH value
4. Pleural fluid cholesterol level >55 mg/dL

LDH, lactate dehydrogenase.

TABLE 37.2

INDICATIONS FOR FLEXIBLE AND RIGID BRONCHOSCOPY IN PEDIATRIC PATIENTS

Flexible Bronchoscope	Rigid Bronchoscope
Stridor sleep-associated airway obstruction	Foreign body (present or suspected)
Persistent hoarseness	Hemoptysis
Unexplained persistent cough	Biopsy
Unexplained or persistent wheezing	Patient for whom FB is indicated but are:
Recurrent or persistent pneumonia	■ Nonintubated and uncooperative and,
Persistent atelectasis	therefore, FB is not possible
Interstitial lung disease	■ Neonates and young infants on mechanical
Suspected congenital anomalies	ventilation, in whom a flexible bronchoscope
Suspected airway compression	cannot pass through the endotracheal tube
Bronchial toilet for therapeutic or diagnostic	without compromising oxygenation and
purposes	ventilation
Evaluation of tracheostomy	

FB, flexible bronchoscope.

effusion is milky in appearance, a chylothorax should be suspected and triglycerides measured in both the pleural fluid and the serum for comparison.

Pleural fluid analysis is also helpful in assessing the need for a tube thoracotomy in cases of empyema. If the pH of the pleural fluid is >7.20, its glucose level is >40 mg per dL, and its lactate dehydrogenase (LDH) level is <1,000 IU per L, the effusion associated with the parapneumonic process is in the exudative stage, and no further therapeutic intervention is usually recommended. However, if the pleural effusion increases in size or the patient remains or becomes febrile, a repeat thoracentesis is recommended. If the repeat pleural fluid analysis reveals pleural fluid, which is grossly purulent, has a pH <7.20, a glucose level <40 mg per dL, and an LDH level of >1,000 IU per L, or if the Gram stain result is positive for microorganisms, tube thoracostomy is recommended.

Bronchoscopy

The differences between rigid bronchoscopy (RB) and flexible bronchoscopy (FB) are the size, flexibility, auxiliary instrumentation, optics, and type of sedation used in each of the procedures. The flexible bronchoscope is sized according to the outer diameter (e.g., 3.5 mm), and the patient must breathe around the bronchoscope. The rigid bronchoscopes are sized according to their internal diameter; therefore, a 3.5-mm rigid bronchoscope has a 4 to 4.5 mm outer diameter and is large enough to allow the patient to breathe through them. Rigid bronchoscopes as small as 2.5 mm are currently available. The rigid bronchoscope allows the passage of various instruments through the lumen. This includes suction catheters, forceps for biopsies and extractions of foreign bodies, and Fogerty catheters for tamponade of the bleeding vessels. In the

pediatric FB, one is limited to the use of the suction channel's lumen (1.2 mm internal diameter), and very few instruments can be passed through it. The glass-rod fiber-optic telescope, which is passed through the rigid bronchoscope, provides the best optical performance. These telescopes are available in various sizes (the smallest being a 2.5 mm) with various wide angles (80 and 70 degrees) in its tip. The advantage of the optics in the flexible bronchoscope is the flexibility. This allows visualization of areas that the rigid bronchoscope may not reach, such as the apices of the lung, and also allows a study of the dynamics of the airways, especially the upper airways. The flexible bronchoscope can be used with mild sedation and local anesthesia in most cases, with the patient breathing normally. RB is commonly done under general anesthesia. This is the preferred procedure to investigate the posterior aspect of the larynx and upper trachea for tracheoesophageal fistula (H-type), biopsies, therapeutic excision of tissue from the airways, and foreign body extraction, and when bleeding from the airways is expected during the procedure and in a ventilated patient in whom the flexible bronchoscope cannot be passed through the endotracheal tube (ETT). Both techniques should be available for the pediatric patient and individualized on the basis of the clinical condition. The indications for FB and RB in the pediatric age-group are summarized in Table 37.2.

Techniques

The standard pediatric FB consists of a flexible shaft through which two bundles of glass fibers and one suction channel of 1.2-mm diameter pass. Light is brought to the tip of the bronchoscope by one bundle of fiber-optic glass, and the other bundle carries the image. The distal 2 to 2.5 cm of the instrument is flexible. The suction channel is used to suction, irrigate the airway, perform bronchial lavage,

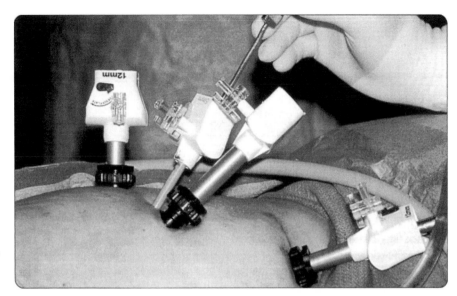

Figure 37.3 Video-assisted thoracic surgery (VATS) is especially helpful for peripheral pulmonary or pleural lesions. (From Bone RC, Campbell GD, Payne DK. *Bone's atlas of pulmonary and critical care medicine.* Philadelphia, PA: Lippincott Williams & Wilkins;2002:98.)

and pass a cytology brush, a very small grasping forceps or basket. It is possible to perform FB in the ICU, operating room, or in a bronchoscopy suite. In the nonintubated patient, the nasal insertion route is predominantly used because it is more comfortable for the patient and is the easiest route of access to the trachea.

In patients who are already intubated, the flexible bronchoscope can be introduced through an ETT adapter. The flexible bronchoscope may be a tight fit within the ETT, therefore, an assistant is necessary to stabilize the ETT and prevent its downward displacement. FB can also be performed safely through a laryngeal mask airway. Children with a tracheostomy may be examined through the tracheostomy tube or directly through the stoma once the tracheostomy tube has been removed. The procedure may also be performed from the nose or mouth to determine the end of the tracheal cannula or to examine the airway either with or without the tracheostomy tube in place.

Flexible bronchoscopes can also be useful during difficult intubations. This is especially true in children with oropharyngeal and cervical spine abnormalities. The 3.5-mm bronchoscope may be used to insert a 4.5-mm ETT. For ETT with sizes ≤4.5 mm, there are bronchoscopes with an outer diameter of 2.2 mm. To secure the airway properly, first pass the tip of the flexible bronchoscope through the tube, insert the tip through the nose and larynx, and then thread the ETT down through the larynx and into the trachea. Bronchoscopy also helps identify the position of the tip of the tube and its required distance from the carina.

A common technique used in pediatric patients undergoing FB is lavage. It may be used for diagnostic and treatment purposes. The lavage fluid for diagnostic purposes is examined for organisms (i.e., bacteria, fungi, and viruses) and cytology. The removal of secretions and plugs from within the airway can also be augmented by lavage.

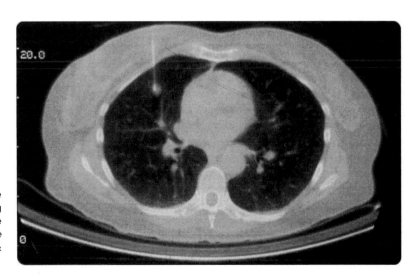

Figure 37.4 The use of transthoracic needle aspiration is particularly useful for peripheral lung lesions. (From Bone RC, Campbell GD, Payne DK. *Bone's atlas of pulmonary and critical care medicine.* Philadelphia, PA: Lippincott Williams & Wilkins;2002:98.)

Topical anesthesia is essential throughout the FB. Two percent lidocaine liquid or gel without preservative is commonly used. The maximum safe dose is 4 mg per kg. Its action lasts for approximately 20 minutes. Lidocaine may be instilled directly into the nose before the procedure and then on the airway mucosa through the suction channel. For bronchoscopy through the nares, phenylephrine 0.5%, xylometazoline 0.1%, or oxymetazoline 0.05% can be helpful in vasoconstricting the mucosa of the nares and in allowing the easier passage of the flexible bronchoscope.

Complications

Ongoing assessment of the patient is essential to detect problems or complications. Communication with an awake patient is also helpful in limiting anxiety. The frequency of complications during bronchoscopic procedures, flexible or rigid, is low. Complications can include hypoxemia, hypercapnia with acidosis, arrhythmias, laryngospasm, bronchospasm, infection, pneumothorax, hemoptysis, direct trauma to the nasal tissue or larynx, and subglottic edema with stridor. Hypoxemia can be prevented by providing adequate oxygen during the FB and monitoring the patient with a continuous pulse oximeter. Another major cause of hypoxia is from hypoventilation secondary to sedatives. Therefore, sedatives should be given in incremental doses to avoid oversedation. Hypercapnia is more difficult to monitor, but if attention is given to air entry during the procedure and the procedure is performed rapidly, it is possible to avoid this complication.

Pediatric FBs or RBs are generally not done in a completely sterile environment. *Pseudomonas*, mycobacteria, and fungi are commonly reported pathogens; however, iatrogenic infections from bronchoscopy are uncommon. Attention to adequate cleaning and disinfection of the bronchoscope between use is essential.

Thoracoscopy

Recent advances in video technology have allowed the development of thoracoscopy, or video-assisted thoracic surgery (VATS), for the diagnosis and management of pleural and parenchymal lung disease (see Fig. 37.3). During this procedure, a rigid scope with a distal lens is inserted through a trocar into the pleura. This allows the operator to manipulate under direct vision the other biopsy instruments passed through the separate, small intercostal incisions into the pleural space. The biggest advantage of thoracoscopy is that the pleura or lung can be inspected visually and biopsied under direct observation. These procedures are helpful in the diagnosis of exudative pleural effusions of uncertain etiology, decortication of complicated parapneumonic effusions, pleurodesis of malignant pleural effusions, biopsy of pleural or peripheral parenchymal lung lesions, and resection of blebs or bullae in pneumothoraces. This procedure is much less invasive than the traditional thoracotomy performed for lung biopsy and has largely replaced "open lung biopsy."

Transthoracic Needle Aspiration

A transthoracic needle aspiration involves inserting a thin-walled 23- or 25-gauge aspiration needle under local anesthesia percutaneously into a specific lung lesion under the guidance of CT scan or fluoroscopy (see Fig. 37.4). This procedure enables the aspiration of fluid or cells for cytologic or microbiologic analyses, although one of the limitations of this technique is the small amount of clinical material obtained.

The potential risks of this procedure include intrapulmonary bleeding and the creation of a pneumothorax with collapse of the underlying lung. Contraindications to needle aspiration are a bleeding diathesis, pulmonary

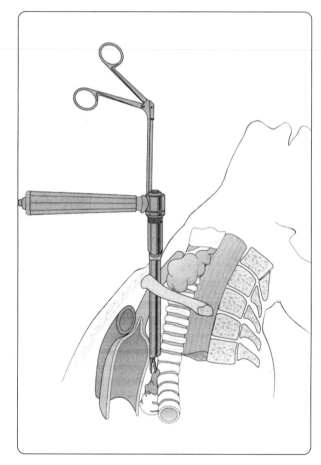

Figure 37.5 Mediastinoscopy. Mediastinoscopy is an invasive, yet safe, procedure that can be used to identify malignant lymph nodes in the superior mediastinum. Mediastinal lymph node metastasis usually denotes unresectability. The introduction of mediastinoscopy has reduced the frequency of staging thoracotomies from 30%–50% to 5%–15%. (From Bone RC, Campbell GD, Payne DK. *Bone's atlas of pulmonary and critical care medicine.* Philadelphia, PA: Lippincott Williams & Wilkins; 2002:99.)

hypertension, suspected pulmonary vascular lesions, and the presence of blebs or bullae in the immediate vicinity of the potential biopsy site.

Mediastinoscopy, Mediastinotomy, Pleural Biopsy, and Open Lung Biopsy

Additional diagnostic procedures in children include mediastinoscopy, mediastinotomy, pleural biopsy, and open lung biopsy. All these are invasive procedures performed under general anesthesia by a qualified surgeon. Mediastinoscopy (through a suprasternal approach) and mediastinotomy (through a parasternal approach) are the two major procedures used to obtain specimens from masses or nodes in the mediastinum (see Fig. 37.5). They are usually performed to provide a histologic diagnosis for suspected lung tumors and to assess the spread of disease to mediastinal structures. Pleural biopsies are particularly helpful in diagnosing pleural effusions secondary to tuberculosis or malignancy. Because pleural biopsies remove parietal pleura, which are supplied by arterioles under systemic pressure, the presence of a coagulopathy represents a relative contraindication to this procedure.

CONCLUSION

In summary, close collaboration between clinicians and radiologists can help ensure that the optimal procedure to obtain the needed information is performed in the critically ill child.

RECOMMENDED READINGS

1. Bar-Zohar D, Sivan Y. The yield of flexible fiberoptic bronchoscopy in pediatric intensive care patients. *Chest.* 2004;126:1353–1359.
2. Gates RL, Caniano DA, Hayes JR, et al. Does VATS provide optimal treatment of empyema in children? A systematic review. *J Pediatr Surg.* 2004;39:381–386.
3. Copley SJ, Padley SP. High-resolution CT of paediatric lung disease. *Eur Radiol.* 2001;11:2564–2575.
4. Culver DA, Gordon SM, Mehta AC, et al. Infection control in the bronchoscopy suite. *Am J Respir Crit Care Med.* 2003;167: 1050–1056.
5. Kim OH, Kim WS, Kim MJ, et al. US in the diagnosis of pediatric chest diseases. *Radiographics.* 2000;20:653–671.
6. Muller NL. Computed tomography and magnetic resonance imaging: Past, present and future. *Eur Respir J Suppl.* 2002;35:3s–12s.
7. Quasney MW, Goodman DM, Billow M, et al. Routine chest radiographs in pediatric intensive care units. *Pediatrics.* 2001;107: 241–248.
8. Segura RM. Useful clinical biological markers in diagnosis of pleural effusions in children. *Paediatr Respir Rev.* 2004;5(Suppl A): S205–S212.

Asthma

Regina Okhuysen-Cawley   *James B. Fink*

Acute severe asthma is a common cause of severe respiratory distress and failure in the pediatric intensive care unit (PICU). Asthma is caused by a complex interplay of genetic, immunologic, and neurohumoral factors. Although fatal asthma is uncommon in children, significant morbidity may be observed. This chapter discusses the current management of acute asthma in children admitted to the PICU.

Although patients with previously mild intermittent disease may develop severe exacerbations, several subpopulations are at particular risk for life-threatening events: African American adolescent boys with poor socioeconomic support, patients with a history of episodes requiring PICU admission, those with severe atopy, those with blunted perception of bronchoconstriction, changes in their corticosteroid regimens, and a pronounced diurnal variation in their pulmonary function. The lack of recognition of an attack's severity by the patient, family, or health care provider may lead to tragedy in this acute illness.

PATHOPHYSIOLOGY OF LIFE-THREATENING ASTHMA

The immunologic aspects of asthma are complex and are detailed elsewhere.[1] Factors contributing to airway obstruction include bronchoconstriction, epithelial cell injury–mediated neurogenic inflammation with loss of smooth muscle reactivity, inflammatory cell infiltration, and luminal obstruction due to secretions and cellular debris. Progressive dynamic hyperinflation eventually leads to altered mechanical functioning during breathing and results in respiratory muscle fatigue. Nonhomogeneous airflow obstruction causes an inequality of ventilation and perfusion and leads to hypoxemia. Superimposed atelectasis or pneumonia may create a true shunt and more pronounced hypoxia. Pulmonary edema develops in extreme cases. A combination of increased right ventricular afterload and decreased left ventricular preload causes a fall in cardiac output.[2] The radiographic findings associated with these pathophysiologic states and their associated complications are shown in Figure 38.1.

PATTERNS OF LIFE-THREATENING ILLNESS

The most common pattern of life-threatening illness is the insidious development of progressive airway edema on a baseline of increased airway tone. Precipitants for this type of episode include viral and *Mycoplasma* infections. A pattern of respiratory failure that is increasingly recognized in pediatrics is termed *acute asphyxic asthma*. These patients develop acute respiratory failure within minutes of the sudden onset of dyspnea. They commonly have the previously mentioned risk factors. Histologic features in the lungs of these patients include a sudden influx of neutrophils and T cells in addition to the eosinophils and macrophages seen in patients in whom asthma has stabilized. Often, patients with acute asphyxial asthma present with acute cardiorespiratory arrest or with evidence of hypoxic–ischemic encephalopathy following a prolonged arrest.[3]

EVALUATION

A rapid triage should determine the severity of airflow obstruction. The general appearance, respiratory rate and pattern, degree of tachycardia, and oxygen saturation should be continually assessed. Markers of severe distress include lethargy or agitation, orthopnea, markedly fragmented speech, severe retractions with accessory muscle use and thoracoabdominal dissociation, and progressive desaturation on continuous pulse oximetry. Air movement may be so poor as to result in a silent chest. Extreme tachycardia is a risk factor for myocardial ischemia in the

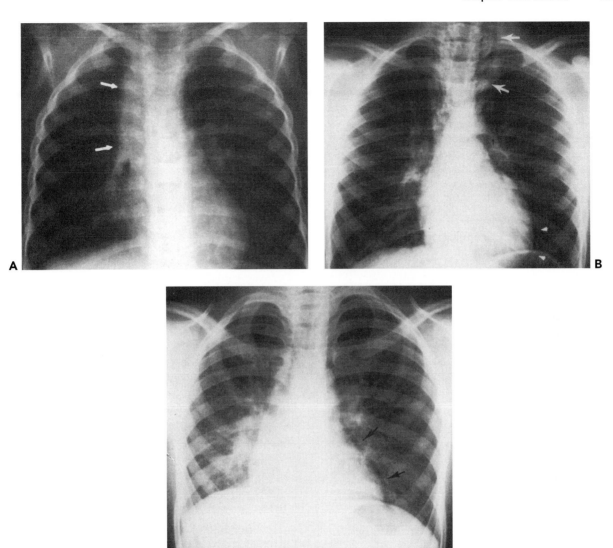

Figure 38.1 Pulmonary complications. **A:** Sublobar atelectasis. A child with asthma having an acute asthma attack; note the area of apparent consolidation in the right paratracheal region (*arrows*). This represents the collapse of one portion of the right upper lobe. A subtler finding assisting interpretation is that the minor fissure is slightly elevated. **B:** A child with asthma having pneumomediastinum with air surrounding the small triangular thymus gland (*T*), extending as linear sheaths into the neck and superior mediastinum (*upper arrows*) and extending along the lower left cardiac edge (*lower arrows*). **C:** Medial pneumothorax. Note the thin strip of free air along the left cardiac border (*arrows*). The finding represents a medial pneumothorax and should not be confused with pneumomediastinum or pneumopericardium. (From Swischuk L. *Emergency radiology of the acutely ill or injured child*. 2nd ed. Philadelphia, PA: Lippincott Williams & Wilkins; 1986;63:77–79.)

adolescent, whereas bradycardia is indicative of imminent cardiopulmonary arrest. Although the estimation of pulsus paradoxus is more difficult in children, it is possible to observe variations in the amplitude of the pulse waveform through oximetry and the quality of the child's radial pulse with respiration. Peak flow maneuvers, a common technique for following airway obstruction in the outpatient settings, may cause an acute deterioration in respiratory function and should be avoided in distressed patients.

Other etiologies for wheezing, such as congenital or acquired causes of airway obstruction in infants and toddlers, and vocal cord dysfunction in older children, must be considered. Patients with congestive heart failure or myocarditis may present with wheezing. The diagnosis of acute severe asthma should be promptly reconsidered in children displaying signs of poor cardiac output or failing to quickly improve with treatment. A chest radiograph is indicated in all acutely ill patients. Arterial blood gas analyses may be necessary in select patients. Respiratory alkalosis is often evident early in the course, but as the airway obstruction continues, the carbon dioxide levels may normalize or become elevated. Normal P_{CO_2} levels in a severely tachypneic and distressed patient can be a harbinger of respiratory failure. Hypoxemia is common. Metabolic acidosis may be present because of dehydration, lactic acid production caused by increased respiratory muscle work, or impaired cardiac output.

PHARMACOTHERAPY

Oxygen therapy is necessary for all patients to control hypoxemia. Oxygen may be administered through a mask, nasal cannula, oxygen tent, or tubing merely held in front of the child's face. Some patients requiring simple or non-rebreather face masks may benefit from low-flow oxygen through a supplemental nasal cannula with trimmed prongs if they exhibit rapid desaturation when the mask is off their face. Inhaled bronchodilators are the first line of therapy and should be delivered with oxygen because β-agonists may increase ventilation and perfusion mismatch by blunting hypoxic pulmonary vasoconstriction. A blender should be used with simple and non-rebreather face masks to minimize oxygen toxicity, facilitate weaning, and prevent absorption atelectasis. Short-acting β_2-agonists, typically albuterol, are the most common agents aerosolized for the treatment of acute bronchospasm. Treatments can be given on an intermittent or continuous basis, although most patients requiring intensive care unit (ICU) admission warrant continuous therapy. Continuous delivery of albuterol, in dosages of up to 20 mg per hour, has been shown to be safe and effective. This drug can be delivered through a mouthpiece, a mask, or in-line in ventilated patients. Albuterol solutions in dilutions and volumes utilized for unit dosing have also been instilled directly into the endotracheal tube in extreme emergencies. Tremors, restlessness, nausea, and vomiting are common side effects of β_2-agonists.

Ipratropium bromide, through its action on muscarinic receptors, acts synergistically with β-agonists. It is devoid of systemic effects, although it can cause mydriasis with loose-fitting delivery devices. Children are typically given 250 to 500 μg every 6 to 8 hours. Although response to an increased dosage of albuterol has been reported, there is no reported benefit to an increased dosage of ipratropium.

Subcutaneous β-agonists such as epinephrine and terbutaline can be used in the initial management of dyspnea in children, who may calm down with improved airflow and may subsequently accept nebulized medications. Although intravenous albuterol, known as salbutamol outside the United States, is deemed highly effective, the only intravenous β-agonist currently available in the United States is terbutaline. Although less selective than albuterol, it is also an effective, although costly, intervention. Most clinicians begin a continuous infusion of 0.4 to 5 μg/kg/minute of terbutaline after an initial loading dose of 10 to 20 μg per kg. Significant tachycardia, tremor, a decrease in diastolic pressures, and lactic acidosis are common. Prolongation of

the QT interval may be observed with any β-agonist, and the risk of dysrhythmia may increase in the presence of hypokalemia. Although clinically significant cardiac toxicity is probably more common in the adult population, the potential for myocardial ischemia and dysrhythmias should be considered in children, particularly in adolescents with other risk factors such as electrolyte disturbances. Following electrocardiographic changes, cardiac enzyme levels, such as troponin, may be helpful in determining whether patients on terbutaline infusions or those who complain of chest pain are experiencing myocardial ischemia.

Steroids, typically methylprednisolone, are necessary to control the inflammatory component of the disease, may decrease mucus production, and enhance upregulation of β-receptors. Patients are typically started on high dosages of 4 to 6 mg/kg/day, which can be rapidly tapered to minimize adverse effects and drug interactions.

It is unclear how magnesium sulfate decreases airway resistance, but it appears to mitigate calcium-mediated bronchoconstriction, modulate smooth muscle excitability, and mediate the activation of adenyl cyclase. Therefore, it may be an important adjunct to other therapies in severely ill patients.[4] Most protocols in children and adults describe bolus dosages of 25 to 50 mg per kg delivered intravenously over 20 minutes, or doses up to 2 g in adult-sized patients. Some clinicians use continuous infusions of magnesium sulfate in dosages of up to 20 mg/kg/hour, although this may result in hypermagnesemia and require additional laboratory monitoring. Aminophylline may have some unique effects regarding diaphragmatic function and airway inflammation, but it is a weak bronchodilator with a narrow therapeutic index and many drug interactions. Its use has fallen out of favor.

Helium–oxygen (heliox) mixtures are of theoretical benefit in severe asthma by decreasing the work of breathing, improving the diffusion of carbon dioxide, and promoting laminar gas flow in constricted airways, which in turn may improve the transport of aerosolized bronchodilating agents to the affected areas. Heliox administration loses its effectiveness if high levels of oxygen (e.g., >50%) are required. The reduced gas density of helium may affect the performance of ventilators, including the measurement of delivered volumes and alarms. Additionally, when heliox is used to drive a nebulizer, it may reduce aerosol output by >50%, requiring appropriate adjustments.[5]

With intermittent or continuous high-dose bronchodilator therapy, most patients show improvement within a few hours of admission to the PICU. As the child recovers, nebulized bronchodilator administration can be weaned from continuous to every 2 hours and then to every 4 hours until the home regimen is reached. Patients with severe symptoms should not be allowed anything by mouth until frank improvement is noted. Distraction and the reassuring presence of a parent may be beneficial to help allay anxiety in the acute phase.

VENTILATORY SUPPORT

Indications for invasive mechanical support include cardiopulmonary arrest and overt respiratory failure. In most instances, the decision to proceed with intubation is a difficult one and considers the clinical situation, the presence of comorbidity, and the need for transport.

Noninvasive positive-pressure ventilation has an important role in the management of lower airway obstruction and is easy to institute in older children. Young children and those with cognitive impairment may benefit from a trial of noninvasive ventilation, although they may require cautious sedation with agents such as ketamine to facilitate the tolerance of uncomfortable devices. Sedation should be reserved for mechanical ventilation unless constant monitoring by experienced staff is available. The decision to provide a trial of noninvasive mechanical support should prompt preparation for intubation.[6]

Intubation of patients with severe asthma remains one of the most stressful procedures performed in the PICU. Acute deterioration in cardiorespiratory function due to relative hypovolemia, decreased vascular tone with the onset of sedation and analgesia, and decreased preload with the onset of positive-pressure ventilation can occur during intubation, and precautions should be taken to limit complications. An isotonic fluid bolus may be given before intubation for intravascular volume expansion, and additional volume should be readily available in the peri-intubation period. Topical anesthesia with nebulized 1% lidocaine (1 to 2 mL) may be provided. Preoxygenation with a non-rebreather face mask can be started while preparations for intubation are being made. The most experienced individual available should perform the procedure with full stomach precautions.

Pretreatment with atropine will prevent bradycardia during airway instrumentation and will decrease airway secretions, particularly if ketamine is used. Glycopyrrolate is an alternative in older children. Histamine-releasing drugs such as morphine and atracurium should be avoided. Ketamine has an intrinsic bronchodilator effect and is less likely to cause hypotension. It also produces a dissociated state of analgesia and sedation that will facilitate airway management. Small doses of a benzodiazepine such as midazolam may be given with the ketamine. Etomidate is another useful option but lacks any intrinsic analgesic effect and has a very short half-life.

The largest bore endotracheal tube that can be safely placed should be used. Cuffed endotracheal tubes may be utilized, particularly in children who have a subacute presentation with a significant inflammatory component.

The goals of mechanical ventilation are to ensure adequate oxygenation and to provide support while the underlying pathology resolves. Dynamic hyperinflation and ventilator-associated morbidity may be decreased by controlling tidal volumes and ventilatory rates, an approach known as *permissive hypercarbia*, given the respiratory acidosis that is commonly observed.

Most children with acute, severe asthma display prolonged time constant physiology. Superimposed processes may precipitate an acute lung injury pattern. Most authors advocate using short inspiratory times, fast inspiratory flow rates, low frequencies, and a prolonged expiratory time. It is important to select optimal levels of positive end-expiratory pressure (PEEP) to aid exhalation, decrease dynamic hyperinflation and atelectasis, enhance surfactant distribution and function, and minimize shear stress.

Some patients, particularly those presenting with an acute asphyxial pattern, improve very rapidly and may need only supportive modes such as pressure support ventilation or volume support ventilation. Most children have relatively fixed airway obstruction. The ideal mode of ventilating such children is not yet known, but the use of decelerating flow pressure–limiting modes such as pressure-regulated volume control (PRVC) may be advantageous in that these modes theoretically provide for more homogeneous medical gas distribution and may thereby enhance oxygenation while limiting peak airway pressures. Pressure control ventilation is widely available, but ventilation may be compromised. Additionally, it typically requires deeper levels of sedation, with neuromuscular blockade in some instances. Continuous graphics monitoring during mechanical ventilation may be helpful in quantifying the degree of dynamic hyperinflation and dyssynchrony and may assist in determining the optimal ventilator settings.[7] Matching inspiratory and expiratory times and flow patterns with mechanical ventilation is often extremely difficult with severe asthma before reduction in airway obstruction. It is not unusual for oxygenation and ventilation to deteriorate temporarily immediately after inhibition. Improvement occurs with recruitment and optimized ventilator settings.

The delivery of bronchodilators may be reduced during mechanical ventilation. The efficiency of standard jet nebulizers is reduced to <3%, requiring larger doses than those used before intubation. Ultrasonic and electronic micropump nebulizers deliver approximately 13% of the dose through the endotracheal tube.

The use of high-frequency oscillation, although counterintuitive, may be of use in select patients presenting with a bronchiolitis-type clinical picture. Patients described in the literature and observed in practice typically require high amplitudes to compensate for the increased attenuation, a low frequency, and a mean airway pressure adjusted as necessary to maintain oxygenation. The expiratory phase may be prolonged to maximize the active exhalation characteristic of high-frequency oscillatory ventilation (HFOV).[8] Interactive ventilator modes such as volume support ventilation may expedite weaning. Extubation should occur when clinically indicated because the continued presence of the endotracheal tube acts as an irritant in the airway. Some children may benefit from chest physiotherapy.

Intrapulmonary percussive ventilation with albuterol may help clear residual atelectasis.

MANAGEMENT OF REFRACTORY DISEASE

Additional modalities to be considered include the use of inhaled anesthetic agents such as isoflurane. Hypotension can be corrected with isotonic fluid infusion or dopamine. Sedation (and neuromuscular blocking agents) can be decreased during the treatment and will need to be adjusted when isoflurane is discontinued.[9] Inhaled nitric oxide usually improves oxygenation and has a modest beneficial effect on ventilation. Documentation of this technique in life-threatening asthma is limited; however, a trial of therapy is relatively easy to implement in most ICUs.[10] Some clinicians use heliox mixtures during ventilation. Extracorporeal life support (ECLS) should be considered before the onset of severe hypoxemia or a significant complication of therapy. It may also be helpful in the event of an acute deterioration in respiratory function. Survival with ECLS is very high in patients with asthma, and the morbidity associated with this invasive therapy is minimized with the application of venovenous techniques. Bronchoscopy is generally contraindicated, but a therapeutic procedure, which may include lavage, may be necessary for mechanical obstruction due to bronchial casts or tenacious secretions resistant to recombinant human deoxyribonuclease (rhDNase)[11] or other mucolytics. External chest compression to assist in exhalation has been described in patients whose condition is deteriorating with extreme hyperinflation.

MANAGEMENT OF RELATED MORBIDITY

Although hypercarbia into the mid-100–mm Hg range is generally well tolerated, it has been implicated in neurologic events in older children, including increased intracranial pressure, subarachnoid hemorrhage, and cranial nerve palsies. Bicarbonate infusion is of dubious benefit in managing respiratory acidosis. Agents such as tromethamine may be considered in patients who are profoundly acidemic.

Many PICUs have protocols in place to decrease described morbidities that have been observed in mechanically ventilated patients with asthma, such as myopathy, exposure keratopathy, gastrointestinal hemorrhage, deconditioning, foot drop, pressure ulceration, and deep venous

thrombosis. These problems may be associated with neuromuscular blockade and bed rest. These protocols should be implemented as soon as possible after intubation. Myopathy appears to be more common when high-dose steroids and steroidal-based neuromuscular blocking agents such as vecuronium and aminoglycosides are used concurrently. Hyperglycemia and electrolyte abnormalities such as hypokalemia and hypermagnesemia may be contributing factors that can be identified and corrected. It is reasonable to monitor urinary myoglobin or creatine phosphokinase (CPK) in sicker patients at risk for rhabdomyolysis.

Strongly suspected or confirmed infections should be treated aggressively. Nosocomial infections may be minimized by paying attention to detail, including hand washing, early institution of transpyloric enteral nutrition, and use of sterile technique for all procedures. Posttraumatic stress disorder, opioid and benzodiazepine habituation, and altered sleep patterns may complicate longer PICU stays.

Mortality due to life-threatening asthma may be decreasing in the adult population and should be increasingly rare in children. It is prudent to include a pulmonary medicine consultation in the patient's care plan before discharge from the PICU.

REFERENCES

1. Bochner BS, Undem BJ, Lichtenstein LM. Immunological aspects of allergic asthma. *Ann Rev Immunol.* 1994;12:295–335.
2. Werner HA. Status asthmaticus: A review. *Chest.* 2001;119:1913–1929.
3. Maffei FA, Van der Jagt EW, Powers KP, et al. Duration of mechanical ventilation in life-threatening pediatric asthma: Description of an acute asphyxial subgroup. *Pediatrics.* 2004;114:762–767.
4. Silverman RA, Osborn H, Runge J, et al. IV magnesium sulfate in the treatment of acute severe asthma. *Chest.* 2002;122:489–497.
5. Abd-Allah SA, Rogers MA, Terry M, et al. Helium-oxygen therapy for acute severe asthma requiring mechanical ventilation. *Pediatr Crit Care Med.* 2003;4(3):353–357.
6. Thill PJ, McGuire JK, Baden HP, et al. Noninvasive positive pressure ventilation in children with lower airway obstruction. *Pediatr Crit Care Med.* 2004;5(4):337–342.
7. Sarnaik AP, Daphtary KM, Meert KL, et al. Pressure controlled ventilation in children with severe status asthmaticus. *Pediatr Crit Care Med.* 2004;5(2):133–138.
8. Duval EL, Van Vught AJ. Status asthmaticus treated by high frequency oscillatory ventilation. *Pediatr Pulmonol.* 2000;30(4):350–353.
9. Wheeler DK, Clapp CR, Ponaman ML, et al. Isofluorane therapy for status asthmaticus in children: A case series and protocol. *Pediatr Crit Care Med.* 2000;1(1):55–59.
10. Nakagawa TA, Johnston SJ, Falkos SA, et al. Life-threatening status asthmaticus treated with inhaled nitric oxide. *J Pediatr.* 2000;137(1):119–122.
11. Durward A, Forte V, Shemie S. Resolution of mucus plugging and atelectasis after intratracheal rhDNase therapy in a mechanically ventilated child with refractory status asthmaticus. *Crit Care Med.* 2002;28(2):560–562.

Disorders of the Lung Parenchyma

39

Angela T. Wratney   Ira M. Cheifetz   James D. Fortenberry   Matthew L. Paden

---

The main function of the respiratory system is to provide adequate oxygen and remove carbon dioxide. In the setting of acute respiratory failure, the lungs are unable to preserve adequate gas exchange. Subsequently, tissue oxygen delivery can be impaired, and/or ventilation becomes inadequate resulting in hypercapnia and potential acidosis.

RESPIRATORY DISTRESS AND RESPIRATORY FAILURE

Respiratory distress and respiratory failure are clinical diagnoses of a pulmonary system that is no longer capable of providing normal gas exchange without artificial support. The term *respiratory distress* indicates that the patient is utilizing compensatory mechanisms to preserve adequate gas exchange. *Respiratory failure* is a late clinical finding resulting from the failure of these compensatory mechanisms to preserve adequate gas exchange or to ensure adequate oxygen delivery. As most pediatric cardiopulmonary arrests have their origin in the respiratory system, failure to recognize and treat respiratory distress/failure in a timely manner can have significant adverse outcomes.

The signs of respiratory distress include increased effort and/or decreased effectiveness of respiration. Physical signs of increased respiratory effort include tachypnea, tachycardia, and increased work of breathing (i.e., subcostal and supraclavicular retractions). In the setting of respiratory disease, associated with a variable degree of hypoxemia or hypercarbia, compensatory mechanisms to restore normal gas exchange may become increasingly apparent. Patients may present with effortful breathing associated with nasal flaring, grunting, or increased use of accessory muscles of respiration. Increased inspiratory or expiratory force may cause retractions (supraclavicular, subcostal, or intercostal),

and paradoxic breathing may be noted (abdomen retracts upon inspiration and expands upon expiration).

Some children will present with effortless tachypnea resulting from an increased respiratory drive caused by metabolic acidosis or central nervous system disease. Children with neuromuscular disease may not manifest the typical clinical signs of agitation or vigorous respiratory muscle use; therefore, it is imperative to have a higher level of suspicion for respiratory disease in these patients. Patients with neuromuscular disorders also warrant an appreciation for their limited respiratory reserve.

The patient with respiratory distress may also demonstrate changes in the presence or quality of breath sounds on auscultation. Decreased breath sounds and diminished air entry in the setting of increased respiratory effort suggest worsening respiratory disease. Patients who present with upper airway obstruction may present with acute agitation secondary to hypoxia. Patients who present with a weak cough, inability to control secretions, or an incompetent gag reflex have little capacity to protect their airway. These patients may require immediate and urgent airway support.

Respiratory disease in pediatric patients can rapidly progress from respiratory distress to acute respiratory failure with a significant impairment in gas exchange. Although respiratory failure is classically described by arterial blood gas values (PaO_2 <60 mm Hg and/or $PaCO_2$ >50 mm Hg), it is best recognized by the physician as a clinical syndrome marked by a progression of the signs and symptoms of respiratory distress. Infants and children are particularly prone to developing respiratory failure secondary to: (a) smaller airway caliber resulting in a greater resistance to airflow, (b) greater chest wall compliance resulting in chest wall retractions with forceful inspiratory effort resulting in paradoxical breathing and a restriction of lung capacitance, (c) greater propensity for rapid fatigue of the respiratory muscles and diaphragm, and (d) greater predisposition to develop apnea in the neonate.

The hallmark of acute respiratory disease is usually hypoxia in the pediatric patient. Hypoxia results from impaired gas exchange secondary to hypoventilation, airway obstruction, ventilation–perfusion mismatch, diffusion abnormalities (although clinically very rare), hemoglobinopathies, and congenital cardiac lesions (intracardiac right-to-left shunting).

Despite the etiology of respiratory illness, a typical clinical picture results in tachypnea, hypocapnia, and hypoxia associated with the physical signs of respiratory distress. Clinical evaluation should involve a search for the underlying cause of hypoxia and respiratory distress/failure as well as for signs of impaired cardiorespiratory reserve. An evaluation, which reveals progressive deterioration or signs of inability to maintain adequate respiratory effort, indicates the need for greater level of monitoring, intervention, and support.

Evaluation of respiratory distress should include an assessment of capacity for airway control, congenital or acquired anatomic airway abnormalities, and signs of obstructed airflow. Airway control refers to providing a patent air passage from the nose/mouth to the lungs and the ability to protect the airway from aspiration of food or saliva. This latter ability requires an intact central nervous system and oropharyngeal motor control. Anatomic airway defects may be visualized by an examination of the palate, the chin to mandibular distance, and the ability to open the mouth widely.

Airway obstruction may be indicated by the presence of stridor, a high-pitched sound. Stridor is usually heard on inspiration, indicating increased airflow resistance in the upper airway. Stridor upon inspiration and expiration (biphasic stridor) is indicative of an extrathoracic airway obstruction. Hoarseness may indicate trauma or inflammation of the vocal cords.

Physical assessment of breathing involves noting the presence or absence, quality, location, characteristics, and symmetry of breath sounds on auscultation of the lung fields. Generalized limited air entry or movement may indicate hypoventilation or airway obstructive disease. Respiratory disease is indicated by the absence of breath sounds (consolidation) or by an abnormal quality of breath sounds present in particular lung regions. Auscultation may reveal wheezes, rhonchi, rales, or crackles. Wheezing indicates airway obstruction, usually bronchospasm, of the lower airways and a prolonged expiratory time may be noted. Rales usually indicate alveolar fluid. Crackles may indicate the opening and closing of atelectatic alveoli with respiratory effort. Rhonchi are harsh, bronchiolar sounds resulting from secretions partially occluding airflow. These may disappear with forceful expiratory effort or cough. Appreciation for the symmetry or asymmetry of findings

may localize the affected lung region and may indicate the need for further evaluation and imaging. It should be noted that auscultation of the infant and small child may be remarkably normal despite pathologic findings on a chest x-ray (CXR).

Worsening respiratory status or impending respiratory failure may be noted by decreased air entry, significant anxiety, depressed level of consciousness, hypoventilation, or failure to improve upon serial examination.

Cyanosis is not frequently present on physical examination. Bluish discoloration of the skin does not occur until the deoxygenated hemoglobin exceeds 4 to 5 g per dL. Anemia may mask cyanosis owing to the decreased total amount of hemoglobin.

Physical examination may also include a bedside evaluation of pulmonary function to track changes in respiratory capacity with intervention. Peak flow testing is easily performed at the bedside and it provides a numeric assessment of the peak expiratory force. Comparison of the patient's best expiratory effort with normative values and with previous performance can aid in the assessment of worsening lower respiratory disease. This maneuver may be difficult to perform in children, especially those with significant respiratory distress, and is rarely performed routinely in the pediatric intensive care unit (PICU).

Negative inspiratory force (NIF) measurements may be obtained to assess the respiratory function of the chest wall and inspiratory muscles. NIF <-20 cm H_2O indicates significant impairment of inspiratory capacitance. A normal NIF measurement is -75 to -100 cm H_2O, and a forceful cough to clear the airway is thought to occur at -25 cm H_2O.

An evaluation of the cardiac status of a patient with respiratory distress is essential. Physical examination should note the quality of end-organ perfusion—capillary refill time, temperature of the peripheral extremities, and presence of compensatory mechanisms to improve cardiac output (e.g., tachycardia or increased systemic vascular resistance), urine output, and mental status.

A CXR is an important tool in the initial evaluation for the underlying etiology of respiratory distress, and serial examinations can assess the effect of interventions on the progression of disease (see Fig. 39.1). Unfortunately, the CXR does not often reveal an etiology for the disease process and many films only reflect generic changes consistent with pulmonary insult. Similarly, the CXR findings typically lag behind the clinical assessment and, therefore, do not adequately and immediately assess the therapeutic benefit of interventions. Nonetheless, CXRs are routinely obtained and do provide a great deal of information to rule out certain disease entities (e.g., pneumothorax) or to indicate pathologic conditions (e.g., pleural effusions, elevated diaphragm, rib fractures, or aspirated foreign body).

To avoid missing pathology, evaluation of the CXR should involve consideration of film quality, presence of rotation, and a systematic consideration of the chest

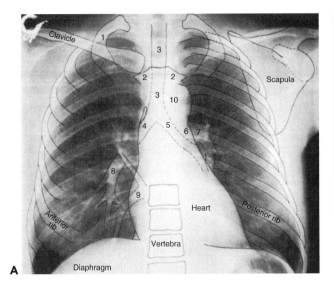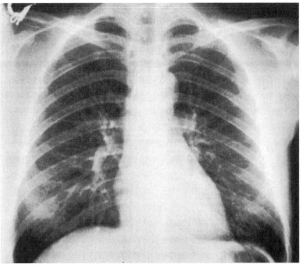

Figure 39.1 **A:** Posteroanterior chest radiograph with overlay of structures noted. *1.* First rib. *2.* Upper manubrium. *3.* Trachea. *4.* Right main bronchus. *5.* Left main bronchus. *6.* Main pulmonary artery. *7.* Left pulmonary artery. *8.* Right interlobar pulmonary artery. *9.* Right pulmonary vein. *10.* Aortic arch. **B:** Same radiograph without overlay. (From George RB, Light RW, Matthay MA, et al., eds. *Chest medicine: Essentials of pulmonary and critical care medicine.* 4th ed. Philadelphia, PA: Lippincott Williams & Wilkins; 2004.)

structures: (i) integrity of the airways, (ii) lung field markings, (iii) pleural space, (iv) bones, (v) soft tissues, (vi) cardiac silhouette, (vii) pulmonary vascular markings, (viii) overall symmetry, (ix) diaphragm, and (x) evaluation of proper placement of all tubes, wires, and catheters. It is also particularly informative to compare with previous films for appropriate interpretation of findings. Mediastinal shifting may occur owing to volume loss (shifting toward the affected side) or owing to mass effect (shifting away from the affected side).

The CXR may be remarkably normal despite significant pulmonary disease. This may commonly occur in the setting of aspiration, hypoplastic left-sided heart disease, radiolucent foreign body aspiration, early acute chest syndrome (ACS), and in young patients. Decubitus films may be used to evaluate the layering of pulmonary effusions or to detect gas trapping which occurs with foreign body aspiration into a main bronchus.

No particular laboratory test is critical during an acute respiratory crisis; the laboratory values rarely indicate an unknown process or immediately change resuscitation management. When obtained, the arterial blood gas provides the best assessment of the adequacy of gas exchange. Evaluation of the arterial blood gas will aid in the assessment of the acuteness of onset of disease, oxygen tension, and limits of ventilatory reserve. Although capillary blood samples may be used, they are not reliable measures of arterial oxygenation, especially in the poorly perfused patient. Venous blood gases are generally only helpful as an indicator of venous oxygen saturation, a surrogate for cardiac output, when drawn from an intrathoracic central vessel.

An arterial blood gas may have a PaO_2 that is anywhere between 60 and 200 mm Hg (see the oxyhemoglobin saturation curve), whereas the saturation as measured by pulse oximetry reads 90% to 95%. Pulse oximeters may indicate a hemoglobin saturation that is unchanged despite a large reduction in the arterial oxygen tension. The PaO_2 may also be used to calculate the A-a gradient supporting clinical concerns for impaired alveolar–arterial gas exchange.

The arterial blood gas will not be accurate in the setting of an abnormal hemoglobin level. PaO_2 refers to the dissolved gas and not to the portion bound to the hemoglobin. In the case of a hemoglobinopathy, a calculated oxygen saturation level from the PaO_2 using the oxyhemoglobin saturation curve will be falsely high, despite a severe deficit in tissue oxygen delivery. Therefore, the actual functional saturation of hemoglobin in this situation must be measured by co-oximetry. Co-oximetry measures four different wavelengths of light emittance and measures the oxy-, carboxy-, and deoxyhemoglobin concentration directly.

Management of the patient with respiratory distress/failure includes an assessment of airway, breathing, and circulation. Prompt cardiopulmonary resuscitation is vital to restore adequate systemic oxygen delivery. Identification and targeted therapy for the underlying etiology and elimination of any potential source for exacerbation of the disease is a critical first step in treatment.

When therapeutic measures do not result in the expected improvement, the clinician must evaluate exacerbating factors including increased oxygen demand (e.g., fever, seizures, shivering, or excessive work of breathing) or the presence of intrathoracic disease, impairing resuscitation

PULMONARY PARENCHYMAL DISEASES CAUSING CRITICAL ILLNESS IN CHILDREN

Infectious

Pneumonitides
  Bacterial
  Viral
  Fungal
  Atypical
  Mycobacterial
  Parasitic
Parapneumonic processes
  Pleuritis
  Empyema

Noninfectious

Acute respiratory distress syndrome
Aspiration pneumonitis
  Hydrocarbons
  Gastric aspiration
  Chemical
  Near-drowning
Inhalation injury
Autoimmune vasculitides
Acute chest syndrome/sickle cell disease
Acute exacerbation of chronic lung disease

(e.g., pneumothorax, pleural effusions, chest wall injury, or impaired cardiac filling). Adequate resuscitation often involves multiple therapeutic interventions, each of which must be prioritized with the benefits and risks of each therapy considered.

Manifestations of pulmonary parenchymal disorders can be categorized as primarily infectious or noninfectious in nature (see Table 39.1). Common conditions that result in respiratory compromise and require care in the PICU are discussed in the subsequent text.

ETIOLOGIES OF PARENCHYMAL LUNG DISEASE

Infectious Etiologies

The infectious agents responsible for pneumonia and lower respiratory tract infection (LRTI) can be divided into bacterial, viral, fungal, mycobacterial, and atypical causes. Incidence of specific pathogens differs by age (see Table 39.2). Further details about the pathophysiology of these diseases can be found in Chapter 3.3. For the intensivist, identification of the pathogen involved in the critical illness, and institution of timely and appropriate antimicrobial therapy is of vital importance in limiting organ damage.

Bacterial Pneumonias

Patients presenting with streptococcal disease may be observed to have lobar consolidation on chest radiography, although a pattern of bronchopneumonia may also be present in children (see Fig. 39.2).

Staphylococcal pneumonia is a common cause of ventilator-associated and nosocomial pneumonia. However, it also occurs as a community-acquired disease, especially in the setting of a precedent or coexisting viral infection such as influenza. This is likely due to the influence of viral hemagglutinins, which inhibit neutrophil and monocyte activation, subsequently predisposing the patient to bacterial superinfection.

Chest radiography classically shows a lobar consolidation, and the presence of pneumatoceles, pleural effusion, air fluid levels, or areas suspicious for necrosis should increase suspicion for staphylococcal pneumonia (see Fig. 39.3). Treatment has changed remarkably over the past decade, with the increasing prevalence of strains of methicillin resistant *Staphylococcus aureus* (MRSA). Vancomycin-intermediate and vancomycin-resistant strains have also rarely been reported. For serious invasive disease where *Staphylococcus* is considered, empiric therapy should start with vancomycin until culture and antibiotic sensitivities are known.

Pseudomonas aeruginosa is the most common and deadly cause of bacterial nosocomial pneumonia in the PICU (see Fig. 39.4). *Pseudomonas* infection is also more common in patients with cystic fibrosis, tracheostomy dependence, and immunocompromise. In patients with mechanical ventilation support, the presence of fever, increasing ventilatory support, and change in secretions should alert the clinician to the possibility of the presence of nosocomial pneumonia. Appropriate cultures collected by direct aspiration, protected brush specimen, or bronchiolar lavage should be sent for evaluation. The presence of gram-negative rods with many white cells and few epithelial cells is indicative of gram-negative nosocomial pneumonia, and oxidase positive testing implicates *Pseudomonas* species.

The development of antibiotic resistance in *Pseudomonas* species has made empiric therapy considerations more difficult. *Pseudomonas* species generally harbor extended spectrum β-lactamase activity, and serious or life-threatening infections should not be treated with an antipseudomonal synthetic penicillin alone.

The atypical pneumonias include infections caused by *Mycoplasma pneumoniae*, *Chlamydia pneumoniae*, and *Legionella pneumophila*. They are a common cause of pneumonia in the age-group of schoolgoing children, demonstrating fever, persistent cough (which can last for weeks after the infection has cleared), hypoxia, myalgias, and rales on auscultation. While generally appearing less ill than other bacterial pneumonitides, infected patients can require intensive care admission because of significant hypoxia or complications from their disease.

TABLE 39.2

ETIOLOGY AND TREATMENT OF INFECTIOUS PNEUMONIA BY AGE

	Age				
	0–4 wk	**4–8 wk**	**8–12 wk**	**12 wk–4 y**	**5 y–Adolescence**
Etiology (in order of prevalence)	Group B *Streptococcus*, gram-negative enteric bacteria, *Listeria monocytogenes*	*Chlamydia trachomatis*, viruses (RSV, parainfluenza), *Streptococcus pneumoniae*, *Bordetella pertussis*, group B *Streptococcus*, gram-negative enteric bacteria, *Listeria monocytogenes*	*Chlamydia trachomatis*, viruses (RSV, parainfluenza), *Streptococcus pneumoniae*, *Bordetella pertussis*	Viruses (RSV, parainfluenza, influenza, adenovirus, rhinovirus), *Streptococcus pneumoniae*, *Haemophilus influenzae* (*nontype B*), *Moraxella catarrhalis*, group A *Streptococcus*, *Mycoplasma pneumoniae*, *Mycobacterium tuberculosis*	*Mycoplasma pneumoniae*, *Chlamydia pneumoniae*, *Streptococcus pneumoniae*, viruses (RSV, parainfluenza, influenza, adenovirus, rhinovirus), *Mycobacterium tuberculosis*
Initial inpatient treatment	Neonatal pneumonia or sepsis: ceftriaxone or cefotaxime plus ampicillin	Neonatal pneumonia or sepsis: ceftriaxone or cefotaxime plus ampicillin	For *Streptococcus pneumoniae*: see next column	Penicillin or ampicillin or cefuroxime, cefotaxime or ceftriaxone, clindamycin, vancomycin until alternative susceptible agents are identified	Macrolides, cefuroxime plus macrolides, macrolides plus cefotaxime or ceftriaxone or clindamycin, vancomycin

RSV, respiratory syncytial virus.
Modified from Lichenstein R, Suggs AH, Campbell J. Pediatric pneumonia. *Emerg Med Clin North Am.* 2003;21:437–451.

Diagnosis of mycoplasmal disease is usually made with the combination of the clinical picture along with serologic testing, although cold agglutinins are not specific. Treatment includes supportive care and use of macrolides or doxycycline. Mycoplasmal disease can cause a wide range of complications, including arthritis, hemolysis, Stevens-Johnson syndrome, pericardial effusions, myocarditis, and both infectious and postinfectious encephalitis. Antibiotic therapy has not been conclusively shown to treat these nonpulmonary complications.

Patients presenting with interstitial infiltrates and hypoxemia out of proportion to the severity of radiographic disease should raise suspicion for *Pneumocystis carinii* pneumonia (PCP) infection. In infants, PCP may be the first presentation for human immunodeficiency virus (HIV) infection. Any patient presenting with PCP should be screened for HIV unless known to be HIV positive already. Diagnosis can be established by bronchoscopy or even deep lavage of secretions and adequate staining for PCP. Treatment of pneumonia with appropriate antibiotics and early institution of high-dose corticosteroids have improved outcome in these patients.

L. pneumophila is a rare cause of pediatric pneumonia, but severe disease can necessitate mechanical ventilation,

particularly in immunosuppressed children. Immunocompetent children with pneumonia may also develop pericarditis, and immunodeficient children may develop more severe pneumonia and extrapulmonary disease manifestations. Diagnosis is based on a high index of clinical suspicion, particularly in children with a history of exposure to travel, hot tubs, or hospitalization. Serologic tests and direct fluorescent antigen methods are available, as well as a *Legionella* urinary antigen test which has very good sensitivity and specificity when compared to culture. Treatment should be instituted initially with intravenous azithromycin, which can be converted to an oral form once improvement is seen.

Respiratory Syncytial Virus

Respiratory syncytial virus (RSV), an enveloped, single-stranded, negative-polarity RNA paramyxovirus, is one of the most common causes of respiratory tract infection in children. Although RSV is endemic in the United States, there is marked seasonal occurrence of the cases primarily between November and May with some regional variation. Infants are most likely to develop symptoms severe enough to require PICU admission with RSV most typically producing lower airway obstruction, apnea, or pneumonia.

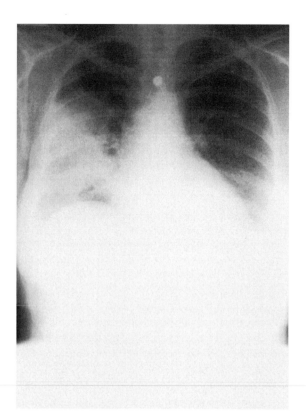

Figure 39.2 Pneumococcal pneumonia with right lower lobe consolidation and left lobe bronchopneumonia. (From George RB, Light RW, Matthay MA, et al., eds. *Chest medicine: Essentials of pulmonary and critical care medicine.* 4th ed. Philadelphia, PA: Lippincott Williams & Wilkins; 2004.)

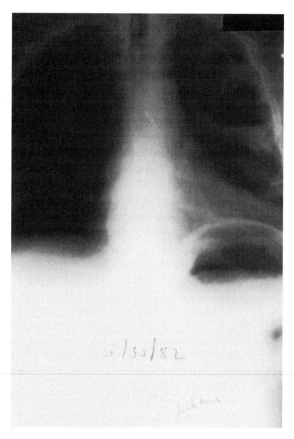

Figure 39.3 Necrotizing lung cavities due to *Staphylococcus aureus.* (From George RB, Light RW, Matthay MA, et al., eds. *Chest medicine: Essentials of pulmonary and critical care medicine.* 4th ed. Philadelphia, PA: Lippincott Williams & Wilkins; 2004.)

Risk factors for increased morbidity and mortality from RSV include prematurity, congenital heart disease, and infant chronic lung disease (CLD). Confirmation of RSV can be made with the use of available rapid testing immunosorbent assays using samples from nasal washings. Specific diagnosis may be helpful for cohort purposes but does not affect specific therapy.

Lower airway obstruction due to bronchiolitis is the most common form of RSV infection requiring intensive care unit (ICU) admission and may be superimposed with pneumonia. Increasing amounts of airway inflammation and edema, increased mucus secretion, and sloughing of respiratory epithelium contribute to the lower airway obstruction. Affected patients demonstrate marked respiratory distress, tachypnea, hypoxia, and chest wall retractions. Physical examination may reveal rhinorrhea, a palpable liver edge from lung hyperinflation, inspiratory rales, and end-expiratory wheezing. Bradypnea with continued work of breathing, grunting respirations, and alteration in the level of consciousness are all signs of an impending respiratory failure. Chest radiography demonstrates hyperinflation and patchy perihilar atelectasis.

Apnea is a well-known finding of RSV infection, particularly in premature infants, and is an indication for PICU admission. Affected infants may demonstrate apnea even before parenchymal findings. On the basis of polysomnography studies, the apnea may be centrally mediated and may involve signaling from pulmonary nerves through the γ-aminobutyric acid (GABA) and substance P pathways. If the apnea causes cardiovascular instability, frequent bradycardia, or does not self-terminate with additional high-flow nasal cannulas or continuous positive airway pressure (CPAP), intubation will be required.

Typical findings of RSV pneumonia include tachypnea, coryza, fever, and cough. Usual criteria for hospital admission include hypoxia, inability to feed, severely increased work of breathing, and dehydration. Respiratory distress is a result of alveolar filling and consolidation. However, other factors including discrete infiltrates on chest radiography and severe hypoxia due to the ventilation–perfusion mismatch may also cause symptoms of distress. Hypoxia can worsen with the administration of inhaled β_2-agonists owing to the blunting of hypoxic vasoconstriction and increased ventilation–perfusion mismatch.

Treatment of RSV bronchiolitis and pneumonia consists primarily of providing oxygen and supportive care.

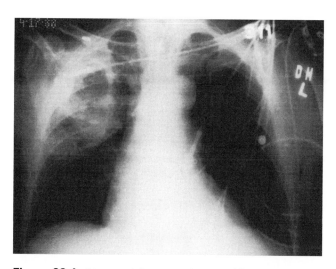

Figure 39.4 Nosocomial pneumonia caused by *Pseudomonas aeruginosa* in a patient treated for a long term with steroids. (From George RB, Light RW, Matthay MA, et al., eds. *Chest medicine: Essentials of pulmonary and critical care medicine.* 4th ed. Philadelphia, PA: Lippincott Williams & Wilkins; 2004.)

Aerosolized β-adrenergic agonists and epinephrine in patients with RSV may be useful in a small subset of patients with RSV who show clinical response to initial doses. Corticosteroids have not shown efficacy in decreasing hospital length of stay in patients with RSV, although some physicians advocate their use in patients with coexisting asthma or reactive airway disease. Noninvasive positive pressure ventilation can also be used in patients with increased distress in an effort to avoid intubation. Ribavirin remains the only U.S. Food and Drug Administration (FDA)-approved drug for treating RSV infection, but its efficacy is uncertain; ventilator–drug interactions are significant and it is not currently used in most institutions. Ribavirin may have a role in immunocompromised patients with severe RSV disease. Although bacterial superinfection is uncommon, empiric antibiotic use should be considered in patients, particularly with signs of concomitant sepsis, pending culture results. An endotracheal aspirate for Gram stain and culture can be helpful to evaluate for secondary bacterial infection.

Relatively few patients with RSV will require intubation even with significant initial distress. Ventilator management must be individualized to specific patient response. Ventilator strategies generally address airway obstruction by employing lower ventilator rates and maximizing expiratory time. Typically, intubated infants with RSV will require intubation for 7 to 10 days, and severity of illness leading to death has become increasingly less common. Some patients, however, develop severe pneumonia and may require alternative ventilator support with oscillatory ventilation or other methods. Although patients with RSV may develop increased air trapping with oscillatory ventilation or require frequent separation from oscillatory support to remove endotracheal secretions, successful use of high frequency oscillatory ventilation (HFOV) in patients failing conventional mechanical ventilation has been obtained. In a similar fashion, other adjunct therapies such as surfactant administration or inhalation of nitric oxide have also shown benefit in some patients, although no specific criteria to outline which of the patients may best benefit from these therapies exist. Rarely, patients develop severe disease refractory to conventional support and are placed on extracorporeal life support. Overall survival in patients with RSV who require extracorporeal-membrane oxygenation (ECMO) is fairly good.

Pertussis

Bordetella pertussis is an organism that generally causes airway irritation and spasmodic cough but can progress to severe respiratory dysfunction and death. Although successful vaccination for pertussis exists, unfounded concerns over the adverse effects related to this vaccination have caused some parents to withhold vaccination in their children. This has led to fears in some countries, especially in Europe, that a pertussis epidemic may occur in the future if the no-vaccine trend continues. Children who are vaccinated against pertussis develop a less severe course of illness if they contract pertussis. Waning immunity following childhood vaccination has caused recent debate about whether a booster vaccine should be given in older childhood or not. Young infants may contract pertussis before vaccination when exposed to siblings or other family members with the disease. The characteristic paroxysms of coughing can lead to feeding intolerance, apnea, or bradycardia. Although usually successfully treated with supportive care, pertussis can progress to severe pneumonia, cause fatal myocardial damage, or result in severe neurologic dysfunction. It remains as one entity that has a high mortality when multiple-organ dysfunction develops, despite the use of alternative therapies such as oscillatory ventilation or extracorporeal life support.

Influenza

Influenza viruses are negative-sense single-stranded RNA viruses, and types A and B are responsible for most illnesses. The complications of influenza in children often require care in a PICU. Mortality increases in the presence of prematurity, congenital cardiac disease, and immunocompromise. Clinical diagnosis of influenza is relatively straightforward in older children, with prominent fever, body aches, and upper respiratory symptoms, but may be more difficult to ascertain in infants and younger children. Less common presentations of influenza include tracheobronchitis, myocarditis, rhabdomyolysis, Reye syndrome, and encephalitis. The most common complication of influenza is superinfection with bacterial pathogens, notably with the *Staphylococcus* species. Superinfection with Panton-Valentine leukocidin-containing *S. aureus* species in adolescents and young adults with influenza can produce fulminant respiratory failure and shock, with a reported 75% mortality rate.

Supportive treatment including mechanical ventilation can be required. Amantadine or rimantadine may offer some antiviral treatment of influenza, inhibiting influenza M2 proteins and preventing viral uncoating, but must be initiated rapidly after onset of symptoms for benefit. A newer class of neuroaminidase inhibitors could benefit some critically ill patients and may be considered for use in immunocompromised patients.

Other Viral Infections

Adenovirus, specifically types 3 and 7, can cause a rapidly evolving acute life-threatening pneumonia with necrosis, pulmonary hemorrhage, and subsequent bronchiolitis obliterans. Survival is dependent on the degree of pulmonary necrosis elicited. Treatment in the immunocompetent patient largely consists of supportive care and mechanical ventilation. The use of ribavirin, ganciclovir, cidofovir, and intravenous immunoglobulin has been considered in immunocompromised children.

Human metapneumovirus (HMPV) is a recently identified pathogen that produces a spectrum of disease similar to RSV. Diagnosis of HMPV is currently by a polymerase chain reaction-based method and is not widely available. Treatment is supportive and similar to that of patients with RSV.

Hantaviruses, a rodent-borne family of viruses found predominantly in the Americas, can cause fulminant pulmonary edema and parenchymal injury, with death generally associated with cardiogenic shock. Disease is seen more frequently in those years with increased rainfall and abundant crop harvests, thereby leading to increased rodent populations and their proximity to humans. Approximately 80% of reported Hantavirus (Sin Nombre) infections in the United States occur in children and pediatric mortality (33%) differs little from adults. Diagnosis can be made on the basis of clinical symptoms, a history of exposure to rodents or to their droppings, and results of serologic testing. Findings of hemoconcentration, thrombocytopenia, leukocytosis, absence of granules in neutrophils, and increased immunoblastic lymphocyte counts also suggest Hantavirus infection. Pulmonary artery catheter monitoring may be helpful in differentiating the cardiogenic shock of Hantavirus from septic shock and guiding supportive therapy. Therapy with ribavirin early in the course of the disease may offer improvement.

Fungal Pneumonias

Fungal pneumonias are essentially a disease of the immunocompromised child. *Candida* species are known components of upper respiratory flora and are often found in nasopharyngeal or endotracheal tube samples from both immunocompetent and immunocompromised individuals, making it difficult to differentiate colonization from infection. *Candida* pneumonia can occur either as a primary pulmonary infection or as a disseminated pneumonia if infection occurs through hematogenous spread. Empiric treatment may be necessary in a symptomatic immunosuppressed child. Treatment choice will be dependent on the species of *Candida* isolated and typical sensitivity patterns.

Aspergillus pneumonia, usually caused by *Aspergillus fumigatus*, is increasingly identified in immunocompromised patients with neutropenia. In solid organ or bone marrow transplant patients, mortality can approach >75%. Invasive aspergillosis occurs after inhalation of the spores, and characteristically is associated with large areas of pulmonary necrosis secondary to direct blood vessel invasion by the organism and subsequent thrombosis. Clinical signs include persistent fever and relatively mild respiratory distress. Classic chest radiography findings of wedge-shaped pleural-based densities indicate advanced stage of the disease. Suspicion of invasive pulmonary aspergillosis in a patient with neutropenia should lead to prompt use of bronchoscopy to confirm the diagnosis, and empiric treatment should begin as early as possible with an amphotericin B-containing product or itraconazole. *Aspergillus* can also produce allergic bronchopulmonary aspergillosis or aspergilloma in patients with cystic fibrosis.

Mucormycosis is an unusual infection that occurs primarily in immunocompromised patients. It has a high rate of invasion into blood vessels and can often result in tissue necrosis because of the occlusion of blood supply.

In nonimmunocompromised patients, organisms such as *Histoplasmosis*, *Blastomycosis*, and *Coccidioidomycosis* are also found. Because these organisms tend to be endemic to certain areas of the country, knowledge of local agents and the patient's travel history are important.

Mycobacterial Pneumonia

While rates of disease have declined in the United States, *Mycobacterium tuberculosis*, an aerobic acid-fast bacillus, must be considered in critically ill patients presenting with pulmonary disease of uncertain etiology. When tuberculosis is suspected, patients, family members, and close contacts should be placed in a negative pressure room under respiratory isolation according to the hospital infection control policy. Disseminated pulmonary tuberculosis can produce respiratory failure, and patients may have associated mycobacterial meningitis with severe central nervous system symptoms.

Parapneumonic Infectious Processes

Development of a pleural collection of purulent exudate may occur spontaneously but is usually associated with bacterial pneumonia. Empyema is most typically associated with staphylococcal or streptococcal lung infections. An empyema may be severe enough to produce respiratory failure. Adequate treatment requires drainage in addition to appropriate antibacterial coverage. Primary drainage with decortication has been advocated, and use of video-assisted thoracoscopy offers a less invasive approach to management. Improved drainage of empyema with the instillation of agents such as tissue plasminogen activator or urokinase through the thoracostomy tube into the pleural space has been described. Concerns over potential induced bleeding or introduction of air or contaminated material from the thoracostomy tube must be considered.

Noninfectious Processes

Acute Respiratory Distress Syndrome

Acute respiratory distress syndrome (ARDS) represents a generalized parenchymal pulmonary response to a broad array of insults (see Table 39.3). The insults may represent a primary process affecting the lung such as a chemical aspiration, or a secondary response to a distant or generalized trigger.

Revision of the term *adult* to *acute* in ARDS by the 1994 American–European Consensus Conference emphasized the understanding that children demonstrate a similar generalized lung response to that of adults. ARDS is currently defined as a subset of acute lung injury (ALI). Both entities include acute onset of respiratory symptoms, bilateral infiltrates on CXR, and pulmonary artery wedge pressure <18 mm Hg or the absence of clinical evidence of left atrial hypertension.

ARDS (as a subset of ALI = Pao_2/Fio_2 ratio of <300 mm Hg) also requires the presence of a Pao_2/Fio_2 ratio of <200 mm Hg irrespective of positive end-expiratory pressure used.

TABLE 39.3

CAUSES OF ACUTE RESPIRATORY DISTRESS SYNDROME IN CHILDREN

Direct Lung Injury
Common
Pneumonia
Aspiration of gastric contents
Less common
Pulmonary contusion
Fat emboli
Near-drowning
Inhalation injury
Reperfusion pulmonary edema

Indirect Lung Injury
Common
Sepsis
Severe trauma with shock
Less common
Cardiopulmonary bypass
Drug overdose
Acute pancreatitis
Massive blood transfusions

Applying the consensus conference criteria, ARDS has been reported to occur in approximately 0.7% to 4.2% of patients admitted to PICUs. The relatively low incidence of ARDS makes it difficult to perform outcome studies even by utilizing multicenter trials. In one recent multicenter trial of nine large PICUs, by screening all children on mechanical ventilation it was found that ARDS was demonstrated in only 23 (7.6%) of 303 eligible patients.

Multiple causes exist for ARDS to occur in children (Table 39.3), either through direct lung injury or by inducing a secondary or "downstream" response from a distant insult. Systemic sepsis remains the most common secondary cause of ARDS in children. Each of these causes has been associated with triggering the intrinsic lung response that produces ARDS. This inflammatory response has been associated with activation of multiple pathways. Cellular responses have been implicated, with neutrophil-mediated injury being the most studied. Humoral response with release of excessive proinflammatory and inadequate anti-inflammatory cytokines is demonstrated. Coagulation pathways have also been implicated. *In vitro* blockade of these responses has demonstrated the ability to inhibit development of typical ARDS injury. ARDS results from a combination of these responses, the impairment and overwhelming of lung repair, and mechanisms of resolution of lung inflammation.

ARDS has been the subject of intense efforts to improve outcome with a variety of interventions. However, by its heterogenous nature, the syndrome has eluded a "magic bullet." A general trend toward gentler ventilation with lower tidal volumes and permissive hypercapnia has proven to be the most effective in improving outcomes, and is discussed elsewhere in the text. The primary approach involves maintaining adequate oxygenation and ventilation while avoiding exacerbating lung trauma. HFOV offers an alternative approach in the patient failing conventional ventilation, although benefits of earlier use remain uncertain. Attempts to provide pharmacologic blockade of the initial inflammatory response has proven unsuccessful *in vivo*. Corticosteroids are not effective during the exudative phase, but a small study has suggested potential benefit if administered during a period coincident with fibroproliferation. Inhaled nitric oxide can induce acute improvements in oxygenation in pediatric ARDS because of its pulmonary vasodilatory effect, but has not been shown to affect overall outcome. Prone positioning also improves ventilation–perfusion matching, but improvements in mortality or length of stay have not been demonstrated. Recent studies have suggested potential benefits in decreasing mortality with intratracheal institution of bovine surfactant.

It is possible that while no single therapy impacts outcome, a cumulative effect may accrue from introducing multiple interventions. Overall, survival in adult ARDS has shown significant improvement over the past 15 years. Comparative outcome data in children is lacking. However, a database of more than 8,000 patients with ARDS from the Pediatric Critical Care Study Group found an overall mortality of 52% in 1991, whereas recent smaller studies from 2003 to 2004 found a mortality of 22% to 28% in children meeting consensus conference ARDS criteria. These results suggest a positive impact of changes in ventilation techniques, targeted ARDS interventions, and overall improvements in pediatric intensive care. Limited long-term outcome studies have also shown nearly complete resolution of pulmonary function abnormalities in pediatric ARDS survivors.

Acute Chest Syndrome/Sickle Cell Disease

The lung can be both acutely and chronically affected by sickle cell disease (SCD). The ACS has been reported to occur in 15% to 43% of all patients with SCD and to be responsible for up to 25% of SCD deaths. ACS is defined as the appearance of a new pulmonary infiltrate as seen in the CXR, in association with fever, cough, tachypnea, and chest pain in a patient with SCD. ACS is usually associated with a vaso-occlusive crisis, which may be precipitated by an infection, including chlamydial, mycoplasmal, and viral infections. Infarction and fat embolism are seen in a significant number of patients with ACS. Clinically it is difficult to differentiate specific cause. Optimal pain control, oxygen, empiric antibiotics, simple packed red blood cell transfusion, and aggressive pulmonary toilet with incentive spirometry may be helpful in decreasing the progression of ACS. However, patients failing to improve with these measures generally require intensive care admission. Exchange transfusion is indicated in patients with ACS not responding to the above measures in order to avoid high post-transfusion hemoglobin concentration and to maximize lowering of sickle hemoglobin fraction. Noninvasive positive pressure face mask ventilation may avoid intubation. However, ACS may progress to multilobar disease indistinguishable from ARDS, and similar mechanical ventilation maneuvers may be necessitated. ECMO has been successfully employed in children failing other support. Corticosteroids may have some benefit in decreasing ACS length of stay. Whether the current interest in inhaled nitric oxide as a therapy for patients with SCD will prove to be of great benefit is yet to be determined. Preliminary data on relief of pulmonary hypertension associated with ACS, decrease in sickling of cells, and improvement of microvascular flow with exposure to inhaled nitric oxide is intriguing. A multi-institutional trial evaluating the effects of pulsed inhaled nitric oxide in patients presenting with pain crisis is currently under way.

Autoimmune Vasculitides

A variety of autoimmune diseases can produce severe respiratory insufficiency. Systemic lupus erythematosus and scleroderma can produce diffusion defects. Wegener

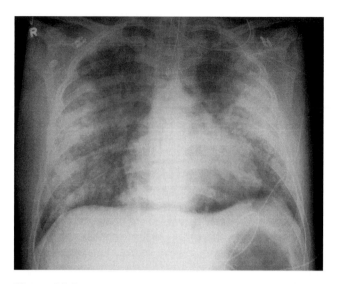

Figure 39.5 Bilateral pulmonary hemorrhage in an adolescent with Wegener granulomatosis.

granulomatosis and similar conditions are associated with antineutrophil cytoplasmic antibodies, which may lead to intrapulmonary deposition of antigen–antibody complexes. These processes may frequently manifest diffuse pulmonary infiltrates and prominent pulmonary hemorrhage that can be life-threatening (see Fig. 39.5). Therapy with immunosuppressive agents is likely necessary in addition to supportive ventilation. Use of extracorporeal techniques such as plasmapheresis or ECMO in severe cases of conditions such as Wegener condition have been reported with successful outcomes. Of interest, despite the frequent association of autoimmune diseases and pulmonary hemorrhage, continued bleeding even with patients requiring systemic heparinization during extracorporeal support is uncommon.

Aspiration Pneumonitides

Aspiration of a variety of substances can induce severe pneumonitis and respiratory failure. Most commonly, aspiration of gastric contents can occur either as a primary event, often in conjunction with gastroesophageal reflux in infants, or as a secondary event in a patient with altered mental status and impairment of protective airway reflexes. Aspiration of activated charcoal during attempted decontamination of a toxic ingestion can produce an injury greater than the toxicity of the ingested agent being treated, and caution in use is emphasized. Aspiration of hydrocarbons can produce profound chemical pneumonitis, even with relatively small exposure to these agents. Aspiration of fresh or salt water occurs with near-drowning, inducing a pneumonitis that is associated with impairment of surfactant production irrespective of the type of water ingested. A relatively small amount of water ingestion may produce a significant injury, and the process may be a greater result of inflammatory response to produce ARDS, or from ischemia-reperfusion lung injury due to cardiorespiratory arrest in drowning.

Treatment of aspiration pneumonitis is supportive and may require significant ventilatory support. Because surfactant impairment may occur in each of these settings, exogenous surfactant therapy has been suggested but is not proven to be specifically effective. Neither prophylactic antibiotics nor corticosteroids are recommended. If evidence of bacterial infection such as fever, purulent tracheal secretions, or leukocytosis develops, antibiotic choice should include coverage of anaerobic organisms.

Lung Disease in Immunosuppressed Patients

Increasing numbers of children require immunosuppression because of chemotherapy and transplantation. They are at significant risk for pulmonary complications, including opportunistic and hospital-acquired infections, graft versus host responses, and idiopathic pulmonary syndrome with fibrosis. Early experience with respiratory failure in immunosuppressed children suggested that requirement for mechanical ventilation presaged a dismal outcome. More recent reported experience suggests that advances in general intensive care may be leading to improved survival in children with oncologic diseases or following bone marrow transplantation. Therapy in these patients should take into account potential opportunistic pathogens such as *P. carinii* and *L. pneumophila*.

Pulmonary Embolus

The diagnosis of pulmonary embolus has been rare in children, although heightened awareness that deep venous thrombosis (DVT) occur in children with perhaps more frequency than previously considered has led to an increase in pulmonary embolism (PE) as a differential diagnosis in patients with hypoxia and dyspnea without known etiologies. Respiratory alkalosis concomitant with hypoxemia is a hallmark of pulmonary embolus. The classic wedge-shaped lesion on CXR may be present. Improved differentiation of PE on spiral computed tomography (CT) or magnetic resonance imaging (MRI) can also be diagnostic. Elevated pulmonary artery pressures and signs of right ventricular dysfunction by echocardiogram may also be helpful. Newer diagnostic tests such as D-dimers may replace other measures of coagulation and fibrin breakdown such as fibrinogen and split products. The prevalence of the use of central venous catheters and the associated thrombosis that can occur should increase suspicion for pulmonary embolus in select patients. Examination for DVT by physical examination and ultrasonography should be conducted. Attention to prophylaxis for DVT by heparin, low-molecular-weight heparin or other means should be addressed in postpubertal patients who are bedridden or in patients at high risk for venous stasis from underlying conditions. The prompt identification and proper treatment of PE may be aided by the adoption of guidelines

or pathways for workup and treatment of this disorder in the PICU.

Acute Manifestations of Chronic Lung Disease in Infants

CLD, defined as supplemental oxygen requirement at 30 days of age in association with chest radiographic abnormalities, is the most common adverse respiratory outcome in premature infants, particularly those below 28 weeks gestational age at birth. Inflammatory injury characterizes the development of CLD. Typically, prolonged mechanical ventilation with evidence of barotrauma was thought most likely to predispose to CLD. However, increasing numbers of very low birth weight infants with minimal ventilator exposure have developed CLD, perhaps related to poor alveolar growth and impaired pulmonary remodeling together with infection and patent duct arteriosus presence. Pulmonary hypertension can complicate untreated or undertreated CLD of infancy.

Infants with CLD can develop acute respiratory failure in association with relatively mild viral insults, aspiration events from reflux, or stimuli inducing a pulmonary hypertensive crisis. Mechanical ventilation is frequently required and it may be difficult to wean patients owing to poor compliance and significant air trapping. Airway hyper-responsiveness is treated with inhaled β agonists, and inhaled anticholinergics can also be helpful due to the enhanced parasympathetic tone in these infants. Corticosteroids are potentially useful due to the chronic inflammatory component of disease and superimposed airway response. Diuretics may also be useful to reduce acute increases in the chronic interstitial edema seen in these patients.

RECOMMENDED READINGS

1. Bentham JR, Shaw NJ. Some chronic obstructive pulmonary disease will originate in neonatal intensive care units. *Paediatr Respir Rev.* 2005;6:29–32.
2. Bernard GR, Artigas A, Brigham KL, et al. The American-European consensus conference on ARDS. *Am J Respir Crit Care Med.* 1994;149:818.
3. Fackler J. Acute respiratory distress syndrome. In: Rogers M, ed. *Textbook of pediatric intensive care.* Baltimore, MD: Williams & Wilkins; 1996:197–233.
4. Kaplan SL. Review of antibiotic resistance, antibiotic treatment and prevention of pneumococcal pneumonia. *Paediatr Respir Rev.* 2004;5(Suppl A):S153–S158.
5. Lichenstein R, Suggs AH, Campbell J. Pediatric pneumonia. *Emerg Med Clin North Am.* 2003;21:437–451.
6. Long S. *Principles and practice of pediatric infectious diseases,* 2nd ed. Oxford, UK: Elsevier; 2002.
7. Randolph AG, Meert KL, O'Neill ME, et al. The feasibility of conducting clinical trials in infants and children with acute respiratory failure. *Am J Respir Crit Care Med.* 2003;167:1334.
8. Siddiqui AK, Ahmed S. Pulmonary manifestations of sickle cell disease. *Postgrad Med J.* 2003;79:384.
9. Sinaniotis SA. Viral pneumoniae in children: Incidence and aetiology. *Paediatr Respir Rev.* 2004;5(Suppl A):S197–S200.
10. Ware LB, Matthay MA. The acute respiratory distress syndrome. *N Engl J Med.* 2000;342:1334.

Pulmonary Hypertension

40

Asrar Rashid   D. Dunbar Ivy

Until recently, the primary manifestations of pulmonary hypertension encountered in the pediatric intensive care unit (PICU) were related to persistent pulmonary hypertension (PPHN) of the neonate or secondary pulmonary hypertension from respiratory disease and hypoxia. With the advent of improved cardiac surgery techniques, diagnostic tools, and treatments, many patients with pulmonary hypertension who would have died from their disease are now being admitted into the PICU. Because the mortality remains high, these patients require careful assessment, monitoring, and treatment. This chapter focuses on the primary and secondary causes, diagnosis, and treatment of patients with pulmonary hypertension including the recent advances in targeted pharmacologic therapies that impact morbidity and mortality.

NEONATAL PULMONARY HYPERTENSION

Neonatal pulmonary hypertension is the oldest recognized and studied form of pulmonary hypertension in the ICU. Newborns whose pulmonary vascular resistance (PVR) remains high after birth can develop "PPHN." The usual triggers for PPHN include lung parenchymal disorders that result in hypoxia (meconium aspiration, pneumonia), lung hypoplasia occurring with congenital diaphragmatic hernia, infections such as that caused by group B streptococcus, and nonpulmonary conditions such as hyperviscosity.

Diagnosis

All patients with suspected PPHN should have four extremity blood pressures, chest radiograph, and cardiac echocardiogram performed to rule out structural heart disease. Chest radiograph often reveals clear lung fields and reduced pulmonary vascular markings, unless a parenchymal lung process is present. Echocardiogram may demonstrate shunting at the level of the foramen ovale and ductus arteriosus, a dilated right ventricle or right atrium, and tricuspid regurgitation. A hyperoxia test, performed by simultaneous sampling of arterial blood from the right radial artery and the umbilical artery catheter (UAC), is helpful to distinguish PPHN from cardiac defects. Cardiac lesions associated with poor pulmonary blood flow do not show an increase in arterial saturation at high concentrations of oxygen, whereas infants with PPHN will often show an increase in oxygenation such as a Pa_{O_2} difference of >20 mm Hg between the right artery and UAC if right-to-left ductal shunting is present.

Treatment

Although in the past PPHN was treated with aggressive hyperventilation and high concentrations of oxygen, current strategies focus on providing adequate cardiac filling pressures, preventing and treating metabolic acidosis, and providing prompt treatment of any underlying trigger. In the past, infants failing to improve with conventional medical therapy may have been treated with extracorporeal life support (extracorporeal-membrane oxygenation [ECMO]) with good success. Since the advent of inhaled nitric oxide (iNO), however, the need for ECMO has been reduced and many infants respond to the pulmonary vasodilating effects of iNO with improved oxygenation.

Resolution of PPHN often occurs within a few days once the underlying disease is treated and the normal reduction in pulmonary arterial pressure and muscularity occurs. Most infants with recovery from PPHN will do well over the long term. A more specific discussion of the treatment of PPHN can be found in texts focusing on neonatal physiology.

RESPIRATORY DISEASE

Lung disease is an important factor in the etiology of pulmonary hypertension in some patients. Alveolar hypoxia results in pulmonary vessel vasoconstriction, whereas hypoxia in the systemic circulation results in vessel dilation. The capacity of the pulmonary vasculature to constrict in hypoxic lung areas helps direct blood to better ventilated zones, thereby improving ventilation–perfusion matching. The PaO_2 of pulmonary artery blood can also reduce PVR, although this effect is minor compared to the role of alveolar hypoxia. While the exact mechanism of hypoxic vasoconstriction is yet to be defined, there is evidence to suggest the role of potassium channels within pulmonary vascular smooth muscle.

Hypoxic pulmonary vasoconstriction can increase pulmonary pressure and lead to right ventricular hypertrophy or right-sided heart failure. Right ventricular function is usually normal until the disease progresses in severity. The diagnosis of elevated pulmonary pressures can be made by echocardiogram or by the placement of pulmonary artery catheters. Despite the controversy on the use of pulmonary artery catheters, they may be helpful, especially in the early stages of disease when fluid shifts and impaired cardiac function make it difficult to assess cardiac output and the effects of therapy. As with neonatal PPHN, the prevention and treatment of metabolic acidosis and the resolution of the underlying lung disease are important to limit ongoing pulmonary hypertension. The use of systemic vasodilating agents such as milrinone and dobutamine may be helpful, whereas more specific agents such as iNO may also benefit some patients. Limiting further lung injury by use of "gentle ventilation" with low tidal volume, pressure-limited ventilation, or high-frequency ventilation may also reduce pulmonary hypertension by improving hypoxemia and reducing cytokine release.

Patients with severe respiratory failure that require mechanical ventilation are also at risk for elevations in PVR and pulmonary artery pressure (PAP). In addition to hypoxia and ventilator-induced lung injury resulting in cytokine release, the inflation status of the lung also affects PVR. When the lung is at functional residual capacity (FRC), PVR is lowest. Over or underinflation of the lung, then, can result in increased PVR. Positive end-expiratory pressure (PEEP) can help to maintain FRC and alleviate hypoxemia in patients with lung disease, thereby reducing PVR. However, high levels of PEEP may increase PVR by compressing resistance vessels near alveoli if they become overexpanded. This effect may be minimized with severe parenchymal disease whereby patients may tolerate even high levels of PEEP without any adverse effects on PVR in this condition. In severe cases of respiratory disease, diffuse lung injury results in fibrosis and may lead to irreversible pulmonary hypertension from a loss of pulmonary capillary surface areas. Bronchopulmonary dysplasia in infants surviving prematurity and lung disease is an increasing cause of pulmonary artery hypertension. Patients with ongoing pulmonary hypertension may also develop cor pulmonale, evidenced by right ventricular hypertrophy, over time. The finding of cor pulmonale carries a poor prognosis.

The treatment of cor pulmonale depends on the etiology and severity of the lung disease. Nocturnal oxygen administration may alleviate hypoxia without hypercapnia. In patients with cystic fibrosis, calcium channel blockers (CCBs) have not shown proven effectiveness and may worsen oxygenation.[1,2] In some patients with severe pulmonary hypertension and cor pulmonale, lung transplantation may be an option when medical therapy fails. For this reason, the use of lung transplantation in cystic fibrosis has increased over the last few years.

PRIMARY PULMONARY HYPERTENSION AND PULMONARY HYPERTENSION RELATED TO CARDIAC DISEASE

Previously, the diagnosis of pulmonary hypertension in children carried a poor prognosis. In a 1965 series of 35 patients with primary pulmonary hypertension, none survived for more than 7 years. Further, 22 out of 35 (63%) died in the first year after the onset of symptoms.[3] In a 1995 case series of 18 patients, the prognosis was still poor with a median survival of 4 years.[4] Recent advances in the understanding of vascular biology and the normal and hypertensive pulmonary circulations have led to a broader pharmaceutical armamentarium against pulmonary hypertension. As a result, preliminary studies have been promising. For example, there was 90% survival at 4 years in children with severe idiopathic pulmonary hypertension treated with prostacyclin.[5]

Pulmonary hypertension may be idiopathic or primary without an underlying cause, or secondary to a specific disease process. Idiopathic pulmonary arterial hypertension (IPAH) is a rare and poorly understood condition that is diagnosed by excluding conditions that are responsible for secondary pulmonary hypertension. Without appropriate treatment, the natural history of IPAH is progressive and fatal. In contrast, the natural history of pulmonary hypertension from congenital heart disease has a broad range of survival, ranging from months to decades.

The selection of appropriate therapies is complex, requiring familiarity with the disease process, complicated delivery systems, dosing regimens, medication complications, and side effects. This section discusses the current diagnosis and treatment of children with primary and secondary pulmonary hypertension.

Definition

Pulmonary hypertension is defined as a mean PAP >25 mm Hg at rest, or >30 mm Hg during exercise.[6] In 1998, the World Health Organization (WHO) proposed a new classification of pulmonary hypertension, which was updated in 2003 (see Table 40.1). This classification is appropriate to both the pediatric and adult age-group.

Diagnostic Evaluation

The most successful strategy in the treatment of moderate to severe pulmonary hypertension is to treat the underlying cause, and therefore the workup of pulmonary hypertension involves a complete history and examination (see Table 40.2) and extensive evaluation (see Table 40.3)

TABLE 40.1
WHO CLASSIFICATION OF PULMONARY HYPERTENSION

1. Pulmonary arterial hypertension
   1.1 Idiopathic pulmonary hypertension
   1.2 Familial
   1.3 Related to:
       (a) Collagen vascular disease
       (b) Congenital systemic-to-pulmonary shunts
       (c) Portal hypertension
       (d) HIV infection
       (e) Drugs/toxins
           (1) Anorexigens
           (2) Other
   1.4 Persistent pulmonary hypertension of the newborn
   1.5 Pulmonary veno-occlusive disease
2. Pulmonary hypertension with left heart disease
   2.1 Left-sided atrial or ventricular heart disease
   2.2 Left-sided valvular disease
3. Pulmonary hypertension associated with disorders of the respiratory system and/or hypoxemia
   3.1 Chronic obstructive pulmonary disease
   3.2 Interstitial lung disease
   3.3 Sleep disordered breathing
   3.4 Alveolar hypoventilation disorders
   3.5 Chronic exposure to high altitude
   3.6 Neonatal lung disease
   3.7 Alveolar-capillary dysplasia
   3.8 Others
4. Pulmonary hypertension due to chronic thrombotic and/or embolic disease
   4.1 Thromboembolic obstruction of proximal pulmonary arteries
   4.2 Obstruction of distal pulmonary arteries
       (a) Pulmonary embolism (thrombus, tumor, and/or parasites)
       (b) *In situ* thrombosis
       (c) Sickle cell disease
5. Miscellaneous
   (e.g., sarcoidosis)

HIV, human immunodeficiency virus.

TABLE 40.2
HISTORY AND EXAMINATION

History	Diet pill use; contraceptive pill; methamphetamine use
	Onset and length of pulmonary hypertension
	Family history of pulmonary hypertension
	Prior cardiac and other surgeries
	Living at high altitude
Symptoms	Chest pain; dyspnea; shortness of breath; syncope
Physical examination	Loud second heart sound; systolic murmur of tricuspid regurgitation or diastolic murmur of pulmonary insufficiency; palpable second heart sound; peripheral edema; jugular venous distension

aiming to exclude all known etiologies of pulmonary hypertension (Table 40.1). IPAH is defined as a diagnosis of exclusion.[5] A retrospective study of 84 cases of pulmonary hypertension classified the new diagnoses according to IPAH, familial or owing to anorexigenic use. Survival in these patients at 1, 2, and 3 years was 87%, 75%, and 61%, respectively. Multivariate analysis showed that belonging to the African American or Asian descent was associated with an increased risk of death. Higher serum albumin, cardiac index, and acute vasoreactivity were independently associated with improved survival.[7]

History and physical examination should be undertaken with attention to etiology (Tables 40.1 and 40.2). Symptoms may include exertional dyspnea, reduced exercise tolerance, orthopnea, atypical chest pain, and hemoptysis. Syncope in this condition is a worrisome sign of end-stage disease. Special situations may predispose to the development of pulmonary arterial hypertension. For example, we have recently described a case series of children who lived at an altitude and presented with high-altitude pulmonary edema (HAPE). These children were subsequently found to have chronic pulmonary hypertension. Therefore, all children living at an altitude who present with HAPE should be screened for pulmonary hypertension.[8]

Noninvasive diagnostic studies are important in the evaluation of pulmonary hypertension (Table 40.3). Cardiac catheterization is important to evaluate PAP and resistance, as well as to determine reactivity of the pulmonary vasculature. Further, because respiratory disease is an important cause of pulmonary hypertension, extensive evaluation of the lung should be undertaken.

Congenital Heart Disease

A variety of congenital cardiac lesions cause pulmonary hypertension (see Table 40.4). The age at which these lesions cause irreversible pulmonary vascular disease varies.

TABLE 40.3

DIAGNOSTIC EVALUATION OF PULMONARY HYPERTENSION

Chest radiograph (signs of cardiomegaly and enlarged pulmonary arteries)
ECG (right ventricular hypertrophy and ST-T changes)
Echocardiogram (Right ventricular hypertrophy, exclude congenital heart disease,
     quantify right ventricular systolic pressures)
Cardiac catheterization with acute vasodilator testing (Evaluate pulmonary artery pressure and resistance and degree of pulmonary reactivity)
Liver evaluation
    Liver function tests with γ-glutaryl transferase
    Abdominal ultrasound (portopulmonary hypertension)
    Hepatitis profile
Complete blood count, urinalysis
Hypercoagulable evaluation
    DIC screen
    Factor V Leiden
    Antithrombin III
    Prothrombin mutation 22010
    Protein C
    Protein S
    Anticardiolipin IgG/IgM
    Russell viper venom test lupus anticoagulant
Collagen vascular workup: looking for autoimmune disease
    Antinuclear antibody with profile (DNA, Smith, RNP, SSA, SSB, centromere, SCL-70, CRP)
    Rheumatoid factor
    Erythrocyte sedimentation rate
    Complement
Lung evaluation
    Pulmonary function tests with DLCO/bronchodilators (to exclude obstructive/restrictive disease)
    Sleep study and pulse oximetry (degree of hypoxia or diminished ventilatory drive)
    CT/MRI scan of chest (evaluation of thromboembolic disease or interstitial lung disease)
    Ventilation–perfusion test
    Lung biopsy
Six-minute walk test/cycle ergometry
HIV test
Thyroid function tests
Toxicology screen (cocaine/methamphetamine)
    Consider brain natriuretic peptide, uric acid, and von Willebrand factor

DIC, disseminated intravascular coagulation; ECG, electrocardiogram; IgG, immunoglobulin G; IgM, immunoglobulin M; RNP, ribonucleoprotein; CT, computed tomography; MRI, magnetic resonance imaging; DLCO, diffusing capacity of lung for carbon monoxide.

In general, patients with ventricular septal defect or patent ductus arteriosus do not develop irreversible pulmonary vascular changes before the age of 1 to 2. Children with Down syndrome may have an increased risk of pulmonary hypertension. Furthermore, infants with an atrial septal defect or ventricular septal defect with chronic lung disease have an increased risk for the early development of severe pulmonary vascular disease. Patients with atrioventricular

TABLE 40.4

CARDIAC LESIONS ASSOCIATED WITH PULMONARY HYPERTENSION

Left-to-Right Shunts

VSD
Atrioventricular septal (canal) defect
Patent ductus arteriosus
Atrial septal defect
Aortopulmonary window

Increased Pulmonary Venous Pressure

Cardiomyopathy
Coarctation of the aorta (left ventricular diastolic dysfunction)
Hypoplastic left heart syndrome
Shone complex
Mitral stenosis
Supravalvar mitral ring
Cor triatriatum
Pulmonary vein stenosis/veno-occlusive disease
Total anomalous pulmonary venous return

Cyanotic Heart Disease

Transposition of the great arteries
Truncus arteriosus
Tetralogy of Fallot (pulmonary atresia/VSD)
Univentricular heart (high-flow $\pm$ restrictive atrial septum)

Anomalies of the Pulmonary Artery or Pulmonary Vein

Origin of a pulmonary artery from the aorta
Unilateral "absence" of a pulmonary artery
Scimitar syndrome

Palliative Shunting Operations

Waterston anastomosis
Potts anastomosis
Blalock-Taussig anastomosis

VSD, ventricular septal defect.

septal defect may develop irreversible pulmonary vascular disease earlier than patients with other left-to-right shunt lesions.

Patients with cyanotic congenital cardiac lesions may also develop pulmonary hypertension. Hypoxia with increased shunting is a potent stimulus for the rapid development of pulmonary vascular disease. Examples include transposition of the great arteries, truncus arteriosus, and univentricular heart with high flow. Total correction of many cardiac lesions in the first months of life may prevent the late development of pulmonary hypertension. Finally, palliative shunting operations for certain cardiac anomalies designed to increase pulmonary blood flow may lead to the development of pulmonary hypertension.

Eisenmenger Syndrome

Eisenmenger syndrome describes pulmonary hypertension with a reversed central shunt.[9] In general, the term

Eisenmenger syndrome is used for shunts that are distal to the tricuspid valve. Elevated PVR, and bidirectional or right-to-left shunting through a systemic-to-pulmonary connection, such as a ventricular septal defect, patent ductus arteriosus, univentricular heart, or aortopulmonary window characterize this syndrome. The shunt is initially left-to-right, but as the underlying condition continues to increase PVR, shunt reversal occurs, leading to cyanosis, and erythrocytosis. In general, the prognosis of patients with Eisenmenger syndrome is much better than for patients with IPAH. Syncope, right-heart failure (RHF), and severe hypoxemia have been associated with a poor prognosis. Phlebotomy may be utilized in Eisenmenger syndrome and should be reserved for temporary relief of major hyperviscosity symptoms or to improve perioperative hemostasis. Noncardiac operations on patients with Eisenmenger syndrome are associated with a high mortality rate, and should be managed by a multidisciplinary team experienced in the care of patients with pulmonary hypertension.

Idiopathic Pulmonary Arterial Hypertension

Primary or IPAH is a rare disease, which occurs most frequently in young adult women.[10] IPAH is characterized by progressive and sustained elevations of pulmonary artery pressure without a defined etiology. Six percent to twelve percent of cases of IPAH may be familial in origin with an autosomal dominant pattern of inheritance involving the phenomenon of genetic anticipation.[11,12] The gene for familial primary pulmonary hypertension is chromosome 2q33. Diverse germline heterozygous mutations to this gene lead to defects in the bone morphogenetic protein receptor-II (BMPR-II).[13-15] In turn, this can result in uncontrolled proliferation of vascular smooth muscle.[16,17] More than 50 disease-causing defects in the gene encoding BMPR-II have been reported; however, many have been identified in patients with no family history of pulmonary arterial hypertension owing to the low penetrance of these mutations.[13-15,18-23] BMPR-II is a type II receptor of the transforming growth factor (TGF)-β family of cytokines, members of which are considered essential for the cellular process of proliferation, differentiation, and apoptosis.[24] Mutations of the type I receptor activin receptor-like kinase-1 (ALK-1) may rarely cause pulmonary hypertension, and so far, no link has been found between ALK-1 and BMPR-II.[25,26]

Clinical and genetic screening of first-degree relatives may help to identify at-risk individuals early in their course. Clinical screening includes a chest x-ray, electrocardiogram (ECG), echocardiogram, and possibly exercise testing. Genetic screening involves analysis for BMPR-II mutations. However, the absence of the mutation does not exclude IPAH.[17]

Thromboembolic Disease

Thromboembolic disease as a cause of pulmonary hypertension in children is uncommon. However, an accurate diagnosis is essential for treatment.[27] Predisposing factors include collagen vascular disease, hypercoagulation disorders (Table 40.1), bacterial endocarditis, and a right atrial shunt (cerebral ventricular) for hydrocephalus. Similarly, the use of oral contraceptive agents may cause hypercoagulation leading to pulmonary thromboembolic phenomena. The diagnosis involves a high index of suspicion, and evaluation by ventilation–perfusion scanning and computed tomography (CT) scanning. In adults with chronic thromboembolic pulmonary hypertension, pulmonary thromboendarterectomy improves survival and quality of life.

Therapeutic Considerations

General Principles

Most children with mild pulmonary hypertension do not require treatment other than treatment of the underlying etiology. Therefore, a complete evaluation for the causes of pulmonary hypertension is important. Other general principles include avoidance of pregnancy and use of birth control pills in age appropriate patients.

Operability

In patients with congenital heart disease, the timing of surgery depends upon several factors. These include age, lesion, vasoreactivity at cardiac catheterization, findings on lung biopsy, and pulmonary wedge angiography.[28-30]

Vasodilator Therapy

Despite appropriate surgical correction, pulmonary hypertension and pulmonary vascular disease may progress. As vasoconstriction is an important component in the development of medial hypertrophy, vasodilators are frequently used to decrease PAP, improve cardiac output, and potentially reverse some of the pulmonary vascular changes noted in the lung. A long-term strategy for the treatment of pulmonary hypertension is shown in Figure 40.1.

Ideally, vasodilator responsiveness should be assessed in a controlled situation such as the cardiac catheterization unit to determine whether the pulmonary vasculature is responsive to intervention. A positive response is defined by assessing the change of cardiac and pulmonary catheter data to vasodilators (see Table 40.5).[31] The younger the child at the time of testing, the greater the likelihood of acute pulmonary vasodilation in response to vasoreactivity testing.[32] Many oral and inhaled vasodilators have been used for the testing of vasodilator responsiveness.[30,33]

Nitric Oxide

The use of newer vasodilator agents, particularly nitric oxide, has been an important advance in determining vasoreactivity. iNO therapy improves gas exchange and selectively lowers PVR in several clinical diseases, including idiopathic pulmonary hypertension and congenital heart disease.[30,33-40] iNO bypasses the damaged endothelium

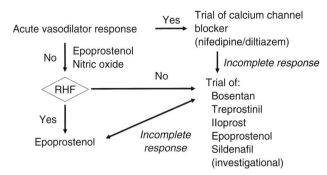

Figure 40.1 Algorithm for the long-term treatment of pediatric pulmonary arterial hypertension. Children who respond acutely (see text) to vasodilator testing with nitric oxide or epoprostenol should initially be treated with CCBs, such as nifedipine or diltiazem. Children who do not respond to acute vasoreactivity testing should be treated with other forms of therapy. In the presence of a nonreactive pulmonary vasculature and RHF, continuous intravenous epoprostenol should be initiated. In the absence of RHF, other agents may be trialed first. Bosentan, treprostinil, iloprost and sildenafil have been studied and approved for treatment of pulmonary arterial hypertension. Other investigational drugs, such as sitaxsentan and ambrisentan, are being assessed. For patients with severe disease, combination therapy may be considered but has not been well studied. RHF, right heart failure.

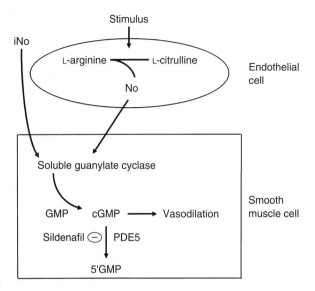

Figure 40.2 Inhaled nitric oxide (iNO) bypasses the damaged endothelium seen in pulmonary hypertensive disorders, and diffuses to the adjacent smooth muscle cell, where it activates soluble guanylate cyclase resulting in an increase in cyclic guanosine 3′,5′-monophosphate (cGMP) and vasodilation. Phosphodiesterase type 5 (PDE5) degrades cGMP within vascular smooth muscle, and may limit vasodilation. Sildenafil blocks (-)PDE5 causing vasodilation. GMP, guanylic acid; NO, nitric oxide.

in pulmonary hypertensive disorders, and diffuses to the adjacent smooth muscle cell, where it activates soluble guanylate cyclase resulting in an increase in cyclic guanosine 3′,5′-monophosphate (cGMP) and vasodilation (see Fig. 40.2). Currently, either nitric oxide or prostacyclin is recommended as the agent of choice for evaluating pulmonary vasoreactivity (Fig. 40.1).

Recent studies have begun to explore the role of long-term use of nitric oxide in the treatment of pulmonary hypertensive disorders.[36,41,42] Although iNO therapy causes sustained decreases in PVR, adverse hemodynamic effects may complicate iNO therapy after abrupt withdrawal.[43,44] Inhibition of phosphodiesterase-5 (see later), which degrades cGMP within vascular smooth muscle, causes vasodilation and may attenuate the rebound effect (see Fig. 40.3).[45,46]

TABLE 40.5
POSITIVE RESPONSE TO VASODILATORS

Patients responding positively to acute vasodilator testing are defined as those who demonstrate all of the following:
1. Decrease in the mean pulmonary artery pressure and resistance by 20%, or greater, with a fall to near normal levels
2. Experience no change or an increase in their cardiac index
3. Exhibit no change or a decrease in the ratio of pulmonary vascular resistance to systemic vascular resistance
4. Exhibit normal right atrial pressure and cardiac output

Calcium Channel Blockers

The use of CCBs to evaluate vasoreactivity may be problematic because these drugs can reduce cardiac output.[32] In addition, such deleterious effects may be prolonged because of the relatively long half-life of CCBs. Consequently, elevated right atrial pressure and low cardiac output are contraindications to acute or chronic calcium channel blockade.

Our approach is to perform an acute trial of CCB therapy only in those patients who are responsive to iNO or prostacyclin. Patients who do not have an acute vasodilatory response to short-acting agents and who are then placed on CCB therapy are unlikely to benefit from this form of therapy.[31] At least 60% of children with severe pulmonary hypertension are unresponsive to acute vasodilator testing, and are candidates for other forms of therapy, other than calcium channel blockers.

Children who are acute responders to CCB have a long-term risk of treatment failure on CCB. Therefore, there is a need for close follow-up, including serial vasodilator testing and transplant evaluation before treatment failure.[47] The strategy for CCB usage has been associated with a 5-year survival rate of 97% for acute responders.[31] However, at the extended 10-year follow-up of the CCB acute responders, the survival rate was only 81% and the treatment success was only 47%.[47]

Prostacyclin

Adults with IPAH and children with congenital heart disease demonstrate an imbalance in the biosynthesis of

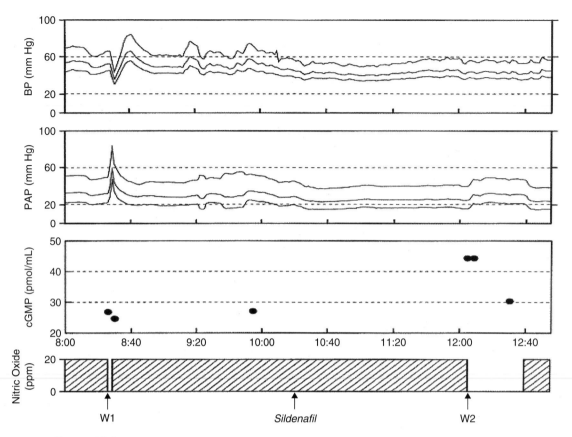

Figure 40.3 Withdrawal of inhaled nitric oxide (iNO) in postoperative congenital heart disease causes a rebound effect with associated rise in pulmonary artery pressure (PAP) and fall in systemic blood pressure (BP). Reinitiation of iNO returns hemodynamics to baseline. Sildenafil increases cGMP and blunts the rebound effect after repeat withdrawal of NO. W1, withdrawal one; W2, withdrawal two (Atz AM, Wessel DL. Sildenafil ameliorates effects of iNO withdrawal. *Anesthesiology*. 1999;91:307–310.)

thromboxane A_2 and prostacyclin. Likewise, adults and children with severe pulmonary hypertension show diminished prostacyclin synthase expression in the lung vasculature.[48] Prostacyclin administered over the long term, utilizing intravenous epoprostenol, improves survival and quality of life in adults and children with primary pulmonary hypertension (see Fig. 40.4).[31,47,49] Recent studies have shown an improved outcome in patients who were previously poor candidates for CCBs, or thought to be candidates only for lung transplantation. Survival in these patients has markedly improved using the targeted approach to therapy outlined in the preceding text. Using this strategy, 5-year survival in patients with primary pulmonary hypertension who were not candidates for CCB therapy may be higher than 80% in children.[31]

The use of prostacyclin in patients with congenital heart disease is promising.[50] Disadvantages of prostacyclin analogs, such as epoprostenol, include the dose-dependent side effects of the drug (nausea, anorexia, jaw pain, diarrhea, musculoskeletal aches, and pains) and side effects due to the method of delivery. The drug must be given through a central line and therefore potential complications include clotting, hemorrhage, cellulitis, and sepsis. In addition, the product is delivered by continuous infusion; an abrupt cessation may cause acute deterioration and death in some cases. In patients with residual shunting, continuous prostacyclin may result in worsening cyanosis and complications of cerebrovascular accidents.

Alternative Delivery Routes for Prostacyclin Analogs

Success of epoprostenol (a synthetic analog of natural prostacyclin) therapy coupled with limitations of its delivery has led to the utilization of prostacyclin analogs with alternative delivery routes.

Treprostinil, a subcutaneous prostacyclin analog, has a half-life of 45 minutes with a similar side effect profile as that of prostacyclin. Importantly, it can also cause pain and erythema around the infusion site thereby limiting its usefulness in young children. Treprostinil has been tested in a multicentre international placebo-controlled randomized study and was found to have beneficial effects on hemodynamics and exercise tolerance, the latter being dose dependent.[51] A study of intravenous treprostinil is under way.

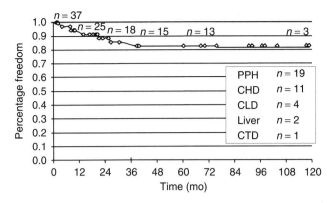

Figure 40.4 Kaplan-Meier curves of freedom from death or transplant with long-term prostacyclin treatment in children with pulmonary hypertension at the Children's Hospital Heart Institute/Pediatric Heart Lung Center, Denver, Colorado. PPH, primary pulmonary hypertension; CHD, congenital heart disease; CLD, chronic lung disease; Liver, liver disease; CTD, connective tissue disease.

An inhaled prostacyclin analog, iloprost, has undergone initial trials with significant beneficial effects on symptomatology and quality of life.[52] Iloprost has a half-life of 20 to 25 minutes and therefore six to nine inhalations a day are required to be clinically effective. The advantage of an inhaled prostacyclin is that it can cause selective pulmonary vasodilation without affecting systemic blood pressure (see Fig. 40.5). Additionally inhaled prostacyclin analogs can improve gas exchange and pulmonary shunt in cases of impaired ventilation–perfusion by redistributing pulmonary blood flow, from nonventilated to ventilated, aerosol-accessible lung regions.[53] A recent randomized controlled trial of aerosolized prostacyclin therapy was shown to improve oxygenation in children with acute lung injury.[54] Inhaled iloprost was recently approved in the United States and has been approved in Europe.

Beraprost, an orally active prostacyclin analog, is fast acting and has a half-life of 35 to 40 minutes; it has beneficial effects, which may be attenuated with increasing length of treatment.[55]

Endothelins

Another target for treatment of pulmonary hypertension is the vasoconstrictor peptide endothelin (ET). The ETs are a family of isopeptides consisting of ET-1, ET-2, and ET-3. ET-1 is a potent vasoactive peptide produced primarily in the vascular endothelial cell, but it may also be produced by smooth muscle cells. Two receptor subtypes, ET_A and ET_B mediate the activity of ET-1. ET_A receptors on vascular smooth muscle mediate vasoconstriction. ET_B receptors on smooth muscle cells mediate vasoconstriction, whereas ET_B receptors on endothelial cells cause release of nitric oxide or prostacyclin (PGI_2) and act as clearance receptors for circulating ET-1 (see Fig. 40.6). ET-1 expression is increased in the pulmonary arteries of patients with pulmonary hypertension. Bosentan, a dual ET receptor antagonist, lowers PAP and resistance, and improves exercise tolerance in adults with pulmonary arterial hypertension.[56] In children with pulmonary arterial hypertension related to congenital heart disease or IPAH, bosentan lowered pulmonary pressure and resistance, and was well tolerated (see Fig. 40.7).[57] Bosentan has been used in adults with Eisenmenger physiology with good effect.[58]

Bosentan, has been successfully used in children on long-term epoprostenol therapy. Specifically, concomitant use of Bosentan allowed for a decrease in epoprostenol and its associated side effects, and discontinuation of epoprostenol in some children with normal PAP.[59] Recent work has shown that Bosentan may be used as a first-line

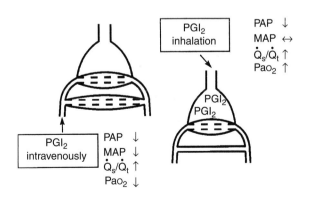

Figure 40.5 Both intravenous and inhaled prostacyclin lower mean pulmonary artery pressure (PAP). However, inhaled prostacyclin has a selective effect without lowering mean arterial pressure (MAP), intrapulmonary shunt (Qs/Qt), or arterial oxygen content (Pao_2). PGI_2, prostacyclin (From Max M, Rossaint R, Inhaled prostacyclin in the treatment of pulmonary hypertension. *Eur J Pediatr.* 1999;158(suppl 1):523–526.)

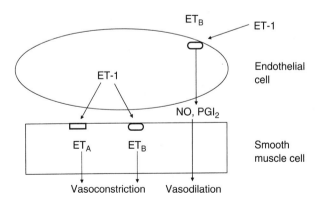

Figure 40.6 Endothelin-1 (ET-1) is a potent vasoactive peptide produced primarily in the vascular endothelial cell, but it may also be produced by smooth muscle cells. Two receptor subtypes, ET_A and ET_B mediate the activity of ET-1. ET_A receptors on vascular smooth muscle mediate vasoconstriction. ET_B receptors on smooth muscle cells mediate vasoconstriction, whereas ET_B receptors on endothelial cells cause release of nitric oxide (NO) or prostacyclin (PGI_2) and act as clearance receptors for circulating ET-1.

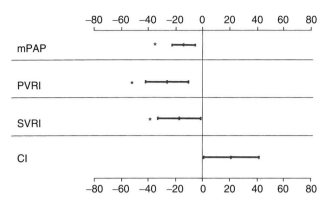

Figure 40.7 Percent change in hemodynamics after 12 weeks of treatment in children with pulmonary hypertension treated with Bosentan, a dual endothelin receptor antagonist. Bosentan significantly lowered mean pulmonary artery pressure (mPAP), pulmonary vascular resistance index (PVRI), systemic vascular resistance index (SVRI), but not the cardiac index (CI). (Barst RJ, et al. Pharmacokinetics, safety, and efficacy of Bosentan in pediatric patients with pulmonary arterial hypertension. *Clin Pharmacol Ther.* 2003;372–382.)

agent for advanced pulmonary hypertension resulting in prolonged survival.[60]

Selective ET_A receptor blockade is also possible using sitaxsentan, an ET receptor antagonist with high oral bioavailability, with a long duration of action, and with a high specificity for the ET_A receptor. Sitaxsentan may benefit patients with pulmonary arterial hypertension by blocking the vasoconstrictor effects of ET_A receptors while maintaining the vasodilator/clearance functions of ET_B receptors. Sitaxsentan given orally for 12 weeks was seen to have beneficial effects on exercise capacity and cardiopulmonary hemodynamics in patients with pulmonary arterial hypertension that was idiopathic, related to connective tissue disease or congenital heart disease.[61] Further studies using selective ET_A receptor blockade in postoperative congenital heart disease[62,63] have been reported.

Phosphodiesterase-5 Inhibitors

Specific phosphodiesterase-5 inhibitors, such as sildenafil, also have a role in the treatment of pulmonary hypertension.[64–66] These drugs promote an increase in cGMP levels and therefore cause pulmonary vasodilation (Fig. 40.2). Sildenafil is as effective a pulmonary vasodilator as iNO and may be preferred because it does not increase pulmonary wedge pressure.[5,67] Sildenafil may also be useful in the setting of iNO therapy withdrawal (Fig. 40.3),[68] in postoperative pulmonary hypertension,[68,69] or in the presence of pulmonary hypertension related to chronic lung disease.[70] In the acute postoperative setting, sildenafil may worsen oxygenation[68,71] In other patients with pulmonary hypertension, sildenafil may reduce right ventricular mass, and improve cardiac function and exercise capacity in patients with pulmonary arterial hypertension, WHO functional class III.[72] Studies examining the use

of such oral phosphodiesterase-5 inhibitors over the long term are ongoing.

Anticoagulation

Anticoagulation may be required because some causes of pulmonary hypertension may be associated with low cardiac output leading to sluggish blood flow through the pulmonary artery, which may predispose to the development of pulmonary thrombi. In adults with IPAH, use of warfarin improves survival. However, the long-term use of anticoagulation has not been studied widely in children, but is usually recommended. The use of anticoagulation agents in patients with Eisenmenger syndrome is controversial. In primary pulmonary hypertension, the aim is to keep the international normalized ratio (INR) between 1.5 and 2.0. Risks of anticoagulation in other forms of pulmonary hypertension must be weighed against advantages.

Atrial Septostomy

The general indications for atrial septostomy include pulmonary hypertension refractory to chronic vasodilator treatment[73] and in symptomatic low cardiac output states. Syncope and intractable RHF are indications for patients who are treated with vasodilators if the patients remain refractory. Risks associated with this procedure include a worsening of hypoxemia with resultant right ventricular ischemia and worsening right ventricular failure, increased left atrial pressure, and pulmonary edema.

Transplantation

For patients who do not respond to prolonged vasodilator treatment, or with certain lesions, such as pulmonary vein stenosis, lung transplantation may be offered.[74–76] Cystic fibrosis accounts for most lung transplants, with primary pulmonary hypertension as an indication for transplantation in 14% to 17% of patients. For certain patients, including those with congenital heart disease, heart–lung transplantation may be necessary.

CONCLUSION

Advances in the understanding of the pulmonary vasculature have led to improved survival in children with severe pulmonary hypertension. The timely diagnosis of pediatric pulmonary hypertension is of paramount importance because treatment strategies improve morbidity and mortality. An extensive evaluation is performed in children with severe pulmonary hypertension because the most successful strategy involves treatment of any underlying disorder. Further, a targeted approach to treatment includes acute vasodilator testing at cardiac catheterization to determine long-term therapy. In patients reactive to acute vasodilator testing with short-acting vasodilators, such as iNO, CCBs have been shown to provide effective therapy. For those patients who are not reactive to acute vasodilator testing, one should consider other forms of therapy, such as epoprostenol.

Newer treatment strategies in children include the use of ET receptor antagonists, iNO, prostacyclin analogs, and phosphodiesterase inhibitors. Recent advances have given the clinician more options in the management of a once fatal condition; however, more work is required to understand the role of new treatments for children with pulmonary hypertension in different clinical settings.

REFERENCES

1. Davidson A, Bossuyt A, Dab I. Acute effects of oxygen, nifedipine, and diltiazem in patients with cystic fibrosis and mild pulmonary hypertension. *Pediatr Pulmonol.* 1989;6(1):53–59.
2. Geggel RL, Dozor AI, Fyler DL, et al. Effect of vasodilators at rest and during exercise in young adults with cystic fibrosis and chronic cor pulmonale. *Am Rev Respir Dis.* 1985;131:531–536.
3. Thilenius OG, Nadas AS, Jockin H. Primary pulmonary vascular obstruction in children. *Pediatrics.* 1965;75–87.
4. Sandoval J, Bauerle O, Gomez A, et al. Primary pulmonary hypertension in children: Clinical characterization and survival. *J Am Coll Cardiol.* 1995;466–474.
5. Barst RJ. Recent advances in the treatment of pediatric pulmonary artery hypertension. *Pediatr Clin North Am.* 1999;331–345.
6. Rich S, Dantzker DR, Ayres SM, et al., eds. Primary pulmonary hypertension. Executive summary from the world symposium. *Primary pulmonary hypertension.* World Health Organization; 1998.
7. Kawut SM, Horn EM, Berekashvili KK, et al. New predictors of outcome in idiopathic pulmonary arterial hypertension. *Am J Cardiol.* 2005;199–203.
8. Das BB, et al. High-altitude pulmonary edema in children with underlying cardiopulmonary disorders and pulmonary hypertension living at altitude. *Arch Pediatr Adolesc Med.* 2004;1170–1176.
9. Berman EB, Barst RJ. Eisenmenger's syndrome: Current management. *Prog Cardiovasc Dis.* 2002;129–138.
10. Humbert M, Sitbon O, Simonneau G. Treatment of pulmonary arterial hypertension. *N Engl J Med.* 2004;1425–1436.
11. Rich S, Dantzker DR, Ayres SM, et al. Primary pulmonary hypertension. A national prospective study. *Ann Intern Med.* 1987;216–223.
12. Loyd JE, Butler MG, Foroud TM, et al. Genetic anticipation and abnormal gender ratio at birth in familial primary pulmonary hypertension. *Am J Respir Crit Care Med.* 1995;152:93–97.
13. Lane KB, Machado RD, Pauciulo MW, et al. Heterozygous germline mutations in BMPR2, encoding a TGF-beta receptor, cause familial primary pulmonary hypertension. The International PPH Consortium. *Nat Genet.* 2000;81–84.
14. Deng Z, Morse JH, Slager SL, et al. Familial primary pulmonary hypertension (gene PPH1) is caused by mutations in the bone morphogenetic protein receptor-II gene. *Am J Hum Genet.* 2000:737–744.
15. Thomson JR, Machado RD, Pauciulo MW, et al. Sporadic primary pulmonary hypertension is associated with germline mutations of the gene encoding BMPR-II, a receptor member of the TGF-beta family. *J Med Genet.* 2000;741–745.
16. Newman JH, Wheeler L, Lane KB, et al. Mutation in the gene for bone morphogenetic protein receptor-II as a cause of primary pulmonary hypertension in a large kindred. *N Engl J Med.* 2001;319–324.
17. Trembath RC, Harrison R. Insights into the genetic and molecular basis of primary pulmonary hypertension. *Pediatr Res.* 2003; 883–888.
18. Machado RD, Pauciulo MW, Thomson JR, et al. BMPR2 haploinsufficiency as the inherited molecular mechanism for primary pulmonary hypertension. *Am J Hum Genet.* 2001:92–102.
19. Uehara R, Suzuki H, Kurokawa N, et al. Novel nonsense mutation of the BMPR-II gene in a Japanese patient with familial primary pulmonary hypertension. *Pediatr Int.* 2002;433–435.
20. Humbert M, Deng Z, Simonneau G, et al. BMPR2 germline mutations in pulmonary hypertension associated with fenfluramine derivatives. *Eur Respir J.* 2002;518–523.
21. Rindermann M, Grunig E, von Hippel A, et al. Primary pulmonary hypertension may be a heterogeneous disease with a second locus on chromosome 2q31. *J Am Coll Cardiol.* 2003;2237–2244.
22. Machado RD, Rudarakanchana N, Atkinson C, et al. Functional interaction between BMPR-II and Tctex-1, a light chain of Dynein, is isoform-specific and disrupted by mutations underlying primary pulmonary hypertension. *Hum Mol Genet.* 2003;3277–3286.
23. Morisaki H, Nakanishi N, Kyotani S, et al. BMPR2 mutations found in Japanese patients with familial and sporadic primary pulmonary hypertension. *Hum Mutat.* 2004;632.
24. Massague J, Chen YG. Controlling TGF-beta signaling. *Genes Dev.* 2000;627–644.
25. Trembath RC, Thomson JR, Machado RD, et al. Clinical and molecular genetic features of pulmonary hypertension in patients with hereditary hemorrhagic telangiectasia. *N Engl J Med.* 2001;325–334.
26. Harrison RE, Flanagan JA, Sankelo M, et al. Molecular and functional analysis identifies ALK-1 as the predominant cause of pulmonary hypertension related to hereditary haemorrhagic telangiectasia. *J Med Genet.* 2003;865–871.
27. Auger WR, Channick R, Kerr KM, et al. Evaluation of patients with suspected chronic thromboembolic pulmonary hypertension. *Semin Thorac Cardiovasc Surg.* 1999;11:179–190.
28. Rabinovitch M. Pulmonary hypertension: Pathophysiology as a basis for clinical decision making. *J Heart Lung Transplant.* 1999;18(11):1041–1053.
29. Balzer DT, Kort HW, Day RW, et al. Inhaled Nitric Oxide as a Preoperative Test (INOP Test I): The INOP Test Study Group. *Circulation.* 2002;106(12 Suppl 1):176–181.
30. Rimensberger PC, Spahr-Schopfer I, Berner M, et al. Inhaled nitric oxide versus aerosolized iloprost in secondary pulmonary hypertension in children with congenital heart disease: Vasodilator capacity and cellular mechanisms. *Circulation.* 2001; 544–548.
31. Barst RJ, Maislin G, Fishman AP. Vasodilator therapy for primary pulmonary hypertension in children. *Circulation.* 1999;99(9): 1197–1208.
32. Widlitz A, Barst RJ. Pulmonary arterial hypertension in children. *Eur Respir J.* 2003;155–176.
33. Atz AM, Adatia I, Lock JE, et al. Combined effects of nitric oxide and oxygen during acute pulmonary vasodilator testing. *J Am Coll Cardiol.* 1999;33(3):813–819.
34. Pepke-Zaba J, Heigenbottam HT, Dinh-Xaun AT, et al. Inhaled nitric oxide as a cause of selective pulmonary vasodilatation in pulmonary hypertension. *Lancet.* 1991;338:1173–1174.
35. Ivy DD, Kinsella JP, Wolfe RR, et al. Atrial natriuretic peptide and nitric oxide in children with pulmonary hypertension after surgical repair of congenital heart disease. *Am J Cardiol.* 1996;77(1):102–105.
36. Ivy DD, Parker P, Doran A, et al. Acute hemodynamic effects and home therapy using novel pulsed nasal nitric oxide delivery system in children and young adults with pulmonary hypertension. *Am J Cardiol.* 2003;886–890.
37. Ivy DD, Griebel JL, Kinsella JP, et al. Acute hemodynamic effects of pulsed delivery of low flow nasal nitric oxide in children with pulmonary hypertension. *J Pediatr.* 1998;133(3):453–456.
38. Berner M, Beghetti M, Spahr-Schopfer I, et al. Inhaled nitric oxide to test the vasodilator capacity of the pulmonary vascular bed in children with long-standing pulmonary hypertension and congenital heart disease. *Am J Cardiol.* 1996;77(7):532–535.
39. Atz AM, Wessel DL. Inhaled nitric oxide in the neonate with cardiac disease. *Semin Perinatol.* 1997;25(4):441–455.
40. Wessel DL, Adatia I, Giglia TM, et al. Use of inhaled nitric oxide and acetylcholine in the evaluation of pulmonary hypertension and endothelial function after cardiopulmonary bypass. *Circulation.* 1993;88(5 Pt 1):2128–2138.
41. Channick RN, Newhart JW, Johnson FW, et al. Pulsed delivery of inhaled nitric oxide to patients with primary pulmonary hypertension: An ambulatory delivery system and initial clinical tests. *Chest.* 1996;109(6):1545–1549.

42. Katayama Y, Heigenbottam TW, Cremona G, et al. Minimizing the inhaled dose of NO with breath-by-breath delivery of spikes of concentrated gas. *Circulation.* 1998;98(22):2429–2432.

43. Atz AM, Adatia I, Wessel DL. Rebound pulmonary hypertension after inhalation of nitric oxide. *Ann Thorac Surg.* 1996;62: 1759–1764.

44. Pearl JM, Nelson DP, Raake JL, et al. Inhaled nitric oxide increases endothelin-1 levels: A potential cause of rebound pulmonary hypertension. *Crit Care Med.* 2002;30(1):89–93.

45. Ivy DD, Kinsella JP, Ziegler JW, et al. Dipyridamole attenuates rebound pulmonary hypertension after inhaled nitric oxide withdrawal in postoperative congenital heart disease. *J Thorac Cardiovasc Surg.* 1998;115(4):875–882.

46. Atz AM, Wessel DL. Sildenafil ameliorates effects of inhaled nitric oxide withdrawal. *Anesthesiology.* 1999;91:307–310.

47. Yung D, Widlitz AC, Rosenzweig EB, et al. Outcomes in children with idiopathic pulmonary arterial hypertension. *Circulation.* 2004;660–665.

48. Tuder RM, Cool CD, Geraci MW, et al. Prostacyclin synthase expression is decreased in lungs from patients with severe pulmonary hypertension. *Am J Respir Crit Care Med.* 1999;159(6):1925–1932.

49. Sitbon O, Humbert M, Nunes H, et al. Long-term intravenous epoprostenol infusion in primary pulmonary hypertension: Prognostic factors and survival. *J Am Coll Cardiol.* 2002;40(4):780–788.

50. Rosenzweig EB, Kerstein D, Barst RJ. Long-term prostacyclin for pulmonary hypertension with associated congenital heart defects. *Circulation.* 1999;99(14):1858–1865.

51. Simonneau G. Barst RJ, Galie N, et al. Continuous subcutaneous infusion of treprostinil, a prostacyclin analogue, in patients with pulmonary arterial hypertension: A double-blind randomized, placebo-controlled trial. *Am J Respir Crit Care Med.* 2002;165(6).

52. Olschewski H. Simonneau G, Galie N, et al. Inhaled iloprost for severe pulmonary hypertension. *N Engl J Med.* 2002;347(5): 322–329.

53. Max M, Rossaint R. Inhaled prostacyclin in the treatment of pulmonary hypertension. *Eur J Pediatr.* 1999;S23–S26.

54. Dahlem P, van Aalderen WM, de Neef M, et al. Randomized controlled trial of aerosolized prostacyclin therapy in children with acute lung injury. *Crit Care Med.* 2004;1055–1060.

55. Barst RJ, McGoon M, McLaughlin V, et al. Beraprost therapy for pulmonary arterial hypertension. *J Am Coll Cardiol.* 2003; 2119–2125.

56. Rubin LJ, Badesch DB, Barst RJ, et al. Bosentan therapy for pulmonary arterial hypertension. *N Engl J Med.* 2002;896–903.

57. Barst RJ, Ivy D, Widlitz AC, et al. Pharmacokinetics, safety, and efficacy of bosentan in pediatric patients with pulmonary arterial hypertension. *Clin Pharmacol Ther.* 2003;372–382.

58. Gatzoulis MA, Rogers P, Wei L, et al. Safety and tolerability of bosentan in adults with Eisenmenger physiology. *Int J Cardiol.* 2005;147–151.

59. Ivy DD, Doran A, Claussen L, et al. Weaning and discontinuation of epoprostenol in children with idiopathic pulmonary arterial hypertension receiving concomitant bosentan. *Am J Cardiol.* 2004;943–946.

60. McLaughlin VV, Sitbon O, Badesch DB, et al. Survival with first-line bosentan in patients with primary pulmonary hypertension. *Eur Respir J.* 2005;244–249.

61. Barst RJ, Langleben D, Forst A, et al. Sitaxsentan therapy for pulmonary arterial hypertension. *Am J Respir Crit Care Med.* 2004;441–447.

62. Schulze-Neick I, Li J, Reader JA, et al. The endothelin antagonist BQ123 reduces pulmonary vascular resistance after surgical intervention for congenital heart disease. *J Thorac Cardiovasc Surg.* 2002; 124(3):435–441.

63. Prendergast B, Newby DE, Wilson LE, et al. Early therapeutic experience with the endothelin antagonist BQ-123 in pulmonary hypertension after congenital heart surgery. *Heart.* 1999;82(4):505–508.

64. Prasad S, Wilkinson J, Gatzoulis MA. Sildenafil in primary pulmonary hypertension. *N Engl J Med.* 2000;1342.

65. Kumar S. Indian doctor in protest after using Viagra to save "blue babies". *BMJ.* 2002;181.

66. Michelakis ED, Tymchak W, Noga M, et al. Long-term treatment with oral sildenafil is safe and improves functional capacity and hemodynamics in patients with pulmonary arterial hypertension. *Circulation.* 2003;2066–2069.

67. Michelakis E, Tymchak W, Lien D, et al. Oral sildenafil is an effective and specific pulmonary vasodilator in patients with pulmonary arterial hypertension: Comparison with inhaled nitric oxide. *Circulation.* 2002;105:2398–2403.

68. Schulze-Neick I, Hartenstein P, Li J, et al. Intravenous sildenafil is a potent pulmonary vasodilator in children with congenital heart disease. *Circulation.* 2003;II167–II173.

69. Atz Am LA, Fairbrother DL, Uber WE, et al. Sildenafil augments the effect of inhaled nitric oxide for postoperative pulmonary hypertensive crisis. *J Thorac Cardiovasc Surg.* 2002;628–629.

70. Ghofrani HA, Wiedemann R, Rose F, et al. Sildenafil for treatment of lung fibrosis and pulmonary hypertension: A randomised controlled trial. *Lancet.* 2002;895–900.

71. Stocker C, Penny DJ, Brizard CP, et al. Intravenous sildenafil and inhaled nitric oxide: A randomised trial in infants after cardiac surgery. *Intensive Care Med.* 2003;1996–2003.

72. Wilkins MR, Paul GA, Strange JW, et al. Sildenafil versus Endothelin Receptor Antagonist for Pulmonary Hypertension (SERAPH) Study. *Am J Respir Crit Care Med.* 2005;171(11):1292–1297.

73. Sandoval J, Gaspar J, Pulido T, et al. Graded balloon dilation atrial septostomy in severe primary pulmonary hypertension. A therapeutic alternative for patients nonresponsive to vasodilator treatment. *J Am Coll Cardiol.* 1998;297–304.

74. Boucek MM, Edwards LB, Keck BM, et al. Registry for the International Society for Heart and Lung Transplantation: Seventh official pediatric report–2004. *J Heart Lung Transplant.* 2004; 933–947.

75. Gaynor JW, Bridges ND, Clark BJ, et al. Update on lung transplantation in children. *Curr Opin Pediatr.* 1998;256–261.

76. Clabby ML, Canter CE, Moller JH, et al. Hemodynamic data and survival in children with pulmonary hypertension. *J Am Coll Cardiol.* 1997;554–560.

Disorders of the Chest Wall and Respiratory Muscles

41

Angela T. Wratney   Ira M. Cheifetz

The chest wall and the muscles involved in respiration work in concert to actively expand the thorax and lungs on inspiration and to passively recoil on expiration during tidal breathing (see Table 41.1). Weakness or disruption of the interconnections between the respiratory muscles and the thoracic cage destabilizes the chest wall, resulting in an inefficient respiratory effort. Similarly, abnormal growth of the ribs or curvature of the spine will distort the biomechanical properties of the chest wall.

The respiratory system in the pediatric patient is particularly sensitive to the negative effects of chest wall defects and respiratory muscle weakness. Increased chest wall compliance and higher airway resistance in the neonate and young child result in an inability to compensate for muscle fatigue. In this population, paradoxical motion of the chest wall can occur as respiratory distress increases—the chest wall collapses inward with deep inspiration, restricting maximum lung expansion. With diaphragm dysfunction, inward movement of the abdomen on inspiration forces the diaphragm cranially, restricts chest wall expansion, and limits inspiratory capacity.

Weak inspiratory muscle function produces a restrictive pattern evidenced by decreased vital capacity (VC), total lung capacity, and functional residual volume while preserving forced expiratory capacity. Expiratory muscle weakness, however, decreases expiratory reserve, increases residual volume, and impairs cough. Any inefficiency of the respiratory system contributes to progressive loss of lung compliance, atelectasis, and worsening gas exchange.

Progressive or chronic hypoventilation can result in sleep disorders, daytime ventilatory failure, and impaired airway clearance and cough. These patients are particularly vulnerable to respiratory infections and may progress to respiratory failure due to their limited reserve capacity. Pulmonary function testing is used to assess a patient's respiratory capacity during the course of illness. In general, maximal negative inspiratory pressures less efficient than -20 to -30 cm H_2O signify severe inspiratory muscle weakness and potential for impending respiratory illness. To assess expiratory function, a maximum positive expiratory airway pressure <40 cm H_2O indicates the inability to generate an effective cough. Forced VC less than three times the predicted tidal volume is associated with impaired coughing and subsequent retention of secretions whereas

TABLE 41.1
MUSCLE EFFECTS OF BREATHING

	Inspiration	Expiration
Quiet (primary muscles)	Diaphragm External intercostals	Elastic recoil of lung tissue Surface tension Gravity on ribs Internal intercostals
Forced (secondary or accessory muscles)	Sternocleidomastoids Scalenes Pectoralis major Pectoralis minor Serratus anterior Serratus posterior superior Upper iliocostalis	Abdominals External oblique Internal oblique Rectus abdominus Latissimus dorsi Serratus posterior inferior

respiratory failure may ensue if this value falls below two times the predicted capacity.

Although each disease process has a distinct pathologic entity, the prevention of morbidity associated with various respiratory diseases and the treatment of respiratory failure is in many ways very similar.

CHEST WALL DISORDERS

Congenital Disorders

Pectus Excavatum

Clinical Presentation
Pectus excavatum is a common congenital chest wall deformity occurring in 1 of 300 births with a male predominance. Abnormal bone and cartilage growth of the ribs on each side of the sternum create the concave appearance of the anterior chest wall.

Respiratory Effects
Posterior displacement of the sternum causes lung compression, decreased intrathoracic volume, and cardiac displacement. A restrictive pattern on pulmonary function testing is common, with the severity of sternal compression inversely affecting VC. However, most patients with pectus excavatum have normal exercise tolerance and cardiac function. Chest and back pain are common musculoskeletal complaints, which may arise during adolescence as secondary to rapid bone growth, and poor postural tone. "Poor posture" (i.e., an anterior sloping of the cervicothoracic spine with shoulders slumped forward) is typical of patients with pectus, and this positioning exaggerates the chest wall restriction and can cause various degrees of scoliosis.

Imaging Studies
The severity of the cardiac shift, the posterior displacement of the sternum, and the degree of spinal curvature may be measured on anteroposterior (AP) and lateral chest x-rays (CXR). Computed tomography (CT) of the chest is useful to evaluate causes of significant cardiopulmonary impairment or to provide anatomic detail for operative planning. The CT scan index is derived by dividing the transverse chest diameter by the AP diameter. A CT scan index above 3.2 has been correlated with a severe deformity requiring surgery. An echocardiogram may be obtained to assess cardiac anatomy and function in patients with cardiopulmonary limitations. Pulmonary function testing can measure changes in predicted volumes, gas exchange capacity, and exercise tolerance.

Treatment
Treatment options range from observation for asymptomatic patients to surgical sternal elevation in symptomatic patients to reduce cardiopulmonary compromise. Patients with cardiopulmonary disease or limitations of activity secondary to the posterior displacement of the sternum are strongly considered for surgical repair. Elective pectus repair is more common; adolescents desire cosmetic repair to correct the sunken appearance of the anterior chest wall. Elective repair may also be advised for the patient who will later undergo open heart surgery (such as for mitral valve replacement or other cardiac disease). Open heart surgery may be challenging, if the pectus is unrepaired, due to the extreme leftward displacement of the heart.

Operative repair of the pectus deformity may be done by sternal osteotomy or by a thoracoscopically guided minimally invasive technique. Both have excellent cosmetic results. The former is an extensive surgery requiring anterior chest wall exposure, creation of muscle and skin flaps, and extensive cartilage resection. In the minimally invasive technique, a convex stainless steel support bar is placed directly behind the sternum to force outward displacement. This procedure is ideally performed in patients who are 8 to 12 years of age when the chest wall is still very malleable and stabilization of the bar is easily achieved. Displacement of the retrosternal bar occurs in <2.5% of procedures.

Outcome
Patients with pectus excavatum are able to lead active healthy lives, often without functional impairment. Symptomatic patients with cardiorespiratory limitations should receive pulmonary, cardiac, and surgical consultation. Operative repair restores the aesthetic curvature to the anterior chest wall, but surgical outcomes suggest an unpredictable degree of improvement in pulmonary function testing, exercise tolerance, and increased cardiac index on exertion.

Acquired Disorders

Scoliosis

Clinical Presentation
Scoliosis is a common spinal deformity, broadly defined as >10 degrees lateral displacement of the spine from its central axis (Cobb angle). Progressive spinal curvature may develop in otherwise healthy adolescents or may result from progressive weakness in patients with underlying chronic neuromuscular disease. Although absolute curvature of the spine is an important consideration, rate of curvature progression, age of onset, and relative skeletal maturity are also significant factors for predicting the risk of progressive skeletal deformity and respiratory compromise.

Imaging Studies
Two-dimensional, upright posterior–anterior radiographs of the full spine indicate the degree of lateral curvature using the Cobb method (see Fig. 41.1), which determines the magnitude of the curve angle between the uppermost and lowermost portions of the affected spine. A Cobb angle >10 degrees defines the presence of scoliosis. Cobb angles of 30 to 60 degrees signify mild to moderate scoliosis; more severe scoliosis occurs with Cobb angles of 66 to 136

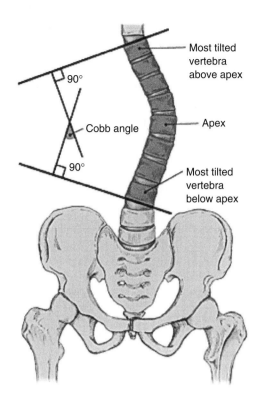

Figure 41.1 Detecting scoliosis: measurement of the Cobb angle. (From Greiner KA. Adolescent idiopathic scoliosis: Radiologic decision-making. *Am Fam Physician.* 2002;65:1817–1823.)

degrees, and very severe deformity exists when the Cobb angle exceeds 100 degrees. The predominant direction (right or left), location, and number of displaced vertebra are also noted. Radiographs of the wrist and hips may be obtained to assess the degree of skeletal maturity. Magnetic resonance imaging (MRI) is indicated for patients with neurologic signs such as severe unexplained headaches, ataxia, or cavus feet.

Respiratory Effects

Progressive deformity of the thoracic cage causes a restrictive pulmonary defect with a reduction of VC. Chest wall compliance is inversely proportional to the Cobb angle and is commonly 25% to 50% of predicted in patients with severe scoliosis. To compensate for decreased thoracic compliance, patients recruit abdominal and expiratory muscles while also increasing rib cage motion to assist in tidal breathing.

The degree of respiratory impairment is not linearly related to the severity of the Cobb angle, as respiratory function is also affected by the length of spinal involvement, the cephalad location of the curve, and the disruption of normal kyphosis. Patients with mild to moderate scoliosis are generally asymptomatic. More severe scoliosis may result in dyspnea on exertion. Patients with severe scoliosis are generally symptomatic, but the clinical variability is tremendous. Many patients with severe scoliosis

have a reduced VC and also have pulmonary hypertension affecting cardiovascular function and exercise tolerance.

In general, Cobb angles >70 degrees affecting more than seven vertebrae and located in the upper thorax are most likely to be associated with severe pulmonary restriction.

Treatment

Treatment of scoliosis may consist of observation, orthosis, or operative intervention. Depending upon the presence of various risk factors (age of onset, Cobb angle, length of spinal involvement, cephalad location, stage of skeletal immaturity, and evidence of restrictive disease on pulmonary function testing), patients may progress through one or all of these treatment options.

No clear guidelines for the surgical management of symptomatic or severe scoliosis exist. The goal of surgical intervention is to prevent progressive respiratory compromise. Clinical outcomes following surgical treatment of idiopathic scoliosis are strongly linked to curve magnitude. A meta-analysis of 173 patients who underwent a Harrington repair suggests a range of improvement in lung function from 2% to 11% of predicted value.

Surgical repair of scoliosis in patients with chronic respiratory failure has resulted in a mixed outcome. The risks of potentially prolonged surgery and significant blood loss in a patient with chronic respiratory failure and limited respiratory reserve must be weighed against the potential benefits. Baydur et al. reported that reconstructive spine surgery in pediatric patients with severe scoliosis associated with restrictive lung disease is well tolerated. Patients with underlying neuromuscular disease or chronic hypoventilation may be palliated with nocturnal mechanical ventilation pre- or postoperatively to support patency of the smaller airways, optimize gas exchange, and ameliorate the cardiorespiratory work of breathing.

Trauma

Flail Chest

Clinical Presentation

A flail chest indicates that a portion of the rib cage has lost continuity with the thorax because of multiple contiguous rib fractures. The chest wall in the infant and child is more compliant and the mediastinum more mobile than in the adult. Therefore, bony fractures signify a high-velocity injury and a high probability of intrathoracic trauma.

Respiratory Effects

The flail segment moves paradoxically with respiratory effort, causing ineffective gas exchange and pain. Abnormal accessory muscle recruitment (i.e., splinting) will occur in an attempt to stabilize the chest wall and muscle connections in the area of the flail segment. Ventilatory function is most affected by closer proximity of the flail segment to the diaphragm and by the severity of the underlying pulmonary contusion.

Treatment

Prolonged ventilatory support may be required because of parenchymal injuries rather than the disturbances caused by the flail chest wall. A pressure bandage placed circumferentially across the chest will stabilize the chest wall and reduce pain. Positive-pressure ventilation may be required to recruit atelectatic lung, restore normal gas exchange, and stabilize the fractures.

Diaphragm Rupture

A significant compressive force to the abdomen and lower chest, because of blunt trauma or lap belt injury, may result in traumatic rupture of the diaphragm. Abdominal contents herniate into the thoracic cavity through the defect, causing potentially life-threatening pulmonary compression. Traumatic rupture may be suspected on radiographic images when the diaphragm is not clearly visualized or when fluid does not completely clear from the pleural space after chest tube placement. All diaphragmatic injuries require operative repair.

Phrenic Nerve Injury

Clinical Presentation

The phrenic nerves arise from the cervical plexus (roots C3, C4, C5) and provide the sole innervation to the diaphragm. Because of its long course, injury to the phrenic nerve may occur due to a number of etiologies such as those occurring during cardiothoracic procedures (transection or stretch, cautery burns, cold damage with topical ice slush hypothermia, or disruption of the vascular supply), associated with a traumatic birth (traction of the phrenic roots and brachial plexus), or during ill-attempted placement of an internal jugular catheter. Diaphragm paralysis should be suspected in newborns with respiratory distress after a difficult or forceps-assisted delivery. Cardiothoracic procedures involving the great vessels are most often associated with an increased risk of phrenic nerve injury. Examples of common procedures include (a) placement or takedown of a systemic-pulmonary artery shunt, (b) pulmonary artery reconstruction, (c) ligation of a patent ductus arteriosus, (d) pulmonary artery banding, and (e) a "redo" sternotomy.

Respiratory Effects

The degree of respiratory compromise inflicted by diaphragmatic injury is dependent on the age of the child and whether the injury is unilateral or bilateral. Motion of the injured diaphragm is paradoxical, moving cephalad with the chest wall during inspiration and expanding into the abdominal cavity with exhalation. With diaphragm weakness or injury, inspiration requires accessory muscle recruitment and increased thoracic effort to expand the lungs. In children younger than 2 years, the chest wall is more compliant than the lungs, causing retraction rather than expansion upon inspiration. This only further restricts ventilatory capacity and increases the work of breathing. Isolated unilateral diaphragm paralysis may be well tolerated in older children and adults but is not well tolerated in infants. Infants will typically manifest respiratory distress and be unable to maintain adequate gas exchange without positive-pressure ventilation. Infants are disadvantaged due to their supine position as well, which exacerbates the restrictive effects of the paralyzed diaphragm on ventilatory capacity. Bilateral diaphragm paralysis is not well tolerated at any age. Infants and small children are at high risk for respiratory failure, whereas adults and older children may be able to overcome alveolar hypoventilation with temporary noninvasive support.

Imaging Studies

Paradoxical motion of the diaphragm may be identified by a chest x-ray, an ultrasonography, fluoroscopy, or phrenic nerve stimulation. CXR indirectly reflect paradoxical motion of the diaphragm by the presence of a raised hemidiaphragm at rest or upon inspiration. Examination must occur during spontaneous respiratory effort; studies performed during positive-pressure assistance (continuous positive airway pressure or mechanical ventilation) are uninterpretable. Ultrasonography and fluoroscopy provide a direct, dynamic assessment of diaphragm movement with respiratory effort. Ultrasonography has the advantage of providing real-time information at the bedside; whereas fluoroscopy requires transport to the radiologic suite and radiation exposure. Diagnosis of bilateral diaphragm paralysis can be challenging as the diaphragms may appear to move with the chest wall or with accessory muscle effort. Electromagnetic stimulation of the phrenic nerve can be done directly (during thoracic procedures) or indirectly (transcutaneously at its cervical origin) providing definitive evidence for nerve function. The absence of diaphragmatic contraction after phrenic nerve stimulation generally indicates complete, irreversible phrenic nerve damage.

Treatment

Potential treatment options include observation, noninvasive or invasive positive-pressure ventilation, and surgical plication of the affected hemidiaphragm. The appropriate therapy for an individual patient may depend on multiple integrated factors that include patient age, degree of respiratory compromise, presumed etiology for injury and likelihood for functional recovery of the phrenic nerve, associated cardiorespiratory compromise, and institutional and individual surgeon preferences.

Because of uncertainty regarding the possibility for functional recovery, 2 to 3 weeks of observation may be preferred for select patients with adequate respiratory reserve. Noninvasive support with continuous positive airway pressure of 5 to 10 cm H_2O can reduce the work of breathing and maintain adequate alveolar ventilation.

Clinical studies in adults indicate that as many as 30% of patients will never regain diaphragmatic function. The potential for spontaneous recovery in children may be even lower. de Leeuw et al. published one of the largest series of children (<1 to 14.4 years of age) with diaphragmatic paralysis following cardiothoracic surgery. One hundred and seventy episodes of diaphragmatic paralysis were identified in 10,395 cardiothoracic operations from 1985 to 1997, an overall incidence of 1.6%. Confirmed recovery of diaphragmatic function was noted in only 15/170 episodes at a median interval of 14 days (range 6 days to 5.2 years). Diaphragmatic plication was performed in 40% of patients at a median of 15 days. At the time of plication, 77% of patients were receiving mechanical ventilation. The median time to extubation was 4 days (range <1 to 65 days) after plication. Younger patients and those receiving mechanical ventilation at the time of evaluation were most likely to have a significantly shorter trial of observation before plication. Therefore, the authors concluded that the potential for spontaneous recovery of diaphragmatic function is very low and the decision to plicate should be based on the respiratory status of the patient.

The optimal timing for surgical plication is unknown and the criteria for determining a failed observation trial are not standardized. Immediate benefits are seen after plication of the affected diaphragm in most patients. Plication decreases the work of breathing, improves efficiency of the respiratory muscles, increases VC, and can enable liberation from mechanical ventilation.

Obesity and Ascites

Morbid obesity (40 kg per m^2) and massive intra-abdominal ascites displace the diaphragm into the chest, restricting respiratory capacity. The associated restrictive lung disease reduces functional residual capacity (FRC), expiratory flow, expiratory reserve volume, and maximal inspiratory pressures to as much as 50% of predicted value. These effects are exaggerated in the supine position. Obese patients also have reduced respiratory system compliance and increased total respiratory resistance due to smaller functional lung volumes and alterations in chest wall mechanics. Respiratory muscle efficiency is reduced in obese patients as evidenced by a markedly increased total body oxygen consumption of 16% (normal: 1% to 3%). Improvement in lung volumes and respiratory muscle function may be seen in patients only after significant weight loss (mean weight loss 23.6%) and may be because of improved chest wall mechanics.

RESPIRATORY MUSCLE DISORDERS

Neuromuscular Disease

Common neuromuscular diseases, presenting symptoms, treatment, and outcomes are shown in Table 41.2. Selected conditions are discussed in more detail in subsequent text.

Duchenne Muscular Dystrophy

Clinical Presentation

Muscular dystrophy (MD) is a group of inheritable disorders characterized by progressive skeletal muscle weakness. As affected muscles degenerate, fat and connective tissue accumulate. Of the nine major types of MD, Duchenne muscular dystrophy (DMD) is the most common, affecting one in 3,500 male infants. DMD is an X-linked recessive defect in the gene coding for dystrophin, the cytoskeletal protein present in skeletal and cardiac muscle. Affected muscle groups fail to show histologic staining for dystrophin. Although it has been extensively studied, very little is actually known about how a deficiency of dystrophin results in muscle weakness.

The onset of weakness may not be fully appreciated in the young child. Children aged 2 to 5 years may be unable to completely close their eyes or raise their eyebrows due to weak orbicularis oculi muscles, and may have difficulty climbing stairs or may "waddle" due to weak hip-flexors. Fatty accumulation in the calf muscles causes pseudohypertrophy and tightening of the Achilles' tendon. Concern may arise when the child begins to "toe walk" in an effort to maintain balance due to progressive weakness of the calf and quadriceps muscles. In the older child (6 to 9 years), exaggerated lordotic posturing develops to overcome weak pelvic and shoulder muscles. Without assistance from these central pelvic-girdle muscles, the child will use the Gowers maneuver to "crawl up" from a squatting position. Classically, the child will roll to a prone position, push up on all fours, and then use his hands to "walk" up his legs and thighs to achieve a standing position.

Progressive muscle weakness, obesity, and progressive spinal deformity restrict lung capacity and increase the risk for respiratory failure. A variable percentage of patients with DMD will also have progressive cardiomyopathy. Death from cardiac or respiratory failure generally occurs by 20 years of age.

Laboratory Testing and Imaging Studies

DMD is confirmed by a serum, creatine phosphokinase (CPK), which is elevated by 50 to 100 times the normal along with evidence of muscle degeneration on biopsy and electromyelogram (EMG). Biopsy of the affected muscle will demonstrate the absence of dystrophin and an accumulation of fat and connective tissue on histologic staining. EMG will detect abnormalities in the nerve conduction and muscle twitch responsivity.

A chest x-ray can be used to evaluate the severity of scoliosis and detect enlargement of the cardiac silhouette. Electrocardiograms and echocardiograms are indicated to rule out conduction and myocardial defects secondary to cardiac muscle involvement.

Respiratory Effects

DMD causes a progressive, restrictive pulmonary system disease by weakening chest wall muscles and distorting the

TABLE 41.2
NEUROMUSCULAR DISEASES

Site	Common Examples	Pathophysiology	Affected Age	Affected Muscle Groups	Respiratory Effects	Treatment[a]	Outcome
Anterior horn cell	Spinal muscular atrophy Type I (Werdnig-Hoffmann disease)	Autosomal recessive Degeneration of anterior horn cell and bulbar motor nuclei	Floppy at birth	Generalized skeletal muscle weakness Bulbar muscle atrophy	Inspiratory and expiratory hypotonia	Supportive care	Death by 18 mo of age
	Spinal muscular atrophy Type II (Kugelberg-Welander disease)	Autosomal recessive Degeneration of anterior horn cell and bulbar motor nuclei	6 to 18 mo of age	Pectoral girdle and proximal muscles	Respiratory muscle hypotonia	Supportive care	Variable; respiratory failure from 2 to mid-20 y of age
Peripheral nerve	Guillain-Barré syndrome	Postinfectious demyelination or complete axonal degeneration Prodromal URI or GE	≥3 y	Ascending, symmetric motor paralysis Distal more than proximal muscle involvement Bulbar palsies Sensory loss Autonomic dysfunction	Variable; MV in 20% of patients Loss of upper airway protective reflexes	IVIg or plasma exchange Corticosteroids not helpful	Good functional recovery
Neuromuscular junction	Myasthenia gravis	Antibodies bind to and destroy Ach receptors	Neonatal infantile or juvenile MG—≥2 y of age	Generalized muscle weakness Proximal more than distal muscle involvement Bulbar palsies Exacerbated by exertion	Dyspnea Acute respiratory failure[b] Prolonged respiratory failure Loss of upper airway protective reflexes	Anticholinesterase agents—neostigmine or pyridostigmine Surgical thymectomy Immunosuppressive agents—steroids, azathioprine, or cyclosporine Short-term immunotherapies (IVIg, plasmapheresis)	Normal functional status Life-long immuno-suppression often needed

		Age of onset	Clinical features		Treatment	Prognosis
Infantile botulism	Irreversible binding of *Clostridium botulinum* toxin at presynaptic mb. to inhibit Ach release	Infant <1 y	Generalized muscle weakness Descending, symmetrical paralysis Bulbar palsies Autonomic dysfunction	Hypotonia Acute respiratory failure	MV required (50%) Human botulinum antitoxin	Prolonged, but good recovery
Muscle cell Duchenne muscular dystrophy	X-linked recessive mutations in dystrophin gene—cytoskeletal protein in skeletal and cardiac muscle	2–5 y	Proximal muscle weakness	Restrictive pulmonary disease Chest wall weakness Scoliosis Obesity	Steroids provide temporary benefit Role of surgical spinal correction unclear NIPPV may provide palliative support	Wheelchair-bound by age 12 y Death by 20 y of age

[a]All patients with neuromuscular diseases (NMD) may benefit from respiratory and supportive care, along with physical and occupational therapy. Disease-specific therapies are listed in the table.

[b]Differential for acute respiratory failure in MG patients includes: (a) myasthenic crisis—antibody-mediated neuromuscular receptor blockade; (b) anticholinesterase therapy toxicity—cholinergic excess; (c) medication-induced toxicity—exacerbation of neuromuscular blockade by aminoglycosides, β-blockers, verapamil, or muscle relaxants.

URI, upper respiratory tract infection; GE, gastroenteritis; MV, mechanical ventilation; IVIg, intravenous immune globulin; Ach, acetylcholine; mb., membrane; NIPPV, noninvasive positive-pressure ventilation.

normal spinal curvature. A combination of weak respiratory muscles, inactivity, obesity, and chest wall deformity results in progressive scoliosis and restrictive lung disease. Many patients, as a result, are wheelchair-dependent in early adolescence. Unfortunately, for each year that a child is wheelchair-dependent, the curvature of the spine increases by 10 degrees. This reduction in VC directly impacts survival. The median survival of patients with DMD who have a VC <1 L is 3 years and a VC <20% predicted implies impending, irreversible respiratory failure.

Treatment

Aggressive respiratory care is required for these patients as the degree of respiratory impairment progresses in an attempt to prevent acute respiratory decompensation. Neuromuscular weakness increases the risk for pneumonia, aspiration, and atelectasis secondary to limited cough strength and muscle strength. Acute infections compound chronic respiratory deficits and may rapidly lead to respiratory failure.

Surgical spinal correction to reduce the degree of scoliosis can make symptomatic improvements in posture and comfort, but it is not clear that these improvements affect pulmonary function. Steroid therapy with prednisone may slow the progression of disease temporarily, but no drug has been found to appreciably affect long-term outcome. Noninvasive mechanical ventilation has sustained adequate gas exchange in patients with neuromuscular disease, but it is not clear that it slows the inevitable progression to respiratory failure or improves survival in these patients.

Myasthenia Gravis

Clinical Presentation

Myasthenia gravis (MG) is a chronic, relapsing and remitting autoimmune disorder that can cause life-threatening periods of weakness. Antibodies bind to and destroy the acetylcholine receptor, thereby impairing neuromuscular transmission. Patients present with generalized weakness, with particularly profound involvement of the proximal limb muscles, the diaphragm, and the neck extensors. Characteristically, muscle weakness is most prominent after bouts of exertion.

MG may be acquired in populations of various ages with differing patterns of muscle weakness and prognosis for response to treatment. Neonatal MG occurs as the result of the transplacental passage of maternal anti–acetylcholine-receptor antibodies from the mother with MG to the fetus. Neonates are severely affected with generalized weakness in the first day of life and improve dramatically with conventional therapy. Complete resolution is expected within the first 6 weeks of life. An infant born to a mother who does not have MG may rarely be affected by one of two types of myasthenic disorders. Congenital MG may present with mild opthalmoplegia and poor feeding within the first few days of life. Although respiratory muscles are rarely

affected, the disease course is unfortunately prolonged and often refractory to therapy. In contrast, infantile MG is associated with periods of marked respiratory depression and apnea and has been incriminated as a rare cause of sudden infant death syndrome. Once identified, symptoms are responsive to conventional therapy, and the disease course subsides after the first 2 years of life.

Most commonly, MG presents in children aged 2 years to adolescence and is known as *juvenile* or *classic* MG. Children present with complaints of diplopia, facial weakness, or clumsiness due to bulbar palsies and extremity weakness. Progressive weakness of the respiratory muscles may result in dyspnea with exercise or at rest. This form is associated with a greater incidence of other autoimmune disorders (10% of patients), such as hyperthyroidism and thyrotoxicosis, and an increased association with collagen vascular disease.

Laboratory Studies

Up to 90% of patients with MG have circulating serum antibodies directed against the nicotinic acetylcholine receptor in the neuromuscular junctions. Ten per cent to 20% of patients have "antibody negative disease" in which the type(s) of circulating anti–acetylcholine-receptor antibodies are not detected by standard laboratory radioimmunoassay. These autoantibodies reduce the number of available acetylcholine receptors at the neuromuscular junction by enhancing endocytosis, destruction, and blockade. The antibody titer does not predict the severity or duration of weakness.

Imaging Studies

Patients with myasthenia gravis may have thymic hyperplasia (85%) or a thymoma (15%), which can be visualized on chest CT scan or MRI. The CXR is a relatively insensitive screening tool to identify a thymoma but may be obtained to identify a potential infectious source as the trigger for an acute exacerbation. Single-fiber EMG classically shows a progressively decremental response of at least 10% in the muscle fiber action potential with repetitive stimulation of the nerve at 3 Hz.

Respiratory Effects

Life-threatening respiratory muscle weakness may result from three potential mechanisms: (a) severe blockade of cholinergic neuromuscular transmission during an acute mysthenic crisis, (b) side effects of medications known to enhance neuromuscular blockade, or (c) cholinergic excess resulting from the medications used to treat MG symptoms.

An acute myasthenic crisis refers to respiratory failure secondary to neuromuscular blockade. The crisis may be triggered secondary to infection, surgery, medication, pregnancy, or idiopathic causes. Patients may initially present with stridor or decreased expiratory efforts. Within days, untreated muscle weakness progresses to respiratory failure requiring mechanical ventilation. The mortality rate of an acute myasthenic crisis is 10%. Not all patients with MG develop limb weakness. Therefore, the presence or severity of peripheral muscle weakness cannot be used to predict the potential for respiratory compromise. Diaphragm weakness may also persist despite the return of normal peripheral strength.

Edrophonium (Tensilon) may be used for diagnostic purposes to identify myasthenic patients with new onset disease. This anticholinesterase has a rapid onset (30 seconds) and short duration (approximately 5 minutes), which relieves the cholinergic blockade to produce a temporary improvement in muscle strength.

A patient with myasthenia may also develop profound weakness with exposure to medications that exacerbate decreased transmission at the neuromuscular junction. The following medications should be avoided in patients with known MG: β-blockers, verapamil, aminoglycosides, and muscle relaxants. The use of epidural and intravenous general anesthetics reduce the intraoperative need for neuromuscular blockade. The depolarizing muscle relaxant, succinylcholine, is not used due to the unpredictability of its effect in patients with myasthenia.

Muscle weakness may also progress due to a cholinergic crisis resulting secondary to the anticholinesterase medications used to treat MG. Cholinergic excess is marked by excessive secretions, lacrimation, bowel and bladder dysfunction, and bronchospasm. The diagnosis is made on improvement of the symptoms after temporary withdrawal of the medication.

Indications for mechanical support in MG include apnea, hypoventilation, severe respiratory muscle fatigue, or inability to clear airway secretions. Respiratory strength measures may be used to indicate changes in muscle strength over time and assess the need for continued ventilatory support.

Treatment

To enhance muscle strength, four methods of treatment may be effective when used alone or in combination: (a) anticholinesterase agents, (b) surgical thymectomy, (c) immunosuppression, and (d) short-term immunotherapies including plasma exchange and intravenous immunoglobulin (IVIg). Acetylcholinesterase inhibitors such as edrophonium, neostigmine, or pyridostigmine inhibit the breakdown of acetylcholine at the neuromuscular junction, thereby enhancing the potential for interaction between acetylcholine and the limited number of junctional acetylcholine receptors. Most patients do not have a sustained response to these agents, and additional treatment is generally required within months of diagnosis.

Surgical thymectomy is recommended for all pediatric patients with generalized MG who are beyond puberty. Thymectomy is recommended because the thymus is believed to be the source of the anti–acetylcholine-receptor antibodies, but the procedure is delayed until puberty to complete the role of the thymus in the normal development

of the immune system. Post-thymectomy, the need for pharmacologic therapy may fluctuate over a period, but many patients require less medication. Thymectomy is associated with improvement in muscle strength in 85% of cases, and 35% of patients appear to have clinical remission within months.

Immunosuppressive therapy is indicated when weakness is not adequately controlled by anticholinesterase drugs. Prednisone, azathioprine, or cyclosporine is initiated in gradually increasing doses to achieve adequate muscle strength. The goal is to provide the least amount of immunosuppressive drug possible and avoid side effects. Prednisone may induce a transient exacerbation of weakness in up to 48% of patients during the first weeks of treatment. Daily high-dose steroid treatment is to be continued for 3 months before the dosage is tapered and modified to an alternate-day regimen to minimize side effects. Azathioprine is used in patients for whom steroids are contraindicated or who have had an insufficient response to steroids, or as an adjunct to permit a reduction in steroid use. Azathioprine may interfere with T-cell production of acetylcholine-receptor antibody. Therapeutic benefit may not be appreciable for as long as 1 year. Cyclosporine blocks T-cell activation and clinical benefit is usually seen within 1 to 2 months. Those patients who benefit from immunosuppressive agents generally require life-long immunosuppressive therapy to maintain functional strength.

Short-term immunotherapies, such as plasmapheresis and IVIg, provide rapid relief of symptoms with maximal improvement within days of treatment. This may provide improved muscle strength in preparation for operative procedures or to decrease the duration of mechanical ventilatory support. The results are sustained for a period of weeks to months, allowing intermittent improvement for patients with otherwise refractory disease. The degree of muscle improvement with plasmapheresis roughly correlates with the reduction in circulating anti–acetylcholine-receptor antibody. The mechanism of action for IVIg is unknown but is speculated to be a blocking antibody approach.

Prognosis

Most patients with MG lead normal lives. However, most of them must take immunosuppressive medication indefinitely despite the risks of adverse effects. Respiratory failure can be prevented with timely intervention, appropriate titration of anticholinesterase and immunosuppressive medications during acute exacerbations, and surgical thymectomy.

Guillain-Barré Syndrome

Clinical Presentation

Guillain-Barré syndrome is an acute inflammatory peripheral neuropathy, which results in demyelination of the affected nerve sheaths (>80% of patients) or complete axonal degeneration (<20% of patients). Patients present with symmetric motor weakness in the lower extremities, predominantly affecting distal greater than proximal muscles, and progressively evolving into an ascending paralysis. Patients complain of paresthesias, numbness, and sensory loss, reflecting the involvement of the peripheral sensory nerve fibers. Affected children may present with nonspecific complaints of lethargy, weakness, or clumsiness with walking. In some patients, bulbar palsies result in cranial nerve weakness affecting the ocular, facial, and pharyngeal muscles. A descending paralysis may follow with the potential for loss of airway protective reflexes. Neurologic symptoms of Guillain-Barré may occur days to weeks after an upper respiratory infection (cytomegalovirus is found in 25% of patients) or bacterial gastroenteritis (*Campylobacter jejuni* is cultured in 66% of patients).

Physical Examination

On neurologic examination, bilateral weakness of the distal muscles in the lower extremities, areflexia, stocking-glove paresthesias, numbness, and loss of vibratory and position sense are prominent in most patients at presentation. Cranial nerve palsies may also present with abnormal phonation and lack of control of the facial and pharyngeal muscles. The respiratory examination may reveal a weak cough or difficulty in swallowing secretions. Autonomic instability in these patients may cause unexpected circulatory compromise with intravenous sedatives or anesthetics.

Laboratory Evaluation

The diagnosis of Guillain-Barré syndrome is made clinically based on history, constellation of clinical findings, and pattern of muscle weakness. Classically, an elevated protein level in the absence of inflammatory cells (albuminocytologic dissociation) is detected in the cerebrospinal fluid in over 90% of patients at some point in the course of the disease. Nerve conduction is delayed, and electromyograms are consistent with lower motor neuron disease.

Respiratory Effects

The progression of weakness proceeds over a variable time frame for each patient. Maximal muscle weakness may be reached in a period of days to weeks after the onset of motor disease, and the duration of muscle weakness may be prolonged. In 20% of patients, severe respiratory failure results in the need for mechanical ventilatory support. Respiratory compromise may be forewarned by the onset of difficulty clearing secretions, weakening of cough and gag reflexes, and alveolar hypoventilation. Bedside pulmonary function testing may include forced or crying VC and maximum negative inspiratory pressure measurements to follow changes over time. Mechanical ventilatory assistance or intubation is considered when: (a) the forced VC is <15 to 20 mL per kg, (b) the maximum negative inspiratory pressure is >-20 to -30 cm H_2O, (c) alveolar hypoventilation generates a $Paco_2$ >50 mm Hg, (d) pulmonary secretions cannot be managed with chest physical therapy, (e) protective airway reflexes are lost, or (f) progressive atelectasis occurs.

Treatment

Plasma exchange and IVIg are of equivalent benefit for children if administered within 2 to 4 weeks of the onset of neuropathic symptoms. Combination therapy does not add further benefit. Corticosteroids are not recommended for the management of Guillain-Barré syndrome.

Prognosis

Most patients are weaned from mechanical ventilation within 2 weeks. Prolonged weaning may be anticipated in those patients with axonal degeneration. Predictors of long-term muscle weakness in children are young age and a rapid progression to maximal weakness. Children who are younger than 9 years and who progress to maximal weakness in <10 days are at particularly increased risk of long-term deficits. In general, children have good functional recovery. In adults, a prolonged plateau time (i.e., time from maximum muscle weakness to the onset of improvement) is predictive of residual motor weakness after recovery.

SPINAL CORD INJURY

Clinical Presentation

The location and severity of spinal cord injury in children is dependent upon age-related anatomic differences and mechanisms of injury. Young children (<2 years of age) are prone to high cervical injuries resulting from birth-related injuries and child abuse secondary to disproportion of the cephalic weight to the poorly developed tone of the cervical musculature. Children younger than 10 years have spinal cord trauma from falls and motor vehicle collisions as well as postinfectious causes. Children at this age are less prone to spine fracture because of the increased elasticity of the spinal ligaments, but may allow for significant disruption of the spinal axis without apparent spinal cord injury without radiographic abnormalities (SCIWORA). Children older than 10 years more typically injure their thoracolumbar spine due to high speed motor vehicle collisions and sports-related trauma.

Respiratory Effects

Respiratory muscle impairment depends on the level of spinal injury. High cervical cord lesions (C1 to C2) are nearly uniformly incompatible with life due to paralysis of the diaphragm, intercostals, scalene, and abdominal muscles. Middle cervical injury (C3 to C5) causes loss of diaphragm, intercostal, and abdominal muscle function. Although the accessory muscles of inspiration remain intact, because of innervation from cranial nerve XI and cervical nerves C2 to C4, most children cannot ventilate effectively. Low cervical cord lesions (C6 to C8) and upper thoracic lesions (T1 to T6) preserve muscle function of the diaphragm and neck. Loss of intercostal and abdominal muscle tone can cause chest wall instability, decreased lung compliance, and diminished FRC. Although unassisted ventilation is expected, expiratory reserve capacity and cough strength can be adversely affected. The inability to generate sufficient intra-abdominal pressure to produce forceful expiration may lead to atelectasis, decreased secretion clearance, and a greater risk for pneumonia.

Imaging

The specific findings associated with spinal cord injury are outlined in Chapter 52. Pulmonary findings with imaging may reveal associated pulmonary contusions, presence of airleak such as pneumothorax that may be associated with rib fractures, or evidence of parenchymal injury from aspiration of gastric contents or blood.

Treatment

Most patients with severe spinal cord injury require mechanical ventilatory assistance partly due to acute muscle paralysis. Intubation is especially challenging and, if performed by inexperienced personnel or with inappropriate technique, further dislocation of the cervical spine may result and extend the spinal cord injury. Because of a variable degree of chest wall trauma, pulmonary parenchymal injury, and denervation of the respiratory muscles, mechanical ventilatory parameters should be individually optimized. Aggressive pulmonary toilet, chest physiotherapy, and postural changes are vital to prevent respiratory compromise.

During the rehabilitation phase, patients with mid or lower cervical injury may learn to augment cough strength through recruitment of the pectoralis major muscle, abdominal binding, and electrical or magnetic stimulation of the abdominal muscles. Bilateral phrenic nerve pacing may be an option for patients who have intact phrenic motor nerves. In adults, variable success from 34% to 80% in avoiding mechanical ventilation with phrenic nerve pacing has been reported. Phrenic nerve pacing is increased slowly over 3 to 4 months to allow for the previously paralyzed muscles to become conditioned and to avoid damage to the diaphragm.

INTENSIVE CARE UNIT MYOPATHY

Acquired muscle weakness (myopathy) and neuromuscular impairment (polyneuropathy with motor and sensory weakness) are increasingly recognized as clinically significant sequelae of critical illness. An acquired myopathy should be considered in the critically ill child (usually with a history of multiorgan system injury) with proximal or generalized weakness and who is difficult to wean from mechanical ventilation.

The mechanism of intensive care unit (ICU) myopathy is not known. Even brief exposure to steroids, particularly the fluorinated compounds (e.g., prednisone, methylprednisolone, and dexamethasone), have been associated with myopathic sequelae. Myopathy may occur in the critically ill patient due to prolonged effects of neuromuscular blockade, immobilization, poor nutrition, and altered metabolism of pharmacologic agents known to potentiate the effects of neuromuscular blockade, such as aminoglycosides, polymyxins, macrolides, calcium channel blockers, β-blockers, procainamide, D-penicillamine, and lithium. CPK levels may be elevated in as many as 50% of patients. Nerve conduction is intact. However, electromyogram studies show decreased spontaneous muscular activity and early recruitment of short-duration motor unit potentials. Most cases of ICU myopathy are reversible; however, full resolution may take weeks to months and require aggressive physical rehabilitation.

Critical illness polyneuropathy also causes generalized weakness, respiratory muscle weakness, and areflexia, but does not affect sensory function. Patients typically have normal muscle strength of the facial and extraocular muscles. Despite degeneration of motor and sensory axons on biopsy, functional recovery is expected.

Treatment

Prevention is the ideal treatment of ICU myopathy. Limiting the use of corticosteroids and muscle relaxants to the lowest effective dose may be helpful. Monitoring for rising CPK levels may provide early detection. In adults, 62% of patients who were difficult to wean from mechanical ventilation had neuromuscular disease severe enough to account for ventilator dependency. The incidence of acquired neuromuscular disease in pediatric patients requiring a prolonged weaning from mechanical ventilation, often with multiple failed extubation attempts, is unknown.

NONINVASIVE VENTILATION

Patients with impaired chest wall mechanics or respiratory muscle weakness may derive benefit from noninvasive ventilation at some point during the course of illness. Noninvasive bilevel positive airway pressure (BiPAP) ventilation has been employed in an attempt to achieve the following goals: (a) avoid endotracheal intubation, (b) relieve dyspnea by unloading respiratory muscles, (c) optimize patient comfort, (d) improve alveolar gas exchange, (e) reduce the length of stay in the ICU, and (f) reduce mortality in progressive neuromuscular disorders.

In patients with chronic hypoventilation, assisted ventilation lowers $PaCO_2$, thereby resetting the sensitivity of the respiratory control center to carbon dioxide. For patients with primary muscle abnormalities, noninvasive ventilation allows chronically fatigued muscles to rest and results in a reduction in the excessive inspiratory contractile efforts.

The ability of noninvasive ventilation to reduce mortality remains unproven. Some authors caution that "prophylactic" ventilatory support for patients may be associated with worse survival outcomes due to a false sense of security offered by this support and a delayed appreciation for respiratory compromise. Not all patients with neuromuscular disease benefit from noninvasive ventilatory assistance. Therapeutic benefit is limited in patients affected with rapidly progressing disease, copious secretions, impaired upper airway reflexes, and in those patients with impending respiratory failure.

SUMMARY

Age-related anatomic differences in the compliance of the lung and chest wall dictate the relative ability to recruit accessory muscles of respiration to compensate for disruption of normal respiratory mechanics. Children younger than 2 years are particularly susceptible to develop respiratory failure in the face of chest wall or respiratory muscle dysfunction. Older children and adolescents may be able to temporarily sustain adequate alveolar ventilation through accessory muscle recruitment. For many neuromuscular disease processes, there is no cure. The goal is to provide aggressive respiratory supportive care to reduce the potential for significant morbidity due to progressive atelectasis, pneumonia, aspiration, and muscle fatigue.

RECOMMENDED READINGS

1. Aldrich TK, Prezant DJ. Adverse effects of drugs on the respiratory muscles. *Clin Chest Med.* 1990;11:177.
2. Black LF, Hyatt RE. Maximal respiratory pressures: Normal values and relationship to age and sex. *Am Rev Respir Dis.* 1969;99:696.
3. Buckingham JM, Howard FM, Bernatz PE, et al. The value of thymectomy in myasthenia gravis: A computer-assisted matched study. *Ann Surg.* 1976;184:453–458.
4. Cahill JL, Lees GM, Robertson HT. A summary of preoperative and postoperative cardiorespiratory performance in patients undergoing pectus excavatum and carinatum repair. *J Pediatr Surg.* 1984;19:430–433.
5. D'Empaire G, Hoaglin DC, Perlo VP, et al. Effect of prethymectomy plasma exchange on postoperative respiratory function in myasthenia gravis. *J Thorac Cardiovasc Surg.* 1985;89:592.
6. de Leeuw M, Williams JM, Freedom RM, et al. Impact of diaphragmatic paralysis after cardiothoracic surgery in children. *J Thorac Cardiovasc Surg.* 1999;118:510–517.
7. Dushay KM, Zibrak JD, Jensen WA. Myasthenia gravis presenting as isolated respiratory failure. *Chest.* 1990;97:232.
8. Eberle E, Brink J, Azen S, et al. Early predictors of incomplete recovery in children with Guillain-Barré polyneuritis. *J Pediatr.* 1975;86:356.
9. Giostra E, Magistris MR, Pizzolato G, et al. Neuromuscular disorder in intensive care unit patients treated with pancuronium bromide. *Chest.* 1994;106:210.
10. Gould L, Kaplan S, McElhinney AJ, et al. A method for the production of hemidiaphragmatic paralysis. Its application to the study of lung function in normal man. *Am Rev Respir Dis.* 1967;96:812.
11. Hadeed HA, Braun TW. Paralysis of the hemidiaphragm as a complication of internal jugular vein cannulation: Report of a case. *J Oral Maxillofac Surg.* 1988;46:40.
12. Hart N, Nickol AH, Cramer D, et al. Effect of severe isolated unilateral and bilateral diaphragm weakness on exercise performance. *Am J Respir Crit Care Med.* 2002;165:1265–1270.
13. Hebra A, Swoveland B, Egbert M, et al. Outcome analysis of minimally invasive repair of pectus excavatum: Review of 251 cases. *J Pediatr Surg.* 2000;35:252–257.
14. Loeffel NB, Rossi LN, Mumenthaler M, et al. The Landry-Guillain-Barré Syndrome. Complications, prognosis and natural history in 123 cases. *J Neurol Sci.* 1977;33:71.
15. Lonstein JE, Carlson JM. The prediction of curve progression in untreated idiopathic scoliosis during growth. *J Bone Joint Surg Am.* 1984;66:1061–1071.
16. McCarthy RE. Disorders of the pediatric and adolescent spine: Management of neuromuscular scoliosis. *Orthop Clin North Am.* 1999;30(3):435.
17. Menkes JH. Diseases of the motor unit. In: *Textbook of child neurology.* Philadelphia, PA: Lea & Febiger; 1975:463.
18. Millichap JG, Dodge PR. Diagnosis and treatment of myasthenia gravis in infancy, childhood and adolescence. *Neurology.* 1960;11:1007–1014.
19. Moore P, James O. Guillain-Barré syndrome: Incidence, management, and outcome of major complications. *Crit Care Med.* 1981;9:549.
20. Nuss D, Kelly RE, Croitoru DP. A 10-year review of a minimally invasive technique for the correction of pectus excavatum. *J Pediatr Surg.* 1998;33:545–552.
21. Papastamelos C, Panitch H, England S, et al. Developmental changes in chest wall compliance in early childhood. *J Appl Physiol.* 1995;78:179–184.
22. Proctor MR. Spinal cord injury. *Crit Care Med.* 2002;30:S489–S499, Supplement.
23. Quigley PM, Haller JA, Jelus KL. Cardiorespiratory function before and after corrective surgery in pectus excavatum. *J Pediatr.* 1996;128:638–643.
24. Roland EH. Muscular dystrophy. *Pediatr Rev.* 2000;21(7):233.
25. Shamberger RC. Congenital chest wall deformities. *Curr Probl Surg.* 1996;33:469–542.
26. Baydur A, Swank SM, Stiles CM, et al. Respiratory mechanics in anesthetized young patients with kyphoscoliosis: Immediate and delayed effects of corrective spinal surgery. *Chest.* 1990;97:1157–1164.

Gases and Drugs Used in Support of the Respiratory System

42

Angela T. Wratney   Ira M. Cheifetz

The main functions of the respiratory system are to provide oxygen and remove carbon dioxide. In the setting of acute respiratory failure, the lungs are unable to adequately perform these essential functions. Impairment in tissue oxygen delivery or inadequate ventilation may cause metabolic or respiratory acidosis, potentially resulting in end-organ injury.

The basis of critical care medicine is to support the function of the cardiorespiratory system to provide optimal systemic oxygen delivery. Intensivists must recognize the therapeutic indications for various types of gases and other medications to restore adequate systemic oxygen delivery and carbon dioxide elimination. This chapter discusses the clinical and therapeutic indications for common respiratory gases (a) normobaric oxygen, (b) hyperbaric oxygen (HBO), (c) hypoxic gas mixtures, (d) exogenous carbon dioxide administration, (e) heliox, (f) inhaled nitric oxide (iNO), and (g) surfactant.

OXYGEN, MONITORING, HYPOXIC GAS OR CARBON DIOXIDE, AND HELIOX

Angela T. Wratney and Ira M. Cheifetz

NORMOBARIC OXYGEN

Oxygen Delivery Systems

Oxygen administration should be initiated immediately for patients with documented hypoxemia or with clinical signs and symptoms of hypoxia. A variety of devices exist for administering supplemental oxygen depending upon the fraction of inspired oxygen concentration (FIO_2) desired (see Table 42.1). Flow characteristics determine whether the oxygen delivery system will be sufficient to meet the inspiratory flow needs of the patient (high-flow systems) or if the flow provided will be insufficient (low-flow systems), causing the patient to entrain a variable quantity of room air. High-flow devices, therefore, have a more stable, measurable delivery of the FIO_2 independent of patient respiratory effort. High-flow delivery devices can be used with masks, tracheostomy collars, nebulizers, and oxygen tents or hoods. Examples of low-flow systems include nasal cannula, simple facemasks, or facemasks with a reservoir (nonrebreather or partial rebreather).

TABLE 42.1

FRACTION OF INSPIRED OXYGEN BY VARIOUS DELIVERY SYSTEMS

	FIO_2 Delivery (%)	Flow Required (L)
Blow-by oxygen	<30	15
Face tent	<40	10–15
Nasal cannula	24–50	<6
Face mask	<60	6–10
Venti mask	<60	Variable
Partial rebreather	<60	15
Partial rebreather with horns or/non-rebreather	~100	15

FIO_2, fraction of inspired oxygen concentration.

Nasal Cannula

Nasal cannulae provide a low flow of oxygen (generally 0.1 to 6 Lpm). FIO_2 delivery ranges between 24% and 50% depending on the patient's inspiratory flow rate, inspiratory volume, entrainment of atmospheric gas, and mixture with exhaled gas in the anatomic dead space. The potential advantage of a nasal cannula is that it is less restrictive than a mask and may be better tolerated by young children.

Face Masks

Simple face masks deliver ranges between 35% and 55% oxygen. The mask fits over the patient's nose and mouth providing a low flow rate between 6 and 10 L per minute. Nonrebreathing face masks incorporate a simple face mask adapted with a reservoir bag and an inflow system for fresh gas infusion to deliver as much as 100% oxygen. Two one-way valves, located between the mask and the reservoir and at the exhalation port, ensure that each inspiratory breath consists of fresh gas and that exhaled gas is eliminated without entrainment of room air. As a safety mechanism, one additional port is kept open to allow the entrainment of room air in the event that the gas flow to the system is interrupted. Partial rebreathing masks are similar to nonrebreathing masks, consisting of a reservoir bag, a mask, and an inflow gas source. However, the system lacks the unidirectional valve between the face mask and the reservoir. Therefore, it does not prevent exhaled carbon dioxide from entering and mixing with the oxygen in the reservoir bag.

Venturi masks are high-flow systems that provide fixed concentrations of 24%, 28%, 31%, 35%, 40%, or 50% oxygen. These concentrations are determined by the manufacturer with the recommended flow rates necessary to generate a specific oxygen-to-air entrainment ratio. The flow velocity of oxygen entering the mask causes the entrainment of air through side ports in the device. Dependable oxygen concentrations are administered as long as the total gas flow exceeds the patient's peak inspiratory flow.

Oxygen Hood and Tent

Oxygen hoods may be used for infants to provide an oxygen-rich environment with easy patient access. Oxygen hoods rest over an infant's head and are small enough to recover the FIO_2 quickly when the seal is disturbed. The gas source is supplied by a high-flow nebulizer device. Within the hood, the oxygen concentration can layer, causing a top-to-bottom gradient of up to 20%. To optimize patient care and avoid heat loss, careful monitoring of the FIO_2 and appropriate heating of the gas source should occur. Oxygen tents allow the patient to move freely within a larger oxygen-rich environment; yet these are unpractical because access to the patient requires frequent disruption of this environment.

Physiologic Shunts

Right-to-left shunts occur when blood passes from systemic veins to systemic arteries without first exchanging gas with the alveoli. This can occur physiologically when blood flow bypasses poorly ventilated alveoli. If supplemental oxygen alone does not improve hypoxia, the patient may benefit from invasive or noninvasive positive pressure ventilation to improve lung volume and V/Q matching. Anatomic shunts may occur secondary to right-to-left intracardiac lesions (i.e., cyanotic congenital heart disease) and are generally unresponsive to supplemental oxygen.

Risks of Oxygen Therapy

Oxygen is highly combustible. The unusual, but finite, risk of fire associated with oxygen in patients requiring high-risk electrical devices (e.g., electrocautery units) can be devastating. Oxygen enrichment refers to any area where the oxygen concentration exceeds 21%. Using oxygen in an underventilated area such as under occlusive drapes (i.e., during sterile procedures) significantly increases the risk of fire.

MONITORING

Pulse Oximetry

The pulse oximeter detects the percent of saturated hemoglobin in the capillary-tissue bed being monitored. The probe contains opposing units: a photodetector with two light-emitting diodes (660 and 940 nm) on one side and a microprocessor on the opposing side. The microprocessor determines the relative absorption of these two light forms by the hemoglobin forms present within the tissue bed. On the basis of the ratio of the absorbance at the two wavelengths, the percentage of saturated hemoglobin is determined. Pulse oximeter algorithms are determined from simultaneous co-oximetry data on healthy volunteers. Standard pulse oximeters report with reliable accuracy ($\pm 2\%$ to 4%) under ideal conditions in the saturation range of 70% to 100%.

Clinical conditions which might alter the reliability of the pulse oximetry reading include poor perfusion, inaccurate pulse determination (i.e., motion artifact), oxygen saturations <70%, and the presence of abnormal hemoglobin. Pulse oximetry will be inaccurate, requiring co-oximetric analysis to determine the true hemoglobin saturation, for patients with severe cyanosis (i.e., saturation <70%) and for those patients with carboxyhemoglobin (COHb) or methemoglobin. The pulse oximeter will display an erroneously high saturation in these cases owing to the pattern of light absorbance of the hemoglobin. Methemoglobin absorbs light almost equally at both wavelengths, and the pulse oximetry technology interprets this absorbance ratio as a saturation of 85%. The greater the percentage of methemoglobin in the bloodstream, the greater the likelihood for the pulse oximeter to read 85%. Therefore, the pulse oximeter does not accurately reflect the true

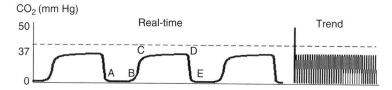

Figure 42.1 Normal capnogram waveform. The capnogram waveform provides information about ventilation in the conducting airways and in the alveolar units. *A–B,* inspiratory baseline; *B–C,* expiratory upstroke; *C–D,* expiratory plateau; *D,* end-tidal carbon dioxide value; *D–E,* inspiration begins.

oxygen saturation nor does it indicate the concentration of methemoglobin.

Pulse oximeters are insensitive to changes in arterial oxygen tension along the flat portion of the oxyhemoglobin curve. Any Pa_{O_2} greater than approximately 80 mm Hg is reflected as a hemoglobin saturation of >98%. Therefore, a large decrease in arterial oxygen tension may occur without a change in the pulse oximeter reading. The presence of biochemical factors (e.g., pH, 2,3-diphosphoglycerate [2,3-DPG] concentration, and temperature) may shift the oxyhemoglobin curve. Under standard conditions, an oxygen saturation of 90% typically reflects a Pa_{O_2} of 60 mm Hg; in the presence of alkalosis, a saturation of 95% may be associated with a $Pa_{O_2} \leq 60$ mm Hg.

Pulse oximetry is designed to detect hypoxemia; however, it is being increasingly used in the intensive care setting to detect periods of hyperoxemia. In the neonatal nursery, the Pa_{O_2} is maintained <80 mm Hg to reduce the risk of retinopathy of prematurity. Similarly, in the care of neonates with ductal-dependent systemic blood flow (e.g., hypoplastic left heart syndrome), oxygen saturations approximately above 85% may indicate excessive pulmonary blood flow. Studies evaluating the performance of pulse oximeters demonstrated a tendency to overestimate actual arterial saturation; therefore, pulse oximetry should not be the sole means of monitoring for clinically significant hyperoxemia.

Capnography

Capnography is the continuous, real-time, graphic display of carbon dioxide concentration in exhaled gas. End-tidal carbon dioxide monitoring can be used to measure the quantity of carbon dioxide present in the exhaled air (partial pressure of end tidal carbon dioxide [P_{ETCO_2}]) by placement of a probe in the nostril of a spontaneously breathing patient or by detection at the proximal end of the endotracheal tube. P_{ETCO_2} is the standard of care for intubated patients in the operating room and is increasingly used in monitoring a patient's respiratory status outside of the operating room. Bedside assessment allows evaluation of both the waveform (capnogram) and the end-tidal carbon dioxide value. The capnogram provides information about ventilation in the conducting airways and the alveolar units. An increasing slope serves as an indicator of increased resistance to exhaled gas flow and increased dead space ventilation (see Fig. 42.1).

End-tidal carbon dioxide is approximately equal to alveolar P_{CO_2} when dead space ventilation is small. As a result, P_{ETCO_2} may substitute for repeated arterial blood gas (ABG) analysis during stable periods of respiratory disease depending on the degree of dead space ventilation. In the presence of significant interstitial lung disease or progressive respiratory compromise, the P_{ETCO_2} may poorly correlate with the Pa_{CO_2} measured by ABG analysis because of increased dead space ventilation. Interpretation of the arterial-P_{ETCO_2} gradient is particularly useful to indicate alveolar–arterial ventilation. Decreased P_{ETCO_2} as compared with Pa_{CO_2} may indicate: endotracheal tube obstruction, inadvertent extubation, excessive endotracheal tube air leak, decreased cardiac output or pulmonary blood flow, increased dead space ventilation, or worsening pulmonary compliance with decreased ventilation.

HYPERBARIC OXYGEN THERAPY

Clinical Indications

HBO is approved for use in the following clinical conditions: decompression sickness, arterial air emboli, carbon monoxide poisoning, and myonecrosis, and gas gangrene of soft tissues (e.g., necrotizing fasciitis).

Principles of Hyperbaric Oxygen

At sea level (i.e., 1 atm) the plasma oxygen concentration is 0.003 mL per dL blood or 3 mL per L. At 3 atm, 100% F_{IO_2} dramatically increases the amount of dissolved oxygen in the blood to 60 mL per L of plasma, which is almost sufficient to supply the oxygen expenditure of resting tissues without the contribution of oxygen bound to hemoglobin. The Pa_{O_2} under these conditions is approximately 2,280 mm Hg ($Pa_{O_2} = 1.0 \times [3.0$ atm $\times 760$ mm Hg]). Therefore, HBO has advantages in the treatment of conditions in which hemoglobin–oxygen binding and oxygen delivery are impaired, including hemoglobinopathies, severe anemia, and carbon monoxide poisoning.

HBO also increases the capillary-tissue oxygen gradient. This may underlie the beneficial properties seen with HBO in promoting angiogenesis and wound healing, bacteriocidal activity against anaerobic organisms, protection against clostridial α toxin, and the ability to restore neutrophil-mediated bacterial killing in previously hypoxic tissues.

HBO also has therapeutic properties in the treatment of decompression illness and arterial gas embolism. On the basis of Boyle Law, the pressure of a gas is inversely proportional to its volume. Therefore, "bubble volume" reduces significantly within the highly pressurized HBO chamber. Reduced bubble size relieves small vessel obstruction and may restore blood flow to compromised, distal tissue beds.

Carbon Monoxide Poisoning

The most common indication for HBO in pediatrics is carbon monoxide poisoning. Carbon monoxide is a colorless and odorless gas produced from incomplete combustion of carbon containing products. Common exposures include structure fires, underventilated heating units, gasoline-powered equipment in enclosed spaces, automobile exhaust, and kerosene heaters and stoves.

Carbon monoxide is toxic because it disrupts hemoglobin-oxygen–carrying capacity and cellular metabolism. Hemoglobin has 240 times the affinity for carbon monoxide than oxygen. Once bound, COHb shifts the oxyhemoglobin curve to the left resulting in decreased oxygen-carrying capacity. Carbon monoxide also affects cellular metabolism by binding to proteins, cytochromes, guanylate cyclase, and nitric oxide synthase.

Acute symptoms of carbon monoxide toxicity include headache, nausea, and ataxia. The clinical spectrum can progress rapidly to pulmonary edema, myocardial ischemia, neurologic impairment, seizures, loss of consciousness, and cardiac arrest. Often, delayed but permanent neuropsychologic impairments may result.

Blood gas analysis is commonly falsely reassuring. The PaO_2 on an ABG is often normal or elevated despite significant hypoxemia. PaO_2 reflects dissolved oxygen and does not reflect the significant derangement of carbon monoxide–bound hemoglobin. Evaluation of the blood gas by co-oximetry is required to detect the elevated COHb concentration and to determine the severity of the abnormal hemoglobin–oxygen saturation. Of note, the COHb level does not reflect the severity of illness nor does it reflect the duration of carbon monoxide exposure. This may result secondary to the often considerable time which lapses between exposure, onset of symptoms, and the laboratory evaluation. Therefore, patients should be treated according to the severity of symptoms, especially neurologic symptoms, rather than solely on the basis of COHb levels.

Indications for Hyperbaric Oxygen Therapy

The Undersea and Hyperbaric Medical Society has recommended HBO therapy for patients with a COHb level $\geq 40\%$ or for specific clinical situations irrespective of the COHb level—a history or sign of either neurologic or cardiac dysfunction (including seizure, syncope, or chest pain suggestive of cardiac ischemia), severe acidosis, and pregnancy.

The half-life of COHb is approximately 5 hours and 20 minutes in room air. This is reduced to 90 minutes with FIO_2 1.0 at 1 atm. At 3 atm, the half-life is reduced even further to 23 minutes. The general belief is that early treatment provides the greatest potential benefit. Therefore, exposed patients should immediately receive 100% oxygen. Prompt referral to an HBO center is recommended for those patients meeting specific criteria. An HBO center may not be readily available, and therefore the decision to transport a critically ill patient to an HBO center versus continuing resuscitation therapy with 100% oxygen can be difficult. Careful consideration must be given to the risk-benefit ratio of the transport.

Risks of Hyperbaric Oxygen Therapy

Side effects of HBO are often mild and reversible but rarely can be severe and life threatening. The toxicity is significantly reduced if pressures do not exceed 300 kPa and the length of each treatment is <120 minutes. Potential risks include fire hazard, seizures, reversible myopia due to oxygen toxicity of the lens, pulmonary oxygen toxicity with decreased lung compliance, trauma to tympanic membranes, sinuses, and lungs, and gas embolization. Airway obstruction may result if trapped air expands, causing alveolar overdistension or rupture. Pulmonary toxicity can be avoided by decreasing the dose and duration of oxygen exposure to avoid damage to the alveolar-capillary membrane. HBO treatment can cause systemic vascular resistance to increase to 30% to 60% resulting in a concurrent decrease in cardiac output. Central nervous system (CNS) toxicity includes seizures, dizziness, muscle twitching, decreased visual fields, or irritability and develops in 1 per 10,000 patients. CNS toxicity reverses on discontinuation of HBO.

Before the HBO therapy, children should be given antipyretics to treat fevers and tympanostomy placement to avoid the risks for seizure and the rupture of tympanic membranes, respectively. Increased metabolic rate during HBO therapy may lead to increased risk of hypoglycemia for patients with diabetes and for patients with Graves disease in whom the increased metabolic rate may increase the risk of oxygen toxicity.

HYPOXIC GAS OR CARBON DIOXIDE ADMINISTRATION

Clinical Indications

Intensive care units which manage patients with single ventricle congenital heart disease may at times use supplemental nitrogen gas (forming a hypoxic gas mixture) or administer exogenous carbon dioxide to increase pulmonary vascular resistance (PVR) in an effort to control the ratio of pulmonary (Q_p) to systemic (Q_s) blood flow. These topics are discussed in detail in the cardiac section (see Chapter 31).

Caution must be taken when delivering hypoxic gas mixtures to patients on mechanical ventilation support. Hypoxic gas mixtures are obtained by nitrogen dilution—the addition of low-flow nitrogen into the ventilator circuit. Administration of nitrogen and compressed air through a mechanical ventilator overrides important safety features. The FiO2 control knob is no longer a control of administered oxygen but rather a control of either air or nitrogen. Therefore, if this knob is inadvertently turned, in either direction, the delivered concentration of hypoxic gas may be significantly altered. Furthermore, commercially available oxygen analyzers do not accurately monitor these lower oxygen concentrations. It is impossible to deliver a hypoxic gas mixture by a ventilator and not override a safety mechanism. Therefore, the technical delivery of a hypoxic gas mixture requires expertise and vigilance to these considerations. For patient safety, clinical examination must be augmented by continuous monitoring of the delivered FiO2 and the measured oxygen saturation, in addition to frequent ABG sampling.

Mechanical considerations with the administration of carbon dioxide are also important. During carbon dioxide administration, minute ventilation must be maintained constant because there is no effect if the patient's respiratory rate increases (i.e., minute ventilation increases) in an attempt to eliminate the exogenous carbon dioxide. Decreases in the ventilator set tidal volume and respiratory rate to achieve hypoventilation may have similar results as exogenous carbon dioxide administration, but if ventilator settings are decreased significantly, arterial desaturation may result secondary to the loss of lung volume. The therapeutic range of exogenous carbon dioxide is 1% to 4% (8 to 30 mm Hg). The quantity of carbon dioxide in room air is 0.03% (0.22 mm Hg). Published nomograms aid in selecting the blender settings required to deliver precise concentrations of oxygen and carbon dioxide through a double-blender system.

HELIOX

Clinical Indications

Helium–oxygen mixtures (heliox) constitute a medical gas therapy with a unique therapeutic application to respiratory processes with high airway resistance or obstructive pathology. Helium is biologically inert; yet because of the extremely low density of the gas, it acquires physiologically advantageous features. Heliox may be used as an adjuvant to improve airflow in patients with excessive work of breathing, to augment the delivery of bronchodilators to obstructed lower airways, and to allow time for the onset of other medical therapies to take effect (i.e., corticosteroids) and/or a disease to follow its path of natural resolution.

Properties of Helium

Helium has the lowest density of any medical gas therapy. Helium (0.179 μP) is approximately one-seventh the density of air (1.293 μP) and oxygen (1.429 μP). By its lower density, helium improves gas flow through airways with high resistance in two ways: (i) improved airflow characteristics in the turbulent areas of narrowed airways and (ii) conversion of turbulent gas flow to a more laminar flow. Laminar flow facilitates gas delivery to the alveoli for efficient gas exchange in the clinical setting.

In narrowed airways with turbulent gas flow, the low density of helium allows greater gas flow at lower driving pressures. This is mathematically defined by the Bernoulli principle

$$Q = \left(\frac{2\Delta P}{\rho} \right)^{1/2}$$

where Q = turbulent gas flow rate, ΔP is the airway driving pressure, and ρ is the gas density. As gas flow becomes less turbulent in the affected airways, flow velocity is reduced, and the flow pattern changes from turbulent to more laminar. This, in turn, is represented by the Reynolds number (Re); a lower Reynolds number indicates gas flow with greater laminar flow characteristics.

$$Re = \frac{2Vr\rho}{\eta}$$

where V is the gas velocity, r is the airway radius, ρ is the gas density, and η is the gas viscosity. A Reynolds number <2,000 predicts laminar flow and >4,000 predicts turbulent flow.

Clinical Applications

In clinical application, the physical properties of heliox may result in a lower resistance to gas flow, increased alveolar oxygen tension, and decreased work of breathing. Heliox has been clinically applied as an adjuvant therapy for patients with obstructive airway disease to reduce turbulent airflow, improve respiratory distress, augment deposition of inhaled bronchodilators, and possibly avert the need for intubation. Heliox has been studied in upper and lower airway obstruction secondary to infection (i.e., croup or epiglottitis), traumatic injury (i.e., direct airway injury or postextubation laryngeal edema), bronchiolitis, and asthma. Many clinical studies, although often limited to small patient numbers, strongly suggest that heliox may have potential therapeutic benefits for select patients. The early application of heliox therapy may provide benefit especially when conventional therapies are implemented but before these therapies achieve full effect (i.e., corticosteroids).

Heliox may also be used as a therapeutic bridge to possibly avert the need for intubation. It seems reasonable to consider heliox as a relatively safe "therapeutic bridge" to allow time for the planning of more definitive respiratory support, the onset of therapeutic medications, or the natural resolution of a disease process. The beneficial effects of heliox occur within minutes of application, and no adverse effects of heliox have been reported. Therefore, a trial for potential therapeutic benefit in the appropriate patient seems advisable. The National Asthma Education and Prevention Program supported the potential benefits of heliox in the treatment of asthma exacerbations, especially as an alternative to intubation.

Under standard conditions, <10% of the nebulized drug reaches the lungs because most of it is deposited in the posterior oropharynx. The associated improved gas flow characteristics of heliox, theoretically, should facilitate delivery of β-agonists further down the tracheobronchiolar tree. Clinical and laboratory studies conducted have conflicting results but suggest that heliox administration may deliver a larger deposition of bronchodilator in the distal airways and improve gas movement as measured by spirometry.

The density of heliox is dependent upon the relative percentage of helium compared to oxygen. However, even those patients with high oxygen requirements (FIO_2 0.80 or greater) may have improved gas exchange with heliox.

Technical Considerations

Helium must always be administered with oxygen. Heliox tanks are commercially available in concentrations of 80:20 (helium:oxygen) and 70:30. Although tanks of 100% helium are available, an interruption in oxygen delivery could possibly result in the accidental administration of a hypoxic gas mixture, including the possibility of delivering 100% helium. Continuous in-line monitoring of inspired oxygen concentration to ensure adequate oxygen delivery to the airways is warranted. Premixed heliox tanks with at least a 20% oxygen concentration avoids this potentially fatal complication.

Heliox can be administered through a face mask or a mechanical ventilator. Nasal cannula administration of heliox is generally ineffective because the flow rate of helium is inadequate. Additionally, administering heliox through a tent is impractical because the helium and oxygen layer with the helium rising to the top. Heliox must be delivered through a closed system because entrainment of room air will contaminate the heliox mixture with air or oxygen, thereby negating the lower density benefit of delivered helium in the delivered gas. Flowmeters and monitoring devices that measure tidal volume on the basis of the nitrogen/oxygen flow and oxygen-calibrated systems must be recalibrated for heliox use. If not calibrated for heliox, the lower density of helium causes the administered flow to be greater than the indicated flow.

Mechanical Ventilation

Heliox delivery through mechanical ventilators may be problematic. Ventilators are designed and calibrated for a mixture of oxygen and air; therefore, adding a gas of a different density, viscosity, or thermal conductivity can affect both the delivered and measured tidal volume.

INHALED NITRIC OXIDE

Emily L. Dobyns and Eva Nozik Grayck

iNO has been used in a variety of diseases to improve oxygenation and lower PVR. The ability to deliver nitric oxide to the lungs as a gas makes nitric oxide a unique and a selective pulmonary vasodilator. When inhaled, nitric oxide distributes itself to the ventilated areas of the lung. Nitric oxide diffuses across the alveolar-capillary membrane to the smooth muscle cells of the adjacent pulmonary vessels. Nitric oxide selectively binds to soluble guanylate cyclase in the vascular smooth muscle cell to activate cyclic guanosine 3′,5′-monophosphate (cGMP), and produce pulmonary vasodilatation (see preceding text). Nitric oxide that diffuses into the bloodstream is rapidly bound to hemoglobin and inactivated, thereby, limiting its effects mainly to the lung. This is in contrast to intravenous vasodilators, which, when administered systemically, can result in systemic hypotension because these agents nonselectively dilate both the pulmonary and systemic vasculatures. In addition, systemic administration of vasodilators dilates both ventilated and unventilated lung units, increasing pulmonary shunt and worsening oxygenation.

CLINICAL APPLICATIONS

The clinical applications of iNO include persistent pulmonary hypertension of the newborn (PPHN), acute respiratory distress syndrome (ARDS), primary and secondary pulmonary hypertension, postoperative cardiac surgery, and post–lung transplantation.

PPHN of the newborn may result from a variety of insults, but common to each is the presence of extrapulmonary right-to-left shunting of blood across a patent ductus arteriosus or foramen ovale due to high PVR. Early studies of brief treatment with nitric oxide demonstrated improved oxygenation in neonates with PPHN. Oxygenation rapidly decreased after discontinuing iNO, and additional therapies were required.

Subsequent pilot studies of continuous inhalation of nitric oxide in neonates with echocardiographic evidence of high PVR with right-to-left shunting showed a sustained improvement in oxygenation without the need for additional therapies. On the basis of these early results, several multicenter randomized trials were conducted to determine the efficacy of iNO in term neonates with PPHN.

The Neonatal Inhaled Nitric Oxide Study (NINOS) was the largest of these trials, in which 235 term neonates were randomized to treatment with iNO or placebo gas. The hypothesis of this trial was that treatment with iNO would decrease mortality and the need for extracorporeal membrane oxygenation (ECMO). Treatment with iNO acutely improved oxygenation and significantly reduced the need for ECMO compared to control infants. However, there was no difference in mortality between treatment groups. Importantly, toxicities associated with nitric oxide, which included methemoglobinemia, high exhaled nitrogen dioxide concentrations, or intracranial hemorrhage, were rare and study gas was not stopped in any patient because of toxicity. On the basis of the results of these trials, the U.S. Food and Drug Administration approved the use of iNO in the treatment of term and near term neonates with clinical or echocardiographic evidence of PPHN.

The role of iNO in the treatment of ARDS is less clearly defined. Unlike PPHN, the predominant mechanism for hypoxemia in ARDS is intrapulmonary shunting due to lung parenchymal disease (edema, inflammation, and others). Rossaint et al. demonstrated that inhalation of nitric oxide acutely improved oxygenation and reduced PVR in adults with severe ARDS. Prolonged treatment with iNO in adult patients with ARDS demonstrated acute, transient improvement in oxygenation, but no difference in mortality, or days alive off ventilator support. *Post hoc* subgroup analysis of the Dellinger study of adults with ARDS demonstrated a higher percentage of patients alive and off mechanical ventilation at 28 days in those treated with 5 ppm iNO compared to placebo. Similar acute but transient improvements in oxygenation have been shown in pediatric patients with acute hypoxemic respiratory failure who were treated with iNO. Mortality in ARDS is most often related to multiorgan failure, so whether these acute and transient improvements in oxygenation will be important in the long-term management of patients with ARDS requires additional studies.

A significant cause of morbidity and mortality following surgical repair of congenital cardiac disease and cardiac transplant is the acute development of pulmonary hypertension which can result in right-sided heart failure and death. In several small studies, postoperative inhalation of nitric oxide selectively reduces PVR and improves right ventricular function and stroke volume. Additionally, a randomized trial of iNO immediately after congenital heart surgery demonstrated a reduction in pulmonary hypertensive crises and earlier extubation in the iNO-treated group compared to placebo.

iNO has also been investigated in post–lung transplant patients to decrease PVR postoperatively and reduce graft failure. In laboratory studies using animal models of ischemia and reperfusion, iNO reduced leukocyte adhesion and distal microvascular constriction. Ischemia-reperfusion injury is a major cause of graft failure in lung transplantation. On the basis of this rationale, adults undergoing lung transplant were randomized to iNO initiated 10 minutes after reperfusion of the lung or placebo. Treatment with iNO had no effect on the outcome of patients following lung transplantation.

In addition to its therapeutic uses, iNO is also used as a diagnostic tool in pediatric and adult patients with pulmonary hypertension from cardiac or pulmonary etiologies. iNO can be used during cardiac catheterization to measure pulmonary vasoreactivity, assess the severity and reversibility of pulmonary hypertension. In these patients, reduction of pulmonary artery pressure or PVR by >20% in response to vasodilating agents predicts a favorable response to oral vasodilators and an improved long-term clinical outcome. iNO has been safely used to assess pulmonary vasoreactivity in both pediatric and adult patients with pulmonary hypertension because it acts rapidly with no observed systemic side effects. This is in contrast to the systemic administration of other vasodilators (prostacyclin, calcium channel blockers) during diagnostic cardiac catheterization, which can result in systemic hypotension, increased intrapulmonary right-to-left shunting, and death. Low-dose iNO delivered through pulsed nasal cannula has also been used in the chronic treatment of pulmonary hypertension.

DOSING

Dosing of nitric oxide has ranged widely in both preclinical and clinical trials. In a randomized, controlled, dose-response trial in neonates with acute hypoxemic respiratory failure, all doses of iNO (5, 20, or 80 ppm) improved oxygenation compared to that of placebo. Treatment with 80 ppm iNO was no more effective than the other doses of iNO studied, but this higher dose of iNO was associated with an increase in methemoglobinemia and high exhaled nitrogen dioxide concentrations. As stated in the preceding text, the inhalation of 5 ppm nitric oxide by adults with ARDS showed better outcomes than placebo in *post hoc* subgroup analysis. These data would support doses between 5 to 20 ppm nitric oxide depending on the patient population and underlying pathophysiology.

Additionally, there can be variability in the clinical response to iNO. The most frequent etiology associated with poor response to iNO is inadequate lung inflation. Other etiologies that should be considered include improper dosing, abnormal pulmonary vascular function or structure, unsuspected anatomic cardiac disease, or myocardial dysfunction.

TOXICITIES, MONITORING, AND COMPLICATIONS

Methemoglobinemia has been reported as a rare complication occurring with inhalation of high concentrations of nitric oxide (>80 ppm). Monitoring methemoglobin levels

4 hours after initiating iNO and every 24 hours of treatment appear to be sufficient. Concentrations of nitrogen dioxide (NO_2) remain low when iNO is delivered in the recommended ranges. Levels of NO_2 are measured using electrochemical sensors.

Abrupt discontinuation of iNO may result in a "rebound response", which is characterized by reductions in oxygenation and an elevation of PVR. Generally, these responses are mild and are a result of brief increases in FiO_2. Postoperative cardiac patients with high pulmonary artery pressures at the time of nitric oxide withdrawal appear to be at the highest risk for rebound.

PHOSPHODIESTERASE INHIBITORS

Nitric oxide activates soluble guanylate cyclase converting guanosine 5′-triphosphate (GTP) to cGMP, resulting in relaxation of the vascular smooth muscle. Hydrolysis of cGMP by cyclic nucleotide phosphodiesterases (PDE) limits the action of cGMP. The isozyme PDE5 has a high affinity for cGMP and is the most active cGMP-hydrolyzing PDE in vascular smooth muscle. Selective inhibition of this isoform with PDE5 inhibitors such as sildenafil and zaprinast is being used to prolong the effects of endogenous nitric oxide. Early studies of diseases with increased pulmonary arterial pressure suggest that oral dosing of sildenafil to inhibit PDE5, lowers pulmonary artery pressure and may be effective in a synergistic manner when combined with iNO.

SUMMARY

iNO decreases PVR and reduces the need for ECMO in term neonates with PPHN. iNO transiently improves oxygenation in patients with ARDS, but whether this acute change results in long-term benefit is currently under further investigation. iNO can be used safely to assess pulmonary vasoreactivity in patients with pulmonary hypertension. It also reduces postoperative pulmonary hypertensive crises in cardiac patients. Dosing and adequacy of lung inflation may be important components in the variability in response to iNO. Inhalation of low-dose nitric oxide appears to be safe. Long-term follow-up of neurodevelopment and lung function is ongoing although the current data are favorable in patients treated with iNO as neonates. Finally, selective PDE5 inhibition may play a role in future treatment of conditions with pulmonary hypertension.

SURFACTANT

Douglas F. Willson

Multiple studies have investigated the use of exogenous surfactant in acute lung injury (ALI). Although surfactant is considered standard therapy for the prevention and treatment of infantile respiratory distress syndrome (IRDS), its use in other types of ALI, remains to be investigated. This section briefly reviews the types of surfactant and the evidence for its use in non-neonatal ALI.

SURFACTANT COMPOSITION AND PHARMACEUTICAL SURFACTANTS

Natural surfactant is a complex mixture of phospholipids, neutral lipids, and protein, with phospholipids being the major component (80% by weight). Each of the components and their balance are important in adsorption, film formation, and film behavior at the alveolar surface.

Four surfactant proteins have been identified: SP-A, B, C, and D. SP-A and SP-D are large, hydrophilic proteins in the collectin family, integral in the innate immune system. SP-B and SP-C are small, hydrophobic proteins present in approximately equal amounts (1% to 2%) and are vital in adsorption (spreading) and film formation. SP-B and SP-C are extracted with the phospholipids in commercial surfactants, whereas the hydrophilic proteins SP-A and SP-D are lost in the extraction process. The presence of SP-B and SP-C is probably the primary reason for the greater efficacy of "natural" surfactants relative to that of the synthetic surfactants. Four types of pharmaceutical surfactants have been studied in animal and human trials (see Table 42.2).

In the United States, currently there are four surfactants that are licensed for clinical use in IRDS: Survanta is a minced bovine lung preparation; Curosurf is a minced porcine lung extract, Exosurf is a synthetic mixture of dipalmitoyl phosphatidylcholine (DPPC) hexadecanol, and tyloxapol; and Infasurf is an unmodified lipid extract of calf lung washings. Differences in surfactant composition are important. The modified natural surfactants are superior to artificial surfactants in improving oxygenation, decreasing mortality, and lowering the incidence of retinopathy and bronchopulmonary dysplasia in human neonates. *In vitro* studies suggest that natural surfactants also better resist inactivation by protein and spread more rapidly at the alveolar surface, probably related to their retention of the hydrophobic surfactant-associated proteins SP-B and SP-C. All surfactants are not equivalent and their efficacy may be critically dependent on the formulation used.

SURFACTANT THERAPY IN ACUTE LUNG INJURY

In the original description of ARDS (adult), Ashbaugh and Petty commented on its similarity to IRDS and described abnormalities in surfactant function. Although surfactant deficiency is common to both conditions, ARDS and other forms of ALI are not simply the "adult" equivalents of

TABLE 42.2
PHARMACEUTICAL SURFACTANTS IN ANIMAL AND HUMAN TRIALS

Type of Surfactant	Description and Characteristics	Brands
Natural (whole)	Recovered intact from lung or amniotic fluid Have excellent surface-active properties but are difficult to manufacture and they carry an infection risk because they cannot be heat sterilized (it denatures the proteins)	None currently available
Modified natural	Sterile lipid extracts of minced lung or alveolar lavage fluid, often modified by the addition or removal of compounds In the lipid extraction process, the hydrophilic SP-A and SP-D are excluded but not the hydrophobic SP-B and SP-C	Survanta, Alveofact, Infasurf, Curosurf
Artificial	Mixtures of synthetic compounds (usually phospholipids) manufactured to resemble the composition and behavior of natural pulmonary surfactant	Exosurf, ALEC
Synthetic natural	Artificial surfactants with genetically engineered surfactant proteins or surfactantlike proteins added	Surfaxin, Venticute

IRDS. As summarized by Jobe and Ikegami, irrespective of whether the initiating event is direct alveolar injury (e.g., aspiration, pneumonia) or indirect lung injury (e.g., sepsis), surfactant may be rendered dysfunctional in ALI by a number of different mechanisms. These mechanisms include:

Surfactant Inhibition: The most consistent surfactant abnormality is inhibition by substances that gain access to the alveolar space after injury to the alveolar-capillary membrane. Albumin, hemoglobin, fibrin, complement, and other serum proteins can be shown *in vitro* to diminish the surface tension–reducing properties of the surfactant by competing with the surfactant for the air–fluid interface and interfering with monolayer formation. Interestingly, the surfactant appears to be unaltered because it can be shown to have normal activity when separated from the protein by simple centrifugation.

Altered Surfactant Metabolism: Animal models of lung injury have shown more rapid conversion of large to small surfactant aggregate forms—a form, which has very poor surface tension lowering properties. Human bronchoalveolar lavage (BAL) specimens from patients with ARDS have shown increased levels of proteases and alterations in surfactant density profiles. Altered composition which reverses with recovery has also been a consistent finding. The relationship of these abnormalities to lung dysfunction is not known, although surfactant isolated from several animal lung injury models has abnormal surface activity.

Decreased Secretion or Recycling due to Alveolar Type II Cell Injury: Animals injured by hyperoxia have decreased incorporation of surfactant precursors into lung tissue, which reverses with recovery. Evidence of damage to alveolar type II cells is more indirect. Surfactant pool size in ALI is inconsistent, with decreased, no change, and increased pool size being reported.

Destruction from Inflammatory Mediators: Inflammation is associated with surfactant dysfunction. Oxygen-free radicals, cytokines, phospholipases, and proteases released by activated leukocytes may inactivate surfactant directly.

Animal Data

Despite unequivocal evidence of surfactant dysfunction in ALI, it does not necessarily follow that replacement will be therapeutic. Animal models of ALI have generally shown a positive response to surfactant replacement determined by the type of injury, the surfactant employed, the timing of administration, method of delivery, and other factors. These models examine the acute response, which is relevant to the surfactant's potential value in humans, but offer limited insight into longer-term efficacy. Ultimately, therapeutic efficacy must be determined by human studies because longer-term outcome cannot be readily addressed in animal models.

TABLE 42.3

CASE SERIES OF SURFACTANT THERAPY IN RESPIRATORY FAILURE

Investigator	N	Patient Population	Etiology of Respiratory Failure	Trade Names	Outcomes
Gunther et al.	27	Adults	ARDS	Alveofact	Improved biochemical and biophysical function
Walmrath et al.	10	Adults	ARDS from sepsis	Alveofact	Improved oxygenation
Spragg et al.	6	Adults	ARDS from multiple causes	Curosurf	Improved oxygenation and biophysical function
Wiswell et al.	12	Adults	ARDS from multiple causes	Surfaxin	Improved oxygenation
Willson et al.	28	Children	ARDS from multiple causes	Infasurf	Improved oxygenation
Creery et al.	2	Infants	Pneumocystis	bLES	Improved oxygenation
Lopez-Herce et al.	20	Children	ARDS and postoperative cardiac	Curosurf	Improved oxygenation
Hermon et al.	19	Children	ARDS and postoperative cardiac	Curosurf or Alveofact	Improved oxygenation
Herting et al.	8	Children	Pneumonia	Curosurf	Improved oxygenation

ARDS, acute respiratory distress syndrome.

Human Studies

The results of human studies of surfactant therapy in (non-IRDS) ALI have been variable. In neonates, surfactant has enjoyed some success in meconium aspiration syndrome and neonatal pneumonia, but its value in congenital diaphragmatic hernia is unclear. Studies in non-neonatal ALI have followed the usual course of initial positive case reports/case series leading finally to randomized prospective studies. As in the initial studies of surfactant in IRDS, however, the first large controlled study in ARDS was definitively negative. Anzueto et al. administered nebulized Exosurf versus placebo to 725 adults with ARDS secondary to sepsis and demonstrated no improvement in oxygenation and no effect on morbidity or mortality. Generalizations from this study are limited, however, by its use of an artificial surfactant, the choice of nebulization as a delivery method, and the very small dose of surfactant administered. Subsequent studies have had mixed but generally more positive results (see Table 42.3). A study of beractant (Survanta), a modified natural surfactant, by Gregory et al. demonstrated a survival advantage for adult patients with ARDS receiving the 100 mg per kg dose, but the study was marred by the lack of blinding and incomplete randomization. The most recent study by Spragg et al. of protein C surfactant (Venticute) in adults with ARDS showed immediate improvement in oxygenation but, disappointingly, no longer-term improvement in duration of mechanical ventilation, lengths of stay, or mortality. *Post hoc* analysis did suggest, however, that the response in ARDS due to "direct lung injury" was quite positive and a prospective study of Venticute in ARDS due to direct lung injury is currently under way.

Pediatric studies have been more encouraging. A small randomized but unblinded trial in children with acute hypoxemic respiratory failure showed that those receiving

calfactant (Infasurf) had immediate improvement in oxygenation and fewer ventilator days and days in intensive care. Luchetti, et al. showed similar benefit using porcine surfactant (Curosurf) in two separate studies in infants with respiratory failure secondary to bronchiolitis. Moller study in children with ARDS showed immediate improvement in

TABLE 42.4

CLINICAL OUTCOMES

	Calfactant (n = 77)	Placebo (n = 75)	p Value
Died (in hospital)	15 (19%)	27 (36%)	0.03
Died without extubation	12 (16%)	24 (32%)	0.02
Failed CMV[a]	13 (21%)	26 (42%)	0.02
ECMO	3	3	NS
Use of nitric oxide	9	10	0.80
HFOV after entry	7	15	0.07
PICU LOS	15.2 ± 13.3	13.6 ± 11.6	0.85
Hospital LOS	26.8 ± 26	25.3 ± 32.2	0.91
Days of oxygen therapy	17.3 ± 16	18.5 ± 31	0.93
Hospital charges	$205 \pm $220	$213 \pm $226	0.83
Hospital charges/d	$7.5 \pm $7.6	$7.9 \pm $7.5	0.74

Numbers in thousands.
[a]Note that some patients had greater than one nonconventional therapy.
CMV, conventional mechanical ventilation; ECMO, extracorporeal membrane oxygenation; NS, not specified; HFOV, high-frequency oscillatory ventilation; PICU, pediatric intensive care unit; LOS, length of stay.
From Willson DF, Thomas NJ, Markovitz BP, et al. Pediatric acute lung injury and sepsis investigators. Effect of exogenous surfactant (calfactant) in pediatric acute lung injury: A randomized controlled trial. JAMA. 2005;293:470–476.

oxygenation and less need for rescue therapy but was underpowered for more definitive outcomes. Most recently, a study by Willson, et al. in pediatric patients with ALI/ARDS showed both immediately improved oxygenation as well as a significant survival advantage for patients receiving calfactant relative to placebo (see Table 42.4).

It should be noted that none of the studies in either adults or children showed significant untoward long-term effects from surfactant administration, although transient hypoxia and some hemodynamic instability during administration are well described. Transmission of infectious agents or allergic reactions has not been reported.

THE FUTURE OF SURFACTANT THERAPY

At present, surfactant replacement is clearly indicated in the prevention and treatment of IRDS but data to endorse its use in other types of ALI is limited. It could be argued that evidence of its dysfunction in ALI/ARDS, favorable effects in animal models, and suggestion of efficacy in some human studies—particularly in the absence of significant untoward effects—make a strong rationale for considering this therapy in any child with acute, severe lung injury. Apart from the considerable expense there is little to discourage its use. Many questions remain to be answered, however, and it would be ideal if some, if not all of these questions were addressed before its indiscriminate adoption.

RECOMMENDED READINGS

1. Abman SH, Griebel JL, Parker DK, et al. Acute effects of inhaled nitric oxide in children with severe hypoxemic respiratory failure. *J Pediatr.* 1994;124(6):881–888.
2. Alvarado M, Hingre R, Hakanson D, et al. Clinical trial of Survanta vs Exosurf therapy in infants <1500 g with respiratory distress syndrome (RDS) [Abstract no. 1865]. *Pediatr Res.* 1993; 33:314.
3. Anderson M, Svartengren M, Bylin G, et al. Deposition in asthmatics of particles inhaled in air or in helium-oxygen. *Am Rev Respir Dis.* 1993;147(3):524–528.
4. Anzueto A, Baughman RP, Kalpalatha KG, et al. Aerolized surfactant in adult with sepsis induced acute respiratory distress syndrome. *N Engl J Med.* 1996;334:1417–1421.
5. Ardehali A, Laks H, Levine M, et al. A prospective trial of inhaled nitric oxide in clinical lung transplantation. *Transplantation.* 2001;72(1):112–115.
6. Ardehali A, Hughes K, Sadeghi A, et al. Inhaled nitric oxide for pulmonary hypertension after heart transplantation. *Transplantation.* 2001;72(4):638–641.
7. Ashbaugh DG, Bigelow DB, Petty TL, et al. Acute respiratory distress syndrome in adults. *Lancet.* 1967;2:319–323.
8. Berkenbosch JW, Grueber RE, Dabbagh O, et al. Effect of helium-oxygen (heliox) gas mixtures on the function of four pediatric ventilators. *Crit Care Med.* 2003;31(7):2052–2058.
9. Bernhard W, Mottaghian J, Gebert A, et al. Commercial versus native surfactants: Surface activity, molecular components, and the effect of calcium. *Am J Respir Crit Care Med.* 2000;162: 1524–1533.
10. Bradley SM, Seismic JM, Adz AM, et al. Hemodynamic effects of inspired carbon dioxide after the Norwood procedure. *Ann Thorac Surg.* 2001;72:2088–2093.
11. Canet J, Sanchis J. Performance of a low flow O₂ Venturi mask: Diluting effects of the breathing pattern. *Eur J Respir Dis.* 1984; 65:68.
12. Centers for Disease Control and Prevention (CDC). Perspectives in disease prevention and health promotion carbon monoxide intoxication–a preventable environmental health hazard. *MMWR.* 1982;31(39):529–531.
13. Chatburn RL, Anderson SM. Controlling carbon dioxide delivery during mechanical ventilation. *Respir Care.* 1994;39:1039–1046.
14. Clark JM, Lambertsen CJ. Pulmonary oxygen toxicity: A review. *Pharmacol Rev.* 1971;23:37.
15. Creery WD, Hashmi A, Hutchinson JS, et al. Surfactant therapy improves pulmonary function in infants with Pneumocystis carinii pneumonia and acquired immunodeficiency syndrome. *Pediatr Polmonol.* 1997;24:370–373.
16. Date H, Triantafillou AN, Trulock EP, et al. Inhaled nitric oxide reduces human lung allograft dysfunction. *J Thorac Cardiovasc Surg.* 1996;111(5):913–919.
17. Davidson D, Barefield ES, Kattwinkel J, et al. Safety of withdrawing inhaled nitric oxide therapy in persistent pulmonary hypertension of the newborn. *Pediatrics.* 1999;104(2 Pt 1):231–236.
18. Day RW, Barton AJ, Pusher TJ, et al. Pulmonary vascular resistance of children treated with nitrogen during early infancy. *Ann Thorac Surg.* 1998;65:1400–1404.
19. Day RW, Tani LY, Minich LL, et al. Congenital heart disease with ductal-dependent systemic perfusion: Doppler ultrasonography flow velocities are altered by changes in the fraction of inspired oxygen. *J Heart Lung Transplant.* 1995;14:718–725.
20. Dechant KL, Faulds D. Colfosceril palmitate: A review of the therapeutic efficacy and clinical tolerability of a synthetic preparation (Exosurf Neonatal) in neonatal respiratory distress syndrome. *Drugs.* 1991;42:877–894.
21. Dellinger RP, Zimmerman JL, Taylor RW, et al. Effects of inhaled nitric oxide in patients with acute respiratory distress syndrome: Results of a randomized phase II trial. Inhaled Nitric Oxide in ARDS Study Group. *Crit Care Med.* 1998;26(1):15–23.
22. DeMello FJ, Haglin JJ, Hitchcock CR. Comparative study of experimental *Clostridium perfringens* infection in dogs treated with antibiotics, surgery, and hyperbaric oxygen. *Surgery.* 1973;73:936.
23. Deneeke SM, and Fanburg BL. et al. Normobaric oxygen toxicity of the lung. *N Engl J Med.* 1980;303:76.
24. Dobyns EL, Anas NG, Fortenberry JD, et al. Interactive effects of high-frequency oscillatory ventilation and inhaled nitric oxide in acute hypoxemic respiratory failure in pediatrics. *Crit Care Med.* 2002;30(11):2425–2429.
25. Dobyns EL, Cornfield DN, Anas NG, et al. Multicenter randomized controlled trial of the effects of inhaled nitric oxide therapy on gas exchange in children with acute hypoxemic respiratory failure. *J Pediatr.* 1999;134(4):406–412.
26. Egan DF. Gas therapy. In: *Fundamentals of respiratory therapy.* 3rd ed. St. Louis, MO: CV Mosby; 1977:117.
27. Emerman CL, Cydulka RK, McFadden ER. Comparison of 2.5 vs. 7.5 mg of inhaled albuterol in the treatment of acute asthma. *Chest.* 1999;115(1):92–96.
28. Frostell C, Fratacci MD, Wain JC, et al. Inhaled nitric oxide. A selective pulmonary vasodilator reversing hypoxic pulmonary vasoconstriction. *Circulation.* 1991;83(6):2038–2047.
29. Ghim M, Severance HW. Ice storm-related carbon monoxide poisonings in North Carolina: A reminder. *South Med J.* 2004; 1060–1065.
30. Ghofrani HA, Wiedemann R, Rose F, et al. Sildenafil for treatment of lung fibrosis and pulmonary hypertension: A randomised controlled trial. *Lancet.* 2002;360(9337):895–900.
31. Gilder H, McSherry C. Phosphatidylcholine synthesis and pulmonary oxygen toxicity. *Biochim Biophys Acta.* 1976;441:48–56.
32. Gluck EH, Onorato DJ, Castriotta R. Helium-oxygen mixtures in intubated patients with status asthmaticus and respiratory acidosis. *Chest.* 1990;98(3):693–698.
33. Gregory TJ, Steinberg KP, Spragg R, et al. Bovine surfactant therapy for patients with acute respiratory distress syndrome. *Am J Respir Crit Care Med.* 1997;155:1309–1315.
34. American Academy of Pediatrics: Committee on Hospital Care. Guidelines and levels of care for pediatric intensive care units. *Crit Care Med.* 1993;7:1077–1086.
35. Gunther A, Schmidt R, Harodt J, et al. Bronchoscopic administration of bovine natural surfactant in ARDS and septic shock: Impact on biophysical and biochemical surfactant properties. *Eur Respir J.* 2002;10:797–804.

36. Gupta VK, Cheifetz IM. Heliox administration in the pediatric intensive care unit: An evidence based review. *Pediatr Crit Care Med.* 2005;6:204–211.

37. Hampson NB, ed. *Hyperbaric oxygen therapy: 1999 committee report.* Kensington, MD: Undersea and Hyperbaric Medical Society; 1999.

38. Hawkins M, Harrison J, Charters P. Severe carbon monoxide poisoning: Outcome after hyperbaric oxygen therapy. *Br J Anesth.* 2000;84:584–586.

39. Hermon MM, Golej J, Burda H, et al. Surfactant therapy in infants and children: Three years experience in a pediatric intensive care unit. *Shock.* 2002;17:247–251.

40. Herting E, Moller O, Schiffman JH, et al. Surfactant improves oxygenation in infants and children with pneumonia and acute respiratory distress syndrome. *Acta Paediatr.* 2002;91:1174–1178.

41. Hollman G, Shen G, Zeng L, et al. Helium-oxygen improves Clinical Asthma Scores in children with acute bronchiolitis. *Crit Care Med.* 1998;26(10):1731–1736.

42. Horbar JD, Wright LL, Soll RF, et al. For the National Institute of Child Health and Human Development Neonatal Research Network. A multicenter randomized trial comparing two surfactants for the treatment of neonatal respiratory distress syndrome. *J Pediatr.* 1993;123:757–766.

43. Huguchi R, Lewis J, Ikegami M. In vitro conversion of surfactant subtypes is altered in alveolar surfactant isolated from injured lungs. *Am Rev Respir Dis.* 1991;145:1416–1420.

44. Humbert M, Sitbon O, Simonneau G. Treatment of pulmonary arterial hypertension. *N Engl J Med.* 2004;351(14):1425–1436.

45. Ichinose F, Roberts JD Jr, Zapol WM. Inhaled nitric oxide: A selective pulmonary vasodilator: Current uses and therapeutic potential. *Circulation.* 2004;109(25):3106–3111.

46. The Neonatal Inhaled Nitric Oxide Study Group. Inhaled nitric oxide in full-term and nearly full-term infants with hypoxic respiratory failure. *N Engl J Med.* 1997;336(9):597–604.

47. Ivy DD, Parker D, Doran A, et al. Acute hemodynamic effects and home therapy using a novel pulsed nasal nitric oxide delivery system in children and young adults with pulmonary hypertension. *Am J Cardiol.* 2003;92(7):886–890.

48. Ivy DD, Kinsella JP, Ziegler JW, et al. Dipyridamole attenuates rebound pulmonary hypertension after inhaled nitric oxide withdrawal in postoperative congenital heart disease. *J Thorac Cardiovasc Surg.* 1998;115(4):875–882.

49. Jaber S, Carlucci A, Boussarsar M, et al. Helium-oxygen in the postextubation period decreases inspiratory effort. *Am J Respir Crit Care Med.* 2001;164(4):633–637.

50. Jobe AH, Ikegami M. Surfactant and acute lung injury. *Proc Assoc Am Physicians.* 1998;110:489–495.

51. Jobes DR, Nicholson SC, Steven JM, et al. Carbon dioxide prevents pulmonary over circulation in HLHS. *Ann Thorac Surg.* 1992;54:150–151.

52. Juurlink DN, Stanbrook MB, McGuigan MA. Hyperbaric oxygen for carbon monoxide poisoning. *The Cochrane Database of Systematic Reviews.* 2004;25:00075320, Accession number.

53. Katz A, Gentile MA, Craig DM, et al. Heliox improves gas exchange during high-frequency ventilation in a pediatric model of acute lung injury. *Am J Respir Crit Care Med.* 2001;164(2): 260–264.

54. Katz AL, Gentile MA, Craig DM, et al. Heliox does not affect gas exchange during high-frequency oscillatory ventilation if tidal volume is held constant. *Crit Care Med.* 2003;31(7):2006–2009.

55. Kinsella JP, Abman SH. High-frequency oscillatory ventilation augments the response to inhaled nitric oxide in persistent pulmonary hypertension of the newborn: Nitric Oxide Study Group. *Chest.* 1998;114(Suppl 1):100S.

56. Kinsella JP, Neish SR, Ivy DD, et al. Clinical responses to prolonged treatment of persistent pulmonary hypertension of the newborn with low doses of inhaled nitric oxide. *J Pediatr.* 1993;123(1):103–108.

57. Kinsella JP, Neish SR, Shaffer E, et al. Low-dose inhalation nitric oxide in persistent pulmonary hypertension of the newborn. *Lancet.* 1992;340(8823):819–820.

58. Kinsella JP, Truog WE, Walsh WF, et al. Randomized, multicenter trial of inhaled nitric oxide and high-frequency oscillatory ventilation in severe, persistent pulmonary hypertension of the newborn. *J Pediatr.* 1997;131(1 Pt 1):55–62.

59. Kress JP, Noth I, Gehlbach BK, et al. The utility of albuterol nebulized with heliox during acute asthma exacerbations. *Am J Respir Crit Care Med.* 2002;165(9):1317–1321.

60. Kudukis TM, Manthous CA, Schmidt GA, et al. Inhaled helium-oxygen revisited: Effect of inhaled helium-oxygen during the treatment of status asthmaticus in children. *J Pediatr.* 1997; 130(2):217–224.

61. Leach RM, Rees PJ, Wilmshurst P. ABC of oxygen: Hyperbaric oxygen therapy. *Br Med J.* 1998;317:1140–1143.

62. Lewis J, Ikegami M, Tabor B, et al. Aerosolized surfactant is preferentially deposited in normal versus injured regions of the lung in a heterogeneous lung injury model. *Am Rev Respir Dis.* 1992;145:A184.

63. Liefer G. Hyperbaric oxygen therapy. *Am J Pract Nurs.* 2001; 101:26–34.

64. Lodato RF. Oxygen toxicity. *Crit Care Clin.* 1990;6:749.

65. Lopez-Herce J, de Lucas N, Carrillo A, et al. Surfactant treatment for acute respiratory distress syndrome. *Arch Dis Child.* 1999;80: 248–252.

66. Luchetti M, Casiraghi G, Valsecchi R, et al. Porcine-derived surfactant treatment of severe bronchiolitis. *Acta Anaesthesiol Scand.* 1998;42:805–810.

67. Luchetti M, Ferrero F, Gallini C, et al. Multicenter, randomized, controlled study of porcine surfactant in severe respiratory syncytial virus-induced respiratory failure. *Pediatr Crit Care Med.* 2002;3:261–268.

68. Lundin S, Mang H, Smithies M, et al. Inhalation of nitric oxide in acute lung injury: Results of a European multicentre study. The European Study Group of Inhaled Nitric Oxide. *Intensive Care Med.* 1999;25(9):911–919.

69. Mahle WT, Clancy RR, Moss EM, et al. Neurodevelopmental outcome and lifestyle assessment in school-aged and adolescent children with hypoplastic left heart syndrome. *Pediatrics.* 2000;105:1082–1089.

70. McPherson SP. Gas regulation, administration and controlling devices. *Respiratory therapy equipment.* 4th ed. St. Louis, MO: CV Mosby; 1990:68.

71. Meade MO, Granton JT, Matte-Martyn A, et al. A randomized trial of inhaled nitric oxide to prevent ischemia-reperfusion injury after lung transplantation. *Am J Respir Crit Care Med.* 2003;167(11):1483–1489.

72. Merritt TA, Hallman M, Spragg R, et al. Exogenous surfactant treatments for neonatal respiratory distress syndrome and their potential role in the adult respiratory distress syndrome. *Drugs.* 1989;38:591–611.

73. Michelakis E, Tymchak W, Lien D, et al. Oral sildenafil is an effective and specific pulmonary vasodilator in patients with pulmonary arterial hypertension: Comparison with inhaled nitric oxide. *Circulation.* 2002;105(20):2398–2403.

74. Miller OI, Tang SF, Keech A, et al. Inhaled nitric oxide and prevention of pulmonary hypertension after congenital heart surgery: A randomised double-blind study. *Lancet.* 2000;356(9240):1464–1469.

75. Moller JC, Schaible T, Roll C, et al. with the Surfactant ARDS Study Group. Treatment with bovine surfactant in severe acute respiratory distress syndrome in children: A randomized multicenter study. *Intensive Care Med.* 2003;29:437–446.

76. Myers TR, Chat burn RL. Accuracy of oxygen analyzers at sub atmospheric concentrations used in treatment of hypoplastic left heart syndrome. *Respir Care.* 2002;47:1168–1172.

77. Myers TR. Therapeutic gases for neonatal and pediatric respiratory care. *Respir Care.* 2003;48:399–422.

78. National Asthma Education and Prevention Program (National Heart Lung and Blood Institute). Guidelines for the diagnosis and management of asthma: Expert panel report 2, Bethesda, MD: US Department of Health and Human Services Public Health Service National Institutes of Health National Heart Lung and Blood Institute; 1997.

79. Notter RH. *Lung surfactants. Basic science and clinical applications.* New York: Marcel Dekker; 2000:16.

80. Pepke-Zaba J, Hingenbottam TW, Dinh-Xuan AT, et al. Inhaled nitric oxide as a cause of selective pulmonary vasodilatation in pulmonary hypertension. *Lancet.* 1991;338(8776):1173–1174.

81. Petty TL, Ashbaugh DB. The adult respiratory distress syndrome: Clinical features, factors influencing prognosis, and principles of management. *Chest.* 1971;60:233–239.

82. Petty TL, Reiss OK, Paul GW, et al. Characteristics of pulmonary surfactant in adult respiratory distress syndrome associated with trauma and shock. *Am Rev Respir Dis.* 1977;115:531–536.

83. Poets CF, Wilken M, Seidenberg J, et al. Reliability of the pulse oximeters in the detection of hyperoxemia. *J Pediatr.* 1993;122:87–90.

84. Prasad S, Wilkinson J, Gatzoulis MA. Sildenafil in primary pulmonary hypertension. *N Engl J Med.* 2000;343(18):1342.

85. Reffelmann T, Kloner RA. Therapeutic potential of phosphodiesterase 5 inhibition for cardiovascular disease. *Circulation.* 2003;108(2):239–244.

86. Riordan CJ, Rand beck F, Storey JH, et al. Effects of oxygen, positive end expiratory pressure, and carbon dioxide on oxygen delivery in an animal model of the univentricular heart. *J Thorac Cardiovasc Surg.* 1996;112:644–654.

87. Roberts JD, Fineman JR, Morin FC, et al. Inhaled nitric oxide in persistent pulmonary hypertension of the newborn. *Lancet.* 1992;340(8823):818–819.

88. Robillard E, Alarie Y, Dagenais-Perusse P, et al. Microaerosol administration of synthetic β-γ-dipalmitoyl-L-α-lecithin in the respiratory distress syndrome: A preliminary report. *Can Med Assoc J.* 1964;90:55–57.

89. Rossaint R, Falke KT, López F, et al. Inhaled nitric oxide for the adult respiratory distress syndrome. *N Engl J Med.* 1993;328(6):399–405.

90. Schaeffer EM, Pohlman A, Morgan S, et al. Oxygenation in status asthmaticus improves during ventilation with helium-oxygen. *Crit Care Med.* 1999;27(12):2666–2670.

91. Sitbon O, Brenot F, Denjean A, et al. Inhaled nitric oxide as a screening agent for safely identifying responders to oral calcium-channel blockers in primary pulmonary hypertension. *Eur Respir J.* 1998;12(2):265–270.

92. Skrinskas GJ, Hyland RH, Hutcheon MA. Using helium-oxygen mixtures in the management of acute upper airway obstruction. *Can Med Assoc J.* 1983;128(5):555–558.

93. Spragg RG, Gilliard N, Richman P, et al. Acute effects of a single dose of porcine surfactant on patients with acute respiratory distress syndrome. *Chest.* 1995;105:195–202.

94. Spragg RG Lewis JF, Walmrath HD, et al. Effect of recombinant surfactant protein C-based surfactant on the acute respiratory distress syndrome. *N Engl J Med.* 2004;351:884–892.

95. Stillwell PC, Quick JD, Munro PR, et al. Effectiveness of open-circuit and oxyhood delivery of helium-oxygen. *Chest.* 1989;95:1222–1224.

96. Tabbut S, Ramamurthy C, Montenegro LM, et al. Impact of inspired gas mixtures on preoperative infants with HLHS during controlled ventilation. *Circulation.* 2001;104:1159–1164.

97. Tobias JD. Heliox in children with airway obstruction. *Pediatr Emerg Care.* 1997;13(1):29–32.

98. Towbin MJ. Respiratory Monitoring. *J Am Med Assoc.* 1990;264:244–251.

99. Van Kaam AH, Haitsma JJ, Kik WA, et al. Response to exogenous surfactant is different during open lung and conventional ventilation. *Crit Care Med.* 2004;32:774–780.

100. Veldhuizen RAW, McCraig LA, Akino T, et al. Pulmonary surfactant subfractions in patients with the acute respiratory distress syndrome. *Am J Respir Crit Care Med.* 1995;152:1867–1871.

101. Vermont Oxford Trials Network. A multicenter randomized trial comparing synthetic surfactant to modified bovine surfactant in the treatment of neonatal respiratory distress syndrome [Abstract no. 1542]. *Pediatr Res.* 1994;35:259.

102. Villanucci S, Marzio D, Scholl M, et al. Cardiovascular changes induced by hyperbaric oxygen therapy. *Undersea Biomed Res.* 1990;17:117.

103. Walmrath D, Gunther A, Ghofrani HA, et al. Bronchoscopic surfactant administration in patients with severe adult respiratory distress syndrome and sepsis. *Am J Respir Crit Care Med.* 1996;154:57–62.

104. Wasiman D, Shupak A, Weisz G, et al. Hyperbaric oxygen therapy in the pediatric patient: The experience of the Israel Naval Medical Institute. *Pediatrics.* 1998;102(5):E53.

105. Werner HA. Status asthmaticus in children: A review. *Chest.* 2001;119(6):1913–1929.

106. Willson DF, Bauman LA, Zaritsky A, et al. Instillation of calf's lung surfactant extract (Infasurf) is beneficial in pediatric acute hypoxemic respiratory failure. *Crit Care Med.* 1999;27:188–195.

107. Willson DF, Jiao JH, Bauman L, et al. Calf's lung surfactant extract in acute hypoxemic respiratory failure in children. *Crit Care Med.* 1996;24:1316–1322, Case series of surfactant in ALI.

108. Willson DF. Calfactant. *Expert Opin Pharmacother.* 2001;2(9):1479–1493.

109. Willson DF, Thomas NJ, Markovitz BP, et al. Pediatric acute lung injury and sepsis investigators. Effect of exogenous surfactant (calfactant) in pediatric acute lung injury: A randomized controlled trial. *JAMA.* 2005;293:470–476.

110. Winters JW, Willing MA, Sanfilippo D, et al. Heliox improves ventilation during high-frequency oscillatory ventilation in pediatric patients. *Pediatr Crit Care Med.* 2000;1(1):33–37.

111. Wiseman LR, Bryson HM. Porcine-derived lung surfactant. A review of the therapeutic efficacy and clinical tolerability of a natural surfactant preparation (Curosurf) in neonatal respiratory distress syndrome. *Drugs.* 1994;48:387–400.

112. Wiswell TE, Smith RM, Katz LB, et al. Bronchopulmonary segmental lavage with surfaxin (KL4-surfactant) for acute respiratory distress syndrome. *Am J Respir Crit Care Med.* 1999;160:1188–1195.

113. Anzueto A, Baughman RP, Kalpalatha KG, et al. Aerolized surfactant in adult with sepsis induced acute respiratory distress syndrome. *N Engl J Med.* 1996;334:1417–1421.

Mechanical Ventilation

43

Mark J. Heulitt   Basem Zafer Alsaatti   Richard T. Fiser   Sylvia Göthberg

INDICATIONS FOR MECHANICAL VENTILATION

There have been no controlled studies elucidating and evaluating the indications for the use of mechanical ventilation in pediatric patients, which has evolved over the last 10 years as we have expanded our knowledge of lung injury caused by mechanical ventilation.[1,2] Also, the use of noninvasive positive-pressure ventilation (NIPPV) has increased, and the need for every patient to be intubated for positive-pressure mechanical ventilation is no longer indicated. The indications for the use of mechanical ventilation are diverse and include both primary respiratory and nonrespiratory causes. These indications are listed in Table 43.1. The decision to place a patient on positive-pressure mechanical ventilation is a combination of clinical judgment, assessing the symptoms and signs of the need for mechanical ventilation, and laboratory tests. Table 43.2 outlines laboratory tests and clinical signs and symptoms of the need for mechanical ventilation. In essence, the decision to place a

TABLE 43.1

INDICATIONS FOR MECHANICAL VENTILATION IN DIFFERENT CLINICAL SITUATIONS

Apnea and impending respiratory arrest
Relief from upper airway obstruction
Acute severe asthma
Neuromuscular disease
Acute hypoxemic respiratory failure
Heart failure and cardiogenic shock
Acute brain injury
Traumatic chest injury
Inability to protect the airway

TABLE 43.2

ASSESSMENT OF THE NEED FOR MECHANICAL VENTILATION

Symptoms	Dyspnea
	Orthopnea
	Increased cough or wheeze
	Somnolence
Signs	Stridor
	Tachypnea
	Use of accessory muscles of respiration
	Retractions
	Prolonged expiratory phase
	Paradoxical abdominal motion on inspiration
	Cyanosis
Laboratory tests	Arterial blood gas measurement
	Pulse oximetric studies
	Chest radiograph
	Measurements of pulmonary mechanics

patient on either invasive or noninvasive positive-pressure mechanical ventilation represents the patient's inability to deal with increased inspiratory loads or to maintain airway patency or gas exchange. Inspiratory loads consist of inertial (e.g., obesity and chest wall density), threshold (e.g., artificial loads placed on airway), resistive (e.g., upper airway obstruction, asthma, and artificial airway), and elastic (e.g., kyphoscoliosis, pulmonary restriction, chest wall trauma, pleural effusions, pneumonia, pulmonary edema, pulmonary fibrosis, and hyperinflation) loads.

DETERMINING THE INITIAL SETTINGS FOR MECHANICAL VENTILATION

After the decision has been made to place the patient on mechanical ventilatory support, it is essential that the settings of the mechanical ventilator be directed toward the indications for ventilatory support. Essentially, mechanical ventilatory support can be subdivided into three phases: acute, maintenance, and weaning. The acute phase of mechanical ventilation is the initial phase, when the clinician matches the patient's disease process with the ventilatory mode and level of support. It is during the acute phase that the clinician must optimize mechanical ventilator support while minimizing potential deleterious effects of positive-pressure mechanical ventilatory support. The initial settings of mechanical ventilatory support depend upon the patient's age and mode of support. Table 43.1 lists the initial settings, which can be subdivided into volume-targeted and pressure-targeted modes. Currently, the selection of ventilator settings is also directed by the clinician's desire to eliminate ventilator-induced lung injury. It is essential for the clinician to recognize that the goal of providing mechanical ventilatory support is not to normalize the patient's blood gas levels at the cost of ventilator-induced lung injury. For patients with obstructive lung disease, such as asthma, this lung protection strategy would include the prevention of high airway pressures and hyperinflation-associated complications. The initial settings would include a lower tidal volume and prolonged exhalation times. Allowing the patient to breathe spontaneously in a support mode is ideal because it would allow the patient to have more control over the exhalation time. However, elevated values of partial pressure of arterial carbon dioxide ($PaCO_2$) may cause agitation in the patient and, therefore, an increase in sedation. The level of positive end-expiratory pressure (PEEP) in patients with obstructive disease has traditionally been set at minimal levels, secondary to the development of auto-PEEP, because of the patient's increased airway resistance with inadequate lung emptying during exhalation. However, some patients may require higher levels of PEEP to match the level of auto-PEEP to splint the airways open, ensuring adequate oxygenation.

Patients with decreased thoracic compliance must have ventilatory settings directed toward lung recruitment to reduce the severity of ventilator-induced lung injury. As discussed in previous sections, this lung protection strategy is primarily accomplished by limiting the distending volume, the change in pressure to distend the alveoli, and the level of end-expiratory pressure. This strategy is directed toward reducing the cyclic collapse and re-expansion of the alveoli due to inadequate levels of PEEP and, therefore, the inability to maintain the alveoli open throughout the respiratory cycle. A proposed strategy toward lung recruitment is outlined in the next section.

LUNG RECRUITMENT

Lung recruitment is a strategy aimed at re-expanding the collapsed lung tissue and then at maintaining high PEEP to prevent subsequent *derecruitment*. To recruit the collapsed lung tissue, sufficient pressure must be imposed to exceed the critical opening pressure of the affected lung. Lung recruitment has gained widespread interest as a tool for the opening of closed lung units. The widespread use of low tidal volumes may increase the risk of reabsorption atelectasis in the basal parts of the lung, which eventually may lead to the consolidation of the affected areas. This atelectatic effect is further enhanced by high inhaled oxygen concentrations. In certain patients, the use of a recruitment maneuver may provide long-term improvement in oxygenation. If the PEEP level can be properly determined and set, the effect will stabilize and further protect the lung by avoiding the cyclic opening and closing of lung units.

The first step is to determine whether this maneuver is appropriate for the patient. Ideal patients for recruitment maneuvers are those with putative acute respiratory distress syndrome (ARDS) in the early phase of the disease (before the onset of fibroproliferation). These patients will continue to be poorly oxygenated in spite of a high fraction of inspired oxygen (FIO_2). Preexisting focal lung disease that may predispose to barotrauma should be regarded as a relative contraindication to the maneuver (e.g., extensive apical bullous lung disease). Patients with "secondary" ARDS (e.g., abdominal sepsis) are thought to be more likely to respond favorably to the maneuver than patients with "primary" lung disease and acute lung injury.

Currently, there are several different methods in clinical use that can accomplish an opening of the collapsed alveoli, and the common denominator for most of these methods is to intermittently apply an increased positive pressure in the lung for a limited time. One method utilizes the graphical display of dynamic inspiratory compliance (Cdyni), which indicates the response of the patient's lung mechanics to each change in applied airway pressure and inspiratory tidal volume. For example, during a stepwise increase of the end-inspiratory pressure (EIP), a corresponding increase in tidal volume (VTi) will occur. Cdyni is defined as:

$$Cdyni = \frac{VTi}{EIP - PEEP}$$

As long as the relative increase in EIP and tidal volume are linear, the Cdyni will appear constant, reflecting the development of the pressure–volume relation in the lung over time. With a continued stepwise increase in EIP, there will eventually be reduced increments in the corresponding tidal volume, which is indicated by a slight decrease in Cdyni. Additional increase in EIP at this point may result in a gradually reducing increment in the tidal volume, accompanied by a decrease in Cdyni.

This pattern may illustrate that the relative frequency of the opening of the collapsed alveoli is reduced relative to the increase in pressure and that further increase in EIP may result in overdistension of the already opened alveoli.

Positive End-Expiratory Pressure Titration

Cdyni may also be a useful parameter to determine the appropriate level of PEEP that may prevent alveolar collapse during expiration. When used for this purpose, Cdyni may help in guiding the titration of effective PEEP. This may be performed by a stepwise decrease of an initial PEEP level, which should be assessed before the recruitment maneuver is being performed. As PEEP is carefully decreased in a stepwise manner, the Cdyni will initially increase with each decrease of the PEEP level, indicating a relief of the overdistended areas in the lung. Subsequently, the Cdyni will reach a plateau, where Cdyni no longer increases when the PEEP level is decreased. With further decrease in the PEEP level, the Cdyni will start decreasing, indicating initial collapse of the alveoli that can no longer be kept open at the current PEEP level.

Effective PEEP should be set 2 to 3 cm H_2O above the indicated collapse pressure as a safety margin after a preceding recruitment maneuver.

Measures of Lung Recruitment

Cdyni can be used as a measure of improvement in lung compliance during lung recruitment; however, other measures should be utilized to ensure recruitment without overdistension of the recruited alveoli. If the lung is recruited, there should be an improvement in oxygenation, pulmonary compliance, and ventilation. It is important for the clinician to not be misled by considering an improvement of oxygenation alone as a measure of lung recruitment. An increase in PEEP can reduce cardiac output and therefore increase partial pressure of arterial oxygen (Pa_{O_2}) despite a decrease in oxygen delivery. The carbon dioxide (CO_2) concentration in expired air depends on alveolar ventilation, cardiac output, and metabolic state. The elimination of CO_2 through expired gas during normal conditions can be calculated from the Brody formula, which predicts CO_2 production during resting conditions:

$$\dot{V}_{CO_2}(\text{elimination/minute}) = \frac{\dot{V}}{\dot{Q}} \times 10 \times BW^{0.75}$$

where V_{CO_2} is exhaled carbon dioxide, V is flow, Q is perfusion, and BW is the body weight.

A measure of CO_2 in the airway is V_{TCO_2}, which can be calculated by dividing $\dot{V}_{CO_2}$ by the respiratory rate. When a stepwise increase of EIP is applied to a collapsed lung, V_{TCO_2} will increase with each pressure step because of the increased ventilation of already opened alveoli and the recruitment of collapsed areas, allowing for additional diffusion of CO_2 from the blood into the alveolar space.

With continued stepwise increase of EIP, V_{TCO_2} will continue to increase to a point where no additional alveoli can be recruited without impeding alveolar blood supply. Alveoli that are already opened could also be overdistended, thereby decreasing the diffusion of CO_2 into the alveoli with a drop in V_{TCO_2}.

POSITIVE END-EXPIRATORY PRESSURE

PEEP can be added to any mode of mechanical ventilation and is produced by a number of different devices regulating the pressure in the expiratory limb of the ventilator circuit. The effect of PEEP is, as a distending pressure, to increase the functional residual capacity (FRC) (volume of gas at the end of exhalation in the lung). By maintaining this pressure above the value that causes the lungs to collapse (closing pressure), atelectasis or alveolar collapse is minimized. The ultimate effect is decreased intrapulmonary shunting of the blood and improved arterial oxygenation.

PEEP increases intrathoracic pressure and therefore has potential hemodynamic consequences by transmitting the applied PEEP to transmural capillary pressure, affecting the right and left sides of the heart. The most dramatic effect of increased PEEP is decreased venous return to the right side of the heart. In children with normal cardiac function, this can easily be compensated for by increasing the intravascular volume by administering isotonic crystalloids or colloids.

MODES OF VENTILATION

Pressure-Controlled Ventilation

Pressure control is illustrated in Figure 43.1. During pressure-controlled ventilation, a pressure-limited breath is delivered during a preset inspiratory time at the preset respiratory rate. The tidal volume is determined by the preset pressure limit. The flow waveform is always decelerating under pressure control. Gas flows into the chest along the pressure gradient. As the alveolar pressure rises with increasing alveolar volume, the rate of flow drops off (as the pressure gradient narrows). The pressure is maintained for the duration of inspiration.

Pressure-controlled ventilation has several advantages. The higher initial flow associated with pressure-controlled ventilation more easily meets the patient's flow demands.

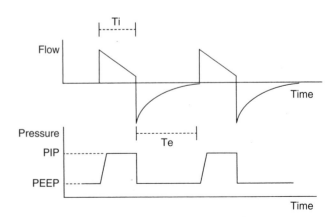

Figure 43.1 Pressure-controlled ventilation. Flow and airway pressure waveforms during pressure-controlled ventilation. Ti, inspiratory time; Te, expiratory time; PIP, peak inspiratory pressure; PEEP, positive end-expiratory pressure.

The peak inspiratory pressure (PIP) during pressure-controlled ventilation is less compared to that of the volume-controlled ventilation for the same tidal volume. During pressure-controlled breaths, the distribution of ventilation may be more even in a lung with heterogeneous mechanical properties. Pressure control is also useful in patients with an air leak; although volume is lost through the leak, the ventilator will continue to attempt to maintain the airway pressure for the duration of the inspiratory phase.

Pressure-controlled ventilation also has several disadvantages. It does not guarantee minute ventilation and, therefore, requires closer observation by the health care provider. The delivered tidal volume will change as the patient's lung mechanics or effort changes. Worsening of the patient's compliance or resistance results in hypoventilation and hypoxia. Conversely, an improvement in patient compliance or an increase in patient effort can lead to a higher tidal volume with alveolar overdistension (volutrauma).

Volume-Controlled Ventilation

Volume-controlled ventilation is illustrated in Figure 43.2. In this mode, the ventilator delivers a preset tidal volume with a constant flow during a preset inspiratory time at the preset respiratory rate. Airway and alveolar pressures are dependent variables and will rise or fall depending upon the changes in lung mechanics or patient effort.

Volume-controlled ventilation includes the following advantages. The clinician has control over minute ventilation and CO_2 clearance, provided there is only a small leak around the endotracheal tube; also, ventilator-induced lung injury due to alveolar overdistension (volutrauma) can be reduced.

Volume control ventilation also has the following disadvantages. The constant flow type of breath delivery in volume-controlled ventilation may not meet the patient's

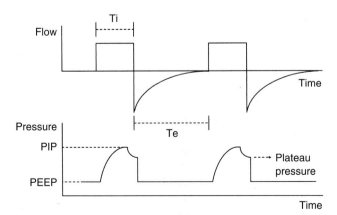

Figure 43.2 Volume-controlled ventilation. Flow and airway pressure waveforms during volume-controlled ventilation. *Ti*, inspiratory time; *Te*, expiratory time; PIP, peak inspiratory pressure; PEEP, positive end-expiratory pressure.

demand and may cause asynchrony between the patient's breathing efforts and the ventilator, leading to an increase in sedation. The PIP is higher in volume-controlled ventilation compared to that in pressure-controlled ventilation for the same tidal volume.

Proportional Assist Ventilation

Proportional assist ventilation (PAV) is designed such that, theoretically, the level of ventilatory support is proportional to patient effort. This mode has been designed to increase or decrease airway pressure by amplifying it proportional to the inspiratory flow and volume. Unlike other modes in which a preset volume or pressure determines the level of support, in PAV, the level of support is determined by an interaction between the patient and the ventilator.

Most of the studies utilizing PAV have been observational, with limited reports in children. In patients supported with PAV, there was a greater variability in tidal volume than that in pressure support ventilation (PSV). However, PAV appears to provide better comfort. Despite some potential advantages, there have been no studies demonstrating outcome benefits. PAV is currently not available in the United States.

Airway Pressure Release Ventilation

Airway pressure release ventilation (APRV) is essentially a high-level continuous positive airway pressure (CPAP) mode that is terminated for a very brief period. The elevated baseline helps in oxygenation, and the timed releases assist in carbon dioxide removal. This mode allows the patient to spontaneously breathe during all phases of the cycle. This is illustrated in Figure 43.3. APRV is different from other modes of ventilation in that it is based on an intermittent decrease in airway pressure, rather than an increase, to provide ventilation. APRV has been successfully used in various forms of respiratory failure and acute lung injury in both adults and children.

In addition to FIO_2, the operator-controlled parameters in APRV mode are: Phigh, Thigh, Plow, and Tlow. Phigh should be set at a level equivalent to the plateau pressure in a conventional mode when transitioning to APRV. If APRV is the first mode to be used, set Phigh at about 20 to 30 cm H_2O and Plow at zero, Thigh is set at about 4 to 6 seconds and Tlow is initially set at about 0.2 to 0.6 seconds. Tlow should then be adjusted on the basis of the expiratory gas flow waveform so that the expiratory flow falls to approximately 25% to 75% of the peak expiratory flow. Generally, Tlow will be shortened in restrictive disease and lengthened in obstructive disease.

The Phigh and Thigh regulate end-inspiratory lung volume and provide a significant contribution to the mean airway pressure (MAP). MAP correlates to mean alveolar volume and is critical for maintaining an increased surface area of open air spaces for diffusive gas movement. As a

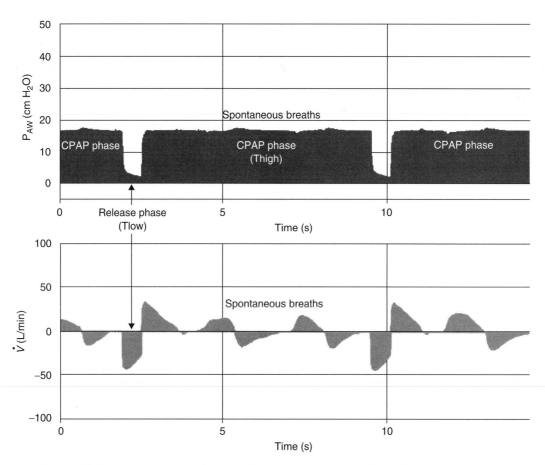

Figure 43.3 Airway pressure release ventilation (APRV). APRV is a form of continuous positive airway pressure (CPAP). The Phigh is equivalent to a CPAP level; Thigh is the duration of Phigh. The CPAP phase (Phigh) is intermittently released to a Plow for a brief duration (Tlow), reestablishing the CPAP level on the subsequent breath. Spontaneous breathing may be superimposed at both pressure levels and is independent of time-cycling. P_{AW}, airway pressure. (From ICON educational supplement 2004.)

result, these parameters control oxygenation and alveolar ventilation. Counterintuitive to conventional concepts of ventilation, the extension of Thigh can be associated with a decrease in Pa_{CO_2} as machine frequency decreases. Plow and Tlow regulate end-expiratory lung volume and should be optimized to reduce airway closure/derecruitment and not be used for primary ventilation adjustment. Generally, to maintain maximal recruitment, most of the Thigh occurs at the Phigh or CPAP level. To minimize derecruitment, the time (Tlow) at Plow is brief. Partial assistance (pressure support or automatic tube compensation [ATC]) can also be added to the spontaneous breaths. When the patient's underlying condition improves, APRV can be gradually weaned by lowering the Phigh and extending the Thigh. The goal is to arrive at straight CPAP.

APRV has the following advantages. Clinical studies have shown that oxygenation and ventilation can be maintained at lower pressures with APRV when compared to conventional ventilatory management. Additionally, improvements in hemodynamic parameters and splanchnic

perfusion have been reported. Because the patient is able to breathe spontaneously throughout the entire respiratory cycle with this mode of ventilation, the need for heavy sedation and neuromuscular blockade is much less than that needed for other methods of ventilation.

APRV, like all other modes, also has some disadvantages. APRV is a form of pressure-controlled ventilation, and therefore, mechanical tidal volume varies according to lung mechanics. Also, the spontaneous breaths during the long inflation period can further increase end-inspiratory lung volume beyond that set by the inflation pressure; therefore, APRV may be less effective as a strategy to limit alveolar overdistension.

Hybrid Techniques

Hybrid techniques, also described as dual-controlled ventilation, are modes that allow the clinician to set a volume target while the ventilator delivers a pressure-controlled breath. Dual control of the breath in these hybrid modes is

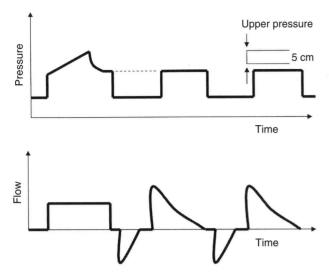

Figure 43.4 Pressure-regulated volume control. In PRVC, the first breath delivered to the patient is a volume-controlled breath. The measured plateau pressure is used as the pressure level for the next breath. The pressure is constant during the set inspiratory time and the flow is decelerating. The set tidal volume is achieved by automatic breath-by-breath pressure regulation. The ventilator adjusts the inspiratory pressure control according to the mechanical properties of the airways/lungs and thorax; the pressure is adjusted to a maximum of 3 cm H_2O per breath. Maximum available pressure is 5 cm H_2O below the preset pressure limit.

designed to be either intrabreath (within a breath) or interbreath (breath-to-breath). Examples of dual-control intrabreath modes are volume-assured pressure support (VAPS) and pressure augmentation. In these modes, the ventilator switches from pressure control to volume control during a single breath. Examples of dual-control interbreath modes are pressure-regulated volume control (PRVC), adaptive pressure ventilation, autoflow, and variable pressure control. In these modes, the pressure limit is increased or decreased automatically to maintain a clinician-selected target volume. Frequently used hybrid modes are discussed in the following sections.

Pressure-Regulated Volume Control

PRVC (or similarly adaptive pressure ventilation, autoflow, volume control, or variable pressure control) is a dual-control breath-to-breath mode (see Fig. 43.4). In PRVC, there is a variable decelerating flow pattern, with breaths being time-cycled. During PRVC, the pressure and volume are regulated. Therefore, all breaths are volume-targeted, with pressure adjusted to reach that volume target. The proposed advantage of this mode is a constant exhaled flow ($\dot{V}_E$) and tidal volume with automatic gradual reduction of the pressure limit as the patient's compliance improves.

Volume-Assured Pressure Support

VAPS and pressure augmentation are described as a dual control within a breath mode, in which the ventilator switches from pressure control to volume control within the breath. In this mode, the clinician chooses a volume target, and the breath begins as a pressure-limited, flow-cycled breath, either spontaneously (pressure support) or mechanically. When inspiratory flow has decelerated to the minimum set level, the delivered volume is measured. If the target volume has been met or exceeded, the breath ends. If the delivered volume has not been met, the volume-assured target breath is transitioned to a volume-targeted breath by prolonging inspiration at the minimum flow and by increasing the inspiratory pressure until the delivered volume has been obtained. The theoretic advantages of these modes are the ability to maintain constant tidal volume and minute volume, with a resultant lower work of breathing (WOB). Again, little evidence is available on its use in infants and children, and there have been no recent studies demonstrating its use.

Support Modes of Ventilation

Pressure Support Ventilation

PSV is a form of mechanical ventilatory support that delivers a clinician-selected amount of positive airway pressure to assist the spontaneous inspiratory effort of an intubated patient. The use of PSV is usually either as a low-level PSV to overcome the airflow resistance associated with the endotracheal tube or as a high-level PSV in the form of a stand-alone ventilatory support mode. The rationale for the use of low-level PSV is that an airflow resistance associated with an endotracheal tube produces an undesirably high pressure-volume (P/V) workload that may compromise comfort and ventilatory function during spontaneous breathing during intermittent mandatory ventilation (IMV) breaths.

Higher levels of PSV can be used as a stand-alone mode by applying the level of inspiratory pressure that is necessary for a desired tidal volume and minute ventilation.

Volume Support Ventilation

Volume support ventilation (VSV) is a volume-targeted mode of ventilation that is essentially pressure supported with tidal volume as a feedback. In this mode, the level of inspiratory pressure is adjusted with each breath to reach a targeted clinician-selected volume. All breaths are patient-triggered, pressure-limited, and flow-cycled.

A retrospective case series by Keenan and Martin, utilizing VSV in infants and children, demonstrated that both PIP and tidal volume were lowered when patients were switched to VSV.[3] This case series illustrates the theoretical advantage of utilizing VSV in weaning pediatric patients. As outlined in the section on "Weaning Mechanical Ventilation," VSV is utilized in patients once they demonstrate that they are ready to be weaned. This is best demonstrated when the patient begins to trigger the ventilator above the set rate. When this happens, the patient's tidal volume is reduced by 15%, and he/she is extubated once the PIP is

≤ 20 cm H_2O; the PEEP is <6 cm H_2O; there is a reversal of the cause for intubation; and there is stability of neurologic (Pediatric Glasgow Coma Score [PGCS] > 10), cardiovascular, and metabolic status. By using the PIP as a guide for extubation, the clinician utilizes an indirect measure of improvement of pulmonary compliance to guide clinical improvement. Also, hybrid modes such as VSV have an advantage in pediatric patients by maintaining a clinician-targeted volume even if there are changes in the patient's airway resistance (e.g., increased secretions) and/or pulmonary compliance (e.g., changes in position).

Closed-Loop Methods

An important factor in successful weaning from mechanical ventilation is the ability of the clinician to manipulate the ventilator so that it responds to the patient's physiologic respiratory demands by providing more or less support, as needed. If the ventilator itself can make these adjustments, on the basis of the patient's physiologic needs and ventilatory pattern, it would provide optimal weaning.[4] Experiments with the concept of closed-loop ventilation have been investigated by other researchers attempting to interface patients and ventilators, using computer-directed algorithms in this way.[5]

Automode

Automode is a patient-interactive mode that uses a computer-directed algorithm to direct both control and support modes, depending on the patient's needs. When automode is enabled, it allows the ventilator to switch between "volume control/volume support" (VC/VS), "pressure control/pressure support" (PC/PS), or "pressure-regulated volume control/volume support" (PRVC/VS), with spontaneously triggered breaths. When automode is activated, the ventilator switches to the corresponding support mode when the patient triggers two consecutive breaths. The ventilator remains in the support mode as long as the patient continues to breathe spontaneously. If the patient stops triggering, the ventilator automatically switches back to the clinician-selected control mode.

Volume-Assured Pressure Support/Pressure Augmentation

VAPS and pressure augmentation are described as a dual control within a breath mode, in which the ventilator switches from pressure control to volume control within the breath. The theoretical advantages of these modes are the ability to maintain constant tidal volume and minute volume, with a resultant lower WOB. Again, little evidence is available on its use in infants and children, and no recent studies demonstrate its use.

Automatic Tube Compensation

ATC utilizes calculated tracheal pressure to compensate for endotracheal tube resistance through a closed-loop control.[6] The calculation for determining tracheal pressure is:

$$\text{tracheal pressure} = \text{proximal airway pressure}$$
$$- (\text{tube coefficient} \times \text{flow}^2)$$

Therefore, the known resistive coefficients of the endotracheal tube and the measurement of instantaneous flow are used to apply pressure proportional to the resistance of the entire respiratory cycle. Theoretically, the interest in ATC has been in eliminating the imposed WOB during inspiration. As previously discussed during the description of PRVC and volume support, there is a theoretical advantage in the use of ATC in pediatric patients with small endotracheal tubes and increased potential for large swings in airway resistance because of the secretions that may limit the amount of support for the patient. The theoretical advantages of ATC are the ability (i) to compensate the WOB imposed by the artificial airway, (ii) to adjust the level of inspiratory flow to meet the patient's demand (similar to PAV), and (iii) to compensate for imposed expiratory resistance to reduce air trapping. However, the advantages are not always realized at the bedside. During expiration, the calculated tracheal pressure is greater than the airway pressure, and, under these conditions, negative airway pressure could reduce expiratory resistance. However, because ATC cannot reduce PEEP to <0 cm H_2O during exhalation, expiratory resistance may not be completely compensated. Also, kinks, bends, or secretions in the endotracheal tube may lead to changes in airflow resistance, again causing incomplete compensation. The evidence for the advantages of ATC is strictly anecdotal, and its role in pediatric patients is yet to be determined.

High-Frequency Ventilation

The theoretical benefits of using very low tidal volumes and very high respiratory rates in the ventilation of patients with acute hypoxemic respiratory failure have been appreciated for approximately 30 years.[5,7–9] During this time, the clinical experience with high-frequency ventilation has grown steadily. Although several different modalities of high-frequency ventilation exist, most clinical experience in neonatal, pediatric, and adult patients has been with the use of high-frequency oscillatory ventilation (HFOV).

Transitioning to High-Frequency Oscillatory Ventilation and High-Frequency Oscillatory Ventilation Strategies

Although the decision regarding when HFOV should be considered for a given patient is extremely individualized, some general concepts can be applied. For a pediatric or adult patient with a diffuse alveolar disease, such as ARDS, a requirement for mean airway pressure (mP_{AW}) >18 to 20 cm H_2O, $F_{IO_2} \geq 0.60$, and PIP ≥ 35 cm H_2O on conventional mechanical ventilation (CMV) should prompt consideration of a transition to HFOV.[10,11] Triggers for transitioning neonates to HFOV typically include substantially lower mP_{AW} and peak airway pressures. Regardless of the specific trigger, both animal and clinical data point to the earlier use of HFOV being more efficacious than the "rescue" usage in all age-groups studied.[10,12–16]

When a patient is transitioned from CMV to HFOV, the power setting, which drives the oscillating diaphragm, is adjusted to produce a ΔP, resulting in a visible chest "wiggle," with chest wall movement being visible from the clavicles to the lower abdomen or pelvis. Some investigators of HFOV in adult patients have suggested that an initial ΔP of "20 + P_{CO_2}" provides a reasonable approximation for beginning HFOV ventilation.[10,17] A range of typical initial frequency settings based on patient weight is shown in Table 43.3. Most commonly, the preset inspiratory/expiratory (I:E) ratio of 1:3 is used initially. Arterial blood gas analysis should be obtained soon after initiation of HFOV. Keeping in mind that pressure is attenuated by the endotracheal tube during HFOV, initial MAP (mP_{AW}) is typically set 3 to 8 cm H_2O above the most recent mP_{AW} used during CMV.[10,15,16,18,19] Two general strategies for HFOV management are commonly accepted—one is the "open lung" strategy for use in patients with diffuse alveolar consolidation, as in ARDS, and the other is a strategy aimed at minimizing preexisting air leak syndromes such as pneumothoraces or bronchopleural fistulae. If a patient with ARDS is to be supported and "open lung" ventilation pursued, a typical management scenario would be to increase the mP_{AW} slowly in 1 to 2 cm H_2O increments until oxygenation has improved to the point of allowing FiO_2 to be gradually reduced to <0.60. Alternatively, the lungs may be exposed to brief periods of very high mP_{AW} as an alveolar recruitment maneuver followed by a return to somewhat lower pressures.[20,21] Data supporting the use of sustained inflation-type recruitment maneuvers to improve lung volume recruitment and oxygenation exist in animal models and neonates with respiratory distress syndrome (RDS) who are supported with HFOV.[20,22–24] More recently, sustained inflation recruitment maneuvers in adult patients with ARDS who are ventilated with HFOV have been shown to significantly improve oxygenation.[25] Pediatric patients may benefit as well from similar recruitment maneuvers, particularly early in the transition to HFOV.[21]

Defining "optimal" lung volume during HFOV with an "open lung" strategy is a rather difficult task. Ideally, one would want to ventilate the patient in the zone of alveolar recruitment, above the closing point on the pressure–volume curve, and to avoid overdistension. In clinical practice, finding this optimal lung volume point is easier said than done. Although Thome et al. demonstrated in preterm infants that the mean lung volume is strongly related to mP_{AW}, this study clearly showed that lung volume could not be accurately predicted by mP_{AW} alone.[24] In practice, mP_{AW} is usually titrated upward till oxygenation improves enough to allow the gradual reduction of FiO_2

TABLE 43.3

TYPICAL INITIAL FREQUENCY SETTINGS BASED ON PATIENT WEIGHT

Patient Weight	Initial Frequency Setting
<2 kg	15 Hz
2–12 kg	10 Hz
13–20 kg	8 Hz
21–30 kg	7 Hz
31–50 kg	6 Hz
>50 kg	5 Hz

below 0.60 or until the chest radiograph shows evidence of lung hyperinflation (more than nine posterior ribs or flattened hemidiaphragms).[26] It is prudent practice to obtain a chest radiograph 1 to 2 hours after transitioning to HFOV to help assess lung recruitment and then to follow chest radiographs at least daily. A recent study by Brazelton et al. presents encouraging data regarding the use of respiratory inductive plethysmography (RIP) to monitor lung volume during HFOV.[27] In this study utilizing swines with saline lavage–induced acute lung injury, lung volumes measured by RIP correlated extremely well with the known lung volumes ($r^2 = 0.78$, p <0.00001) and could often identify critical opening and closing pressures of the injured lung.[27] In addition, electrical impedance tomography holds much promise as a bedside method of measuring regional lung volume changes during HFOV and has been used successfully in an animal model of HFOV.[28,29] It is hoped that these tools will soon be subjected to clinical trials and will prove useful in guiding optimization of mP_{AW} and lung volume in patients ventilated with HFOV.

In the only prospective trial of HFOV use in pediatric patients with severe hypoxemic respiratory failure, Arnold et al. used a similar strategy in patients with preexisting air leak syndromes.[15] MAP was gradually increased to the point at which an oxygen saturation ≥90% could be maintained with an FiO_2 ≤0.60; at this point MAP or pressure amplitude was then aggressively decreased, with oxygen saturation of 85% to 90% being tolerated and FiO_2 being increased as necessary. Once active air leak was resolved, MAP was again incrementally increased as tolerated to gradually reduce FiO_2.[15] In this same study, hypercarbia was tolerated as long as the arterial pH was ≥7.25. An early report of HFOV use in premature infants with pulmonary interstitial emphysema (PIE) noted an 80% survival in patients without septic shock.[30] In a neonatal piglet model of experimental pneumothorax, the air flow through the chest tube, as measured by a pneumotachometer, increased with increasing MAP, amplitude, and inspiratory time, whereas air leak diminished with increasing frequency, supporting the use of higher frequency and lower MAP and amplitudes to minimize air leak.[31]

Addressing hypercarbia after the institution of HFOV is typically achieved in a stepwise manner. First, the endotracheal tube patency and adequate lung recruitment should be verified. Next, ΔP should be increased in 2 to 3 cm H_2O increments until a maximal pressure amplitude is achieved, followed by a decrease in frequency in increments of 0.5 to 1 Hz.[15,19] Some investigators recommend that, following these maneuvers, the endotracheal tube cuff, if present, should be deflated to allow the additional escape of CO_2, with the bias flow being adjusted upward as necessary to maintain MAP.[10,17] Creation of an endotracheal tube cuff leak has been shown in mechanical test lung models to not only enhance CO_2 washout from the trachea but also attenuate transmission of distal oscillatory pressure and volume.[32] Investigators at the Wilford Hall Medical Center currently favor early, as opposed to late, utilization of an endotracheal tube cuff leak to enhance CO_2 elimination during HFOV in large patients, given that this technique could theoretically allow a more "lung-protective" ventilatory approach; that is, the use of lower ΔP and higher frequency with less distal pressure transmission.[10]

Weaning from High-Frequency Oscillatory Ventilation

Although weaning from HFOV is also an individualized process, some basic rules apply. Once a frequency, which allows adequate ventilation, has been found, no change or reduction of frequency is indicated. Rather, for hyperventilation, ΔP is reduced in increments of 1 to 2 cm H_2O. After F_{IO_2} has been gradually decreased to approximately 0.40, MAP is typically decreased in increments of 1 to 2 cm H_2O. Usually, a transition back to CMV is considered when the MAP is <20 to 22 cm H_2O and when the patient can tolerate suctioning. These guidelines are similar to the weaning protocol used by Arnold et al. in the only pediatric, randomized, prospective trial of HFOV.[15] For larger size patients ventilated with the SensorMedics 3100B (Viasys Healthcare, Yorba Linda, CA), the transition back to CMV is often considered when MAP is <24 cm H_2O and oxygen saturation is >88%, with F_{IO_2} ≤0.50.[17,33]

Pediatric Outcomes with High-Frequency Oscillatory Ventilation

After an initial pilot study suggesting the efficacy of HFOV in older pediatric patients with severe hypoxemic respiratory failure,[34] the only prospective, randomized trial of HFOV in this patient population was published by Arnold et al. in 1994.[15] This study was a multicenter trial of HFOV in patients with diffuse alveolar disease or air leak syndrome, with an oxygenation index (MAP × F_{IO_2} × 100 per Pa_{O_2}) >13 for 6 hours, and was designed as a crossover trial if the predefined criteria for treatment failure were met on the initial ventilatory arm to which the patients were randomized.[15] Conventional ventilator management in this study did not target low tidal volumes,

although it allowed some degree of permissive hypercapnia. The HFOV strategy utilized in this study involved fairly aggressive alveolar recruitment. Ultimately, 58 patients were analyzed, and although no differences in survival or length of ventilatory support were seen, significantly fewer patients in the HFOV group required supplemental oxygen at 30 days.[15] Also, the trial noted that failure to improve the oxygenation index at 24 hours after initiation of therapy was highly predictive of mortality.[15] Analysis of the subgroups of this study suggested that HFOV conferred greater benefits to the patients managed solely with HFOV, as opposed to those managed initially with CMV and then by crossing-over to HFOV. This insight lends credence to the idea that earlier use of HFOV in a pediatric population with ARDS is superior to the rescue use.[15,19] A multicenter, descriptive study of HFOV use in pediatric acute hypoxemic respiratory failure was published in 2000.[35] In this study, 232 patients managed with HFOV at ten centers across North America over an 18-month period were analyzed. Patients with and without preexisting lung disease were compared. The study found that patients without preexisting lung disease were significantly more likely to have a favorable response to HFOV than patients with preexisting lung disease.[35] Interestingly, the group with preexisting lung disease also had a significantly longer duration of CMV management before a trial of HFOV, again suggesting that earlier usage of HFOV in the disease process is better.[35] In a multivariate analysis of risk of mortality, only immunocompromise and the oxygenation index at 24 hours were significantly predictive of mortality.[35]

A fascinating retrospective analysis from the Czech Republic provides even more evidence for the superiority of the early use of HFOV as opposed to the rescue use. In this study, 26 consecutive patients older than 1 month with severe hypoxemic respiratory failure/ARDS were managed initially with lung-protective CMV strategies consisting of pressure control or pressure-regulated volume control ventilation with permissive hypercapnia, low tidal volume (<7 mL per kg), high PEEP, and sometimes tracheal gas insufflation (TGI).[36] Patients were changed to HFOV if they failed to respond adequately to the above strategy and were managed on HFOV with aggressive alveolar recruitment. Patients were stratified for the analysis on the basis of duration of CMV before HFOV, with early intervention defined as being within 24 hours. With the two groups evenly matched for severity of hypoxemia (oxygen index [OI] 27 vs. 33) and risk of mortality, this investigation found a 59% survival in early intervention patients versus 13% survival in patients managed with HFOV later in their disease course.[36] Another recently published small case series of pediatric patients with severe acute hypoxemic respiratory failure demonstrated substantial improvement in oxygenation and ventilation parameters when HFOV was instituted early.[37]

Although the use of high-frequency ventilation in lower airway diseases, characterized by air trapping and high airway resistance, was once thought to be contraindicated, some case reports have been published detailing the successful use of HFOV, with its active expiratory phase, in both pediatric bronchiolitis and status asthmaticus. One group reported the successful management of a young girl with severe status asthmaticus with HFOV; the group however cautioned that only centers with considerable HFOV experience should attempt this strategy.[38] Interestingly, in this patient, the investigators noted that adequate MAP was the primary determinant of successful CO_2 elimination, probably because of the opening of collapsed small airways.[38] Two other case series have reported the successful use of HFOV in infants with severe respiratory syncytial virus (RSV) bronchiolitis.[26,39,40] Recently, the group at Duke published its experience with six patients with hemoglobinopathies and acute chest syndrome managed with HFOV.[41] In this disease process, characterized by both ARDS and obstructive mucus airway plugging, the combination of HFOV and aggressive mucus plug removal by bronchoscopy was used successfully in all six patients, with no significant air leak developing.[41]

ADJUNCTS TO MECHANICAL VENTILATION

Noninvasive Mechanical Ventilation

Noninvasive mechanical ventilation (NIV) is defined as the application of positive-pressure ventilation through a face mask or nasal prongs. Outside the neonatal age-group, it is usually applied through a face mask. NIV can be used to prevent endotracheal intubation in patients or as an adjunct after a patient is extubated or to prevent reintubation. NIV can be administered as simple CPAP, so that the patient receives positive pressure, but it offers no assistance to the patient's effort. Today, patients are more commonly placed on a separate NIV device or through a ventilator with PSV.

Tracheal Gas Insufflation

TGI is a method that uses a catheter to introduce a flow of gas into the trachea.[42] A number of techniques have been described. These techniques include the continuous insufflation of oxygen, tracheal oxygen administration, transtracheal jet ventilation, high-frequency jet ventilation, and intratracheal pulmonary ventilation (ITPV). None of these have extensive experience in pediatric patients. ITPV is a method in which a continuous-flow catheter is introduced into the endotracheal tube, with the tip of the catheter placed 1 cm from the carina. The catheter has a reverse-thrust catheter, in which gas exiting the catheter is directed cephalad. The proposed advantage of this technique is to reduce tidal volume and, therefore, alveolar pressure. This technique has been reported in both neonatal and pediatric patients.[43]

Partial Liquid Ventilation

Fuhrman et al. first described partial liquid ventilation (PLV) in 1991.[44] Liquid ventilation has been used in animals with and without lung disease to improve lung function. During liquid ventilation, perfluorocarbons are instilled into the lungs to alter surface tension, recruit and maintain FRC, and improve ventilation–perfusion (V/Q) matching. Perfluorocarbons have a high solubility for oxygen and carbon dioxide, in addition to a low surface tension. In perfluorocarbon-associated gas exchange (PAGE), perfluorocarbons are instilled in the lung at a dose of 15 to 30 mL per kg and are used in parallel with mechanical ventilation. After instillation and establishment of a liquid FRC, gas ventilation with the conventional ventilator is resumed. With PAGE, the perfluorocarbons are oxygenated during inspiration by pushing oxygen down the airway into the liquid-filled alveoli, where it forms bubbles. During exhalation, CO_2 is purged from the perfluorocarbons by the intrinsic elastic recoil of the bubbles, which expels the gas from the lungs. Gas escapes during exhalation because of its lower viscosity and density, and the inertia of the liquid. Recently, there has been evidence that perfluorocarbon may have an anti-inflammatory action. The use of liquid ventilation at this time is experimental. Despite numerous animal studies indicating the benefits of PLV, human data has been limited to case reports and series, with no randomized controlled studies having been published. The early published studies established the feasibility of PLV in patients supported by other means such as extracorporeal membrane oxygenation. Leach et al.[45] presented data in 13 premature infants who failed CMV with improved oxygenation, decreased $PaCO_2$, and improved pulmonary compliance. Survival in the infants who received PLV was 62%. Phase II trials in adults and children have only been published in the abstract form. Despite the potential of this therapy, it has yet to meet the criteria for clinical use.

Prone Positioning

Prone positioning has been shown to have beneficial effects by improving oxygenation and ventilation in patients with ARDS.[46–49] In patients on mechanical ventilation who are in the supine position, the heart, great vessels, and a large portion of the abdominal contents exert traction and forces on the lung. Although the mechanism of improved oxygenation in the prone position is multifactorial, the overall beneficial effect is due to improved V/Q matching and decreased physiologic shunt. Change from the supine to the prone position allows the recruitment of the previously atelectatic dorsal regions of the lung, leading to more homogeneous ventilation. Perfusion, which is relatively gravity-independent, is better matched to ventilation and leads to less V/Q heterogeneity.[50,51] Convincing improvements in outcome have not been shown, and the pediatric literature on the effects of prone positioning is scarce. A recent study of 180 patients stopped after an interim analysis of 94 patients because a higher oxygenation index in the prone group demonstrated no improvement in clinical outcomes in pediatric patients managed with prone positioning.[52]

WEANING MECHANICAL VENTILATION

Weaning from mechanical ventilatory support has traditionally been a mix of science and art. Although there is relative consensus as to when mechanical ventilation should be initiated in the presence of respiratory insufficiency, the management of pediatric patients during recovery from respiratory failure remains largely subjective and is predominately determined by institutional or individual practices or preferences. Weaning patients from mechanical ventilators continues to be one of the most perplexing, yet vital, issues in caring for mechanically ventilated patients, especially critically ill infants and children. Weaning patients from mechanical ventilation requires waiting until the disease process that caused the patient to need assisted ventilation reverses and then successfully decreasing ventilator support to a level that allows for extubation. Successfully weaning patients off the ventilator rapidly is of utmost importance because of the inherent risks involved in such an invasive medical intervention.[53] Restoring patients to a physiologic state of normal spontaneous ventilation is critical to their long-term prognosis.

Clinical Trials of Weaning

There have been a limited number of clinical trials of weaning from mechanical ventilation in pediatric patients. In adult patients, numerous studies have demonstrated the advantage of certain weaning strategies including spontaneous breathing trials and respiratory therapist-driven protocols.

There have been three spontaneous breathing trials to date that were designed to demonstrate the advantage of one weaning strategy in infants and children. Farias et al.[54] studied 257 consecutive infants and children who received mechanical ventilation for at least 48 hours and were deemed ready to undergo a breathing trial by their primary physician. Patients were randomly assigned to undergo a trial of breathing with either a pressure support of 10 cm H_2O or a T-piece. Bedside measurements of respiratory function were obtained immediately before discontinuation of mechanical ventilation and within the first 5 minutes of breathing through a T-piece. The primary physicians were unaware of these measurements; however, the decision to extubate a patient at the end of the breathing trial was made by them. Of the 125 patients in the pressure support group, 99 (79.2%) completed the breathing trial

and were extubated, but 15 of them (15.1%) required reintubation within 48 hours. Of the 132 patients in the T-piece group, 102 (77.5%) completed the breathing trial and were extubated, but 13 of them (12.7%) required reintubation within 48 hours. The percentage of patients who remained extubated for 48 hours after the breathing trial did not differ in the pressure support and the T-piece groups (67.2% vs. 67.4%; $p = 0.97$).

The Process of Weaning

Weaning is a dynamic process that usually begins during patient recovery at some undefined point, determined by the bedside physician. The bias resulting from the physician's decision inevitably decreases the reproducibility of any study and makes the results less reliable for extrapolation to clinical practice. The standard indices for assessing patient "weanability" include the following: (i) The resolution of the etiology of respiratory failure and attainment of stable respiratory status (i.e., decreased FIO_2 and PEEP level; absence of tachypnea with a respiratory rate <60 for infants younger than 12 months, <40 for the preschool and school-aged child, and <30 for adolescents; absence of acidosis [pH <7.35]; or hypercapnia [PCO_2 >60 mm Hg]; the parameters to indirectly assess oxygenation and compliance include PaO_2:FIO_2 ratio >267 [PaO_2 >80 mm Hg on an FIO_2 of 0.3] and oxygen saturation [SpO_2] >94% on an FIO_2 ≤0.5, PIP <20 cm H_2O, and PEEP ≤5 cm H_2O) and adequate respiratory muscle function (acceptable respiratory effort); (ii) hemodynamic stability, including no evidence of shock—this criterion includes good perfusion (e.g., capillary refill <3 seconds), age-appropriate blood pressure (above −2 SD cutoff for age), and good cardiac function (e.g., no requirement of infusions of vasoactive and/or inotropic medications, with the exception of dopamine ≤5 μg/kg/minute); (iii) neurologic function—the patients must be easily arousable to verbal or physical stimulation (e.g., Pediatric Glasgow Coma Score ≥11) and must be capable of moving an uninjured upper and lower extremity against gravity; and (iv) metabolic factors—patients must have acceptable serum potassium, magnesium, and phosphorus concentrations.

The decision to wean the patient may also have an impact on the length of mechanical ventilation. Decision-making by respiratory care practitioners (RCP) has long been felt to have the potential to reduce the length of mechanical ventilation because of the availability of the respiratory therapist at the bedside for frequent patient assessments. Respiratory therapist–driven weaning protocols are being examined as an alternative to current standard practices of weaning.[55,56] It is thought by some health care providers that RCPs may provide an optimal weaning method. RCPs classically perform diagnostic tests such as blood gas analyses, pulse oximetry, end-tidal CO_2 measurements, and airway function screenings; in addition, they have the expertise to interpret the information obtained from these tests. According to one recent study in adults, weaning and extubation of ventilated patients by RCPs reduced the length of mechanical ventilation.[55] In this control trial of 300 adult patients who were randomized to daily screening and spontaneous breathing trials by RCPs, there was a 25% reduction in the median number of days of mechanical ventilation in the intervention group. A study of 223 pediatric patients by Schultz et al.[57] demonstrated a decrease in the total length of ventilation, weaning time, and time to extubation in patients weaned by an RCP-driven protocol versus a physician-directed weaning.

Adjuncts to Weaning

Pharmacologic Agents

The routine administration of corticosteroids is a frequent adjunct to extubation. The anti-inflammatory effects of steroids form the basis of this approach. Two well-designed trials[58,59] in which dexamethasone therapy was provided before extubation in children have unequivocally demonstrated that steroids reduce postextubation stridor. The inferences from these trials were significant because they were truly blinded studies. In contrast to the demonstrated effect on stridor, the effect of corticosteroids on reintubation is unclear. In one of the two studies, 7 of the 32 patients who did not receive steroids required reintubation, in contrast to none of the 31 patients who received steroids. The trend in the other study was in the opposite direction, with 4 of the 77 children who did not receive steroids and 9 of 76 children who received steroids requiring reintubation. It is unclear why these studies demonstrated opposite results. For those who believe that dexamethasone therapy is warranted only if it prevents reintubation, the question remains unanswered. The two trials[59,60] found reintubation rates of >10%.

Heliox

After endotracheal extubation, the upper and total airway resistances may frequently be increased, resulting in a high inspiratory effort to breathe. A few patients, ranging from 5% to 16%, develop postextubation airway obstruction and frank respiratory distress.[61] In addition, a substantial number of patients develop inspiratory distress after extubation, leading to reintubation.[62,63] In these patients, an increase in upper airway and total inspiratory resistance may also lead to respiratory distress. After tracheal extubation, upper and total airway resistances may frequently be increased, resulting in an increase in the inspiratory effort to breathe. As discussed earlier, infants and children have both anatomic and physiologic differences with adults that predispose them to airway edema and dysfunction.

Helium-oxygen (HeO_2) mixture has a low density and a high kinematic viscosity, allowing for a reduction in airway resistance. Some studies showed that this mixture could have beneficial effects in the treatment of upper airway obstruction.[64] The use of HeO_2 mixture in adults[65] and in children[66] with upper airway obstruction has been reported in several anecdotal series and a few studies, and it has become one of the more accepted indications for HeO_2 use.[64] Although the effect of HeO_2 was shown mainly through observational studies, the fact that the immediate improvement obtained with HeO_2 breathing was reversed when it was discontinued even briefly suggested an independent beneficial effect of the gas related to its physical properties.

Noninvasive Mechanical Ventilatory Support

The process of discontinuing mechanical ventilation must balance the risk of complications due to unnecessary delays in extubation with the risk of complications due to premature discontinuation and the need for reintubation. The use of NIPPV is a promising therapy after the failure of extubation but has not yet been shown to reduce the need for reintubation or postintubation mortality.[67] In principle, because most pediatric patients require reintubation owing to poor or excessive effort,[68] noninvasive support may provide the patient with a bridge to extubation. The use of noninvasive ventilatory support in pediatric patients has limitations, primarily because of technical reasons. For noninvasive ventilatory support to function properly, the mask or nasal prongs must be adequately sealed to the patient. Because of the varying physical sizes and the lack of cooperation of pediatric patients, noninvasive mechanical ventilatory support can be difficult in this patient population.

Recognition of Weaning Failure

Failure of weaning can be categorized by increased respiratory load or decreased respiratory capacity. Increased respiratory load is represented by increased elastic load (e.g., unresolved lung disease, secondary pneumonia, abdominal distension, and hyperinflated lungs), increased resistive load (e.g., thickened airway secretions, partially occluded endotracheal tube, and upper airway obstruction), or increased minute ventilation (e.g., pain and irritability, sepsis/hyperthermia, and metabolic acidosis). Decreased respiratory capacity is represented by decreased respiratory drive (e.g., sedation, central nervous system [CNS] infection, traumatic brain injury, and hypocapnia/alkalosis), muscular dysfunction (e.g., muscular catabolism and weakness [malnutrition], and severe electrolyte disturbances), and neuromuscular disorder (e.g., diaphragmatic dysfunction, prolonged neuromuscular blockade, and cervical spinal injury).

Extubation failure with subsequent reintubation in pediatric patients ranges between 14% and 24%.[54,69,70] In a recent study of 632 pediatric patients, the failure rate of planned extubation was 4.9%. The rate of failure increased with the length of time the patients received mechanical ventilation, with patients ventilated for >24 hours having a failure rate of 6.0% and those ventilated for >48 hours having a rate of 7.9%.[71] Predicting extubation outcome in patients is usually based upon clinical judgment. However, attempts have been made to identify specific predictors of extubation failure. The success of these predictors has been mixed. Baumeister et al.[72] adapted adult integrated indexes for pediatric patients by normalizing the tidal volume and dynamic compliance to body weight. Extubation failure was defined as reintubation within 24 hours; the failure rate was 19%. In another study of pediatric patients Venkataraman et al.[68] studied 208 patients ventilated for at least 24 hours and identified the criteria for low risk (<10%) and high risk (25%) of extubation failure on the basis of direct measurements of pulmonary function. For this study, the percentage of patients who required reintubation within 48 hours, excluding those who failed secondary to upper airway obstruction, was 16.3%. Thirty-four of the 208 patients who were studied were reintubated, with an overall failure rate of 16.3%. Of the patients that failed extubation, 65% required reintubation secondary to poor or excessive effort. Extubation failure increased significantly, with decreasing tidal volume indexed to body weight of a spontaneous breath, increasing FiO_2, increasing MAP, increasing oxygenation index, increasing fraction of total minute ventilation provided by the ventilator, increasing peak ventilatory inspiratory pressure, or decreasing mean inspiratory flow.

REFERENCES

1. Heulitt MJ, Anders M, Benham D. Acute respiratory distress syndrome in pediatric patients: Redirecting therapy to reduce iatrogenic lung injury. *Respir Care.* 1995;40:74–85.
2. Heulitt MJ, Desmond B. Lung protective strategies in pediatric patients with ARDS. *Respir Care.* 1998;43(11):952–960.
3. Keenan HT, Martin LC. Volume support ventilation in infants and children: Analysis of a case series. *Respir Care.* 1997;42(3):281–287.
4. Ranieri VM. Optimization of patient-ventilator interactions: Closed-loop technology to turn the century [editorial]. *Intensive Care Med.* 1997;23(9):936–939.
5. Marchak BE, Thompson WK, Duffty P, et al. Treatment of RDS by high-frequency oscillatory ventilation: A preliminary report. *J Pediatr.* 1981;99(2):287–292.
6. Guttmann J, Haberthur C, Mols G. Automatic tube compensation. *Respir Care Clin N Am.* 2001;7:475–501.
7. Lunkenheimer PP, Rafflenbeul W, Keller H, et al. Application of transtracheal pressure oscillations as a modification of "diffusing respiration." *Br J Anaesth.* 1972;44(6):627.
8. Lunkenheimer PP, Frank I, Ising H, et al. Intrapulmonary gas exchange during simulated apnea due to transtracheal periodic intrathoracic pressure changes. *Anaesthesist.* 1973;22(5):232–238.
9. Butler WJ, Bohn DJ, Bryan AC, et al. Ventilation by high-frequency oscillation in humans. *Anesth Analg.* 1980;59(8):577–584.
10. Derdak S. High-frequency oscillatory ventilation for acute respiratory distress syndrome in adult patients. *Crit Care Med.* 2003;31(Suppl 4):S317–S323.
11. Doctor A, Arnold J. Mechanical support of acute lung injury: Options for strategic ventilation. *New Horiz.* 1997;7:359–373.
12. deLemos RA, Coalson JJ, deLemos JA, et al. Rescue ventilation with high frequency oscillation in premature baboons with hyaline membrane disease. *Pediatr Pulmonol.* 1992;12(1):29–36.
13. Gerstmann DR, Minton SD, Stoddard RA, et al. The Provo multicenter early high-frequency oscillatory ventilation trial: Improved pulmonary and clinical outcome in respiratory distress syndrome. *Pediatrics.* 1996;98(6 Pt 1):1044–1057.
14. Courtney SE, Durand DJ, Asselin JM, et al. High-frequency oscillatory ventilation versus conventional mechanical ventilation for very-low-birth-weight infants. *N Engl J Med.* 2002;347(9):643–652.
15. Arnold JH, Hanson JH, Toro-Figuero LO, et al. Prospective, randomized comparison of high-frequency oscillatory ventilation and conventional mechanical ventilation in pediatric respiratory failure. *Crit Care Med.* 1994;22(10):1530–1539.
16. Fort P, Farmer C, Westerman J, et al. High-frequency oscillatory ventilation for adult respiratory distress syndrome–a pilot study. *Crit Care Med.* 1997;25(6):937–947.
17. Derdak S, Mehta S, Stewart TE, et al. High-frequency oscillatory ventilation for acute respiratory distress syndrome in adults: A randomized, controlled trial. *Am J Respir Crit Care Med.* 2002;166(6):801–808.
18. Ferguson ND, Stewart TE. The use of high-frequency oscillatory ventilation in adults with acute lung injury. *Respir Care Clin N Am.* 2001;7(4):647–661.
19. Ventre KM, Arnold JH. High frequency oscillatory ventilation in acute respiratory failure. *Paediatr Respir Rev.* 2004;5(4):323–332.
20. Byford LJ, Finkler JH, Froese AB. Lung volume recruitment during high-frequency oscillation in atelectasis-prone rabbits. *J Appl Physiol.* 1988;64(4):1607–1614.
21. Froese A, Kinsella JP. High-frequency oscillatory ventilation: Lessons from the neonatal/pediatric experience. *Crit Care Med.* 2005;33(Suppl. 3):S115–S121.
22. Kolton M, Cattran CB, Kent G, et al. Oxygenation during high-frequency ventilation compared with conventional mechanical ventilation in two models of lung injury. *Anesth Analg.* 1982;61(4):323–332.
23. Froese AB, Butler PO, Fletcher WA, et al. High-frequency oscillatory ventilation in premature infants with respiratory failure: A preliminary report. *Anesth Analg.* 1987;66(9):814–824.
24. Thome U, Topfer A, Schaller P, et al. Effects of mean airway pressure on lung volume during high-frequency oscillatory ventilation of preterm infants. *Am J Respir Crit Care Med.* 1998;157(4 Pt 1):1213–1218.
25. Ferguson ND, Chiche JD, Kacmarek RM, et al. Combining high-frequency oscillatory ventilation and recruitment maneuvers in adults with early acute respiratory distress syndrome: The Treatment with Oscillation and an Open Lung Strategy (TOOLS) Trial pilot study. *Crit Care Med.* 2005;33(3):479–486.
26. Priebe GP, Arnold JH. High-frequency oscillatory ventilation in pediatric patients. *Respir Care Clin N Am.* 2001;7(4):633–645.
27. Brazelton TB 3rd, Watson KF, Murphy M, et al. Identification of optimal lung volume during high-frequency oscillatory ventilation using respiratory inductive plethysmography. *Crit Care Med.* 2001;29(12):2349–2359.
28. van Genderingen HR, van Vught AJ, Jansen JR. Regional lung volume during high-frequency oscillatory ventilation by electrical impedance tomography. *Crit Care Med.* 2004;32(3):787–794.
29. Wolf GK, Arnold JH. Noninvasive assessment of lung volume: Respiratory inductance plethysmography and electrical impedance tomography. *Crit Care Med.* 2005;33(Suppl 3):S163–S169.
30. Clark RH, Gerstmann DR, Null DM, et al. Pulmonary interstitial emphysema treated by high-frequency oscillatory ventilation. *Crit Care Med.* 1986;14(11):926–930.
31. Ellsbury DL, Klein JM, Segar JL. Optimization of high-frequency oscillatory ventilation for the treatment of experimental pneumothorax. *Crit Care Med.* 2002;30(5):1131–1135.
32. Van de Kieft M, Dorsey D, Morison D, et al. High-frequency oscillatory ventilation: Lessons learned from mechanical test lung models. *Crit Care Med.* 2005;33(Suppl 3):S142–S147.
33. Mehta S, Granton J, MacDonald RJ, et al. High-frequency oscillatory ventilation in adults: The Toronto experience. *Chest.* 2004;126(2):518–527.
34. Arnold JH, Truog RD, Thompson JE, et al. High-frequency oscillatory ventilation in pediatric respiratory failure. *Crit Care Med.* 1993;21(2):272–278.
35. Arnold JH, Anas NG, Luckett P, et al. High-frequency oscillatory ventilation in pediatric respiratory failure: A multicenter experience. *Crit Care Med.* 2000;28(12):3913–3919.

36. Fedora M, Klimovic M, Seda M, et al. Effect of early intervention of high-frequency oscillatory ventilation on the outcome in pediatric acute respiratory distress syndrome. *Bratisl Lek Listy.* 2000;101(1):8–13.

37. Ben Jaballah N, Mnif K, Bouziri A, et al. High-frequency oscillatory ventilation in paediatric patients with acute respiratory distress syndrome-early rescue use. *Eur J Pediatr.* 2005;164(1):17–21.

38. Duval EL, van Vught AJ. Status asthmaticus treated by high-frequency oscillatory ventilation. *Pediatr Pulmonol.* 2000;30(4): 350–353.

39. Duval EL, Leroy PL, Gemke RJ, et al. High-frequency oscillatory ventilation (HFOV) in RSV-bronchiolitis patients. *Respir Med.* 1999;93:435–440.

40. Medbo S, Finne PH, Hansen TW. Respiratory syncytial virus pneumonia ventilated with high-frequency oscillatory ventilation. *Acta Paediatr.* 1997;86:766–768.

41. Wratney AT, Gentile MA, Hamel DS, et al. Successful treatment of acute chest syndrome with high-frequency oscillatory ventilation in pediatric patients. *Respir Care.* 2004;49(3):263–269.

42. Ravenscraft SA. Tracheal gas insufflation: Adjunct to conventional mechanical ventilation. *Respir Care.* 1996;41(2):105–111.

43. Makhoul IR, Bar-Joseph G, Blazer S, et al. Intratracheal pulmonary ventilation in premature infants and children with intractable hypercapnia. *ASAIO J.* 1998;44(1):82–88.

44. Fuhrman BP, Paczan PR, DeFrancisis M. Perfluorocarbon-associated gas exchange. *Crit Care Med.* 1991;19(5):712–722.

45. Leach CL, Greenspan JS, Rubenstein SD, et al. Partial liquid ventilation with perflubron in premature infants with severe respiratory distress syndrome. *N Engl J Med.* 1996;335(11):814–815.

46. Oczenski W, Hormann C, Keller C, et al. Recruitment maneuvers during prone positioning in patients with acute respiratory distress syndrome. *Crit Care Med.* 2005;33(1):54–61.

47. Guerin C, Gaillard S, Lemasson S, et al. Effects of systematic prone positioning in hypoxemic acute respiratory failure: A randomized controlled trial. *JAMA.* 2004;292(19):2379–2387.

48. Gattinoni L, Vagginelli F, Carlesso E, et al. Prone-Supine Study Group. Decrease in PaCO$_2$ with prone position is predictive of improved outcome in acute respiratory distress syndrome. *Crit Care Med.* 2003;31(12):2727–2733.

49. Gattinoni L, Tognoni G, Pesenti A, et al. Effects of prone positioning on the survival of patients with acute respiratory failure. *N Engl J Med.* 2001;345(8):568–573.

50. Pelosi P, Brazzi L, Gattinoni L. Prone position in acute respiratory distress syndrome. *Eur Respir J.* 2002;20:1017–1028.

51. Messerole E, Peine P, Wittkopp S, et al. The pragmatics of prone positioning. *Am J Respir Crit Care Med.* 2002;165:1359–1363.

52. Curley MAQ, Fineman LD, Cvijanovich N, et al. Prone positioning in pediatric acute lung injury. Results of a randomized controlled clinical trial. *Pediatr Crit Care Med.* 2005;6(2):244.

53. Heulitt MJ, Anders M, Benham D. Acute respiratory distress syndrome in pediatric patients: Redirecting therapy to reduce iatrogenic lung injury. *Respir Care.* 1995;40(1):74–85.

54. Farias JA, Retta A, Alia I, et al. A comparison of two methods to perform a breathing trial before extubation in pediatric intensive care patients. *Intensive Care Med.* 2001;27(10):1649–1654.

55. Ely EW, Baker AM, Dunagan DP, et al. Effects on the duration of mechanical ventilation of identifying patients capable of breathing spontaneously. *N Engl J Med.* 1996;335(25):1864–1869.

56. Horst HM, Mouro D, Hall-Jenssens RA, et al. Decrease in ventilation time with a standardized weaning process. *Arch Surg.* 1998; 133:483–489.

57. Schultz TR, Lin RJ, Watzman M, et al. Weaning children from mechanical ventilation: A prospective randomized trial of protocol directed versus physician directed weaning. *Respir Care.* 2001;46(8):772–782.

58. Tellez DW, Galvis AG, Storgion SA, et al. Dexamethasone in the prevention of postextubation stridor in children. *J Pediatr.* 1991;118:289–294.

59. Anene O, Meert KL, Uy H, et al. Dexamethasone for the prevention of postextubation airway obstruction: A prospective, randomized, double-blind, placebo-controlled trial. *Crit Care Med.* 1996;24:1666–1669.

60. Harel Y, Vardi A, Quigley R, et al. Extubation failure due to post-extubation stridor is better correlated with neurologic impairment than with upper airway lesions in critically ill pediatric patients. *Int J Pediatr Otorhinolaryngol.* 1997;39:147–158.

61. Anene O, Meert KL, Uy H, et al. Dexamethasone for the prevention of postextubation airway obstruction: A prospective, randomized, double-blind, placebo-controlled trial. *Crit Care Med.* 1996;24:1966–1969.

62. Epstein SK, Ciubotaru RL, Wong JB. Effect of failed extubation on the outcome of mechanical ventilation. *Chest.* 1997;112:186–192.

63. Epstein SK, Ciubotaru RL. Independent effects of etiology of failure and time to reintubation on outcome for patients failing extubation. *Am J Respir Crit Care Med.* 1998;158:489–493.

64. Manthous CA, Morgan S, Pohlman A, et al. Heliox in the treatment of airflow obstruction: A critical review of the literature. *Respir Care.* 1997;42:1034–1042.

65. Barach A. The use of helium in the treatment of asthma and obstructive lesions in the larynx and trachea. *Ann Intern Med.* 1935;9:739–765.

66. Duncan P. Efficacy of helium-oxygen mixtures in the management of severe viral and post-intubation croup. *Can Anaesth Soc J.* 1979;26:206–212.

67. Esteban A, Frutos-Vivar F, Ferguson ND, et al. Noninvasive positive-pressure ventilation for respiratory failure after extubation. *N Engl J Med.* 2004;350(24):2452–2460.

68. Venkataraman ST, Nadeem K, Brown A. Validation of predictors of extubation success and failure in mechanically ventilated infants and children. *Crit Care Med.* 2002;28(8):2991–2996.

69. Randolph AG, Wypij D, Venkataraman ST, et al. Pediatric Acute Lung Injury and Sepsis Investigators (PALISI) Network. Effect of mechanical ventilator weaning protocols on respiratory outcomes in infants and children: A randomized controlled trial. *JAMA.* 2002;288(20):2561–2568.

70. Farias JA, Alia I, Retta A, et al. An evaluation of extubation failure predictors in mechanically ventilated infants and children. *Intensive Care Med.* 2002;28(6):752–757.

71. Edmunds S, Weiss I, Harrison R. Extubation failure in a large pediatric ICU population. *Chest.* 2001;119(3):897–900.

72. Baumeister BL, el-Khatib M, Smith PG, et al. Evaluation of predictors of weaning from mechanical ventilation in pediatric patients. *Pediatr Pulmonol.* 1997;24(5):344–352.

Extracorporeal Techniques

44

Steven A. Conrad   *Heidi J. Dalton*

Extracorporeal life support (ECLS) is a technique to support patients with severe but potentially reversible cardiac or respiratory failure for whom conventional therapy is inadequate, allowing time for organ recovery. ECLS comprises a family of extracorporeal techniques, the most common of which is extracorporeal membrane oxygenation (ECMO). The extracorporeal circuit is a modification of the heart–lung machine used for intraoperative cardiopulmonary bypass.

ECMO offers an effective means of support to patients, failing other currently available techniques for support of respiratory or cardiac failure. Many patient populations and diagnoses are shown in Tables 44.1 to 44.3 and Figure 44.1 with their outcomes. Although patients with adult respiratory distress syndrome are not shown in Figure 44.1, the diagnoses and outcome are very similar to those seen in pediatric patients. The largest change in non-neonatal ECMO over the past few years is the variety of patients to whom it has been applied. Immunocompromised patients and those with recent trauma, tracheal surgery, burns, smoke inhalation, septic shock, sickle cell disease, and toxic ingestions with cardiopulmonary collapse are types who have received successful ECMO therapy. The multiple exclusion criteria used in the early days of ECMO have now been fairly well eliminated, with each potential patient being considered on a case-by-case basis. Even patients with known bleeding disorders such as hemophilia have received ECMO support successfully. The newest category of ECLS use, designated as *"extracorporeal cardiopulmonary resuscitation (ECPR),"* is in patients during cardiac arrest. The 40% survival observed in these patients makes ECLS a viable option in select patients, especially those in the postoperative period of congenital heart defects repair. Although no specific ECLS criteria have been universally accepted, Table 44.4 illustrates some common parameters assessed during ECLS evaluation. The initiation of ECMO results in several beneficial changes in circulatory function, including lowering pulmonary vascular resistance and reducing right atrial pressure. Improved oxygenation and ventilation allows reduction of ventilatory pressures and breathing rate, which helps limit ventilator-induced lung injury, provides an optimal environment to promote lung healing, and reduces ongoing inflammatory responses in the lung. This may help limit secondary organ dysfunction, which is often an end result of this process. Reduction of intrathoracic pressure from reduced ventilator settings may also improve cardiac function.

THE EXTRACORPOREAL LIFE SUPPORT CIRCUIT

Aspects of the ECLS circuit vary among centers, but the general components are relatively standard. ECLS circuits employ a venous cannula for blood drainage, an optional venous reservoir, a blood pump, an artificial lung, a heat exchanger, and an arterial or venous return cannula (see Figs. 44.2 and 44.3).

Cannulae

Obtaining adequate vascular access for blood drainage and reinfusion is pivotal to adequate extracorporeal support. Neonates and infants require cannulae ranging in size from 8 to 14 French (Fr), with the smaller sizes being used for arterial access. Cannulae in adolescents and adults range in size from 16 to 32 Fr. Because vascular access is the limiting

TABLE 44.1

EXTRACORPOREAL LIFE SUPPORT PATIENT POPULATION AND OUTCOME

Category of Life Support	Number of Cases	Number Survived Because of ECLS	Number Survived to Discharge or Transfer
Neonatal respiratory	19,463	16,623 (85%)	14,942 (77%)
Pediatric respiratory	2,883	1,847 (64%)	1,608 (56%)
Adult respiratory	1,025	610 (60%)	542 (53%)
Cardiac	5,902	3,357 (57%)	2,367 (40%)
ECPR	635	338 (53%)	247 (39%)
Total	**29,908**	**22,775 (76%)**	**19,706 (66%)**

ECLS, extracorporeal life support; ECPR, extracorporeal cardiopulmonary resuscitation.
Data adapted from the International ELSO Registry Report, January 2005, www.elso.med.umich.edu/ Registry.htm Ann Arbor, MI.

factor in obtaining flow, the largest cannulae that can be safely placed in a given vessel are typically used.

Double-lumen cannulae, available in sizes from 12 to 18 Fr, simplify venovenous access in patients up to 10 to 12 kg and can be inserted percutaneously.[1] The cannula has a drainage lumen with two ports; a distal port is positioned in the inferior right atrium and a proximal port is positioned in the superior right atrium. The reinfusion lumen is situated midway between the two drainage ports and ejects the returning blood from the ECLS circuit into the middle of the right atrium directed toward the tricuspid valve. This configuration reduces recirculation.[2] Currently, these cannulae are placed through the right internal jugular vein into the right atrium. Larger double-lumen

TABLE 44.2

NEONATAL AND PEDIATRIC EXTRACORPOREAL LIFE SUPPORT DIAGNOSES AND OUTCOMES

Diagnosis	Total Runs	Average Run Time (h)	Longest Run Time (h)	Survival
Neonatal Patients				
CDH	4,629	233	1,072	2,426 (52%)
MAS	6,663	129	936	6,253 (94%)
PPHN	2,996	145	1,176	2,347 (78%)
RDS	1,388	133	1,093	1,167 (84%)
Sepsis	2,396	138	1,200	1,802 (75%)
Pneumonia	268	211	936	158 (59%)
Air leak syndrome	97	167	656	70 (72%)
Others	1,264	170	1,131	811 (64%)
Pediatric Respiratory				
Viral pneumonia	747	318	1,372	471 (63%)
Bacterial pneumonia	309	265	1,332	171 (55%)
Pneumocystis	22	371	1,144	9 (41%)
Aspiration pneumonia	170	279	2,437	111 (65%)
ARDS, postoperative/trauma	72	223	818	45 (63%)
ARDS, nonpostoperative/trauma	286	294	999	148 (52%)
ARF, not ARDS	608	244	1,483	288 (47%)
Others	720	200	2,239	386 (54%)

CDH, congenital diaphragmatic hernia; MAS, meconium aspiration syndrome; PPHN, persistent pulmonary hypertension; RDS, respiratory distress syndrome; ARDS, acute respiratory distress syndrome; ARF, acute respiratory failure.
Data adapted from the International ELSO Registry Report, January 2005, www.elso.med.umich.edu/ Registry.htm Ann Arbor, MI.

TABLE 44.3

OUTCOME OF EXTRACORPOREAL LIFE SUPPORT IN PATIENTS WITH CARDIAC DISORDERS BY UNDERLYING DISEASE

	Total Number of Patients	Survived	Survival (%)
Congenital heart disease	4,106	1,576	38
Cardiac arrest	141	39	28
Cardiogenic shock	141	60	42
Cardiomyopathy	406	209	51
Myocarditis	170	98	58
Others	880	344	39

Data adapted from the International ELSO Registry Report, July 2004, www.elso.med.umich.edu/Registry.htm Ann Arbor, MI.

cannulae that support adult-sized patients are currently under development.

Blood Pump

Two types of blood pumps are used for ECLS. Historically, the occlusive *roller pump* has provided most of the ECMO support. The roller pump is a positive displacement pump in which the roller compresses tubing against a backing plate as it rotates. Blood flow is related to the tubing diameter and rotation speed.

Centrifugal pumps are nonocclusive and generate flow through a spinning rotor, which is often maintained by magnets within it. Blood enters the cone at the apex and is propelled tangentially to the base of the pump head, where it is expelled. Centrifugal pumps are safer but inherently more likely to produce hemolysis under conditions of inadequate venous drainage, but technologic improvements may reduce this problem.

Venous Reservoir

The venous reservoir, or bladder, acts as a safety device to prevent the development of high negative pressure in the ECMO tubing that can lead to hemolysis or air cavitation. If venous return is lost to the point where the bladder collapses, a servoregulating switch opens and signals the roller-head pump to stop. Once venous return is again adequate, the bladder refills and the switch is deactivated. Newer versions of the bladder incorporate a section of collapsible tubing, which signals the roller-head pump to slow down until adequate filling is obtained and to speed up when venous return is re-established. This may reduce the degree of acute blood flow changes noted with the older style of servoregulation. Some ECLS systems have completely abandoned the bladder box because of improved servoregulation techniques by pressure or flow monitoring.

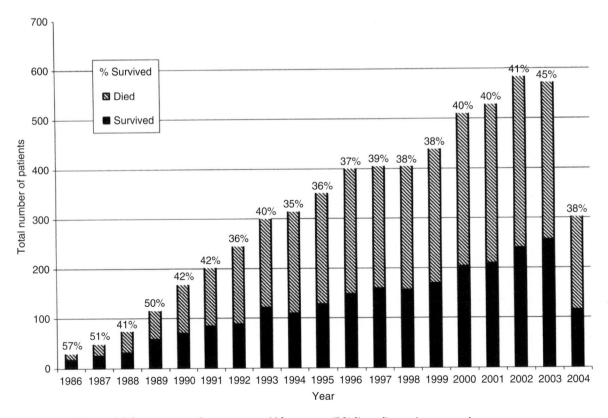

Figure 44.1 Outcome of extracorporeal life support (ECLS) cardiac patients over time.

TABLE 44.4
PARAMETERS USED FOR EXTRACORPOREAL LIFE SUPPORT CONSIDERATION

Severe respiratory failure not responding to conventional therapy[a]

OI >40 or 30–40 consistently

$$OI = \frac{(MAP \times F_{IO_2}) \times 100}{Pa_{O_2}}$$

$P_{AO_2} - Pa_{O_2} > 650$ for >4 h (neonates)

$P_{AO_2} - Pa_{O_2} > 450$ for >4 h (older patients, rarely used currently)

Acidosis and shock (pH <7.25 with hypotension)

Gestational age $\geq$32 wk or weight >2.0 kg

Mechanical ventilation $\leq$10 d

Qs/Qt >0.5

MAP >23 cm H_2O (conventional ventilator) Prolonged MAP >25–30 cm H_2O (high-frequency ventilation)

Barotrauma: persistent air leak

Hypercarbic respiratory failure with hemodynamic compromise or severe acidosis

(pH <7.00)

Acute decompensation with potentially reversible respiratory failure

---

OI, oxygen index; MAP, mean airway pressure; F_{IO_2}, fraction of inspired oxygen; Pa_{O_2}, partial pressure of arterial oxygen; $P_{AO_2} - Pa_{O_2}$, alveolar–arterial difference in partial pressure of oxygen; Qs/Qt, shunt fraction.

[a]May include pressure-limited, low tidal volume approach, trial of inhaled nitric oxide, prone positioning, surfactant, or others.

Artificial Lung

Although the artificial lung used during ECLS provides both oxygen and carbon dioxide gas exchange, it is commonly known as a *membrane oxygenator*. Two types of membrane oxygenators are used for ECLS. The *solid silicone membrane lung* consists of very thin silicone rubber sheets separated by a wire mesh that is spiral wound on a polycarbonate support. Gas flows through the interior of the envelope and blood flows between the turns of the wound silicone sheet. Diffusion of oxygen and carbon dioxide takes place across the membrane, which is permeable to these gases. Silicone membrane lungs have a variable life span but normally function well up to a week or more with ECLS support.

Hollow-fiber oxygenators are constructed of hydrophobic polymer fibers, which contain pores that can range in size from 0.2 to 0.7 μm. Blood flows outside the fibers and gas flows inside. The pores present a direct gas–liquid interface for gas exchange. Although these oxygenators have excellent gas exchange properties, leakage of plasma proteins from microporous pores over time impairs gas exchange and results in membrane failure. The lower priming volume and resistance to blood flow makes these oxygenators easier and faster to prime than the solid silicone membrane lungs. Therefore, the use of hollow-fiber oxygenators for emergency ECLS, called *rapid deployment,* is common. Newer polymers such as polymethylpentene are resistant to plasma leakage but are not available in the United States.

Heat Exchanger

A heat exchanger uses circulating temperature-controlled water to maintain the blood reinfused into the patient at a desired temperature. In addition to maintaining normothermia, the heat exchanger can be used to induce hypothermia. The ease and rapidity in obtaining the desired temperature with ECLS support is a potential benefit to patients who have had a cardiac arrest and in whom hypothermia may offer neuroprotection.

Monitoring Devices

Most ECLS circuits have pressure-monitoring sites, especially on the postoxygenator limb, to prevent tubing rupture or excessive hemolysis. Some centers also monitor premembrane pressure because widening of the difference between pre- and postoxygenator pressures is an early indication of clotting within the membrane lung. Venous saturation monitoring on the venous limb of the ECLS circuit is a simple and useful measure of the adequacy of the balance between oxygen delivery and extraction. Temperature monitoring is also routinely performed within the ECLS circuit and in the patient.

MODES OF EXTRACORPOREAL SUPPORT

There are two major cannulation techniques used for the access of ECLS. To date, *venoarterial* access has provided most of the support, but recently *venovenous* support is gaining popularity in respiratory failure without cardiac dysfunction. The sites for cannulation and the basic principles of support with venoarterial and venovenous ECLS are shown in Table 44.5.

Practical Points: Venoarterial Support

Venoarterial bypass provides both cardiac and pulmonary support. With femoral access, the extent to which the arterialized reinfusion blood flows retrograde up the aorta will be determined by the flow rates and pressure differentials between the antegrade native heart ejection and the ECLS arterial return. Inadequate antegrade flow from femoral cannulation is problematic in the presence of severe pulmonary failure because poorly oxygenated blood returning from the pulmonary circuit will be ejected into the proximal aorta by the left ventricle, resulting in potential myocardial and cerebral hypoxia. Femoral access may result in distal limb perfusion and drainage abnormalities. Monitoring of distal pulses and venous drainage is important. Veno–venoarterial ECLS is a modification in which a third cannula is inserted through the right internal jugular vein to the right atrium. Blood is drained from a femoral venous cannula and returned to both the right

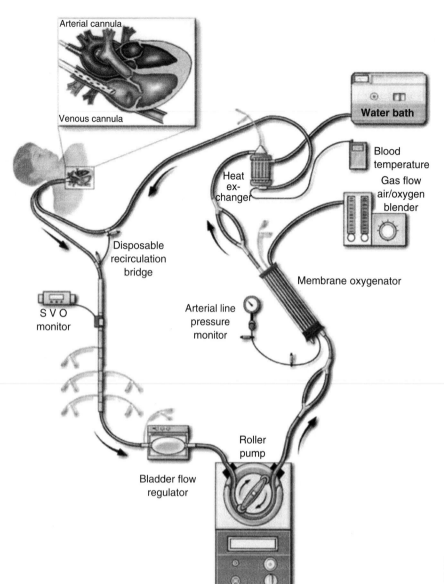

Arterial cannula

Venous cannula

Water bath

Blood temperature

Gas flow air/oxygen blender

Heat ex- changer

Membrane oxygenator

Disposable recirculation bridge

S V O monitor

Arterial line pressure monitor

Roller pump

Bladder flow regulator

Figure 44.2 Venoarterial extracorporeal life support (ECLS) roller-head circuit. SVO, venous oxygen saturation.

atrium and the femoral artery. This type of support is ideal for patients who require pulmonary support, as well as partial cardiac assistance. Venoarterial ECLS increases left-sided heart afterload. Severe left ventricular failure may result in pulmonary edema or hemorrhage. The need for left atrial venting or the creation of an atrial septostomy to allow drainage of the left atrium may be needed.

Venovenous ECLS (see Fig. 44.3) improves myocardial blood flow and oxygenation. This may improve cardiac performance and allow the use of venovenous ECLS for cardiac dysfunction, especially if increased intrathoracic pressure from high ventilator settings is a cause of cardiac dysfunction. Although not yet proven, the avoidance of the need to instrument the carotid artery may reduce neurologic complications or the risk of stroke later in life. Flow is easier to obtain when draining from the right atrium, but the reverse direction is more commonly used

because it is associated with less recirculation and improved systemic oxygenation. A variant of venovenous support (extracorporeal carbon dioxide removal [ECCO$_2$R]) is to both drain and reinfuse blood through the bilateral femoral veins. The drainage cannula is positioned in the low inferior vena cava (IVC), with the reinfusion cannula placed in the opposite femoral vein, and is advanced further up the IVC toward the right atrium. Lower flow rates are used, which are effective for carbon dioxide removal. This mode is useful for hypercapnic states such as severe asthma.

Circuit Priming

Circuit-priming solutions most commonly consist of balanced acetate-buffered electrolyte solution to which albumin and often red blood cells are added. The control of pH is achieved with bicarbonate or tris-hydroxymethyl

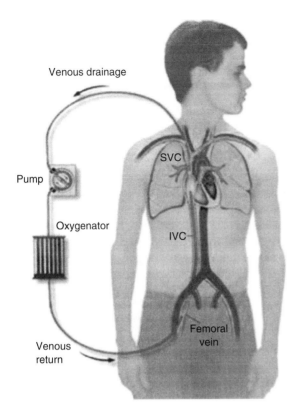

Figure 44.3 Venovenous extracorporeal life support (ECLS) roller-head circuit. SVC, superior vena cava; IVC, inferior vena cava.

aminomethane (THAM). Heparin is added for anticoagulation, and appropriate amount of calcium is added to maintain ionized calcium levels. Using the freshest blood available for priming limits the hyperkalemia noted in the ECLS circuit. Although hyperkalemia can be marked, it rarely results in adverse clinical effects because the potassium level becomes diluted once the circuit blood mixes with the patient's blood volume, which has a lower potassium content unless severe derangements exist in the patient.

Initiation of Extracorporeal Life Support

The procedure is usually performed at the bedside with appropriate sedation, analgesia, and neuromuscular blockade. Lack of spontaneous inspiratory efforts limits the risk of air embolism during cannulation. Immediately before cannula insertion, heparin (50 to 100 units per kg) is administered to ensure anticoagulation. Following cannulation, the circuit is attached to the cannulae. The ECLS flow is increased incrementally to a goal rate of 100 to 200 mL per kg for neonatal patients, whereas older patients may require only 80 to 100 mL per kg to achieve adequate cardiopulmonary support.

Complete bypass of the pulmonary circuit results in high ventilation–perfusion ratios with severe alkalosis and ischemia within the pulmonary bed. The predominant perfusion to the coronary arteries and the myocardium

is from the native left-sided heart ejection, even during venoarterial support.[3] For these reasons, ECLS should be maintained at a "partial" level that provides adequate oxygen delivery to the patient but allows some native blood flow through the lungs. Hemodynamics, oxygenation, and indirect measures of adequate oxygen delivery such as mixed venous saturation, lactate level, urine output, and neurologic function are important indicators that demonstrate whether appropriate support with ECLS has been achieved. Patients with hyperdynamic states such as sepsis may require increased levels of support.

Maintenance of Extracorporeal Life Support

Once ECLS is initiated, the remainder of ECLS support is focused on providing adequate oxygen delivery in an environment that promotes organ healing while minimizing complications.

The adequacy of oxygen delivery during venoarterial support is achieved by targeting the normal mixed venous oxygen saturation, usually measured in the venous drainage limb of the ECLS circuit. Increasing oxygen delivery to the patient is accomplished by increasing bypass flow through the ECLS circuit. For patients with primary respiratory failure, the increased proportion of bypass flow will reduce the amount of blood going through the diseased pulmonary circuit, resulting in a higher level of oxygenation. Arterial saturation during venoarterial ECLS measured in the patient will typically be 90% to 100%. During venovenous support, the mixed venous oxygen saturation measured on the ECLS circuit may not reflect the tissue venous saturation reliably because of the recirculation of well-oxygenated arterial return into the venous cannula. Monitoring of venous saturation at central points outside the right atrium may provide a better indication of overall tissue perfusion. Because venovenous ECLS allows blood to pass through the native cardiopulmonary circuit before systemic delivery, oxygenation obtained by the diseased lungs will be lower than that observed with venoarterial cannulation. Arterial saturations of 80% to 90% are common. Despite the lower observed PaO_2 and saturations during venovenous support, adequate oxygen delivery can be provided. The indirect parameters of balanced oxygen delivery to extraction, such as hemodynamics, lactate level, urine output, and neurologic function, are more useful in venovenous ECLS than focusing on arterial blood gas parameters.

The amount of bypass that can be directed to the ECLS circuit depends on the available venous return, the caliber of the drainage and reinfusion cannulae, and the circuit tubing. The difficulty with obtaining adequate venous return is often due to hypovolemia from low central venous pressures. This can be easily corrected with fluid administration. Correction of anemia by transfusion of blood products will also increase oxygen-carrying capacity. Maintenance of hematocrit values of 30% to 40% is sufficient to sustain adequate oxygen content.

TABLE 44.5

ACCESS SITES AND EFFECTS OF VENOARTERIAL AND VENOVENOUS EXTRACORPOREAL LIFE SUPPORT

	Venoarterial Sites	Venovenous Sites
Cannulation sites	**Cervical:** internal jugular vein to right atrium; right common carotid artery to aortic arch **Femoral:** saphenous or femoral vein to IVC or right atrium; femoral artery to iliac or aorta **Mediastinal:** directly to the right atrium; directly to the aortic arch **Other arterial:** axillary (rarely)	**Single-site cannulation:** internal jugular vein alone (double-lumen cannula) **Two-site cannulation:** jugular vein and femoral vein; bilateral femoral veins to IVC or IVC/RA junction
Oxygenation	Pao_2 80–150 mm Hg; saturation 95%–100%	Pao_2 45–80 mm Hg; saturation 80%–90%
Cardiac effects	Decreases preload, increases afterload; the amount of bypass may affect pulse pressure; coronary perfusion is provided by left ventricular output; bypass may lower PVR and PA pressure	No change in CVP or pulse pressure; normal flow is through cardiopulmonary circuit It may improve coronary oxygen delivery. Improved oxygenation to right ventricle/PA may decrease PVR
Oxygen delivery capacity	High	Moderate
Circulatory support	Partial to complete support, depending on the extent of bypass	No direct effect; improved delivery to coronary and pulmonary circuits may improve cardiac output
Pulmonary Circulation		
Right-to-left shunt	Decreases saturation of blood in aorta	Increases hemoglobin saturation of blood in aorta
Left-to-right shunt	May result in pulmonary congestion and systemic hypoperfusion	May cause pulmonary congestion and systemic hypoperfusion

IVC, inferior vena cava; RA, right atrial; CVP, central venous pressure; Pao_2, partial pressure of arterial oxygen; PVR, pulmonary vascular resistance; PA, pulmonary artery.

Intermittent administration of packed red blood cells to maintain adequate blood volume and hematocrit is frequently needed during ECLS. Platelet sequestration in the ECLS circuit is a constant problem. The platelet count is traditionally maintained between 75,000 and 150,000 per mm^3 to reduce bleeding, although there are now several examples of patients with thrombocytopenia being placed on ECMO where significant bleeding did not occur. Monitoring of the coagulation parameters and administration of fresh frozen plasma or other factors may also be required to limit bleeding.

Patient Care During Extracorporeal Life Support

Adequate nutrition is essential during ECLS. Enteral nutrition is the preferred route when feasible and is well tolerated.[4] Lipids are associated with plasma leakage and a shortened life span of the polypropylene hollow-fiber oxygenators.

Maintaining fluid balance and reducing fluid overload are necessary goals during ECLS. Diuretics promote urine excretion and are often the first line of therapy provided, often by continuous infusion of furosemide. The concentration of fluids to balance intake and output can also be useful. Hemofiltration, as a method to control fluid balance and augment fluid removal, has become common practice in many centers. Other adjunctive extracorporeal therapies such as plasmapheresis or liver support systems have also been used easily and successfully with ECMO.

For patients with respiratory failure, the goal of pulmonary care during ECLS is to minimize ventilator-induced lung injury and to provide an optimal environment for healing. Neonatal patients are often maintained on settings with low peak inspiratory pressure (25 to 30 cm H_2O), a positive end-expiratory pressure (PEEP) of 5 cm H_2O, an intermittent mandatory ventilation rate (6 to 12 breaths per minute), and a fraction of inspired oxygen (FIO_2) of 0.21 to 0.30. Maintaining lung expansion and functional residual capacity with higher levels of PEEP (10 to 15 cm H_2O) have been associated with a shorter duration of ECMO, and this approach is also used in many centers. In older patients, the use of PEEP (5 to 15 cm H_2O) with reduced peak airway pressures (<30 cm H_2O), low ventilator rates (6 to 12 breaths per minute), and low concentrations of inspired oxygen (<40%) is the predominant method of support. The use of pressure support ventilation with continuous positive airway pressure (CPAP) is becoming a more common approach, allowing patients to remain awake, clear the airway secretions better through coughing, and establish a safe respiratory rate and tidal volume.

In patients with barotrauma and persistent air leaks even at low distending airway pressures, the reduction of ventilator settings may not be sufficient to seal the air leak. These patients may be candidates for a period of total lung rest to promote the healing of ruptured parenchyma. This can be accomplished by using low CPAP or by removing the patient from mechanical ventilator support. Often, resolution of alveolar rupture occurs within 48 hours of such treatment. As functional residual capacity falls during this process, the radiograph often becomes opaque. Reinflation of collapsed lungs may be assisted by bronchoscopy, lavage of inspissated secretions, and recruitment maneuvers to expand alveoli and resume mechanical ventilator support.

In severely diseased lungs, manipulation of ventilator settings may have little effect on gas exchange. Oxygenation and carbon dioxide elimination depend on the function of the ECMO circuit. As the lungs heal, compliance and tidal volume increase. Visible lung improvement in the chest radiograph is a simple but often reliable indication that healing is occurring. An increasing concentration of expired carbon dioxide and improvement in systemic oxygenation without increased ECLS flow also demonstrates improved gas exchange within the lung. In patients with pulmonary artery catheters, reduction in pulmonary pressures may also be indicative of resolution of lung injury. These events may signal that the patient can be weaned from ECLS support.

During ECLS, the provision of adequate analgesia and sedation can become difficult, especially in patients with slow recovery who require prolonged ECLS. The most common medications used during ECLS are morphine, fentanyl, midazolam, and lorazepam. Pharmacokinetic studies have noted that the membrane oxygenator may absorb medications, particularly in the early period of ECLS. Patients may also become tolerant to infused medications and may require large increases in dosage to maintain adequate sedation and analgesia. As an alternative to high concentrations of sedative medications, in some centers anesthesia gases are mixed into the membrane oxygenator. Alternatively, maintaining the patient in the awake state limits the need for sedation. This approach has been used successfully in Europe.

Weaning from Extracorporeal Membrane Oxygenation

As the patient recovers respiratory or cardiac function, the amount of ECLS support can be reduced. The bypass provided by ECLS is usually weaned in an incremental manner over time, although some patients may be weaned for a "trial" very quickly, similar to what is done in the operating room at the end of the cardiopulmonary bypass. Goals for oxygenation, supply of carbon dioxide, and maintenance of hemodynamic status are established, and ventilator support is increased but maintained at noninjurious levels as weaning continues.

COMPLICATIONS

The most common complications noted with ECLS for patients with respiratory and cardiac disorders, both mechanical and patient-related, are provided in Tables 44.6 and 44.7. Bleeding remains the most frequently noted adverse event with ECLS because of the requirement for systemic heparinization. Bleeding can occur from many sites, but bleeding into the brain parenchyma often necessitates a decision to discontinue ECLS support. Assessment of neurologic function by clinical examination, head ultrasonography, and computed tomography can provide an ongoing assessment of intracranial hemorrhage. Serial studies can often assist in decision-making processes by demonstrating whether the hemorrhage is expanding.

Attempts to control bleeding should focus on surgical correction, when applicable; reduction of heparin dose; and correction of coagulation or platelet abnormalities by the infusion of blood products and by the use of antifibrinolytic agents (aminocaproic acid) or serine protease inhibitors (aprotinin). Aprotinin has been described to also preserve platelet function, reduce vascular permeability, and decrease the inflammatory response to extracorporeal circulation. Heparin may be discontinued for a certain period, but the risk of developing a clot within the ECLS circuit is high.[5] The use of factor VIIa for intractable bleeding during ECLS has been reported.[6] Although some reports have associated the use of factor VIIa with reduction in bleeding in some reports, others have noted thrombosis both within the patient and in the ECLS circuit, particularly if used concomitantly with other medications such as aminocaproic acid.[7]

LONG-TERM OUTCOME

Most of the information regarding neurologic outcome and ECLS has come from the neonatal respiratory failure population. In one study that evaluated the use of ECMO in

TABLE 44.6

MECHANICAL AND PATIENT-RELATED COMPLICATIONS FOR PATIENTS WITH RESPIRATORY DISORDERS

Complications	Neonatal Respiratory Complications	Pediatric Respiratory Complications	Adult Respiratory Complications
Mechanical			
Oxygenator failure	5.7 (55)	13.8 (44)	18.2 (43)
Tubing rupture	0.7 (74)	3.8 (47)	4.0 (30)
Pump malfunction	1.8 (68)	3.1 (47)	4.1 (37)
Cannula problems	11.1 (70)	14.2 (48)	10.7 (42)
Patient-Related			
GI hemorrhage	1.7 (46)	4.0 (25)	4.3 (26)
Cannula site bleeding	6.1 (68)	9.2 (60)	11.5 (47)
Surgical site bleeding	6.1 (46)	16.0 (47)	22.4 (35)
Hemolysis	12.2 (68)	8.8 (42)	5.3 (28)
Brain death	1.0 (0)	6.0 (0)	3.8 (0)
Seizures: clinically determined	10.9 (62)	7.3 (35)	2.0 (45)

Table entries are in % reported (% survival).
GI, gastrointestinal.
Adapted from the International ELSO Registry Report, July 2004, www.elso.med.umich.edu/Registry.htm Ann Arbor, MI.

neonatal patients, major handicaps were found in 17% of patients by the age of 5 years.[8] Of the ECMO survivors, 13% had intelligence quotient (IQ) scores <70, 6% had motor disability problems, 5% had sensorineural hearing deficits, and 2% had seizure disorders. Another report compared 5-year-old patients who were referred to a children's hospital as neonates for ECMO evaluation. Patients who received ECMO were compared to referrals who recovered without undergoing ECMO. Overall, no differences in IQ, cognitive deficits, seizure disorder, cerebral palsy, or

TABLE 44.7

MECHANICAL AND PATIENT-RELATED COMPLICATIONS FOR PATIENTS WITH CARDIAC DISORDERS

Complications	0–30 d	31 d and <1 y	1 y and <16 y	16 y and More
Mechanical				
Oxygenator failure	7.2 (23)	7.2 (28)	9.1 (37)	16.4 (27)
Tubing rupture	0.7 (31)	1.1 (24)	2.0 (30)	0.9 (20)
Pump malfunction	1.3 (32)	1.9 (26)	2.2 (42)	1.8 (36)
Cannula problems	6.7 (33)	5.9 (35)	6.4 (31)	6.8 (32)
Patient-Related				
GI hemorrhage	0.9 (5)	1.8 (14)	2.8 (23)	2.4 (15)
Cannula site bleeding	6.8 (27)	6.7 (23)	10.7 (44)	12.9 (30)
Surgical site bleeding	31.0 (29)	33.9 (36)	31.3 (42)	31.9 (27)
Hemolysis	10.8 (24)	9.9 (33)	8.5 (35)	8.1 (34)
Brain death	1.3 (0)	5.1 (0)	9.5 (0)	7.9 (0)
Seizures: clinically determined	9.7 (29)	11.0 (24)	6.8 (21)	4.8 (12)

Table entries are in % reported (% survival).
GI, gastrointestinal.
Data adapted from the International ECLS Registry Report, July 2004, www.elso.med.umich.edu/Registry.htm Ann Arbor, MI.

hearing loss were noted between the groups. Parents of 35% of the patients on ECMO and those of 25% of the near-miss group noted behavioral problems.

Information regarding long-term outcomes in older patients is not as well described as in infants. Most centers report outcomes at the time to discharge but do not systematically perform follow-up examination. In one small report of 19 patients (15 pediatric and 4 adult patients) who received ECLS, 58% survived to discharge. Overall, the Pediatric Cerebral Performance Category (PCPC) was normal in 64% (seven patients) of patients, with only one patient (9%) demonstrating moderate disability. Results of the Pediatric Overall Performance Category (POPC) found that 27% (three patients) of patients were normal while 45% (five patients) were mildly disabled, 18% (two patients) had moderate disability, and 9% (one patient) had a severe abnormality (spinal cord injury). More specific long-term evaluation of pediatric and adult patients who recover from ECLS is needed. Further, comparison between ECLS-treated patients and those who receive conventional care should also be performed to assess the impact of ECLS on long-term outcome.

THE FUTURE

The use of extracorporeal devices to support the heart, lung, kidneys, liver, and other organs is growing as advances in technology and the understanding of specific organ failure continue. Clinical experience with extracorporeal life support, advances in cannulation techniques, and support strategies have also led to an increase in ECLS use in patient populations excluded in the past. Careful assessment of long-term outcome in patients with severe illness who receive ECLS, as well as those who do not, is a much needed area of focus for the future. Currently, data suggest that ECLS offers a life-saving therapy that is not associated with inappropriately high levels of poor neurologic and functional outcome. Efforts to make ECLS more efficient, safe, and less labor-intensive should continue.

REFERENCES

1. Reickert CA, Schreiner RJ, Bartlett RH, et al. Percutaneous access for venovenous extracorporeal life support in neonates. *J Pediatr Surg*. 1998;33:365–369.
2. Rais-Bahrami K, Walton DM, Sell JE, et al. Short, improved oxygenation with reduced recirculation during venovenous ECMO: Comparison of two catheters. *Perfusion*. 2002;17:415–419.
3. Kato J, Seo T, Ando H, et al. Coronary arterial perfusion during venoarterial extracorporeal membrane oxygenation. *J Thorac Cardiovasc Surg*. 1996;111:630–636.
4. Scott LK, Boudreaux K, Thaljeh F, et al. Early enteral feedings in adults receiving venovenous extracorporeal membrane oxygenation. *JPEN J Parenter Enteral Nutr*. 2004;28:295–300.
5. Wegner J. Biochemistry of serine protease inhibitors and their mechanisms of action: A review. *J Extra Corpor Technol*. 2003;35(4): 326–338.
6. Verrijckt A, Proulx F, Morneau S, et al. Activated recombinant factor VII for refractory bleeding during extracorporeal membrane oxygenation. *J Thorac Cardiovasc Surg*. 2004;127:1812–1813.
7. Bui JD, Despotis GD, Trulock EP, et al. Fatal thrombosis after administration of activated prothrombin complex concentrates in a patient supported by extracorporeal membrane oxygenation who had received activated recombinant factor VII. *J Thorac Cardiovasc Surg*. 2002;124:852–854.
8. Glass P, Wagner AE, Papero PH, et al. Neurodevelopmental status at age five years of neonates treated with extracorporeal membrane oxygenation. *J Pediatr*. 1995;127(3):447–457.

Neurologic Disorders

Michael J. Bell   *JoAnne E. Natale*

Global/Regional Ischemia

45

Rebecca N. Ichord

Cerebral ischemia occurs in the setting of several distinct clinical conditions that have in common a decrease in oxygen delivery to the brain below the threshold level needed to maintain cellular viability. Global ischemia occurs when systemic hypoxemia or circulatory failure, or both, impair brain oxygen delivery to the ischemic threshold, and is associated typically with such conditions as cardiac or respiratory arrest, septic shock, hypovolemic shock, or strangulation. Focal ischemia occurs when there is a regionally selective failure of cerebral perfusion, or a focal mismatch between substrate delivery and consumption. Focal ischemic injury is typically associated with arterial ischemic stroke (AIS), and also occurs in cerebral venous occlusive disease and sickle cell anemia. In some patients, a global ischemic process such as hypotension leads to a focal infarct as a result of regional differences in perfusion deficit and in ischemic vulnerability within the brain. Although molecular and cellular processes are similar in global and focal ischemia, there are significant differences in clinical manifestations, associated diseases, management, and outcomes.

Cerebral ischemia in infants and children poses unique challenges as compared to adults. Global ischemia in infants and children is most often the end product of respiratory or airway disease, and as such is a mixed injury with hypoxemia, hypercarbia, and hypoperfusion. In contrast, global ischemia in adults is most often purely circulatory owing to cardiac arrest. Similarly, in focal ischemia, the risk factors, clinical manifestations, and potential for recovery are vastly different in children compared to that of adults. These facts, along with the differing responses to ischemia in a developing brain compared to that of a mature brain, make it difficult to extrapolate research findings from adults to infants and children. Hence, there is a critical need for researchers and care providers, both in the basic and clinical sciences, to develop age-specific and disease-specific approaches to understand and treat cerebral ischemia in infants and children.

DEFINITIONS OF ISCHEMIC BRAIN INJURY

Brain injury due to global ischemia has been studied in neonates intensively for many years, but has received less attention in older infants and children. A number of lessons from neonates can be applied to older children, beginning with definitions. Strictly speaking, "global ischemia" refers to a systemic physiologic perturbation leading to failure of brain oxygen delivery, and is distinct from the brain injury caused by an ischemic exposure, which is more precisely referred to as *post-hypoxic–ischemic encephalopathy* (HIE). The nature and severity of the HIE is probably linked to the duration and severity of the ischemic insult. Clinical studies have shown that clinical grading of the acute encephalopathy in neonates is feasible and reliable, and when combined with imaging and electrophysiologic markers of the extent of ischemic injury, provide valid outcome prediction. Clinical grading of HIE is exemplified by Sarnat staging system, which classifies encephalopathy in term newborns as mild, moderate, or severe on the basis of the presence and severity of abnormalities in level of consciousness, tone, neonatal reflex behaviors, seizures, and autonomic function. Infants with mild encephalopathy or moderate encephalopathy of <1-week duration have a low risk of long-term disability, whereas infants with severe encephalopathy of any duration or moderate encephalopathy of >1-week duration have a high risk of disability. A system of clinically grading acute postischemic encephalopathy for prognostic purposes is widely used in adults. The limited data available in children support the utility of an approach to defining HIE with a combination of clinical markers with objective assessments such as electroencephalogram (EEG) or imaging.

Focal ischemia, or stroke, encompasses several distinct cerebrovascular disorders, traditionally defined by clinical criteria, consisting of the sudden onset of an acute focal neurologic deficit localizing to a vascular distribution. So defined, stroke includes ischemic infarction from arterial occlusion or hypoperfusion (AIS), venous infarction related to cerebral sinovenous thrombosis (SVT), and primary intracranial hemorrhage (ICH). The capacity of magnetic resonance imaging (MRI) to identify ischemic injury with high sensitivity and specificity has led to a redefinition of stroke syndromes based on combined clinical and imaging criteria. In this approach, ischemic stroke is viewed as a spectrum of "acute ischemic cerebrovascular syndrome," which includes completed stroke and transient ischemic attacks (TIAs); up to 40% of such cases may in fact have an infarct as observed from imaging studies and are at very high risk of subsequent strokes. The importance of broadening the definition of stroke syndromes to incorporate imaging criteria is even greater in children than in adults. This arises from the fact that infants and very young children do not clinically manifest a focal cerebral ischemic injury in a reliable localizing manner. Until data to the contrary is available, the same redefinition of ischemic stroke should pertain to children as well. Therefore, events resembling TIAs in children should be evaluated and managed with the same level of urgency and completeness as for completed stroke.

EPIDEMIOLOGY: INCIDENCE AND RISK FACTORS

The incidence of ischemic brain injury in children is not precisely known. HIE following global ischemia is estimated to affect <1 per 1,000 live-born term neonates. Population-based incidence figures for pediatric (non-neonatal) HIE are not available. An idea of the magnitude of the problem can be obtained from studies, showing that 1% to 2% of admissions to tertiary care pediatric hospitals involve an episode of cardiopulmonary resuscitation. Incidence estimates for stroke vary depending on whether neonatal stroke, hemorrhagic stroke, and venous thrombosis are included. Data derived from the Canadian Pediatric Stroke Registry estimate the incidence of ischemic stroke at 3.3/100,000/year from birth through 18 years of age, nearly double the estimates from previous decades, and comparable to the incidence of childhood brain tumors. When hemorrhagic stroke is included, the estimated incidence for all strokes in children rises to 6/100,000/year, with approximately one third of all strokes occurring in neonates.

Risk factors for cardiac arrest in children are dominated by congenital heart disease, respiratory failure, and shock. Risk factors for stroke in children are very different from those in adults, where atherosclerosis, hypertension, and diabetes predominate. A recent 22-year consecutive cohort study from the United Kingdom describes risk factor analysis for 212 children with AIS. About half of the cases in this cohort had no known stroke risk factor before presentation (cryptogenic), and the remaining had a known risk factor including congenital heart disease, thrombophilia, or known vasculopathy. After thorough evaluation in the cryptogenic group, risk factors were identified in >96%, which included previously undefined cervical or cranial vasculopathy in 80%. In many cases, multiple risk factors were identified, such as the coexistence of known heart defects with cerebral or cervical vascular lesions or prothrombotic risk factors. Prothrombotic risk factors affect 10% to 18% of childhood ischemic stroke cases, 41% of children with SVT, and 60% to 70% of infants with neonatal stroke.

EVALUATION AND TREATMENT: TIME IS BRAIN

Cerebral ischemic injury syndromes are among the few true emergencies in pediatric neurology. Diagnosis and management should occur in parallel, and are presented as such here. Evidence-based diagnostic and treatment guidelines are not presently available. The guidelines provided here represent a consensus based on data from cohort studies, and the experience and results of trials in adult studies. In all matters of treatment, it is reasonable to assume that the principle of "time is brain" applies equally to children as it does to adults.

Acute Management: Initial Supportive Care

Management of cerebral ischemia begins with early identification of the condition. In the case of global ischemia, this is usually straightforward and obvious. Any child exhibiting neurologic symptoms after resuscitation from an episode of global hypoxia or ischemia can be considered to have experienced some degree of global ischemia. The identification of children having an episode of focal ischemia is much more challenging. Any child with an acute onset of focal neurologic deficit of any duration, or with unexplained altered consciousness, particularly with headache, should be considered to possibly have a cerebrovascular disorder. Other clinical settings to consider stroke syndromes include seizures in a near-term newborn, or in an infant recovering from cardiac surgery.

Upon identification of a child with suspected cerebral ischemia, a series of treatment and diagnostic procedures should be simultaneously activated. Treatment before definitive diagnosis is by necessity supportive, but can be critical to the evolution of the deficit, and should include the following:

1. Ensure airway, oxygenation, and air exchange, providing supplemental oxygen to maintain SaO_2 ≥95%.
2. Monitor cardiopulmonary status continuously, with intermittent frequent checks of blood pressure (BP),

temperature, neurologic status (Glasgow Coma Scale [GCS]), and bedside blood glucose levels.

3. In the case of suspected stroke, restrict activity to bed rest until the clinical deficit is stable or improving (24 to 72 hours) to avoid potential posturally triggered fluctuations in perfusion.

4. Establish IV access and provide maintenance volume with nondextrose-containing isotonic fluids, aiming for normovolemia, and blood glucose levels of 60 to 120 mg per dL.

5. Maintain BP around the 50th percentile for the child's age- or height-related norms. Treatment of hypertension in the setting of acute stroke is controversial. Unless BP is extremely elevated, or suspected to be a cause of acute heart failure, it is generally advised that elevated BP should not be treated with acute BP-lowering agents.

6. Prevent and treat hyperthermia aggressively, aiming for core temperatures <37.0°C.

7. Treat seizures with anticonvulsants, taking care to avoid transient BP depression from rapid dosing.

8. Institute deep vein thrombosis (DVT) prophylaxis for children and adolescents who are seriously immobilized by their deficit.

9. Hold oral intake, pending 24 hours of hemodynamic and respiratory stability, and evaluation of adequate swallowing function by a speech therapist.

While initial supportive care is begun, steps should be taken simultaneously to obtain a diagnosis, which will then guide further management decisions. At the point of triage, appropriate experts in childhood cerebrovascular disorders should be notified promptly about the patient, and decisions made concerning the diagnostic studies to be obtained, and in what time frame, and oversight of the patient's care during imaging studies (especially if this requires sedation), and finally arrangements for transfer of the patient to the appropriate acute care hospital unit.

Acute Management: Initial Diagnostic Studies

Diagnostic evaluation of the underlying causes for global ischemia from respiratory failure or shock is the province of qualified pediatric intensivists, and is not discussed in detail here. For children with suspected stroke syndromes, laboratory studies at the time of admission should include comprehensive chemistry and hematologic profiles, prothrombin time (PT), partial thrombin time (PTT), and international normalized ratio (INR). Other admission diagnostic studies commonly obtained in the setting of acute stroke include urinalysis and electrocardiogram (EKG), and more specific testing as indicated by patient history and exam findings, for example, in case of fever or in a patient with sickle cell anemia. If acute anticoagulation therapy is anticipated, then an expanded thrombophilia evaluation should be considered. The specifics of which studies to obtain should ideally be worked out as part of an institutional stroke protocol involving consultation

TABLE 45.1
LABORATORY EVALUATION FOR THROMBOPHILIA

Laboratory Test	Comments
CBC, PT/PTT	Must be sent before giving heparin
Protein C—functional	Not helpful if patient is on warfarin sodium (Coumadin)
Protein C—immunologic if <6 mo	Normal levels in neonates are based on immunologic test
Protein S—functional and free	Not helpful if patient is on warfarin sodium (Coumadin)
Antithrombin-III	Must be sent before giving heparin
Factor V Leiden mutation	This is not a factor V level
Prothrombin mutation	G20210A genotype prothrombotic
Lupus inhibitor screen	Includes anticardiolipin antibody, anti-2GPI, dRVVT, and TTI
MTHFR gene mutation	C677T genotype prothrombotic
Plasma homocysteine level	High level prothrombotic
Lipoprotein (a)	High level prothrombotic

CBC, complete blood count; PT, prothrombin time; PTT, partial thrombin time; 2GPI, 2-glycoprotein I; dRVVT, diluted Russell viper venom test; TTI, tissue thromboplastin inhibition. MTHFR, methylenetetrahydrofolate reductase.

with pediatric thrombosis experts because these tests and their results are subject to change as research progresses in this area. An example of a list of studies to evaluate for thrombophilia is shown in Table 45.1, and is currently used (or something similar to this) by several pediatric stroke study centers. Current opinion among investigators in childhood stroke is that a broad evaluation for thrombophilia is indicated in all children with thromboembolic cerebrovascular disorders, irrespective of the presence of one or more known risk factors for stroke such as cardiac defects or arterial dissection. While the full treatment and prognostic implications of results of these studies await the results of long-term outcome studies and multicenter trials, it has been observed that children often have multiple stroke risk factors, including thrombophilia. Cardiac evaluation is commonly recommended in children with AIS, and usually involves minimally a transthoracic echocardiogram. Transthoracic echocardiogram may be considered for patients in whom no other major vascular cause is identified, and in whom the transthoracic echo was normal or equivocal.

The key to diagnosis of the extent and nature of cerebral ischemic injury lies in neuroimaging. MRI is far superior to computed tomography (CT) in confirming and characterizing acute ischemic injury, and in defining cerebrovascular abnormalities noninvasively. In most facilities, a CT scan can usually be obtained safely and quickly, and may narrow down the differential diagnosis quickly to a limited number of possibilities that have immediate treatment options. For example, venous thrombosis may appear on a head CT scan in severe cases, and if so should prompt immediate therapy with heparin and urgent venography. If the CT scan is uninformative or nonspecific, then all children with suspected cerebral ischemic injury should have a brain MRI as soon as possible, including vascular imaging as dictated by the clinical suspicion of arterial or venous disease. Repeat imaging will be needed in select patients who develop new or progressive deficits during the first week. Standard angiography should be considered in cases of AIS with equivocal or negative findings on magnetic resonance (MR) vascular imaging, or where no other risk factor is identified.

Acute Management: "Brain Resuscitation and Rescue"

There are no therapies proven to improve the outcome of global cerebral ischemic injury in infants and children. Several clinical trials have suggested that postresuscitation hypothermia may be beneficial for a subset of neonates with HIE, and in adult survivors of cardiac arrest. This treatment has not been tested in children, and is the subject of ongoing intense research. The only proven effective therapy for children with acute stroke is exchange transfusion for children with sickle cell anemia. Most centers that care for patients with sickle cell anemia have in place, procedures for transfusion therapy for acute stroke. In all other children with acute stroke syndromes confirmed by MRI, treatment at present is essentially based on consensus and the judicious and selective application of treatments used in adults. Therapeutic options for children with stroke commonly in use include anticoagulation and antiplatelet agents. Anticoagulation acutely may have a role, provided the initial infarct is nonhemorrhagic in select groups of patients, which is considered to have a high risk of clot propagation (in the case of SVT), or of recurrent embolization: SVT, arterial dissection, cardiogenic embolus. Some centers advocate the use of anticoagulation acutely for AIS related to high-grade stenosis in focal or segmental arteriopathy. Low-molecular-weight heparin (LMWH) has the advantages of ease of administration and predictable effect on coagulation parameters, and a good safety record in children treated for a wide variety of thrombotic conditions. Standard unfractionated heparin has the advantage of being able to be reversed quickly in patients at high risk of hemorrhage or who might need emergency surgery for other problems. Dosage recommendations and monitoring are best worked out in advance as part of an institutional stroke protocol in consultation with local thrombosis specialists.

By the end of the first week after a child has been admitted for a stroke syndrome, most diagnostic studies have been completed, and the patient's clinical deficits have stabilized. Decisions can then be made about secondary preventive treatments, which may include systemic anticoagulation with LMWH or warfarin sodium (Coumadin), or antiplatelet agents, or a definitive procedure such as closure of a patent foramen ovale. The decision to maintain long-term anticoagulation versus antiplatelet agents is individualized depending on the risk factors. Patients with an estimated high risk of stroke recurrence from thromboembolic events should be considered for long-term anticoagulation (e.g., recurrent cardiogenic stroke from fixed structural heart defect, or a patient with a severe permanent thrombophilia), and short-term anticoagulation for 3 to 6 months (arterial dissection, SVT related to head/neck infection). Other patients with known risk factors such as intracranial arteriopathy other than dissection, or with no identifiable risk factors, may be considered for antiplatelet agents. A detailed review of the role of antithrombotic treatment in childhood stroke syndromes is available elsewhere.

Rehabilitation should be started in the acute hospital unit as soon as the patient is hemodynamically stable. Discharge planning needs to start early, leading to a transfer to inpatient rehabilitation or to a home with outpatient rehabilitation. Appropriate family and patient psychosocial supportive services will usually be necessary at all stages of the illness and its treatment.

In occasional cases, there may be a role for two additional interventions for extreme or rare circumstances. Decompressive craniectomy may be both lifesaving and function sparing in adults, and may be even more so in children. Children with large middle cerebral artery stroke syndromes who display rapid deterioration in level of consciousness or progress to signs and symptoms of impending herniation should be considered for this procedure. The second controversial intervention is thrombolysis. Current standard of care for adult stroke involves using IV tissue plasminogen activator (tPA) only for patients 18 years and older meeting strict inclusion criteria, which can be found described in detail in the AHA website. The major limiting factor is that IV thrombolysis must be started within 3 hours of symptom onset, which is defined as the time the patient was last seen in a healthy condition. Children with stroke rarely meet this time limit. The role of thrombolysis for individuals below age 18 is much more controversial. Evidence as to the safety and efficacy of thrombolysis for children with stroke is extremely limited, and that existing for thrombolysis for systemic clots suggests a high risk of hemorrhagic complications. Until such evidence is available, decisions about using thrombolysis for individuals younger than 18 years are probably best handled with extreme caution, and in consultation with an affiliated adult stroke program experienced in the use of thrombolysis in adults.

CONCLUSION

Cerebral ischemic injury is one of the few neurologic emergencies in pediatric medicine, for which there are no proven therapies outside of transfusion for sickle cell anemia. The incidence of global and focal ischemia is highest among neonates, and overall, is similar to that of childhood brain tumors. Morbidity is high, and mortality remains significant. Evaluation and treatment should proceed in parallel, and with the understanding that "time is brain." This begins with clinical suspicion of a cerebral ischemic injury in any child with a new focal neurologic deficit or unexplained acute encephalopathy or post-HIE. It relies heavily on timely and comprehensive brain and vascular imaging, and finishes with evaluation in all patients for underlying cardiac, prothrombotic, and cerebrovascular risk factors. Treatment is initially supportive, aiming to minimize progression of injury by optimizing perfusion and preventing hyperthermia. Judicious and selective use of platelet inhibitors and systemic anticoagulation may limit progression or recurrence in children with thromboembolic and vascular disease. Early and aggressive rehabilitation are necessary to optimize recovery. There is very little data about the safety or efficacy of thrombolysis at present. Long-term follow-up with clinical and neuroimaging assessment are necessary to fully ascertain recurrence rates and support recovery.

RECOMMENDED READINGS

1. Sarnat HB, Sarnat MS. Neonatal encephalopathy following fetal distress. *Arch Neurol.* 1976;33:696–705.
2. Levy DE, Caronna JJ, Singer BH, et al. Predicting outcome from hypoxic-ischemic coma. *JAMA.* 1985;253:1420–1426.
3. Mandel R, Martinot A, Delepoulle F, et al. Prediction of outcome after hypoxic-ischemic encephalopathy: A prospective clinical and electrophysiologic study. *J Pediatr.* 2002;141:45–50.
4. Kidwell CS, Warach S. Acute ischemic cerebrovascular syndrome: Diagnostic criteria. *Stroke.* 2003;34:2995–2998.
5. Slonim AD, Patel KM, Ruttimann UE, et al. Cardiopulmonary resuscitation in pediatric intensive care units. *Crit Care Med.* 1997;25:1951–1955.
6. deVeber G, Roach ES, Riela AR, et al. Stroke in children: Recognition, treatment, and future directions. *Semin Pediatr Neurol.* 2000; 7:309–317.
7. Reis AG, Nadkarni V, Perondi MB, et al. A prospective investigation into the epidemiology of in-hospital pediatric cardiopulmonary resuscitation using the international Utstein reporting style. *Pediatrics.* 2002;109:200–209.
8. Ganesan V, Prengler M, McShane MA, et al. Investigation of risk factors in children with arterial ischemic stroke. *Ann Neurol.* 2003;53:167–173.
9. Gunther G, Junker R, Strater R, et al. Symptomatic ischemic stroke in full-term neonates: Role of acquired and genetic prothrombotic risk factors. *Stroke.* 2000;31:2437–2441.
10. deVeber G, Andrew M. Cerebral sinovenous thrombosis in children. *N Engl J Med.* 2001;345:417–423.
11. Chan AK, deVeber G. Prothrombotic disorders and ischemic stroke in children. *Semin Pediatr Neurol.* 2000;7:301–308.
12. Dix D, Andrew M, Marzinotto V, et al. The use of low molecular weight heparin in pediatric patients: A prospective cohort study. *J Pediatr.* 2000;136:439–445.
13. Monagle P, Chan A, Massicotte P, et al. Antithrombotic therapy in children: The Seventh ACCP Conference on Antithrombotic and Thrombolytic Therapy. *Chest.* 2004;126:645S–687S.
14. Koh MS, Goh KY, Tung MY, et al. Is decompressive craniectomy for acute cerebral infarction of any benefit? *Surg Neurol.* 2000; 53:225–230.
15. Gupta AA, Leaker M, Andrew M, et al. Safety and outcomes of thrombolysis with tissue plasminogen activator for treatment of intravascular thrombosis in children. *J Pediatr.* 2001;139: 682–688.
16. Adams H, Adams R, Del Zoppo G, et al. Stroke Council of the American Heart Association; American Stroke Association. Guidelines for the early management of patients with ischemic stroke: Guidelines update a scientific statement from the Stroke Council of the American Heart Association/American Stroke Association. *Stroke.* 2005;Apr;36(4):916–23.

Disorders of the Muscle

46

JoAnne E. Natale   Michael J. Bell

Traditionally, the term *neuromuscular disorders* refers to those diseases that involve the motor unit. Diseases of the motor unit are classified into motor neuropathies, peripheral neuropathies, disorders of neuromuscular transmission, and myopathies. The hallmark symptom of diseases of the motor unit is weakness, which may affect respiratory or bulbar muscles. Most pediatric neuromuscular diseases are manifest by insidiously progressive or fluctuating weakness. As such, they usually present as nonemergent diagnostic challenges. The pediatric intensivist usually becomes involved for evaluation and treatment of acute weakness and the management of airway compromise or respiratory failure. As discussed in Chapter 7, in addition to the many primary diseases of the motor unit, secondary neuromuscular disorders may evolve during the course of treatment of critically ill children.

The important aspects of evaluation of the infant and child with weakness include defining the distribution of weakness, involvement of cranial nerves, sensory abnormalities, autonomic dysfunction, and bladder and rectal sphincter involvement. In general, acute diseases of the lower motor unit present with symmetric weakness and normal or depressed deep tendon reflexes. In contrast, diseases of the central nervous system (CNS) usually manifest as asymmetry of weakness, hyperreflexia, extensor plantar responses, focal cranial nerve deficits, and/or focal sensory deficits. Patients with acute spinal cord disease, however, may present with symmetric flaccid paraparesis or quadriparesis. Early bladder or bowel sphincter disturbance in a child with acute symmetric paralysis warrants special concern because it may be caused by a compressive myelopathy that needs emergent diagnosis and neurosurgical treatment. Conversely, bulbar weakness in a child with acute quadriparesis places the lesion either rostral to the spinal cord or delineates a more diffuse neuromuscular disorder.

Diseases and conditions that can cause weakness or paralysis leading to respiratory failure are listed in Table 46.1. Although a full explanation of each of these diseases is beyond the scope of this chapter, important examples of disorders within each component of the motor unit will be discussed, including diseases of the spinal cord (acute transverse myelitis [ATM]), anterior horn cell/peripheral nerve (poliomyelitislike flaccid paralysis, spinal muscular atrophy [SMA], tetanus, and Guillain-Barré syndrome [GBS]), neuromuscular junction (myasthenia gravis [MG], toxin-mediated disorders), and muscle (muscular dystrophies, critical illness myopathy).

MYELOPATHIES

Acute Transverse Myelitis

ATM is a focal inflammatory disease of a portion of the spinal cord, which leads to loss of motor, sensory, and autonomic function. Although rare (overall incidence of ATM approximately is 4 cases per 1,000,000), the bimodal distribution of cases includes children from ages 10 to 19 years whereas a second peak occurs in adults. Many systemic diseases can cause focal disorders of spinal cord function, including thrombosis, infections, connective tissue diseases, radiation injury, and mass lesions. Standardized diagnostic criteria for idiopathic ATM were published in 2002 and include development of mixed deficits that can be bilateral (with a definitive sensory level), inflammation of the spinal cord (demonstrable by cerebrospinal fluid [CSF] or magnetic resonance imaging [MRI] findings), a typical course of worsening between 4 hours and 21 days after onset of symptoms, and exclusions of spinal masses or other systemic disorders (see Table 46.2).

Although uncommon, ATM requires rapid recognition and prompt management. Clinical findings generally include bilateral extremity weakness, loss of sphincter control, and loss of sensory levels. A focused history and physical examination should elicit the course of progression and presenting symptoms and lead to exclusions of other possible

TABLE 46.1

NEUROMUSCULAR CAUSES OF ACUTE RESPIRATORY FAILURE

Anatomic Location	Disorder
Spinal cord	*Acute transverse myelitis*
	Spinal cord compression
Lower motor neuron/anterior horn cell	*Poliomyelitislike flaccid paralysis*
	Rabies
	Spinal muscular atrophy[a]
	Tetanus
	West Nile virus flaccid paralysis
Peripheral nerve	Critical illness polyneuropathy/myopathy
	Diphtheria
	Guillain-Barré syndrome[a]
	Heavy metal toxicity (arsenic, lead)
	Porphyria
	Saxitoxin (paralytic shellfish poisoning)
	Thallium intoxication
Neuromuscular junction	*Botulism (infantile)*
	Congenital myasthenic syndromes[a]
	Hypermagnesemia
	Lambert-Eaton myasthenic syndrome
	Myasthenia gravis
	Neuromuscular blocking drugs
	Organophosphate poisoning
	Snake venom
	Tick paralysis
Muscle	Acute quadriplegic myopathy
	Acute electrolyte deficiency (hypokalemia, hypophosphatemia)
	Congenital myopathies
	Central core
	Myotubular
	Nemaline rod
	Critical illness polyneuropathy/myopathy
	Metabolic myopathies
	Acid maltase deficiency
	Carnitine palmityl-transferase deficiency
	Mitochondrial myopathy
	Muscular dystrophies
	Polymyositis/dermatomyositis
	Rhabdomyolysis
	Stonefish mycotoxin poisoning

Italics: conditions described in more detail in the text.
[a]Most common diagnoses to consider in the evaluation of the floppy infant.

TABLE 46.2

DIAGNOSTIC CRITERIA FOR IDIOPATHIC ACUTE TRANSVERSE MYELITIS

Inclusion Criteria

1. Development of sensory, motor, and/or autonomic dysfunction attributable to spinal cord
2. Bilateral signs or symptoms (not necessarily symmetric)
3. Clearly defined sensory level
4. Exclusion of extra-axial compressive etiology by MRI or myelography (CT scan of the spine is inadequate)
5. Inflammation of the spinal cord demonstrated by CSF pleocytosis, elevated IgG, or gadolinium enhancement within 7 d of symptom onset
6. Worsening neurologic dysfunction between 4 h and 21 d after the onset of symptoms

Exclusion Criteria

1. History of radiation to the spine in the previous 10 y
2. Clear arterial distribution of clinical deficit consistent with thrombosis of the anterior spinal artery
3. Abnormal flow voids on the surface of the spinal cord consistent with AVM
4. Serologic or clinical evidence of connective tissue disorder
5. CNS manifestations of syphilis, Lyme disease, HIV, mycoplasma, or other viral infection
6. Brain MRI abnormalities suggestive of multiple sclerosis
7. History of optic neuritis

MRI, magnetic resonance imaging; CT, computed tomography; IgG, immunoglobulin G; CSF, cerebrospinal fluid; AVM, arteriovenous malformation; CNS, central nervous system; HIV, human immunodeficiency virus.
From Transverse Myelitis Consortium Working Group. Proposed diagnostic criteria and nosology of acute transverse myelitis. *Neurology.* 2002;59(4):499–505.

etiologies including trauma. Once adequate respiratory and cardiovascular function is assured, a gadolinium-enhanced MRI of the spinal cord is required to diagnose ATM and to exclude a compressive or traumatic etiology. Management of these neurosurgical emergencies is discussed in Chapter 47. MRI findings consistent with ATM include enhancement of focal segments of the spinal cord after gadolinium contrast. Confirmatory CSF findings include pleocytosis (with a predominance of lymphocytes) and an increase in CSF immunoglobulin G (IgG). Because these CSF markers may be normal in early ATM, the lumbar puncture should be repeated 2 to 7 days after a negative result in CSF study when symptoms remain suggestive for ATM. If spinal cord inflammation is present, the next priority is to determine if it is associated with brain or optic tract demyelination using a gadolinium-enhanced brain MRI. Absence of cerebral demyelination suggests the diagnosis of ATM, whereas more extensive CNS demyelination suggests the diagnosis of multiple sclerosis or acute disseminated encephalomyelitis. Serum testing for known etiologies of ATM [Lyme titers, tests for syphilis (rapid plasma reagent [RPR] or venereal disease research laboratory [VDRL]), and serologic testing for connective tissue disorders] should be performed to diagnose treatable causes of ATM.

Despite standardized diagnostic criteria, immunopathogenic mechanisms leading to idiopathic ATM remain obscure. An antecedent infectious illness has been observed in 30% to 60% of idiopathic cases. Autoimmune mechanisms, such as molecular mimicry and superantigen-mediated disease, account for some cases of ATM. Although it is widely reported that ATM is a postvaccination event, this infrequent association suggests that the two events are not causally related.

Treatment regimens for infectious or connective tissue disorders should be instituted to ameliorate symptoms of ATM. For idiopathic ATM, consensus treatment strategies that improve outcomes have not been identified. On the basis of the immunologic nature of ATM and improved recovery in two small open-labeled studies in children, methylprednisolone is commonly offered to children with acute idiopathic ATM. However, given the limitations of these studies, controlled trials with methylprednisolone, and other immunomodulatory treatments, are worthy of further investigation.

MOTOR NEURONOPATHIES

Spinal Muscular Atrophy

SMA is a family of autosomal recessive disorders characterized by weakness caused by degeneration of anterior horn cells. Three major types of SMA are recognized based on clinical features. The most severe form, SMA I (also known as *acute infantile or Werdnig-Hoffman disease*), begins in the first few months of life and frequently progresses to death from respiratory failure before 2 years of age if mechanical ventilation is not provided. These alert and interactive infants have symmetric proximal and intercostal muscle weakness, absence of deep tendon reflexes, lack of normal muscular development, poor muscle tone, and tongue vermicular movements (erroneously termed *muscle fasciculations*). Chronic juvenile SMA, or type II, usually presents before the age of 18 months with failure to walk. Tremulous movements of the outstretched fingers, termed *polyminimyoclonus*, are frequently observed. Although muscle power remains stable, there is a loss of functionality due to increased linear growth, weight gain, and orthopedic deformity. Life expectancy extends into the third or fourth decade of life. The mildest form of SMA is type III, also known as *Wohlfart-Kugelberg-Welander syndrome*, which generally presents in late childhood or adolescence with proximal weakness, waddling gait, and lumbar lordosis.

All forms of SMA have been linked to chromosome 5q11.2 to 13.3. The survival motor neuron gene (*SMN1*), mapped to this region, is deleted in >98% of individuals with any type of SMA. DNA testing for this mutation is the primary diagnostic test for SMA. Despite the linkage of SMN gene defects to SMA, specific therapies for the various forms of this disorder remain elusive. Because the weakness is generally progressive, limiting the complications of restrictive lung disease, poor nutrition, orthopedic deformities, and pulmonary infections are the care goals for infants and children with SMA. As with any progressive neuromuscular disease, ongoing discussions with the patient's family regarding their preference for invasive or supportive treatment are essential for optimal critical care management. Noninvasive ventilation and tracheostomy have broadened the options available for families of these infants with SMA. If invasive mechanical ventilation is indicated for acute respiratory failure, weaning from mechanical ventilation as soon as possible will limit muscle deconditioning. Ventilation in the prone position may provide benefits to oxygenation, while improving exhalation by splinting the abdominal muscles.

Poliomyelitislike Flaccid Paralysis

Several of the acute motor neuron diseases are well known, but relatively rare. Over 100 cases of vaccination-associated poliomyelitis (VAP) were recognized between 1961 and 1984. Nonetheless, cases of flaccid paralysis caused by coxsackie virus (group A7, A10, B3, and B5), echoviruses (types 2, 6, and 9), adenovirus, mumps, varicella-zoster, and Epstein-Barr virus have been reported. More recently, a poliomyelitislike syndrome caused by mosquito-borne West Nile virus has gained considerable attention, but rarely occurs in young individuals. The clinical features of neurotropic viral infections include fever, meningeal signs, and muscle pain that precede asymmetric flaccid paralysis. Typically, sensation is preserved.

Tetanus

While tetanus is also rare in industrialized nations, it must be considered in the differential diagnosis of children presenting with acute or subacute focal or generalized rigidity. The neurotoxin tetanospasmin that is produced by the anaerobe *Clostridium tetani* blocks glycine-mediated inhibitory synapses surrounding the motor neuron, resulting in anterior horn cell hyper excitability and spontaneous and reflex-elicited motor neuron discharges. Therefore, tetanus is the exception to the rule that neuromuscular diseases present with weakness. Human antitetanus globulin and antibiotics are cornerstones of therapy. Sympathetic hyperactivity may respond to β-blockers and morphine.

PERIPHERAL NEUROPATHIES

Guillain-Barré Syndrome

GBS, an immune-mediated polyneuropathy, is the most common neuromuscular disorder necessitating intensive care unit (ICU) admission and ventilator support. Symptoms include rapidly ascending paralysis that lasts for several weeks or longer. Subtypes are based on clinical features and histopathologic findings. The pathogenesis of GBS is incompletely understood, but likely includes both humoral and cellular immune mechanisms because (i) complement is activated and deposited on myelin sheaths, (ii) antiganglioside or glycolipid antibodies are frequently observed, (iii) cytokines produced from T cells have been reported, and (iv) macrophages invade myelin sheaths. A viral illness, particularly with a herpesvirus, often precedes the onset of symptoms by approximately 1 to 3 weeks.

GBS has been divided into as many as five distinct subtypes, and other unusual presentations have also been described. Acute inflammatory demyelinating polyneuropathy (AIDP) is the classic form of ascending paralysis that is the most common presentation in Europe and the United States. Acute motor axonal neuropathy (AMAN) presents with pure motor symptoms because only motor axons become demyelinated. AMAN is the most prevalent form of GBS in China and affects children and young adults in summer epidemics. An axonal variant that affects both sensory and motor axons is termed *acute motor and sensory axonal neuropathy* (AMSAN). AMSAN affects both sensory and motor axons with a greater sensory component than AIDP and, usually, has a more severe clinical course. Histologically, AMAN and AMSAN are distinguished from AIDP by their lack of T-cell lymphocyte infiltrates. The Miller-Fisher syndrome (MFS) is a distinct form of GBS that is characterized by the triad of ophthalmoplegia, ataxia, and areflexia, and can transition into classical AIDP in a subset of cases. Acute pandysautonomia with selective degeneration of peripheral nerves is associated with autonomic nervous system dysfunction but preserved sensory and motor functions. Lastly, by definition, weakness evolving for longer than 8 weeks excludes a diagnosis of GBS and suggests an alternative diagnosis such as chronic inflammatory demyelinating polyradiculoneuropathy (CIDP).

The diagnosis of GBS is largely based on clinical symptoms as well as ancillary testing. CSF analysis at the end of the first week of illness normally demonstrates an acellular increase in protein concentrations. Recent studies have suggested that the lipopolysaccharide of *Campylobacter jejuni* may mimic the nervous system gangliosides GM_1, GD_{1a}, GD_3, and GT_{1a} and this molecular similarity may be responsible for the production of antiganglioside antibodies observed in GBS. However, only about 50% of patients with GBS demonstrate antibodies against GM_1. Abnormal nerve conduction studies are found in the distribution of clinical symptoms. More extensive electrophysiologic testing, such as measuring differences in axonal excitability, can distinguish between the various subtypes of GBS if required.

Treatment supports cardiovascular and respiratory functioning followed by immunotherapies to mitigate neurologic symptoms. Airway monitoring and support are especially important given the possibility of cranial nerve involvement and the rapidity of symptom progression in some GBS subtypes. Measurement of pulmonary function, including vital capacity, can be used to monitor changes in respiratory muscle mechanics.

Numerous studies have documented the utility of immunomodulatory therapy in GBS. Plasmapheresis is thought to act by removing the causative autoantibodies and complement from the serum by simple serum replacement. Similarly, intravenous immunoglobulin (IVIg) is believed to bind circulating autoantibodies and prevent

their continued activity. Both plasma exchange and IVIg are equally effective in shortening the course of classic demyelinating form of GBS. Either must be administered within the first 7 to 10 days from symptom onset for maximum benefit. Their efficacy in the GBS variants has not been subject to the same scientific scrutiny, but clinical reports support their use. IVIg should also be the preferred treatment when prominent signs and symptoms of dysautonomia, particularly hypotension, are a major component of the clinical picture. In an early controlled trial comparing IVIg to plasma exchange, IVIg (0.4 g/kg/day over 5 days) improved motor function and recovery time better than plasma exchange. Although IVIg and plasma exchange were equally effective in improving motor function at 4 weeks after clinical onset, combination therapy with both IVIg and plasma exchange provided no additional benefit. Similarly, there is no value to adding corticosteroids to either plasmapheresis or IVIg. Finally, 6 days of 2.5 g/kg/day IVIg was far superior to 3 days of IVIg at 1.2 g/kg/day to initiate walking in course of time (84 vs. 131 days) and in decreasing the need for mechanical ventilation. Therefore, current recommendations for symptomatic GBS include either plasmapheresis or IVIg at a dosage of at least 2 g/kg/day.

The prognosis for recovery in children is generally excellent; most children achieve a complete functional recovery within 6 months from the onset of illness. The axonal variants often have a more prolonged recovery.

DISORDERS OF NEUROMUSCULAR TRANSMISSION

Myasthenia Gravis

MG is an immune-mediated disorder that is characterized by the production of autoantibodies against the acetylcholine receptor, producing blockade of transmission at the neuromuscular junction. Although the precise mechanism responsible for the production of these autoantibodies is unclear, the thymus seems to play a role because thymectomy is curative in select patients. MG occurs with a prevalence of 12 to 15 per 100,000, with approximately 10% to 25% of these cases presenting during childhood or adolescence. MG occurs with increased frequency in African Americans and, prior to adolescence, there is an equal distribution of cases in males and females.

MG is purely a motor condition characterized by weakness that worsens with repeated activity. Often, the muscles controlling the eyelid and extraocular movement are the first to be affected. Therefore, diplopia and ptosis are frequent presenting symptoms, and MG should be strongly considered in children with isolated weakness of muscles controlled by the cranial nerves. More relevant, however, to the intensive care pediatrician is myasthenic crisis. Such crises are life-threatening episodes of respiratory or bulbar dysfunction. Myasthenic crisis can be precipitated

TABLE 46.3

SIGNS OF IMPENDING RESPIRATORY FAILURE IN PATIENTS WITH NEUROMUSCULAR DISEASE

Accessory muscle use
Air hunger
Atelectasis
FVC ≤15 mL/kg (or 50% decrease from baseline)
Hypercarbia
Hypoxemia
NIF <20 cm H_2O
PIF <40 cm H_2O
Profound weakness on neck flexion
Paradoxical breathing (sign of diaphragmatic weakness)
Respiratory acidosis (late)
Restlessness, anxiety
Tachycardia
Tachypnea

FVC, forced vital capacity; NIF, negative inspiratory force; PIF, positive inspiratory force.

by infections, pregnancy, surgery, or various drugs. Some common drugs, particularly aminoglycosides, lidocaine, procainamide, and magnesium, can lead to myasthenic crisis and should be avoided when possible in patients with MG. Over 30% of myasthenic crises are idiopathic.

Treatment of MG and myasthenic crisis includes provision of supportive care, elimination of any triggers/exacerbating factors, and maximizing muscular function. Patients in myasthenic crisis need to be monitored carefully for impending respiratory failure using the criteria provided in Table 46.3. Unlike GBS, MG often presents without an orderly progression of ascending symptoms. Therefore, the child's ability to maintain a patent airway and maintain respiratory function must be continually assessed. The best study of ventilator management in myasthenic crisis suggests that using a combination of approaches that includes sigh breaths during ventilation, high positive end-expiratory pressure (PEEP), frequent functioning, and chest physiotherapy is most effective. If muscle relaxants are necessary to facilitate intubation, the dose should be titrated using peripheral nerve monitoring (train-of-four [TOF], as described in Chapter 7). TOF monitoring will also assist in assessing readiness for extubation after surgical procedures in patients with MG. Ventilatory weaning should begin when the patient demonstrates improved strength and triggers have been eliminated. Appropriate strategies include provision of continuous positive airway pressure (CPAP), high-pressure support, and slow weaning over a period of 2 to 3 days.

Treatment options for MG and myasthenic crisis include anticholinesterases, plasmapheresis, IVIg, and corticosteroids. Anticholinesterases increase the amount of acetylcholine within the synaptic cleft by decreasing its catabolism. This transiently improves the transmission of the action potential across the neuromuscular junction and improves muscle function. Plasmapheresis and IVIg have been used to reduce autoantibodies implicated in MG. Corticosteroids theoretically diminish the intrinsic immune reactions responsible for production of the autoantibodies against the acetylcholine receptor. The combination of these options has not been systematically studied. One small study suggests that plasmapheresis may be associated with earlier extubation. Beneficial effects of steroids have been sporadically reported.

Toxin-Mediated Disorders of Neuromuscular Junction

Infantile Botulism

Numerous toxins affecting neuromuscular synaptic transmission are listed in Table 46.1. Infantile botulism is the most common toxin-mediated disorder in infants. The incidence of infant botulism has remained at 60 to 90 cases per year in the United States over the last 20 years. Infants routinely ingest the spores of the clostridial species *Clostridium botulinum*, *C. baratii*, or *C. butyricum*, whose toxins can be released in the gut and then absorbed into the bloodstream when the spores have germinated. As discussed in Chapter 7, toxins from *C. botulinum* cleave presynaptic proteins to prevent acetylcholine release at the neuromuscular junction and at cholinergic synapses in the autonomic nervous system. Clinical manifestations reflect the lack of cholinergic neurotransmission. Characteristic symptoms in affected infants include dry mouth, cranial nerve dysfunction (e.g., poor suck, weak cry, facial diplegia, ptosis, decreased extraocular motility, and sluggish papillary light response with mydriasis), descending paralysis, hypotonia, and protracted constipation. The hypotonia and paucity of movement may last for weeks.

Diagnosis of botulism requires either isolation of toxin from stool or electrodiagnostic studies. Identification of toxin in stool is confirmatory; however, it may take 2 weeks to obtain the results of this bioassay. As recent data demonstrate a beneficial effect of botulism immune globulin (BIG) when administered early in the course of infantile botulism, rapid electrodiagnostic confirmation is indicated. Nerve conduction studies show normal sensory nerve conduction velocity and normal sensory nerve potential amplitude. Motor nerve studies reveal normal nerve conduction velocity with low amplitude compound muscle action potentials. Low-rate (2 Hz) repetitive stimulation may elicit an electrodecremental response. The hallmark of botulism (as in other presynaptic disorders of neuromuscular transmission) is a pathologic facilitation of the compound muscle action potential to high-frequency (20 to 50 Hz) repetitive stimulation. To further enhance diagnostic certainty, tests to exclude other causes of hypotonia, particularly neuroimaging and electroencephalogram (EEG), should also be obtained.

Although hypotonic infants with botulism are usually afebrile, initial treatment may include antibiotics for other infections (sepsis, pneumonia). In such cases, aminoglycosides should be avoided because they potentiate botulinum neuromuscular blockade and increase the risk for respiratory failure. Until recently, treatment of infant botulism was confined to nonspecific supportive strategies used for all neuromuscular disorders. In 2003, human BIG was approved by the U.S. Food and Drug Administration (FDA) for use in infant botulism. The FDA reported results of a controlled clinical trial in 59 infants with laboratory-confirmed infant botulism. Compared to placebo, BIG administered within the first 3 days of hospital admission reduced average length of hospital stay from 5.7 to 2.6 weeks (p <0.0001), reduced length of pediatric intensive care unit (PICU) stay from 3.6 to 1.3 weeks (p <0.01), reduced average time on mechanical ventilation from 2.4 to 0.7 weeks (p <0.01), and reduced the average number of weeks of tube feeding from 10 to 3.6 weeks (p <0.01). With timely diagnosis and appropriate supportive care, the prognosis for full recovery after infantile botulism is excellent.

Tick Paralysis

Although tick paralysis is an uncommon etiology of acute paralysis, the rapid reversal of clinical effects by simply removing the tick highlights the importance of recognizing this syndrome. This is especially true because ticks are often found in areas where detection is difficult, such as the scalp, nose, ear canal, or perineum. Paralysis has been related to the bite of at least 43 different species of female ticks and appears to be produced by inhibition of acetylcholine release at the neuromuscular junction. Clinically, symptoms begin 2 to 6 days after tick attachment, with listlessness and fatigue, followed by ascending symmetrical paralysis and areflexia 1 to 2 days later. Sensory symptoms have also been reported.

MYOPATHIES

Critical Illness Myopathy and Muscular Dystrophies

Disorders of muscular strength are becoming more widely recognized in critically ill children, and critical illness myopathy and the muscular dystrophies are among the most common etiologies. As discussed in more detail in Chapter 7, critical illness neuropathy and myopathy are common in adults and appear to be under-recognized in children with increasing numbers of cases being described. Although critical illness neuropathy is closely associated with recovery from sepsis, critical illness myopathy can follow any severe respiratory illness and is closely associated with the use of high-dose corticosteroids. Flaccid weakness of extremities, diminished muscle mass, and decreased

respiratory effort are the common physical findings of critical illness myopathy. Histologic analysis reveals disorganization of the muscle fibers, often with necrosis. Electrophysiologic studies show reduction or absence of compound muscle and sensory action potentials, fibrillations, and loss of motor potentials with maximal efforts. Muscle biopsy is required for conclusive diagnosis. There are no specific therapies for critical illness myopathy and symptoms improve over several weeks to months.

The dystrophinopathies are a family of X-linked recessive disorders resulting from mutation in the dystrophin gene. With an incidence of 1 in 3,500 live male births, Duchenne muscular dystrophy (DMD) is the most common dystrophinopathy. Skeletal muscle weakness in DMD progresses relentlessly, often with the inability to ambulate by age 12. Development of kyphoscoliosis along with respiratory muscle weakness produces a restrictive respiratory pattern. In addition to skeletal muscle, 90% of patients with DMD have abnormalities on electrocardiogram (EKG), and many have cardiomyopathy with poor ejection fraction (see Chapter 32). Diagnosis of DMD is based on myopathic signs and symptoms, highly increased serum creatine kinase (CK) levels, myopathic changes on electromyogram (EMG), and absence of dystrophin in muscle biopsy.

Children with DMD rarely present with acute onset of muscular weakness. The pediatric intensivist tends to encounter patients with muscular dystrophy when their muscle disorder limits their ability to recover from surgery or from respiratory or cardiovascular complications of their muscle disease. Therefore, critical care management of children with DMD often involves decisions to support respiratory effort noninvasively (CPAP, PEEP, bilevel positive airway pressure [BiPAP]), invasively (endotracheal intubation), or permanently (tracheostomy). When considering muscle relaxation to facilitate intubation or surgery, succinylcholine is contraindicated in individuals with dystrophinopathies because of the risk of hyperkalemic cardiac arrest and rhabdomyolysis. Cardiovascular function should be considered for both prognostic reasons and as a clinical consideration when procedures are performed.

Recognition of Respiratory Failure in Neuromuscular Disease

Individuals with acute or chronic neuromuscular disease most commonly develop respiratory failure from bulbar and respiratory muscle weakness/paralysis and/or pulmonary complications such as pneumonia, or pulmonary embolism. Together, these problems can compromise upper airway function and diminish tidal volume leading to respiratory failure. A more detailed discussion of the pathophysiology of respiratory failure in neuromuscular disease is found in Chapter 41. Early recognition of imminent respiratory failure can avoid the inherent risks of emergent airway management. Assessment focuses on evaluating airway patency, respiratory muscle strength, and gas exchange. Difficulty with swallowing secretions or hoarse voice signals problems with the upper airway. Paradoxical abdominal movement is a sign of diaphragmatic weakness, and is generally accompanied by intercostal muscle retractions. Useful clinical signs of impending respiratory failure are listed in Table 46.3. In older children and adolescents, bedside spirometry measurements are useful for repeated quantitative assessment of respiratory muscle strength.

Respiratory failure is a potentially life-threatening complication of acute or decompensated chronic neuromuscular disorders. Ventilatory support can be provided with invasive or noninvasive modalities. A discussion of proper selection of ventilatory modes, and strategies for weaning from mechanical ventilation are found in Chapter 53.

GENERAL CRITICAL CARE MANAGEMENT ISSUES

Patients with neurogenic respiratory failure are at increased risk of ICU complications including ventilator-associated pneumonia, deep vein thromboses (DVT), atelectasis, and skin breakdown. Strategies to limit these complications include the use of noninvasive ventilation, semirecumbent positioning, mouth care, H_2-blockers, judicious application of PEEP, prone positioning, age and risk-appropriate DVT prophylaxis, and use of mechanical inexsufflator cough assist device and intrapulmonary percussive ventilation to improve mucus clearance.

RECOMMENDED READINGS

1. Varelas PN, Chua HC, Natterman J, et al. Ventilatory care in myasthenia gravis crisis: Assessing the baseline adverse event rate. *Crit Care Med.* 2002;30:2663–2668.
2. Transverse Myelitis Consortium Working Group. Proposed diagnostic criteria and nosology of acute transverse myelitis. *Neurology.* 2002;59(4):499–505.
3. Birnkrant DJ, Pope JF, Eiben RM. Management of the respiratory complications of neuromuscular diseases in the pediatric intensive care unit. *J Child Neurol.* 1999;14:139–143.
4. Dalakas MC. Intravenous immunoglobulin in autoimmune neuromuscular diseases. *JAMA.* 2004;291:2367–2375.
5. Finder JD, Birnkrant D, Carl J, et al. Respiratory care of the patient with Duchenne muscular dystrophy: ATS consensus statement. *Am J Respir Crit Care Med.* 2004;170:456–465.
6. Fox CK, Keet CA, Strober JB, et al. Recent advances in infant botulism. *Pediatr Neurol.* 2005;32:149–154.
7. Henderson RD, Lawn ND, Fletcher DD, et al. The morbidity of Guillain-Barré syndrome admitted to the intensive care unit. *Neurology.* 2003;60:17–21.
8. Laghi F, Tobin MJ. Disorders of the respiratory muscles. *Am J Respir Crit Care Med.* 2003;168:10–48.
9. MacDuff A, Grant IS. Critical care management of neuromuscular disease, including long-term ventilation. *Curr Opin Crit Care.* 2003;9:106–112.
10. Mathews KD. Muscular dystrophy overview: Genetics and diagnosis. *Neurol Clin.* 2003;21:795–816.
11. Miske LJ, Hickey EM, Kolb SM, et al. Use of the mechanical inexsufflator in pediatric patients with neuromuscular disease and impaired cough. *Chest.* 2004;125:1406–1412.
12. Rabinstein AA, Wijdicks EF. Warning signs of imminent respiratory failure in neurological patients. *Semin Neurol.* 2003;23:97–104.

Neurological Emergencies

47

Roger J. Packer   *Derek A. Bruce*

Focal nontraumatic lesions of the central nervous system (CNS) cause neurologic damage by a variety of different mechanisms, including compression and/or destruction of specific areas of the brain or spinal cord tissue, obstruction of cerebrospinal fluid (CSF) outflow, demyelination, and disruption of CNS vasculature resulting in hemorrhage or ischemia. These lesions are often associated with edema, intensifying the degree of dysfunction and/or CSF obstruction. There may also be secondary damage due to cerebral herniation. This chapter focuses on the presentation and management of tumors that affect the CNS, although similar neurologic deficits can be caused by other processes, including abscesses, focal infectious cerebritis and encephalitis, cerebrovascular accidents, focal manifestations of neurometabolic diseases, and acute demyelinating conditions.

Clinical presentation is dependent on the location and size of the lesion, the amount of surrounding edema, and the proximity to CSF pathways. However, the rapidity of the growth of the lesion and the age of the patient also significantly impact the signs and symptoms seen. Infants with mass lesions notoriously present with nonspecific findings including lethargy, enlarging head circumference, abnormal eye movements, and retardation or deterioration of psychomotor development, prior to the recognition of focal neurologic deficits.

INTRACRANIAL TUMORS

Brain tumors are the second most common form of childhood cancer and the leading cause of morbidity and mortality from cancer in children. Unlike the situation in adults, most childhood brain tumors are primary CNS lesions. Metastatic tumors, primarily because of neuroblastoma and less frequently sarcoma, may arise, but make up <5% of all tumors. Primary CNS tumors encompass a vast array of different histologies and occur

in approximately 3.5 per 100,000 children at risk per year. They may present at any point during childhood, but tend to be more frequent in the first decade of life, with approximately 20% of patients developing symptoms before the age of 2 years. Diagnosis has been simplified with the routine availability of magnetic resonance imaging (MRI); however, histologic confirmation is required for most lesions, with specific exceptions.

Infratentorial Tumors

Approximately 50% of all childhood brain tumors will arise in the posterior fossa. Four major subtypes of childhood brain tumors constitute most infratentorial tumors: medulloblastomas, cerebellar astrocytomas, ependymomas, and brain stem gliomas (see Table 47.1).

Medulloblastomas, the most common form of malignant childhood brain tumors, constitute approximately 40% of all posterior fossa tumors. Medulloblastomas usually arise from the roof of the fourth ventricle and typically present with a 2- to 4-month history of headaches, vomiting, and truncal unsteadiness. Neuroradiographically, they are characteristically enhancing masses, filling the fourth ventricle with resultant obstructive hydrocephalus in over 80% of patients. There may be infiltration of the brain stem. Approximately 5% to 10% of patients will present more explosively because of hemorrhage within the tumor, with the acute onset of severe headaches, vomiting, and obtundation. Twenty percent to 35% of patients with medulloblastoma will have disseminated the disease at the time of diagnosis to either intracranial sites or the spinal subarachnoid space. However, dissemination is usually asymptomatic.

Cerebellar astrocytomas also constitute approximately 40% of all childhood posterior fossa tumors. Cerebellar astrocytomas, which typically arise in the lateral hemispheres of the cerebellum, usually present with a 3- to 6-month

TABLE 47.1
CHILDHOOD COMMON INFRATENTORIAL MASS LESIONS

	Incidence	Peak Age	Presentation	Neuroradiographic Features	Management	Special Features
Medulloblastoma	40% of all posterior fossa tumors	3–5 y; second peak 7–8 y	Headache; nausea; vomiting; midline ataxia	Hyperdense mass on CT scan; enhancing, often homogeneously; hydrocephalus up to 80%	External ventriculostomy; corticosteroids; surgical resection	75% + survival; dissemination at diagnosis in up to 33%; posterior fossa mutism postoperative in 20%–30%
Cerebellar astrocytoma	40% of all posterior fossa tumors	5–10 y	Lateral cerebellar finding; headaches; nausea; vomiting later	Cyst with mural nodule; 75% with hydrocephalus	± external ventriculostomy; corticosteroid; surgical resection	20% midline/solid; >95% cure for pilocytic
Brain stem gliomas	10%–20% of all posterior fossa	Any age; usually >5 y	Multiple cranial nerve palsies; motor and cerebellar impairment	Diffuse nonenhancing pontine lesion with contiguous spread; 30% or less with hydrocephalus	Corticosteroids; stabilization; if hydrocephalus, CSF divergence; surgery for focal lesions	Diffuse lesions: 90% die within 18 mo; focal lesion: better prognosis
Ependymomas	10%–20% of all posterior fossa	Peaks in those <3 y	Like medulloblastoma; often sixth, seventh, and eight cranial nerve palsies	Usually enhancing inhomogeneously; may be laterally placed; approximately 50% hydrocephalus	External ventriculostomy; corticosteroids; Resection	Variable survival: 40%–80%; often postoperative cranial nerve palsies
Demyelinating masses	Rare	Any age—usually somewhat older	Acute onset focal cerebellar deficits; headaches	Hypodense mass with peripheral enhancement; usually no hydrocephalus	Corticosteroids; ± biopsy	May be part of acute disseminated encephalomyelitis
Stroke	Rare	Any age—usually somewhat older	Acute onset focal cerebellar deficits; headaches	Hypodense mass with peripheral enhancement; usually no hydrocephalus	Corticosteroids of questionable utility; mannitol; surgical decompression if uncontrolled local edema	Usually of unclear etiology
Cerebellar hemorrhage	Rare	Any age	Acute onset focal cerebellar deficits; hydrocephalus	Hyperintense cerebellar mass	Corticosteroids; control ICP; surgical evacuation; MRI or arteriogram	May be difficult to separate from hemorrhagic medulloblastoma

CT, computed tomography; CSF, cerebrospinal fluid; ICP, intracranial pressure; MRI, magnetic resonance imaging.

history of unsteadiness involving one side of the body with associated dysmetria. Within 2 to 3 months, headaches, nausea, vomiting, and truncal unsteadiness develop because of the growth of the tumor toward the midline and secondary obstruction of CSF pathways. Neuroradiographically, cerebellar astrocytomas most commonly are cystic lesions with an enhancing mural nodule. Most cerebellar astrocytomas are histologically low-grade pilocytic tumors. Solid midline lesions, presenting more like medulloblastomas, arise in approximately 10% to 20% of patients.

Brain stem gliomas constitute 20% of childhood posterior fossa tumors. Occurring in children of all ages, they are somewhat more common later in childhood and present with the insidious development of multiple cranial nerve findings, motor impairment, unsteadiness, and dysmetria. Neuroradiographically characterized as diffuse lesions that most commonly involve the pons, often with contiguous involvement of the medulla, midbrain, and other CNS sites; these tumors are usually histologically grade II or grade III astrocytomas. Hydrocephalus is present in less than one third of patients at diagnosis. Approximately 20% of brain stem gliomas are histologically lower grade and carry a better prognosis. These include tumors that, although intrinsic to the brain stem, are partially cystic or solid (most likely pilocytic astrocytomas), tectal masses usually presenting with hydrocephalus due to the obstruction of the third ventricle, and cervicomedullary masses that are posteriorly exophytic from the brain stem.

Ependymomas constitute 15% to 20% of all childhood posterior fossa tumors and tend to occur in younger children, especially those younger than 5 years. Ependymomas may clinically mimic either a slow growing form of medulloblastoma or a more aggressive form of cerebellar astrocytoma. They also have a predilection for the cerebellopontine angle, resulting in multiple cranial nerve deficits including seventh and eighth nerve palsies. Hydrocephalus is present in well over half the patients by the time of diagnosis.

Emergency Management of Posterior Fossa Tumors

As is the case for most mass lesions of the CNS, the initial step in emergency management is the control of intracranial pressure (ICP). Most patients will require the initiation of corticosteroids, usually dexamethasone, at an initial intravenous bolus dose of 1 mg per kg followed by a maintenance dose of 1 to 2 mg/kg/day in divided doses (initial maintenance dose may be as high as 10 mg, four times daily, but usually 4 mg, four times daily, is adequate). For those patients with hydrocephalus, emergency CSF diversion may be required. For patients with hydrocephalus, and signs of increased ICP such as papilledema, sixth nerve palsy, decreased level of consciousness, or decerebrate posturing emergency, diversion of the CSF may be required. This has usually been done by ventriculostomy and external ventricular drainage but currently is often handled by performing

an endoscopic third ventriculostomy and leaving an external drain for pressure monitoring. The risk of upward herniation of the posterior fossa contents because of lowering the supratentorial pressure is a rare complication of acute CSF drainage, but is more likely with cystic tumors. The presentation is of deteriorating consciousness, unilateral or bilateral III nerve palsy similar to the symptoms of downward transtentorial herniation, after CSF drainage. The clue to the diagnosis is that removing more CSF results in continued worsening of the child's neurologic condition. About 24 to 72 hours later, the CSF diversion is followed by tumor resection. Especially in children with cystic tumors and suppressed consciousness or pressure waves (episodic severe headache, bradycardia, intermittent visual loss with the headache), steroids are unlikely to have much effect on the local raised pressure, and emergency tumor resection may be required. CSF drainage and monitoring is continued after surgery until it is clear that CSF flow is adequate. With the current treatment, <50% of patients will require permanent CSF diversion procedure. Following surgery, there is often postoperative edema and corticosteroids are maintained for a few days and then carefully tapered.

Surgical tumor removal is not only required for diagnosis, but is a critical component of management for children with medulloblastomas, ependymomas, and cerebellar astrocytomas. Total surgical resection improves the outcome for children with cerebellar astrocytomas, medulloblastomas, and ependymomas. Children with diffuse intrinsic brain stem gliomas can be reliably diagnosed on the basis of neuroradiographic features. Histologic confirmation is usually not necessary and brain stem surgery is associated with increased, transient, and, at times, permanent neurologic deficits. Patients with tectal brain stem gliomas can often be managed for years with CSF diversion alone.

Following surgery, especially for patients with medulloblastoma, but also at times for patients with other forms of large, predominantly midline posterior fossa tumor, there may be development of the delayed onset (usually 12 to 24 hours after surgery) of mutism, hypotonia, supranuclear cranial nerve palsies, alterations in consciousness, and severe emotional liability. This syndrome, of unclear etiology, possibly due to cerebellar damage, has been termed *the posterior fossa mutism syndrome*. It is distinct from direct damage to the brain stem, secondary to the tumor or surgery, which is not characterized by mutism and is more likely to present with multiple cranial nerve findings, motor difficulties, and cerebellar dysfunction. Onset of the posterior fossa cerebellar mutism syndrome may be explosive, and it usually lasts weeks. Some degree of residual damage is present in over 50% of patients. Another postoperative syndrome, aseptic meningitis, commonest after astrocytoma resection, is believed to be a chemical meningitis following surgery. Aseptic meningitis has been associated with relatively rapid withdrawal of corticosteroids following surgery; it is usually self-limited, and has to be differentiated from postoperative bacterial meningitis by CSF sampling.

Supratentorial Central Nervous System Tumors

Supratentorial CNS tumors can be best considered as located in three relatively distinct areas of the brain; the diencephalic (chiasm/hypothalamic/thalamic) region, the pineal region, and the cerebral cortex.

The most common suprasellar tumors are gliomas (predominantly low grade), craniopharyngiomas, and germinomas. Diencephalic gliomas constitute approximately 40% of all lesions in this region, tend to present insidiously with visual difficulties including decreased visual acuity, complex visual field loss, and nystagmus. Neuroradiographically they are characterized by relatively diffuse lesions, which may enhance and often infiltrate posteriorly along the visual pathway. Depending on the extent, they may also cause focal neurologic deficits by infiltration into the thalamic region. In young children, especially those younger than 2 years, diencephalic gliomas notoriously result in the "diencephalic syndrome," which includes failure to thrive despite apparent normal caloric intake. Many of these patients will also have, on closer examination, associated visual or other neurologic deficits. Most diencephalic gliomas are low grade and hydrocephalus is present in <20% of patients at the time of diagnosis. Children with neurofibromatosis type 1 are at a higher likelihood of developing visual pathway gliomas, especially those involving the optic nerves and chiasm. They tend to have a more indolent form of disease. These tumors rarely present as emergencies, but when they do, it is usually because of acute intracranial hypertension due to hydrocephalus.

Children with craniopharyngiomas classically present with heterogeneous masses that have both cystic and solid components arising in the suprasellar region. They manifest visual difficulties including unilateral visual loss with associated contralateral temporal visual field loss in eccentric lesions and, in midline lesions, bitemporal hemianopsias. Hydrocephalus, due to distortion and obstruction of the third ventricular outflow, is present in approximately half of the cases. Endocrinologic deficits occur in as many as 90% of patients at diagnosis and the most common initial finding is growth hormone deficiency, although other deficits such as hypothyroidism may be present.

Suprasellar germinomas are the third most common form of tumor arising in this region of the brain and may, despite their histologic aggressivity, present with diabetes insipidus or with a long-standing history of other endocrinologic problems. Other processes such as histiocytosis may also arise in a similar fashion in the suprasellar region. Emergency presentation is usually related to sudden visual loss from tumor compression of the optic nerves and chiasm or hydrocephalus.

Approximately 5% to 10% of all childhood brain tumors occur in the pineal region. The classic presentation of pineal region masses is the "Parinaud syndrome" due to tectal compression, which includes pupils that react better to light than accommodation, retraction or convergence nystagmus, limitations of upgaze, and lid retraction. A wide variety of different tumor types may arise, including germinomas, mixed germ cell tumors, pineoblastomas, and gliomas, and they cannot be reliably separated on neuroradiographic grounds. Although most lesions will require surgery for definitive diagnosis, mixed germ cell tumor can be diagnosed by elevations of α-fetoprotein and β-human chorionic gonadotropin (β-HCG) in CSF, and choriocarcinomas can be diagnosed by elevation of β-HCG.

Cortical childhood brain tumors are predominantly high-grade or low-grade gliomas, although other tumor types may occur, such as cortical primitive neuroectodermal tumors and ependymomas (see Fig. 47.1). Low-grade cortical gliomas arise in any region of the cortex and usually present with seizures, nonspecific headaches and, somewhat less frequently, focal neurologic deficits. Higher-grade gliomas are more likely to be associated with focal neurologic deficits and headaches early in the course of illness, and less frequently, seizures. Both tumor types may have surrounding edema, but high-grade tumors are more likely to have significant amounts of edema with a shift of the brain and symptoms and signs of increased ICP. Supratentorial primitive neuroectodermal tumors comprise 2% to 3% of primary childhood brain tumors and tend to occur early in life. They present explosively with focal neurologic deficits secondary to the tumor and associated edema, at times with hemorrhage into the tumor. Choroid plexus neoplasms, comprising 2% to 3% of childhood brain tumors, may constitute up to 20% of all CNS tumors during the first year of life. Both choroid plexus carcinomas and papillomas are most likely to arise in the lateral ventricles, but may arise in the fourth or third ventricles. Papillomas classically present with symptoms of increased ICP and hydrocephalus. The hydrocephalus is due probably to both overproduction of CSF and possible poor reabsorption. Choroid plexus carcinomas, which are more infiltrative, may present with hydrocephalus, especially due to the obstruction of one horn of the lateral ventricle, but they may also result in focal neurologic deficits due to invasion directly into brain parenchyma.

Young children, especially those younger than 1 year, may develop a massive intracranial tumor that may look aggressive on computed tomography (CT) scan or MRI, but are remarkably histologically benign. Tumor types such as the dysembryonic neuroepithelial tumor (DNET) and desmoplastic infantile glioma or gangliogliomas may cause remarkably little in the way of focal neurologic deficits in infants, despite their large size on diagnosis.

Emergency Management of Supratentorial Tumors

The emergency management of supratentorial brain tumors is dependent on the location of the tumor, its size, and associated edema. As is the case for infratentorial tumors, patients usually require the immediate initiation of corticosteroids, and for those patients with focal obstruction of

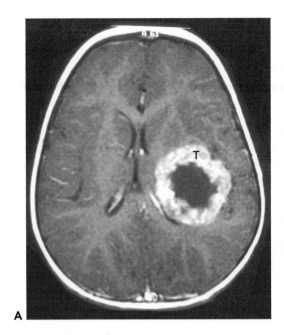
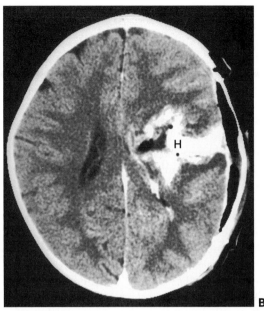

Figure 47.1 A: This magnetic resonance image of a 2-year-old child shows a large enhancing mass (*T*) in the left temporoparietal area. **B:** Immediately after surgery to remove the rhabdoid neuroepithelial tumor, the patient had sustained hypertension and awakened slowly from her anesthesia with a mild right hemiparesis. This computed tomography scan shows hemorrhage (*H*) in the tumor bed. With blood pressure control and observation, the patient recovered to a normal level of consciousness, with resolution of her hemiparesis over several days. (From Litofsky NS, Recht LD. Neurologic problems in the intensive care unit. In: Irwin RS, Rippe JM. eds. *Intensive care medicine*, 5th ed. Philadelphia, PA: Lippincott Williams & Wilkins; 2003:1900.)

CSF (trapped ventricles), temporary CSF diversion may be required, followed by attempts at removal of the tumor to open up CSF pathways. For patients with primary intra-ventricular tumors, surgery may be easier through dilated ventricles, and immediate surgery is undertaken without an attempt at external CSF drainage. Occasionally, patients will present in extremis due to the mass effect of tumor and associated edema. Such children will require endo-tracheal intubation, hyperventilation and/or mannitol for control of increased ICP prior to definitive treatment. If the ICP cannot be controlled or progressive signs of neu-rologic deterioration occur, emergency tumor resection is required. The routine use of antiepileptics in those patients with cortical tumors, without a history of seizures prior to surgery, is controversial. Patients may be placed on anticon-vulsants immediately before surgery (phosphenytoin at 18 to 20 mg per kg, intravenously, followed by maintenance intravenous) and then intravenous or oral phenytoin in the postoperative period for a variable duration.

SPINAL CORD MASS LESIONS

Mass lesions of the spinal cord may result in rapid neu-rologic deterioration either due to direct compression of spinal cord tissue or mass related arterial and/or venous obstruction. A variety of different mass lesions may cause spinal cord compromise and include traumatic injuries; intramedullary hemorrhage (because of arteriovenous malformations); epidural, intradural, and intramedullary spinal cord tumors; focal inflammatory or postinflam-matory myelitis; and intramedullary or extramedullary abscesses.

Spinal cord lesions are best conceptualized as extradu-ral, extramedullary intradural, or intramedullary. Signs and symptoms are obviously most dependent on the region of the spinal cord involved, but are also dependent on the age of the child and rapidity of tumor growth. Tumors that compress the main body of the spinal cord will result in back pain and weakness, with resultant paresis that, de-pendent on the portion of the cord involved, is usually a paraparesis or a quadriparesis. There may be sensory abnor-malities, which may be difficult to discern in a sick, irritable child. A band or belt of dysesthesia is a major warning sign of spinal cord involvement, and sensory levels must be carefully searched for. Bowel and bladder dysfunction oc-curs in nearly 50% of patients on diagnosis, but are more often the presenting sign of masses that involve the conus medullaris. In primary conus medullaris lesions there is also a mixture of lower and upper motor neuron weakness of the lower extremities. Masses in the cauda equina region tend to be present a bit less explosively with low back pain, radicular pain, weakness of one or both lower extremities, and later bowel and bladder difficulties. This discussion will deal predominantly with spinal cord intramedullary and extramedullary tumors and transverse myelitis.

Approximately one third of all childhood spinal cord tumors will be extradural, and most of these will be metastatic lesions. The most common metastatic lesion is neuroblastoma, although sarcomas and lymphomas are not infrequently seen. Metastatic childhood spinal cord tumors present with localized back pain in 80% to 90% of patients, with some degree of focal neurologic impairment. Approximately half the children will have abnormal spine radiographs. MRI has greatly simplified the diagnosis of such lesions and is also useful in determining the extent of lesions.

Intradural extramedullary lesions comprise approximately one fourth of mass lesions involving the spinal cord. Neurofibromas, schwannomas, dermoids, and epidermoids are the most common histologic subtypes.

Astrocytomas, both benign and malignant, comprise most of the intramedullary tumors. Both high-grade and low-grade intramedullary primary spinal cord tumors tend to present with focal neurologic impairment with some degree of back pain; however, onset may be very insidious due to the infiltrating nature of the lesions, especially low-grade gliomas. Ependymomas present similarly to infiltrative spinal cord gliomas.

Emergency Management of Spinal Cord Tumors

Outcome for children with spinal cord tumors, especially extramedullary tumors, is highly dependent on the degree of neurologic compromise present at the time of intervention. Those patients who are ambulatory and have good neurologic function at the time of diagnosis and emergency treatment tend to maintain function. For those patients with significant motor deficits at diagnosis, time is of essence, as intervention within the first 24 hours of neurologic compromise is associated with better outcome and regaining of neurologic function. The time frame outlined is predominantly based on the adult experience with metastatic lesions and children may have neurologic recovery even when deficits are present for >24 hours.

In almost all cases, the first step in management is the use of corticosteroids, usually dexamethasone, at an intravenous bolus of 2 mg per kg, up to 50 to 100 mg, followed by the use of dexamethasone at 1 to 2 mg/kg/day in divided doses. Following stabilization of the patient, emergency spinal decompression is usually indicated for patients with extradural masses, especially in patients with possible metastatic disease without a known primary. In certain circumstances, as in children with known primary disease with neuroblastoma and lymphoma and minimal to moderate neurologic dysfunction, treatment with emergency radiation or chemotherapy can be used instead of emergency surgical decompression and tumor removal.

Although there is a degree of urgency for treating patients with intramedullary tumors, these tumors tend to be more infiltrative and surgical intervention, including decompression and removal of the tumor, may result in minimal acute benefit and possibly even neurologic worsening. Radical resection of lower grade tumors, especially low-grade gliomas, has resulted in long-term disease control and restoration of function in patients; however, this has been predominantly shown in centers with significant experience in the management of such lesions. Radical surgery for malignant astrocytomas of the spinal cord has not been associated with a significant improvement in outcome. Intramedullary ependymomas are usually treated by surgical resection. If total resection is not achieved then some form of adjuvant therapy is required.

Transverse Myelitis

Transverse myelitis is an acute inflammation and demyelination of the spinal cord and is thought to be autoimmune in pathogenesis. The illness tends to present relatively acutely and may progress for 1 to 2 days. At onset, there is often back pain, dependent on the level of cord involvement including monoparesis, paraparesis, quadriparesis, sensory abnormalities, and bowel and bladder involvement. Acutely there is usually flaccidity of the involved limbs with areflexia followed by, in the ensuing days or weeks, increased tone and hyper-reflexia.

Diagnosis is usually confirmed on the basis of neuroradiographic features of a swollen spinal cord, with a variable degree of enhancement. The lesion may be difficult to separate on neuroradiographic findings alone from a primary intrinsic tumor, and the presence of other demyelinating lesions within the brain or other parts of the spinal cord may be useful in making the diagnosis. CSF analysis is at times nonspecific, but may be helpful and reveal a mild to moderate pleocytosis (usually <100 cells) with a slightly elevated protein and a normal spinal fluid glucose.

Emergency Management of Transverse Myelitis

Management of transverse myelitis is usually symptomatic. The disease may be the initial manifestation of multiple sclerosis, but in probably <20% of cases transverse myelitis will be the first manifestation of this chronic illness. Patients need to be closely followed up for ascension of the lesion and respiratory impairment. Although high-dose corticosteroids are often utilized for transverse myelitis, their efficacy has never been proven in a randomized trial. There are presently studies underway for evaluating the efficacy of intravenous immunoglobulins (IVIg) and/or plasmapheresis in the management of transverse myelitis.

Altered Mental Status

48

Leticia Manning Ryan   *Stephen J. Teach*

Various medical and traumatic conditions can cause altered mental status and coma in children. Coma is caused by a disruption of global neuronal function or by direct injuries to areas within the brain stem that are responsible for wakefulness and is defined as "a state of profound unconsciousness from which one cannot be aroused." The common causes of coma in children are listed in Table 48.1. Several of these conditions are discussed in detail in other chapters of this text: stroke and intracerebral hemorrhage (see Chapter 45), central nervous system (CNS) tumors (see Chapter 47), CNS infections (see Chapter 49), status epilepticus (see Chapter 50), and traumatic brain injury (see Chapter 52). This chapter focuses on the causes of encephalopathy that require intensive care, in particular, (a) metabolic coma, (b) collagen vascular diseases leading to coma, (c) toxin-induced coma, (d) acute hydrocephalus from failure of a ventricular shunt, and (e) hypertensive encephalopathy. In addition, this chapter discusses the diagnostic approach and management of the critically ill child who develops a sudden deterioration in consciousness.

CAUSES OF ALTERED MENTAL STATUS AND COMA

Many metabolic abnormalities may alter the level of consciousness by diffusely depressing the cerebral arousal. Hypoglycemia is one of the most common nonstructural causes because it causes altered mental status by depriving the brain of its primary utilizable substrate. The blood glucose level at which the symptoms of hypoglycemia develop varies among individuals, but coma with isoelectric electroencephalogram (EEG) is almost uniform when the blood glucose level is <10 mg per dL. In hypoglycemic coma, the low glucose delivery is not the cause of neuronal death, rather, the endogenous excitatory neurotoxins released by the brain produce neuronal cell membrane rupture. Abnormalities in serum electrolytes, including sodium, calcium, magnesium, and phosphorus,

---

TABLE 48.1

MAJOR ETIOLOGIC CATEGORIES OF ACUTELY ALTERED CONSCIOUSNESS IN CHILDREN

Acute hydrocephalus
Infections
Metabolic disorders
Psychiatric disorders
Seizures
Toxic exposures
Trauma
Tumors
Vascular disorders

---

and acid–base disturbances can cause abnormal brain functioning by altering the neuronal ionic environment. Acute or chronic azotemia can lead to stupor or even coma because of inadequate clearance of endogenously produced toxins, such as urea itself, phenols, aromatic hydroxy acids, amines, and myoinositol. Similarly, hepatic dysfunction and failure can lead to coma because of the accumulation of neurotoxins, such as ammonia and medium-chain fatty acids, and because of a breakdown in serotonergic and glutaminergic neurotransmission within the brain.

Impaired consciousness and coma are common presenting features of hyperglycemic syndromes, such as diabetic ketoacidosis (DKA) and hyperosmolar nonketotic hyperglycemia syndrome (HNHS). In addition, HNHS may present with neurologic findings such as delirium, seizures, or transient hemiparesis. In both these conditions, the altered mental status is attributed to hyperglycemia and hyperosmolarity rather than acidosis. Coma rarely occurs when the measured serum osmolarity is <340 mOsm per L or when the effective serum osmolarity is <320 mOsm per L. Often, mental status changes improve as metabolic derangements are corrected, and cerebral edema is an exceedingly rare complication during the correction of

HNHS in adults. However, DKA-associated cerebral edema may worsen during the initial phase of therapy, presumably because of a too-rapid correction of hyperglycemia.

Collagen vascular diseases, including systemic lupus erythematosus (SLE), are characterized by both small and large vessel arteritis. In these disorders, both inflammatory and noninflammatory, thrombotic vasculopathy in the cerebral arterial system contributes to alterations in mental status by localized hypoperfusion or alterations in cerebral metabolism. Up to one third of patients with SLE have CNS involvement, although the other etiologies for these neurologic symptoms (e.g., cerebral vascular accidents, seizure, infection, hypertensive crises, or intracerebral hemorrhage) must be considered.

Exogenous toxins may impair cerebral function directly through neuronal effects or indirectly by causing hypoxia, electrolyte or acid–base abnormalities, enzyme inhibition, or seizures. Drugs or other toxins (a) taken as part of a child's routine care (benzodiazepines or antiepileptics, narcotics, and others), (b) taken as an intentional overdose of a prescribed medication (e.g., salicylates and antidepressants), (c) accidentally ingested (e.g., hydrocarbons, organophosphates, and lead), or (d) taken as a recreational agent (e.g., γ-hydroxybutyrate, heroin, cocaine, and alcohol) can lead to coma.

Children with brain injuries may require diversions of ventricular fluid because of inadequate absorption of cerebrospinal fluid (CSF). Malfunction of these shunts results in acute hydrocephalus and, ultimately, coma. The risk for shunt failure is greatest in the first months after placement of these shunts, and obstruction of the proximal portion of the shunt may occur as a result of valve occlusion, progressive infection, increased viscosity of CSF, or migration of the shunt tip into the brain parenchyma. Distal obstruction also may result from disconnection of the shunt tubing, migration of the catheter outside its intended space, or obstruction of drainage by local CSF collection.

Acute hypertensive encephalopathy arises in a patient with hypertension and is characterized by diffused cerebral dysfunction, including headaches, confusion, vomiting, and convulsions, sometimes leading to coma. Rapid intervention to reduce the accompanying increased intracranial pressure is required because the syndrome often does not remit spontaneously.

DIAGNOSIS

Clinical Manifestations or Presentation

Because the differential diagnosis of coma is so large and varied, a thorough history and physical examination is essential for the prompt diagnosis and treatment of disorders affecting the mental status. More efficient and specific therapeutic interventions to correct the CNS dysfunction will result from a directed investigation of the cause of the encephalopathy.

Metabolic etiologies of altered mental status vary greatly depending on the age of the child. For example, in infancy, hypoglycemia may become manifest during severe sepsis or illnesses, leading to dehydration and shock. In older children, hypoglycemia can occur as a result of ingestion of oral hypoglycemic agents. In addition to encephalopathy, the clinical manifestations include seizures and irritability. DKA can present in children of all ages with polyuria, polydypsia, weight loss, nausea and emesis (see Chapter 12). The clinical manifestations of electrolyte imbalances (i.e., seizures, confusion, weakness, muscle spasms) can be nonspecific, but helpful in raising clinical suspicion. Systemic conditions, such as renal and hepatic failure and collagen vascular disorders, will present with characteristic signs and symptoms. Pediatric toxic ingestions often do not present with a clear history of exposure followed by the onset of symptoms; a list of medications present in the home should be obtained and reviewed.

Hypertensive encephalopathy should be suspected in any child with elevated blood pressure in the presence of acute CNS dysfunction. Several important clinical considerations of hypertensive encephalopathy may help exclude other causes of altered mental status: (a) symptoms of generalized brain dysfunction tend to develop over time (12 to 24 hours); (b) focal neurologic findings are unusual, unless there is associated bleeding; (c) papilledema almost always is noted and, if absent, should raise a suspicion of another etiology; and (d) compared with an acute CNS bleed, the mental status improves rapidly with treatment.

Physical Examination

A complete physical examination should be performed in all children with coma to assess the degree of altered consciousness and the associated neurologic findings. Although originally designed to assess traumatic brain injury, the Glasgow Coma Scale is commonly used to describe the mental status in children. The findings consistent with neurologic emergencies, including Cushing triad (bradycardia, hypertension, and altered respirations), abnormalities in brain stem function, and papilledema, must be determined promptly.

Many metabolic disorders have characteristic physical examination findings. The clinical signs of hypoglycemia include jitteriness and tachycardia. The classic examination findings of DKA include the fruity breath odor of ketosis, hyperventilation (i.e., Kussmaul respirations), and dehydration. The Chvostek sign (i.e., contraction of the facial muscles in response to percussion over the facial nerve) may be elicited in cases of hypocalcemic tetany. The symptoms of many of the metabolic disorders in newborns include characteristic odors of bodily fluids. The clinical manifestations of renal failure and liver failure are discussed in Chapter 56 and 63, respectively. A helpful distinguishing feature of diffuse encephalopathy is the preservation of the pupillary light reflex.

In cases of CNS vasculitis, many physical findings may be elicited, but few are specific. Rashes, arthritis, and other inflammatory changes such as pericarditis and pleuritis may be present, but the ultimate diagnosis of the disorder normally requires serologic testing. In addition to mental status changes, focal neurologic findings may be present as a result of cerebral ischemia or infarction.

Toxin-induced coma can cause characteristic changes in vital signs and physical examination findings. The constellation of signs and symptoms may be characteristic of a particular toxin (toxidrome). For instance, the anticholinergic toxidrome is characterized by tachycardia, hyperthermia, altered mental status, mydriasis, dry mucous membranes, decreased bowel sounds, and urinary retention. Physical examination findings may also suggest ventricular shunt failure and hydrocephalus including a full and tense fontanelle, rapid enlargement in head circumference, increased prominence of the scalp veins, split sutures, sunset sign, and a hyper-resonant sound when the skull is percussed (Macewen sign). Hydrocephalus may also be accompanied by unilateral or bilateral cranial nerve palsies, and a head tilt may occur also as a result of a cranial nerve palsy or cerebellar tonsillar herniation. Swelling along the shunt track may be due to CSF tracking and is also indicative of obstruction.

Imaging Studies

The general approach to a coma of unclear etiology in a child should include urgent computed tomography (CT) scan of the brain. The metabolic etiologies of coma do not require imaging studies unless the diagnosis is in question or there is clinical suspicion of secondary cerebral edema. In cerebritis secondary to collagen vascular disease, magnetic resonance imaging (MRI) and CT scans with contrast may identify both small and large vessel arteritis, as well as parenchymal ischemic changes. Imaging studies are not typically helpful in toxin-induced coma, except to rule out other causes. A plain film of the abdomen may identify the presence of radio-opaque pill fragments, such as iron. A noncontrast head CT scan should be obtained if the diagnosis is uncertain or if there is a clinical suspicion of secondary cerebral edema or hemorrhage. In contrast, ventricular shunt failure is diagnosed using a noncontrast head CT scan and compared with previous scans taken when the shunt was functioning. If there is CT evidence of acute hydrocephalus or a strong clinical suspicion for malfunction, a plain radiographic "shunt series" should be obtained. In most cases (approximately 80%), these studies identify shunt malfunction. If hypertensive encephalopathy is suspected, an MRI should be performed to confirm the diagnosis.

Laboratory Tests

Screening laboratory studies are required for children with coma that cannot be diagnosed by history, physical examination, and neuroimaging. In infants with possible inborn errors of metabolism, testing the serum for amino acids and urine for organic acids will aid in making the diagnosis. In children with suspected collagen vascular diseases, severe active disease may be manifested by decreased levels of serum complement (C3 and C4) and the presence of antibodies to double-stranded DNA. However, there is presently no laboratory study that confirms the diagnosis of cerebritis in these patients. In SLE, the measurement of immunoglobulin G (IgG) index (CSF IgG/serum IgG) divided by the albumin index (CSF albumin/serum albumin) estimates the extent of IgG synthesis within the blood–brain barrier. Although this measurement is increased in a variety of infections, it also indicates severe CNS involvement in SLE. Although there is no toxicology panel that is completely exhaustive, the toxicologic screening for agents normally abused can be helpful in determining some of the causes of coma in children. Specific drug levels can be obtained for other common agents, such as acetaminophen, aspirin, ethanol, iron, and anticonvulsants. Other metabolic laboratories may enable the identification of patterns characteristic of certain ingestions (i.e., serum glucose level, electrolytes, serum osmolarity, arterial blood gas values, liver function panel, and heavy metals content in urine). Additionally, an electrocardiogram (EKG) should be obtained to detect rhythm and interval changes.

TREATMENT

Management

Stabilization of the airway and maintenance of cardiovascular function are the primary supportive issues. In metabolic coma, electrolyte abnormalities should be corrected and the underlying disorder treated. Patients with other conditions such as renal and hepatic failure and collagen vascular disease require therapy for the primary disorder and correction of the secondary manifestations. In CNS vasculitis, intravenous corticosteroid therapy should be initiated. Adjunctive agents such as cyclophosphamide or plasmapheresis may also be beneficial. Until the infection is definitively excluded as the etiology, broad-spectrum antibiotics should be considered.

Treatment of toxin-induced coma often includes gastrointestinal decontamination, including gastric lavage, activated charcoal, and/or whole bowel irrigation, as appropriate to the specific agent. Therapeutic trials of naloxone and flumazenil and empiric administration of thiamine may be appropriate. If the toxin is known or strongly suspected, specific treatment protocols and antidotes, if available, may be employed. Controlled lowering of blood pressure for hypertensive encephalopathy includes infusion of titratable agents including vasodilators, such as nicardipine, nitroprusside, and labetalol.

Prognosis

The prognosis of pediatric patients presenting with altered mental status reflects both the underlying process and the course of the illness, including the duration and extent of the neurologic insult. Serial neurologic examinations are fundamental to the prognosis. Persistent absence of response to painful stimuli and/or the absence of pupillary light response is/are sensitive predictors of poor outcome.

No individual adjunct study definitively determines prognosis. Serial EEGs may provide useful prognostic information, particularly in neonates. Somatosensory-evoked potentials (SEP) may have a role in the prediction of neurologic outcome. Limited studies have shown that bilaterally absent SEP is predictive of poor outcome and that normal SEP bilaterally is predictive of good outcome. The use of magnetic resonance spectroscopy (MRS) and/or MRI can be considered in selective circumstances to detect subtle metabolic and structural defects. Their utility as a single tool to determine prognosis has not been proven.

SUDDEN NEUROLOGIC DETERIORATION IN CRITICALLY ILL CHILDREN

Infants and children admitted to intensive care units are at risk for neurologic decline because of either their underlying critical illness or the therapeutic interventions (see Table 48.2). Delay in the diagnosis of neurologic complications increases the risk of morbidity and mortality. In this section, an approach to the evaluation of the critically ill infant or child with acute neurologic deterioration is presented.

An important fundamental clinical imperative is the need for frequent neurologic assessment in all critically ill patients. As experience is gained with new neuromonitoring techniques such as continuous EEG, near infrared spectroscopy, brain tissue Po_2, and transcranial Doppler ultrasonography (see Chapter 7), these may contribute significantly to improved detection of altered neurologic status. The essential elements of neurologic examination should include an assessment of the level of arousal, ability to follow commands and respond to environmental stimulation, pupillary size and reactivity, response to painful stimuli, and general muscle strength and tone. The practice of daily sedation "holidays" in many intensive care units provides an opportunity to obtain a neurologic assessment that most closely reflects the patient's true neurologic status without compromising patient comfort and safety.

When an acute change in consciousness is noted, the approach should take into consideration the patient's age, coexisting organ dysfunction, current medications and their dosing schedule, and metabolic status. Worsening of their primary disorder often causes neurologic deterioration in patients presenting with acute CNS disease. In children without primary CNS disease, an acute change in mental status is more often due to drug toxicity, metabolic disturbances, or nonconvulsive status epilepticus. A lumbar puncture to diagnose nosocomial CNS infection is rarely indicated unless the patient has had a recent neurosurgery, shows clinical signs of meningitis or encephalitis, or is immunocompromised. The diagnosis of nonconvulsive status epilepticus is most accurately made with an EEG. For patients with focal neurologic findings, or unexplained impairments in arousal, a noncontrast CT scan should be obtained. Diffusion-weighted MRI can reveal abnormalities such as hypertensive encephalopathy, vasculitis, cerebral venous thrombosis, or fat embolism that are not detected by conventional CT scan.

TABLE 48.2

SUDDEN DETERIORATION IN NEUROLOGIC STATUS ASSOCIATED WITH SELECT CONDITIONS AND INTENSIVE CARE UNIT INTERVENTIONS

Underlying Condition	Neurologic Change
Cardiac surgery	Stroke, nonconvulsive status epilepticus
Orthopedic surgery	Fat embolism
Solid organ transplantation	Stroke, seizures, drug-induced encephalopathy, CNS opportunistic infection
Bone marrow transplantation	Intracranial hemorrhage, seizures, drug-induced encephalopathy, CNS opportunistic infection
Cancer	Intracranial hemorrhage, CNS infection
Intracranial surgery	Seizure, bleeding, edema, CNS infection
Traumatic brain injury	Intracranial hypertension, bleeding, seizures, CNS infection, edema, herniation, hydrocephalus
Stroke	Stroke progression, bleeding, seizures, edema, herniation
CNS tumor	Edema, hydrocephalus, herniation, bleeding
Diabetic ketoacidosis	Cerebral edema, herniation
Hepatic failure	Cerebral edema, herniation
Renal dialysis	Dialysis disequilibrium syndrome
Anticoagulation/thrombolysis	Intracranial hemorrhage
Central venous cannulation	Cerebral air embolism, stroke

CNS, central nervous system.

RECOMMENDED READINGS

1. Abbruzi G, Stork CM. Pediatric toxicological concerns. *Emerg Med Clin North Am.* 2002;20:223–247.
2. Barnes NP, Jones SJ, Hayward RD, et al. Ventriculoperitoneal shunt block: What are the best predictive clinical indicators? *Arch Dis Child.* 2002;87:198–201.

3. Garton HJL, Piatt JH. Hydrocephalus. *Pediatr Clin North Am.* 2004; 51:305–325.

4. Jennekens FGI, Kater L. The central nervous system in systemic lupus erythematosus. Part 1. Clinical syndromes: A literature investigation. *Rheumatology.* 2002;41:605–618.

5. King D, Avner JR. Altered mental status. *Clin Pediatr Emerg Med.* 2003;4:171–178.

6. Kirkham FJ. Non-traumatic coma in children. *Arch Dis Child.* 2001;85:303–312.

7. Mokhlesi B, Corbridge T. Toxicology in the critically ill patient. *Clin Chest Med.* 2003;24:689–711.

8. Trubel HK, Novotny E, Lister G. Outcome of coma in children. *Curr Opin Pediatr.* 2003;15:283–287.

Central Nervous System Infections

49

Andrew M. Bonwit

Direct infections of the central nervous system (CNS) present significant risks for both severe morbidity and mortality in children of all ages. Survivors are often left with permanent impairments that limit their development and functioning as adults.

ACUTE BACTERIAL MENINGITIS

Epidemiology and Causative Agents

Widespread vaccination against *Haemophilus influenzae* Type b led to a precipitous fall in the incidence of this agent, as well as a major change in the distribution of causative agents. *H. influenzae* Type b was the leading bacterial pathogen in children in 1985 (55% of cases compared to only 20% for *Streptococcus pneumoniae*), but by 1995, *S. pneumoniae* was the most common and *H. influenzae* Type b was the fifth most common (*Neisseria meningitidis*, group B streptococcus and *Listeria monocytogenes*). Because of the success of vaccination programs and an increasing number of individuals with immunodeficiencies, the median age of patients with meningitis has increased in the last decade from 15 months to 25 years.

Clinical Presentation

Meningitis should always be considered when a patient presents with altered mental status and fever. Acute bacterial meningitis can present as (i) a steadily progressive illness over a period of 2 to 5 days, (ii) a more rapid illness progressing over 24 to 48 hours, or (iii) a fulminant disease with progression to shock within hours of the first symptoms (see Fig. 49.1). The classic signs of meningitis are fever, lethargy, irritability, decreased or altered level of consciousness, and nuchal rigidity. Additional signs may include vomiting, restlessness, seizures, a bulging fontanel, headache, and photophobia. Petechial rashes are associated with *N. meningitidis*, but have also occurred because of *S. pneumoniae* or *H. influenzae* (see Fig. 49.2).

Predisposing Factors

Bacterial meningitis is most commonly a sporadic disease occurring in previously healthy individuals, but anatomic and immunologic conditions increase susceptibility. Fractures of the cribriform plate of the basilar skull, anatomic or functional asplenia, or infection with human immunodeficiency virus (HIV) can all predispose to infection with *S. pneumoniae*. Deficiencies of the terminal components of complement increase the risk of infection with *N. meningitidis*. Dermal sinus tracts in the lumbosacral spine can lead to meningitis caused by gram-negative enteric flora. CNS surgery or penetrating head trauma can predispose to infections with skin flora.

Diagnostic Studies

Examination of the cerebrospinal fluid (CSF) is essential for definitive diagnosis. Lumbar puncture should be performed immediately on suspicion, provided the clinical condition is permissive. Relative contraindications to lumbar puncture are hemodynamic instability, uncontrolled coagulopathy, or intracranial hypertension related to mass lesions. Empiric antibiotic therapy should be instituted as quickly as possible. A rapid Gram stain of the CSF can guide initial therapy. The likelihood of bacterial meningitis increases in direct proportion to the total CSF white blood cell (WBC) count. For children older than 12 months, a CSF WBC count >5 cells per mL should be considered abnormal, whereas in neonates, a normal CSF WBC may range as

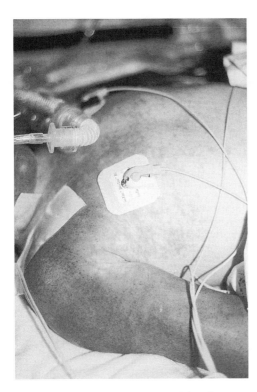

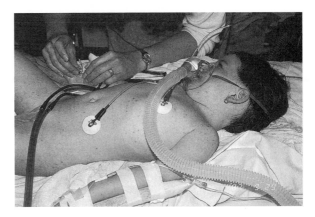

Figure 49.2 Infection with *Neisseria meningitidis*. This young boy is in the early course of a meningococcal infection. He has scattered petechiae, some of which have reached the size of small purpura. Meningococcemia can progress rapidly in many cases. (From Fleisher GR, Ludwig S, Baskin M. *Atlas of emergency medicine.* Philadelphia, PA: Lippincott Williams & Wilkins; 2004: 180.) (See color Figure 49.2.)

Figure 49.1 Purpura fulminans in a child with pneumococcal sepsis. The syndrome of purpura fulminans most commonly occurs in severe sepsis caused by *Neisseria meningitidis* but may also be seen with other organisms, as illustrated by this patient. The characteristic appearance consists of blotchy confluent purple discoloration, which is superimposed on gray, poorly perfused skin. (From Fleisher GR, Ludwig S, Baskin M. *Atlas of emergency medicine.* Philadelphia, PA: Lippincott Williams & Wilkins; 2004: 181.) (See color Figure 49.1.)

high as 32 cells per mL. CSF protein is increased and CSF glucose decreased in bacterial meningitis, but these findings can lack sensitivity except at extreme ranges. When lumbar puncture is initially deferred, delayed examination of the CSF can suggest meningitis with the use of indirect tests for bacterial cell products (latex antigen tests of the CSF for *H. influenzae* Type b, *S. pneumoniae*, *N. meningitidis* and group B streptococcus). This is particularly important for suspected cases of *H. influenzae* Type b and *N. meningitidis* because close family and health care contacts require prophylactic antibiotics. Neuroimaging of the brain should be performed in children with altered levels of consciousness or focal findings suggestive of mass lesions.

Treatment and Complications

Empiric treatment of meningitis is based on the likely organisms, their susceptibility patterns, and the penetration of the antibiotics past the blood–brain barrier. For children older than 2 months, third-generation cephalosporins have activity against most isolates of *S. pneumoniae* and have good penetration into the CSF. These agents also effectively

treat *H. influenzae* and *N. meningitidis*. Over the past two decades, there has been a notable increase in the percentage of clinical isolates of *S. pneumoniae* with decreased susceptibility to penicillins and cephalosporins. Vancomycin should be added based on local susceptibilities.

Infants younger than 2 months are at increased risk for meningitis from group B streptococcus, *L. monocytogenes* and gram-negative organisms (*Citrobacter, Enterobacter* in particular). Because of the lack of data on clinical outcome, cephalosporins should not be considered adequate single agent treatment of group B streptococci. *Listeria* sp. is routinely resistant to cephalosporins, and gram-negative organisms have a variable degree of susceptibility to penicillins and cephalosporins. Therefore, combinations of synthetic penicillins and aminoglycosides are routinely used. If infection with *Enterobacteriaceae* with extended-spectrum β-lactamases or inducible β-lactamases is suspected, treatment with carbapenems may be required.

Corticosteroids, particularly dexamethasone, may improve outcomes by decreasing the host inflammatory response to infection. The most definitive studies demonstrated a salutary effect on the outcome caused by *H. influenzae* Type b and, to a lesser extent, *S. pneumoniae*. The treatment benefit was associated with administration of steroids before or with the start of antibiotic therapy. Contrasted with this beneficial effect, corticosteroid therapy can have detrimental effects for the patient with bacterial meningitis by decreasing the permeability of the blood–brain barrier to some antibiotics, notably vancomycin.

Common complications related to bacterial meningitis are seizures, cerebral edema, cerebral infarction, electrolyte abnormalities, sinus thrombosis, subdural empyema, and coma. Routine intracranial pressure monitoring has not shown to improve clinical outcomes. Mitigation of secondary injuries by monitoring the child's mental status, assessing airway reflexes, and avoiding hypotension and hypoxia are important to maximize clinical outcomes.

TUBERCULOUS MENINGITIS

Epidemiology and Clinical Presentation

Tuberculosis surged in incidence in the mid-1980s, partly because of an increased prevalence of the disease in patients with HIV/acquired immunodeficiency syndrome (AIDS). Primary transmission of *M. tuberculosis* is usually from droplets into the respiratory tract, although cutaneous and gastrointestinal transmission may occur. The period from the time of initial infection to positive skin testing varies from 2 to 10 weeks, with manifestations of symptoms delayed for years. Symptoms generally develop over weeks in children. Differentiation between bacterial and tuberculous meningitis (TBM) can be difficult. TBM should be considered in children with several weeks of low-grade fever, malaise, headache, progressive signs of meningeal irritation (vomiting, worsened headache, neck stiffness), or focal neurologic deficits. Additionally, TBM should be considered when bacterial meningitis is suspected without conclusive culture results, or empiric antimicrobial therapy does result in anticipated clinical improvement.

Diagnosis and Treatment

TBM is only definitively diagnosed after examination of CSF. In general, modest increases in CSF WBC (up to 1,500 cells per mL), increased CSF protein and decreased CSF glucose are classic findings in children with TBM. However, there is considerable variability within these findings. Skin testing can detect whether the child has been exposed to *M. tuberculosis*, although only half of all patients with TBM will have positive reactions. Negative skin tests may reflect anergy to antigens because of overwhelming infection or immunodeficiency. Computed tomography (CT) scan or magnetic resonance (MR) images showing inflammation of basilar brain structures or granulomatous lesions within the parenchyma may be helpful. In a small series of 20 patients, 68% and 58% of patients exhibited either enhancement of basilar brain structures or parenchymal lesions, respectively. Growth of *M. tuberculosis* from CSF has been the "gold standard" for diagnosing TBM but may take between 2 to 5 weeks. Recently, polymerase chain reaction (PCR) of CSF for *M. tuberculosis* has greatly increased the rapidity of diagnosis to days.

If TBM is likely, empiric treatment should be provided with isoniazid, rifampin, pyrazinamide, and streptomycin while awaiting the results of the culture and PCR testing. If an organism is isolated from any source, adjustments for antimicrobial resistance should be made. The duration of therapy for TBM is 2 months of treatment with all four agents (or agents selected based on drug sensitivities),

TABLE 49.1
SCORING SYSTEM FOR TUBERCULOUS MENINGITIS

Symptom	Score
Mental status	
Lethargic	1
Obtunded but somewhat responsive	2
Comatose	3
Seizures	
Controlled	1
Uncontrolled with therapy	2
Muscle tone increased	1
Any focal neurologic deficits	1
Any cranial nerve abnormality	1
Total score	8

Adapted from Saitoh A., Pong A, Waecker NW Jr, et al. Prediction of neurological sequelae in childhood tuberculous meningitis: A review of 20 cases and proposals of a novel scoring system. *Pediatr Infect Dis J.* 2005;24:207–212.

followed by 10 months of isoniazid and rifampin. Adjuvant therapy with dexamethasone has recently been advocated based on a randomized trial of 545 patients treated with dexamethasone for 6 weeks. There was significant improvement in mortality (31% vs. 41%, relative risk [RR] = 0.69), but no reduction in severe disability was noted between the treated and nontreated groups at 9 months. These findings were consistent across subgroups stratified for severity of injury and the presence of HIV disease.

Complications and Outcome

All of the complications related to acute bacterial meningitis are common in TBM. Recently, a TBM acute neurologic (TBAN) score (see Table 49.1) has been developed, with a score ≥4 used as a threshold to predict poor outcome. The overall outcome for children with TBM remains relatively bleak, with 55% of children expected to have moderate to severe neurologic impairment or death.

INVASIVE FUNGAL DISEASE OF THE CENTRAL NERVOUS SYSTEM

Epidemiology and Causative Agents

With increased use of invasive catheters, more potent antibacterial therapies, and increasing use of immunosuppressive agents, fungal infections are increasing in frequency. Primary CNS fungal infections, defined as infections in immunocompetent hosts, are relatively rare and often associated with systemic disease. Secondary CNS fungal infections occur in immunocompromised hosts, including in children with HIV/AIDS, those undergoing cancer chemotherapy, and after organ transplantation. Seeding of the CNS from hematogenous infection and extension of fungal disease from the cranium are the major routes of transmission.

There are relatively few fungi that can cause primary CNS infection. *Cryptococcus neoformans* and *Coccidioides imitans* are the most common. *C. neoformans* is an encapsulated yeast that is present in soil, bird excreta, and trees and has a unique predilection for the CNS. The four serotypes (A to D) exhibit geographic specificity and can cause meningitis in the immunocompetent host. Initial infection with *C. neoformans* usually results from inhalation and formation of a nidus in the lung, producing a lung–lymph node reaction that limits the spread. It can remain dormant for years, leading sequentially to the bloodstream and CNS infection at a time when cellular immunity is diminished. *C. imitans* is a dimorphic yeast that is endemic to the southwestern United States and Mexico. This soil organism normally causes subclinical or self-limited pulmonary infection. Primary disseminated infection can occur, involving the skin, subcutaneous tissue, bone, and the meninges in up to 50% of the cases.

Candida and *Aspergillus* species are the most common fungal agents responsible for secondary infections. *Candida albicans* is the most ubiquitous of the Candida pathogens, yet *C. tropicalis*, *C. lusitaniae* and *C. parapsilosis* are increasingly frequent. In several series, *C. albicans* was the most common fungus isolated from the CSF in premature infants, and represented approximately 2% of all the positive CSF cultures in children younger than 14 years. Infants and children with systemic candidemia appear to be at an increased risk of *Candida* meningitis compared to adults. In a small series, 8 of 40 children with candidemia developed meningitis, whereas this complication is rarely reported in adults. Disorders of phagocytic capabilities of WBC such as myeloperoxidase deficiency, chronic granulomatous disease, and prolonged neutropenia have increased risk. Implantable shunts are also a risk factor. Children with HIV/AIDS do not appear to be at an increased risk of candidal meningitis.

Aspergillus infections of the CNS are only approximately 5% of the cases, but are increasingly found as occult infections at autopsy. *Aspergillus fumigatus* is the main pathogen, but *A. flavus*, *A. versicolor* and *A. terreus* can also cause the disease in humans. When cellular immunity is reduced, *Aspergillus* invades the blood vessel wall including vessels within the CNS. Aspergillus meningoencephalitis is relatively rare. Children undergoing chemotherapy or recipients of solid organ or bone marrow transplants (especially during periods of acute rejection of the graft) are especially at risk.

Diagnosis, Treatment, and Prognosis

The presentation and diagnosis of fungal meningitis is usually a more subacute course of the disease than acute bacterial meningitis. Invasive fungal disease should be suspected with immunodeficiency syndromes, and cerebral infarction (*Aspergillus* sp.) in children with immunodeficiency. Characteristically, there are moderate increases in CSF WBC counts (50 to 300 per mL). The Gram stain of CSF may demonstrate yeast, and India ink staining will specifically diagnose *C. neoformans* and related organisms. As with TBM, fungal meningitis should be strongly suspected when bacterial cultures are negative. Fungal pathogens can be isolated following normal incubation of CSF (*C. albicans* within 2 to 3 days) when the fungal load is $>10^6$ colony-forming units (CFU) per mL. PCR detection of specific fungi is also commercially available. Diagnosis of *Aspergillus* infection has been greatly aided by PCR against the galactomannan antigen (a cell membrane protein) in the serum. In a recent study, PCR diagnosis of *Aspergillus* CNS disease occurred 45 days prior to definitive culture evidence of disease. Neuroimaging has not been helpful in all cases, but has some utility in diagnosing *Aspergillus*-induced infarctions or other parenchymal lesions. In rare instances, definitive diagnosis can be confirmed by either biopsy or cisternal puncture of the lateral ventricle to obtain CSF in sufficient quantities to increase diagnostic sensitivity.

The mainstay of systemic antifungal agents is amphotericin B, or one if its derivatives. Synergistic activities between amphotericin B and flucytosine have been suggested against *Candida* species. Fluconazole or other azole derivatives have shown efficacy against *Candida* as well and may be better tolerated. *Aspergillus* infection may require surgical excision to eradicate the focus, followed by long-term amphotericin administration. *Coccidioides* requires lifelong therapy with fluconazole, even in immunocompetent hosts.

The prognosis for candidal meningitis is among the best in this group. In a study of adults with HIV and candidal meningitis, mortality was 31%. Premature infants with candidal meningitis had a much higher mortality (61%) than older children with neurosurgical causes of candidal meningitis (11%). Aspergillus infection in the CNS is almost universally fatal. In one series, the survival period from the time of diagnosis was only 6 days. In adults with HIV, mortality from cryptococcal meningitis is approximately 40% in several series.

BRAIN ABSCESS, EPIDURAL ABSCESS, AND SUBDURAL EMPYEMA

Epidemiology and Causative Organisms

These abscesses can occur (i) by hematogenous spread of septic emboli (e.g., as a complication of cyanotic congenital heart disease or infected thrombus), (ii) by direct extension of oropharyngeal infections (e.g., otic, sinus, or odontic infection), or (iii) because of head trauma. The site and responsible pathogen for the abscess depends largely on

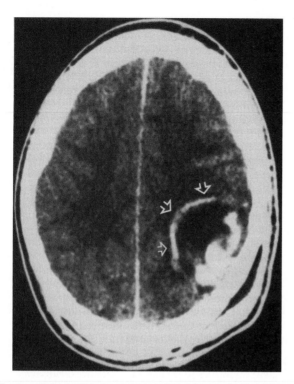

Figure 49.3 A hypodense mass with a well-defined enhancing rim (*arrows*), characteristic of a brain abscess, developed 2 weeks after this 14-year-old child fell on a nail. (From Rogers MC. *Textbook of pediatric intensive care.* 2nd ed. Philadelphia, PA: Lippincott Williams & Wilkins; 2002.)

than one third of all cases, although headache, fever, and emesis are among the most common symptoms. Between 25% and 50% of children present with either altered mental status, seizures, or focal neurologic symptoms. Meningeal symptoms are uncommon. Radicular pain and signs of spinal cord compression can portend a subdural empyema of the spinal cord and should be treated as a neurosurgical emergency. Blood cultures should be obtained because persistent bacteremia may accompany the abscess. However, CSF cultures are rarely positive.

Combinations of third-generation cephalosporins with agents that eradicate anaerobes (clindamycin, metronidazole) are generally required for therapy. Resistant *Staphylococcal* sp. may require vancomycin. Early neurosurgical drainage is generally required for drainage. Reaccumulation or development of new collections may require repeated interventions. Other short-term complications, should the abscess rupture into the CSF, include intracranial hypertension, seizures, altered mental status, syndrome of inappropriate antidiuretic hormone (SIADH), and meningitis.

The prognosis from focal abscesses within the CNS depends upon the location of the lesion primarily. Lesions amenable to surgical excision can be self-limited illnesses that are associated with full recovery. Overall mortality rates in adult series report 14% to 18% mortality of all cases, increasing to 75% in patients presenting in coma. Similar series in children have not been reported.

which pathogenic mechanism causes the infection. Septic emboli from congenital cyanotic heart disease cause multiple abscesses, especially in the middle cerebral artery distribution, with *Staphylococcus aureus* and *Streptococcal* sp. predominating. Extension of sinus or odontic infections usually results in abscesses within the frontal lobe or subdural space from anaerobic and aerobic streptococcal species (*Enterobacter* sp, *S. aureus* or anaerobes). Otic sources of infection lead to abscesses located within the temporal lobes or cerebellum and typically grow mixed flora (including anaerobes, *Streptococcal, Enterobacteraciae,* and *Pseudomonal* sp). Organisms causing abscesses following head trauma generally represent skin flora.

Diagnosis, Treatment, and Prognosis

Diagnosis of brain abscesses virtually always requires neuroimaging (see Fig. 49.3). The triad of headache, fever, and focal neurologic deficit is observed in less

RECOMMENDED READINGS

1. Bonadio WA. The cerebrospinal fluid: Physiologic aspects and alteration associated with bacterial meningitis. *Pediatr Infect Dis J.* 1992;11:423–432.
2. Feigin RD, Schneider JH. Bacterial meningitis beyond the newborn period. In: McMillan JA, DeAngelis CD, Feigin RD, et al., eds. *Oski's pediatrics: Principles and practice.* 3rd ed. Philadelphia, PA: Lippincott Williams & Wilkins; 1999:855–863.
3. Feigin RD, McCracken GH, Klein JO. Diagnosis and management of meningitis. *Pediatr Infect Dis J.* 1992;11:785–814.
4. Gottfredsson M, Prefect JR. Fungal meningitis. *Semin Neurol.* 2000; 20:307–322.
5. Mamidi A, DeSimone JA, Pomerantz RJ. Central nervous system infections in individuals with HIV-1 infection. *J Neurovirol.* 2002;8: 159–167.
6. Saez-Llorens X, McCracken GH Jr. Acute bacterial meningitis beyond the neonatal period. In: Long SS, Pickering LK, Prober CG, eds. *Principles and practice of pediatric infectious diseases.* 2nd ed. Philadelphia, PA: Churchill Livingstone; 2003:264–271.
7. Schneider E, Castro KG. Tuberculosis trends in the United States. *Tuberculosis.* 2003;83:21–29.
8. Thwaites GE, Nguyen DB, Nguyen HD, et al. Dexamethasone for treatment of tuberculous meningitis in adolescents and adults. *N Engl J Med.* 2004;351:1741–1751.

Status Epilepticus

50

Tammy Noriko Tsuchida   Steven L. Weinstein   William Davis Gaillard

DEFINITION

Status epilepticus (SE) is defined as a "seizure of sufficient duration to provide an enduring epileptic condition" (1964). The minimum seizure duration required for the diagnosis of SE has evolved downward from 1 hour to 30 minutes and, as per recent proposals, to 5 minutes. Evolution to shorter times has been based on animal models demonstrating decreased physiologic compensation and brain injury after 30 minutes of continuous generalized tonic–clonic seizure activity despite optimal ventilation. Proponents of earlier treatment have noted that typical seizures last <2 minutes in adults and children. However, in a prospective study of 428 children with first febrile seizures, 13% had seizures for >10 minutes, 9.3% >15 minutes, and 5.1% >30 minutes. Although the pharmacologic treatment of seizures after shorter periods may be justified, the currently accepted definition of SE is that it is the continuous seizure activity lasting at least 30 minutes or two or more seizures without full recovery of consciousness during the interictal period.

CLASSIFICATION AND CLINICAL FEATURES

Broadly, SE can be subdivided into generalized convulsive status epilepticus (GCSE) and nonconvulsive status epilepticus (NCSE) subtypes. NCSE can occur with both generalized (atypical absence) and partial (complex partial) epilepsy and is clinically distinct from GCSE in its lack of limb jerking movements. In GCSE, the seizure typically starts with a brief tonic phase followed by clonic jerking of all extremities (evolving over time from low-amplitude, fast-frequency to high-amplitude, low-frequency movements). GCSE can also consist primarily of tonic stiffening. Untreated GCSE can evolve into more subtle movements

(such as slight finger or face twitches or nystagmus-type eye movements) as the seizure continues and, eventually, there may be no movement associated with the electroencephalogram (EEG) changes. This subtle form, termed *subtle GCSE*, can be a sign of increased severity of the epileptic focus. It can occur late in the convulsion or as the first sign when there is a severe insult. Similar to the clinical appearance, the EEG can change as the SE progresses. With overt convulsions, discrete electrographic seizures can progress to epileptiform discharges that wax and wane. This electrical activity may evolve to monotonous rhythmic continuous discharges and then to periodic bursts of epileptiform discharges (PEDs) separated by periods of background flattening that increase over time. These EEG patterns may be accompanied by convulsions, subtle GCSE, or no movements. PEDs portend a significant brain injury and can also occur in patients without a preceding SE.

EPIDEMIOLOGY

The incidence of GCSE varies from 10 to 61 per 100,000 in population-based studies in the United States and Europe. There can be significant racial differences (whites, 20 episodes per 100,000; and nonwhite, 57 per 100,000) for reasons that are unclear. SE exhibits a bimodal age distribution, with the highest rates in toddlers (<5 years) and older individuals (>55 years) and with a remarkably increased incidence in children younger than 1 year (135 to 155 per 100,000).

The causes of SE in children can be subdivided into categories: (i) acute symptomatic (occurring during an illness with neurologic insult or metabolic dysfunction), (ii) remote symptomatic (a preexisting condition known to increase seizure risk such as intracranial lesion or mental retardation), (iii) febrile, and (iv) cryptogenic (no identifiable etiology) or idiopathic (previously indicated as having no identifiable etiology but currently indicating a genetic etiology). In a large series involving two large centers, the following diseases were determined to be the cause of SE: febrile (28%), central nervous system (CNS) infection (8%), other acute symptomatic diseases (20%) (metabolic disorder, trauma, hypoxia, systemic infection), remote symptomatic disease (24%), cryptogenic disease (15%), and progressive neurologic disease (5%). In another study, SE was caused by (a) non-CNS infections with fever (52%) (including febrile seizures), (b) low anticonvulsant drug level (21%), and (c) stroke (10%). SE also exhibits an age distribution in relation to etiology. In the first year of life, the acute symptomatic etiologies account for half the cases of SE. In contrast, febrile seizures are the cause of SE in two third of the children in their second year of life, whereas children older than 5 years are more likely to have remote symptomatic or cryptogenic etiologies for SE.

PHYSIOLOGY AND OUTCOME

The physiologic responses of the body to prolonged seizures have been studied primarily in animal models and can involve every organ system. Initially, there is a massive sympathetic neurotransmitter release that can result in hypertension, tachycardia, hyperglycemia, and cardiac arrhythmias. Poor pulmonary function can result after a loss of airway reflexes or as a result of neurogenic pulmonary edema. The combination of diminished ventilation with lactate production from contracting muscles can lead to profound acidosis. In adults and animals, hyperpyrexia can result from the muscle contractions of GCSE alone or in combination with a febrile cause of SE. Increased white blood cell (WBC), both in serum and in cerebrospinal fluid (CSF), has been described in adults as a result of GCSE. As GCSE becomes prolonged (>30 minutes), compensatory mechanisms of the brain and hemodynamic and other systems begin to fail, resulting in shock and hypoperfusion of end organs. Rhabdomyolysis has been described and can lead to renal failure or cardiac arrhythmias. Other systemic abnormalities include intravascular coagulation, endocrine failure, and autonomic dysfunction.

Mortality from SE in children ranges from 3% to 11% and is most closely linked to the etiology. In contrast, seizure duration (>1 hour) and anoxia are predictive of mortality in adults with SE. In children, acute symptomatic GCSE is consistently associated with the highest mortality rates, whereas children with febrile SE have minimal mortality and no morbidity even in cases where SE lasts for more than an hour. Morbidities associated with SE include development of epilepsy, and motor and cognitive disabilities.

It is difficult to determine what contribution the underlying etiology, seizure activity, or systemic effects of seizure activity has toward neurologic injuries following SE. Determining this relationship is central to evaluating when and whether to treat electrographic SE. In adult baboons, hippocampal neuronal degeneration occurs after 30 minutes of GCSE even if there is good circulatory support. The mechanism for this injury is speculated to be secondary to changes resulting from the electrically active neurons themselves. As mentioned in Chapter 7, the neurotransmitter glutamate activates postsynaptic receptors (both N-methyl D-aspartate [NMDA] and non-NMDA). This activation leads to increased intracellular calcium levels and apoptotic cell death. These effects are mitigated by NMDA antagonists, suggesting a primary role for glutamate in this process. It is notable that GCSE in immature rodents (roughly equivalent to a human newborn) does not result in overt neuronal injury. However, there is a lower threshold for provoking a second seizure and an increased severity of injury with this second seizure that may be mediated by changes in γ-aminobutyric acid (GABA) and glutamate receptor expression. In adult animal models, systemic factors such as hypoxia, hypoglycemia, lactic acidosis, and hyperpyrexia can exacerbate injury from SE.

TREATMENT

As mentioned earlier, there is controversy about how aggressively to treat SE. Generally, rapidity in treating seizures is related to risks of neurologic injury or risks of causing seizures to become refractory. For instance, because atypical absence SE carries a minimal risk for any serious sequelae, the decision to treat these findings needs to be weighed against the potential side effects of pharmacologic agents. Similarly, focal motor SE (epilepsia partialis continua or EPC) has low morbidity. Because this condition is notoriously refractory to treatment with anticonvulsants, seizure treatment could result in more harm to the patient than the seizure itself. Treatment of GCSE with pharmacologic agents is always warranted because the risk of severe neurologic and systemic complications is significant relative to the minor risks of drug therapy. However, immediate intervention for complex partial seizures is more controversial because the neurologic sequelae vary from no change to memory impairment and may reflect the underlying etiology rather than the damage from the seizure itself.

There is evidence to suggest that increased duration of epileptic activity is associated with refractory SE. In rodents, electrical stimulation of the hippocampus for 30 to 60 minutes produces self-sustained complex partial seizures. The increasing duration of SE in these models decreases pharmacologic treatment efficacy. Clinically, studies have shown that low-dose benzodiazepine therapy is more effective when treatment is started earlier. The mechanism for this effect may involve alterations in NMDA and GABA-A receptors, with increased tonic stimulation, but this hypothesis has not been confirmed.

Initial Management

The treatment of SE involves stabilizing ventilation and circulation, halting the epileptic activity and diminishing potential complications. As with all critical illnesses, maintenance of an intact airway, adequate ventilation, oxygenation, and circulatory function is of primary concern. As the neurologic condition is being assessed, complications of SE such as hypoxia, hypoglycemia, lactic acidosis, hyperpyrexia should be monitored and corrected. Mechanical ventilation should be instituted if the child is unable to maintain oxygenation or is deemed to be at increased risk for aspiration because of diminishment of airway reflexes. Because the utilization of multiple pharmacologic treatments for SE can precipitate respiratory insufficiency, vigilant monitoring of these parameters should be maintained until the epileptic activity is resolved.

Because outcomes and treatment decisions will be linked to the etiology of SE, determination of the cause of SE is important (see Table 50.1). Laboratory testing for glucose, electrolytes, calcium, and magnesium, and liver and renal function tests should be performed. If the patient has refractory SE or if there is a suspicion on the basis of history and examination, antiepileptic drug levels, complete blood count, cultures, toxicologic screens, and other laboratory tests should be obtained. Imaging studies should be obtained if there are physical signs of intracranial hypertension (papilledema or evolving pupillary abnormalities), if there is clinical suspicion of a lesion that would cause mass effect within the cranial cavity, or if the patient has unexplained refractory GCSE. If meningitis is suspected, a lumbar puncture should be performed (see Chapter 49).

TABLE 50.1
ETIOLOGIES OF STATUS EPILEPTICUS

Acute

Increased or decreased glucose levels
Infection
Intracranial bleeding (trauma, stroke, tumor, vascular malformation)
Hypoxia, asphyxia
Stroke
Intracranial mass
Non-AED overdose (INH, stimulant)
AED overdose
AED noncompliance
Alcohol withdrawal
Metabolic disorder

Nonacute

Epilepsy: idiopathic or remote symptomatic
Remote symptomatic
Neurodegenerative

AED, antiepileptic drug; INH, isoniazid.

Benzodiazepines are currently the first-line therapy for rapid cessation of convulsive seizures that last longer than 5 minutes (see Table 50.2). Intravenous lorazepam or rectal diazepam is generally considered the first line of therapy because of their rapid onset of action. Controversy exists between these two choices because data comparing these two options is lacking. Lorazepam causes lesser degrees of respiratory depression and, theoretically, should have a longer duration of action (8 to 24 hours for lorazepam compared to 30 minutes for diazepam). One randomized study in children did not demonstrate a difference between intravenous lorazepam and diazepam but there was a trend for rectal lorazepam preventing seizure recurrence more often than rectal diazepam. Although intravenous lorazepam is preferred, rectal diazepam gel may be easier to deliver when access is a problem. If epileptic activity continues after one or two adequate doses of a benzodiazepine, additional, longer-acting agents are required. It is prudent to use therapies with a low morbidity when the duration of GCSE is <30 minutes because mortality and morbidity for this population is extremely low. Further, because 5% of febrile seizures last longer than 30 minutes and this benign entity represents 25% to 65% of seizures in children younger than 5 years, using therapies with high morbidity would expose some children to unnecessary risks. First-line therapies for most seizures are phenytoin or phenobarbital because of the intravenous route of administration and minimal significant side effects of these agents. Other anticonvulsant medications with favorable side effect profiles have not been extensively used in humans. Fosphenytoin is now recommended over phenytoin because of a decreased incidence of cardiovascular side effects and soft-tissue injury. Fosphenytoin achieves peak brain levels within 15 minutes when given intravenously and within 20 to 30 minutes after intramuscular administration. Care should be taken to avoid excessive dosing because it has a narrow therapeutic range and is epileptogenic at supratherapeutic concentrations. Phenobarbital has several disadvantages compared to fosphenytoin in that it is more sedating, takes longer to reach peak brain concentrations (20 to 60 minutes), and is more likely to cause respiratory depression, particularly when combined with benzodiazepines. As such, phenobarbital is frequently given after fosphenytoin has failed to resolve the epileptic activity. In the first 30 minutes of GCSE treatment, the patient should receive one benzodiazepine and two fosphenytoin doses, and, if GCSE continues, the patient should be started on phenobarbital. If both the first-line agents fail to resolve SE, the causes of SE that will respond only to specific therapies should be reconsidered (i.e., infection, increased intracranial pressure, hypoglycemia, hyperglycemia, isoniazid overdose, or pyridoxine deficiency/dependency) and emergent brain imaging should be obtained.

A single randomized, double-blind trial (performed in adult patients) comparing lorazepam, phenobarbital,

TABLE 50.2
POTENTIAL OPTIONS FOR PHARMACOLOGIC TREATMENT OF STATUS EPILEPTICUS

Medication	Dose	Rate	Side Effects
Initial Therapy			
Lorazepam	0.03–0.1 mg/kg IV	<2 mg/min	Hypotension, respiratory depression, depressed level of consciousness
Diazepam	0.3 mg/kg IV 0.5–0.7 mg/kg rectal	IV over 2–5 min to prevent apnea	Hypotension, respiratory depression, depressed level of consciousness
Fosphenytoin	15–20 mg/kg up to 25 mg/kg PE IV or IM	150 mg PE/min	Hypotension, cardiac arrhythmias
Phenobarbital	15–20 mg/kg up to 30 mg/kg or serum concentration of 15–45 mg/L	1 mg/kg/min (maximum 2 mg/kg/min child, 100 mg/min adult)	Hypotension, respiratory depression, depressed level of consciousness
Valproate (remains experimental)	20 mg/kg IV followed by 1 mg/kg/h or 24 mg/kg divided q8h (maintain serum concentration ~75 mg/L; >100 mg/L during q4h dosing)	6 mg/kg/min	Hypotension, fatal hepatotoxicity
Pyridoxine	50–100 mg IV bolus followed by 15–30 mg/kg/d PO q.d. (pyridoxine-dependent seizures)		Apnea, sleepiness, floppy (up to 24 h), rare dorsal root ganglionopathy if dosage ≥2 g/d
Refractory Seizures			
Diazepam	0.01–0.1 mg/kg/min or to effect		Hypotension, respiratory depression, depressed level of consciousness
Midazolam	0.15–0.2 mg/kg loading dose followed by 1–18 μg/kg/h or to effect		Respiratory suppression (less common)
Phenobarbital high-dose	Dosing b.i.d. to achieve increased serum concentration (up to 70 mg/L)		Respiratory suppression but develops tolerance
Pentobarbital	2–10 mg/kg loading dose up to 20 mg/kg followed by 0.5–5 mg/kg/h or to effect	over 1 h (2–10 mg/kg load) over 2 h (20 mg/kg load)	Cardiac suppression, hypotension, poor cardiac output, immune suppression, respiratory suppression
Thiopental	5 mg/kg loading dose followed by 5–10 mg/kg/h or to effect	Load over 2 min	Hypotension, immune suppression, respiratory suppression
Lidocaine	100 mg or 1–3 mg/kg loading dose followed by 4–10 mg/kg/h (1.5–3.5 mg/kg/h adult)		Cardiovascular dysfunction, paradoxical convulsions at higher levels (>15–20 μg/mL)
Propofol	3–5 mg/kg loading dose followed by 1–15 mg/kg/h or to effect		Propofol infusion syndrome in children

Readers are encouraged to confirm dosing rates with standard pharmacologic references.
IV, intravenous; IM, intramuscular; PO, by mouth; PE, phenytoin equivalents.

diazepam plus phenytoin, and phenytoin for the treatment of GCSE was performed. All therapies were equivalent in resolving SE, except phenytoin alone, possibly explained by the prolonged infusion time of this drug, which is now replaced with fosphenytoin. It is of interest that, in some animal models, phenytoin is not as effective as diazepam or phenobarbital in stopping prolonged SE. Recently, intravenous valproate has been advocated for the resolution of SE, with some promising results. Valproate has shown efficacy with a low side effect profile in adults and children with SE. This should be considered as a first-line medication for patients already on valproate and for children in whom a generalized epilepsy syndrome is suspected. In these children, nonconvulsive seizures and NCSE can be provoked by phenytoin. Larger series of trials are needed for this agent because side effects such as hypotension have been sporadically reported. In addition, there is a 1:600 risk of fatal hepatotoxicity from anticonvulsant polytherapy in children as old as 2 years and younger. This may be due to impairment of fatty acid oxidation from carnitine depletion. Because of this, valproate should be avoided in children with suspected inborn errors of metabolism.

Some would suggest more aggressive treatment during the first 30 minutes in children with a decreased ability to compensate for the physiologic perturbations of GCSE. Systemic abnormalities in animal models contribute to brain injury in SE, and one adult study had found increased mortality from combined stroke and SE. Some of these conditions may include brain tumor, trauma, stroke, sickle cell disease, congenital heart disease, or inborn errors of metabolism.

Management of Refractory Status Epilepticus

Refractory SE is variably defined both in terms of length of time and number of medications used to treat GCSE before cessation of epileptic activity. Although no standard definition of refractory SE is agreed upon, most consider SE to be refractory when seizures do not respond to treatment with benzodiazepine, phenytoin, *and* phenobarbital in a timely manner (usually 30 to 60 minutes). Refractory SE requires more aggressive therapy with anesthetics; higher-dose anticonvulsants; and, eventually, pharmacologic suppression of brain activity. Evidence favoring this aggressive approach includes (i) animal data suggesting irreversible brain injury after 30 minutes of GCSE, (ii) self-sustained seizure activity after 30 to 60 minutes of SE in animals, (iii) increasing risk of systemic complications related to prolonged SE, and (iv) a study of adults and children in which individuals with seizures lasting 30 minutes or more had a higher mortality.

Treatment of refractory SE includes the institution of high-dose therapy to pharmacologically suppress brain activity followed by the institution of long-acting agents to prevent SE recurrence upon withdrawal of the suppressive agents. Suppression of brain activity is intended to halt the firing of the abnormal epileptic focus for a given period, theoretically breaking the feedback of seizure activity and excitotoxicity within the focus. The depth of suppression of electrical activity can vary from being complete (flat EEG) to burst suppression, in which there are variable durations of electrical silence ("suppression") between episodes of electrical activity on the EEG ("burst"). A greater duration of the suppression is indicative of a greater degree ("depth") of cerebral suppression. Burst suppression can be achieved using a variety of agents including pentobarbital, phenobarbital, propofol, high-dose benzodiazepines, or other anesthetic agents. These therapies generally need to

be delivered as continuous intravenous infusions to obtain sufficient brain concentrations for prolonged suppression of brain electrical activity. Ideally, continuous EEG monitoring should be in place to constantly monitor whether the desired level of cerebral suppression has been achieved.

The depth of suppression (depth of burst suppression or total suppression) and duration of suppressive therapies (number of days of suppression) is generally tailored to individual children and has not been systematically studied. A meta-analysis of pentobarbital, propofol, and midazolam used in adults found a mean duration of 30 to 96 hours for these suppressive therapies. Individuals may require therapy for substantially longer period to prevent the recurrence of SE. In a study of childhood SE, the average duration of thiopentone-based burst suppression was 48 hours. Regardless of the duration of suppressive therapy, achieving adequate brain concentrations of other anticonvulsants during this period is imperative. Once therapeutic concentrations of these longer-acting agents are achieved, the suppressing agent can be slowly weaned over days, using lack of seizure recurrence as a measure of success. Most reports suggest maintaining the usual therapeutic doses of long-acting anticonvulsants, but supratherapeutic concentrations such as phenytoin concentrations >20 μg per mL and phenobarbital >40 μg per mL may be necessary.

There are relatively few studies comparing the efficacy of agents used to achieve burst suppression. A meta-analysis comparing diazepam, midazolam, thiopental, pentobarbital, and isoflurane demonstrated equal efficacy for all agents except diazepam, which was inferior. Mortality was less frequent in the midazolam-treated children, yet this may be related to the etiology of SE because these children had the fewest symptomatic etiologies. Therefore, with this relative equivalence of these agents, the choice for individual children is made on the basis of common side effects.

Barbiturates have been used for decades to achieve burst suppression. Of the barbiturates, phenobarbital is the longest-acting, pentobarbital is intermediate-acting, and thiopental the shortest. Because of this, thiopental and pentobarbital must be delivered as continuous infusions to maintain sufficient brain concentrations, whereas phenobarbital can be administered intermittently. All barbiturates can affect cardiovascular performance, with decreases in preload, afterload, and contractility noted on increasing doses. Bolus doses of thiopental may produce hypotension to a larger degree than other barbiturates. Barbiturates at high doses have immunosuppressant effects, but the clinical relevance of this finding is unclear. Children on high-dose phenobarbital in one study became tolerant to the respiratory depressant effect and could be extubated with supratherapeutic serum concentrations.

Benzodiazepine infusions, particularly with midazolam, have become an important tool in inducing burst suppression for refractory SE. Cardiovascular side effects of midazolam are mild and less severe than those related to barbiturates. However, tachyphylaxis is very common, and in one review in adults, 24- to 48-hour treatment with midazolam at constant doses resulted in breakthrough seizures requiring a several-fold dose increase to re-establish control of seizure activity. Prolonged therapy with midazolam or lorazepam can result in significant accumulation of the preservatives propylene and ethylene glycol, respectively. Metabolic acidosis with an osmolar gap can result from prolonged high-dose benzodiazepine therapy.

General anesthetics are among the most potent agents that affect cerebral activity and can be used to treat refractory SE. Propofol has been increasingly used in adults with SE because it has a decreased rate of tachyphylaxis compared to midazolam and causes fewer cardiovascular side effects than pentobarbital. In children, its use has been more limited because of reports of propofol infusion syndrome. In this syndrome, severe metabolic acidosis (secondary to impaired fatty acid oxidation), lipemia, rhabdomyolysis, and cardiovascular collapse have been reported. Inhaled anesthetics such as halothane and isoflurane have also been used to treat refractory SE. However, the delivery of these agents is problematic and severe cardiac arrhythmias limit their usefulness. Lidocaine was also used in the past, but its use has been difficult because of adverse effects on cardiovascular function and provocation of seizures at levels >15 to 20 μg per mL.

There is no data to support the use of a particular maintenance anticonvulsant medication. Selection of a particular anticonvulsant can be based on available routes of administration and lack of drug interactions. A patient may be maintained on phenytoin if the levels during initial treatment are inadequate. Initially administered phenobarbital may be continued because there is increasing efficacy with increasing levels and it has the additional benefits of having a long half-life, minimizing fluctuations in anticonvulsant level as suppressant therapy is tapered. Alternatives include medications such as topiramate and levetiracetam, which are not hepatically metabolized and, are therefore, unlikely to result in adverse drug interactions. Valproate level is not affected by pentobarbital or midazolam but can increase levels of both these medications. It may be difficult to increase carbamazepine to adequate levels in children treated with pentobarbital because of interactions with metabolizing enzymes within the liver. Theoretically, oxcarbazepine levels are not affected by pentobarbital or midazolam, but this has not been studied in humans. Carbamazepine, oxcarbazepine, phenytoin, and fosphenytoin can all decrease midazolam levels because they are inducers of the metabolic pathway of midazolam, and because of this these agents may not be the ideal choices.

As the clinical signs of seizures abate, the signs of subtle GCSE and NCSE must be diagnosed and treated. The clinical features of subtle GCSE may be slight movements of the eyes, face, or limbs, whereas NCSE may manifest with subtle eye movements or solely unexplained unresponsiveness. In children with refractory SE or suspected subtle GCSE or NCSE, an EEG is required to confirm that seizures have been successfully treated. Further, an EEG can help distinguish between subtle GCSE and atypical absence SE provoked by phenytoin. If there is no EEG access, empiric treatment can be initiated. Resumption of a normal level of consciousness would suggest that the patient had been in NCSE.

FUTURE DIRECTIONS: NEUROPROTECTION

Because outcomes in children with SE are related primarily to etiology, the future should be directed at protecting neurons from the acute insult in addition to seizure-related injury. There appears to be some overlap in ischemia and seizure mechanisms of injury in that both appear to occur through excitotoxic mechanisms. Research into the mechanisms of injury from ischemia, head trauma, and infection will help determine future modes of neuroprotection. In addition, because there can be significant neuronal loss from the seizure itself in animal models, mechanisms that can block the glutamatergic excitotoxic cascade may improve outcomes after SE. The clinically used NMDA antagonist ketamine can prevent neuronal injury when given after 75 minutes of continuous clonic jerking in a rodent model, even if seizures continue clinically or electrographically. In one rodent model of limbic SE (similar to the human NCSE), treatment within 1 hour of SE using phenobarbital or the NMDA antagonist MK-801 prevented the development of epilepsy rather than leading to the cessation of electrographic seizure. Antagonism of another glutamate receptor, the amino-3-hydroxy-5-methyl-4-isoxazole propionic acid (AMPA) receptor, may be useful in ameliorating neuronal loss after SE. In one study, AMPA receptor blockade with topiramate prevented neuronal loss without stopping seizures. In addition, unlike other anticonvulsant agents, it does not cause neuronal injury in infant rodent models.

In the future, larger trials on well-characterized agents used to treat SE will be required to maximize the clinical outcomes, with guidance from information gleaned from animal models. Because phenobarbital is more efficacious than phenytoin in seizure cessation in rodents, relatively simple clinical trials could test this hypothesis in children. Efficacy and effect of newer anticonvulsants such as valproate, topiramate (Topamax), and levetiracetam on outcomes need to be determined, especially because some of these agents have additional theoretical neuroprotective benefits.

CONCLUSION

SE is a common disorder in children and represents complex neurophysiologic processes. Prolonged GCSE can result in neuronal damage, and this can be exacerbated by systemic abnormalities. Current treatment is based on balancing the risks of injury from SE against the morbidities of the therapies. More studies are needed to evaluate the efficacy of treatments for SE, particularly refractory SE. Future therapies should be directed both at improving efficacy of seizure cessation and at blocking the pathways that cause neuronal injury.

RECOMMENDED READINGS

1. Bittigau P, Sifringer M, Ikonomidou C, et al. Antiepileptic drugs and apoptosis in the developing brain. *Ann NY Acad Sci.* 2003;993:103–114, discussion 123–124.
2. Bleck TP. Management approaches to prolonged seizures and status epilepticus. *Epilepsia.* 1999;40 Suppl 1:S59–S63, discussion S64–S66.
3. Cascino GD. Nonconvulsive status epilepticus in adults and children. *Epilepsia.* 1993;34(Suppl 1):S21–S28.
4. Claassen J, Hirsch LJ, Emerson RG, et al. Treatment of refractory status epilepticus with pentobarbital, propofol, or midazolam: A systematic review. *Epilepsia.* 2002;43:146–153.
5. Gilbert DL, Gartside PS, et al. Efficacy and mortality in treatment of refractory generalized convulsive status epilepticus in children: A meta-analysis. *J Child Neurol.* 1999;14:602–609.
6. Holmes G. Seizure-induced neuronal injury: Animal data. *Neurology.* 2002;59:S3–S6.
7. Kahriman M, Minecan D, Kutluay E, et al. Efficacy of topiramate in children with refractory status epilepticus. *Epilepsia.* 2003;44(10):1353–1356.
8. Kaplan PW. No, some types of nonconvulsive status epilepticus cause little permanent neurologic sequelae (or: "The cure may be worse than the disease"). *Neurophysiol Clin.* 2000;30:377–382.
9. Klitgaard H, Pitkanen A. Antiepileptogenesis, neuroprotection, and disease modification in the treatment of epilepsy: Focus on levetiracetam. *Epileptic Disord.* 2003;5(Suppl 1):S9–S16.
10. Leszczyszyn DJ, Pellock JM. Status epilepticus. In: Pellock JM, Dodson WE, Bourgeois BFD, eds. *Pediatric epilepsy : Diagnosis and therapy.* New York: DEMOS; 2001:275–289.
11. Manno EM. New management strategies in the treatment of status epilepticus. *Mayo Clin Proc.* 2003;78:508–518.
12. Ramsay RE. Treatment of status epilepticus. *Epilepsia.* 1993;34(Suppl 1):S71–S81.
13. Riviello JJ Jr, Holmes GL. The treatment of status epilepticus. *Semin Pediatr Neurol.* 2004;11:129–138.
14. Sanchez RM, Jensen FE. Maturational aspects of epilepsy mechanisms and consequences for the immature brain. *Epilepsia.* 2001;42:577–585.
15. Shneker BF, Fountain NB. Assessment of acute morbidity and mortality in nonconvulsive status epilepticus. *Neurology.* 2003;61:1066–1073.
16. Treatment of convulsive status epilepticus. Recommendations of the Epilepsy Foundation of America's Working Group on Status Epilepticus. *JAMA.* 1993;270:854–859.
17. Wasterlain CG, Fujikawa DG, Penix L, et al. Pathophysiological mechanisms of brain damage from status epilepticus. *Epilepsia.* 1993;34(Suppl 1):S37–S53.
18. Young GB, Jordan KG, Doig GS, et al. An assessment of nonconvulsive seizures in the intensive care unit using continuous EEG monitoring: An investigation of variables associated with mortality. *Neurology.* 1996;47:83–89.
19. Yu KT, Mills S, Thompson N, et al. Safety and efficacy of intravenous valproate in pediatric status epilepticus and acute repetitive seizures. *Epilepsia.* 2003;44(5):724–726.
20. Zhang G, Raol YH, Hsu FC, et al. Effects of status epilepticus on hippocampal GABAA receptors are age-dependent. *Neuroscience.* 2004;125:299–303.

Brain Death

51

I. David Todres

Death by neurologic criteria has been recognized internationally, yet a worldwide consensus on diagnostic criteria is lacking. In the United States, brain death is defined as the cessation of brain function, including the brain stem. On the basis of this definition, the American Academy of Pediatrics established guidelines in 1987 for determining brain death in infants and children. Despite these guidelines and more recent statutes that legally recognize death by neurologic criteria, brain death remains a complex and controversial topic in health care.

HISTORICAL PERSPECTIVE

The first report of the state that is now recognized as brain death appeared in 1959. French neurologists Mollaret and Goulon described a condition referred to as *le coma dépassé*, that is, a state beyond coma. These patients were totally unresponsive and had absent deep tendon and cranial nerve reflexes, apnea, and isoelectric electroencephalogram (EEG). They reported that this state was different from other comatose states but did not refer to it as death. In 1968, an *ad hoc* committee of the Harvard Medical School published clinical guidelines that shaped the development of the criteria for brain death. The term used by the committee to define the condition of brain death was *irreversible coma*, a potentially confusing term because this state is usually applied to a patient in a vegetative condition. The Harvard criteria consisted of the following requirements: (i) absence of receptivity and responsivity, (ii) absence of movements, (iii) absence of elicitable reflexes, (iv) apnea, and (v) isoelectric EEG. All the tests needed to be repeated 24 hours later, and if no changes were noted, brain death was declared.

In 1981, the President's Commission for the Study of Ethical Problems in Medicine and Biomedical and Behavioral Research developed guidelines for the determination of brain death. These guidelines established two fundamental criteria for death: (i) irreversible cessation of circulation and respiratory function or (ii) irreversible cessation of all functions of the entire brain, including the brain stem. Therefore, death can be declared without cardiac arrest. All the states in the United States have enacted the legislation accepting this definition of death. The President's Commission cautioned the use of these guidelines in children younger than 5 years, reflecting uncertainty in recovery from prolonged coma and limited experiences in this determination with younger children. Seeking to remedy the exclusion of children younger than 5 years, a task force established guidelines in 1987 for the determination of brain death in infants and children. Emphasis was placed on relatively longer observation periods (the younger the child, the longer the observation period) and the need for confirmatory tests (see Table 51.1). Infants younger than 7 days were excluded because of the lack of evidence to guide recommendations. Formal guidelines for the determination of brain death in neonates younger than 7 days have not been developed.

CLINICAL DIAGNOSIS

Epidemiology

The overall incidence of brain death in older infants and children ranges from 1% to 2% of admissions to pediatric intensive care units (PICUs). The percentage of patients who are brain-dead compared to the total number of patients who have died in PICUs ranges from 11% to 33%.

Proximate History to Determine the Cause of Brain Death

The first step in the diagnosis of brain death is to identify the unequivocal, irreversible causative event responsible for the clinical state of the child. A major cause of brain death is the result of a hypoxic insult to the brain. This may arise from breathing a hypoxic mixture (e.g., near-drowning, smoke inhalation) or following a failure of the cerebral circulation to deliver the required oxygen for

TABLE 51.1

GUIDELINES FOR THE DETERMINATION OF BRAIN DEATH IN CHILDREN

History

Determination of the proximate cause of coma to ensure the absence of remediable or reversible conditions (toxic and metabolic disorders, sedatives or hypnotic drugs, paralytic agents, hypothermia, hypotension, and surgically remediable conditions have to be excluded)

Physical Examination Criteria

The three cardinal findings in brain death are coma or unresponsiveness, absence of brain stem reflexes, and apnea

1. Coma or unresponsiveness
2. Absence of brain stem reflexes
    a. Midposition or fully dilated pupils (drug effect should be excluded); no response to light
    b. Absence of spontaneous, oculocephalic ("doll's eye"), and caloric (oculovestibular) indirect eye movements
    c. Absence of movement of bulbar musculature and corneal, gag, cough, sucking, and rooting reflexes
    d. Absence of spontaneous respiratory movements (apnea) with standardized testing
3. Absence of hypothermia or hypotension
4. Flaccid tone and absence of spontaneous or induced movements, excluding spinal cord–mediated reflexes
5. Examination should be consistent for brain death throughout the period of observation and testing

Observation Period According To Age

7 d–2 mo:	Two examinations and EEGs 48 h apart
2 mo–1 y:	Two examinations and EEGs 24 h apart; a repeat examination and EEG are unnecessary *if* a radionuclide angiogram shows no cerebral blood flow
More than 1 y:	Two examinations 12–24 h apart; laboratory testing (EEG, cerebral blood flow studies) is not required; however, observation period may be reduced *if* EEG shows electrocerebral silence or radionuclide studies demonstrate no cerebral blood flow

EEG, electroencephalogram.
Adapted from Task Force for the Determination of Brain Death in Children. Guidelines for Determination of Brain Death in Children. *Pediatrics.* 1987;80:298.

metabolism (e.g., cardiac arrest, post-traumatic cerebral edema, or sudden infant death syndrome). Infection (e.g., meningitis) may cause loss of brain stem reflexes but may leave the cortical function intact and be associated with complete recovery. Metabolic causes (e.g., overdose of barbiturates) may also be reversible. A clear history of the events leading to a state suggestive of brain death is critical for determining the proximate cause of the coma. A computed tomographic (CT) scan is often essential for determining the cause of brain death. However, the CT scan may be normal in children with fulminant meningitis, and the examination of cerebrospinal fluid is diagnostic.

Neurologic Evaluation

Prerequisites for Clinical Examination

The neurologic examination is the standard method for determining brain death. The guidelines for the determination of brain death in children provide a standardized protocol for performing the examination to establish brain death. However, to ensure the validity of the clinical examination, certain criteria must be met before conducting the examination. First, neuromuscular blocking drugs or sedatives affect the interpretation of the clinical examination and must be excluded. Train-of-four peripheral nerve stimulation should elicit four unattenuated twitches

(see Chapter 7 for discussion of train-of-four). If there is evidence of partial neuromuscular blockade, the administration of neostigmine along with atropine will reduce pharmacologic weakness. Laboratory testing can reveal the presence of sedatives, and when rapidly available, the measurement of blood levels will assist in clarifying whether the drug is blunting responses during the clinical examination. Even low blood concentrations of sedatives may have a profound impact on the neurologic examination, particularly in those individuals nearing brain death. Delaying brain death evaluation until at least four half-lives have passed or waiting for 48 hours after administration of the drug can lessen the confounding effect of sedatives. Second, complicating medical conditions that may confound the clinical assessment must be excluded, particularly severe acid–base or electrolyte disturbances. Profound endocrine imbalances, such as hypo- or hyperthyroidism, cortisol deficiency, or diabetes insipidus, should also be treated before brain death is determined. Third, the core body temperature must exceed 32°C for the determination of coma and evaluation of brain stem reflexes; however, the temperature must be ≥36.5°C when performing the apnea test. Fourth, the systolic blood pressure must be maintained above the lower limit of normal for the given age. Fifth, evidence for drug intoxication or poisoning should be ruled out. Therefore, the clinical determination of brain death requires that these confounding conditions are met to eliminate the possibility of a false-positive test.

For the diagnosis of brain death, the whole brain (i.e., cortical and brain stem) has to be evaluated. The key features of the clinical brain death evaluation include the presence of coma, absence of brain stem reflexes, and apnea that persists over time. Age-dependent intervals between examinations are defined in the guidelines of the American Academy of Pediatrics.

Cerebral Unresponsiveness

The depth of coma, or cerebral unresponsiveness, is assessed by the presence or absence of motor responses, including eye opening, to a noxious stimulus. Noxious stimuli include a loud voice and standardized painful stimuli, such as pressing on a finger nail bed or on the supraorbital ridge. Spontaneous movements and reflexes have been described in patients with brain death, confirmed by ancillary testing, and should not be misinterpreted as evidence of brain stem function. Examples of spinally mediated movements observed independent of noxious stimulation include spontaneous movements of limbs, respiratorylike movements including shoulder elevation and adduction or back arching, flexion of the trunk to a partial sitting position (so-called Lazarus sign), deep tendon reflexes, triple flexion responses, or Babinski sign.

Brain Stem Evaluation

Examination of the brain stem involves the assessment of cranial nerve reflex pathways in the pons and medulla. A detailed description of the cranial nerve examination in children is found in Chapter 7. For the diagnosis of brain death, pupils are in midposition (4 to 9 mm), with no constrictive response to bright light. When the eyes are held open, there should be no spontaneous ocular movement, including nystagmus. Ocular movements should be absent when the head is turned rapidly from midposition to 90 degrees bilaterally (oculocephalic reflex) for brain death. However, do not perform the oculocephalic reflex in patients in whom there is a concern for spinal cord injury; rather, perform the oculovestibular test (cold calorics). First confirm whether the tympanic membranes are intact and free from cerumen or blood. Elevate the head 30 degrees and maintain midline position. Irrigate the tympanic membrane with 30 to 50 mL of ice water over 60 seconds while observing eye movements. Continue observing for an additional minute. After waiting for 5 minutes, repeat the test on the opposite tympanic membrane. There will be no eye movement in brain death, but with an intact brain stem, the eyes should deviate toward the cold, irrigated ear. Confounding factors for oculovestibular testing include exposure to ototoxic drugs and trauma to the petrous bone.

Apnea Test

Once the absence of brain stem reflexes has been confirmed, the documentation of apnea under controlled conditions completes the clinical brain death evaluation. Apnea signifies the loss of the final brain stem structure to be affected in the rostral-to-caudal progression of brain death. The apnea test involves observing respiratory effort in response to hypercapnia and acidosis without producing hypoxia. The formal test for apnea is performed in the following manner. Preoxygenate the patient with 100% oxygen for 20 minutes before beginning the test. Adjust the ventilator to produce partial pressure of arterial carbon dioxide ($Paco_2$) between 40 and 45 mm Hg to minimize the time off the ventilator and to reduce the risk of severe hypoxemia. Adjust a non–self-inflating resuscitation bag using 100% oxygen to deliver the continuous positive airway pressure (CPAP) equal to the level of the positive end-expiratory pressure (PEEP) that the patient is receiving by the ventilator. This will decrease the potential of lung derecruitment and hypoxemia. Detach the ventilator circuit from the endotracheal/tracheostomy tube and immediately attach the bag to the airway. Observe the patient closely for respiratory movements. Measure partial pressure of arterial oxygen (Pao_2), $Paco_2$, and pH at 5-minute intervals. As $Paco_2$ increases at a rate of 3 to 4 mm Hg per minute, the apnea tests generally last 10 to 15 minutes. If the patient becomes significantly hypoxemic (O_2 saturation <90%) during testing, the systolic blood pressure becomes hypotensive for age, or cardiac arrhythmia develops, immediately draw an arterial blood sample and reconnect the ventilator. Apnea is present if respiratory movements are absent and the final arterial blood gas shows a $Paco_2$ of 60 mm Hg or a value 20 mm Hg higher than the pretest baseline value. If respiratory movements are observed, the apnea test result is negative, and the clinical diagnosis of brain death is not supported. When respiratory movements are not observed and blood gas values do not meet the criteria or the test is aborted because of complications, the apnea test is indeterminate and additional confirmatory testing is necessary.

Performance of an apnea test places the patient at risk for complications, most commonly hypotension, pneumothorax, and cardiac arrhythmia. In adults, complications occur in 26% of apnea tests. Unfavorable conditions present before the apnea test, including no preoxygenation, acid–base or electrolyte abnormalities, increase the risk of complications (odds ratio 3.65, 95% confidence interval, 1.64 to 8.14).

Ancillary Tests

Brain death is a clinical diagnosis. However, ancillary testing must be performed in patients in whom the clinical history is uncertain or specific components of clinical testing cannot be reliably performed or evaluated; for example, severe facial trauma, preexisting pupillary abnormalities, sleep apnea, or severe pulmonary disease resulting in severe chronic retention of CO_2. Ancillary tests include the tests for brain electrical activity (EEG and evoked potentials) and cerebral blood flow (cerebral angiography, radionuclide imaging, transcranial Doppler [TCD]).

Electroencephalogram

The appropriateness of the EEG in confirming the clinical diagnosis of brain death is generally accepted in the United States but is considered nonessential in the United Kingdom. However, in the evaluation for brain death, the EEG must be considered with the criteria of establishing the proximate cause, ensuring the absence of reversible conditions, and performing a clinical examination consistent with brain death. Because brain stem activity cannot be assessed with EEG, it must not be considered as a diagnostic tool on its own (i.e., the sole determinant of brain death).

The American Electroencephalographic Society has established guidelines to improve the validity and increase the sensitivity of EEG recording to determine brain death. The diagnosis of brain death requires at least 30 minutes of continuous recording that adheres to the minimal technical criteria for the 16-channel EEG recording. However, it should be noted that the interpretation of the EEG for a diagnosis of electrocerebral silence (ECS) is fraught with technical difficulties, particularly in pediatric patients for whom there are no official guidelines for recording ECS. The guidelines established for adults are difficult to apply to the young child, such as the requirement that interelectrode distance should be 10 cm or more, an impractical requirement in infants because of their small head size. Electrical artifacts may make the tracing unsatisfactory for diagnostic purposes; however, recent advancements in electrical shielding in newer EEG monitors have improved the quality by reducing instrumentation errors.

Although hypothermia and hypotension affect the clinical detection of true brain death, their effects on EEG criteria are less pronounced. The standards for valid EEG interpretation require a core temperature of $32°C$; however, in children, the complete loss of EEG activity does not occur until the core temperature is below $18°C$. On the other hand, the degree of hypotension that correlates with ECS has not been documented. Therefore, blood pressure standards for EEG interpretation are the same as those required for a valid clinical evaluation of brain death.

Barbiturates are employed in the management of intracranial hypertension and status epilepticus specifically to induce ECS. The precise blood concentrations at which barbiturates produce ECS is unknown and is likely confounded by patient factors such as age, hepatic function, and pharmacogenomics. Furthermore, a study in adults demonstrated residual toxic levels of barbiturates in the postmortem state despite the absence of these agents in the serum in the premorbid state. Given the unpredictable and potentially confounding relationship between the subtherapeutic blood barbiturate concentration and its effect on EEG, some advocate the practice of confirming brain death with radionuclide brain blood flow studies.

Studies of brain death in pediatric patients demonstrated that the clinical criteria used in adults could be applied to children older than 3 months. In addition, the studies reported that a single EEG demonstrating ECS was sufficient to confirm brain death. However, the role of the EEG in determination of brain death in the newborn is problematic because it may not correlate with the neurologic examination or cerebral blood flow studies. Specifically, persistent EEG activity has been documented in infants with clinical and radionuclide evidence of brain death. One approach recommended by Volpe is a 72-hour observation period for neonates younger than 7 days and a diagnosis of brain death only when a cause for the coma is unequivocally established. In spite of its limitations in the youngest infants, the EEG remains valuable in confirming brain death when combined with clinical examination and other ancillary studies.

Measurements of Cerebral Perfusion

Cerebral Angiography

Nonfilling of intracerebral arteries by cerebral angiography is the gold standard for ancillary tests used to confirm brain death. Despite its sensitivity, technical limitations including patient transfer, prolonged study time, risk of radiocontrast nephropathy, and invasiveness limit cerebral angiography to those situations in which other ancillary tests fail to confirm brain death. Conventional four-vessel angiography may document no intracerebral filling at the carotid bifurcation or circle of Willis when intracranial pressure exceeds arterial systolic pressure. Usually, the external carotid circulation remains patent while filling of the superior sagittal sinus may be delayed. Similar vascular evaluation is performed using magnetic resonance angiography (MRA).

Radionuclide Imaging

Radionuclide cerebral angiography using the technetium 99 m–hexamethyl propyleneamine oxime (^{99m}Tc-HMPAO) brain scan is used as a confirmatory test for brain death in children, defined by the absence of isotope uptake in the brain parenchyma. Specifically, the absence of cerebral perfusion using the technique of radionuclide angiography is valuable confirmatory evidence of cerebral death, although sagittal sinus activity may be seen, reflecting the drainage of emissary veins. In addition, some authors have argued that this test is a valid diagnostic procedure for the detection of brain death in infants and even neonates. Indeed, Goodman and others have suggested that absence of cerebral blood flow alone is sufficient to diagnose brain death, even in the absence of other testing. A significant advantage of radionuclide imaging studies is that they may be performed at the bedside, an especially important advantage because the patient is usually in an ICU with maximal therapy pending the diagnostic evaluation by the scan.

Transcranial Doppler Ultrasonography

TCD ultrasonography provides a bedside, noninvasive assessment of cerebral blood flow in the middle cerebral and vertebral arteries. An absence of the diastolic peak or reverberating flow with small peaks in early systole is suggestive of brain death. However, the initial absence of Doppler signals cannot be interpreted as being consistent with brain death because 10% of patients may not have adequate temporal insonation windows.

Other Imaging Modalities

Xenon CT scan, *positron emission tomography* (PET), *magnetic resonance imaging* (MRI), *magnetic resonance spectroscopy* (MRS), and MRA provide assessments of cerebral blood flow and are discussed in detail in Chapter 7. However, limited availability, cost, and requirement for specialized facilities make these tests less relevant for making decisions about brain death diagnoses.

Evoked Potentials

Somatosensory evoked potential (SEP) has been used to corroborate the diagnosis of brain death in adults. The bilateral absence of the N20-P22 response on median nerve stimulation measured over the parietal sensory cortex is supportive of brain death. These findings have not been validated in children.

Observation Periods

The task force proposed three sets of guidelines for the observation period and the use of ancillary testing to confirm the state of brain death (Table 51.1). Although some commentators have pointed to what they consider shortcomings in the guidelines, particularly with reference to the recommended observation periods, the guidelines have not been revised to date.

ATTITUDES OF THE PUBLIC TO THE CONCEPT OF BRAIN DEATH

Much of the ambiguity in accepting brain death as the death of the individual stems from the fact that brain-dead patients demonstrate features previously associated with life, such as a pulse and warm skin. However, they also possess some characteristics associated with death, but these are exhibited by individuals in a persistent vegetative state, such as unawareness of the self and environment. Clarification of the difference between brain death and persistent vegetative state is important in educating the family as they go through the process of accepting the death of their loved one. An example from the United Kingdom illustrates how the confusion over these states created parental distrust of the ICU team when artificial ventilation was withdrawn following the declaration of brain death of a child. The media's reporting of clinical cases of brain death has also contributed to misunderstandings of this concept. An example of this is when a 13-year-old had "died" after being taken off "life support" despite the

fact that death had been declared by brain death criteria 1 week earlier.

Cultural and religious perspectives are reflected in the attitudes of the family and the public to the concept of brain death. Several Western religions have accepted the concept of brain death. For example, in August 2000, Pope John Paul II formally endorsed brain death as being fully consistent with Roman Catholic teachings. Although some orthodox rabbis have stated that brain death is compatible with Jewish law because it is the physiologic equivalent of decapitation and most Jews accept brain death, it remains unacceptable for other orthodox Jews. Recently, Islam has supported the concept of brain death as true death in the context of considering organ transplantation. Internationally, both India and Japan have seen some acceptance of the concept in spite of religious and cultural resistance.

In spite of the general acceptance of brain death in the United States, some religious resistance persists, recognized, for example, by New York, requiring allowance for "reasonable accommodation to an individual's religious or moral objections to the use of neurologic criteria to diagnose death." In these situations, physicians can continue ventilatory support without aggressive treatment, anticipating cardiac arrest within a few days. However, this issue is controversial and no clear consensus about appropriate management is yet available.

PHYSICIANS' ATTITUDES TOWARD THE CONCEPT OF BRAIN DEATH

Many health care professionals remain confused about the medical and legal definitions of brain death. In spite of the fact that they are identical and, for example, are recognized so by the American Academy of Pediatrics, American Academy of Neurology, and the American Bar Association, when asked if they would diagnose brain death in a clinical scenario that clearly meets the criteria, 82% of neurologists and 73% of pediatric intensivists indicated that they would. However, only 17% of neurologists and 56% of pediatric intensivists indicated that they would declare the patient brain-dead when specifically asked to consider the medicolegal aspects of the case. In a more recent study, Harrison AM and Botkin JR found that only 36% of pediatric residents and 39% of pediatric attendings correctly defined brain death. Interpretation of a clinical scenario and knowledge of testing criteria were also far from complete. Despite some of its shortcomings and criticisms, determination of death using brain death criteria has now been in clinical practice for nearly four decades and is generally accepted worldwide.

RECOMMENDED READINGS

1. Ashwal S, Schneider S. Brain death in children: Part I. *Pediatr Neurol.* 1987;3:5–11.

2. Ashwal S, Schneider S. Brain death in children: Part II. *Pediatr Neurol*. 1987;3:69–77.

3. Ad Hoc Committee of the Harvard Medical School to Examine the Definition of Brain Death. A definition of irreversible coma. *JAMA*. 1968;205:337–340.

4. Fackler JC, Troncoso JC, Bivoa FR. Age-specific characteristics of brain death in children. *Am J Dis Child*. 1988;142:999–1003.

5. Farrell MM, Levin DL. Brain death in the pediatric patient: Historical, sociological, medical, religious, cultural, legal and ethical consideration. *Crit Care Med*. 1993;21:1951.

6. Goudreau JL, Wijdicks EFM, Emery SF. Complications during apnea testing in the determination of brain death: Predisposing factors. *Neurology*. 2000;55:1045–1048.

7. Harrison AM, Botkin JR. Can pediatricians define and apply the concept of brain death? *Pediatrics*. 1999;103(6):e82.

8. Quality Standards Subcommittee of the American Academy of Neurology. Practice parameters: Assessment and management of patients in the persistent vegetative state. *Neurology*. 1995;45: 1012–1014.

9. Task Force for the Determination of Brain Death in Children. Guidelines for the determination of brain death in children. *Pediatrics*. 1987;80:298–300.

10. Uniform Determination of Death Act, 12 Uniform Laws Annotated (ULA) 589 (West 1993 and West Supp. 1997).

11. Wijdicks EFM. Diagnosis of brain death. *N Engl J Med*. 2001; 344:1215–1221.

Brain and Spinal Cord Trauma

52

JoAnne E. Natale   Michael J. Bell

Trauma is the leading killer of children in the United States, and traumatic brain injury (TBI) accounts for over 50% of those deaths. The Centers for Disease Control and Prevention (CDC) estimates that over 3,000 children die each year because of TBI, and many thousands of survivors will endure lifelong disabilities. Spinal cord injuries are considerably less common, accounting for approximately 5% of all such injuries. However, young children are particularly prone to high cervical injuries; among children younger than 2 years, 80% of spinal cord injuries occur in this vulnerable anatomic region and potentially lead to quadriplegia. Injury prevention strategies have helped to reduce the incidence of central nervous system (CNS) trauma in children, but the concerted effort of intensivists, neurosurgeons, and trauma surgeons is required to maximize clinical outcome.

The systematic study of childhood head and spinal cord injury is currently in its infancy. Recently, guidelines have been published in an effort to standardize practice within the United States. Importantly, these guidelines were developed largely as extrapolations from adult studies combined with expert opinion. This chapter will discuss primary injuries and prevention of secondary injuries using various treatment strategies for children with traumatic brain and spinal cord injury.

PRIMARY INJURIES

Direct injuries to the brain or spinal cord are termed *primary injuries*. In general, fractures of bones (fractured skull, fractured vertebrae or cartilaginous disks), contusions to nervous system tissue, shearing injuries to the white matter, and collections of extra-axial blood (subdural, subarachnoid, and epidural hematomas) are considered primary injuries (see Figs. 52.1 and 52.2). Early therapies

to alleviate these problems and diminish their potential impact are important to maximize overall outcome. In a large series, investigators using the Traumatic Coma Data Bank (TCDB) found that children younger than 4 years had (i) significantly more evacuated subdural hematomas, (ii) a higher incidence of trauma from assaults, and (iii) a dramatically poorer survival (including a mortality of >60% for children younger than 1 year) compared to younger children and adolescents. Speculation regarding the poor survival of infants and toddlers has varied widely. Infants have larger head-to-body surface area ratios and greater forces may be exerted on critical brain structures during assaults (a major category of infant trauma). The brain of an infant has considerably greater water content and decreased myelination compared to older children and this may affect outcome. Lastly, since an infant's brain is growing rapidly, there are likely to be critical differences in brain metabolism that might affect outcome in some manner.

Bony fractures commonly occur after brain trauma in infants (up to 40%) as well as older children (up to 70%). However, except for depression of brain parenchyma or risks for localized infection, there are few complications of these injuries. Bony fractures within the spinal canal have a greater likelihood to cause permanent impairment of function because of the relatively small size of the spinal canal. Fractures of the atlanto-occipital-axis structures can cause spinal cord transection at the foramen magnum and death. Dislocations of vertebral bodies into the spinal canal can cause permanent motor and/or sensory impairments at any spinal cord segment. For these reasons, vigilance in manipulation of the spine is essential during management.

Contusions to the cerebral cortex or spinal cord are mixtures of live cells, dead cells, and debris from hematogenous elements. Contusions occur when the brain is directly impacted by an object or when it is thrust

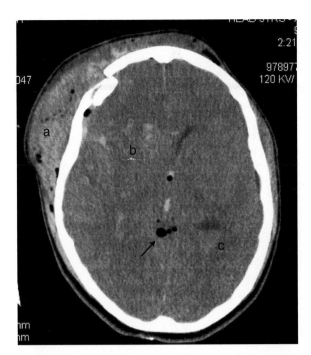

Figure 52.1 Computed tomography (CT) scan of an adolescent with severe traumatic brain injury. Depressed fracture of right frontal bone, with overlying subgaleal hematoma (*a*). Contusion with intraparenchymal hemorrhage in right hemisphere (*b*) with mass effect (midline shift to left, obliteration of right lateral ventricle). Layering of blood in occipital horn of left lateral ventricle (*c*). Air (*black arrow*) is present in numerous locations.

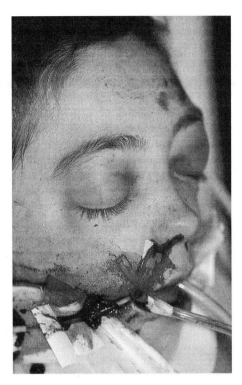

Figure 52.2 "Raccoon eyes" secondary to severe closed head injury with basilar skull fracture. (From Fleisher GR. *Atlas of emergency medicine.* Philadelphia, PA: Lippincott Williams & Wilkins; 2004:388.) (See color Figure 52.2.)

into the opposite direction toward the cranium (*contre coup* contusions). Contusions to the cortex are the most common, with frontal and occipital regions predominating.

Shear injury to the white matter occurs when forces applied to the skull result in disruption of the long white matter tracts that connect different regions of the brain or connect the brain to the peripheral nervous system through the spinal cord. Several descriptive terms have been used including "inner cerebral trauma," "diffuse degeneration of the white matter," and most recently, "diffuse axonal injury (DAI)." DAI occurs in >50% of severe TBI and is associated with an increased risk of intracranial hypertension in the delayed periods. The main histologic feature of DAI is disruption of axons and white matter tracts seen microscopically.

Extra-axial collections of blood can occur in any of the potential spaces within the brain or spinal cord. Epidural hematomas are caused by injury of penetrating arteries resulting in blood collecting in the extradural space (see Fig. 52.3). This collection can cause compression of the normal brain adjacent to the injury and can lead to rapid onset of symptoms including coma and herniation. Subdural hematomas are always associated with lacerations of the brain parenchyma. Blood collects from injuries to bridging veins resulting in a space-occupying lesion between the dura and the brain surface. Subdural hematomas carry a poorer prognosis than epidural hematomas because of the

damage to the underlying brain. Subarachnoid hemorrhage results from bleeding into the subarachnoid space. Ordinarily, the amount of blood within the subarachnoid space is relatively small and does not lead to significant changes on cerebral compliance. However, in adults, subarachnoid hemorrhage is associated with an increased risk of delayed vasospasm and stroke. It is unclear if this association exists in children.

SECONDARY INJURIES

The current dogma suggests that when primary injuries are not avoided, minimization of secondary injuries is the therapeutic goal to maximize patient outcomes. Some of the known secondary injuries believed to adversely affect outcomes are intracranial hypotension, hypoxia, and hyperthermia. These factors are common to both brain and spinal cord trauma. Abrupt movement of the spine is a potential cause for secondary injury after spinal cord trauma injury and is associated with unstable spinous elements.

Intracranial Hypertension

Contused cortex and abnormal collections of blood within the cranium can grow in size and alter the homeostasis of the pressure-to-volume relationship within the

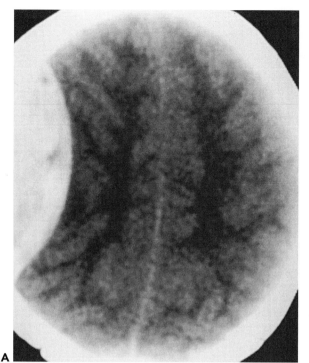 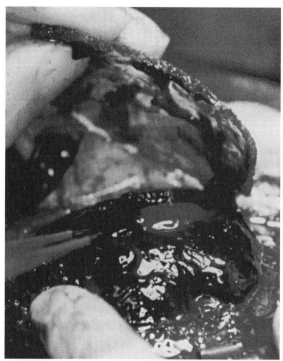

Figure 52.3 Epidural hematoma. This 8-year-old boy presented after a sledding accident. He had no loss of consciousness but complained of headache and vomiting. **A:** A computed tomography scan of the head shows the classic biconvex hyperdensity of an epidural hematoma. He proceeded to the operating room where a large mass of clotted blood **(B)** was removed. (From Fleisher GR. *Atlas of emergency medicine.* Philadelphia, PA: Lippincott Williams & Wilkins; 2004:391.)

brain (see Chapter 7). Specifically, as the masses enlarge, compensatory mechanisms are sequentially activated including increased absorption of cerebrospinal fluid (CSF), displacement of CSF into the spinal canal, and decreased cerebral blood volume in the venous system. Once these mechanisms are exhausted, further increases in cranial volume leads to increased pressure within the cranial vault (intracranial hypertension) until the pressure rises to such an extent to decrease the arterial blood volume in the brain. This leads to cerebral infarction and herniation syndromes.

In addition to simply predicting herniation events, it became clear that intracranial hypertension was itself a secondary injury. In the early 1990s, several groups demonstrated that adults who developed intracranial hypertension (intracranial pressure [ICP] >20 or 25 mm Hg depending on the study) had poor outcomes. Both, the number of incidents of intracranial hypertension and the degree of intracranial hypertension, seemed to have predictive power. Today, competing hypotheses involve the limitation of intracranial hypertension and the augmentation of cerebral perfusion pressure (CPP). As mentioned earlier in this text, CPP is equal to the difference between mean arterial pressure (MAP) and ICP. Competing strategies have emerged to either maintain CPP above an arbitrary limit (70 mm Hg in adults and 60 mm Hg in children) or ICP below the arbitrary limit of 20 mm Hg.

Currently, the published guidelines consider both these thresholds as recommendations but not standards.

There are many therapeutic strategies that can be employed to either raise CPP or lower ICP (see Table 52.1). Choice of individual strategies can vary among institutions and among investigators. In general, selection of therapies (such as CSF drainage, mannitol, and hypertonic saline) with the most favorable risk-to-benefit ratios are initiated more routinely than others (hyperventilation, barbiturate coma, decompressive craniectomy). In severe cases, patients will require many (if not most) of these strategies to prevent herniation and minimize instances of intracranial hypertension or decreased CPP.

Recently, CPP-directed management recommended by the Brain Trauma Foundation has been questioned from investigators in Europe. The Lund protocol (named for Lund University Hospital in Sweden) asserts that intracranial hypertension can be most effectively managed by decreasing the cerebral blood volume rather than maintaining an arbitrary CPP. As the blood–brain barrier loses its volume-regulating ability after trauma, increases in MAP (and CPP) will cause a net filtering of fluid from the vascular compartment into the brain itself. This shift will lead to increased swelling and decreased cerebral compliance. As an alternative, the Lund protocol recommends maintaining plasma oncotic pressure, using antihypertensive

TABLE 52.1

CONVENTIONAL STRATEGIES TO LOWER INTRACRANIAL PRESSURE OR RAISE CEREBRAL PERFUSION PRESSURE AFTER TRAUMATIC BRAIN INJURY

	Proposed Mechanism	Potential Deleterious Side Effect(s)
Therapeutic Goal: Lower ICP		
Mannitol	a. Immediate: changes in blood viscosity leading to decreased cerebral blood volume b. Prolonged (h): increasing serum osmolarity leads to net water flow from within the brain into serum	a. Hypotension if inadequate fluid resuscitation b. Case reports of renal failure with serum osmolarity >320 OSM
Hypertonic saline (NaCl)	Increase in serum osmolarity leads to net water flow from within the brain into serum	Renal failure not reported yet, limited experience at extreme concentrations of serum Na
Hyperventilation	Decrease in cerebral blood volume as a function of decreased cerebral blood flow	Areas of brain that are hypoperfused may experience worsened ischemia and potential infarction
Cerebrospinal fluid drainage	Decrease CSF volume in the cranium, thereby restoring volume–pressure relationship within the cranial vault	Requires ventriculostomy-based ICP monitor; may be technically challenging if swelling is pronounced
Sedation/muscle paralysis	Decreased cerebral blood flow by decreasing cerebral metabolism; ultimately affecting cerebral blood volume	Short-term: effects of narcotics on cerebral compliance Long-term: withdrawal from narcotics, chronic weakness/myopathy from paralytics
Pharmacologic coma (barbiturates, propofol, benzodiazepine, or others)	Dramatically decrease cerebral blood flow by decreasing cerebral metabolism; ultimately affecting cerebral blood volume	Hemodynamic instability, direct myocardial depressants, shock, and cardiovascular collapse
Induced hypothermia	Decreased temperature will lower cerebral metabolism, leading to decreases in cerebral blood flow and cerebral blood volume	Potential for cardiac dysrhythmias, coagulation disturbances
Therapeutic Goal: Raise CPP		
Fluid resuscitation with hypertonic solutions	Increasing preload, improving cardiac performance and MAP, ultimately leading to increase in CPP	Risk of pulmonary edema, fluid overload, increased risk of pneumonia
Institution of vasopressors (agonists—dopamine, norepinephrine, phenylephrine; epinephrine; vasopressin)	Increasing contractility and afterload to improve cardiac performance, leading to increase in MAP and CPP	Effect of vasopressors in injured brain unknown
Induced hypertension	By increasing MAP greater than normal, areas of brain with intact autoregulation will experience vasoconstriction; the sum of this vasoconstriction will allow more potential space for swelling to occur without concomitant rise in ICP	In areas without intact autoregulation, cerebral blood flow will be passive leading to increases in cerebral blood volume (thereby leading to increased ICP and decreased CPP)
Decompressive craniectomy	Removal of skull will allow brain to herniate outward, improving perfusion to the area of brain at risk	Ischemia around edges of bone due to compression; increased risk for infection; long-term data limited

ICP, intracranial pressure; CPP, cerebral perfusion pressure; CSF, cerebrospinal fluid; MAP, mean airway pressure, hours.

therapies to limit capillary leak and reducing CPP to approximately 60 mm Hg for adults and 40 to 50 mm Hg for children. This approach resulted in good outcomes in Sweden. However, its replicability in other adult centers or in significant numbers of children after TBI has not been established.

Hypotension and Hypoxia

Hypotension and hypoxia have been associated with adverse clinical outcome in a number of clinical studies. It has been hypothesized that imposing the additional stress of either limited perfusion or limited oxygen delivery to injured regions causes potentially viable cells to die, thereby extending the injury. This "penumbra" is more clearly defined in response to cerebral infarction (see Chapter 45) but likely exists in traumatic contusions as well. As MAP reaches a critically low level (thought to be approximately 50 mm Hg in adults), cerebral blood flow decreases linearly. At this extreme portion of the cerebral autoregulation curve, cerebral arterioles are maximally dilated. The relationship between hypoxia and cerebral blood flow is more complex. Although it is clear that isolated arterioles vasodilate in response to hypoxia in *ex vivo* preparations, the clinical parameter most indicative of this effect in humans is still unclear. PaO_2, oxygen delivery, and oxygen carrying capacity thresholds have been proposed without universal acceptance.

Dozens of clinical studies have shown that the most extreme version of hypoxia and hypotension, traumatic cardiac arrest, results in meaningful survival in <5% of children and adults. In the aforementioned data from the TCDB, the group with the greatest amount of documented hypotension (0 to 4 years) had the worst clinical outcome. Other groups have demonstrated in adults that every episode of hypotension and hypoxia decreases the chances of good neurologic outcome.

Hyperthermia

Although the routine use of hypothermia has not proven to be effective in improving overall outcome (see Chapter 7), the deleterious effects of hyperthermia are clear. Increase in body temperature is associated with increase in cerebral metabolism. This increase in cerebral metabolic demand can lead to two untenable conditions: (i) Early after injury, cerebral blood flow may be inadequate for tissue needs at a baseline. When additional metabolic demands cannot be met with increased blood flow, infarction of penumbral regions begins. (ii) When cerebral blood flow *can* be increased to meet metabolic demand, increase in blood flow will be associated with increase in cerebral blood volume and ultimately intracranial hypertension.

In either instance, cerebral hemodynamic function is disturbed by hyperthermia, effects that could be minimized by adequate temperature control. Importantly, it should be remembered that brain temperature is greater than body temperature in general (between 0.5°C and 2°C).

Unstable Spinal Cord Injuries

The spinal cord snugly fits into the spinal canal because of simultaneous bone and cord growth during development. Figure 52.4 displays the normal relation of the bony structures of the cervical spine. Forces applied either to the head or the torso can damage spinal ligaments or bony processes in close proximity to either somatic nerves or the spinal cord itself. During stabilization and treatment, bony fragments can damage the cord and ruptured ligaments may impair the blood supply to the cord if a patient is moved

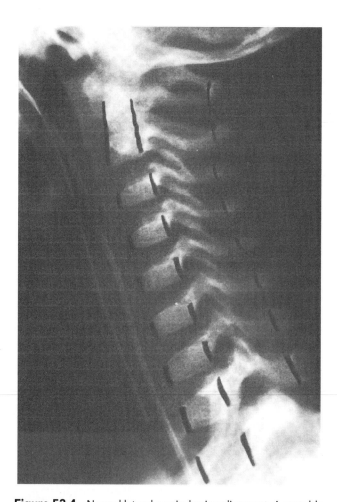

Figure 52.4 Normal lateral cervical spine alignment. A portable lateral cervical spine radiograph obtained in the emergency department on an injured child must show all seven cervical vertebra and the cervicothoracic junction. Three curvilinear lines are followed in assessing alignment. These are, from anterior to posterior, the anterior body line, the posterior body line, and the laminar junction line (each marked on the radiograph with a wax pencil). (From Rogers MC. *Textbook of pediatric intensive care.* 3rd ed. Philadelphia, PA: Lippincott Williams & Wilkins; 1996.)

with an unstable spinal fracture. Because of this, a high index of suspicion should be maintained for occult spinal cord instability until definitive testing can be obtained.

MANAGEMENT OF BRAIN AND SPINAL TRAUMA

Initial Stabilization

The initial management of the child having brain and spinal cord trauma is identical to the management of all critically ill children. Assessment of the adequacy and patency of the airway is the first priority. Consideration should be made for children with neck trauma for two independent reasons. First, occult fractures should be assumed, in most cases, and cervical spine immobilization should be maintained.

Additionally, the potential for airway fractures or edema that may manifest as swelling of glottic and supraglottic structures must be assessed. Pre-emptive intubation should be performed if the risk of swelling is significant. Adequacy of breathing and air movement should be assessed, with special considerations for possible traumatic injuries to the chest cage (pneumothorax, flail chest). Cardiovascular function should be examined with considerations of potential blood loss from other traumatic injuries, cardiac contusions from blunt chest trauma, and shock from generalized hypovolemia.

Neurologic assessment using the Glasgow Coma Scale (GCS) score is a rapid and reliable method for assessing levels of consciousness (described in detail in Chapter 7). Published guidelines suggest that patients with GCS scores <8 have a high risk of intracerebral injury and would benefit from early endotracheal intubation. Additionally, a decrease in the level of consciousness (GCS decreases by more than three points) is another indication for endotracheal intubation to maintain oxygenation and acid–base balance. Once initial stabilization is completed, a full neurologic examination should be performed to determine all potential injuries. These findings should be confirmed by appropriate neuroimaging studies to determine if any surgical intervention is indicated.

Intensive Care Management

Once initial stabilization and operative interventions are completed, standard critical care to monitor for complications related to head injuries are required. As mentioned earlier, intracranial hypertension can develop as brain swelling worsens and compensatory mechanisms are overcome. ICP monitoring should be instituted when intracranial hypertension is likely based on (i) abnormal level of consciousness without other sufficient justification (i.e., medications), (ii) abnormal neurologic examination, (iii) abnormal computed tomography (CT) scan, and (iv) the discretion of the neurosurgeon. In anticipation of instituting therapies for intracranial hypertension, invasive hemodynamic monitors (arterial catheters, central venous pressure catheters, pulmonary artery catheters) should be considered. Therapies mitigating intracranial hypertension (Table 52.1) should be instituted according to the experience of the clinical team. Prophylaxis for seizures and appropriate electrophysiologic monitoring should be performed.

Pharmacologic therapies for spinal cord injury are currently more advanced than for brain injuries. Although no pharmacologic agents have proven beneficial in brain trauma, several studies have demonstrated that high-dose methylprednisolone therapy for spinal cord injury improves recovery of function in adults. This practice has been adopted by some for the care of injured children because serious complications have not been observed in large adult series. The exact mechanism of action of the steroids is unclear, but hypotheses implicating a decrease in the inflammatory response, decreased scar formation, and reduced free radical release have been postulated.

The other systems of the body can have profound effects on neurologic outcome of patients with brain and spinal cord trauma. There are many aspects of ventilator management that alter cerebral hemodynamic parameters and potentially, neurologic outcome. As mentioned earlier, alterations of arterial pH and Pco_2 have direct effects on cerebral blood flow, and prevention of hypoxia is an important goal to avoid secondary injuries. Maintaining these parameters at the lowest possible intrathoracic pressure will diminish resistance to venous drainage of the brain leading to improvement in intracranial compliance. Strategies to avoid ventilator-associated pneumonia may have particular benefit to patients with brain injuries, because the hyperthermic inflammatory response to infection may be deleterious to injured neurons and glia.

The cardiovascular system can be affected by neurologic injuries as well as the therapies used to treat these problems. Injury to the cervical spinal cord can cause spinal shock, a condition with decreased endogenous catecholamine production marked by hypotension due to decreased vasomotor tone and contractility. Conversely, massive injury to brain structures or prolonged seizures can result in increased catecholamine release and concomitant decrements in cardiovascular function because of increased afterload. Therapies such as mannitol and barbiturates can have effects on preload and global cardiac performance, respectively. Because of the fragility of the cardiovascular system, rigorous hemodynamic monitoring should be maintained to anticipate periods of instability.

Traumatically injured children are at risk for nutritional deficiencies. Energy expenditure can increase up to 80% greater than basal needs for isolated head injury alone. Because of this dramatic increase in energy requirements, current guidelines suggest a goal of 130% to 160% of resting metabolic expenditure beginning by 72 hours after injury and reaching full replacement by 7 days. Glucose metabolism can be affected by multiple processes in the traumatically injured child. High-dose steroids and diabetes insipidus (DI) (because of hypothalamic dysfunction) can lead to hyperglycemia. Since hyperglycemia has been associated with poor outcome in adults, maintaining euglycemia appears to be the most rationale strategy at this time. Sodium and water balance can be altered both by trauma and by therapeutic interventions. Hyponatremia may result from the syndrome of inappropriate secretion of antidiuretic hormone (SIADH) or cerebral salt wasting, whereas hypernatremia may arise from DI or because of hypertonic saline administration.

The hematologic system can be affected by traumatic injury in several ways. The brain contains a high concentration of tissue factor. When the brain is lacerated or the parenchyma is exposed to the bloodstream, activation of coagulation cascades can result, leading to consumption coagulopathy. This coagulopathy can potentially exacerbate bleeding within hematomas or in extracranial sites of bleeding. Traumatically injured children are at risk for acute anemia from blood loss suffered at the time of the injury. There are no published recommendations regarding a target hematocrit for either adults or pediatric patients following CNS trauma. However, given that oxygen delivery is determined in large part by hematocrit, the risks and benefits of red cell transfusions need to be considered, with most clinicians keeping the hematocrit close to 30%. The incidence of deep vein thromboses is increased in children with both TBI and spinal cord injury, particularly those who are postpubertal. Pneumatic stocking placement carries little risk and can prevent these potentially life-threatening complications.

TRAUMA RESEARCH AND FUTURE DIRECTIONS

Improvements in clinical outcome of children after traumatic brain or spinal cord injury can produce lifelong benefits to children. Most of the clinical trials in trauma research have been conducted in adults. Yet the results of these trials may have some relevance to childhood injury because adult trauma victims tend to be of relatively young age. Of the clinical trials, mitigating excitotoxic injury, modulating the immune response, and testing the neuroprotective effects of hypothermia have been tested most comprehensively and these will be summarized in the subsequent text.

Excitatory amino acids, such as glutamate, are released after a variety of injuries to the brain including trauma. Glutamate release increases cerebral metabolic needs by two mechanisms: (i) binding of glutamate to its receptor causes increased neuronal firing and activity and (ii) glutamate release in the synaptic cleft must be reabsorbed by glial cells in an energy-consuming process. It is theorized that injured brain cannot compensate for this increased metabolic requirement in the acute stages of injury. Preclinical studies of glutamate antagonists showed reduction of neuronal cell loss and improved neurologic outcome after trauma in several species. In humans, the most commonly used glutamate antagonist in preclinical trials, MK-801, was found to have unacceptable neuropsychiatric side effects. Therefore, other glutamate antagonists, namely, solfotel, cerestat, and CP 101 to 606 were used. Over 400 patients were enrolled in a phase II trial with CP 101 to 606 without observing significant clinical improvement over placebo, despite the ability of the drug to be concentrated within brain tissue (brain concentrations more than four times the serum concentration). This pattern is common to all of the glutamate antagonists and has been a major disappointment in translating animal data to adults after trauma. This excitotoxic response appears to be more vigorous in immature animal models of injury and therefore, strategies antagonizing glutamate may be more effective in treating traumatic injuries in children compared to adults. Studies targeting this mechanism may hold promise for treating such children.

Inflammation plays an important role in brain and spinal cord trauma. The inflammatory response is believed to contribute to toxicity of neurons and glia and a variety of agents were used to modulate this response. Initially, high-dose corticosteroids were postulated to be beneficial for their ability to decrease edema from cranial tumors and established their efficacy in preclinical testing. After multiple, well-controlled trials, corticosteroids did not show substantial benefit and were implicated in worsening the outcome. Tirilazad, an aminosteroid, was tested in over 1,700 patients after TBI, and a clear benefit for all subgroups could not be determined. However, patients with intracerebral hematomas and those with lowest GCS scores seemed to show improvement with Tirilazad compared to placebo. It is possible that the beneficial effects of immune suppression of the inflammatory response is outweighed by the increased risk of secondary complications (hospital acquired pneumonia, sepsis, and others) of these powerful agents. In lieu of these studies, more focused modulation of the immune response may be successful in diminishing the neurotoxic effects without incurring these side effects.

Hypothermia has had a long history of use and disuse after TBI. As described in Chapter 7 (Neuroscience of Critical Care), hypothermia is thought to decrease the metabolic activity of the brain in times of decreased blood flow, thereby minimizing damage. Hypothermia may also have effects on the various enzymatic reactions in these cells, because these reactions are temperature dependent. Regardless, it is clear that a main advantage of hypothermia is that it acts on a wide variety of harmful cascades simultaneously. A single-center trial of hypothermia showed significant benefit at 3 and 6 months as measured by the Glasgow Outcome Scale score. Clifton's multicenter randomized, controlled trial failed to confirm this beneficial effect. Proponents of hypothermia point out that a single center in this trial had much greater fluid resuscitation volumes in patients with hypothermia compared to patients with hypothermia in other centers and this increased mortality. However, publication of this trial clearly has dampened the enthusiasm for hypothermia as a standard therapy. Children may tolerate hypothermia better due to fewer comorbid conditions (relatively minimal incidence of atherosclerotic heart disease, stroke, and others) and younger patients were benefited most in the Clifton trial by hypothermia. Recently, a phase II trial of hypothermia in children after TBI was completed showing its safety. Trials to prove its efficacy in children will be needed.

The future of trauma research will be multifaceted. Maximizing the prehospital care of traumatically injured children can decrease the incidence of secondary events at a critical period. Aggressively monitoring children after traumatic injuries (with brain microdialysis, interstitial brain oxygen tension, or other devices discussed in Chapter 7) may detect occult disorders prior to permanent injury. Refinement of established treatment paradigms might lead to improvements in clinical outcome. Development of novel pharmacologic agents to alter the brain or spinal cord milieu after trauma is an ongoing process and may lead to significant advances in the future. And lastly, testing these hypotheses in children seems the most effective way to determine their clinical efficacy in this vulnerable patient population.

RECOMMENDED READINGS

1. Adelson PD, Bratton SL, Carney NA, et al. Guidelines for the acute medical management of severe traumatic brain injury in infants, children and adolescents. *Pediatr Crit Care Med.* 2003;4(Suppl 3):S1–S75.
2. Bracken MB, Shephard MJ, Collins WF, et al. Administration of methylprednisolone for 24 or 48 hours or tirilazad mesylate for 48 hours in treatment of acute spinal cord injury. *JAMA.* 1997;277:1597–1604.
3. Dias MS. Traumatic brain and spinal cord injury. *Pediatr Clin North Am.* 2004;51:271–303.
4. Frewen TC, Sumabat WO, Del Maestro RF, Cerebral blood flow, metabolic rate and cross-brain oxygen consumption in brain injury. *J Pediatrics.* 1985;107:510–513.
5. Gupta AK, Al-Rawi PG, Hutchinson PJ, et al. Effect of hypothermia on brain tissue oxygenation in patients with severe head injury. *Br J Anaesth.* 2002;88:188–192.
6. Hlatky R, Valadka AB, Goodman JC, et al. Patterns of energy substrates during ischemia measured in brain by microdialysis. *J Neurotrauma.* 2004;21:894–906.
7. Imberati R, Bellinzona G, Langer M. Cerebral tissue PO2 and SjvO2 changes during moderate hyperventilation in patients with severe traumatic brain injury. *J Neurosurg.* 2002;96:97–102.
8. Muizelaar JP, Marmarou A, De Salles AA, et al. Cerebral blood flow and metabolism in severely head-injured children. *J Neurosurg.* 1989;71:63–71.
9. Narayan RK, Michel M, Ansel B, et al. Clinical trials in head injury. *J Neurotrauma.* 2002;19:503–557.
10. Grande PO. The 'Lund Concept' for treatment of severe brain trauma: A physiological approach. In: Vincent J-L, ed. *Yearbook of intensive care and emergency medicine.* Berlin, Germany: Springer-Verlag; 2004:806–820.
11. Raghupathi R. Cell death mechanisms following traumatic brain injury. *Brain Pathol.* 2004;14:215–222.

Sedation for Procedures and Mechanical Ventilation in Children with Critical Illness

53

Yewande J. Johnson   *Julia C. Finkel*

The goals of providing sedation and analgesia in the pediatric intensive care unit (PICU) include alleviating pain, ensuring patient safety, managing of opioid induced tolerance, and preventing hyperalgesia. Monitoring sedation along with the judicial use of anxiolytics, analgesics, *N*-methyl-D-aspartate (NMDA) antagonists, α_2-adrenoreceptor agonists, and other pharmacologic adjuncts are essential in providing a multimodal regimen. This chapter discusses strategies to achieve these goals as well as approaches for an effective postoperative analgesia for the critically ill child.

MONITORING CONTINUOUS SEDATION

Adequate sedation is necessary to provide patient comfort, to prevent ventilator asynchrony and self-extubation, to protect vascular access, and to facilitate recovery during critical illness. However, oversedation may have deleterious side effects such as exacerbating hemodynamic instability and promoting tolerance. In order to titrate anxiolytics and analgesics to individual patient needs, sedation scores should be utilized. Sedation scales used in pediatric populations include modified Ramsay Sedation Scale, COMFORT, and Motor Activity Assessment Scale (see Table 53.1). The COMFORT Scale is the most comprehensively validated scale, using eight physiologic and behavioral variables. Sedative infusions should be titrated to achieve specific sedation score levels based on clinical condition. Additional sedative boluses given should be given as needed for stimulating activities and procedural sedation.

SEDATIVE AGENTS

Benzodiazepines

Benzodiazepines are the most frequently used sedatives in the pediatric intensive care setting. All benzodiazepines have the property of causing hypoventilation when combined with an opioid or other sedating agents. Caution should be taken when administering benzodiazepines to spontaneously ventilating patients and to neonates. Diazepam, lorazepam, and midazolam are the three most commonly used benzodiazepines available in intravenous formulations.

Midazolam

Unlike diazepam and lorazepam, midazolam is water soluble, which permits absorption after intranasal, rectal, and intramuscular administration. Such an option for midazolam administration is useful in infants and children who lack intravenous access, yet require minimal sedation, or for acute treatment of active seizures. Given as a bolus of 0.05 to 0.1 mg per kg IV, midazolam has a rapid onset (1 to 2 minutes) and short duration of action (1 to 4 hours). Intravenous infusions may be started at 0.05 mg/kg/hour incrementally increasing to adequate levels of sedation.

TABLE 53.1

SCALES USED TO MEASURE SEDATION AND AGITATION

Motor Activity Assessment Scale: Sedation Goal = 2–3

Dangerously agitated	6
Agitated	5
Restless and cooperative	4
Calm and cooperative	3
Responsive to touch or name	2
Responsive only to noxious	1

Ramsay Sedation Scale: Sedation Goal = 4

Anxious, agitated, and/or restless	1
Cooperative, oriented, and tranquil	2
Responds to command only	3
Brisk response to light glabellar tap or loud auditory stimulus	4
Sluggish response to light glabellar tap or loud auditory stimulus	5
No response to light glabellar tap or loud auditory stimulus	6

COMFORT Scale

Alertness

Deeply asleep	1
Lightly asleep	2
Drowsy	3
Fully awake and alert	4
Hyperalert	5

Calmness/agitation

Calm	1
Slightly anxious	2
Anxious	3
Very anxious	4
Panicky	5

Heart rate

Heart rate below baseline	1
Heart rate consistently at baseline	2
Infrequent elevations of 15% or more above baseline (1–3 during observation period)	3
Frequent elevations of 15% or more above baseline (more than three during observation period)	4
Sustained elevation of 15% or more	5

Facial tension

Facial muscles totally relaxed	1
Facial muscle tone normal, no facial muscle tension evident	2
Tension evident in some facial muscles	3
Tension evident throughout facial muscles	4
Facial muscles contorted and grimacing	5

Mean arterial blood pressure

Blood pressure below baseline	1
Blood pressure consistently at baseline	2
Infrequent elevations of 15% or more above baseline (1–3 during observation period)	3
Frequent elevations of 15% or more above baseline (more than 3 during observation period)	4
Sustained elevation of 15% or more	5

(continued)

Respiratory response

No coughing and no spontaneous respiration	1
Spontaneous respiration with little or no response to ventilation	2
Occasional cough or resistance to ventilator	3
Actively breaths against ventilator	4
Coughs or regularly fights ventilator, coughing, or choking	5

Muscle tone

Muscle totally relaxed, no muscle tone	1
Reduced muscle tone	2
Normal muscle tone	3
Increased muscle tone and flexion of fingers and toes	4
Extreme muscle rigidity	5

Physical movement

No movement	1
Occasional, slight movement	2
Frequent, slight movements	3
Vigorous movements limited to extremities	4
Vigorous movements including torso and head	5

Metabolism of midazolam is through the cytochrome P-450 CYP3A with excretion by the kidney. This cytochrome isoform reaches adult levels between 3 to 12 months of age. The pharmacokinetics of midazolam may be unpredictable in hepatic or renal failure. Drugs that are metabolized through the same pathway (e.g., fentanyl, erythromycin, calcium channel blockers) may decrease the hepatic clearance of midazolam and therefore intensify its effects.

Lorazepam

Lorazepam has a relatively slow onset of action (5 to 15 minutes). Bolus dosing of 0.02 to 0.06 mg per kg IV has a duration of action from 2 to 6 hours. Usual infusion dosing of lorazepam ranges from 0.01 to 0.1 mg/kg/hour. Hyperosmolarity and anion gap acidosis has been observed with continuous infusions of lorazepam secondary to its preservative propylene glycol. This preservative in toxic quantities may also lead to renal dysfunction, cardiac arrhythmias, seizures, intravascular hemolysis, and central nervous system (CNS) depression. Toxicity due to propylene glycol should be considered if the patient is experiencing an unexplained metabolic acidosis, high anion gap (>15), and elevated osmolal gap (>10 mOsm per L).

Diazepam

The pharmacologic properties of diazepam discourages its use as a long-term sedative in the intensive care unit (ICU). For example, the hydrophobic nature of diazepam leads to precipitation when added to intravenous fluids, thereby precluding administration by continuous infusion. However, diazepam may be useful as a bolus agent. Diazepam bolus dose ranges from 0.03 to 0.1 mg per kg IV and has an onset of action in 1 to 2 minutes. The sedative effects last 6 to 12 hours with an elimination half-life of up to 37 hours.

Diazepam's active metabolite, desmethyldiazepam, is slowly metabolized and may cause oversedation with repeated dosing. On the other hand, this prolonged activity can provide therapeutic benefits in select patients such as children who require background anxiolysis.

Barbiturates

The use of barbiturates in the intensive care setting is generally limited to bolus administration as a sedative for intubation, as an infusion to induce coma for refractory status epilepticus, or the treatment of increased intracranial pressure (ICP). The risks of long-term barbiturate infusion, including depression of cardiac contractility myocardial depression and immunosuppression must be weighed against their benefits.

Thiopental

In the ICU, thiopental is most frequently used for rapid sequence intubation. A dose of 3 to 5 mg per kg is taken up by the brain in less than a minute. Rapid redistribution after a single dose accounts for rapid termination of its affects. Peripheral venodilation produces a transient decrease in blood pressure. This is compensated by an increase in heart rate. In patients with poor cardiac function, hypotension, and/or hypovolemia, thiopental should be used cautiously.

Chloral Hydrate

Chloral hydrate has been a popular drug for procedural sedation in children. It is not recommended for continuous ICU sedation because of the potential toxicities of repetitive dosing. Chloral hydrate's metabolites, trichloroethanol and trichloroacetic acid, are both pharmacologically active. The half-lives of these metabolites are over 10 hours in preschool-aged children and may last over 40 hours in premature neonates, causing prolonged sedation. The accumulation of high concentrations of trichloroacetic acid may lead to metabolic acidosis and renal failure. In neonates, chloral hydrate and its metabolites interfere with the binding of bilirubin to albumin leading to hyperbilirubinemia.

Ketamine

The NMDA antagonist ketamine has the desirable properties of providing sedation and analgesia without causing hypoventilation. Doses of 0.5 to 2 mg per kg IV can be used to provide 20 to 60 minutes of sedation for procedures. Infusions of ultralow dose ketamine at 0.1 to 0.2 mg/kg/hour may also prevent tolerance by its NMDA antagonist properties. Analgesia is accomplished at significantly higher doses secondary to noradrenergic mechanisms (reviewed in Chapter 8). The drug can also attenuate withdrawal symptoms. In addition, ketamine is the only agent proven to reverse the hyperalgesic state. Metabolism of ketamine is through the cytochrome P-450 system with the active metabolite norketamine being formed. Norketamine is one third to one fifth as potent as ketamine. Because ketamine is a potent cerebral vasodilator, patients with intracranial disease processes may be vulnerable to increased ICP with bolus administration. Ketamine provides central sympathetic stimulation that may result in increased systemic and pulmonary arterial pressures, heart rate, and cardiac output. It also has direct negative cardiac inotropic effects; however, this is usually not seen secondary to the dominant central sympathetic activity except in patients who are catecholamine depleted, such as those with chronic heart failure. Furthermore, the ketamine molecule is structurally similar to phencyclidine, which may account for the reports of visual, auditory, and tactile illusions associated with its use. These illusions may be prevented with the concomitant use of benzodiazepines.

Dexmedetomidine

The α_2-adrenergic agonist dexmedetomidine provides sedation, amnesia, and analgesia with minimal effects on ventilation. Because it is eight times more selective for the α_2-receptor than clonidine, it allows for a greater degree of hemodynamic stability in the critically ill patient. Although systematic clinical trials are still needed to determine the safety of dexmedetomidine in the pediatric population, preliminary studies have demonstrated its efficacy in a variety of clinical settings. Dexmedetomidine has been used without adverse side effects to provide sedation for mechanical ventilation as well for procedural sedation. The drug has also been used in the intensive care setting as part of a rapid benzodiazepine and opioid weaning regimen. Dexmedetomidine also has been shown to reduce postoperative opioid requirements by 66%. The short redistribution half-life of 6 minutes necessitates administration by infusion. A loading dose of 1 μg per kg should be given slowly (over 10 to 15 minutes) to prevent the transient hypertension that may occur secondary to higher doses acting as agonists at peripheral α_2-receptors. The recommended maintenance dosing range is 0.2 to 0.7 μg/kg/hour IV. The most common side effects are hypotension and bradycardia induced by vagal stimulation. Relative contraindications include preexisting severe bradycardia, atrioventricular (AV) conduction disorders, reduced ejection fraction (<30%), hypotension, and hypovolemia. Biotransformation occurs in the liver into three inactive metabolites through cytochrome P-450 CYP2A6. Excretion is primarily through the urine. It remains unknown whether patients become tolerant to dexmedetomidine.

MONITORING ANALGESIA

Agitation in the ICU may be a manifestation of inadequately controlled pain. Inadequate analgesia will cause physiologic stress to the patient, potentially raising metabolic rate and oxygen requirements. In addition to providing pain relief, analgesics are also adjuncts for sedation in the mechanically ventilated patient. Monitoring analgesia in the critically ill pediatric patient is often difficult because they may be preverbal, unable to communicate secondary to nature of illness or concomitant use of sedatives, or receiving neuromuscular blockade. For patients who are not sedated or mechanically ventilated, traditional pediatric pain scales such as FACES, VAS (Visual Analog Scale), FLACC (Faces-Legs-Activity-Cry-Consolable), OPS (Objective Pain Scale) may be appropriate. For most intensive care patients, a pain scoring system that is based on physiologic and behavioral indicators must be used. The Cardiac Analgesic Assessment Scale (CAAS) is such a scale, and has been validated for postoperative pediatric cardiac patients.

Daily interruption of sedative and analgesic drug infusions appears to provide benefits to the critically ill adult patient. These "wake up tests" decrease both the amount of time spent on the ventilator and the length of stay in the ICU. In addition, physical examination during the awake period provides an opportunity to detect changes in neurologic status that would be otherwise masked during periods of deeper sedation. However, reducing administration of sedative to allow a ventilated infant or child to "wake up" poses risks to the security of monitoring lines and the endotracheal tube, which are more difficult to manage than in adults. Nonetheless, if patient safety can be assured, such periods of lowered sedative administration will likely reduce the risk of oversedation that lengthens the time on the ventilator and length of stay in the PICU.

ANALGESIC AGENTS

Opioids

Opioids are the most commonly used analgesics in mechanically ventilated patients. As observed with the use of benzodiazepines, opioids may cause hypoventilation, particularly when used in combination with other sedatives, in neonates and infants. On the other hand, opiate receptor antagonists, such as naloxone, rapidly reverse opiate-induced hypoventilation, and should be available anytime opiates are administered as an analgesic in the critical care setting.

Morphine

Morphine is considered to be the prototype opioid analgesic. A dose of 0.01 to 0.15 mg per kg administered IV has a peak effect within 15 to 30 minutes. The half-life of morphine ranges from 3 to 7 hours. The usual intravenous infusion range is 0.07 to 0.5 mg/kg/hour. For procedural and breakthrough analgesia, the recommended dose is 0.01 to 0.15 mg per kg. Morphine decreases sympathetic nervous system tone in peripheral veins and may

also decrease systemic blood pressure by causing bradycardia and histamine release. To minimize the hypotension caused by morphine administration, volume status must be optimized and the drug administered slowly if given by bolus. The metabolism of morphine occurs primarily through glucuronidation in the liver and kidneys. The primary metabolite (accounting for 75% to 85% of morphine metabolism), morphine-3-glucuronide, is known to have excitotoxic effects. This metabolite, not the parent compound, is most likely responsible for the neuro-excitatory side effects (myoclonus, allodynia, seizures) exhibited in patients receiving morphine. Morphine-6-glucuronide is an active metabolite (accounting for 5% to 10% of morphine metabolism) that has a potency and duration greater than that of its parent compound.

Fentanyl

Fentanyl is a synthetic opioid with a potency 100 times greater than morphine. It is structurally most similar to meperidine. Because of its extreme lipid solubility, its onset of action is faster and has a greater potency than morphine. When given intravenously, fentanyl has an onset of action <30 seconds. Although the half-life ranges from 1.5 to 6 hours, rapid redistribution to skeletal muscle, fat, and other inactive sites accounts for its short duration of action. The usual infusion range is 0.7 to 10 μg/kg/hour. For procedural and breakthrough pain, the recommended dose is 0.35 to 1.5 μg per kg. Chest wall rigidity may be seen with rapid injection of high doses. In contrast to morphine, fentanyl does not cause histamine release. Bradycardia may be seen when given in high doses. Otherwise few cardiovascular side effects are seen with administration. As with other highly potent opioids with high binding affinities (i.e., remifentanil, sufentanil), fentanyl quickly induces tolerance.

Hydromorphone

Hydromorphone is a derivative of morphine with a potency approximately seven times greater. Although its duration of action is slightly shorter than morphine, hydromorphone does not cause histamine release and has no active metabolites. However, an inactive metabolite, hydromorphone-3-glucuronide, is known to have excitotoxic effects manifested by agitation. The usual infusion range is 7 to 15 μg/kg/hour. Doses of 10 to 30 μg per kg IV may be given every 1 to 2 hours for breakthrough pain.

Methadone

Methadone is a synthetic opioid that has a prolonged duration of action (>24 hours). The long half-life accounts for its frequent use in opioid weaning regimens. Its analgesic half-life is considerably shorter (8 to 12 hours). When given as an analgesic, doses of 0.05 to 0.1 mg per kg may be administered every 6 to 8 hours with minimal possibility of prolonged sedation. Methadone may also be used to reverse tolerance to morphine through desensitization of the δ-opioid receptor and through NMDA antagonist properties. The oral bioavailability of 80% to 90% allows for a straightforward conversion between intravenous and oral formulations. Since methadone is the least dialyzable opioid, it is an attractive option for hemodialysis patients.

Techniques to Avoid Opioid Tolerance and to Manage Withdrawal

Iatrogenic opioid tolerance approaches 60% in the neonatal intensive care unit (NICU)/PICU population. The use of adjuvants for those on opioid therapy will lessen the incidence. In patients who are able to receive nonsteroidal anti-inflammatory drugs (NSAIDs), combining opioids with NSAIDs provides opioid sparing secondary to synergism at the potassium channel. As stated in the preceding text, using ketamine in concert with opioids may prevent tolerance by decreasing the need for escalation of opioids. NMDA antagonists may also be used to attenuate withdrawal symptoms. Combining opioids with an ultralow dose of the μ opioid receptor antagonist naloxone 0.1 to 0.5 μg/kg/hour slows the onset of tolerance by blocking the mechanism for supersensitization. Opioid rotational schedules and α_2-adrenergic agonists (clonidine, dexmedetomidine) are also current techniques to avoid opioid tolerance and manage withdrawal. In patients with conditions amenable to neuraxial techniques (e.g., rib fractures), epidural analgesia may be used to avoid IV opioids and induce tolerance.

POSTOPERATIVE PAIN MANAGEMENT

Patients are commonly admitted to the PICU for postoperative care if they have undergone a complex procedure or have significant medical comorbidities. This section will present a multimodal pharmacologic approach to safe and effective acute postoperative pain management in these high-risk infants and children.

Nonopioid Analgesics

Acetaminophen

Long recognized for its ability to relieve mild pain, acetaminophen is a useful adjuvant to opioid therapy in the postoperative period. New higher dosing recommendations for rectal acetaminophen have demonstrated good analgesia with opiate sparing effects at serum acetaminophen concentrations of 10 to 20 μg per mL. Acetaminophen is administered in an initial loading dose of 40 mg per kg per rectum (PR) (often given in the operating room), followed by up to three doses of 20 mg per kg PR every 6 hours.

Nonsteroidal Anti-Inflammatory Drugs

Nonselective NSAIDs are also useful adjuvants to opiate therapy. However, their effects on platelet function and subsequent potential for postoperative bleeding have limited their widespread use in the PICU. With analgesic properties in the absence of inhibition of platelet function, cyclooxygenase-specific inhibitors (cyclooxygenase-2 [COX-2]) have the potential to be useful nonopiate analgesics. Nonetheless, with limited data on the use of COX-2 and the lack of an intravenous formulation available in the United States, these agents have yet to find a place in the postoperative pain management for critically ill infants and children.

Opioid Analgesics

Patient-Controlled Analgesia

Intravenous patient-controlled analgesia (PCA) has provided safe and effective postoperative analgesia for adults for many years. Recently, this analgesic strategy has been successfully extended to adolescents and children as young as 4 years old. Despite the encouraging safety profile, wellknown side effects of opiates can be present in pediatric patients using PCA. Patients with obstructive sleep apnea are at risk for respiratory compromise when using PCA, a particularly relevant consideration as the prevalence of this condition is increasing in children. As mentioned in the preceding text, the addition of acetaminophen or NSAIDs to IV PCA has been shown to decrease opiate requirements and opiate-related adverse effects.

Epidural/Caudal Analgesia

Intraoperatively, epidural anesthesia decreases the need for systemically delivered anesthetics and is mainly used in procedures involving structures below the level of the umbilicus. Similarly, continuation of epidural analgesics in the postoperative period can provide analgesia without potentially detrimental sedative effects of systemic opiates. Results of retrospective studies suggest that pediatric patients who received epidural analgesia after Nissen fundoplication had shorter hospital stays than those receiving systemic opiates. Epidural analgesia can be administered as a continuous infusion or as patient-controlled epidural analgesia.

Despite these benefits, epidural drug delivery has recognizable risks. Bupivacaine, the most common choice for a local anesthetic agent for epidural delivery, can produce convulsions and cardiac arrhythmias when free serum levels are high. Since neonates and infants have immature hepatic metabolism and lower concentrations of serum binding proteins, particularly α_2-acid glycoprotein, they are at increased risk for local anesthetic accumulation and toxicity. Because lidocaine levels are more easily obtained, some centers prefer the use of this agent to bupivacaine, particularly in younger patients. Serious complications of epidural analgesia including infection, permanent neurologic deficit, and respiratory depression, are rare. Newer epidural analgesic strategies combining local anesthetics with opioids, NMDA antagonists, or clonidine may be indicated in patients with impaired hepatic metabolism or those requiring longer-term administration.

Attention to sedation and analgesia is a critical component of care for the infant and child with critical illness. A growing range of pharmacologic agents broadens the approaches for analgesia and sedation in critically ill children who are at particularly high risk for untoward side effects due to their underlying organ immaturity or dysfunction. Proper monitoring is essential to ensure appropriate dosing based on changing clinical status and end-organ function. Multimodal approaches are often indicated for the critically ill child who poses additional challenges for postoperative pain management.

ACKNOWLEDGMENT

Supported in part by grant 1 U10HD045993-02, National Institute of Child Health and Development, Bethesda, MD.

RECOMMENDED READINGS

1. Ambul B, Hamlett KW, Marx CM, et al. Assessing distress in pediatric intensive care environments: The COMFORT scale. *J Pediatr Psychol.* 1992;17(1):95–109.

2. American Academy of Pediatrics, Committee of Drugs, Committee on Environmental Health. Use of chloral hydrate for sedation in children. *Pediatrics.* 1993;92(3):471–473.

3. Anand KJ, Arnold JH. Opioid tolerance and dependence in infants and children. *Crit Care Med.* 1994;22(2):334–342.

4. Crain SM, Shen KF. Antagonists of excitatory opioid receptor functions enhance morphine's analgesic potency and attenuate opioid tolerance/dependence liability. *Pain.* 2000;84(2–3):121–131.

5. Dean M. Opioids in renal failure and dialysis patients. *J Pain Symptom Manage.* 2004;28(5):497–504.

6. DeWildt SN, de Hoog M, Vinks AA, et al. Population pharmacokinetics and metabolism of midazolam in pediatric intensive care patients. *Crit Care Med.* 2003;31(7):1952–1958.

7. Finkel JC, ElRefai A. The use of dexmedetomidine to facilitate opioid and benzodiazepine detoxification in an infant. *Anesth Analg.* 2004;98(6):1658–1659.

8. Hemstatpat K, Monteith GR, Smith D, et al. Morphine-3-glucuronide's neuro-excitatory effects are mediated via indirect activation of N-methyl-D-aspartic acid receptors: Mechanistic studies in embryonic cultured hippocampal neurons. *Anesth Analg.* 2003;97(2):494–505.

9. Luginbuhl M, Gerber A, Schnider TW, et al. Modulation of remifentanil-induced analgesia, hyperalgesia, and tolerance by small-dose ketamine in humans. *Anesth Analg.* 2003;96(3):726–732.

10. Murray MJ, Peruzzi WT, Lumb PD, et al. Clinical practice guidelines for sustained use of sedatives and analgesics in the adult critically ill patient. *Crit Care Med.* 2002;30(1):119–141.

11. Suominen P, Caffin C, Linton S, et al. The cardiac analgesic assessment scale (CASS): A pain assessment tool for intubated and ventilated children after cardiac surgery. *Paediatr Anesth.* 2004;14(4):336–343.

Renal Disorders

Robert E. Lynch

Fluid Management and Electrolyte Disturbances

54

Alok Kalia   Amita Sharma

SODIUM

Sodium and its attendant anions are the primary contributors to extracellular fluid (ECF) tonicity. An excessive increase or decline in the plasma sodium concentration leads to osmotically driven water gradient across the cell membrane. Sodium disorders have been discussed in detail in Chapters 11 and 15 and will only be briefly reviewed here.

Hyponatremia is defined as a serum Na concentration of 135 mEq per L or lower. Acute hyponatremia places the individual at risk for cerebral edema. Brain cells compensate for the decline in plasma osmolality by extruding electrolytes (4 to 6 hours) and organic osmolytes (24 to 48 hours), and reducing intracellular fluid (ICF) osmolality. Rapid correction of compensated hyponatremia increases the risk for osmotic demyelination syndrome; for example, central pontine myelinolysis. The conditions associated with hyponatremia can be categorized as follows: (i) Hypovolemic hyponatremia (sodium loss with relative water excess) includes diarrhea, third-space losses, cutaneous losses, diuretic therapy, salt-wasting renal tubular disease (interstitial nephritis, obstructive uropathy), bicarbonaturia (renal tubular acidosis, renal bicarbonate excretion as compensation for nasogastric suction or chronic vomiting), mineralocorticoid deficiency, and cerebral salt wasting. (ii) Euvolemic hyponatremia (normal or slightly elevated water content with decreased sodium content) includes syndrome of inappropriate secretion of antidiuretic hormone (SIADH), ecstasy use, glucocorticoid deficiency, hypothyroidism, near drowning in freshwater, and long-distance runners who replace sweat losses with liberal intake of hypotonic rehydration solutions. (iii) Hypervolemic hyponatremia (increased sodium content with a greater increase in water retention) includes congestive

TABLE 54.1
CAUSE OF HYPONATREMIA

Normal total body water and sodium (hyperosmolar hyponatremia)
  Hyperglycemia[a]
  Mannitol, glycerol therapy
Increased total body water and sodium (edema-forming states)
  Congestive heart failure
  Nephrosis
  Cirrhosis
  Acute renal failure
Decreased total body water and sodium (hypovolemic states)
  Gastrointestinal losses (vomiting, diarrhea, fistulae)
  Renal losses (diuretics, renal tubular acidosis, primary interstitial disease)
  Adrenal (mineralocorticoid deficiencies)
  Third-space losses (ascites, burns, pancreatitis, peritonitis)
Increased total body water but normal total body sodium
  Syndrome of inappropriate antidiuretic hormone secretion
  Water intoxication
  Miscellaneous (rest osmostat, hypothyroidism, glucocorticoid deficiency)
  Pseudohyponatremia
  Extreme hyperlipidemia or hyperproteinemia

[a]For every 100-mg/dL increase in plasma glucose concentration above normal, there is a corresponding decrease in plasma sodium concentration of approximately 1.6 mEq/L.
From Fleisher GR. *Atlas of emergency medicine.* Philadelphia, PA: Lippincott Williams & Wilkins; 2004:298.

cardiac failure, nephrotic syndrome, hepatic cirrhosis, and renal insufficiency with an inability to excrete adequate free water (see Table 54.1).

The workup generally includes urine osmolality and urine sodium. Maximally dilute urine (osmolality <100 mosmol per L) indicates appropriate free water excretion (excessive free water intake or a reset osmostat, as seen in a form of SIADH) and urine osmolality >100 mosmol per L indicates impaired free water excretion (i.e., reduction in effective ECF volume, SIADH, hypothyroidism, and cortisol deficiency). Urinary sodium concentration of <15 mEq per L signifies avid sodium reabsorption (extrarenal sodium loss or decreased effective ECF), and a urinary sodium concentration of >15 mEq per L generally signifies SIADH or renal sodium loss.

Hypernatremia is defined as a serum sodium concentration exceeding 145 mEq per L, usually indicating a deficit of free water or, less commonly, administration of excessive sodium. Maintenance of hypernatremia requires an inability to ingest free water and/or excrete concentrated urine. Acute hypernatremia may lead to a significant decline in brain volume with tearing of emissary veins and thrombosis of cerebral vessels. If hypernatremia persists for more than 48 hours, brain cells begin to accumulate osmotically active molecules and reclaim some of the lost water. A rapid decline in the serum Na level in this compensated state may lead to cerebral edema. Etiologies of hypernatremia can be categorized as follows: (i) Hypernatremia associated with a deficit of free water and normal or reduced total body sodium content results from central or nephrogenic diabetes insipidus, osmotic diuresis, profuse sweating, profuse diarrhea, primary hypodipsia, or inadequate provision of free water. (ii) Hypernatremia associated with high total body sodium content results from sodium excess, dialysis against high sodium concentration dialysate, salt water drowning, and excessive ingestion of sodium chloride (see Table 54.2).

TABLE 54.2

CAUSES OF HYPERNATREMIA

Increased total body sodium or increased total body sodium
  greater than increased total body water
    Sodium poisoning (accidental; sodium bicarbonate therapy)
    Hyperaldosteronism (rare in children)
Normal total body sodium; "pure" water loss
    Insensible losses: respiratory and skin
    Renal (central and nephrogenic diabetes insipidus)
    Inadequate access to water
Decreased total body sodium less than decreased total body
  water
    Extrarenal (gastrointestinal)[a]
    Renal (osmotic diuretics; glucose, mannitol, urea)
    Obstructive uropathy
Normal total body sodium and water with abnormal central
  osmotic regulation of water balance
    Essential hypernatremia

[a]In diarrheal states, hypernatremia usually results from a combination of relatively greater water than sodium losses coupled with relatively greater sodium than water replacement.
From Fleisher GR. *Atlas of emergency medicine.* Philadelphia, PA: Lippincott Williams & Wilkins; 2004:299.

POTASSIUM

Although ECF potassium represents only 2% of total body potassium, change in serum potassium concentration is the most important variable affecting the transcellular potassium gradient. This gradient is a critical determinant of the normal function of the heart, nervous system, and skeletal and smooth muscles. Hypokalemia is defined as a serum potassium concentration of <3.5 mEq per L. Hypokalemia is caused by (i) transcellular shifts (metabolic alkalosis, insulin administration, β_2-adrenergic agonists, recovery from diabetic ketoacidosis, hyperglycemia, rapid cell proliferation in leukemias, lymphomas, hypothermia, massive transfusion with washed potassium-depleted blood, hypokalemic periodic paralysis), (ii) gastrointestinal losses (nasogastric suctioning/vomiting, chronic diarrhea; villous adenomas, chronic laxative abuse), and (iii) *renal losses* (mineralocorticoid excess, Cushing syndrome, congenital adrenal hyperplasia [11β hydroxylase and 17α hydroxylase deficiency], Liddle syndrome, syndrome of apparent mineralocorticoid excess, diuretic therapy, persistent metabolic acidosis, renal tubular acidosis, Bartter syndrome, Gitelman syndrome, and magnesium deficiency).

Mild hypokalemia (2.5 to 3.5 mEq per L) may be treated with oral supplementation unless there are continuing losses indicating the likelihood of a further decline. A level of <2.5 mEq per L may be treated by potassium chloride usually infused intravenously at a rate of 0.25 to 0.5 mEq/kg/hour with cardiac monitoring. Hypokalemia should be corrected before the correction of acidosis; and refractory hypokalemia may require magnesium supplementation.

Hyperkalemia is defined as a serum potassium level >5.5 mEq per L. Etiologies include (i) pseudohyperkalemia (e.g., hemolysis, leucocytosis, thrombocytosis); (ii) redistribution hyperkalemia (i.e., rhabdomyolysis, tumor lysis, massive hemolysis, diabetic ketoacidosis); and (iii) impaired renal excretion of potassium (renal dysfunction, Addison disease, congenital adrenal hyperplasia, pseudohypoaldosteronism types I and II, type IV renal tubular acidosis, and drugs such as potassium sparing diuretics, angiotensin-converting enzyme inhibitors and angiotensin II blockers, β-blockers, cyclosporine, nonsteroidal anti-inflammatory agents).

Severe hyperkalemia is a medical emergency (see Table 54.3). Therapy is directed at minimizing membrane depolarization, shifting potassium into cells, and promoting potassium loss. If significant electrocardiogram (EKG) abnormalities are present, intravenous calcium should be administered as calcium antagonizes the membrane actions of hyperkalemia. The usual dose is 10% calcium gluconate (0.45 mEq Ca^{2+} per mL) 50 to 100 mg per kg or 10% calcium chloride (1.36 mEq Ca^{2+} per mL) 10 to 25 mg per kg infused over 2 to 3 minutes. The effect is rapid but lasts only for 30 to 60 minutes. The dose can be repeated if there is no change in the EKG. Infusion of glucose

ACUTE RENAL FAILURE: EMERGENCY TREATMENT OF HYPERKALEMIA

1. Serum K 5.5–7.0 mEq/L (normal EKG): 1 g/kg Kayexalate orally or rectally[a]
2. Serum K >7.5 mEq/L or >7.0 mEq/L with abnormal EKG[b]:
   Step 1. 0.5 mL/kg calcium gluconate as 10% solution over 2–4 min with EKG monitoring; stop when pulse rate decreases by 20 beats/min or to <100 beats/min
   Step 2. 3.3 mL/kg sodium bicarbonate as 7.5% solution
   Step 3. 1 mL/kg glucose as 50% solution; if hyperkalemia persists, infuse 20%–30% glucose solution with 0.5 U/kg regular insulin; keep blood sugar <300 mg/dL
3. Serum K persistently >6.5 mEq/L: dialysis

K, potassium; EKG, electrocardiogram.
[a]Kayexalate exchanges 1 mEq potassium for 1 mEq sodium and lowers serum potassium by approximately 1 mEq/L within 4 hours. It can be administered orally with food or beverage, by nasogastric tube, or rectally in 10% glucose/water (1 g in 4 mL) or in 20% sorbitol (50–100 mL). It must be retained for at least 30 minutes.
[b]Serum potassium >7.0 with a normal electrocardiogram can be treated as outlined in step 1.
From Fleisher GR. *Atlas of emergency medicine*. Philadelphia, PA: Lippincott Williams & Wilkins; 2004.

(1 g per kg) and insulin (0.2 U per g of glucose) infusion will result in a fall in the serum potassium concentration of 0.5 to 1.5 mEq per L starting within 15 to 30 minutes. The peak effect occurs at 60 minutes and lasts for several hours. Sodium bicarbonate is a useful adjunct in the presence of significant acidosis. β_2-adrenergic agonists administered have rapid action but their efficacy remains limited. Finally, forced saline diuresis (by a loop diuretic) or a cation exchange resin such as sodium polystyrene sulfonate (Kayexalate) can enhance excretion by renal or gastrointestinal tract respectively. Sodium polystyrene sulfonate (Kayexalate) (1 g per kg) is administered orally in 70% sorbitol or as a retention enema. An effect is seen in approximately 2 hours. Dialysis may be required in patients with reduced renal function.

CALCIUM

Hypocalcemia is defined as a serum calcium concentration of <8.5 mg per dL or an ionized calcium level of <1.00 to 1.13 mmol per L. In patients with hypoalbuminemia, total serum calcium level will be low while the ionized calcium level may be normal. Etiologies include (i) loss of ionized calcium from ECF (sepsis, rhabdomyolysis, hyperphosphatemia acute pancreatitis, osteoblastic metastases, hungry bone syndrome, respiratory alkalosis, citrate or alkali administration), (ii) disturbances of parathyroid hormone (hypoparathyroidism, Di George syndrome, parathyroidectomy, pseudohypoparathyroidism, hypomagnesemia), (iii) vitamin D deficiency, and (iv) chelation hypocalcemia (hyperphosphatemia, massive blood transfusions, high plasma oxalate, or lactate level). Clinical manifestations relevant to the intensive care unit (ICU) include laryngospasm, Trousseau sign, Chvostek sign, seizures, and EKG (prolonged QT interval, heart block, or ventricular fibrillation).

Symptomatic patients should be given 10% calcium gluconate (100 to 200 mg per kg) or 10% calcium chloride (20 mg per kg) over 5 to 10 minutes. Too rapid an infusion can cause cardiac arrest. A bolus dose often needs to be followed by a continuous infusion. Calcium supplementation should precede correction of acidosis to prevent a further decline in the ionized calcium level. In patients with associated hyperphosphatemia, the phosphorus needs to be corrected before treating the hypocalcemia to avoid soft-tissue calcification. Resistant hypocalcemia may require concomitant therapy for magnesium or potassium deficiency.

Hypercalcemia is defined as a serum calcium level exceeding 11 mg per dL. The upper limit of normal ionized calcium is approximately 1.30 mmol per L. Etiologies include increased (i) bone resorption (primary hyperparathyroidism, malignancy, thyrotoxicosis, immobilization, vitamin A overdose, hyperthyroidism, paraneoplastic syndrome), (ii) increased intestinal absorption (milk-alkali syndrome, vitamin D overdose, hypervitaminosis A, sarcoidosis), and (iii) increased renal absorption (thiazide diuretics, familial hypocalciuric hypercalcemia). Most patients are asymptomatic. Very high serum calcium levels may be accompanied by confusion, weakness, abdominal cramping, anorexia, nausea, vomiting, constipation, pancreatitis, and renal failure. EKG findings include a shortened QT interval, wide T wave, and first-degree atrioventricular block.

Treatment of hypercalcemia is directed toward the underlying cause. If the serum calcium level exceeds 13 mg per dL, forced saline diuresis (with a loop diuretic) is often effective within 6 to 12 hours in patients with normal renal and cardiac function. Thiazide diuretics should be avoided. In patients with renal or heart failure, removal of calcium is best achieved by hemodialysis using a low calcium bath. In cases of persistent hypercalcemia, concomitant measures aimed at reducing bone resorption should be initiated. Bisphosphonates reduce calcium mobilization from the bone; both oral and parenteral preparations are available. Calcitonin, which reduces calcium loss from the bone and increases renal excretion, can lower the serum calcium level as much as 1 to 2 mg per dL within 2 to 4 hours, but tachyphylaxis rapidly occurs. Calcitonin is best utilized as an adjunct to bisphosphonates for rapid calcium reduction while waiting for the latter to become effective. Glucocorticoids are helpful in reducing intestinal calcium absorption in patients with sarcoidosis or vitamin D toxicity.

PHOSPHORUS

Hypophosphatemia is defined as serum phosphate concentrations <2.5 mg per dL. Etiologies include (i) enhanced cellular uptake (parenteral alimentation, refeeding syndrome, hungry bone syndrome, postparathyroidectomy, diabetic ketoacidosis being treated, intravenous glucose infusion, elevated catecholamine levels, and recovery from metabolic acidosis or respiratory alkalosis), (ii) inadequate intake or intestinal absorption, and (iii) excessive renal phosphate excretion (hyperparathyroidism, Fanconi syndrome, X-linked or autosomal dominant hypophosphatemic rickets, tumor-induced osteomalacia, acetazolamide, metolazone, osmotic diuresis, *cis*-platinum therapy, and renal transplantation in patients with severe secondary hyperparathyroidism). Mild to moderate hypophosphatemia has no symptoms. A serum phosphate concentration of <1.0 mg per dL may lead to confusion, weakness, muscle pain, rhabdomyolysis, hemolysis, congestive cardiac failure, and respiratory failure.

Acute severe hypophosphatemia should be treated with parenteral infusion of sodium or potassium phosphate (1 mL contains 94 mg phosphate, 4 mEq sodium, or 4.4 mEq of potassium). Five to 10 mg per kg of phosphate may be administered initially over 6 hours, followed by a maintenance infusion of 15 to 45 mg/kg/day. Hypocalcemia is a potential complication of intravenous phosphorus infusion. If the potassium salt is used, the infusion rate should not exceed the recommended rate for potassium administration. Once the serum phosphorus exceeds 2 mg per dL, oral therapy may be initiated at the rate of 30 to 90 phosphorus (P) mg/kg/day with potassium phosphate (Neutraphos) (each capsule contains 250 mg P, 7 mEq Na and K). Diarrhea is a common complication of oral phosphorus therapy.

Hyperphosphatemia is defined as serum phosphorus level >7 mg per dL. Etiologies include (i) decreased phosphate excretion (chronic renal failure, hypoparathyroidism, acromegaly, thyrotoxicosis, administration of bisphosphonates), (ii) phosphate shift from the ICF to the ECF (tumor lysis syndrome, rhabdomyolysis, acute hemolysis, lactic acidosis), (iii) increased phosphate load (sodium phosphate enemas with renal insufficiency or reduced gut motility), and (iv) pseudohyperphosphatemia. Laboratory error may be seen in patients with hyperglobulinemia, hyperlipidemia, hemolysis, and hyperbilirubinemia. Hyperphosphatemia is usually asymptomatic. Hypotension and congestive cardiac failure have been described with severe hyperphosphatemia.

If renal function is intact, renal phosphate excretion can be augmented by intravenous saline followed by a loop diuretic. In patients with renal failure, phosphate binding drugs or dialysis should be utilized. Hyperphosphatemia is usually accompanied by hypocalcemia, and therapy may need to be directed at the latter.

MAGNESIUM

Hypomagnesemia is defined as a serum level of <1.7 mg per dL. Etiologies include (i) redistribution (acute pancreatitis, catecholamine excess, thyrotoxicosis, insulin administration, hungry bone syndrome, metabolic alkalosis), (ii) reduced intake, (iii) increased intestinal losses, and (iv) increased renal losses (loop and thiazide diuretics, volume expansion, hypercalcemia, renal tubular acidosis, nephrotoxic drugs, during recovery from acute tubular necrosis, renal transplantation, postobstructive diuresis, Bartter syndrome, Gitelman syndrome, primary renal magnesium wasting). Severe hypomagnesemia may be accompanied by depression and apathy, paresthesias, tremors, tetany, muscle spasms, muscle weakness, myoclonic jerks, seizures, vertigo, delirium, and coma. Chvostek and Trousseau signs may be positive. Atrial fibrillation, coronary artery spasm, increased susceptibility to digoxin-induced arrhythmias and ventricular fibrillation have also been described.

Symptomatic patients and those with a serum magnesium level of <1 mg per dL should receive magnesium intravenously, usually with magnesium sulfate. The initial dose is 25 to 50 mg per kg (maximum 2 g) diluted to 10 mg per mL and given over 15 to 30 minutes with cardiac monitoring. The rate of infusion should not exceed 150 mg per minute. The dose can be repeated every 4 to 6 hours for a total of four doses. Once the serum magnesium level is in the safe range, oral administration with magnesium salts should be initiated if possible. Refractory hypomagnesemia may require correction of hypokalemia and hypocalcemia.

Hypermagnesemia is defined as a serum magnesium level exceeding 3 mg per dL. Etiologies include (i) redistributive (extensive soft-tissue injury, trauma, shock, sepsis, cardiac arrest, severe burns, adrenal insufficiency, hypothyroidism, theophylline intoxication, hypothermia), (ii) reduced excretion (renal insufficiency) in combination with an increased exogenous load (antacids, enemas), and (iii) increased load (prolonged retention of magnesium containing cathartics, Epsom salts poisoning, laxative abuse). Clinical manifestations of severe hypermagnesemia include paresthesias, muscle weakness, hyporeflexia, vasodilatation, and flushing. Hypotension, lethargy, respiratory depression, flaccid quadriplegia, coma, and cardiac arrest have been described with levels approaching 10 mg per dL.

Calcium gluconate or chloride should be administered parenterally to symptomatic patients with severe hypomagnesemia. Administration of saline along with a loop diuretic will promote renal excretion of magnesium. Hemodialysis should be considered in patients with reduced renal function.

RECOMMENDED READINGS

1. Moritz ML, Ayus JC. The pathophysiology and treatment of hyponatremic encephalopathy: An update. *Nephrol Dial Transplant.* 2003; 8(12):2486–2491.
2. Khatwa UA, Kin LL. An unusual case of hypernatremia: A diagnostic challenge. *Pediatr Crit Care Med.* 2004;5(5):511–512.

3. Ethier JH, Kamel KS, Magner PO, et al. The transtubular potassium concentration in patients with hypokalemia and hyperkalemia. *Am J Kidney Dis.* 1990;5(4):309–315.
4. Rastergar A, Soleimani M. Hypokalemia and hyperkalemia. *Postgrad Med J.* 2001;77:759–764.
5. Kamel KS, Charles W. Controversial issues in the treatment of hyperkalemia. *Nephrol Dial Transplant.* 2003;18:2215–2218.
6. Ziegler R. Hypercalcemic crisis. *J Am Soc Nephrol.* 2001;12:S3–S9.
7. Agus ZS. Hypomagnesemia. *J Am Soc Nephrol.* 1999;10(7):1616–1622.
8. Subramanian R, Khardori R. Severe hypophosphatemia: Pathophysiological implications, clinical presentation and treatment. *Medicine.* 2000;79(1):1–8.

55

Maintenance and Support of Kidney Function in Critical Illness

Mohammad Ilyas   *Eileen N. Ellis*

The incidence of acute renal failure (ARF) in critically ill patients is variable and has been reported between 3% to 25% in adults, depending on the population studied and the criteria used to define ARF. As many as 8% to 24% of infants admitted to neonatal intensive care units (ICUs) develop ARF. There is a mortality rate as high as 50% in adult patients with hospital-acquired ARF. However, when ARF occurs in association with multiple organ dysfunction, mortality rates can be much higher, varying in published series between 40% and 90%. The etiology of pediatric ARF in the ICU has shifted in recent decades with advancements in pediatric critical care. The underlying causes include congenital heart disease, malignancy and tumor lysis syndrome, hemolytic uremic syndrome, acute tubular necrosis (ATN), nephrotoxins, bone marrow and solid organ transplantation, and sepsis. Children develop severe and life-threatening ARF associated with multiple organ dysfunction often early in their ICU course. More than 80% of deaths occur within 7 days of diagnosis of ARF with multiple organ dysfunction. The most important risk factors for ARF are often present on admission and most commonly include acute circulatory and respiratory failure.

Many attempts have been made to prevent ARF in the ICU setting, and fluid administration is considered an initial measure in this regard. The incidence of ARF in patients with burns and trauma has decreased by prompt resuscitation with adequate volumes of crystalloid fluid. Maintenance of adequate fluid balance remains a mainstay of prevention of ARF in both pediatric and adult patients with burns, trauma, and other types of volume depletion. Care must also be taken to prevent resuscitation fluid overload while maintaining fluid balance, although with the availability of mechanical ventilation and renal replacement therapy, it is better to err on the side of generous fluid resuscitation.

Fluid resuscitation in patients with burns requires special consideration. In a recent review of pediatric patients with burns, the overall mortality rate was 9% and approximately 25% of nonsurvivors had refractory shock. The greatest fluid losses in patients with burns occur in the first 24 hours after the burn and therefore, initial resuscitation is most important. Several of the more common resuscitation formulas use a total 24-hour fluid requirement of approximately 4 mL/kg/% burn body surface area plus maintenance fluids in pediatric patients with burns. Half of this fluid is usually given over the first 8 hours and the remainder over the next 16 hours.[1] Crystalloids are recommended for the first 24 hours with colloids added following that. Adequacy of fluid resuscitation is monitored by measurement of urine output, pulse, blood pressure, and respiratory rate. The end point for adequate fluid resuscitation is urine output of 1 to 1.5 mL/kg/hour in children, although urine output of 0.5 mL/kg/hour may be acceptable if serum creatinine is stable. Recently, investigators have been concerned about suprafluid resuscitation in patients with burns with as much as 8 mL/kg/% burn body surface area given. This supraresuscitation appears to be related to increased opioid administration. Excessive fluid resuscitation has complications such as tissue edema, tissue hypoxia, and abdominal or extremity compartment syndrome. Therefore, fluid resuscitation in this group of patients is complex and requires close monitoring to avoid ARF while preventing the complications of fluid overload.

In every ICU patient, the first goal in prevention or treatment of hypotension is providing adequate volume through fluid resuscitation. Once adequate fluid has been administered, blood pressure should be maintained with the use of inotropes and vasopressors because maintenance of adequate blood pressure, and hence adequate renal perfusion pressure and renal blood flow, is critical to prevention of ARF and to survival.[2] Although vasoconstrictors might decrease renal blood flow, in clinical studies of sepsis in adults, norepinephrine has been shown to increase renal blood flow and improve renal function.[3] Recent studies have shown that catecholamine-resistant hypotension in distributive shock may respond to administration of vasopressin. The rise in blood pressure with vasopressin is significant enough that catecholamines can often be decreased.[4] Despite these results, randomized trials with vasopressin demonstrating improved outcomes or studies in critically ill children are still lacking. It was also long believed that "low-dose" dopamine, regardless of blood pressure, was beneficial in the prevention of ARF, but many recent studies have conclusively shown that this therapy plays no role in preventing ARF in critically ill patients.

Other pharmacologic agents, including diuretics, mannitol, calcium-channel blockers, and atrial natriuretic peptide (ANP), have been used in an attempt to prevent ARF. There is minimal evidence to support the use of mannitol or calcium-channel blockers in the prevention of ARF. Loop diuretic administration may result in diuresis and help in fluid management, but there is no evidence of actual improvement in renal function with the use of these agents.[5] The efficacy of the diuresis produced by either continuous infusion or intermittent administration of furosemide has been compared in critically ill pediatric patients with renal sufficiency. Despite discrepant results, it appears that continuous infusion may be more efficacious in producing diuresis in hemodynamically unstable patients, although intermittent administration may be preferred in cardiovascularly stable patients.[6] Several recent studies have also been completed analyzing the combined effects of furosemide, mannitol, and dopamine or furosemide and dopamine with mixed results.

ANP has been shown to increase glomerular filtration rate independent of renal blood flow and increase natriuresis, but high doses of ANP can result in hypotension that could cause further renal tubular damage and decreased glomerular filtration rate. Despite the possible beneficial effects of ANP, most clinical studies have not shown any benefit to renal function in critically ill patients; however, one recent study of patients who had cardiopulmonary bypass found that long-term infusion of ANP resulted in improved renal function and decreased need for dialysis.[7]

Studies of the use of brain natriuretic peptide (BNP) show promise in adults with severe sodium retention, but utility in children remains to be demonstrated.

Drug administration plays an additional role in the prevention of ARF. Certain nephrotoxins should be avoided in the setting of marginal renal function in the ICU if possible. These include aminoglycosides, amphotericin B, vancomycin, and others. However, these medications are frequently required for the underlying disease process of the patient. Estimation of renal function in critically ill children becomes quite important and may require more than serum creatinine as a measure of renal function. Once renal function is estimated, drugs with renal metabolism or toxicity can then be dosed according to the degree of renal dysfunction and drug levels monitored if necessary (see Chapter 59).

TUMOR LYSIS SYNDROME

Tumor lysis syndrome is a life-threatening process in which rapid destruction of tumor cells results in hyperuricemia, hyperphosphatemia, hyperkalemia, hypocalcemia, and often ARF. Tumor lysis syndrome most often occurs in patients with lymphoproliferative malignancies as they are exposed to chemotherapy or radiation, but it can occur spontaneously. Risk factors for the development of tumor lysis syndrome include large tumor burden, elevated lactate dehydrogenase, extensive bone marrow involvement, high tumor sensitivity to chemotherapy, and preexisting renal dysfunction. The metabolic derangements of tumor lysis syndrome can begin within hours of administration of chemotherapy. After beginning chemotherapy, the patient at risk for tumor lysis should be monitored carefully for hyperkalemia, hyperphosphatemia, hypocalcemia, and hyperuricemia.

Classic prophylaxis for tumor lysis syndrome in the at-risk patient aims at decreasing the formation and increasing the renal clearance of uric acid. This is accomplished by slow introduction of chemotherapy, adequate hydration, allopurinol therapy, and alkalization of urine. Aggressive hydration should begin as early as possible prior to the administration and continue 2 to 3 days after the administration of chemotherapy. Patients at risk for the development of fluid overload and compromised cardiac function should be carefully monitored during fluid therapy. In addition to fluid administration, the treatment and prevention of hyperuricemia includes urinary alkalinization to increase the solubility of uric acid and prevent the intratubular precipitation of uric acid. The goal is to raise the urine pH to >7.0. This can often be accomplished by infusing 0.45% normal saline with 5% dextrose to which 50 to 75 mmol per L sodium bicarbonate has been added. Urine pH should be monitored to maintain the desired alkalinity.

Tumor lysis syndrome releases purine nucleic acids that are metabolized into uric acid resulting in hyperuricemia. Allopurinol is an inhibitor of xanthine oxidase, the enzyme responsible for conversion of hypoxanthine to xanthine and then to uric acid as the end product of purine metabolism. Oral preparations of allopurinol have been available since the 1960s and their administration has decreased uric acid production in patients at risk for tumor lysis syndrome. An intravenous form of allopurinol has recently become available for patients who are unable to take oral medications or in whom intravenous administration is preferred. A recent study showed that intravenous administration of allopurinol decreased uric acid levels in 95% of pediatric patients who had elevated uric acid levels, and prevented the increase of uric acid levels in 92% of pediatric patients with normal pretreatment uric acid levels.[8] However, the effectiveness of allopurinol is limited by its slow onset of action, ability to trigger allergic reactions, and significant drug interaction with common chemotherapeutic agents.

In addition to limiting production of uric acid with allopurinol, uric acid can be converted into a more soluble form to facilitate excretion. Urate oxidase oxidizes uric acid into allantoin, which is five times more soluble than uric acid. Urate oxidase has been available in Europe since the 1970s but its use has been limited by the high incidence of anaphylaxis. Recently, a recombinant form of urate oxidase, rasburicase, has been developed. In pediatric patients at high risk for tumor lysis syndrome, use of rasburicase has resulted in decreased uric acid levels and decreased need for dialysis.[9] Therefore, rasburicase has been found to be efficacious and well-tolerated in the prevention of tumor lysis syndrome.

When prevention and conventional management of tumor lysis syndrome fails and the patient has severe electrolyte disorders or ARF, dialysis therapy is indicated and should be started quickly and aggressively. Intermittent hemodialysis is often preferred because of more efficient clearance of solutes accumulated in tumor lysis syndrome as well as rapid correction of the metabolic derangements. However, experience with continuous renal replacement therapies in the treatment of tumor lysis syndrome is generally favorable. The continuous nature of the therapy may offer advantages over intermittent therapy in select patients. Continuous renal replacement therapy has also been utilized as a prophylactic adjunct to the treatment of pediatric patients at high risk for tumor lysis syndrome.

CONTRAST-INDUCED NEPHROPATHY

Contrast-induced nephropathy (CIN) has become a significant source of morbidity and mortality with the increased use of iodinated contrast media in diagnostic imaging and interventional procedures, especially in critically ill patients. It is most commonly defined as ARF occurring within 48 hours of exposure to intravascular radiographic contrast material when renal failure is not attributable to other causes. CIN most commonly causes a nonoliguric, asymptomatic, transient decline in renal function. More severe renal dysfunction with oliguric renal failure may occur. Although the incidence of CIN varies markedly in studies due to differences in the definition of renal failure, an incidence of 14.5% was seen in a large epidemiologic study. Much higher incidence is reported in patients with diabetic nephropathy. Despite lack of exact rates of incidence, CIN remains an important source of morbidity in hospitalized patients and has been found to result in excessive mortality rates, independent of other risk factors.[10]

Various patient factors have been noted to increase the risk of CIN. These include preexisting renal dysfunction; diabetes mellitus with renal insufficiency; administration of nephrotoxic drugs including cyclosporin A, aminoglycosides, amphotericin, and nonsteroidal anti-inflammatory drugs; sepsis; and reduced intravascular volume.[11] Risk is also increased with the administration of large contrast doses and multiple injections of contrast media within 72 hours. Use of low osmolarity contrast media may reduce the risk of CIN, but this has been shown only in adult studies of patients with preexisting renal dysfunction when the contrast was given intra-arterially.[10]

Prevention of CIN begins with recognition of patients with specific risk factors who require contrast administration. The most important risk factor is preexisting renal dysfunction. An adequate estimate of renal function in infants and children must be obtained prior to administration of contrast media. If a patient has preexisting renal dysfunction, careful consideration of the risks and benefits of the procedure must be carried out prior to administration of the minimally effective dose of contrast media. Use of lower osmolarity contrast agents may also decrease the risk of CIN. Nephrotoxic drugs should also be avoided prior to administration of the contrast media.

Several studies in adult patients have shown that administration of IV fluids before and during the procedures requiring contrast media reduced CIN. Hydration should begin several hours prior to use of the contrast media and continue for several hours following the procedure. Administration of sodium bicarbonate hydration may be superior to saline administration in prevention of CIN.[11] Despite the lack of large controlled randomized trials or studies in children, hydration prior to contrast administration appears to be an appropriate strategy.

Because there is some evidence that reactive oxygen species play a role in the development of CIN, an antioxidant, N-acetylcysteine, has been studied as a prevention of CIN with mixed results. Because of a positive outcome in some studies, favorable side effect profile, and low cost, N-acetylcysteine has gained favor as a preventive therapy, particularly in high-risk groups. Two recent meta-analyses have reviewed many of the same studies using N-acetylcysteine to prevent CIN in adult patients with chronic renal insufficiency but have described conflicting results. Despite the lack of conclusive evidence or data in children, use of N-acetylcysteine, either orally in two doses the day before and the day of the contrast procedure or IV in doses of 150 mg per kg over 30 minutes before the contrast procedure, has gained popularity.

Removal of contrast media after a procedure by hemodialysis and hemofiltration has been studied. Hemodialysis does not prevent the development of CIN in comparison to saline hydration and patients receiving hemodialysis are more likely to have reduced renal function and require additional hemodialysis. However, a recent study comparing the role of prophylactic hemofiltration and saline hydration in patients with chronic renal failure undergoing coronary interventions to prevent the development of CIN found that serum creatinine increase over baseline was significantly lower in the hemofiltration group. Further, in-hospital events, requirement of temporary renal replacement therapy, and mortality was higher in the group receiving saline hydration. Although these results are encouraging, high cost and increased intensity of care required for hemofiltration limit its use in this setting.

RHABDOMYOLYSIS

Rhabdomyolysis is a systemic metabolic disorder caused by leakage of muscle cell constituents into the blood following the necrosis of skeletal muscle. In rhabdomyolysis, massive amounts of myoglobin are released and, once the binding proteins are saturated, myoglobin is filtered by the glomeruli resulting in ARF. The exact mechanism of ARF in rhabdomyolysis is unknown, but the three possible mechanisms include renal vasoconstriction, renal tubular obstruction due to precipitation of pigment, and myoglobin-associated tubular cytotoxicity. Rhabdomyolysis is detected by an increased serum creatine kinase, increased serum and urine myoglobin, and can be suspected by a urinalysis showing dark colored urine or positive dipstick for blood but few red blood cells on microscopic examination.

Acute rhabdomyolysis may be caused by trauma and crush injury or muscle necrosis from ischemia, inflammation, viral infection, strenuous muscle exercise, electrical current, hyperthermia, spider bites, or exposure to drugs and toxins. The common offending drugs include alcohol, amphetamine, cocaine, phencyclidine (PCP), 3, 4-methylenedioxymethamphetamine (ecstasy), statins, corticosteroids, diuretics, and narcotics. Various electrolyte abnormalities result from rhabdomyolysis including hyperkalemia, hypocalcemia, and hyperphosphatemia. ARF is the most important complication of rhabdomyolysis and fortunately is less common in children than adults with rhabdomyolysis. In a retrospective review of 18 pediatric patients with rhabdomyolysis, the most frequent cause was acute viral encephalopathy/encephalitis, followed by status epilepticus and status asthmaticus.[12] More than 70% of

these patients had evidence of multiple organ dysfunction and 50% had ARF. The presence of dehydration, massive muscular necrosis, and metabolic acidosis were contributing factors for the development of ARF in children with rhabdomyolysis.[12] In children, rhabdomyolysis can also be chronic in nature as seen with certain congenital muscle disorders that usually start during childhood. They should be suspected if muscular weakness or myoglobinuria recurs frequently or is seen in situations not likely to cause rhabdomyolysis in healthy children.

The primary goal in the management of patients with rhabdomyolysis is to prevent factors that are associated with ARF such as volume depletion, tubular obstruction, acidosis, and free radical release. Intravenous fluid therapy to increase urine flow is essential to prevent the development of ARF. Commonly, intravenous fluids consist of 0.45% normal isotonic saline with 5% dextrose to which 50 to 75 mmol per L of sodium bicarbonate is added and are administered at 1.5 to 2 times the maintenance fluid needs. Addition of bicarbonate to intravenous fluids helps prevent acidosis, hyperkalemia, and precipitation of myoglobin in tubules. Urine pH should be monitored during bicarbonate administration with a goal of maintaining urine pH >7.0. If good urine output has been established, addition of mannitol has been recommended to increase renal blood flow and glomerular filtration rate, act as an osmotic agent to reduce interstitial fluid accumulation, increase urine flow, and scavenge free radicals. Loop diuretics are not usually recommended, because although these may increase tubular flow and decrease the risk of precipitation of myoglobin in tubules, they may also increase aciduria and calcium losses. A recent retrospective review of adult patients with rhabdomyolysis failed to show any benefit of administration of bicarbonate and mannitol in the prevention of ARF, the need for dialysis, or mortality.[13] Until there is further study in this area, bicarbonate and mannitol fluid therapy are still generally recommended. If hyperkalemia or ARF ensue despite these measures, renal replacement therapy is indicated.

The main strategies for prevention of renal insufficiency in the critically ill pediatric patient are aimed at excellent clinical care with maintenance of adequate blood pressure and renal perfusion. These include adequate fluid administration, use of inotropes and vasopressors, avoidance of nephrotoxic drugs, and possibly maintenance of euglycemia. If, despite these preventive strategies, ARF should develop, various forms of renal replacement therapy are available for the critically ill pediatric patient. Early initiation of renal replacement therapy may improve survival.[2]

REFERENCES

1. Hettiaratchy S, Papini R. Initial management of a major burn: II—assessment and resuscitation. *BMJ.* 2004;329:101–103.
2. Goldstein SL, Somers MJG, Baum MA, et al. Pediatric patients with multiorgan dysfunction syndrome receiving continuous renal replacement therapy. *Kidney Int.* 2005;67:653–658.

3. Redl-Wenzl EM, Armbruster C, Edelmann G, et al. The effects of norepinephrine on hemodynamics and renal function in severe septic shock states. *Intensive Care Med.* 1993;19:151–154.

4. Dunser MW, Mayr AJ, Ulmer H, et al. The effects of vasopressin on systemic hemodynamics in catecholamine-resistant septic and postcardiotomy shock: A retrospective analysis. *Anesth Analg.* 2001;93:7–13.

5. Shilliday IR, Quinn KJ, Allison MEM. Loop diuretics in the management of acute renal failure: A prospective, double-blind, placebo-controlled, randomized study. *Nephrol Dial Transplant.* 1997;12:2592–2596.

6. Klinge J. Intermittent administration of furosemide or continuous infusion in critically ill infants and children: Does it make a difference? *Intensive Care Med.* 2001;27:623–624.

7. Sward K, Valsson F, Odencrants P, et al. Recombinant human atrial natriuretic peptide in ischemic acute renal failure: A randomized placebo-controlled trial. *Crit Care Med.* 2004;32:1310–1315.

8. Smalley RV, Guaspari AL, Haase-Statz S, et al. Allopurinol: Intravenous use for prevention and treatment of hyperuricemia. *J Clin Oncol.* 2000;18:1758–1763.

9. Goldman SC, Holcenberg JS, Finklestein JZ, et al. A randomized comparison between rasburicase and allopurinol in children with lymphoma or leukemia at high risk for tumor lysis. *Blood.* 2001;**97**:2998–3003.

10. Gleeson TG, Bulugahapitiya S. Contrast-induced nephropathy. *Am J Radiol.* 2004;183:1673–1689.

11. Merten GJ, Burgess WP, Gray LV, et al. Prevention of contrast-induced nephropathy with sodium bicarbonate: A randomized controlled trial. *JAMA.* 2004;291:2328–2334.

12. Watanabe T. Rhabdomyolysis and acute renal failure in children. *Pediatr Nephrol.* 2001;16:1072–1075.

13. Brown CV, Rhee P, Chan L, et al. Preventing renal failure in patients with rhabdomyolysis: Do bicarbonate and mannitol make a difference? *J Trauma-Injury Crit Care.* 2004;56:1191–1196.

Acute Renal Failure

56

Craig William Belsha

Acute renal failure (ARF) is characterized by an abrupt decline in kidney function over hours to days, leading to a decreased ability to regulate water, electrolyte, and acid–base balance.[1] Although decreased urine output accompanies the development of ARF in many patients, the urine output may be normal or even increased in others. The causes of ARF are often classified within these three groups: prerenal (reversible renal vasoconstriction), intrinsic renal, and postrenal (obstructive) failure[2,3] (see Table 56.1). The pathophysiology of individual causes of renal failure within these categories is reviewed in Chapter 8.

ARF may occur in 5% of hospitalized pediatric patients and in up to 8% of children following open cardiac surgery.[4] The major etiologies of ARF may vary by age-group, population, and hospital setting. A recent review in a US tertiary children's hospital showed that renal ischemia (21%), nephrotoxic medications (16%), and sepsis (11%) were leading causes of ARF, with ischemia being most common in children aged 5 years or less and nephrotoxins being most common in older children.[5] Hemolytic uremic syndrome, discussed in Chapter 57, has also been a common cause of renal failure in some pediatric centers.

DIAGNOSIS

The use of blood urea nitrogen (BUN) or serum creatinine as markers for the presence of ARF have limitations in that glomerular filtration rate (GFR) may fall by as much as 50% before serum creatinine rises because of increased tubular secretion of creatinine in renal failure. Also, a relatively large change in the serum value of creatinine in patients with preexisting chronic renal failure may represent a relatively less change in their actual renal function than in individuals without preexisting renal dysfunction.

Although there is no common definition for ARF in the pediatric age-group, the Acute Dialysis Quality Initiative (ADQI) group recently proposed a classification scheme for ARF in adults.[6] The acronym RIFLE includes three severity

TABLE 56.1

CAUSES OF ACUTE RENAL FAILURE[a]

Prerenal
  Decreased cardiac output (cardiogenic shock)
  Decreased intravascular volume (hemorrhage, dehydration, "third-spacing")
Renal
  Primary renal parenchymal disease
    Vascular (acute glomerulonephritis, hemolytic uremic syndrome)
    Interstitial (pyelonephritis, drug-induced)
  Acute tubular necrosis
  Ischemic injury
  Nephrotoxic injury (antibiotics, uric acid)
  Pigmenturia (myoglobinuria, hemoglobinuria)
Postrenal
  Obstructive uropathy
    Posterior urethral valves
    Intra-abdominal tumor
    Nephrolithiasis (rare)
      Renal vein thrombosis (rare outside the neonatal period)

[a]Major pediatric causes of acute renal failure are in parentheses.
From Fleisher GR. *Atlas of emergency medicine.* Philadelphia, PA: Lippincott Williams & Wilkins; 2004.

levels (*R*isk of renal dysfunction when serum creatinine level is increased 1.5 times the normal level, *I*njury to the kidney when serum creatinine level is increased two times the normal level, *F*ailure of kidney function when serum creatinine level is increased three times the normal level) and two clinical outcomes (*L*oss of kidney function and *E*nd-stage kidney disease).

Clinical Evaluation

History and physical examination are important in determining the etiology of ARF in children. The signs and symptoms at presentation can also be combined to provide

TABLE 56.2

ACUTE RENAL FAILURE PRESENTING SYMPTOMS AND SIGNS

Symptoms	Signs	Likely Diagnosis
Nausea, vomiting	—	Gastroenteritis (ATN)
Diarrhea	Dehydration, shock	Gastroenteritis (ATN)
Hemorrhage	Shock	ATN
Fever	Petechiae, bleeding	Sepsis, DIC (ACN)
Melena	—	HUS
Sudden pallor	—	HUS
Grand mal seizures	—	HUS
Fever, chills	Flank tenderness	Pyelonephritis
Fever, skin rash	Erythema multiforme, purpura	AIN
—	—	HSP nephritis
Sore throat	Hypertension	PSGN
Pyoderma	Edema	PSGN
Grand mal seizures	Congestive heart failure	PSGN
Trauma	Muscle tenderness	Myoglobinuria
Myalgia	Myoedema	Myoglobinuria
Antibiotics, diuretics	—	Nephrotoxic acute renal failure
Variable urine output	Suprapubic mass	OU

ATN, acute tubular necrosis; DIC, disseminated intravascular coagulation; ACN, acute cortical necrosis; HUS, hemolytic uremic syndrome; AIN, acute interstitial nephritis (hypersensitivity nephritis); HSP, Henoch-Schönlein purpura; PSGN, poststreptococcal glomerulonephritis; OU, obstructive uropathy.
From Fleisher GR. *Atlas of emergency medicine.* Philadelphia, PA: Lippincott Williams & Wilkins; 2004.

useful information about the etiology and differential diagnosis of the renal failure (see Table 56.2). Symptoms suggestive of the presence of prerenal ARF may include diarrhea, vomiting, hypotension, and oliguria. Signs of dehydration such as dry mucous membranes, depressed anterior fontanel, tachycardia, or orthostatic hypotension may also favor the presence of prerenal azotemia. Fluid overload, hypertension, or symptoms suggestive of uremia, such as fatigue, weakness, nausea, vomiting, loss of appetite, itching, or confusion may suggest intrinsic or postrenal failure. Postrenal or obstructive ARF may occur in the presence of a history of urinary tract infection, stones, and poor urinary stream or an enlarged bladder detected on examination.

Acute tubular necrosis (ATN), a common cause of intrinsic ARF, may be found following recent cardiovascular surgery or other ischemic insults or detected by a history of recent exposure to nephrotoxic medications, chemotherapeutic agents, or radiographic contrast media. A history of fever and rash may suggest interstitial nephritis

or glomerulonephritis. Other systemic symptoms such as arthritis or hemoptysis suggest a multisystem illness such as vasculitis. A prior history of bloody diarrhea and the presence of pallor may be seen with hemolytic uremic syndrome. In the hospitalized patient, careful chart review is helpful in identifying possible etiologies for ARF, but it may be difficult to determine which of several possible causes is the actual etiology of ARF.

Laboratory Tests

The ratio of BUN to creatinine is often elevated ($>20:1$) in prerenal conditions. Other causes for an elevation in BUN may include gastrointestinal bleeding, use of systemic corticosteroids, catabolism caused by the underlying medical condition, or a high-protein diet. An elevation in the creatinine level that exceeds the elevation in BUN level suggests rhabdomyolysis, malnutrition, or liver disease.

Urinary volume is often <200 mL/m^2/day or <1 mL/kg/hour in children with oliguric ATN. Nonoliguric ATN is common and has various causes, including nephrotoxic antibiotic-induced ARF. Anuria, defined as complete cessation of urinary output other than a few milliliters of urine per 8-hour nursing shift, should suggest a diagnosis other than ATN, the most easily reversible one being obstruction. Vascular events should be a consideration in a patient with abrupt anuria; such events include renal vein or renal artery thrombosis. A vascular event would have to affect both kidneys to cause total anuria in a patient with two functioning kidneys. Polyuria, defined as an excessive urine volume in the presence of rising BUN and/or creatinine level(s) may be seen with some causes of intrinsic ARF or following relief from obstruction.

The urine of a patient with acute glomerulonephritis is often tea-colored or rusty in appearance, whereas the urine of a patient with hemoglobinuria or myoglobinuria may be pink in color. Red blood cells would be seen on urine microscopy in the former case, but these are absent in the latter case. The urinalysis in a patient with prerenal ARF may show concentrated urine with a specific gravity of 1.020 or higher and the presence of hyaline and finely granular casts. Mild proteinuria (trace to 2+) or microscopic hematuria (1 to 2+) may be seen in prerenal azotemia. Heavy proteinuria, however, would indicate glomerulonephritis. Hyaline and fine granular casts may be seen in prerenal azotemia, but coarse granular and red blood cell casts are seen frequently in glomerulonephritis.

Urinary indices are often used to differentiate prerenal azotemia from ATN. In prerenal ARF, the concentrating ability is intact, urine osmolality is elevated to >500 mOsm per kg, and the ratio of urine to plasma osmolality is also >2. In contrast, in the presence of intrinsic ARF, the renal concentration ability is often impaired, leaving a lower urine osmolality of >350 mOsm per kg and a urine to plasma osmolality ratio of >1. The urine sodium concentration is low in prerenal ARF (>10 mEq per L in children and >30 mEq per L in newborns) but is often higher in intrinsic ARF (<60 mEq per L). The kidney failure index (KFI), determined by the urine sodium level divided by the urine to plasma creatinine ratio, has been suggested to be a better way of distinguishing between prerenal (<1 in children and <2.5 in newborns) and intrinsic renal failure (>2 in children and >2.5 in newborns).

$$(KFI) = \frac{U_{Na}}{(U_{Cr}/P_{Cr})}$$

The fractional excretion of sodium (FE$_{Na}$) is also useful in distinguishing among these conditions, although exceptions exist and the recent use of diuretics makes interpretation difficult. This parameter is calculated as FE$_{Na}$ = ($U_{Na} \times P_{Cr} \times 100$)/($U_{Cr} \times P_{Na}$), where U_{Na} represents the urinary sodium concentration, P_{Na} the plasma sodium concentration, U_{Cr} the urine creatinine concentration, and P_{Cr} the plasma creatinine concentration. In children with renal hypoperfusion, the FE$_{Na}$ is <1%, and in intrinsic ARF, it is >2.5%. A higher cutoff value (>2.5% to 3%) for intrinsic ARF has been suggested in preterm infants owing to their greater normal urinary Na losses. The fractional excretion of urea nitrogen (FE$_{UN}$) has been proposed as a more sensitive test in adults to distinguish between prerenal and intrinsic ARF even in a patient who has received diuretics. It is calculated as FE$_{UN}$ = ($U_{UN} \times P_{Cr} \times 100$)/($U_{Cr} \times BUN$), where U_{UN} is the urine urea nitrogen level, BUN is the blood urea nitrogen, U_{Cr} the urine creatinine concentration, and P_{Cr} the plasma creatinine concentration. A FE$_{UN}$ of <35% supports prerenal azotemia, whereas a value of >50% suggests intrinsic renal failure.

Imaging and Other Studies

Renal imaging may be especially helpful in the evaluation of ARF in children to establish the presence of both kidneys, evaluate renal size, rule out urinary tract obstruction, and evaluate renal blood flow. Renal ultrasonography is noninvasive, may be performed at the bedside of critically ill patients, and can provide information about the renal parenchyma and collection system. Doppler flow ultrasonography is helpful in evaluating renal arterial and venous blood flow but requires significant operator skills to be used effectively. Radionuclide methods are available for assessing renal blood flow and excretory (secretory) function. Blood flow studies can be used to determine whether renal blood flow is occurring and, if so, whether the blood flow to the two kidneys is symmetrical.

Renal biopsy is rarely required for ARF occurring in the hospital setting from nephrotoxic medication injury or preceding hypotension. Biopsy would be indicated when a patient is suspected of having rapidly progressive glomerulonephritis or acute interstitial nephritis or to distinguish ATN from acute rejection in renal transplantation patients with primary nonfunction of the graft following transplantation.

TREATMENT

A number of metabolic and clinical abnormalities are associated with renal failure (see Table 56.3). Therefore, the goals of therapy in children with ARF are to (i) correct any existing fluid and electrolyte imbalance, (ii) provide adequate nutrition, (iii) control blood pressure, (iv) use specific therapies as indicated in the underlying etiology of ARF, and (v) avoid additional renal insults to enhance renal outcome. Blood pressure control is reviewed in Chapter 5 and the role of renal replacement therapy in ARF in Chapter 58.

"Maintenance" fluid calculations are often not applicable in the setting of ARF. Fluid therapy should be based on the patient's needs to replace existing fluid deficits and to provide for insensible and ongoing losses through urine, stool, chest, or nasogastric (NG) tube or ostomy. Insensible losses can be estimated as 400 mL/m^2/day but may be greater in preterm infants or in febrile or tachypneic patients. Insensible losses can be replaced by sodiumfree solutions. The measurement of urine or body fluid electrolytes is often helpful in guiding the replacement of ongoing losses.

Hyponatremia is a common electrolyte abnormality that develops usually as a result of fluid overload. If the serum sodium level is >120 mEq per L, fluid restriction or water

TABLE 56.3

METABOLIC AND CLINICAL ABNORMALITIES IN END-STAGE RENAL FAILURE

Anemia
    Decreased erythropoietin production
    Hemolysis
    Blood loss (bleeding tendency)[a]
Cardiovascular
    Congestive heart failure[a]
    Uremic pericarditis[a]
Fluid, electrolyte, acid–base balance
    Reduced free-water clearance, obligatory isothermia[a]
    Potassium balance lost when glomerular filtration rate
    10 mL/min, hyperkalemia common[a]
    Metabolic acidosis (increased anion gap)[a]
Vitamin D/calcium metabolism
    Hypocalcemia, hyperphosphatemia[a]
    Secondary hyperparathyroidism
    Osteomalacia (aluminum bone disease)
Immune function
    Increased risk of infection[a]
    Impaired host defense (white blood cell function)
Neurologic function[a]
    Inability to concentrate, loss of memory
    Headache, drowsiness, coma
    Weakness, tremors, seizures
    Peripheral neuropathy
    Autoimmune dysfunction (sweating, swings in blood pressure)

[a]Improved with dialysis.
From Fleisher GR. *Atlas of emergency medicine*. Philadelphia, PA: Lippincott Williams & Wilkins; 2004.

removal by dialysis will usually correct the hyponatremia. If the serum sodium is <120 mEq per L, the child is at increased risk for the development of hyponatremic seizures, and correction with hypertonic saline to the serum sodium level of approximately 125 mEq per L should be considered. The amount of sodium needed is estimated by the formula: $[(125 - Na_c)\,(Wt)\,(0.6)] = mEq\ Na$, where Na_c is the current serum Na concentration, Wt is the weight in kilograms, and 0.6 is the percentage of weight that represents the total body water. This sodium replacement is typically given over several hours and overcorrection of the hyponatremia needs to be avoided.

Hyperkalemia (>6.5 mEq per L) with T-wave elevation on the electrocardiogram requires prompt treatment to avoid the development of cardiac arrhythmias. Calcium (20 mg per kg as calcium chloride or 100 mg per kg as calcium gluconate) infusion may help stabilize cell membranes and decrease the risk of arrhythmias. Calcium administration does not change the serum potassium level. Intravenous glucose and insulin (0.1 U per kg of regular insulin and 0.5 g per kg of glucose [2 mL per kg of 25% glucose]) may help lower serum potassium level acutely by shifting the potassium into the intracellular space. β-Adrenergic antagonists such as albuterol may also assist in lowering the potassium acutely in situations in which intravenous access is not available. The ion exchange resin sodium polystyrene sulfonate (Kayexalate) may be given as 1 g per kg body weight, either orally or rectally, to lower the serum potassium level. This medication is typically placed in sorbitol or dextrose solution to enhance potassium excretion from the body.

Because the kidneys regularly excrete acids generated by diet and metabolism, metabolic acidosis is a common abnormality in patients with ARF. Respiratory compensation may help partially correct this acidosis; however, patients with neurologic or respiratory problems may be compromised in this ability and develop severe acidosis. Hypocalcemia is another common abnormality in patients with ARF. As metabolic acidosis increases the fraction of the total calcium that is free (ionized calcium), the correction of metabolic acidosis will lower the ionized calcium level, potentially leading to the development of hypocalcemic seizures or tetany. Hyperphosphatemia is another common abnormality in ARF and should be treated with dietary phosphate restriction and with oral calcium carbonate or calcium acetate. Hypercalcemia may occur with the use of calcium-containing phosphate binders and potentially lead to metastatic calcification when the product of calcium and phosphorus is elevated (>70). Sevelamer hydrochloride, a non–calcium-containing phosphate binder, has been effective in limited pediatric studies.

"Renal-dosage" dopamine (1 to 3 μg/kg/minute) has been widely used in an effort to improve diuresis and renal function, although few pediatric studies have been conducted to evaluate the safety and efficacy of this therapy in ARF.[7] The practice remains controversial because several clinical trials in adults have failed to show a benefit in patient survival/outcome or the delay/reduction in the need for dialysis. The Surviving Sepsis Campaign Management Guidelines Committee recommends against the use of low-dose dopamine for renal protection.[8]

Diuretics are often used in the setting of ARF to increase urine volume, control fluid balance, and enhance the delivery of nutrition. While augmenting urine volume, mannitol may increase intratubular urine flow and limit intratubular obstruction by debris. It may also reduce cellular swelling and damage. A lack of response to mannitol therapy, however, may lead to congestive heart failure or pulmonary edema and hyperosmolality. Few controlled trials have been conducted with mannitol; the one in children following cardiovascular surgery has suggested some benefit, but additional study is needed.[1] Loop diuretics such as furosemide increase urine flow rate and may decrease intratubular obstruction, inhibit Na^+/K^+ adenosine triphosphatase, and limit oxygen consumption in injured tubules. Their use may be associated with electrolyte abnormalities, the potential for decreased renal perfusion, worsening renal function, and the risk for ototoxicity. Recent studies suggest that continuous dosing of loop diuretics is advantageous as compared with intermittent dosing in critically ill patients because of a more controlled diuresis and less alteration in hemodynamic stability.

Prompt and adequate nutrition is important to the management of children with ARF. Enteral feedings should be provided if the gastrointestinal tract is functional. In newborns and infants, PM60/40 formula can be utilized, whereas older children should be provided a diet low in potassium and phosphorus with sufficient carbohydrates to avoid the breakdown of endogenous protein for glucose. Protein intake should not be excessive but should be provided to meet the nutritional needs, depending on the patient's condition, and may be increased with additional losses during peritoneal dialysis and hemofiltration.

PROGNOSIS

The outcome for children and adolescents with ARF depends on the underlying condition. Survival is better for those with primary renal causes of ARF such as glomerulonephritis or hemolytic uremic syndrome as opposed to those developing ARF following cardiovascular surgery or with multiorgan dysfunction syndrome (MODS).[9,10] Patients older than 1 year are more likely to survive than younger infants. Additional factors increasing the risk for mortality in some studies include hypotension, use of pressors, or the need for renal replacement therapy or mechanical ventilation. Renal recovery is often excellent in some conditions (e.g., ATN, acute interstitial nephritis), but significant residual damage may be present in others (e.g., hemolytic uremic syndrome, cortical necrosis, and rapidly progressive glomerulonephritis). Patients with residual damage may initially show improvement in renal function only to later have progressive loss of kidney function with hyperfiltration and development of proteinuria, hypertension, and chronic renal failure.

REFERENCES

1. Filler G. Acute renal failure in children. *Paediatr Drugs.* 2001; 3:783–792.
2. Schrier RW, Wang W, Poole B, et al. Acute renal failure: Definitions, diagnosis, pathogenesis, and treatment. *J Clin Invest.* 2004;114:5–14.
3. Lameire N, Van Biesen W, Vanholder R. Acute renal failure. *Lancet.* 2005;365:417–430.
4. Andreoli SP. Acute renal failure: Clinical evaluation and management. In: Avner E, Harmon W, Niaudet P, eds. *Pediatric nephrology.* Philadelphia, PA: Lippincott Williams & Wilkins; 2004: 1233–1251.
5. Hui-Stickle S, Brewer ED, Goldstein SL. Pediatric ARF epidemiology at a tertiary care center from 1999 to 2001. *Am J Kidney Dis.* 2005;45:96–101.
6. Bellomo R, Ronco C, Kellum JA, et al. Acute renal failure – definition, outcome measures, animal models, fluid therapy and information technology needs: The Second International Consensus Conference of the Acute Dialysis Quality Initiative (ADQI) Group. *Crit Care.* 2004;8:R2004–RR212.
7. Prins I, Plötz FB, Uiterwaal CSPM, et al. Low-dose dopamine in neonatal and pediatric intensive care: A systemic review. *Intensive Care Med.* 2001;27:206–210.
8. Dellinger RP, Carlet JM, Masur H, et al. Surviving sepsis campaign guidelines for management of severe sepsis and septic shock. *Crit Care Med.* 2004;32:858–871.
9. Williams DM, Sreedhar SS, Mickell JJ, et al. Acute kidney failure, a pediatric experience over 20 years. *Arch Pediatr Adolesc Med.* 2002;156:893–900.
10. Goldstein SL, Somers MJG, Baum MA, et al. Pediatric patients with multi-organ dysfunction syndrome receiving continuous renal replacement therapy. *Kidney Int.* 2005;67:653–658.

Hemolytic Uremic Syndrome

57

Ellen G. Wood

Hemolytic uremic syndrome (HUS) is characterized by microangiopathic hemolytic anemia, thrombocytopenia, and acute renal failure (ARF). First described in 1955 by Gasser, the overall mortality has dramatically decreased from 90% in 1955 to approximately 5% today.[1] It continues to be one of the most common causes of ARF, particularly in young children. In a recent prospective study of HUS in Germany and Austria, 72% of patients were younger than 5 years. Annual incidence rates ranged from 0.4 to 0.7 cases per 100,000 children younger than 15 years and from 0.5 to 1.7 cases per 100,000 children younger than 5 years. Median age of patients was 2.9 years (range 1.4 to 5.6 years). Forty-nine percent (188 of 388) of cases occurred from June to September.[2] Despite the almost explosive increase in knowledge regarding diarrhea (+) HUS over the past two decades, HUS remains a challenge for the intensivist and the nephrologist, and is a major public health concern. It can affect virtually all organ systems at unexpected times and with unusual presentations.

DIAGNOSIS

Clinical/Laboratory Findings

HUS is characterized by the sudden onset of pallor, decreased activity, and an ill appearing child. Volume status may be low, normal, or expanded. A microangiopathic hemolytic anemia is uniformly present, with numerous fragmented red blood cells (RBCs) on peripheral smear, typically a negative Coombs test, and a very elevated lactate dehydrogenase (LDH). There may be a mild elevation of indirect bilirubin and a decreased haptoglobin level. Associated with the microangiopathy is thrombocytopenia, usually severe, with platelet count averaging approximately

40,000 per mm^3 on presentation. Leukocytosis, reported in 20% to 25%, has been associated with a worse outcome. Renal involvement ranges from isolated hematuria and proteinuria to oligoanuric acute renal failure. Over 50% of patients require some form of renal replacement therapy for an average of 10 days before the recovery of renal function. The severity of anemia and thrombocytopenia do not correlate with the severity of renal involvement.[1–3]

Although the kidney is most commonly affected, numerous other organs may also be involved. The central nervous system (CNS) may be affected in as many as 20% to 25% of patients.[2] Manifestations include lethargy, irritability, seizures, hemiparesis, cortical blindness, coma, and stroke.[1,2,4] Patients with CNS involvement have been reported to have an increased risk of death.[1,5] Gastrointestinal tract (GI) involvement is generally divided as HUS with diarrhea (diarrhea [+] HUS) or without diarrhea (diarrhea [−] HUS). GI tract involvement is more likely with diarrhea (+) HUS, although vomiting is commonly seen as a prodromal finding in atypical diarrhea (−) HUS. At the time of the presentation of diarrhea (+) HUS, vomiting, crampy abdominal pain, and diarrhea may be resolving, or may still be prominent features. More serious GI complications include intussusception, bowel necrosis, and bowel perforation with septicemia. Bowel stricture can occur as a late complication.[1,2,4,5] In diarrhea (+) HUS, more severe colitis has been reported to be predictive of neurologic involvement and prolonged renal failure.[1] Pancreatic involvement with elevation of serum lipase and amylase has been reported in as many as 20% of patients. Transient or permanent diabetes mellitus has been reported in 4% to 15% of cases, and pancreatic pseudocyst has recently been described.[1,4,5] Elevated transaminases with an enlarged liver are common. While hypertension occurs commonly during the course of HUS, more severe cardiac involvement is rare. However, severe myocardial dysfunction can result in a potentially fatal outcome.[1,4,5] Recent reports suggest that cardiac troponin I (cTnI) may be a sensitive predictor of the severity of cardiac involvement.[6] Pleural effusion is the most common pulmonary finding. Primary lung involvement is rarely seen although pulmonary microthrombi have been described at autopsy. Pulmonary hemorrhage is even less common. It is primarily seen in drug-induced HUS, but has been recently reported in a patient with diarrhea (+) HUS.[1,4,5]

Signs and Symptoms

Hemolytic Uremic Syndrome with Diarrhea

Diarrhea (+) HUS accounts for 90% of cases of HUS.[1-3] The association of Shiga toxin (Stx)–producing *Escherichia coli* (STEC) was described in 1983. Reports from large outbreaks suggest that HUS will develop in approximately 5% to 10% of those infected with STEC. STEC infection most commonly presents as crampy abdominal pain and watery diarrhea without fever, progressing to bloody diarrhea in >50% of cases. The incubation period after inoculation is generally 2 to 5 days. HUS develops in those affected approximately 1 week after the onset of diarrhea.[1-4] However, recent studies suggest that endothelial injury has already occurred in patients who go on to develop HUS within the first 2 to 4 days of the onset of diarrhea. Two toxins have been studied extensively, Stx1 and Stx2. HUS occurs more often in individuals infected with Stx2. There are currently approximately ten Stx2 gene variants, with Stx2c being most commonly associated with HUS. The functional receptor for Stx1 and Stx2 is the neutral glycolipid globotriaosylceramide (Gb3). Gb3 receptors are present within the cytoplasmic membranes of susceptible cells. Often Stx1 and Stx2 are both isolated. Stx1 has a higher binding affinity for Gb3 and probably competes with Stx2 for binding sites. Stx2 binds more slowly but also dissociates at a slower rate. This may be of importance in Stx2 being more likely to induce vascular damage. In the piglet model, which develops severe CNS symptoms of HUS, animals infected with the STEC strain 0157:H7 containing both Stx1 and Stx2 developed neurologic complications 33% of the time versus 90% in those infected with an Stx2-producing strain of 0157:H7. The kidney endothelium has abundant Gb3 receptors and a high blood flow, which likely explains its particular susceptibility to injury. In addition to direct endothelial injury from Stx, release of cytokines from damaged cells appears to be of importance. Interleukin-6, interleukin-8, and tumor necrosis factor-α have been implicated.[1,7] By the time of presentation with HUS, STEC are often no longer present in the stool. Isolation rates dramatically drop by the end of the first week to the 20% to 30% range.[1-4]

Patients with leukocytosis >20,000 per mm^2 are more likely to have a positive stool culture for STEC.[1,4,5] In studies where culture as well as measurement of antibodies to 0157 lipopolysaccharide were undertaken, approximately 80% of patients in the United States were diagnosed as having STEC infection as the etiology of HUS. *E. coli* 0157 is the only STEC that can be easily identified by stool culture in most clinical labs. Non-0157 strains, identified by the Centers for Disease Control and Prevention (CDC) between 1983 and 1999, include serogroup 026 in 22% and 0111 in 14%.[3] In a recent prospective study from Germany and Austria, non-0157 strains were reported in 43% of 394 children with HUS. Disease was more severe in the cases with 0157 strains.[2] Cattle are the major reservoir for STEC. Despite increased public health efforts to prevent STEC infection, there has not been a decrease in infection rates thus far. Undercooked hamburger is well known to be a common source. Other reported sources have included unpasteurized milk, other foods contaminated by cattle such as unpasteurized apple cider and alfalfa sprouts, contaminated lake water, and the rails and soil of pastures in petting zoos. A recent outbreak of STEC infection was traced to exposure to a fairground building, where cultures of sawdust and rafters grew STEC 6 to 42 weeks after the outbreak. *E. coli* 0157 was probably dispersed through the air in some of those infected.[1-5]

Hemolytic Uremic Syndrome without Diarrhea

Diarrhea (−) HUS has been defined as microangiopathic anemia, thrombocytopenia, and ARF in the absence of diarrhea, implying the absence of STEC infection. It accounts for approximately 10% of HUS cases.[1,8] Urinary tract infection caused by STEC, producing HUS, technically falls into this classification since it is diarrhea (−). Generally, however, diarrhea (−) HUS is associated with a variety of etiologies (see Table 57.1) including other infectious agents, genetic forms, drug-induced causes, and autoimmune disease.[8] These patients have a varied presentation. In general, there is a more insidious onset, which may be characterized by upper respiratory symptoms, fever, and/or vomiting. Rapid onset of oliguria is less common. In genetic forms, recurrence or relapse is often seen. This group also has a high risk of end-stage renal disease with recurrence after renal transplant. Most reports have been retrospective in nature with small numbers of patients. A recent report describes 27 patients identified during enrollment of patients with HUS in a multicenter prospective study of SYNSORB-Pk between 1997 and 2001.[8] Complete data was available in 24 patients. Male:female ratio was 1.7; 17 of 24 (71%) were white, median age was 2 years, younger than in the diarrhea (+) group (median age of 4.2 years). Two thirds had a prodromal febrile illness lasting approximately 5 days. Seventeen of 24 patients (71%) required dialysis. Three of these (12.5%) did not recover renal function; the mean duration of dialysis for the remaining patients was 40 ± 27 days. Serious nonrenal complications were more common than in patients with diarrhea (+) HUS (91% versus 18%). Hypertension developed in 71%, cardiomyopathy with heart failure in 3 of 24 (12.8%) and

TABLE 57.1

ETIOLOGIES OF ATYPICAL DIARRHEA (−) HEMOLYTIC UREMIC SYNDROME

Infection Induced

Streptococcus pneumoniae
Group A streptococcus
Human immunodeficiency virus

Genetic Forms

Factor H deficiency
von Willebrand factor cleaving protease (ADAMTS13) deficiency
Intracellular defects of vitamin B_{12} metabolism
Membrane cofactor protein deficiency
Idiopathic autosomal recessive disease
Idiopathic autosomal dominant disease

Drug Induced

Cyclosporine, tacrolimus
Sirolimus
Mitomycin C, cisplatin, bleomycin
Ticlopidine
Quinine

Autoimmune Disease

Systemic lupus erythematosus
Antiphospholipid syndrome

seizures in 3 of 24 (12.8%). The most common etiology of HUS in this group was infection with *Streptococcus pneumoniae* which was isolated from blood, cerebrospinal fluid (CSF), or pleural fluid in 9 of 24 (38%) patients. In a review of reported cases of pneumococcal-induced HUS, an incidence of empyema as high as 51% has been reported. Other etiologies were too infrequent to analyze.

S. pneumoniae-induced HUS was first described in 1971. Its frequency has been reported by several authors to be increasing in recent years. In one recent study, 0.6% of children with invasive pneumonococcal infections developed HUS. The pneumococcus produces a circulating neuraminidase, which cleaves N-acetyl neuraminic acid from the glycoproteins on the cell membrane of RBCs, platelets, and glomerular capillary walls. Different strains likely produce different amounts. This exposes the Thomsen-Freidenreich antigen (T-antigen), which can react with immunoglobulin M (IgM) antibodies normally circulating against the T-antigen. Intravascular hemolysis ensues.[8,9] In a recent study, 6 of the 10 patients with pneumococcal-induced HUS were positive for RBC T-antigen activation.[9] Numerous groups have reported higher mortality rates from pneumococcal-induced HUS, ranging from 29% to 50% of patients.[8,9] The recent prospective study group surprisingly had no deaths from pneumococcal-induced HUS although hospitalization was longer.[8]

Imaging Studies

Renal ultrasound shows echogenic kidneys, sometimes enlarged, often with loss of corticomedullary differentiation. Blood flows in the acute phase may show decreased or absent diastolic flow with elevated resistive indices (RI). An improvement in RIs has been reported as predictive of impending improvement of renal function. Computed tomography (CT)/magnetic resonance imaging (MRI) in patients with neurologic symptoms have been reported to most often show abnormalities of the basal ganglia. A recent study reported changes in the dorsolateral portion of the lentiform nucleus to be the most characteristic finding. Abnormalities have also been seen in the thalamus, cerebellum, and brainstem. Subtle changes are clearly better demonstrated by MRI. The most predictive abnormality for long-term neurologic residua is a hemorrhagic component within a lesion.[10]

Pathology

The diagnosis of HUS is usually made on clinical and laboratory findings. Occasionally, renal biopsy is warranted. Patients with diarrhea (+) HUS most often have thrombotic microangiopathy of the glomerular capillaries and preglomerular arterioles with edema of endothelial cells, and widening of the subendothelial space. Glomerular capillaries contain RBCs, platelets, and fibrinogen. In severe cases, often with prolonged anuria, patchy or diffuse cortical necrosis may be seen. In patients with diarrhea (−) HUS, an arterial microangiopathy is more often seen rather than a glomerular lesion, affecting arterioles and interlobular arteries. Intimal edema, necrosis of arteriolar walls, luminal narrowing, and thrombosis are seen. Glomeruli appear ischemic and shrunken, often with wrinkling of the glomerular basement membrane. This lesion is more commonly seen in the presence of severe hypertension.[1]

TREATMENT

Despite numerous approaches to specific therapies for HUS, there is currently no definitive therapy other than supportive care for patients with diarrhea (+) HUS. Fresh frozen plasma (FFP) and/or plasmapheresis have/has been reported to benefit certain patients with diarrhea (−) HUS.[1-5,8] Supportive therapy and early dialysis have resulted in a dramatic fall in mortality.[1,4,5,8,9] Careful attention to fluid and electrolyte disturbances is of utmost importance. Once adequate volume replacement has been achieved, use of insensible losses plus replacement of urine output and other losses may be required. In patients with oliguria, the use of loop diuretics can be tried. Doses as high as 6 mg per kg intravenously have been tried as well as continuous infusion of furosemide.[5] Total parenteral nutrition may be needed because of intolerance to oral feedings.

RBC transfusions have been given in 37% to 75% of patients in various studies.[1-5,8,9] Recommendations in patients with *S. pneumoniae*-induced HUS have been to use only washed RBCs, because transfusion of blood products containing plasma can theoretically worsen the manifestations of HUS due to the presence of anti–T IgM antibodies in plasma.[8,9] There is no definitive data to support or refute these recommendations. Platelets have been transfused in 16% to 55% of patients, usually only for clinical bleeding or for surgical procedures. Routine platelet transfusions are generally avoided because of the potential risk of worsening the thrombotic process.[1-5,9] The need for dialysis has been reported in 50% to 60% patients.[1,2,4,5] Use of peritoneal dialysis has been most often reported, although contraindicated in patients with particularly severe colitis. Both hemodialysis and continuous hemofiltration have also been used. A combination of dialysis modalities is often required.[1,2,4,5,8]

Patients who develop CNS involvement require careful attention to detection and control of seizures. Cerebral edema is a common feature of severe CNS involvement. Strategies to decrease intracranial pressure may be indicated.[4,5] Use of mannitol in this situation is limited in those patients with renal failure because severe hyperosmolality can result. Hypertonic saline would be an acceptable alternative therapy.

Inotropic agents may be required in patients with significant cardiomyopathy. Extracorporeal-membrane oxygenation has been successfully used for life-threatening cardiac involvement as reported by Thomas et al. in 2004.[11] Hypertension may respond to decrease in intravascular volume in the presence of volume overload. However, antihypertensives may be required in addition.[1,4,5,8]

A recent randomized trial found no benefit of pulsed intravenous methylprednisolone as an anti-inflammatory therapy in these patients.[1] No benefit of FFP infusions or of plasmapheresis has been reported in diarrhea (+) HUS.[1] Plasmapheresis has been occasionally used in patients with particularly severe extrarenal manifestations, although there is no controlled data to support its use in these situations. Both FFP and plasmapheresis have been beneficial in patients with rare familial and genetic etiologies for HUS as well as in occasional patients with HUS from *S. pneumonia*.[1,5,8,9] Some patients with frequent relapses can be controlled with ongoing FFP infusions or plasmapheresis on a regular basis given weekly to monthly.

The use of antibiotics in patients with STEC infection remains controversial. A recent meta-analysis could not implicate the use of antibiotics in increasing the risk for development of HUS, concluding that the impact of this treatment is still unknown.[1] Three potential therapeutic approaches are being investigated in the hope that one or more of these therapies will show benefit to the patient with STEC-induced HUS. They include treatment with: (i) synthetic toxin binders, (ii) "probiotic" bacteria expressing Gb3 on their cell surface, and (iii) monoclonal

antibodies against Shiga toxin.[1,7] The first synthetic toxin binder to be used in humans, Synsorb-Pk had the trisaccharide of Gb3 receptor covalently bound to a silicon-based material. Children were enrolled in a prospective randomized trial from 1997 to 2001. The study was terminated early because of lack of benefit in the treatment group compared to the placebo group.[1,8] More recently, several more potent toxin binders (molecularly engineered polymers of Gb3) have been reported, one called *Super Twig*, another Synthetic Gb3 polymers. These agents show much higher affinity for Stx1 and Stx2 compared with Synsorb-Pk. Both agents have been protective in animal models of HUS. The effectiveness of these agents may depend on how early diagnosis and subsequent therapy can be instituted.[1,7] Recently, a nonpathogenic strain of *E. coli* and nonpathogenic *Neisseria* strain have been engineered to produce a lipopolysaccharide terminating in the Gb3 receptor. These probiotic bacteria bind Stx1 and Stx2 with much greater affinity than Synsorb-Pk, and can prevent lethal disease in mice. The same concerns as with synthetic toxin binders apply to these agents regarding need for very rapid diagnosis and treatment, likely within the first 2 to 3 days of onset of diarrhea. Maximum toxin production experimentally occurs during the logarithmic growth phase of the bacteria; once the stationary phase of growth is reached, no further toxin is produced. Despite the early production of toxin, circulating toxin or toxin bound to neutrophils has been detected for up to 1 week after diagnosis of STEC-induced diarrhea. Given this data, evaluation of these new approaches and trials of monoclonal antibodies appear to be warranted. From experimental studies, in mice and piglets, it appears that monoclonal antibodies directed against the A subunit of Stx2 are superior in protection from lethal disease. The A subunit causes inhibition of protein synthesis while the B pentamer chains are responsible for toxin binding to the target cell. These antibodies have protected piglets when given after the onset of diarrhea.[1,7] Phase I, II, and III trials are planned to determine pharmacokinetics in humans, and then to determine whether treatment of children presenting with bloody diarrhea can prevent HUS. Studies are also planned to use higher doses of these agents to treat children with HUS to determine whether the clinical course can be modified.[1,7]

REFERENCES

1. Tzipori S, Sheoran A, Akiyoshi D, et al. Antibody therapy in the management of Shiga toxin-induced hemolytic uremic syndrome. *Clin Microbiol Rev*. 2004;17:926–941.
2. Gerber A, Karch H, Allerberger F, et al. Clinical course and the role of Shiga toxin–producing Escherichia coli infection in the hemolytic uremic syndrome in pediatric patients, 1997–2000, in Germany and Austria: A prospective study. *J Infect Dis*. 2002;186:493–500.
3. Banatvala N, Griffin PM, Greene KD, et al. The United States National Prospective Hemolytic Uremic Syndrome Study:

Microbiology serologic, clinical, and epidemiologic findings. *J Infect Dis.* 2001;183:1063–1070.

4. Brandt JR, Fouser LS, Watkins SL, et al. Escherichia coli O 157: H7-associated hemolytic uremic syndrome after infection of contaminated hamburgers. *J Pediatr.* 1994;125:519–526.

5. Siegler RL. Spectrum of extra renal involvement in post diarrheal hemolytic-uremic syndrome. *J Pediatr.* 1994;125:511–518.

6. Askiti V, Hendrickson K, Fish AJ, et al. Troponin I levels in a hemolytic uremic syndrome patient with severe cardiac failure. *Pediatr Nephrol.* 2004;19:345–348.

7. Karmali MA. Prospects for preventing serious systemic toxemic complications of Shiga toxin—producing Escherichia coli infections using Shiga toxin receptor analogues. *J Infect Dis.* 2004; 189:355–359.

8. Constantinescu AR, Bitzan M, Weiss L, et al. Non–enteropathic hemolytic uremic syndrome: Course. *Am J Kidney Dis.* 2004; 43:976–982.

9. Cochran JB, Panzarino VM, Maes LY, et al. Pneumococcus-induced T–antigen activation in hemolytic uremic syndrome and anemia. *Pediatr Nephrol.* 2004;19:317–321.

10. Steinborn M, Leiz S, Rudisser K, et al. CT and MRI in hemolytic uremic syndrome with central nervous system involvement: Distribution of lesions and prognostic value of imaging findings. *Pediatr Radiol.* 2004;34:805–810.

11. Thomas NJ, Messina JJ, DeBruin WJ, et al. Cardiac failure in hemolytic uremic syndrome and rescue with extracorporeal life support. *Pediatr Cardiol.* 2005;26(1):104–106.

Renal Replacement Therapy

58

Stuart L. Goldstein

In general theoretical terms, acute renal failure (ARF) is defined as the sudden loss of the kidneys' ability to regulate fluid and electrolyte homeostasis. The determination of a practical ARF definition to guide patient management, however, has been hampered in both adult and pediatric populations by relying on serum creatinine concentration as the principal marker of renal function. Serum creatinine concentration is a less ideal ARF marker because of many reasons. First, serum creatinine does not differentiate the nature, type, and timing of the renal insult. Second, changes in serum creatinine concentrations often lag behind the changes in glomerular filtration rate (GFR). Third, dialysis readily clears serum creatinine, rendering its levels useless in the assessment for improving renal function once dialysis has begun. Recently, a consensus conference of nephrologists and intensivists has proposed a multidimensional ARF definition, termed *the RIFLE* (Risk, Injury, Failure, Loss, End-Stage Renal Disease) criteria, on the basis of differing degrees of GFR and urine output changes. The use of such criteria will be helpful in guiding decisions to initiate and terminate renal replacement therapy for patients with ARF, as well as to refine the epidemiology of ARF.

Provision for appropriate renal replacement therapy for pediatric patients with ARF requires special considerations that are not commonly encountered in the care of adult patients. Pediatric patients with ARF may range in weight from a 1.5-kg neonate to a 200-kg young adult. In addition, disease states that may require acute renal replacement therapy in the absence of significant renal dysfunction, such as inborn errors of metabolism or postoperative care of an infant with congenital cardiac defects, are more prevalent in the pediatric setting. Optimal care for the pediatric patient requiring renal replacement therapy demands an understanding of the causes and patterns of pediatric

ARF and multiorgan dysfunction syndrome (MODS) and a recognition of the local expertise with respect to the personnel and equipment resources.

PEDIATRIC ACUTE RENAL FAILURE EPIDEMIOLOGY

Advancements and improvements in the care for critically ill neonates, infants with congenital cardiac disease, and children with bone marrow or solid organ transplantation have lead to a dramatic broadening of pediatric ARF epidemiology. Although multicenter epidemiologic pediatric ARF data do not exist, single-center data from the 1980s report hemolytic uremic syndrome, other primary renal causes, sepsis, and burns as the most prevalent causes leading to pediatric ARF. More recent single-center data detail the underlying causes of pediatric ARF in large cohorts of children and demonstrate an epidemiologic shift in instances where ARF is more often a comorbidity of another underlying disease or systemic process. Bunchman et al.[1] reported data from 226 children with ARF treated with renal replacement therapy, with the most common causes being congenital heart disease, acute tubular necrosis (ATN), and sepsis. A more recent study evaluating all-cause pediatric ARF revealed that it more commonly results as a comorbidity or as a result of nephrotoxic treatment of another systemic illness.[2]

Until recently, most pediatric ARF treatment studies were limited to review articles. Such a dearth of pediatric data may result, in part, from the relatively recent changes noted in the clinical spectrum of pediatric ARF, as given in the preceding text, and the increased use of continuous renal replacement therapy (CRRT) to treat more critically ill children with ARF.

RENAL REPLACEMENT THERAPY

The classic indication for initiating renal replacement therapy is to remove hazardous levels of accumulated solutes or fluids from patients with ARF. Data supporting the initiation of renal replacement therapy earlier to prevent worsening solute or fluid accumulation are emerging and are discussed later in the chapter. Currently, three renal replacement modalities exist: intermittent hemodialysis (IHD), peritoneal dialysis (PD), and CRRT.

Renal replacement therapy process is driven by two concepts: clearance and fluid removal (ultrafiltration [UF]). Solute clearance during renal replacement therapy is accomplished by two mechanisms: diffusion down a concentration gradient across a semipermeable membrane and convection of solute driven by fluid removal. UF is controlled in IHD and CRRT by creating a transmembrane hydrostatic pressure and, for PD, by increasing the oncotic pressure of the dialysis fluid instilled intraperitoneally. Table 58.1 provides a summary of different dialytic techniques and the underlying physical principles.

IHD requires a vascular access, usually in the form of a dual-lumen venous hemodialysis catheter, a water source, a reverse osmosis water treatment system to make the dialysis fluid, a hemodialysis machine, and trained dialysis personnel. IHD treatments typically last for 3 to 4 hours, although, in a prolonged IHD therapy, termed *sustained low-efficiency dialysis (SLED)*, treatment times last up to 12 hours. Circuits receive heparin for anticoagulation, which is dosed on the basis of bedside activated clotting times. Complications of hemodialysis include bleeding, hypotension, and access problems (see Table 58.2).

PD does not require intravascular catheter, but rather a catheter placed into the peritoneal cavity. The advantage of PD over intermittent dialysis (ID) and CRRT is that no anticoagulation and no specifically trained dialysis personnel are needed. However, PD is a less efficient and less predicable modality with respect to solute and fluid removal. PD complications include catheter blockage, leakage along the tunnel, peritoneal-to-pleural dialysis fluid leak, and bacterial peritonitis.

CRRT has many advantages in supporting the critically ill patient with ARF. UF rates are lower than IHD because the therapy is provided continuously. Therefore, CRRT is better suited for patients with hemodynamic instability. In addition, UF rates can be adjusted with changes

TABLE 58.1

DIALYSIS MODALITIES

Technique	Dialyzer	Physical Principle
Hemodialysis		
Conventional	Hemodialyzer	Concurrent diffusive clearance and UF
Sequential UF/ clearance	Hemodialyzer	UF followed by diffusive clearance
UF	Hemodialyzer	UF alone
Hemofiltration		
SCUF	Hemofilter	Arteriovenous UF without a blood pump
CAVH	Hemofilter	Arteriovenous convective transport without a blood pump
CAVHD	Hemofilter	Arteriovenous hemodialysis without a blood pump
CAVHDF	Hemofilter	Arteriovenous hemofiltration and hemodialysis without a blood pump
CVVH	Hemofilter	Venovenous convective transport with a blood pump
CVVHD	Hemofilter	Venovenous hemodialysis with a blood pump
CVVHDF	Hemofilter	Venovenous hemofiltration and hemodialysis with a blood pump
Peritoneal Dialysis		
Intermittent	None	Exchanges are performed for 10–12 h every 2–3 d
CAPD	None	Manual exchanges are performed daily during waking h
CCPD	None	Automated cycling device performs exchanges nightly

UF, ultrafiltration; SCUF, slow continuous ultrafiltration; CAVH, continuous arteriovenous hemofiltration; CAVHD, continuous arteriovenous hemodialysis; CAVHDF, continuous arteriovenous hemodiafiltration; CVVH, continuous venovenous hemofiltration; CVVHD, continuous venovenous hemodialysis; CVVHDF, continuous venovenous hemodiafiltration; CAPD, continuous ambulatory peritoneal dialysis; CCPD, continuous cycling peritoneal dialysis.
From Irwin RS, Rippe JM. *Intensive care medicine.* Philadelphia, PA: Lippincott Williams & Wilkins; 2003.

TABLE 58.2

DIALYSIS COMPLICATIONS

Hemodialysis

Hypotension
Cramps
Bleeding
Leukopenia
Arrhythmias
Infections
Hypoxemia
Pyrogen reactions
Dialysis dysequilibrium syndrome
Angioaccess dysfunction
Technical mishaps
   Incorrect dialysate mixture, contaminated dialysate, air
     embolism, spallation

Hemofiltration

Bleeding
Thrombosis of hemofilter
Technical mishaps
   Incorrect dialysate mixture, incorrect replacement solution,
     contaminated dialysate, air embolism
Hemolysis
Angioaccess dysfunction
Hypotension
Congestive heart failure

Peritoneal Dialysis

Peritonitis
Catheter infections
Catheter dysfunction
Abdominal pain
Visceral perforation
Pleural effusion
Respiratory failure
Technical mishaps
   Inappropriate dialysate composition, contaminated dialysate

From Irwin RS, Rippe JM. *Intensive care medicine.* Philadelphia, PA: Lippincott Williams & Wilkins; 2003.

in fluid administration rates, which allows for a more consistent level of net fluid removal. CRRT provision requires a hemodialysis catheter, but the available dialysis/hemofiltration fluids are made with industry-standard sterile solutions, either provided in the final concentration by the manufacturer or made from a concentrate on site in the pharmacy. Another advantage of CRRT over hemodialysis is the availability of regional citrate anticoagulation. With this method, the circuit is anticoagulated with a citrate infusion that lowers the ionized calcium level to <0.5 mmol per L. A calcium infusion is provided to the patient to maintain a normal patient serum calcium level. Therefore, only the circuit is anticoagulated, whereas with standard heparin anticoagulation, the patient also runs the risk of systemic anticoagulation.

Transition from the use of adaptive CRRT equipment[3,4] to hemofiltration machines with volumetric control allowing for accurate UF flows has likewise led to a change in the prevalence patterns of the pediatric renal replacement therapy modality. Accurate UF and blood flow rates are crucial for pediatric CRRT because the extracorporeal circuit volume can comprise >15% of a small pediatric patient's total blood volume, and small UF inaccuracies may represent a large percentage of a small pediatric patient's total body water. Polls of the US pediatric nephrologists demonstrate increased CRRT use over PD as the preferred modality for treating pediatric ARF. In 1995, 45% of pediatric centers ranked PD and 18% ranked CRRT as the most common modality used for initial ARF treatment. In 1999, 31% of centers chose PD, versus 36% of centers that reported CRRT, as their primary initial modality for ARF treatment.[5]

SPECIFIC PEDIATRIC PATIENT POPULATIONS

The Critically Ill Pediatric Patient

Survival rates for critically ill children with ARF receiving renal replacement therapy have been fairly consistent from 1978 through 2001. The overall reported patient survival ranges from 52% to 58%. In the last decade, survival rates stratified by the renal replacement therapy modality have also been stable; survival rates for patients receiving hemodialysis (73% to 89%) are higher than those receiving PD (49% to 64%) or CRRT (34% to 42%),[1,2,6,7] which suggests that patients receiving IHD are more clinically stable than those receiving either PD or CRRT.

Unfortunately, many issues plague the pediatric ARF outcome literature, which include a relative lack of prospective study and the inconsistent use of methods to control the severity of patient's illness in the outcome analysis; few studies have considered the effect of a clinical variable on the outcome. Pediatric patients receiving CRRT and requiring pressors do appear to have an increased mortality rate compared to those without pressor need.

Few pediatric outcome studies have used a standardized scoring system to control for patient illness severity. Higher Pediatric Risk of Mortality (PRISM) scores have correlated with increased actual mortality in a limited number of patients.

A more recent study[6] examined the outcome of 22 critically ill children who received only venovenous CRRT modalities, and it used the PRISM score to control for illness severity at intensive care unit (ICU) admission and CRRT initiation. Neither the mean PRISM scores at the time of pediatric intensive care unit (PICU) admission nor the time of CRRT initiation differed between the survivors and nonsurvivors. Of the clinical variables studied (GFR, pressor number, mean airway pressure, patient size, or percentage fluid overload), only the degree of percentage fluid overload at the time of CRRT initiation differed between survivors (16.4% ± 13.8%) and nonsurvivors (34.0% ± 21.0%, $p = 0.03$), even when controlled for severity of illness by PRISM score using a multiple regression model. Subsequent single-center reports and a multicenter study[8] confirm the finding that the degree of fluid overload at CRRT initiation is an independent risk factor for mortality. These data, coupled with the predilection for early multiorgan system failure and death in critically ill children with ARF, argue for early and aggressive initiation of CRRT. Although the mean PRISM scores were not different between survivors and nonsurvivors, controlling for patient illness severity using PRISM scores was essential for mitigating concerns that the patients who received more fluid before CRRT initiation were more ill and, therefore, had a higher risk of mortality. Further study of a much larger cohort, using PRISM or other illness severity scoring systems, is clearly warranted to substantiate the findings of our relatively small study.

Infants

Infants and neonates with ARF present unique problems for renal replacement therapy provision. As noted earlier, the delivery of hemodialysis or CRRT to these small patients entails a significant portion of their blood volume to be pumped through the extracorporeal circuit. Therefore, extracorporeal hemodialysis and CRRT circuit volumes that comprise >10% to 15% of patient blood volume should be primed with the whole blood to prevent hypotension and anemia. Because the prime volume is not discarded, it is important to not reinfuse the blood into the patient at the end of the treatment to prevent volume overload and hypertension. When whole blood comes into contact with an AN69 membrane, commonly found in CRRT circuits, a syndrome termed *the bradykinin release syndrome* can occur, which leads to significant hypotension in the patient. This phenomenon may be mitigated by a bolus dose of calcium and sodium bicarbonate during CRRT initiation.

Acute PD requires much less technical expertise, expense, and equipment compared to IHD and CRRT. PD catheters can be placed quickly and easily. Initial dwell volumes should be limited to 10 mL per kg of patient body weight to minimize intra-abdominal pressure and the potential for fluid leakage along the catheter tunnel. Although PD may have a less efficient solute removal than hemodialysis or CRRT, its relative simplicity and minimally associated side effects allow for renal replacement therapy provision in settings lacking pediatric dialysis specific support and personnel.

CRRT has been prescribed since the mid-1980s for the treatment of ARF in critically ill infants. The first CRRT modalities were arteriovenous in configuration because the extracorporeal volumes were small in these circuits and

UF was driven by patient perfusion pressure, thereby reducing the risk of hypotension from too much UF. As mentioned before, the introduction of more accurate machines with volumetric control has increased the use of venovenous modality CRRT in pediatric patients, including neonates and infants. In an early neonatal outcome study in 1991 reporting patients who received either continuous arteriovenous hemofiltration (CAVH) or continuous venovenous hemofiltration (CVVH), Zobel noted that technical problems occurred only with CVVH. Symons et al. reported data from a more recent retrospective multicenter study evaluating the CVVH course for 90 infants >10 kg from 1993 through 2001, which demonstrated very few technical complications using newer CVVH machinery. Infant survival rate for patients receiving CRRT has also been consistent over the last decade at 35% to 38%, which is similar to the survival rates noted in the preceding text for older pediatric patients, although patients <3 kg exhibited a trend toward worse survival (24%) when compared to infants >3 kg (41%).[9]

FUTURE STUDIES

The recent epidemiologic pediatric ARF data presented in this chapter has demonstrated the need and laid the groundwork for future prospective pediatric study. Because pediatric ARF is relatively rare, a multicenter study will be required to enroll a sufficient number of patients for appropriate statistical analysis. Currently, a group of 13 US pediatric centers, the Prospective Pediatric Continuous Renal Replacement Therapy Registry Group (ppCRRT Registry),[10] is gathering data with respect to critically ill children who receive CRRT. The ppCRRT Registry aims to provide insight into the potential clinical factors that affect pediatric patient outcome, compare the efficacy of different anticoagulation protocols, assess specialized patient populations including those with metabolic disorders and bone marrow transplantation, and evaluate the efficacy and effects of CRRT cytokine removal. Future endeavors will include the assessment of CRRT pharmacokinetics, broadening the scope to include all pediatric patients with ARF and performing prospective randomized trials to evaluate the effect of CRRT dose and modality upon patient outcome.

REFERENCES

1. Bunchman TE, McBryde KD, Mottes TE, et al. Pediatric acute renal failure: Outcome by modality and disease. *Pediatr Nephrol.* 2001;16:1067–1071.
2. Hui-Stickle S, Brewer ED, Goldstein SL, et al. Pediatric ARF epidemiology at a tertiary care center from 1999 to 2001. *Am J Kidney Dis.* 2005;45:96–101.
3. Bunchman TE, Donckerwolcke RA. Continuous arterial-venous diahemofiltration and continuous venovenous diahemofiltration in infants and children. *Pediatr Nephrol.* 1994;8:96–102.

4. Bunchman TE, Maxvold NJ, Kershaw DB, et al. Continuous venovenous hemodiafiltration in infants and children. *Am J Kidney Dis*. 1995;25:17–21.
5. Warady BA, Bunchman T. Dialysis therapy for children with acute renal failure: Survey results. *Pediatr Nephrol*. 2000;15:11–13.
6. Goldstein SL, Currier H, Graf C, et al. Outcome in children receiving continuous venovenous hemofiltration. *Pediatrics*. 2001; 107:1309–1312.
7. Maxvold NJ, Smoyer WE, Gardner JJ, et al. Management of acute renal failure in the pediatric patient: Hemofiltration versus hemodialysis. *Am J Kidney Dis*. 1997;30:S84–S88.
8. Goldstein SL, Somers MJ, Baum MA, et al. Pediatric patients with multiorgan dysfunction syndrome receiving continuous renal replacement therapy. *Kidney Int*. 2005;67:653–658.
9. Symons JM, Brophy PD, Gregory MJ, et al. Continuous renal replacement therapy in children up to 10 kg. *Am J Kidney Dis*. 2003;4(5):984–989.
10. Goldstein SL, Somers MJ, Brophy PD, et al. The Prospective Pediatric Continuous Renal Replacement Therapy (ppCRRT) registry: Design, development and data assessed. *Int J Artif Organs*. 2004; 27:9–14.

Renal Pharmacology

59

Douglas L. Blowey   *James D. Marshall*

The renal system plays an essential role in the disposition of many therapeutic agents and adverse intoxicants encountered by infants and children in the intensive care unit (ICU). Renal dysfunction is an exceedingly common root cause or secondary finding in critical illness.

Potentially irreversible nephron damage may result from the appropriate pharmacotherapeutics that are necessary to manage a life-threatening disease, from iatrogenic misadventures, or from a combination of the two. A change in renal function may critically alter drug disposition. Carefully calculated dosing regimens, and possibly renal replacement therapy, should be initiated to accommodate the current and expected level of renal dysfunction, thereby avoiding effects adverse to many organ systems. While managing complex pharmacotherapeutics, a failure to clearly identify the therapeutic goal or to account for changes in drug disposition associated with renal failure can culminate in drug toxicity or inadequate treatment.

DRUG DISPOSITION

Understanding and using the relationship between the amount of drug administered and the clinical effect is the goal of rational therapeutics. The "LADMER" system describes this relationship: *L*iberation of drug from the dosage form; *A*bsorption into the systemic circulation, *D*istribution throughout the body; *M*etabolism in various systems; *E*xcretion from the body; and the *R*esponse or effect. The LADMER elements provide the basis for achieving the desired therapeutic drug concentration while avoiding unnecessary toxicity. Renal dysfunction and other recognized variables (e.g., age, mass and relative proportion of body fat or water, genetic idiosyncrasy, metabolic rate, and the health of other organ systems) might affect any LADMER variable.

Pharmacokinetics provides a mathematical description of the movement of drugs or drug metabolites through the various interactive body systems. The complementary science of pharmacodynamics describes the magnitude of a drug's response at its site of action and is more familiar to practitioners. Although complete pharmacokinetic compendia are available,[1] a highly detailed knowledge is not necessary to guide most ICU therapeutics. A working knowledge of the normal and abnormal parameters describing the disposition and effects of all agents employed during treatment is however essential when treating a critical child with renal disease.

Absorption

Absorption of drugs into the systemic circulation is primarily affected by the route of administration. When the drug is given intravenously, its absorption is considered complete in most cases, and renal insufficiency generally has no effect. Notable exceptions are the several important "prodrugs," agents that, as administered, are inert, requiring activation by a metabolic chemical alteration before becoming effective (e.g., fosphenytoin, chloramphenicol). Drugs administered *through* the gastrointestinal tract, intramuscularly, subcutaneously, topically, or intraperitoneally must be absorbed across tissues, which are subject to pathophysiologic variation (e.g., absorptive surface integrity, local pH, circulation, edema, and gastric and intestinal transit time) secondary to renal disease and associated critical illnesses. For example, scarring of the peritoneal cavity secondary to peritonitis may limit the absorption of drugs delivered in peritoneal dialysate. In this instance, drug absorption may range dramatically from increased to normal to nonexistent. As a basic assumption, ICU practitioners understand that only a fraction of the total dose of any nonintravenously administered agent and some prodrugs will be absorbed, and the fraction absorbed (F_a) is expressed as a proportion without units of measure.

$$F_a = \frac{\text{Dose}}{(Cp_{max} \times V_d)}$$

where F_a is the fraction absorbed, Cp_{max} is the maximal plasma concentration after a dose is fully absorbed, and V_d is the distribution volume.

The impact of renal failure on the fraction absorbed must be considered if pathophysiologic changes, which might cause a deviation from "normal," are obvious or if therapeutic failure is discovered. Understanding the factors that influence the fraction absorbed will lead to improved administration regimens. Some consequences of renal disease that may influence the fraction absorbed are listed in Table 59.1.

Distribution

As a drug enters the systemic circulation, it eventually distributes into tissue reservoirs. Relative drug partitioning among the various body tissues depends on factors including drug pK_a, plasma pH, degree of free drug binding to plasma proteins and tissue constituents, perfusion of tissue beds, concentration gradients across semipermeable membrane systems, and partitioning of the drug to fat or water (lipo- or hydrophilicity). Although some drugs are actively concentrated into certain tissues to the benefit or detriment of the patient, most drugs do not generally "seek" a tissue with active sites or receptors but are distributed through the body by physical forces.

TABLE 59.1

POTENTIAL CHANGES IN DRUG DISPOSITION WITH KIDNEY FAILURE

Parameter	Effect	Mechanism
Absorption	Decreased	Altered gastric pH
		Delayed gastric emptying
		Edema of intestinal absorptive surfaces
		Uremia-induced nausea and vomiting
		Subcutaneous edema
		Muscle wasting
		Drug interactions (phosphate binders, adsorptive resins, etc.)
Distribution	Increased	Expansion of body water
		Increased free (unbound) drug fraction
Metabolism	Decreased	Inhibition of cytochrome P-450 metabolism
		Drug interaction
		Direct inhibition by "uremic" milieu
	Increased	Induction of cytochrome P-450 metabolism
Excretion	Decreased	Decreased GFR
		Decreased tubular secretion
		Drug interaction
		Competition with "uremic" substances

GFR, glomerular filtration rate.

It is useful to summarize the effect of these numerous interactive forces by estimating the distribution volume (V_d), expressed in units of liters per kilogram.

$$V_d = \frac{(\text{Dose} \times e^{-k_e \times t_i})}{Cp_0}$$

where k_e is the elimination rate constant = elimination half-life/natural log 2, t_i is the infusion time, and Cp_0 is the plasma concentration at end-infusion.

The distribution volume relates plasma drug concentration to the total amount of drug in the body, and the result, when compared to body water, helps determine whether a drug is distributed primarily within the systemic circulation or to extravascular sites. The distribution volume is a hypothetical value with no true anatomic correlate. A large distribution volume implies that most of the drug present in the body resides *outside* the vascular space, whereas a small volume of distribution suggests that the opposite is true. In another view, the distribution volumes of agents that are effective at sites relatively distant from the bloodstream are larger, whereas those that are effective in highly perfused tissues may be smaller. Drugs that typically distribute into body water have distribution volumes of around 1 L per kg and, if not highly protein-bound in plasma, tend to reside in tissues (e.g., aminoglycosides, vancomycin). Regardless of the hydrophilicity, drugs that avidly bind to plasma proteins (e.g., albumin, α_1-acid glycoprotein) are restricted in their distribution to extravascular sites because, generally, only the protein-unbound (i.e., "free") drug is able to pass through intact membranes and interact with receptors at a site of action. Highly protein-bound drugs are typically characterized by small distribution volumes. For example, phenytoin is highly bound to albumin (90% to 95%) and has a small distribution volume (0.7 L per kg).

Renal disorders commonly encountered in critical care can dramatically affect the distribution volume, an effect that may result in therapeutic failure (Table 59.1). Edema, common to many forms of renal dysfunction, dramatically expands the distribution volume of agents such as aminoglycosides and vancomycin that preferentially distribute into body water. In these cases, a failure to quantify edema and increase the expected distribution volume, accordingly, will lead to underestimating the loading dose, with consequent delay of therapeutic effect. Chronic, severe renal disease or substantial nephrosis may lead to severe plasma protein deficiencies, such that the free, effective fraction of a highly protein-bound drug becomes relatively larger than normal. This results in an expanded distribution volume for highly protein-bound agents and, unless a reduced total dosing strategy is implemented, exposes the patient to potential toxicity. Similarly, uremia can induce changes in albumin structure, such that acidic drugs may be bound less avidly. The elimination of agents that have small distribution volumes because of avid protein binding is limited to the unbound fraction. As a clinical problem, dialytic therapy cannot be expected to reduce the total body burden of such agents rapidly. Therefore, treatment must be continued for an extensive period to prevent "rebound" elevation of the free fraction as the bound fraction reequilibrates.

The clinician finds the distribution volume to be objectively useful when calculating the loading drug dose, expressed in mg per kg, necessary to achieve instantaneous, effective, therapeutic serum drug concentration:

$$\text{Loading dose} = (Cp_{des} - Cp_{meas})V_d$$

where Cp_{des} is the plasma concentration desired, Cp_{meas} is the plasma concentration measured, and V_d is the distribution volume.

As discussed, the distribution volume chosen during loading dose calculation may require a fractional increase or decrease from normal, depending on influencing clinical variables. Once a proper loading dose has been given, a therapeutic plasma concentration will be achieved and the patient would have been optimally treated for the moment. Thereafter, the clinician may design further dosing strategies at greater leisure in consideration of other critical pharmacokinetic parameters.

Biotransformation

Biotransformation may be defined as the physicochemical conversion of a drug molecule to a new chemical moiety, a "metabolite." Many biotransformation processes are *de facto* steps toward detoxification in which the change decreases or eliminates drug activity. However, drug metabolites may be generated that have significant pharmacologic activity,[2,3] toxic properties,[4] and a disposition profile different from the parent drug.

Most tissues, including those in the kidney, possess the ability to biotransform drugs through cytochrome-mediated, oxidation–reduction or hydrolysis reactions or through conjugation with any of the several endogenous chemical substrates. These processes render the drug less active and more water- or fat-soluble. Quantitatively, the hepatic and gastrointestinal systems are by far the most important organs of drug metabolism. In fact, relatively few drug biotransformation profiles are substantially altered by renal disease or failure. Imipenem, high levels of which are toxic to the central nervous system, is dependent on the renal tissue for metabolism and the kidney for elimination. More commonly, other tissues produce potentially toxic accumulation of active drug metabolites that are dependent on the renal system for elimination. For example, whereas meperidine biotransformation proceeds unaltered in renal failure, the active and central nervous system–toxic metabolite normeperidine accumulates with repeated dosing and increases the risk of seizures in patients with renal failure.[4] Finally, nephrotoxicity may be caused by the limited, yet critical, intrinsic renal metabolism of a parent drug into a toxic intermediate that can induce local tissue damage. For example, a highly reactive intermediate metabolite generated by cytochrome-mediated hydroxylation of acetaminophen during acute

or chronic intoxication lethally binds sulfhydryl groups of local proteins, causing necrosis and contributing to renal failure. The potential changes in drug metabolism in children with kidney failure are listed in Table 59.1.

Elimination

Of the fraction of drug absorbed after administration, the amount of drug and drug metabolite eliminated from the body is a sum of elimination by the renal, hepatobiliary–intestinal, exocrine (salivary, mammary, sweat glands), and pulmonary systems. Although some or all of these systems may contribute to the elimination of any particular agent, the kidney is generally the most important. Various renal processes including glomerular filtration, active tubular secretion, and renal tubular reabsorption affect drug elimination.

Unless limited by size or charge, the unbound portion of circulating drug or metabolite is filtered through the glomeruli at a rate equal to the glomerular filtration rate (GFR). For drugs that are primarily eliminated by glomerular filtration, the rate of elimination mirrors the renal function, as measured by standard clinical tests (e.g., creatinine clearance). As such, when intrinsic glomerular health or systemic renal perfusion declines during critical illness, reduced drug elimination rate may result in corresponding accumulation and toxicity.

The active renal tubular secretion of drugs and drug metabolites by relatively nonspecific transport systems in the proximal tubule can contribute substantially to the amount of drug eliminated by the kidney. Driven by high-energy metabolic processes, renal tubular activity is exquisitely sensitive to perfusion and substrate delivery. As such, disorders that result in acute tubular necrosis will directly affect secretion-mediated clearance. The renal tubular secretion of a drug, a capacity-limited process, may be inhibited by other drugs or endogenous substrates that employ the same transport systems such as the competitive inhibition of tubular secretion of penicillin by probenecid.[5]

Reabsorption is the passive diffusion of nonionized (noncharged) drug from the filtrate into the renal tubular cell and, thereby, back into the systemic circulation. Therefore, tubular reabsorption may be considered as opposing total elimination. Relatively alkaline urine, pH >7.5, favors the ionized form of acidic drugs and limits reabsorption, whereas reabsorption of basic drugs is enhanced in basic urine because the nonionized form of the drug is favored. This concept is used clinically to manipulate the elimination of some toxins[6] or therapeutic agents. The potential changes in renal elimination in children with kidney failure are listed in Table 59.1.

The pharmacokinetic parameter of clearance mathematically objectifies the concept of elimination. Clearance refers to the blood volume that would have to be completely freed of drug over time to account for the observed elimination rate. Total clearance (Cl_{total}), which may be expressed as

L/kg/hr, is the clearance rate observed by studying the overall disposition of the drug through the body, whereas renal clearance (Cl_{renal}), expressed in the same units, denotes the fraction of total clearance rate due to renal activity alone.

$$Cl_{total} = (V_d)(k_e)$$

where Cl_{total} is the total clearance, V_d is the distribution volume, and k_e is the elimination rate constant, which is elimination half-life/natural log 2.

The clinical significance of decreased kidney function on a drug-dosing regimen is a function of the therapeutic index of the drug, renal clearance as compared to total clearance, and the potential decline or improvement in those renal functions that are responsible for a drug's renal clearance. Often, the most difficult task is to obtain an accurate measurement of renal function. During pharmacokinetic modeling in critically ill patients, perhaps the most important and commonly employed renal function test relates to the volume of water and accompanying solute that is filtered through the glomeruli per unit time, the GFR, which is estimated by measuring the rate at which the kidney removes a substance from the blood or the renal clearance of that substance. The measured substance may be an endogenous compound such as creatinine, an exogenous compound that is specifically administered to measure the GFR (e.g., inulin, isotope, iothalamate), or a compound primarily eliminated by glomerular filtration that is administered as part of clinical care (e.g., gentamicin). The clearance of creatinine is corrected for body surface area. Creatinine clearance (C_{cr}), expressed as mL/min/1.73 m², is calculated by measuring the amount of creatinine in an accurately timed urine collection and a midcollection plasma creatinine.

$$C_{cr} = \frac{\left[\begin{array}{c} \text{Urine Cr (mg/dL)} \\ \times \text{ (Urine volume (mL)/Time (minute))} \end{array} \right]}{\text{Plasma Cr (mg/dL)}} \times \frac{1.73 \text{ m}^2}{\text{BSA (m}^2)}$$

Creatinine clearance is low at birth and rapidly rises during the first 2 weeks of life, followed by a steady rise until adult values are reached by 8 to 12 months, and tables of age-related normal values are readily available.[7]

Although not as accurate as a timed urine collection, creatinine clearance can be estimated by measuring the child's serum creatinine and length.[8]

$$C_{cr} = \frac{\text{Length (cm)} \times K}{\text{Plasma Cr (mg/dL)}}$$

where K represents the creatinine production rate and varies with age—0.45 for a term newborn, 0.55 for a child, and 0.7 for an adolescent boy. It is important to understand that the normal relationship among serum creatinine, length, and GFR is altered in the presence of muscular disease and malnutrition or in clinical settings in which the serum creatinine is rapidly changing (e.g., acute renal failure, recovery from renal failure, and dialysis). In these situations, a timed urine collection is required for an accurate estimate of the GFR.

Once the renal clearance of creatinine has been quantified, the renal clearance of several drugs commonly used to treat the critically ill may be estimated. Aminoglycosides and vancomycin have narrow therapeutic indices, yet the clearance of these agents is primarily by glomerular filtration. Unrecognized reduced renal clearance may lead to ototoxic and nephrotoxic accumulation when subtle renal disorders with reduced GFR occur.

DIALYSIS

The impact of dialysis on drug disposition is determined largely by the extent of drug removal by dialysis. During dialysis, the systemic drug clearance encompasses renal, hepatic, and other intrinsic clearance pathways plus the additional clearance provided by dialysis. In general, drug removal is considered clinically significant when >25% of the administered dose is removed by dialysis. The failure to recognize the extent of drug removal and to provide supplemental dosing can result in underdosing. Drug elimination during dialysis occurs by diffusion and convection. The contribution of each process to the clearance varies among the different dialysis modalities. Diffusion is the movement of a drug across a dialyzer membrane or peritoneal membrane from a higher to a lower drug concentration. Although drug usually moves from the blood compartment to the dialysis fluid, it can be absorbed from the dialysis fluid when the drug concentration of the dialysis fluid exceeds the serum drug concentration, such as with the intraperitoneal administration of antibiotics during the treatment of peritonitis. Convection is the movement of drug across the dialyzer membrane or peritoneal membrane that occurs with the flow of an ultrafiltrate.

Dialysis removes only the free drug from the body because the drug bound to plasma proteins and other cellular constituents does not cross the dialyzer membrane or peritoneal membrane and is poorly removed by any form of dialysis. The efficiency of drug removal is the greatest by hemodialysis, medium by continuous renal replacement therapies (CRRT), and least by peritoneal dialysis. Although drug removal by CRRT and peritoneal dialysis is less efficient than that by hemodialysis, the total drug removal may be equivalent because CRRT and peritoneal dialysis are performed for a longer period.

CLINICAL APPROACH: PHARMACOLOGIC MANAGEMENT OF THE CRITICALLY ILL PATIENT WITH RENAL DISEASE

Perhaps the most common, costly, and avoidable iatrogenic complications occurring in the pediatric intensive care unit (PICU) arise from indiscriminate prescribing of

TABLE 59.2
STRATEGY FOR DRUG DOSING IN KIDNEY FAILURE

1. Review medication administration record
2. Determine whether there are any active or toxic metabolites and the degree of elimination by kidney
3. Estimate kidney function
4. Determine the percentage of drug elimination by the kidney
    a. If <25%: adjustment unlikely to be needed
    b. If >25%: adjustment may be needed
5. Adjust dose or dosing interval using "dosing adjustment factor" or published guidelines
6. If patient is receiving dialysis, evaluate the need for supplemental dosing
7. Monitor pharmacodynamic response
8. Monitor pharmacokinetic response (i.e., therapeutic drug monitoring, when available)
9. Consider clinical pharmacology or pharmacy consultation

pharmaceutical agents. One can frequently discover the source of unexpected morbidity simply by reviewing the medication administration record for improper dosing regimens, clinical circumstances, and drug interactions.

Much of this needless burdening could be avoided by using relatively noncomplex mental tools and excellent data sources that are freely available to both prescribers and those who prepare and administer pharmaceutical agents.

In critically ill infants and children with renal failure, and the subset who are receiving some form of dialysis, an individualized systematic approach (see Table 59.2) using the available adult and pediatric data on drug disposition in renal failure is required to design a drug administration regimen that maximizes the effectiveness of therapy while minimizing the potential for adverse effects. Familiarity with reference texts (e.g., Pediatric Drug Handbook,[9] Physician's Desk Reference, Micromedex) and the ability to rapidly perform computerized literature searches for information on drug disposition are needed. When renal disease is a component of the overall illness, an estimate of the relative contribution of renal clearance to the total drug elimination and the possible indirect influence of renal disease on other disposition parameters should be sought. Each agent to which the patient is exposed should be checked against the others for potential drug interactions. A list of treatment agents that are potentially nephrotoxic should be compiled. Finally, physical examination may reveal signs of disorders that might influence drug disposition, such as edema, kwashiorkor, jaundice, and systemic abnormalities such as poor cardiac output, hepatorenal syndrome, and hormonal imbalances that might influence renal function.

In each case in which information indicates a possible relationship between renal function and drug disposition, and if there is a suspicion of renal disease, the design of a successful therapeutic regimen begins with an estimate of the child's residual renal function. Although children receiving dialysis by definition have very poor renal function, it is inappropriate to assume that there is no renal elimination because many children maintain a significant amount of residual renal function. Failure to account for the continued renal elimination of drug may result in insufficient drug dosing and therapeutic failure. If one assumes that drug protein binding, distribution, and metabolism are not altered to a clinically significant degree in renal failure, an assumption that is likely true for most drugs, then a dosing adjustment factor (Q) can be estimated using the following equation:

$$Q = 1 - \left[\text{Fraction renal elimination} \times \left(1 - \frac{\text{Child's } Cl_{cr}(\text{mL/minute/1.73 m}^2)}{\text{Normal } Cl_{cr}(\text{mL/minute/1.73 m}^2)} \right) \right]$$

The appropriate dose amount or dosing interval for a child with reduced kidney function is generated by applying the dosing adjustment factor to either the normal dose amount ($Q \times$ normal dose = adjusted dose) or the normal dosing interval (normal dosing interval/Q = adjusted dosing interval). For example, the total gentamicin clearance is approximately 90% because of renal clearance. In a patient who requires gentamicin therapy, if creatinine clearance is 50% of normal, then a normal total daily dose of gentamicin must be multiplied by a Q value of 55% to avoid accumulation.

The dosage adjustment factor described in the preceding text estimates the changes in elimination associated with renal failure but does not account for any additional clearance by dialysis. Supplemental drug doses may be required to replace dialysis-induced drug losses. Whether a change is made in the dose amount, dosing interval, or both depends on the therapeutic goal and relationships between drug concentrations and clinical response *versus* toxicity. A pharmacodynamic assessment, possibly coupled with therapeutic drug monitoring before, during, and after dialysis or other treatments that will likely change drug disposition immediately or over time (e.g., extracorporeal-membrane oxygenation [ECMO], cardiopulmonary bypass), should be performed to check the adequacy of pharmacologic predictions.

Once the prescribed drug-dosing schedule has been adjusted for renal failure, a supplemental dose or dosing adjustment may be required for children receiving dialysis when >25% of drug is removed during the dialysis procedure. Supplemental dosing is given to replace the amount of drug removed by dialysis and may be achieved as a partial of the full dose administered after hemodialysis or as an increase in the dosing amount or frequency in children receiving peritoneal dialysis or CRRT. When possible, routine maintenance drugs should be provided after hemodialysis. Guidelines for drug dosing during dialysis are available in selected references.[10]

Of course, many pediatric patients present challenging pharmacotherapeutic issues to the clinician, and the tools of a simplified approach are rapidly exhausted. A pediatric clinical pharmacologist or pharmacist may be able to bring more knowledge and skill, or perhaps simply better access to critical data, to the bedside and assist the practitioner with individualized dosing regimens and monitoring.

REFERENCES

1. Ritschel W, Kearns GL. *Handbook of basic pharmacokinetics.* 5th ed. Washington, DC: American Pharmaceutical Association; 1999.
2. Bauer TM, Ritz R, Haberthur C, et al. Prolonged sedation due to accumulation of conjugated metabolites of midazolam. *Lancet.* 1995;346(8968):145–147.
3. Ball M, McQuay HJ, Moore RA, et al. Renal failure and the use of morphine in intensive care. *Lancet.* 1985;1(8432):784–786.
4. Szeto HH, Inturrisi CE, Houde R, et al. Accumulation of normeperidine, an active metabolite of meperidine, in patients with renal failure of cancer. *Ann Intern Med.* 1977;86(6):738–741.
5. Odugbemi T. An open evaluation study of sulbactam/ampicillin with or without probenecid in the treatment of gonococcal infections in Lagos. *Drugs.* 1988;35(Suppl 7):89–91.
6. Prescott L, Balali-Mood M, Critchley J, et al. Diuresis or urinary alkalinisation for salicylate poisoning. *Br Med J.* 1982;285: 1383–1386.
7. Arant BS Jr. Developmental patterns of renal functional maturation in the human neonate. *J Pediatr.* 1978;92(5):705–712.
8. Schwartz G, Brion LP, Spitzer A. The use of plasma creatinine concentration for estimating glomerular filtration rate in infants, children, and adolescents. *Pediatr Clin North Am.* 1987;34(3): 571–590.
9. Taketomo CK, Hodding JH, Kraus DM. *Pediatric dosage handbook.* 11th ed. Hudson, OH: Lexi-comp; 2004.
10. Veltri MA, Neu AM, Fivush BA, et al. Drug dosing during intermittent hemodialysis and continuous renal replacement therapy: Special considerations in pediatric patients. *Paediatr Drugs.* 2004;6(1):45–65.

Gastrointestinal Disorders

David M. Steinhorn   *Jonathan S. Evans*

Gastrointestinal Bleeding

60

Franziska Mohr   Marsha Kay

Gastrointestinal (GI) hemorrhage is a common presenting symptom in pediatric patients. Bleeding can occur anywhere along the highly vascularized GI tract and the clinical presentation may vary from chronic occult blood loss to acute life-threatening hemorrhage. The differential diagnosis for GI blood loss varies with age, location of bleeding site, and associated symptoms. The incidence of GI bleeding in children in the outpatient setting is not known. Published data is limited to children in the pediatric intensive care unit and reports indicate that upper GI hemorrhage occurs in 10% to 25% of critically ill children.[1]

DIFFERENTIAL DIAGNOSIS

Upper Gastrointestinal Bleeding in Neonates and Infants

Hematemesis and melena occur uncommonly in the neonatal period (see Table 60.1). Critically ill newborns having sepsis, respiratory failure, congenital heart disease, asphyxia, or intraventricular hemorrhage can develop GI bleeding due to gastritis or gastroduodenal ulcerations within the first few days of life. In the neonatal intensive care unit (NICU), up to 20% of all patients develop signs of GI bleeding.[2] Mechanical ventilation, delayed or abnormal delivery, and hypotension after birth are the primary risk factors for developing significant mucosal erosions. Stress-induced lesions can be found in up to 53% of patients on mechanical ventilation in the NICU, making these infants candidates for prophylactic gastroprotective treatment.[2] Upper GI bleeding has been described in up to 1.5% of healthy full-term newborns and often presents within the first 24 to 48 hours of life. Endoscopy reveals gastritis or gastric ulcers as the source of bleeding

TABLE 60.1

DIFFERENTIAL DIAGNOSIS: UPPER GASTROINTESTINAL HEMORRHAGE

Acutely Ill Patient	Clinically Stable Patient
Neonates and Infants	
Vitamin K deficiency	Swallowed maternal blood
Vascular malformations	Stress ulcer
Congenital blood dyscrasias	Gastritis, esophagitis
Duplication cyst	Maternal NSAID use
Coagulopathy due to septicemia	Nasogastric tube irritation
Aortoesophageal fistula	Mallory-Weiss tear
Toddlers and School-Aged Children	
Esophageal varices	Gastritis, esophagitis
Vascular malformations	Mallory-Weiss tear
Duplication cyst	Peptic ulcer disease
Aortoesophageal fistula	Pill esophagitis
Dieulafoy	Foreign body
Peptic ulcer with high-risk stigmata	Duplication cyst
Adolescents	
Gastric or duodenal ulcer	Gastritis, esophagitis
Esophageal varices	Mallory-Weiss tear
Dieulafoy lesion	Pill esophagitis
Aortoesophageal fistula	

NSAID, nonsteroidal anti-inflammatory drug.

in most cases. Esophagitis can be present in up to 38% of patients and duodenal ulcers have been described occasionally.[3] Coagulopathy leading to hemorrhage can be seen with overwhelming sepsis, maternal idiopathic thrombocytopenic purpura, von Willebrand disease, hemophilia, use

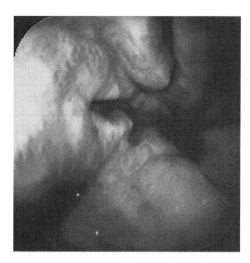

Figure 60.1 Endoscopic view of moderate-sized esophageal varices with multiple red marks. (From Yamada T, Alpers DH, Laine L, et al., eds. *Atlas of gastroenterology*, 3rd ed. Philadelphia, PA: Lippincott Williams & Wilkins; 2003.) (See color Figure 60.1.)

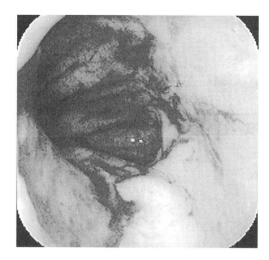

Figure 60.2 Endoscopic view of an oozing distal esophageal ulcer. (From Yamada T, Alpers DH, Laine L, et al., eds. *Atlas of gastroenterology*, 3rd ed. Philadelphia, PA: Lippincott Williams & Wilkins; 2003.) (See color Figure 60.2.)

of nonsteroidal anti-inflammatory drugs (NSAIDs), or vitamin K deficiency. Newborns with fat malabsorption (e.g., pancreatic insufficiency), altered bowel flora from antibiotic use, lack of vitamin K prophylaxis or liver failure, and infants who are exclusively breastfed are at increased risk of developing hemorrhagic disease of the newborn from vitamin K deficiency. Additionally, acid peptic disease becomes an increasingly common diagnosis in this age-group.

Upper Gastrointestinal Bleeding in Children

Many of the etiologies discussed for neonates and infants should be considered in the differential diagnosis of upper GI hemorrhage in toddlers and school-age children (Table 60.1). Peptic disorders such as esophagitis, gastritis, gastric ulcer, duodenitis, or duodenal ulcer are the most frequently identified etiologies. Primary peptic ulcer disease related to *Helicobacter pylori* is rarely seen in this age-group and almost all ulcers occur secondary to multisystem disease.[1] Acute hematemesis in young children should trigger careful abdominal examination for signs of extrahepatic portal hypertension such as hepatomegaly or splenomegaly. In extrahepatic portal hypertension, esophageal and gastric varices develop early in life in most cases and frequently present with hematemesis before the age of 5 years (see Fig. 60.1). In a patient with painless hematemesis, a Mallory-Weiss tear is an important diagnostic consideration. Dieulafoy lesion can present in toddlers and school-age children with massive recurrent upper GI hemorrhage.

Upper Gastrointestinal Bleeding in Adolescents

The aforementioned entities can present in adolescents (Table 60.1), although bleeding originates in this age-group most commonly from peptic ulcer disease. Medication history can be helpful in patients presenting with bleeding from esophagitis, because bleeding may be associated with the use of aspirin, NSAIDs, ferrous sulfate, potassium, quinidine, alendronate, or tetracyclines. Pill-induced esophagitis can, in rare cases, ulcerate and perforate into adjacent organs including the left atrium or major vessels and result in uncontrollable hemorrhage (see Fig. 60.2). Adolescents can present with Mallory-Weiss tears, Dieulafoy lesion, or variceal bleeding. Chronic liver disease as the etiology for portal hypertension is more prevalent in this age-group.

Specific Lesions

Esophagitis, Gastritis, and Peptic Ulcer Disease

Erosive esophagitis leading to bleeding is frequently caused by severe gastroesophageal reflux disease and is often associated with neuromuscular disease or hiatus hernia. Acid suppression with either H_2-receptor antagonists or proton pump inhibitors is indicated to decrease the inflammatory response and allow for mucosal healing. In some cases, additional treatment with prokinetic agents such as metoclopramide is warranted. Viral esophagitis may present with hematemesis and is typically caused by herpes simplex virus, cytomegalovirus, or occasionally varicella-zoster virus. It should be considered in the immunocompromised host presenting with odynophagia or dysphagia not responding to acid suppression therapy. Eosinophilic esophagitis is an increasingly recognized entity that occasionally presents with bleeding from mucosal ulcerations. The hallmark of the disease is inflammation of the mucosa due to eosinophilic infiltrates that may be associated with food allergies.

Peptic ulcer disease is one of the most common causes of mucosal bleeding in children although the incidence is much lower in the pediatric population than in adults. In children younger than 10 years, almost all ulcers are associated with contributing risk factors such as antibiotic use, underlying inflammatory bowel disease, NSAID use, or stress from severe head injury, burns, sepsis, major surgery, or associated with coagulopathy. Peptic ulcer disease in adolescent patients without additional risk factors is usually based on *H. pylori* infection. Ulcers are frequently located in the duodenal bulb and can present with significant hematemesis or melena due to their close proximity to the large gastroduodenal blood vessels. Treatment may consist of a combination of acid suppression and *H. pylori* eradication therapy for primary peptic ulcer disease or acid suppression and treatment of the underlying pathology in cases of secondary peptic ulcer disease. In some cases, endoscopic as well as medical treatment for bleeding mucosal lesions is required.

Mallory-Weiss Tear

The typical presentation of a Mallory-Weiss tear is hematemesis, often with a preceding history of retching. Episodes of forceful vomiting, hiccupping or coughing, as well as trauma from vigorous use of oropharyngeal suction or passage of a nasogastric tube can result in mucosal lacerations that may lead to significant hemorrhage. Bleeding from these lesions is usually self-limited and seldom requires therapeutic intervention. Confirmation of the suspected diagnosis can be achieved by endoscopy. Longitudinal lacerations close to the esophagogastric junction are the hallmark of the diagnosis. Treatment with acid suppression and barrier agents like sucralfate can help promote the healing process.

Varices

Bleeding from esophageal or gastric varices is an uncommon but potentially life-threatening cause of severe GI hemorrhage in children. Varices develop as a complication of portal hypertension due to underlying liver disease or from extrahepatic causes such as cavernous transformation of the portal vein. The rise of portal pressure causes development of collateral vessels and portosystemic shunting. Shunts develop at the gastric cardia, between the coronary veins and esophageal veins, in the abdominal wall from the umbilical vein, in the anal canal between the inferior mesenteric and inferior hemorrhoidal veins, and from the gastric, splenic, and adrenal veins to the renal vein. If the hepatic venous pressure gradient increases to >12 mm Hg, esophageal varices start to develop.[4] Forty percent to 70% of children with liver cirrhosis due to biliary atresia develop varices before the age of 5 years and 90% of children with cirrhosis caused by cystic fibrosis will develop varices on average within 3 years of the first sign of liver disease. The lifetime bleeding risk from varices for children with liver cirrhosis is thought to be 22%, but increases to 38% in those with known varices due to liver cirrhosis. In patients with extrahepatic portal hypertension, the lifelong risk of

bleeding from varices is even higher at 80%, with 50% of episodes of first bleeding occurring before the age of 5 years.

Dieulafoy lesion

A Dieulafoy lesion is an uncommon cause of hematemesis in children. Affected patients usually present with massive hematemesis, melena, or hematochezia without associated pain or systemic symptoms. The bleeding originates from a small abnormal submucosal artery that may be congenital in origin and is typically located in the proximal stomach. It erodes through the mucosa and causes significant bleeding.

Angiodysplasia

In children, angiodysplasia occurs most frequently as part of hereditary hemorrhagic telangiectasia (Rendu-Osler-Weber syndrome). Bleeding occurs from lesions in the small intestine. Although episodes are frequently self-limited, bleeding can be massive and difficult to control. Additional causes of visceral telangiectasia in pediatric patients include Turner syndrome, Fabry disease, von Willebrand disease, and *c*alcinosis, *R*aynaud phenomenon, *e*sophageal motility disorders *s*clerodactyly, and *t*elangiectasia (CREST) syndrome, and lesions occur anywhere in the alimentary tract.

Others

Bezoars and ingested foreign bodies can cause mucosal erosions and ulceration. When a foreign body is lodged in the esophagus for a prolonged period, it may result in deep ulcerations and tissue necrosis leading to perforation into adjacent structures. The most severe complication is an aortoesophageal fistula, a rare cause of massive GI hemorrhage associated with high rates of morbidity and mortality. This has been described after prolonged nasogastric intubation, especially in children with right aortic arch as well as after cardiac or aortic surgery. Hemobilia, defined as bleeding into the biliary ducts, can present with hematemesis, melena, or hematochezia. It can derive from a ruptured hepatic artery aneurysm, crush injury to the liver, massive hepatic necrosis, or after liver biopsy. The treatment is directed at the underlying pathology.

Lower Gastrointestinal Bleeding in Neonates and Infants

In neonates and infants, a wide variety of diseases can present with hematochezia (see Table 60.2).

An important cause of rectal bleeding in neonates and infants is necrotizing enterocolitis. Most patients with this condition are preterm infants usually in the NICU presenting with abdominal distension, vomiting, and signs of systemic illness before the bleeding occurs. Midgut volvulus and enterocolitis associated with Hirschsprung disease are potential life-threatening etiologies for rectal bleeding in the newborn period. In both conditions, bleeding occurs late in the illness. Infectious enterocolitis can present at any age. The pathogens identified most commonly in patients presenting with bloody diarrhea are *Salmonella, Escherichia coli, Shigella, Campylobacter,* and *Clostridium difficile.* In children younger than 2 years, the presence of *C. difficile* toxin in the stool can be a normal finding in healthy individuals and may not represent the etiology of the rectal bleeding. Intussusception and Meckel diverticulum may also present in infants.

Lower Gastrointestinal Bleeding in Children

Most of the etiologies for rectal bleeding discussed in the preceding text may also present in toddlers and school-aged children (Table 60.2). A common bleeding source in children older than 1 year is a colonic polyp. Recurrent episodes of painless hematochezia are the typical presentation. Meckel diverticulum, duplication cysts, infectious colitis, and anal fissures present commonly in this age-group. Occasionally, massive upper GI bleeding due to peptic ulcer disease or vascular malformation can present

TABLE 60.2

DIFFERENTIAL DIAGNOSIS: LOWER GASTROINTESTINAL HEMORRHAGE

Acutely Ill Patient	Clinically Stable Patient
Neonates and Infants	
Necrotizing enterocolitis	Swallowed maternal blood
Infectious colitis	Dietary protein intolerance
Malrotation with volvulus	Anorectal lesions
Disseminated coagulopathy	Duplication cyst
Vitamin K deficiency	Meckel diverticulum
Duplication cyst	Vascular malformations
Meckel diverticulum	
Vascular malformations	
Congenital blood dyscrasias	
Intussusception	
Toddlers and School-Aged Children	
Meckel diverticulum	Anal fissures
Vascular malformations	Polyps/polyposis syndrome
Intussusception	Infectious colitis
Hemolytic uremic syndrome	Inflammatory bowel disease
Ischemic colitis	Henoch-Schönlein purpura
Neutropenic colitis/typhlitis	Lymphoid nodular hyperplasia
Duplication cyst	Vascular malformations
	Meckel diverticulum
	Duplication cyst
Adolescents	
Ischemic colitis	Anal fissures
Vascular malformations	Polyps/polyposis syndrome
Duplication cyst	Infectious colitis
Neutropenic colitis/typhlitis	Inflammatory bowel disease
Infectious colitis	Hemorrhoids
Inflammatory bowel disease	

with hematochezia because the cathartic effect of blood decreases the intestinal transit time significantly. In the setting of an acutely ill child presenting with a history of acute gastroenteritis and bloody stool, hemolytic uremic syndrome should be considered. Acute colitis develops in approximately 50% of patients and is often seen with toxin producing *E. coli* (0157:H7). Inflammatory bowel disease can also present in this age-group. Vascular malformations include arteriovenous malformations, hereditary hemorrhagic telangiectasia, and intestinal cavernous hemangiomas. In the immunocompromised patient, lower GI hemorrhage is seen with neutropenic colitis or typhlitis. In this scenario, the diagnosis should be established by computed tomography (CT) scan as colonoscopy carries a high risk for complications including perforation.

Lower Gastrointestinal Bleeding in Adolescents

The differential diagnosis of rectal bleeding in adolescents comprises many of the previously listed disorders, but is most frequently associated with colitis (Table 60.2). Infectious causes can be identified in many cases of adolescents with bloody diarrhea. Polyps can be the etiology of lower GI bleeding although isolated polyps are less common after the onset of puberty. Polyps can occur either as isolated benign polyps, or as part of a number of polyposis syndromes including familial adenomatous polyposis, juvenile polyposis coli, Peutz-Jeghers syndrome, hereditary nonpolyposis colorectal cancer, and Turcot syndrome.

Specific Lesions

Infectious Colitis

In children presenting with acute lower GI hemorrhage and associated altered bowel movements, GI infection should be suspected. The most important bacterial pathogens leading to bloody diarrhea are *Salmonella, Shigella, Campylobacter,* or *E. coli. C. difficile* is another important pathogen inducing bacterial colitis particularly in patients with a prior history of antibiotic use or hospitalization or in those who are immunocompromised. In addition, parasitic infections should be considered in patients with recent history of foreign travel, exposure to contaminated water sources, or elevated peripheral eosinophil count, although most are not associated with rectal bleeding. In the immunocompromised host, viral infections or infections due to other agents can cause significant colitis, leading to rectal bleeding. Cytomegalovirus has been reported as a cause of life-threatening hemorrhage due to colitis in a patient with immunodeficiency syndrome. *Mycobacterium avium intracellulare* can present with diarrhea and small bowel ulceration, especially in immunocompromised hosts. Diagnosis of infectious colitis can frequently be made by stool cultures and stool evaluation for ova and parasites. Occasionally, when no organism can be identified, colonoscopy and biopsy may be required. Most bacterial infections are self-limited and do not require antibiotic treatment in all but the immunosuppressed patients. Pseudomembranous colitis due to *C. difficile* is an exception. Left untreated, this can lead to significant morbidity and can result in complications including toxic megacolon and colonic perforation. The preferred first-line therapy is metronidazole, but some patients may require treatment with oral vancomycin for eradication. Addition of a probiotic appears to be helpful in management of this pathogen.

Inflammatory Bowel Disease

Up to 25% of all patients with inflammatory bowel disease present before the age of 20 years. Some patients with this condition can present with massive and life-threatening hemorrhage, often following a "herald" bleed. Treatment consists of a combination of anti-inflammatory and immunosuppressive therapy, nutrition support, and in some cases antibiotic treatment if coinciding bacterial infections such as *C. difficile* are suspected.

Meckel Diverticulum/Duplication Cysts

Meckel diverticulum is the most common cause of small bowel hemorrhage in children. This congenital remnant of the omphalomesenteric duct is present in approximately 2% of all patients. Ectopic gastric mucosa can be found in 90% of bleeding Meckel diverticula and the diverticulum is usually located within 2 feet of the ileocecal valve. Children commonly present with painless hematochezia before the age of 2 years. Bleeding from intussusception of the diverticulum with resultant ischemia has also been described. In children with suspected ectopic gastric mucosa, the diagnosis can be made with the technetium-99m pertechnetate scan. Once identified, surgical excision of the lesion is the treatment of choice. Duplication cysts are the second most common source of bleeding in the small bowel. They arise mainly from the mesenteric border of the small bowel, but can be present anywhere in the GI tract. As in Meckel diverticulum, bleeding is usually painless and originates from ectopic gastric mucosa or ischemic injury due to intussusception. Diagnosis is made through nuclear medicine scan or CT scan although some cases are diagnosed at the time of surgery. Treatment is surgical resection.

Vascular Malformations

In addition to hereditary hemorrhagic telangiectasia and visceral telangiectasia associated with Turner syndrome, Fabry disease, von Willebrand disease or CREST syndrome, hemangiomas are a known cause of hematochezia. Diffuse cavernous hemangiomas, when present in the GI tract, are usually located in the jejunum. Associated hemangiomas of the skin can aid in the diagnosis. Bleeding from these lesions is uncommon in children older than 2 years. Blue rubber bleb nevus is a condition of multiple cavernous hemangiomatous malformations occurring in the skin and

throughout the GI tract and may present with bleeding or intussusception. Arteriovenous malformations are mainly located in the right colon and may also be found in patients with hereditary hemorrhagic telangiectasia.

Others

Occult or gross blood in the stool is found in 25% to 50% of patients with Henoch-Schönlein purpura. Intussusception is a rare but potentially life-threatening complication.

DIAGNOSTIC EVALUATION

Laboratory

It is imperative to determine whether this in fact represents GI blood loss. Stool samples that contain blood will turn the guaiac test rapidly positive. False-positive results can occur after ingestion of peroxidases from plants (melons, radishes, turnips, and horseradish), red meat, and iron preparations. False-negative results can be seen with consumption of large doses of ascorbic acid. A complete blood count, partial prothrombin, and partial thromboplastin time as well as type and cross match are usually indicated. Additional tests including aspartate aminotransferase, alanine aminotransferase, γ-glutamyl transpeptidase, bilirubin, blood urea nitrogen (BUN), creatinine, albumin, and total protein can be helpful. In patients presenting with hematochezia, measuring BUN/creatinine ratio has been shown as useful in distinguishing upper from lower GI hemorrhage. A ratio >30 has a sensitivity of 98% for upper GI bleeding.[5]

Imaging

Diagnostic radiology is of limited value in the initial evaluation. In children with suspected foreign body ingestion, bowel perforation, or obstruction, a plain radiograph can be helpful. Barium contrast examination is useful in identifying esophageal strictures, malrotation of the gut, or intussusception, but is inferior to endoscopy in diagnosing mucosal lesions such as esophagitis, gastritis, or peptic ulcer disease, because the contrast in the GI tract can make visualization of the mucosa more difficult. Ultrasonography is helpful when liver disease, portal hypertension, or large vascular abnormalities are suspected, and is often performed after endoscopy when active bleeding has subsided.

CT scan or magnetic resonance imaging (MRI) may be used to evaluate for mass lesions and vascular malformations once the patient has been stabilized and no acute deterioration is anticipated.

Nuclear Medicine

When endoscopy and contrast studies have failed to establish a diagnosis, scintigraphy can aid in identifying the bleeding source. Technetium 99m sulfur colloid detects active bleeding rates as low as 0.05 to 0.1 mL per minute. The tracer has a half-life of <2.5 minutes and is concentrated in the reticuloendothelial system. Intermittent bleeding or slow blood loss can be missed during the short time interval between injection and clearance of the tracer. Another disadvantage is the inability to identify lesions in areas that are superimposed by the liver or spleen, as tracer is concentrated in both organs. The tagged red blood cell (RBC) scan can be used to identify lesions that are actively bleeding at the time of imaging. Patient's RBCs labeled with technetium-99m pertechnetate remain in the circulation for up to 24 hours after injection. Delayed imaging increases the sensitivity of the test as intermittent bleeding episodes are more likely to be captured. Studies in adults have shown negative imaging during the first 3 hours after injection followed by positive scans on delayed imaging in up to 73% of patients.[6]

Meckel diverticulum is diagnosed with technetium-99m pertechnetate injected intravenously. It loosely binds to plasma proteins and accumulates in functional gastric mucosa including the stomach and ectopic locations. There is a relatively high false-positive and false-negative rate of up to 20%.

When endoscopy and scintigraphy do not identify a bleeding source, angiography can be useful to not only determine the site of hemorrhage but also to intervene therapeutically either by embolization or infusion of vasoconstrictive agents such as vasopressin. Angiography detects blood loss at a rate of 0.5 mL per minute or more and is therefore less sensitive than scintigraphy. In adults, angiography can successfully establish the diagnosis in 71% of patients with an acute bleeding episode, but only in 55% of patients with chronic blood loss.

Endoscopy

Endoscopy is the preferred diagnostic tool in the evaluation and treatment of patients with acute GI hemorrhage. Endoscopy is able to determine the site of bleeding in up to 80% of cases for upper GI bleeding and up to 40% of cases for bleeding sources distal to the ligament of Treitz. In addition, endoscopy provides information regarding the likelihood of rebleeding and means of immediate intervention. Complication rates for emergency endoscopies are higher than those associated with elective endoscopies.

Only approximately 5% of patients experience recurrent bleeding from an unidentified source.[7] When additional diagnostic steps are unsuccessful or if small bowel lesions are suspected, capsule endoscopy offers valuable information. In adult series, capsule endoscopy successfully identified a bleeding source in 92% of patients with ongoing obscure overt bleeding who had negative results on upper and lower endoscopy, but only in 44% of patients with occult bleeding and 12.9% with remote episodes of obscure overt bleeding. In two recent pediatric studies, capsule endoscopy

identified a bleeding source in 75% to 80% of children with obscure occult GI hemorrhage. The main complication of the investigation is that the capsule can become lodged in a stricture, fistula, or diverticulum.

TREATMENT

Medical Treatment

A nasogastric tube should be passed in almost all cases of upper GI bleeding. This allows for the removal of gastric content, as well as residual blood, and early detection of renewed bleeding. Gastric lavage with iced water with or without epinephrine was used in the past, but benefit has not been established; the procedure carries the risk of hypothermia and therefore this therapy is no longer performed. In patients with mucosal erosions or ulcerations such as esophagitis, gastritis, duodenitis, gastric ulcer, duodenal ulcer, and Mallory-Weiss tear, treatment options include neutralization of gastric acid as well as decrease of its production. At a gastric pH of 4 or greater, acid has been suppressed sufficiently to prevent further damage and allow for healing. The use of antacids should be limited in patients with renal impairment because of potential toxicity. H_2-receptor antagonists prevent release of gastric acid and are often the first-line therapy because injectable forms are widely available. H^+/K^+ ATPase blockers inactivate the proton pump and thereby inhibit the release of gastric acid with greater potency and longer lasting effect than H_2-blockers. Intravenous forms have recently become available for use. Sucralfate is a basic aluminum salt that is viscous at acid pH and forms a protective layer that selectively adheres to the ulcer base. It has no antacid properties and its main side effect is constipation secondary to the aluminum content. In the clinical setting, a combination of H_2-blocker or proton pump inhibitor with sucralfate is often used.

Somatostatin

Somatostatin is an amino acid peptide that inhibits vasodilatory GI peptides including glucagon, vasoactive intestinal peptide (VIP), and substance P. It decreases azygous blood flow by selective vasoconstriction of the splanchnic system, thereby lowering portal pressure. Bolus injections of the drug cause rapid and significant decrease in splanchnic flow and show significant effect on controlling acute bleeding episodes when compared to placebo in studies conducted in adult patients. The recommended dosage is one to three bolus injections of 250 μg per bolus followed by a continuous infusion of 3 to 5 μg/kg/hour (maximum 250 μg per hour).[8] Side effects are less severe compared to vasopressin and include hyperglycemia, gall bladder stasis, flushing, nausea, dyspepsia, bradycardia, and steatorrhea. Blood glucose levels should therefore be monitored closely in children on somatostatin therapy.

Octreotide

Octreotide is a synthetic analog of somatostatin, which decreases splanchnic blood flow with a longer half-life than somatostatin. It has an inconsistent effect on the hepatic venous pressure gradient and intravariceal pressure, but leads to significant reduction in azygous blood flow. The recommended dose for pediatric patients is a bolus of 1 μg per kg (maximum 50 μg) followed by a continuous infusion of 1 to 2 μg/kg/hour (maximum 50 μg per hour).[9,10] The infusion is tapered 24 to 48 hours after cessation of bleeding and can be readministered if rebleeding occurs. Randomized controlled trials have shown better control of bleeding with fewer side effects using octreotide compared to vasopressin.[11] Bleeding ceases in up to 71% of children with portal hypertension, but renewed bleeding occurs in up to 52% after stopping therapy. In children with bleeding that is unrelated to portal hypertension, octreotide therapy successfully terminates initial bleeding episodes in 50%, with rebleeding in up to 29% of patients after stopping of therapy.[12] The greatest reduction in bleeding can be achieved when octreotide is used in combination with endoscopic treatment.

Vasopressin

Vasopressin binds to the V_1 receptor of vascular smooth muscle cells leading to vasoconstriction in the mesenteric arterial system. This decreases portal venous inflow and therefore reduces portal venous pressure. Because of the risk of significant side effects and the availability of superior alternatives, vasopressin is no longer the drug of choice for pharmacologic control of acute GI hemorrhage.

Endoscopic Therapy

In the management of acute GI bleeding in children, a variety of endoscopic techniques are available to achieve hemostasis. Lesions that are particularly at risk for severe bleeding include deep ulcers of the lesser curvature of the stomach or those in the posterior duodenal bulb because of close proximity to large blood vessels. When treating high-risk lesions, surgical intervention should be immediately available, because torrential bleeding that is uncontrollable through endoscope may develop. Studies in adults have shown an increased risk for rebleeding (up to 50% or more) in patients with an ulcer with evidence of active bleeding, an ulcer with visible vessel at its base, and vascular malformations. These lesions, when identified, should be treated endoscopically if possible.

A variety of endoscopic injection therapies are available including hypertonic saline, epinephrine mixed with either normal or hypertonic saline, and absolute ethanol. Complications of injection therapy include ischemia, rebleeding, and perforation. Complications following sclerotherapy of esophageal varices range from superficial to deep ulcerations and rarely perforation. Esophageal strictures are reported at a rate of 5% to 20% in most pediatric case series. Ischemic spinal cord injury, mediastinitis, and esophageal dysmotility have been reported infrequently following injection therapy. Band ligation is another technique to stop varix bleeding.

Coagulation devices include thermocoagulation and the argon plasma coagulator (a noncontact endoscopic thermal coagulator).

REFERENCES

1. Cochran EB, Phelps SJ, Tolley EA, et al. Prevalence of, and risk factors for, upper gastrointestinal tract bleeding in critically ill pediatric patients. *Crit Care Med.* 1992;20(11):1519–1523.
2. Kuusela AL, Maki M, Ruuska T, et al. Stress-induced gastric findings in critically ill newborn infants: Frequency and risk factors. *Intensive Care Med.* 2000;26:1501–1506.
3. Lazzaroni M, Petrillo M, Tornaghi R, et al. Upper GI bleeding in healthy full-term infant; a case-control study. *Am J Gastroenterol.* 2002;97:89–94.
4. Garcia-Tsao G, Groszman RJ, Fisher RL, et al. Portal pressure, presence of gastroesophageal varices and variceal bleeding. *Hepatology.* 1985;5:419–424.
5. Kay M, Wyllie R. Gastrointestinal hemorrhage. In: Wyllie R, Hyams J, eds. *Pediatric gastrointestinal and liver disease.* 3rd ed. London: Elsevier Science; In Press.
6. Zettinig G, Staudenherz A, Leitha T. The importance of delayed images in gastrointestinal bleeding scintigraphy. *Nucl Med Commun.* 2002;23:803–808.
7. Schilling D, Grieger G, Weidman E, et al. Long-term follow up of patients with iron deficiency anemia after a close endoscopic examination of the upper and lower gastrointestinal tract. *Z Gastroenterol.* 2000;38:827–831.
8. Kiernan PJ. Treatment of variceal bleeding. *Gastrointest Endosc Clin N Am.* 2001;11:789–812.
9. Heikenen JB, Pohl JF, Werlin SL, et al. Octreotide in pediatric patients. *J Pediatr Gastroenterol Nutr.* 2002;35:600–609.
10. Siafkas C, Fox VL, Nurko S. Use of Octreotide for the management of severe gastrointestinal bleeding in children. *J Pediatr Gastroenterol Nutr.* 1998;26:356–359.
11. D'Amico G, Pagliaro L, Bosch J. Pharmacological treatment of hypertension: An evidence based approach. *Semin Liver Dis.* 1999;19:475–505.
12. Eroglu Y, Emerick KM, Whithington PF, et al. Octreotide therapy for control of acute gastrointestinal bleeding in children. *J Pediatr Gastroenterol Nutr.* 2004;38:41–47.

Reflux and Other Motility Disorders

61

Victor M. Pineiro-Carrero

Gastrointestinal (GI) motility disorders are common in the critically ill child. The patients often present with abdominal distension, vomiting, and intolerance to feeding or they can exhibit respiratory symptoms. The control of GI motility is mediated by a complex interaction of neural and hormonal input that exerts stimulatory and inhibitory action on the GI tract. GI motor activity is controlled by the enteric nervous system with extrinsic modulation by the central nervous system through autonomic afferent and efferent fibers (see Chapter 9).

Approximately half of all mechanically ventilated patients have fewer migrating motor complexes, antral hypomotility, and decreased gastric emptying. Several factors in critically ill patients can account for these observed changes. Head injury, abdominal surgery, sepsis, hyperglycemia, recumbent position, and narcotics all contribute to decreased GI motility. The disturbed GI function in these patients gives rise to impaired absorption of drugs and nutrients. In addition, delayed gastric emptying may lead to gastric bacterial overgrowth and gastroesophageal reflux, placing these patients at increased risk of pulmonary aspiration, pneumonia, and sepsis. This chapter will discuss some of the common disorders of esophageal, GI, and colonic motility in the critical care patient.

DISORDERS OF DEGLUTITION

Patients with impaired mental status may develop oropharyngeal dysphagia (difficulty in swallowing). Respiratory complications of impaired swallowing include apnea and bradycardia, choking episodes, chronic noisy breathing, reactive airway disease, chronic or recurrent pneumonia, bronchitis, and atelectasis. Aspiration of oral contents may occur directly, that is, in association with a swallow or it may also occur after an episode of gastroesophageal reflux.

Unfortunately, in the swallowing-impaired child, it may be difficult to detect aspiration based on clinical signs and symptoms alone because "silent aspiration" (aspiration without coughing, gagging, and choking) may occur.[1]

Videofluoroscopy, or the modified barium swallow, is the procedure of choice to evaluate the swallowing function by visualizing the transit of barium-impregnated liquids and pureed foods through the oral cavity, pharynx, and esophagus. This study provides objective evidence of abnormal oral and pharyngeal coordination and detects episodes of aspiration, all of which help identify children in whom oral feeding may be contraindicated. In general, treatment recommendations are based on the patient's ability to swallow, nutritional status, and the presence of gastroesophageal reflux. Often a nasogastric tube or a feeding gastrostomy is used to prevent recurrent aspiration in patients with dysphagia.

GASTROESOPHAGEAL REFLUX

Gastroesophageal reflux is defined as the passive movement of gastric contents into the esophagus. Gastroesophageal reflux disease (GERD) comprises the pathologic sequelae or severe symptoms caused by gastroesophageal reflux. GERD is the most common esophageal disorder affecting infants and children and is very common in the critically ill patient. GERD may lead to esophageal and GI symptoms, including regurgitation, vomiting, chest pain, heartburn, odynophagia (painful swallowing), or dysphagia. It can also cause multiple extraesophageal symptoms, also known as extraesophageal reflux disease (EERD), leading to respiratory disease, hoarseness, sinusitis, and chronic cough. In most patients, GERD is caused by inappropriate transient relaxation of the lower esophageal sphincter. Nevertheless, a recent study in adults has demonstrated that gastroesophageal (GE) reflux in mechanically ventilated patients is predominantly due to very low or absent lower esophageal sphincter pressure.[2] In addition, delayed gastric emptying and abnormal esophageal peristalsis may contribute to the development of GERD. Pain is often a symptom of esophagitis, represented by crying in young infants and heartburn in the older child. Distinctions between odynophagia and dysphagia may be difficult in young children but can be useful to narrow the differential diagnosis between inflammatory conditions and motor abnormalities of the esophagus. The severity of clinical findings depends on the frequency and duration of the reflux, the noxiousness of the refluxed material, and the esophageal mucosal protective mechanisms (mostly secondary peristalsis). Most episodes of regurgitation are not associated with nausea, retching is rare, and expulsion is not forceful or complete. Occasionally, regurgitation of gastric contents to the hypopharynx leads to vomiting with forceful expulsion of gastric contents. Nocturnal reflux leads to more severe symptoms because it occurs at a time when protective esophageal clearance functions and salivation are less active. Nocturnal GERD is associated with increased incidence of complications of GERD, extraesophageal manifestations, Barrett esophagus, and adenocarcinoma.[3]

Extraesophageal Reflux Disease

GERD may cause upper and lower respiratory tract symptoms. Many respiratory diseases, in turn, may worsen GERD. Gastroesophageal reflux is probably a significant factor in asthma exacerbation and probably a causative factor for many patients with asthma. Patients with asthma have a higher prevalence of GERD symptoms than control subjects, and they also associate reflux symptoms with asthma symptoms. Proposed mechanisms that explain how GERD alters airway reactivity leading to bronchospasm include a vagally mediated reflex, a local axonal reflex, heightened bronchial reactivity, and microaspiration. Epidemiologic evidence suggests that GERD is associated with increased incidence of sinusitis, laryngitis, asthma, pneumonia, and bronchiectasis. Chronic hoarseness, chronic cough, and chronic sinusitis have also been associated with GERD. Infantile apnea may occur as a response of the upper airway to gastroesophageal reflux, whereas the bronchospasm of asthma may be seen as a lower airway response to reflux in the older child, and GERD may play an important role in select cases.[4]

Diagnosis

The diagnostic evaluation of GERD includes radiography, endoscopy with esophageal biopsy, esophageal pH monitoring, and more recently the combined pH and esophageal impedance measurements. Radiography is useful to evaluate for anatomic abnormalities. Endoscopy with biopsy is the best method to evaluate for evidence of esophagitis in the patient with unexplained pain, occult GI bleeding, or hematemesis. Nuclear scintigraphy can detect nonacid reflux episodes but is difficult to quantitate and cannot be temporally correlated to extraesophageal symptoms. Esophageal pH monitoring provides a quantitative measurement of acid reflux, which can be associated with other events like cough or apnea. Nevertheless, it does not detect episodes of nonacid reflux. Although esophageal pH testing is considered to be the "gold standard" for identifying gastroesophageal reflux (GER), it has a sensitivity and specificity of approximately 90% and is not a perfect test. A wireless esophageal pH system has been developed, which allows monitoring up to 48 hours without the use of an intranasal catheter, so that patients are less likely to alter their daily activities and/or diet. Also nonacid reflux, undetectable with pH monitoring, may have an impact. There is limited data on nonacid reflux and its effect on the lung. Nonacid GER can be measured by esophageal impedance monitoring, which has not been used in most studies. Simultaneous esophageal pH and intraluminal impedance provides a quantitative method to evaluate acid and nonacid reflux and to correlate these episodes to other symptoms. These two tests may be complementary when performed simultaneously, but they are difficult to analyze, and the lack of pediatric age normative data currently limit their use.[5]

The diagnosis of individual patients suspected of EERD is difficult. Other ancillary diagnostic methods that can be used include videofluoroscopy, scintigraphy to diagnose aspiration (particularly the salivagram), and laryngobronchoscopy. Laryngoscopy is useful to evaluate for the presence of posterior glottic edema, erythema, and nodules. Bronchoscopy, with bronchoalveolar lavage for lipid-laden macrophages or trypsin, is useful to assess presence of aspiration. Polysomnography concurrent with esophageal pH monitoring (usually including electrocardiography, nasal airflow, and respiratory efforts by chest wall impedance) is used to identify apneic episodes (particularly obstructive ones) that are temporally associated with acid reflux episodes.

Treatment

Conservative measures include thickening the feedings and elevating the head of the bed. A recent meta-analysis of studies done in infants and children younger than 2 years determined that thickened feedings reduce the regurgitation severity and decrease the episodes of vomiting whereas positioning therapy is not effective.[6] Antacid therapy, either H_2-receptor antagonists or proton pump inhibitors, is the mainstay of therapy. When GERD is responsible for extraesophageal presentations, the therapy must be aggressive, usually requiring a trial of high-dose proton pump inhibitors to alter the respiratory symptoms. Twice-daily proton pump inhibitors maintained for at least 3 months are recommended. Intravenous proton pump inhibitors are now available for use in children, although there are no studies documenting their advantage over enteral formulations. Fundoplication surgery seems to provide better results, and the best surgical results in adults are obtained in patients with nocturnal asthma, onset of reflux symptoms before pulmonary symptoms, evidence of laryngeal inflammation, and a good response to medical treatment. However, the complication rate for fundoplication is greater in children with respiratory disease or in the high-risk patients discussed in the subsequent text.

High-Risk Groups

Patients with a history of prematurity, particularly those with bronchopulmonary dysplasia, and children with neurologic disorders are at risk for severe GERD and for significant extraesophageal symptoms. Predisposing factors in children with neurologic disorders include increased gastric pressure mediated by spasticity, chronic supine posture with poor esophageal clearance, and possibly impaired GI motility. Erosive esophagitis, strictures, Barrett esophagus, and EERD are all more common in children with neurologic disorders. Patients in these two groups are frequently encountered in the intensive care unit (ICU) and pose a dilemma for evaluation and treatment, especially when they require long-term enteral feedings that may predispose them to aspiration pneumonia and other respiratory events. Patients with esophageal atresia have abnormal esophageal peristalsis and are also at high risk for severe GERD, occasionally leading to erosive esophagitis and distal esophageal strictures.[7]

Other Esophageal Motility Disorders

Other disorders of esophageal motility are rarely encountered in the ICU. Achalasia is the most recognized motor disorder of the esophagus. The term achalasia means "failure to relax" and describes a cardinal feature of this disorder; a poorly relaxing lower esophageal sphincter. In addition, there is lack of propagation of esophageal contractions that result in aperistalsis. These abnormalities lead to the functional obstruction of the esophagus and the symptoms of dysphagia, regurgitation, chest discomfort, and, eventually, weight loss. The esophagogram demonstrates a dilated esophagus with lack of peristaltic waves and a narrow gastroesophageal junction, the "bird beak sign." A detailed description of this disorder is beyond the scope of this chapter and has been reviewed recently.[8] Other hypomotility disorders are seen in patients with scleroderma and patients with long-standing diabetes mellitus. More often, they present with symptoms of dysphagia or GERD.

GASTROPARESIS

Delayed gastric emptying is a common finding in the critically ill patient. Gastric emptying is slowed by duodenal distension, acidification, or perfusion with fat and protein. In the critically ill patient, gastric emptying is delayed by increased gastric acid secretion or by the use of enteral formulas that are hyperosmolar or high in fat or protein concentration. The diagnosis is suspected in a patient with abdominal distension, vomiting, and intolerance to feedings. The upper GI series may show delayed gastric emptying and/or gastroesophageal reflux but is otherwise normal. A gastric emptying scan can confirm the diagnosis but is often not practical in the ICU setting. Occasionally, an upper endoscopy is indicated if there is evidence of hematemesis or suspicion of inflammatory lesions of the proximal GI tract.

Treatment

The treatment options include administering prokinetic agents or bypassing the stomach by instituting transpyloric feedings. Enteral feedings are often poorly tolerated in critically ill patients due to impaired GI motility. Enteral feeds may be delivered into the stomach or the small bowel, depending on the position of the feeding tube within the GI tract. A recent randomized trial in children compared gastric versus small-bowel feedings. It showed that small-bowel feeds allow a greater amount of nutrition to be successfully delivered to critically ill children. Nevertheless, small-bowel feeds did not prevent aspiration of gastric contents. Whether feeding into the small bowel alters the incidence of aspiration remains controversial. A recent meta-analysis of adult trials was unable to demonstrate any clinical benefit from small-bowel feeding compared to gastric feeding. Placement of a small-bowel feeding tube may be difficult to accomplish at the bedside. A variety of techniques for placing tubes beyond the pylorus have been described including the use of stylets, weighted tube tips, and prokinetic drugs, especially intravenous erythromycin. Small-bowel feeding tubes can also be placed using fluoroscopy or endoscopy. Prokinetic agents have the potential for overcoming GI dysmotility in the critical care setting. Unfortunately, the drugs currently available are not very effective. Metoclopramide promotes gastric emptying by acting as an antagonist to the inhibitory actions of dopamine in the gut. Erythromycin, a macrolide antibiotic, promotes motility of the proximal GI tract by activating motilin receptors on enteric nerves and smooth muscle. Erythromycin is more powerful than metoclopramide and it has been shown to be safe. Gastric electrical stimulation is a promising therapeutic option that is in the early stages of development.[9]

INTESTINAL ILEUS

Ileus refers to the functional inhibition of propulsive bowel activity with failure of aboral movement of intestinal contents in the absence of mechanical obstruction. Ileus may be categorized into postoperative, inflammatory, metabolic, neurogenic, and drug-related causes. Each of these categories is a relatively common cause of ileus in hospitalized patients. Following most abdominal surgeries or injuries, the motility of the GI tract is transiently impaired. Resolution of ileus following uncomplicated laparotomy follows a consistent temporal sequence with complete resolution within 2 to 3 days. The clinical consequences of ileus include postoperative discomfort, delay in nutrition, and prolongation of immobilization. In the critical care setting, ileus is often caused by the presence of intra-abdominal infection, systemic conditions (e.g., sepsis), or drugs (e.g., narcotics). The duration of the operation, degree of intestinal manipulation, performance of an enterotomy or even vagotomy, does not appear to influence the duration of postoperative ileus.

The principal clinical findings include poorly localized abdominal pain, abdominal distension, nausea, vomiting, and obstipation. These clinical manifestations may be difficult to distinguish from those associated with mechanical bowel obstruction. The absence of bowel sounds is not a consistent feature of nonobstructive ileus. Differentiation of ileus from mechanical obstruction is usually possible based on the entire clinical scenario and the presence of gas in the stomach, small intestine, and colon on plain abdominal radiography. In the past, a contrast study of the small bowel was often used in ruling out mechanical obstruction in cases in which plain abdominal radiographs are equivocal. Prompt passage of barium through the small intestine and colon confirmed the absence of mechanical obstruction and was consistent with the diagnosis of ileus. More recently, computed tomography (CT) scanning has replaced the use of contrast studies. CT scan offers the additional benefit of delineating other intra-abdominal inflammatory processes, such as abscess and pancreatitis that may contribute to nonmechanical bowel dysfunction. The passage of CT scan contrast into the colon within 4 hours excludes small-bowel obstruction and favors ileus as the etiology of a patient's intestinal dysmotility.

The treatment of ileus following uncomplicated laparotomy involves limiting oral intake, maintaining intravascular volume, and correcting electrolyte abnormalities, particularly hypokalemia. If accompanied by abdominal distension, nausea, or vomiting, a nasogastric tube should be placed. If ileus is prolonged (>3 to 5 days), a thorough search for electrolyte disturbances, drugs, or sepsis should be made. Review of the patient's medications may reveal drugs known to be associated with impaired intestinal motility, especially opiates. Measurement of serum electrolytes may demonstrate hypokalemia, hypocalcemia, hypomagnesemia, or other electrolyte disturbances commonly associated with ileus. CT scan may demonstrate the presence of an intra-abdominal abscess or other evidence of peritoneal sepsis, as well as the presence of postoperative obstruction. Supportive treatment of patients with ileus includes meticulous management of volume and

electrolytes, as well as parenteral nutritional support until the ileus resolves. Prokinetic agents including erythromycin and somatostatin analogs have not been helpful.

ACUTE MEGACOLON

Isolated colonic motility disorders are less frequent in the critically ill child. Acute megacolon may occur in children with severe ulcerative colitis (toxic megacolon), infectious colitis, in response to acute distal obstruction (e.g., volvulus), or associated with a chronic distal obstruction (e.g., Hirschsprung disease). Acute megacolon also rarely occurs in children without obvious colonic disease or mechanical obstruction. In these instances, the pseudo-obstruction is localized to the colon and is known as Ogilvie syndrome. The precise cause of acute colonic pseudo-obstruction is unknown; however, most patients have a coexisting problem such as recent trauma or surgery. Acute megacolon should be suspected in a child with sudden abdominal distension and evidence of isolated colonic dilatation on abdominal plain films. It should be considered in a patient with severe inflammatory bowel disease or an infant with a history of constipation. Occasionally, the patient is recovering quite uneventfully from surgery performed a few days previously and is already eating a regular diet. The abdomen becomes grossly distended and breathing becomes difficult, but there are no peritoneal signs and the white blood cell count is normal. An abdominal x-ray shows massive gaseous distension of the colon. Usually, the small bowel is not seen. The cecal diameter at this point in the course is often more than 7 cm and may reach 10 cm in the older patient.[10]

Treatment

Oral feedings should be withheld, parenteral fluids started, and a nasogastric tube passed. A water-soluble contrast enema can be done to exclude mechanical obstruction and confirm pseudo-obstruction. A hyperosmolar water-soluble enema offers the advantage of promoting colonic evacuation. Once confirmed, acute colonic pseudo-obstruction is treated aggressively with a rectal decompression tube, although caution must be taken in a patient with colitis due to the risk for perforation. Any associated metabolic or electrolyte abnormalities (e.g., hypokalemia) should be corrected. In adults, treatment with erythromycin or neostigmine has been reported to help. For those patients who do not respond to medical therapy but continue to have a normal white blood cell count and no fever or peritoneal signs, the next step is colonoscopic decompression if the cecum remains massively distended (>11 cm in the adult). Gas and liquid stool are aspirated continuously while little additional air (or carbon dioxide) is insufflated. Patients with acute or chronic colitis require broad-spectrum antibiotics. As many as 20%, however, require operation because of colonic dilatation that is refractory to medical therapy. An operation is advisable for patients with a cecal diameter >11 or 12 cm (in adults) and intractability to medical and/or endoscopic management. The most useful and efficacious approach is tube cecostomy, either by conventional open, percutaneous, or, more recently, laparoscopic techniques. Moreover, if at any time a patient manifests fever, leukocytosis, or peritoneal signs, abdominal exploration is mandatory.

REFERENCES

1. Garg BP. Dysphagia in children: An overview. *Semin Pediatr Neurol.* 2003;10(4):252–254.
2. Nind G, Chen WH, Protheroe R, et al. Mechanisms of gastroesophageal reflux in critically ill mechanically ventilated patients. *Gastroenterology.* 2005;128:600–606.
3. Hassal E. Decisions in diagnosing and managing chronic gastroesophageal reflux disease in children. *J Pediatr.* 2005; 146(Suppl 3):S3–S12.
4. Gold BD. Asthma and gastroesophageal reflux disease in children: Exploring the relationship. *J Pediatr.* 2005;146(Suppl 3): S13–S20.
5. Wenzl TG. Investigating esophageal reflux with the intraluminal impedance technique. *J Pediatr Gastroenterol Nutr.* 2002;34: 261–268.
6. Craig WR, Hanlon-Dearman A, Sinclair C, et al. Metoclopramide, thickened feedings, and positioning for gastro-oesophageal reflux in children under two years. *Cochrane Database Syst Rev.* 2004; 18:CD003502.
7. Kovesi T, Rubin S. Long-term complications of congenital esophageal atresia and/or tracheoesophageal fistula. *Chest.* 2004; 126:915–925.
8. Pineiro-Carrero VM, Sullivan CA, Rogers PL. Etiology and treatment of achalasia in the pediatric age group. *Gastrointest Endosc Clin N Am.* 2001;11:387–408.
9. Vandenplas Y, Hauser B, Salvatore S. Current pharmacological treatment of gastroparesis. *Expert Opin Pharmacother.* 2004;5: 2251–2254.
10. DiLorenzo C, Hyman PE. Gastrointestinal motility in neonatal and pediatric practice. *Gastroenterol Clin North Am.* 1996;25: 203–224.

Gastrointestinal Trauma

62

Riccardo A. Superina   *Lisa P. Abramson*

Abdominal trauma should be suspected in any child with injury to the torso regardless of the mechanism. Overall mortality and morbidity from abdominal trauma is low, and a majority is treated nonoperatively. Previous studies from the National Pediatric Trauma Registry (NPTR) demonstrate that 8% to 12% of children who sustain blunt trauma have an abdominal injury and >90% survive. Of the reported deaths obtained from the NPTR, only 22% were related to abdominal trauma.

TABLE 62.1

STANDARD CRITERIA FOR A POSITIVE DIAGNOSTIC PERITONEAL LAVAGE

- 10 mL gross blood return with lavage catheter aspiration
- >100,000 red blood cells/mm^3
- >500 white blood cells/mm^3
- Bile, bacteria, or vegetable matter on microscopic evaluation
- Amylase level >175 IU/dL

DIAGNOSTIC MODALITIES

Computed tomography (CT) scan use has increased in the initial evaluation of the pediatric trauma patient. Advantages of CT scanning include accurate identification of solid organ injuries and decreasing the need for operative exploration or invasive testing. The high-resolution spiral CT scans with intravenous contrast have allowed better staging of solid organ injuries by demonstrating vascular and parenchymal enhancement more accurately than previous scanners. Enteral contrast is not necessary in the acute trauma setting and should be avoided secondary to concerns for aspiration. The greatest limitation of CT scanning in regard to intra-abdominal injury is in identifying hollow viscous injuries. Some associated findings would include pneumoperitoneum, thickened bowel wall, bowel wall enhancement, and free fluid not in association with solid organ injury. Contraindications to CT scans are penetrating injuries that require operative intervention and hemodynamic instability.

Diagnostic peritoneal lavage (DPL) is used less commonly because the availability and accuracy of less invasive diagnostic techniques have increased. DPL is invasive, painful, and associated with a nontherapeutic laparotomy rate of 20% to 40%.[1] It is performed by a small vertical infraumbilical incision after decompression of the bladder and stomach. The midline fascia is incised and a pediatric peritoneal catheter is directed into the pelvis. Aspiration of the catheter for gross blood is performed. If no gross blood is evident, then 10 mL per kg of normal saline is instilled into the peritoneal cavity. It is then allowed to passively drain and aliquots are sent to the laboratory for cell count and Gram stain (see Table 62.1). DPL remains very accurate for the detection of hemoperitoneum but may miss retroperitoneal injuries such as pancreatic transections or contusions. A positive DPL may lead to an unnecessary laparotomy as most hemodynamically stable children with solid organ injury can be treated nonoperatively. DPL may play a role in excluding an intra-abdominal source of bleeding in a hemodynamically unstable child with a massive head injury that needs neurosurgical intervention. It may also help when evaluating children at high risk for bowel injury such as victims of lap belt injuries with negative CT scans and neurologic impairment, making clinical evaluation difficult.

Focused abdominal sonography for trauma (FAST) examinations are currently being investigated to determine its efficacy in children. Thus far, low sensitivities and specificities secondary to solid organ injury without hemoperitoneum limit this modality for use in children.[2] A finding of free fluid may indicate a solid organ injury but does not identify the extent of the injury, and the absence of free fluid on ultrasonography does not exclude intra-abdominal injury. There may be a use for FAST scans in the multiply-injured hemodynamically unstable child to assist in prioritizing operative intervention.

The role of laparoscopy is still being evaluated in the pediatric population. In the adult literature, the sensitivity of laparoscopy is similar to DPL but the specificity is improved allowing for more accurate identification of the injury. Laparoscopy has been inconclusive regarding its utility in making the diagnosis or the decision for laparotomy. It may be possible to perform definitive repair at the time of laparoscopy as demonstrated in several case reports with one jejunal perforation and one gall bladder rupture.[3,4]

SOLID ORGAN INJURY

Spleen and liver are the two most commonly injured organs in blunt abdominal trauma accounting for two third of the overall injuries. Standard of care is nonoperative management of isolated liver and splenic injuries in hemodynamically stable children. The success rate for nonoperative management of isolated blunt splenic and liver injury is >90% at pediatric trauma centers. Conservative treatment of liver and spleen injury has been proven to

TABLE 62.3
LIVER INJURY SCALE

Grade		Injury Description
I	Hematoma	Subcapsular, nonexpanding <10% surface area
	Laceration	Capsular tear, nonbleeding, <1 cm parenchymal depth
II	Hematoma	Subcapsular, nonexpanding, 10%–50% surface area: intraparenchymal, nonexpanding, <2 cm diameter
	Laceration	Capsular tear, active bleeding: 1–3 cm parenchymal depth, <10 cm length
III	Hematoma	Subcapsular, >50% surface area or expanding, ruptured subcapsular hematoma with active bleeding; intraparenchymal hematoma >2 cm or expanding
	Laceration	>3 cm parenchymal depth
IV	Hematoma	Ruptured intraparenchymal hematoma with active bleeding
	Laceration	Parenchymal disruption involving 25%–50% of hepatic lobe
V	Hematoma	Parenchymal disruption involving >50% of hepatic lobe
	Laceration	Juxtahepatic venous injuries
VI	Vascular	Hepatic avulsion

Adapted from the American Association for the Surgery of Trauma www.aast.org.

TABLE 62.2
SPLENIC INJURY SCALE

Grade		Injury Description
I	Hematoma	Subcapsular, nonexpanding <10% surface area
	Laceration	Capsular tear, nonbleeding, <1 cm parenchymal depth
II	Hematoma	Subcapsular, nonexpanding, 10%–50% surface area: intraparenchymal, nonexpanding, <2 cm diameter
	Laceration	Capsular tear, active bleeding: 1–3 cm parenchymal depth that does not involve a trabecular vessel
III	Hematoma	Subcapsular, >50% surface area or expanding, ruptured subcapsular hematoma with active bleeding; intraparenchymal hematoma >2 cm or expanding
	Laceration	>3 cm parenchymal depth or involving trabecular vessels
IV	Hematoma	Ruptured intraparenchymal hematoma with active bleeding
	Laceration	Laceration involving segmental or hilar vessels producing major devascularization (>25% of spleen)
V	Hematoma	Completely shattered spleen
	Laceration	Hilar vascular injury that devascularizes spleen

Adapted from the American Association for the Surgery of Trauma www.aast.org.

be safe in head injured patients and the overall outcome was improved in those children who did not undergo operative intervention. Operative intervention is reserved for patients who have hemodynamic instability, >50% blood volume replacement, and other associated life-threatening intra-abdominal injures. The mainstay for diagnosing these injuries is CT scan, which allows the injury to be graded (see Tables 62.2 and 62.3). CT scanning is highly accurate in identifying the injuries, but there is a poor correlation with injury severity and grade. Most surgeons rely on physiologic signs of ongoing hemorrhage as indicators of surgical need rather than the CT scan grading (see Fig. 62.1).

Nonoperative management of children with blunt splenic trauma included fewer blood transfusions, shorter length of hospital stay, and lower mortality rates. In addition, special consideration is taken in children due to the immunologic function of the spleen and the potential development of postsplenectomy sepsis in asplenic children. The spleen plays an active role in clearing encapsulated bacteria such as pneumococcus, *Haemophilus influenzae*, and meningococcus. The greatest risk for postsplenectomy sepsis is in the first 2 years after splenectomy and in children younger than 5 years. The incidence of sepsis after splenectomy for trauma is 85 times higher than in the normal population.

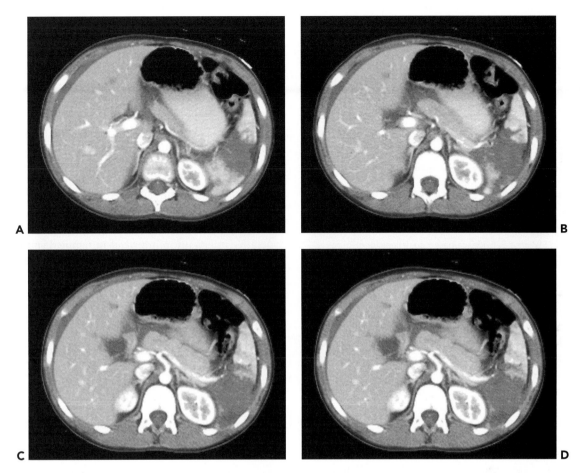

Figure 62.1 An 8-year-old boy presented to the emergency department after a sledding injury complaining of abdominal pain. He was hemodynamically stable and underwent computed tomography (CT) scan, which demonstrates a Grade IV splenic laceration. He did well with conservative management and was discharged home without requiring blood transfusion.

Despite agreement on nonoperative management, there is wide discrepancy in the management of these injured children. In an attempt to make care more uniform, the American Pediatric Surgical Association (APSA) Trauma Committee published consensus guidelines regarding the need for intensive care unit (ICU) admission, length of stay, the need for imaging, and physical activity restriction after injury on the basis of grading of the injury (see Table 62.4).[5] These guidelines were prospectively analyzed and found to have significant reduction in the length of ICU stay, the total length of hospitalization, follow-up imaging, and the interval to restart physical activity within each grade of injury.[6] Another prospective study utilized a standardized treatment algorithm based on hemodynamic status rather than grading of injury.[7] Exploratory laparotomy is performed for those children who fail conservative measures. Total splenectomy is performed for exsanguinating hemorrhage and in multiply-injured patients. Splenorrhaphy may be possible due to the segmental blood supply of the spleen. Topical hemostatic agents may be applied or lacerations may be oversewn.

If total splenectomy is performed, the child should be immunized with vaccines for pneumococcus, *H. influenzae*, and meningococcus. Some advocate routine administration of vaccines in patients undergoing conservative management for splenic lacerations in the event that they may require future splenectomy if nonoperative management fails.

In contrast to splenic trauma, blunt hepatic injury is the most frequent cause of death in children sustaining blunt abdominal trauma (see Fig. 62.2). Surgical intervention for liver lacerations occurs more commonly due to severe hemorrhage from the intrahepatic vasculature or the vena cava. Most liver lacerations to the parenchyma may be controlled with electrocautery or direct ligation of bleeding vessels. Initial management to control life-threatening hemorrhage is direct compression of the liver, compression of the porta hepatis (Pringle maneuver), and packing of deep lacerations. Cases of severe life-threatening hemorrhage with physiologic derangements such as metabolic acidosis, hypothermia, and coagulopathy are treated with staged surgical treatment. This includes perihepatic packing, temporary

TABLE 62.4

GUIDELINES FOR RESOURCE UTILIZATION IN ISOLATED SPLEEN OR LIVER INJURY BASED ON COMPUTED TOMOGRAPHY SCAN GRADE

	I	II	III	IV
ICU d	None	None	None	1
Hospital stay	2	3	4	5
Imaging (pre- or postdischarge)	None	None	None	None
Activity restriction (wk)	3	4	5	6

ICU, intensive care unit.
Adapted from Stylianos S. Evidence-based guidelines for resource utilization in children with isolated spleen or liver injuries. *J Pediatr Surg.* 2000;34:164–169.

abdominal closure, and transfer to the ICU for aggressive resuscitation. Re-exploration occurs after the physiologic and metabolic issues have been addressed and hemostasis with or without resection is attempted. Additional modalities such as angiography with embolization and endoscopic biliary stenting should be considered.

Pancreatic trauma occurs less frequently, secondary to its retroperitoneal location, and comprises 3% to 12% of intra-abdominal injuries in children. Injury results from a deceleration injury, causing the gland to fracture as it crosses the vertebral column. Diagnosis may be difficult on routine CT scans and may require thin cuts through the region of the pancreas with intravenous contrast bolus. Magnetic resonance cholangiopancreatography (MRCP) and endoscopic retrograde cholangiopancreatography (ERCP) may show more details of the ductal anatomy, but are not useful in the acute phase of the evaluation and resuscitation. Serum amylase and lipase levels do not correlate with the extent of injury or predict the need for operative intervention. Hyperamylasemia may occur with salivary gland injury, bowel injury, and closed head injury. Pancreatic contusions without major ductal disruption frequently heal with nonoperative management. Treatment consists of withholding enteral nutrition and starting hyperalimentation until the pain resolves. Nasogastric decompression may be necessary for the associated ileus and for relief of gastric distension. Ultrasonography or CT scan follow-up is necessary to document healing in children with persistent symptoms. If a major ductal injury is detected, early operative intervention improves outcome. If nonoperative management is attempted, there is a 45% to 100% rate of pancreatic pseudocyst formation with the majority resolving over time. However, the duration of hospitalization and need for hyperalimentation increases in this group. Complete pancreatic transection requires distal pancreatectomy and wide drainage.

HOLLOW VISCOUS INJURY

Hollow viscous injuries may be difficult to diagnose on initial evaluation and may require a combination of clinical acumen and judicious investigations. The most common mechanism of injury is motor vehicle collisions. Restrained passengers of a collision with enough force to result in visible abdominal wall contusions (seat belt sign) and vertebral column fracture have up to a 50% risk of intestinal injury. This results from rapid deceleration against the fixation of improperly placed two point restraints allowing the force

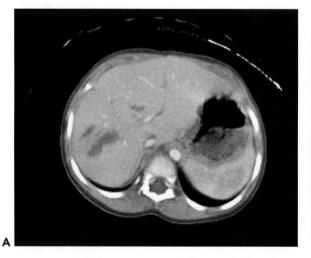
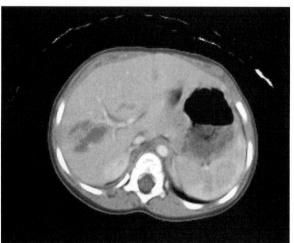

Figure 62.2 A 5-year-old boy was the backseat passenger in a moderate speed motor vehicle collision. No significant physical findings other than vague upper abdominal tenderness. Computed tomography (CT) scan demonstrated a Grade II liver laceration. He was admitted to the ward and managed nonoperatively.

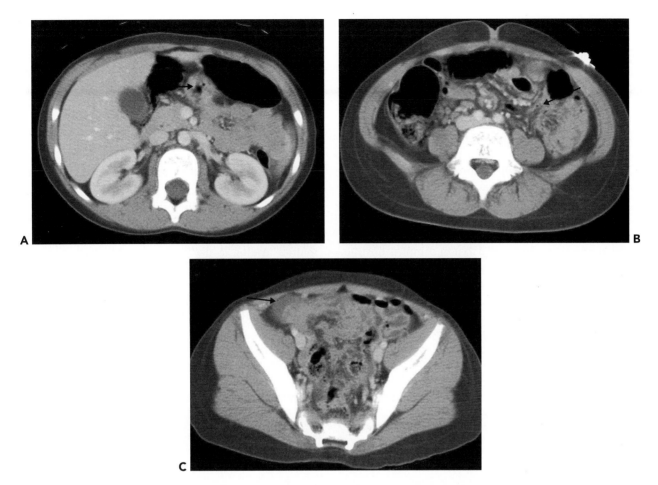

Figure 62.3 A 5-year-old girl restrained in the backseat with a lap belt during a high speed motor vehicle collision. She presented with normal hemodynamics and mild lower abdominal ecchymosis. She underwent a computed tomography (CT) scan which demonstrated thickened loops of bowel (*arrow A*), small areas of free air in the mesentery (*arrow B*), and free fluid without solid organ injury (*arrow C*). She underwent exploratory laparotomy and was found to have a perforation in an area of devascularized jejunum, which was resected. She had an uneventful recovery.

to be transmitted to the abdominal wall, which compresses the bowel between the restraint device and the vertebral column. The deceleration leads to tears in the bowel or in the mesentery at fixed points such as the ligament of Treitz and the ileocecal valve. Mesenteric injuries can lead to areas of ischemia with resultant perforation. Blow-out areas occur because of compression against a distended loop of bowel.

The diagnosis of hollow viscous injury can be difficult and may result in delayed diagnosis. Initial physical examination may reveal abdominal wall ecchymosis and no evidence of peritonitis in up to 50% of patients. Children with occult intestinal injury had changes in temperature, heart rate, and urine output that was different from those without injury as the time from injury increased. No specific laboratory tests are diagnostic. However, leukocytosis was reported to have 85% sensitivity and 55% specificity for occult intestinal injury when done more than 6 hours after injury.[8] Most stable children will undergo additional evaluation for suspected bowel injuries.

Initial plain films will only document pneumoperitoneum in less than one third of patients with intestinal injury. Abdominal CT scanning is the preferred method for evaluating the stable patient with suspected intra-abdominal injury (see Fig. 62.3). However, diagnosis of bowel injury with CT scan remains difficult and may be suggested only by free fluid without solid organ injury. Pneumoperitoneum is often not present or may be very subtle adjacent to the injured loop of bowel. Additional findings of bowel wall thickening and mesenteric fat stranding are suggestive of injury. In the neurologically injured patient, the diagnosis is more difficult and a continued high index of suspicion must be maintained. DPL or diagnostic laparoscopy may be necessary if clinical deterioration occurs. An algorithm has been proposed to guide the diagnosis and management of children with suspected hollow viscous injury in an attempt to reduce the delay in diagnosis.[1]

Gastric injuries from blunt force trauma are caused by compressive force in a patient with a full stomach.

Diagnosis is difficult as free air is not often seen. A nasogastric tube positioned outside of the normal gastric contour is diagnostic. Surgical intervention starts with laparotomy and mobilization of the stomach. The lesser curve and posterior surfaces must be closely inspected to avoid a missed injury. These perforations are oversewn with a two-layer closure and a nasogastric tube is left in place for several days.

Duodenal injuries are difficult to manage secondary to their anatomic association with the pancreas and extrahepatic biliary system. Blunt force trauma to the epigastrium results in an intramural hematoma in most duodenal injuries. The child may present with mild epigastric discomfort and emesis, which persists. CT scanning may demonstrate the hematoma, or upper gastrointestinal series will reveal duodenal narrowing with partial to near complete obstruction (see Fig. 62.4). Nonoperative management consists of nasogastric decompression and hyperalimentation for 1 to 3 weeks. Most hematomas resolve in 10 days and ultrasonography can be used to follow resolution. Full-thickness duodenal injuries may be identified on a CT scan, with extravasation of air or enteral contrast material into the retroperitoneal space. These injuries must be repaired operatively with primary closure if minimal tissue destruction is present. Care must be taken not to narrow the lumen and wide drainage is performed. A variety of techniques may be employed if primary closure cannot be achieved, including using a loop of jejunum to patch the defect, and temporary pyloric exclusion. Primary duodenal closure is not recommended if the injury is more than 24 hours old. Duodenal-tube drainage and feeding-jejunostomy-tube placement is a more conservative approach.

Perforation of the small intestine or colon may result from forceful compression of distended bowel resulting in perforation along the antimesenteric border. Mesenteric injuries leading to devascularized segments of intestines require resection with primary anastomosis. Under extreme circumstances, a small bowel anastomosis is not performed at initial exploration secondary to severe associated injuries or questionable bowel viability that will require second look laparotomy. Colon injuries may be repaired primarily or with resection and anastomosis in the absence of

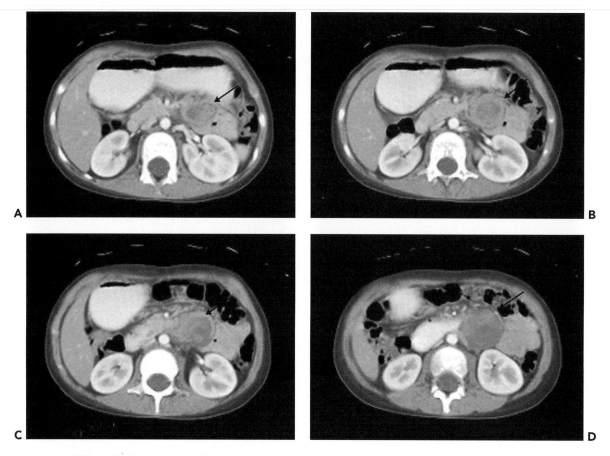

Figure 62.4 A 9-year-old boy presented after a fall over his handlebars with epigastric pain and profuse emesis. Computed tomography (CT) scan revealed a large duodenal hematoma with failure of contrast to progress beyond. He was treated nonoperatively with hyperalimentation, nasogastric decompression, and nothing by mouth (NPO) until bowel function has resumed. He was discharged home with no further problems 10 days postinjury.

shock and/or significant fecal contamination. Otherwise, a diverting colostomy may be required.

Rectal injuries in children result from accidental falls in a straddle position onto sharp or blunt objects, or secondary to sexual abuse. These injuries are frequently diagnosed with an examination under anesthesia. Rectal perforations typically require proximal diversion with an end colostomy, presacral drainage, and rectal wash out. The rectal injury itself should be primarily repaired with a layered closure after debridement of devitalized tissue.

Penetrating trauma in children is much less common and occurs in only 5% of injured children. Treatment of penetrating trauma differs only in the indications for laparotomy. Gunshot wounds that penetrate the peritoneal cavity must undergo laparotomy due to the dissipation of high kinetic energy. Stab wounds below the nipple line and above the inguinal ligament are managed selectively. If there is hemodynamic instability, peritoneal signs, or unexplained blood loss, immediate laparotomy is undertaken. If the patient is stable, wound exploration can be done under local anesthesia in a cooperative child or under general anesthesia in younger patients. Simple observation may also be appropriate in a child with no evidence of a more significant underlying injury. If there is suspicion that the peritoneum has been violated, then several options exist. Some surgeons advocate diagnostic laparoscopy to detect injury to the intra-abdominal organs and potentially repair any damage, or convert to laparotomy. Others would use DPL as the screening tool to determine which patients require laparotomy, using 50,000 red blood cells per mm^3,

stool, bacteria, or increased amylase levels as the criteria. Triple contrast CT scanning for penetrating torso trauma has been shown to have 97% sensitivity and 98% specificity in detecting intra-abdominal injuries in the adult population.[9] Similar studies in children are not available at this time but may provide a less invasive means to determine which child will benefit from laparotomy.

REFERENCES

1. Bruny JL, Densard DD. Hollow viscous injury in the pediatric patient. *Semin Pediatr Surg*. 2004;13:112–118.
2. Coley BD, Mutabagani KH, Martin LC, et al. Focused abdominal sonography for trauma (FAST) in children with blunt abdominal trauma. *J Trauma*. 2000;48:902–906.
3. Gandhi RR, Stringel G. Laparoscopy in pediatric abdominal trauma. *J Soc Laparoendosc Surg*. 1997;1:349–351.
4. McKinley AJ, Mahomed AA. Laparoscopy in a case of pediatric blunt abdominal trauma. *Surg Endosc*. 2002;16:358.
5. Stylianos S. Evidence-based guidelines for resource utilization in children with isolated spleen or liver injuries. *J Pediatr Surg*. 2000; 34:164–169.
6. Stylianos S. Compliance with evidence-based guidelines in children with isolated spleen or liver injury: A prospective study. *J Pediatr Surg*. 2002;37(3):453–456.
7. Mehall JR, Ennis JS, Saltzman DA, et al. Prospective results of a standardized algorithm based on hemodynamic status for managing pediatric solid organ injury. *J Am Coll Surg*. 2001;193: 347–353.
8. Harris HW, Morabito DJ, Mackersie RC, et al. Leukocytosis and free fluid are important indicators of isolated intestinal injury after blunt trauma. *J Trauma*. 1999;46:656–659.
9. Shanmuganathan K, Mirvis SE, Chiu WC, et al. Penetrating torso trauma: Triple-contrast helical CT in peritoneal violation and organ injury—a prospective study in 200 patients. *Radiology*. 2004; 231:775–784.

Hepatic Failure

63

David M. Steinhorn

Acute liver failure is a relatively rare and potentially fatal medical emergency. The pathophysiology is still incompletely understood, leaving the clinician with few specific treatments beyond symptomatic management. Common etiologies include infections, toxins, metabolic disorders, infiltrative diseases, autoimmune hepatitis, and ischemic or irradiation damage, although a significant proportion of cases are cryptogenic.[1] For the pediatric intensivist, the mainstay of therapy consists of supportive measures, with a focus on prevention or treatment of complications and early consideration for liver transplantation.

The definition of liver failure is the loss of vital functions that encompass (i) synthesis of serum proteins including clotting factors and albumin, (ii) bile production and excretion, (iii) detoxification of organic anions, metabolism and storage of glucose and fatty acids, and (iv) elimination of ammonia and other by-products of energy utilization. The significant compromise of these functions implies loss of a critical mass of hepatocytes. "Hyperacute" indicates encephalopathy within 10 days of the onset of jaundice, and acute or "fulminant" liver failure indicates the onset of encephalopathy and coagulopathy within 8 weeks of the onset of liver disease in the absence of preexisting liver disease.[1,2]

EPIDEMIOLOGY

The incidence of acute liver failure in childhood is estimated to be 2,000 cases per year in the United States. A specific etiology is often not determined. The cause of acute liver failure in children is age-dependent,[1,3] with viral hepatitis probably the most common cause in all age-groups. Severe hepatitis due to echovirus and adenovirus is seen almost exclusively in the neonatal population. Liver failure can be a manifestation of overwhelming herpes infection in the newborn or immunocompromised patient. Metabolic liver disease and familial erythrophagocytosis are most commonly found in infants. Acute hepatitis A and B infections are the most common cause in school-aged children. Many of the cases of presumed viral hepatitis in the United States cannot be linked to a known viral pathogen. These cases, referred to as *nontypeable* or *indeterminate hepatitis*, are likely secondary to an as yet unidentified virus. Drug-induced liver disease is more common in older children, especially secondary to intentional acetaminophen overdose. Overall survival is 81% at 3 weeks following presentation with 32% of those requiring liver transplant.

CLINICAL PRESENTATION

In most cases of hepatic failure admitted to the pediatric intensive care unit (PICU), there is overt clinical evidence of hepatic dysfunction with hypoglycemia, coagulopathy, and encephalopathy. Jaundice may develop later, particularly in metabolic diseases. The clinical onset of symptoms may occur within hours or weeks. For most pediatric patients with acute liver failure, there is no history of major medical problems or obvious exposure to hepatitis or toxins.

MANAGEMENT

There is no specific therapy for acute, end-stage liver failure except hepatic replacement. Management is directed toward hepatic support, treatment of acquired infections, early consideration for liver transplantation, and prevention and treatment of complications. The key elements in managing patients before transplantation are (i) meticulous medical support and (ii) rapid referral to a transplant center. Until a diagnosis is made, it is assumed that all children are infectious and that all blood, excretions, and secretions are infectious.

The initial physical examination should determine hepatic, cerebral, cardiovascular, respiratory, renal, and

TABLE 63.1

CLINICAL STAGES OF HEPATIC ENCEPHALOPATHY

Stage	Asterixis	EEG Changes	Clinical Manifestations
I (prodrome)	Slight	Minimal	Mild intellectual impairment, disturbed sleep–awake cycle
II (impending)	Easily elicited	Usually generalized slowing of rhythm	Drowsiness, confusion, coma, inappropriate behavior, disorientation, mood swings
III (stupor)	Present if patient co-operative	Grossly abnormal slowing	Drowsy, unresponsive to verbal commands, markedly confused, delirious, hyperreflexia, (+) Babinski sign
IV (coma)	Usually absent	Appearance of δ waves, decreased amplitudes	Unconscious, decerebrate or decorticate response to pain present (IV$_A$) or absent (IV$_B$)

EEG, electroencephalogram.
Adapted from Trey C, Davidson CS. The management of fulminant hepatic failure. *Prog Liver Dis.* 1970; 2:282–298.[4]

acid–base status. The patient's level of consciousness and degree of hepatic coma are generally categorized as in Table 63.1. Evidence of chronic liver disease or other signs that may suggest an etiology, such as Kayser-Fleischer rings, prominent abdominal veins, cataracts, and needle marks should be established. Liver size and consistency should be determined and documented. The initial laboratory evaluation includes baseline investigations as outlined in Table 63.2. In particular, an abdominal ultrasonography may indicate liver size and patency of hepatic and portal veins, particularly if liver transplant is being considered.

The goal of fluid therapy is to maintain hydration and renal function while not provoking cerebral edema. Maintenance fluids consist of at least 10% dextrose in 0.25 N saline, and intake should be 75% of normal maintenance requirements unless cerebral edema develops. A total sodium intake of 0.5 to 1 mmol/kg/day is usually adequate. Potassium requirements may be large, 3 to 6 mmol/kg/day, as guided by the serum concentration. Patients are at risk for hypophosphatemia and may benefit from intravenous phosphate. Attempts should be made to maintain urinary output using loop diuretics in large doses (furosemide at 1 to 3 mg per kg every 6 hours), dopamine (2 to 5 μg/kg/minute) and colloid/fresh frozen plasma (FFP) to maintain adequate preload and renal perfusion. Hemofiltration or dialysis may be indicated. Hemoglobin should be maintained >10 g per dL for

oxygen delivery. The coagulopathy should be managed conservatively; the massive fluid requirements for FFP may result in fluid overload requiring renal replacement therapy.

It is customary to prescribe vitamin K (2 to 10 mg IV) although it is not usually effective. H$_2$-antagonists and antacids should be administered prophylactically. The role of *N*-acetylcysteine (70 mg per kg 4-hourly) in the management of acute liver failure, other than because of acetaminophen poisoning, may be beneficial and carries low risk.[5] Broad-spectrum antibiotics are only prescribed if sepsis is suspected or liver transplantation is anticipated.

The role of parenteral nutrition is controversial. The main aims are (i) to maintain blood glucose (>40 mg per dL) and (ii) ensure sufficient carbohydrates for energy metabolism to minimize catabolism. Protein intake should be reduced to 1 to 2 g/kg/day. If enteral nutrition is not possible, parenteral nutrition should be provided within 2 to 3 days, as it may be 7 to 10 days before full normal diet is resumed following transplantation.

In evaluating patients with altered mental status from liver failure, a computed tomography (CT) scan is probably not useful early in encephalopathy, but may provide information on cerebral edema or irreversible brain damage later in the disease. Electroencephalogram (EEG) monitoring may be helpful especially if seizures are suspected. Serial examinations and blood ammonia are essential to follow the progress of hepatic encephalopathy.

TABLE 63.2

INITIAL INVESTIGATIONS IN ACUTE HEPATIC FAILURE

- ■ Baseline essential investigations
  - ● Biochemistry
    - ● Bilirubin, transaminases, alkaline phosphatase
    - ● Albumin
    - ● Creatinine, urea, and electrolytes
    - ● Calcium, phosphate
    - ● Ammonia
    - ● Acid–base, lactate
    - ● Glucose
  - ● Hematology—CBC, differential, platelets
    - ● PT, PTT
    - ● Factors V or VII
- ■ Blood group cross-match
- ■ Septic screen with appropriate cultures (*NO* lumbar puncture)
- ■ Radiology
  - ● Chest x-ray
  - ● Abdominal ultrasonography
  - ● Head CT scan or MRI (if cause of encephalopathy not certain)
- ■ Neurophysiology
  - ● EEG (if seizures suspected or cause of encephalopathy not certain)
- ■ Diagnostic investigations
  - ● Serum
    - ● Acetaminophen levels
    - ● Cu, ceruloplasmin (>3 y)
    - ● Autoantibodies (if autoimmune etiology suspected) Immunoglobulins
    - ● Amino acids
    - ● Hepatitis A, B, C, E
    - ● EBV, CMV, HSV
    - ● Leptospira (if clinically relevant)
    - ● Other viruses (adeno, echo)
  - ● Urine
    - ● Toxic screen
    - ● Amino acids, succinylacetone
    - ● Organic acids
    - ● Reducing sugars

CBC, complete blood count; PT, prothrombin time; PTT, partial thromboplastin time; CT, computed tomography; MRI, magnetic resonance imaging; EEG, electroencephalogram; EBV, Epstein-Barr virus; CMV, cytomegalovirus; HSV, herpes simplex virus.

PREVENTION AND MANAGEMENT OF COMPLICATIONS

Hypoglycemia

Hypoglycemia (blood glucose <40 mg per L) develops in most children due to (i) failure of hepatic glucose synthesis and release, (ii) hyperinsulinemia (due to failure of hepatic degradation), (iii) increased glucose utilization (due to anaerobic metabolism), and (iv) secondary bacterial infection. It may contribute to central nervous system (CNS) and other organ dysfunction. Frequent glucose monitoring and intravenous glucose (10% to 50% dextrose) are required. Patients typically require 5 to 8 mg/kg/minute

of dextrose. Clinicians should avoid excessively high rates of glucose infusion because increased insulin production, secondary to excess glucose infusion, leads to increased glucose need and net lipogenesis, which can be avoided by permitting the blood glucose to remain between 40 and 60 mg per L. Profound, refractory hypoglycemia often represents an agonal state.

Coagulopathy and Hemorrhage

Profound disturbances in hemostasis develop secondary to failure of hepatic synthesis of clotting and fibrinolytic factors, reduction in platelet numbers and function, and/or disseminated intravascular coagulation (DIC). The coagulation factors synthesized by hepatocytes include factors I (fibrinogen), II (prothrombin), V, VII, IX, and X. The prothrombin time is the most clinically useful measure of hepatic synthesis of clotting factors and prolongation often precedes other clinical evidence of hepatic failure. Administering vitamin K (2 to 10 mg IV) ensures the sufficiency of this essential cofactor, but rarely improves coagulation. Since the prothrombin time depends on the availability of factor VII, which has a shorter half-life ($t_{1/2}$ approximately 4 to 7 hours) than other factors and decreases more rapidly than other liver-derived clotting factors, it is a more sensitive indicator than other clinical indicators. Fibrinogen concentrations are usually normal unless DIC is present. Decreased levels of factor XIII may contribute to poor clot stabilization. Thrombocytopenia ($<80 \times 10^9$ per L) occurs less commonly in children than in adults. Severe thrombocytopenia, requiring platelet transfusion, suggests hypersplenism, DIC, or aplastic anemia. DIC is present in almost all patients, indicating ongoing clot deposition and dissolution, most probably as a consequence of tissue necrosis in the liver. DIC is rarely significant, but can contribute to organ damage. The administration of concentrates containing activated clotting factors may predispose to DIC.

The goal of therapy is the prevention of life-threatening bleeding and not the maintenance of normal coagulation time. Oozing from needle puncture sites and line insertion is common, whereas pulmonary or intracranial hemorrhage may be terminal events. Life-threatening coagulopathy should be corrected with FFP, cryoprecipitate, and platelets as needed. Administration of recombinant factor VIIa reliably corrects this coagulation defect in patients with acute liver failure for a period of 6 to 12 hours and may be useful in preparation for invasive procedures.[6] In the very small infant, recombinant factor VIIa may provide significant hemostasis with less volume loading. In general, mild to moderate coagulopathy (prothrombin time <25 seconds) requires no therapy except support for procedures. Marked coagulopathy (prothrombin time >40 seconds) should be corrected (10 mL per kg of FFP every 6 hours) to prevent the risk of bleeding, particularly intracranial hemorrhage. If major bleeding occurs, correction is attempted using 15 to 20 mL per kg FFP every 6 hours, or continuous infusions at a rate of 3 to 5 mL/kg/hour. Double-volume exchange transfusion or plasmapheresis may temporarily improve coagulation and DIC, and control hemorrhage. Platelet counts should be maintained above 50×10^9 per L by infusion of platelets.

Prevention of Gastrointestinal Hemorrhage

High-dose H_2-antagonists (ranitidine 1 to 3 mg per kg 8-hourly) or proton-pump inhibitors (omeprazole 10 to 20 mg/kg/day) should be administered intravenously and sucralfate (1 to 2 g 4-hourly) may be given to reduce gastritis or stress ulceration. Prevention of gastrointestinal hemorrhage may also prevent further hyperammonemia.

Encephalopathy

Acute hepatic encephalopathy may be exacerbated by sepsis, gastrointestinal bleeding, electrolyte disturbances, or sedation, particularly benzodiazepine administration. The evolution and progression usually occurs over days. In rare cases, the encephalopathy may progress rapidly with coma and fatal cerebral edema developing within hours. Elective ventilation should be considered if the encephalopathy progresses compromising the airway or if respiratory distress occurs.

Although the role played by ammonia in the development of encephalopathy is controversial, therapy to reduce ammonia production or accumulation is indicated (see Fig. 63.1). The components of therapy are (i) restriction of dietary protein, (ii) enteral antibiotics, (iii) enteral lactulose, (iv) continuous hemofiltration, and (v) controlling the complications of acute liver failure that contribute to ammonia accumulation.

In the early stages of hepatic encephalopathy, measures are taken to minimize the formation of nitrogenous substances in the intestine. A cathartic, such as sodium-free magnesium sulfate and/or a nonabsorbable disaccharide (lactulose 1 to 2 mL per kg every 4 to 6 hours) may be administered. Neomycin (50 to 100 mg/kg/day) may also be used to prevent ammonia production if diarrhea, secondary to lactulose, is a problem. Protein intake should be limited to 0.5 to 1 g/kg/day in this phase to limit ammonia production.

If sedation is required, short-acting barbiturates or opiates can be safely utilized, but benzodiazepines should be avoided. There are potential therapeutic implications related to the γ-aminobutyric acid (GABA) receptor, which has been implicated in encephalopathy. Flumazenil, a benzodiazepine antagonist, may produce temporary reversal of hepatic encephalopathy.[7] Administration is followed within minutes by a clinical response, which may last for several hours. A lack of response to flumazenil may indicate a poor prognosis.

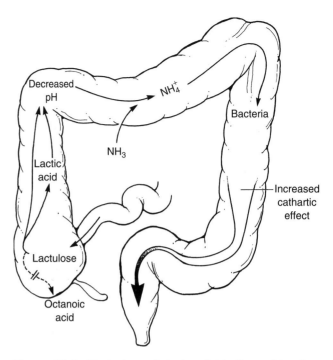

Figure 63.1 Mechanisms of the beneficial effects of lactulose in hepatic encephalopathy. Bacterial fermentation results in an increased transformation to lactic acid and short-chain fatty acids, while decreasing the formation of medium-chain fatty acids such as octanoic acid and favoring catharsis. The resultant reduction in intestinal pH favors the passage of ammonia into the intestinal lumen, with conversion to ammonium ion. Bacteria incorporate NH_4^+ for their own metabolism. (From Yamada T, Alpers DH, Laine L, et al. *Atlas of gastroenterology*, 3rd ed. Philadelphia, PA: Lippincott Williams & Wilkins; 2003.)

Cerebral Edema

Cerebral edema may develop between stage III and stage IV encephalopathy. Brain death associated with cerebral edema is the most frequent cause of death in acute liver failure and contributes to reduced survival after liver transplantation.[8] The diagnosis and management of cerebral edema associated with hepatic failure is analogous to that utilized for other forms of cytotoxic cerebral edema (see Chapter 7).

Renal Dysfunction

Renal insufficiency complicates the course in 75% of children[9] and may be due to prerenal azotemia, acute tubular necrosis, and functional renal failure. Functional renal failure (hepatorenal syndrome) is the most common cause of renal insufficiency. Features include sodium retention (urinary sodium concentration <20 mmol per L), normal urinary sediment, and reduced urinary output (<1 mL/kg/hour). The etiology is multifactorial, and electrolyte imbalance, sepsis, and hypovolemia all play a part. Although functional renal failure recovers quickly after liver transplantation, acute tubular necrosis may severely complicate the postoperative management. Up to 50% of patients require hemodialysis or continuous renal replacement therapy (CRRT); however, renal function returns to normal after successful liver transplantation.

Ascites

Ultrasonography examination in the pretransplant assessment has demonstrated excess peritoneal fluid in most patients, probably due to acute portal hypertension from lobular collapse, vasodilatation, poor vascular integrity, and reduced oncotic pressure. Clinically evident ascites occurs in less than half the patients but may be a site for secondary infection, necessitating paracentesis in septic patients without an obvious focus of infection. Therapy is not indicated, other than the correction of oncotic pressure with albumin and general fluid management. Paracentesis may be indicated if peritonitis is suspected or if the intra-abdominal pressure leads to impaired renal perfusion. However, paracentesis is frequently associated with dramatic intravascular volume shifts as ascites reaccumulates and may predispose to peritonitis.

Secondary Bacterial and Fungal Infections

Most adults and 50% of children develop significant infection,[10] which may be related to impairment of cellular and humoral immune systems. The organisms most often implicated are gram positive (*Staphylococcus aureus*, *S. epidermidis*, and streptococci), presumably of skin origin, but gram-negative bacteria and fungal infections are also observed. Nosocomial infections are common. Broad-spectrum antibiotics should be started at the first suspicion of sepsis, as the signs may be subtle. Prophylactic antifungals such as amphotericin (1.5 mg/kg/day) or fluconazole (3 to 6 mg/kg/day) may be effective, although potentially nephrotoxic.

EXTRACORPOREAL HEPATIC SUPPORT

Transplantation may not be available in short enough time to prevent irreversible complications. Therefore, therapies have been developed over the last decade intended to temporize and support adult patients having acute fulminant hepatic failure or so-called acute or chronic hepatic failure. They utilize a single vascular access with a clearance, against a charcoal filter, of toxins resulting from hepatic failure.[11] Such techniques have been used less frequently in pediatrics and to date there is no pediatric literature to support this therapy. Attempts to create extracorporeal artificial liver systems utilizing living hepatocytes in various configurations have shown promise; however, as yet unsolved technical problems have limited the utility and wide-spread availability of this approach to research centers only.

Alternately, many programs have used CRRT. CRRT targets several important goals in managing patients with liver failure. It provides a means of optimizing fluids and electrolytes, provides improved fluid balance if large volumes of fluid are needed, permits the provision of optimal nutritional support, and greatly enhances ammonia clearance. Data to date have shown that small molecular weight solute (e.g., urea) can be cleared equally effectively between continuous venovenous hemofiltration (CVVH) and continual venovenous hemodiafiltration (CVVHD).[12] Personal experience has also shown that ammonia can be equally cleared by CVVH and CVVHD. Because of the underlying coagulopathy, such patients may require little or no anticoagulation.[13] However, prolonged clotting times resulting from liver failure are due to decreased factor levels rather than to direct anticoagulation. Therefore, some patients may have a confusing coagulation status in which they appear "anticoagulated" based upon clotting times, yet have a tendency to be hypercoagulable partially due to depressed levels of anticlotting factors. In patients with failing hepatic function, citrate is poorly metabolized and may accumulate over time if it is used as an anticoagulant.

LIVER TRANSPLANTATION

Liver transplantation should be considered in all children who develop a stage III or IV hepatic coma, as mortality in this group exceeds 70%.[1] Transplantation is indicated for all forms of acute liver failure. It is also appropriate for some inborn errors of metabolism. Transplantation using a living donor can accelerate the process and is associated with better outcome in the setting of acute liver failure.

The highest mortality is seen in children with indeterminate hepatitis, particularly those with a rapid onset of coma and progression to stage III or IV hepatic coma, a shrinking liver, falling transaminases associated with an increase in bilirubin, and coagulopathy. Such children should be immediately considered for transplantation. In practical terms, it is appropriate to list for emergency liver transplantation all children who have reached stage III hepatic coma. Relative contraindications for transplantation include untreated sepsis, human immunodeficiency virus (HIV) infection, and the presence of vascular thrombosis. Absolute contraindications include progressive terminal extrahepatic disease, irreversible or rapidly degenerative CNS disease, intestinal failure, or untreatable metastatic diseases.

REFERENCES

1. Pineiro-Carrero VM, Pineiro EO. Liver. *Pediatrics*. 2004;113(4): 1097–1106.
2. Baker A, Alonso E, Aw M, et al. Hepatic failure and liver transplant: Working Group Report of the Second World Congress of Pediatric Gastroenterology, Hepatology, and Nutrition. *J Pediatr Gastroenterol Nutr*. 2004;39:S632–S639.

3. Sokol RJ. Fulminant hepatic failure. In: Balistreri WF, Stocker JT, eds. *Pediatric hepatology.* New York: Hemisphere Publishing; 1990:315–362.
4. Trey C, Davidson CS. The management of fulminant hepatic failure. *Prog Liver Dis.* 1970;2:282–298.
5. Sklar G, Subramaniam M. Acetylcysteine treatment for non-acetaminophen-induced acute liver failure. *Ann Pharmacother.* 2004;38:498–500.
6. Brown J, Emerick K, Brown D, et al. Recombinant factor VIIa improves coagulopathy caused by liver failure. *J Pediatr Gastroenterol Nutr.* 2003;37:268–272.
7. Bansky G, Meier PJ, Riederer E, et al. Effects of the benzodiazepine receptor antagonist flumazenil in hepatic encephalopathy in humans. *Gastroenterology.* 1989;97:744–750.
8. Jalan R. Intracranial hypertension in acute liver failure: Pathophysiological basis of rational management. *Semin Liver Dis.* 2003; 23:271–282.
9. Bihari DJ, Gimson AE, Williams R. Cardiovascular, pulmonary and renal complications of fulminant hepatic failure. *Semin Liver Dis.* 1986;6:119–128.
10. Rolando N, Harvey F, Brahm J, et al. Prospective study of bacterial infection in acute liver failure: An analysis of fifty patients. *Hepatology.* 1990;11:49–53.
11. Sauer I, Goetz M, Steffen J, et al. In vitro comparison of the molecular adsorbent recirculation system (MARS) and single-pass albumin dialysis (SPAD). *Hepatology.* 2004;39:1408–1414.
12. Maxvold N, Smoyer W, Custer J, et al. Amino acid loss and nitrogen balance in critically ill children with acute renal failure: A prospective comparison between classic hemofiltration and hemofiltration with dialysis. *Crit Care Med.* 2000;28:1161–1165.
13. Emre S, Schwartz ME, Shneider B, et al. Living related liver transplantation for acute liver failure in children. *Liver Transpl Surg.* 1999;5(3):161–165.

Gastrointestinal Failure

64

David M. Steinhorn

Intestinal failure occurs sporadically and appears most prominently in the medical literature dealing with the short bowel syndrome in children[1] and adults.[2] Intestinal failure is defined as a condition in which inadequate digestion or absorption of nutrients, fluids, and electrolytes lead to malnutrition or dehydration.[3] In pediatrics, such conditions are associated with failure to thrive and often diarrhea or feeding intolerance as the primary manifestations of nutritional failure. Additionally, intestinal failure is a frequent finding in children admitted to the pediatric intensive care unit (PICU), resulting from both acutely acquired and chronic conditions. Intestinal failure routinely complicates many diseases treated in the PICU, necessitating the use of modified enteral feeding regimens or parenteral nutrition. The importance of nutritional support in patients with intestinal failure extends beyond simply providing nutrition to the body. Nutritional support during recovery from critical illness is essential to prevent atrophy of the epithelium and to maintain integrity of the immune barrier function of the bowel.

In developing countries, intestinal failure results most commonly from gastrointestinal infections including parasites, viruses, and bacterial processes. In industrialized countries, severe congenital disease or diseases acquired in early infancy, which require long-term parenteral nutrition, predominate. It is perhaps ironic that much of the acquired intestinal failure in early infancy results from the success in treating sick newborns and infants having intra-abdominal vascular catastrophes. Children with severe intestinal failure represent an important group of chronically ill children with limited therapeutic options. They often require frequent admission to the PICU and are an emotionally and ethically difficult group of patients to treat.

ETIOLOGY OF INTESTINAL FAILURE

Infectious causes of acute, acquired intestinal failure are seen in developed countries and are commonly dealt with by general pediatricians or gastroenterologists. Intestinal failure presenting to the pediatric intensivist generally represents complications of massive resection (short bowel syndrome), congenital diseases of the epithelium (microvillus atrophy, epithelial dysplasia, tufting enteropathy), or neuromuscular diseases involving the gastrointestinal tract such as long-segment Hirschsprung disease or intestinal pseudo-obstruction. Occasionally, patients with active inflammatory bowel disease are admitted to the PICU for assistance with complex management issues including nutritional difficulties, fluid and electrolyte problems, and sepsis or systemic inflammatory response syndrome involving several organ systems.

Acquired Diseases of the Epithelium

Most cases of acquired epithelial disease are infectious or immune in origin. Most viral infections are self-limited and require only supportive care, whereas bacterial and parasitic infections may require specific antimicrobial therapy. Autoimmune disorders are a separate class of epithelial injury and require specific therapies to control the mucosal inflammation and chronic systemic disease that often accompanies it. Hypersensitivity to various constituents of food, such as cow's milk protein or gluten, tend to be self-limited if the offending agent can be identified and eliminated from the diet. Finally, ischemic injury to the intestine as may occur after shock, cardiopulmonary bypass or arrest, and trauma will require variable periods of recovery to ensure the readiness of the intestine for the reintroduction of feeding. Given the 7- to 10-day life span of the enterocytes and the delicate nature of villous and microvillous absorptive surface, recovery of normal digestive and absorptive function may require as much as 10 to 14 days of conservative support involving the use of modified enteral formulas or parenteral nutrition. The brush border enzyme activity recovers at variable rates, with lactase activity being one of the last to return. Therefore, lactose should be reintroduced into the diet at a later time.

Congenital Diseases of the Epithelium

Congenital epithelial diseases include tufting enteropathy, epithelial dysplasia, and microvillous inclusion disease. They are generally not compatible with recovery and require prolonged parenteral nutrition or small bowel transplantation.

Intestinal Pseudo-Obstruction

Intestinal pseudo-obstruction is a poorly understood condition associated with the intolerance of enteral nutrition due to profound dysregulated intestinal motility. It has generally not been amenable to surgical or pharmacologic intervention and commonly becomes a fatal condition secondary to toxic megacolon or recurrent bacteremia and sepsis. The only management is with parenteral nutrition and concerted efforts to keep the bowel decompressed and free of stagnant material. Limited experience with bowel transplant exists in this group of patients, but it may be the only alternative to achieve enteral nutritional support.

Short Bowel Syndrome

The incidence of short bowel syndrome in the general pediatric population is difficult to estimate; however, in a retrospective study of 875 children receiving parenteral nutrition for more than 3 months between 1975 and 2000 at University of California, Los Angeles, 78 (9%) children had a residual jejunoileal segment ≤75 cm due to surgical resection or congenital malformation.[4] Very short small bowel was defined as 15 to 38 cm of residual jejunoileal small bowel and ultrashort small bowel as <15 cm as measured along the antimesenteric border distal to the ligament of Treitz. Poor prognostic markers included residual length <15 cm, removal of the ileocecal valve, resection of >50% of the colon, or the development of cholestasis. The absence of an ileocecal valve was associated with 100% mortality in patients with <15 cm of small bowel; whereas, survival was 75% in those patients when the ileocecal valve was present.

The diseases that may lead to massive loss of small bowel include congenital atresias, midgut volvulus, abdominal wall defects, vascular catastrophes from volvulus or thromboembolism, long-segment Hirschsprung disease (aganglionosis), trauma, and necrotizing enterocolitis (NEC) in the neonate. Additional loss of intestinal mass may be seen occasionally following resection for inflammatory bowel disease or tumors, although this scenario is much less common in children than in adults.

CLINICAL SIGNS OF PATIENTS WITH INTESTINAL FAILURE

The clinical presentation of patients with intestinal failure is dependent upon (i) the degree of malabsorption produced by loss of intestinal mass or epithelial function, and (ii) the mechanism of dysfunction. For example, patients with gluten-sensitive enteropathy may present with profound diarrhea, weight loss, and failure to thrive, which is usually amenable to enteral rehabilitation. Patients with active inflammatory bowel disease may present with bloody, mucoid diarrhea and malabsorption as well as cramping pain, anemia, and generalized malaise with weight loss. They may require both enteral and parenteral nutritional rehabilitation in addition to therapies directed at the underlying inflammatory process.

The gastrointestinal tract has important endocrine and immunologic roles in addition to the roles of digestion and absorption. The loss of intestinal barrier function against bacterial translocation or the development of dysregulated mucosal inflammation can lead to profound systemic illness.

The duodenum extends from the pylorus to the ligament of Treitz and is structurally similar to the jejunum but also contains bicarbonate-secreting glands that aid in neutralizing gastric acidity and in permitting the action of pancreaticobiliary secretions. The duodenum and proximal jejunum are the primary sites of carbohydrate, protein, and water-soluble vitamin and micronutrient absorption (see Chapter 9). Sodium absorption in the proximal small intestine is coupled to the absorption of other nutrients such as glucose. The junctions between cells in the proximal small bowel permit the relatively rapid flux of water and solutes back into the lumen in contrast to the distal small bowel and colon. The upper gut is also the site of production of several gastrointestinal hormones in response to nutrients entering the lumen. The hormones influence the autonomic nervous system and gut motility, regulate the rate of digestion, and promote further growth of the bowel, that is, "trophic effect." The distal small bowel including the distal jejunum and ileum are important sites for lipid and fat-soluble vitamin absorption. Additionally, the distal ileum is the specific site for bile salt resorption (enterohepatic circulation) and vitamin B_{12} absorption. Therefore, the loss of the terminal ileum is associated with depletion in the bile salt pool, which is one of the hallmarks of the short bowel syndrome. Inadequate bile salts are associated with a reduced ability to absorb long-chain (C14 to 20) fatty acids.

INTESTINAL ADAPTION

Intestinal adaption refers to a process in which there are both structural and functional changes in the remaining intestine. It is a complex process depending upon the specific areas of bowel loss and the presence of ostomies or anastomoses.[3,5] Structural adaption refers to the increase in size and surface area. Functional adaptation generally refers to a slowing in transit time, which permits greater absorption of nutrients. The ileum appears to be more capable of undergoing structural adaptive changes while the jejunum manifests primarily functional adaptation. Additionally, increased appetite (hyperphagia) represents a compensatory mechanism to improve the net absorption of nutrients.

The importance of enteral nutrients to the process of bowel adaptation cannot be overemphasized. Atrophy of the epithelium and associated absorptive mechanisms develops when the epithelium is deprived of luminal nutrients and the demand on the epithelium for absorption is reduced. The luminal nutrients are thought to exert their so-called trophic effect through (i) direct stimulation of the epithelial cells leading to hyperplasia, (ii) stimulation of trophic hormone release in the gastrointestinal tract, and (iii) stimulation of trophic secretions from the pancreaticobiliary tract. It has been difficult to demonstrate the superiority of one enteral nutrient over another in supporting adaption, for example, dipeptides versus glucose; however, it appears that the absorptive work demanded of the epithelial cells is an important stimulus. Animal studies suggest that the trophic effect for macronutrients proceeds in the order of free fatty acids > long-chain triglycerides > protein or polysaccharide.[3] The provision of trophic feedings has become a standard in many PICUs without evidence of an increased risk of NEC or other complications.

Hormones and growth factors play a major role in intestinal adaptation. They exert their effects through both paracrine and remote actions. The factors that have been best studied in humans include enteral glutamine supplementation, growth hormone, and glucagonlike-peptide-2.[1,3] An understanding of the full effects of these factors is rudimentary at present and beyond the scope of this book. The interested reader is referred to recent reviews for additional information.[2,3,5]

From a clinical perspective, bowel adaptation occurs in three phases after massive bowel resection. The first phase lasts several weeks and is characterized by large fluid and electrolyte losses lasting up to several weeks after resection. The second phase is associated with an emphasis on nutritional considerations. It is during the second phase that enteral tolerance increases and the dependence upon parenteral nutrition decreases. The third phase is one of relative equilibrium in which no further adaptive changes occur.

MANAGEMENT OF PATIENTS WITH INTESTINAL FAILURE

As in other aspects of critical care, it is axiomatic that the underlying pathology must be corrected and nonviable tissue removed to maximize the potential for recovery. This approach lies at the core of intensive care unit (ICU) management and is essential to reduce the secondary morbidity of multiple organ dysfunction syndrome (MODS). Volume resuscitation and the correction of major fluid and electrolyte imbalances should proceed according to

conventional practice. In the initial phase of management following massive bowel loss, large losses of fluids and associated electrolytes may occur and require appropriate correction. Total parenteral nutrition must be implemented to minimize the loss of lean body mass associated with major abdominal surgery and physiologic stress, and to preserve the residual intestinal mass to whatever extent possible, thereby promoting healing and immune competence. Liver disease associated with short bowel syndrome and the reliance upon parenteral nutrition are the greatest morbidities deriving from intestinal failure. Disruption of the enterohepatic circulation, bacterial overgrowth with repeated portal endotoxemia, and hepatocyte toxicity caused by the intravenous infusion of amino acids and hypertonic dextrose all contribute to liver disease.

Parenteral nutrition with appropriate amino acid solutions, developed for neonates, containing taurine should be provided with intralipids to limit the need for glucose and to provide essential fatty acids. The cycling of parenteral nutrition, which permits a period of 4 to 8 hours of reduced glucose infusion is thought to be beneficial by reducing the hyperinsulinemic state associated with hypertonic dextrose infusion and minimizing hepatic steatosis. Stimulation of the enterobiliary axis through the introduction of enteral long-chain fats or breast milk and the provision of low rates of trophic feedings containing osmolality <310 mOsm per L make up the additional adjuncts to management in the acute postresection phase. Rates in infusion of trophic enteral feedings typically start off as low as 0.5 to 1.0 mL/kg/hour to provide limited nutrients to the proximal gut.

During the subsequent phase of management, continuous enteral feedings should be given through nasogastric or gastrostomy tube to provide a continuous source of stimuli to the enterocytes as intestinal adaptation progresses. Gradual increases in the rate of feeding may be made as the patient demonstrates improved tolerance of the nutrient load. Clinicians should be aware of the potential for bacterial overgrowth that undermines attempts at advancing enteral intake. Bacterial overgrowth is a frequent complication leading to translocation of bacteria, mucosal injury, and further malabsorption. It is manifested by anorexia, vomiting, abdominal distension, and failure to thrive. In addition, it is an additional risk factor for liver disease associated with parenteral nutrition and short bowel syndrome. Close cooperation between the gastroenterology service and the intensivist is important to minimize mishaps and injudicious nutrient prescription.

Ultimately, 75% to 90% of infants and children with short bowel syndrome will survive the loss of large portions of the intestine. The remaining small intestine can adapt even when <15 cm of jejunum remains. The presence of an ileocecal valve and >50% of the colon remaining improves the chances of survival. In patients with 40 to 80 cm of remaining small intestine and intact ileocecal valve, 80% were weaned from parenteral nutrition within 1 year.[1]

SURGICAL MANAGEMENT OF SHORT BOWEL SYNDROME

Several surgical approaches have been developed for patients with short bowel syndrome. Procedures that reverse a loop of bowel to slow transit have been used with some success. Tapering enteroplasty reduces the caliber of the bowel, minimizing the potential for stasis and bacterial overgrowth. Longitudinal intestinal lengthening may be used in select patients with dilated loops to reduce the caliber and increase the length of the bowel.[6]

Patients with life-threatening intestinal failure or associated liver disease may undergo isolated or double organ transplantation as a lifesaving option. Nearly 1,000 small bowel transplants with and without liver transplantation have been performed according to the International Intestinal Transplant Registry (www.intestinaltransplant.org) with approximately two third occurring in children. An overall 3-year survival appears to be approximately 50%. Death typically occurs due to infection (50%), which is a common complication of small bowel transplants, MODS (25%), or lymphoma (10%). Although the prognosis continues to improve yearly as centers develop greater experience and expertise with the procedure, it still is one of the more difficult transplantation procedures, demanding considerable postoperative resources and management. The pediatric intensivist may be called upon to participate in the management of patients following small bowel transplantation, and may see the same patients readmitted on multiple occasions for treatment of the recurrent bacteremia that occurs until mucosal integrity is regained during the 3- to 6-month critical postoperative period.

REFERENCES

1. Goulet O, Ruemmele F, Lacaille F, et al. Irreversible intestinal failure. *J Pediatr Gastroenterol Nutr.* 2004;38:250–269.
2. Buchman A, Scolapio J, Fryer J. AGA technical review on short bowel syndrome and intestinal transplantation. *Gastroenterology.* 2003;124:1111–1134.
3. DiBaise J, Young R, Vanderhoof J. Intestinal rehabilitation and the short bowel syndrome: Parts 1 & 2. *Am J Gastroenterol.* 2004; 99(7,9):1386–1395;1823–1832.
4. Quiros-Tejeira R, Ament M, Reyen L, et al. Long-term parenteral nutritional support and intestinal adaption in children with short bowel syndrome: A 25-year experience. *J Pediatr.* 2004;145: 157–163.
5. Weale A, Edward A, Bailey M, et al. Intestinal adaptation after massive intestinal resection. *Postgrad Med J.* 2005;81:178–184.
6. Bianchi A. Longitudinal intestinal lengthening and tailoring: Results in 20 children. *JR Soc Med.* 1997;90:429–432.

Nutritional Support in Critical Illness

65

Donald E. George   *Laura T. Russo*   *David M. Steinhorn*

Critical illness places increasing demands on the body's nutritional requirements. These conditions promote a catabolic state and negative nitrogen balance. (See Chapter 2 for an extensive discussion of the endocrine and cytokine changes mediating the catabolic state.) Nutritional care of severely ill children and infants has improved considerably over the last three decades largely through an increased understanding of nutritional biochemistry and the physiologic response to stress and trauma. However, the feeding of the critically ill child has not been subjected to extensive trials and there are few evidence-based clinical guidelines. Many recommendations are derived based on data from adult critical care units.

Nutritional support is likely to have only a modest effect on survival although it has a central role in reducing morbidity and accelerating recovery. The deleterious effects of undernutrition on wound healing and immune function must be weighed against the harmful effects of overfeeding including the risks of aspiration, hyperglycemia, and infection. There are striking differences between adults and children (especially neonates) in body composition, protein stores, and energy requirements. Although supporting the nutrition and metabolic needs of children have contributed to the care for patients with very complex diseases, they have also created morbidities such as parenteral nutrition–associated cholestasis, catheter-associated infections, and hyperglycemia.

NUTRITIONAL ASSESSMENT

The existence of chronic malnutrition, as well as the development of acute malnutrition during critical illness, may complicate the response to therapies or impair recovery (see Table 65.1). The nutritional assessment should include

TABLE 65.1

CLASSIFICATION OF MALNUTRITION: WATERLOW CRITERIA

Acute malnutrition:
$$\frac{\text{Actual weight (kg)} \times 100}{\text{Expected weight (kg) for height (cm)} \text{ at 50th percentile}}$$

Stage 0 (normal) >90%
Stage I (mild) 81%–90%
Stage II (moderate) 70%–80%
Stage III (severe) <70%

Chronic malnutrition:
$$\frac{\text{Actual height (cm)} \times 100}{\text{Expected height (cm) for age} \text{ at 50th percentile}}$$

Stage 0 (normal) >90%
Stage I (mild) 90%–95%
Stage II (moderate) 85%–89%
Stage III (severe) <85%

Body mass index $= \dfrac{\text{Actual weight (kg)}}{[\text{Actual height (m)}]^2}$

subjective assessments including specific gastrointestinal problems, previous growth history, changes in body weight, and dietary intake. The objective assessment should include data from clinical, anthropometric, and laboratory evaluations. Objective assessments of nutritional status include growth indices, weight, and Tanner stage. The determination of body mass index (BMI) for children older than 2 years provides important information regarding the nutritional status. In children younger than 2 years, the weight-for-age and weight-for-length is most useful (Table 65.1).

Anthropometric measurements including mid-arm circumference and skin fold determination are useful as they reflect body composition. Potential errors in interpretation are primarily related to changes in body water.

Laboratory assessment of nutritional status can be quantitatively accomplished by measuring the visceral protein pool, the acute-phase protein pool, and the nitrogen and energy expenditures. The pool of proteins in the plasma, interstitial space, and some intracellular proteins represent a relatively labile pool of protein referred to as the *visceral protein pool*. Specific visceral proteins including albumin, transferrin, and prealbumin are helpful in assessing both the initial status and the response to therapy. Serum proteins may be decreased during acute critical illness in the absence of preceding malnutrition. Through the loss of endothelial barrier function, large molecules, such as albumin, move into the extravascular space, lowering their concentration without a concomitant decrease in the total body pool of albumin. Albumin, which has a large pool size and a long half-life (21 days), does not accurately reflect the nutritional status during catabolic states and may be skewed by changes in fluid status. Shorter half-life serum proteins, such as prealbumin (2 days) and transferrin (7 days), reflect nutritional status and respond more quickly to changes in the anabolic state. Prealbumin is also a good marker for the visceral protein pool. When followed longitudinally, the return of previously depressed levels of visceral proteins represents the abatement of physiologic stress or improvement in nutrition.

The body's response to acute physiologic stress tends to be similar whether the inciting event is sepsis, ischemia-reperfusion, trauma, burns, or other inflammatory conditions (see Chapter 2). There is a constellation of aberrations that tend to be both predictable and profound. There is the activation of the hypothalamic-pituitary axis and of the sympathetic nervous system with elevation of growth hormone, endogenous catecholamines, glucagon, and cortisol; and an increase in gluconeogenesis and insulin and growth hormone resistance. Unremitting gluconeogenesis occurs through the release of glycerol and amino acids from the periphery, with their conversion to glucose in the liver and kidney. Hyperglycemia is frequently associated with this state. Activation of the immune system and increased cytokine production can elicit dramatic systemic inflammatory responses through proinflammatory mediators (see Chapter 3.2).

The body's response to withholding feeding, that is, starvation, in healthy individuals is different from that seen during periods of high physiologic stress when nutrient intake is absent (see Table 65.2). In simple starvation, the body's regulatory mechanisms for sparing lean tissue and utilizing triglycerides as the primary energy source is intact. With decreased nutrient intake, an otherwise healthy individual will rely on ketone bodies derived from the breakdown of fat stores to provide energy. Protein stores are relatively spared as the decrease in insulin output allows the use of ketones as fuel, especially for the brain. Protein catabolism is readily suppressed by providing exogenous amino acids or glucose and fat.

TABLE 65.2
COMPARISON OF NUTRIENT METABOLISM IN STARVATION VERSUS SEPSIS/TRAUMA

	Starvation	Sepsis/Trauma
Protein breakdown	+	+++
Hepatic protein synthesis	+	+++
Amino acid oxidation	+	+++
Ureagenesis	+	+++
Gluconeogenesis	+	+++
Energy expenditure	Reduced	Increased
Mediator activation	Low	High
Hormone counter-regulatory capacity	Preserved	Poor
Ketonemia	+++	+
Loss of body stores	Gradual	Rapid
Primary fuels	Fat	Amino acids, glucose, triglycerides

+, increased; +++, very increased.
Adapted from Barton R, Cerra FB. The Hypermetabolism, multiple organ failure syndrome. *Chest*. 1989;96:1153–1160.

In contrast, the breakdown of protein is a central theme in the body's response to stress. The conversion of certain amino acids to glucose and the oxidation of others in peripheral tissues leads to the liberation of large quantities of amino-nitrogen that would become toxic if not for its efficient conversion to urea. Protein catabolism rates can be increased as much as twofold, and since synthesis does not keep pace, a state of negative nitrogen balance ensues. A major consequence of physiologic stress is the net depletion of protein, both structural (e.g., skeletal muscle mass), and functional (e.g., plasma proteins, enzyme systems, antibodies). Total urinary nitrogen losses in critically ill children may be as high as 0.3 g/kg/day, which represents the loss of up to approximately 1.8 g/kg/day of protein. During critical illness or stress, protein breakdown is not readily suppressed; however, the rate of protein synthesis is increased when patients are given adequate calories and amino acids.

ENERGY EXPENDITURE

The energy needs of patients are dependent on their resting metabolic rate, degree of illness, physical activity, and need for growth. Resting energy expenditure (REE) encompasses the basal metabolic rate plus diet-induced thermogenesis (heat generated by the consumption of food). Injury or illness markedly alters energy needs. A catabolic state proportional to the degree of injury occurs suppressing somatic growth. Children are frequently sedated and their activity level is reduced. Further, they are in a temperature-controlled environment and insensible energy losses are reduced. Patients who are mechanically ventilated have a reduced work of breathing.

Indirect calorimetry relies on the measurement of the volume of oxygen consumed (Vo_2) and the volume of carbon dioxide produced (Vco_2), and usually a correction factor based on the urinary nitrogen excreted to calculate energy production. Although indirect calorimetry has limitations, it has helped elucidate that patients with similar clinical appearances may have widely differing metabolic rates when adjusted for age and weight.

Ideally, nutrition should be targeted to support basal metabolic requirements and limit protein loss. In healthy children, REE is approximately 70% of total energy expenditure. Diet-induced thermogenesis makes up only approximately 5% of REE. In general, the REE of critically ill patients tends to be higher than of healthy children, but their activity levels are lower. To account for these alterations, caloric amounts equal to measured energy expenditure or basal energy requirements should be provided. Overfeeding is of no benefit in maintaining lean body mass and results in the synthesis of excess fat. This may induce hepatic steatosis and impaired liver function, and increase the risk of hyperglycemia. Additionally, the synthesis of fat increases CO_2 production, which may contribute to ventilatory compromise. Increase in energy requirement during acute illness and following physiologic stress tend to mirror elevated protein needs.

PRESCRIBING NUTRITIONAL SUPPORT

Nutritional support is employed to minimize the loss of lean body mass and support the synthesis of critical visceral proteins. Nutritional support should be initiated as soon as the patient is hemodynamically and metabolically stable. During most of the acute critical illnesses, it is unreasonable to anticipate significant somatic growth, and the energy required for other activities is markedly decreased. The requirement for nutrients can be divided into the macronutrients consisting of water, protein, carbohydrate, and fat, and the micronutrients consisting of minerals, vitamins, and trace elements. The vitamins and trace elements play key roles as essential cofactors in protein synthesis and intermediary metabolism.

Fluids and Electrolytes

Fluid and electrolyte needs for most patients can be estimated based on body weight, as is commonly prescribed in hospitalized infants and children, and as relevant to their critical care illness.

Protein

An adequate supply of exogenous amino acids is of paramount importance. Although neither glucose nor amino

TABLE 65.3

PROTEIN REQUIREMENTS (G/KG/D)

	Acute Phase (First 3–5 d)	Convalescent Phase (After 5 d)
Infants/children <7 y	1.5–2.5	–2.0–3.0
Children >7 y	1.5–2.0	1.5–2.5

acids will stop the protein breakdown in the stressed patient, amino acid supplementation does improve protein balance through increased protein synthesis. The high rate of protein turnover during critical illness is associated with an increase in urea production and urinary nitrogen losses that may amount to as much as 1 to 2 g/kg/day of protein equivalent. Protein must be administered in amounts sufficient to replace losses, synthesize new tissue and visceral protein, and for some energy utilization. Protein requirements are shown in Table 65.3. Furthermore, calories should be provided in sufficient quantity to ensure that protein can be used for synthesis rather than as an energy substrate (see Table 65.4). The calorie to nitrogen ratio derives from the concept that protein should be used for synthesis of functional and structural molecules rather than used as energy. For a typical healthy individual, the ratio of nonprotein calories to nitrogen ranges from 250 to 350:1. During illness, the ratio may be lower in the range of 100 to 200:1.

Carbohydrate

Carbohydrate serves predominantly as an energy source. The carbon backbone of the sugars also provides the basis for synthesis of many of the nonessential nutrients in the body. The caloric density of common dietary carbohydrate is generally 4 kcal per g except for dextrose solutions, which provide 3.4 kcal per g because of energy lost through the process of hydration in solution. In general, the cellular energy requirements of most critically ill children and adults

TABLE 65.4

TARGET GOALS FOR NONPROTEIN CALORIES (KCAL/KG/D)

	Acute Phase (First 3–5 d)	Convalescent Phase (After 5 d)
All children (<10 kg)	50–80	80–120
Children (1–7 y and >10 kg)	45–65	75–90
Children (>7 y)	30–50	30–75

can be met through the infusion of 5 to 8 mg/kg/minute of dextrose. This range represents approximately 25 to 40 kcal/kg/day of carbohydrate calories and is a close first approximation of basal energy expenditure seen in many hospitalized children. In healthy, nonstressed individuals, ketosis ensues when glucose entry into the circulation falls below 1.5 to 2 mg/kg/minute. Infusion of >10 to 12 mg/kg/minute of glucose results in net lipogenesis and excess carbon dioxide production. Hyperglycemia in stressed patients is due to several factors including increased gluconeogenesis, decreased insulin release, increased insulin resistance, as well as carbohydrate intake. When hyperglycemia develops in the face of *appropriate* rates of glucose infusion, it has become routine to administer insulin as a continuous infusion. Well-controlled studies in critically ill adults support the control of serum glucose in critically ill patients in a narrow euglycemic range.

Fat

Lipid metabolism is generally accelerated by illness and physiologic stress and is a prime source of energy. Hepatic production of ketones is increased, although less than during starvation. During periods of high physiologic stress, triglyceride levels are frequently elevated due to decreased peripheral clearance related to impaired lipoprotein lipase activity, increased generation of triglycerides from excess carbohydrate infusions and, elevation of lipolytic hormones. Typically, 20% to 30% of the caloric intake should be derived from fat. Further, linoleic and linolenic acids are essential fatty acids and must be provided. Patients on enteral feedings may tolerate medium-chain triglycerides (MCT), following bowel injury or with right-sided heart failure, better than long-chain fats. MCT are absorbed directly into the portal circulation avoiding the complex absorptive process needed to digest long-chain fats. Formulas developed for patients with biliary disease typically contain a greater content of MCT and many of the formulas developed for patients with absorption difficulties provide a significant portion of the triglyceride in the form of MCT.

Intravenous fat should be infused as a 20% emulsion in infants to provide a concentrated calorie source (2 kcal per mL) as well as to supply essential fatty acids and lipid that is critical for central nervous system development and cell membrane repair. The usual intake is 2.5 to 3.5 g/kg/day. As little as 0.5 g/kg/day will supply sufficient essential fatty acids. Intravenous fat emulsions are administered continuously unless rising plasma triglyceride levels suggest inadequate clearance. To assess clearance, a minimum period of 4 hours without lipid infusion is needed to approximate the actual triglyceride level. Administration of excess lipid has been associated with several complications including hyperlipemia, bacteremia, decreased oxygenation, and increased infection rates. Although not validated

TABLE 65.5
MICRONUTRIENTS

Weight (kg)	Copper	Zinc	Manganese	Chromium
<3	20[a]	300[a]	10[a]	0.2[a]
3–25	20[a]	100[a]	10[a]	0.2[a]
>25	1 mg/d	2.5–5 mg/d	0.25 mg/d	10 mg/d

[a]μg/kg/d

by clinical trials, it is common practice to restrict the administration of intravenous fat emulsion to 30% to 40% of calories and a maximum of 4 g/kg/day.

Micronutrients

Multivitamin preparations are provided either as unit doses in parenteral nutrition or as multivitamin supplement in the standard formulas. Occasionally, additional vitamins or trace elements will be required for specific deficiency states or diseases, but fine-tuning of micronutrients other than minerals and electrolytes has been difficult to achieve clinically. Current recommendations are given in Table 65.5. The use of pharmacologic doses of vitamins and trace minerals is controversial. Excess is clearly a health risk and further studies are needed.

Refeeding Syndrome

There is a small subset of patients who may actually be harmed by aggressive nutritional support. These patients include children with long-standing eating disorders and those who have been starved due to neglect or environmental circumstances. Decompensation occurs in the first few days following the institution of aggressive nutritional support. The involutional changes that occur with chronic starvation include depression of REE, loss of muscle mass including thinning of the myocardium (marasmic cardiomyopathy), and depletion of body pools of phosphate, potassium, and other critical minerals and electrolytes. The clinical features of refeeding syndrome include rhabdomyolysis, leukocyte dysfunction, respiratory failure, cardiac failure, hypotension, arrhythmias, seizures, coma, and sudden death.

With the institution of nutrition, either by enteral or parenteral route, metabolic activity rises and may exceed the heart's capacity to perform work leading to cardiac failure. In addition, with the restitution of intracellular adenosine triphosphate (ATP) synthesis under the control of insulin, serum levels of critical minerals (phosphate, magnesium, calcium), and electrolytes (potassium) may fall leading to arrhythmias, muscle weakness, and respiratory failure.

Special Considerations

Children with inborn errors of metabolism require care that is tailored to their specific metabolic lesion. Their nutritional needs are best determined by a clinician or dietitian experienced in the management of children with metabolic disorders (see Chapter 16). Patients with renal insufficiency should receive nutrition that is optimized to achieve wound healing, without excessive concern for the increase in blood urea. In general, the increased nitrogen load is handled through dialysis so that optimal nutrition can be provided to promote recovery. With liver failure, provision of calories significantly above energy expenditure results in hyperglycemia, increase in infectious complications, and can nullify the benefits of feeding. Many patients with liver failure are malnourished and have low levels of serum albumin. Severe protein restriction should be avoided. In a patient with hepatic encephalopathy, restriction to 1.0 g/kg/day may be reasonable. The use of high branched-chain amino acid formulas remains controversial. Patients with fulminant hepatic failure require a steady infusion of glucose to avoid hypoglycemia.

Immunonutrition

Considerable attention is currently focused on the use of modified nutrition support regimens to modify the inflammatory response and reduce the secondary organ system dysfunction. A number of nutrients have been shown to improve outcome or minimize nitrogen loss during critical illness in specific populations of adult patients. Glutamine supplementation in critical illness continues to be a controversial subject. Glutamine may not have a direct immunostimulatory action; rather, it is a fuel for rapidly replicating cells such as enterocytes and immune cells. It also serves in multiple biologic functions such as nitrogen processing, visceral protein synthesis, and ammonia production. Arginine is promoted as an immune modulator, although concern has been raised that under certain conditions it may be associated with adverse outcomes. It stimulates the release of growth hormone, insulin, and secretin. Conversion of arginine to ornithine through arginase shuttles nitrogen to urea, and ornithine is involved in polyamine synthesis. Arginine also has trophic effects on the thymus gland. It may promote the formation of nitric oxide. ω-3 Fatty acids may be provided in the form of fish oil or canola oil. They do not have direct immunostimulatory effect but have an indirect effect by competing with ω-6 fatty acids. ω-6 Fatty acids are involved in the cyclooxygenase pathway generating proinflammatory cytokines that may lead to immunosuppression. Upon activation of the cyclooxygenase pathway, ω-3 fatty acids lead to the formation of compounds with much less biologic activity and therefore much less immunosuppressive effect. Trials are under way in critically ill children to determine the benefit of such formulas in the pediatric setting.

ROUTE OF ADMINISTRATION

Enteral Nutrition

Nutrition should be provided through the gastrointestinal tract whenever possible. Enteral feeding has several advantages including maintenance of gut motility, improved mesenteric blood flow, support of gut-associated lymphoid tissue, the release of trophic factors from the gut and pancreas that maintain enterocyte mass and function, and cost. In addition, enterocytes derive a significant portion of their nutrient and energy requirements directly from the luminal contents. Often, continuous drip feedings can begin within hours. In most cases, initiating feedings on the second hospital day is feasible and should be started as a continuous infusion at a rate of approximately 1 mL/kg/hour and advanced every 4 to 6 hours as tolerated. The provision of even small amounts of nutrient (i.e., *trophic* feedings) is thought to provide a number of benefits. Visceral blood flow is improved if 10% to 20% of predicted needs are delivered enterally, and the immune function of the gut improves when 20% to 30% of calories are enteral.

During acute critical illness, continuous drip feedings tend to be better tolerated than bolus feedings, especially in patients with respiratory distress. Transpyloric feeding may minimize the risk of gastroesophageal reflux and aspiration. For young infants, the availability of breast milk is the optimal nutrient source. In older children, the formula for most critically ill children should be lactose free, have some of the fat provided as MCT, and contain easily absorbed proteins, that is, di- and tripeptides (see the preceding text). Most of the currently available formulas developed for children conform to these recommendations. No single formula meets all needs and a wide variety of products are available. Lower osmolarity enteral formulas may reduce the possibility of diarrhea from excess osmotic load to the gut and facilitate absorption. Once an acceptable rate is achieved, caloric density may be increased as tolerated. Problems and remedies due to enteral feeding are illustrated in Table 65.6.

Parenteral Nutrition

The principles and goals of parenteral support during critical illness are the same as with enteral feeding; support the protein synthetic response and provide metabolic support. The benefits of parenteral nutrition carry significant risks in electrolyte and acid–base disturbance, cholestasis, excess carbon dioxide production, and increased risk of bacterial and fungal infection. Venous access is a major limitation. Peripheral parenteral (i.e., not into a large vein) must be relatively dilute. Dextrose concentration can be 12.5% in younger children and 10% in older children. Central venous access allows the use of more concentrated solution.

Because of concerns about tolerance, it is common practice to initiate parenteral support at less than goal

TABLE 65.6
ENTERAL FEEDING INTOLERANCE

Problem	Possible Reason	Possible Remedy
Diarrhea, malabsorption	Delivery too fast	Decrease delivery rate
	High osmotic load	Reduce volume
	Mucosal injury	TPN, continuous low rate drip to allow bowel recovery
	Substrate intolerance	Use elemental formula, especially Disaccharide-free with MCT
Gastric retention/ gastroesophageal reflux	Hypertonic formula	Decrease osmolarity, dilute
	High long-chain fat content	Change to MCT-containing formula
	Hypodynamic gut	Positioning right-side down, consider prokinetic agent: metoclopramide (Reglan), enteral opiate antagonist
Abdominal distension	Ileus, constipation	Rule out surgical abdomen, rule out constipation Add bulking agent or stool softener

TPN, total parenteral nutrition; MCT, medium-chain triglycerides.

rate and increase support over several days. This allows monitoring for metabolic effects such as hyperlipidemia, hyperglycemia, and acidosis. One technique is to order the nutrient solution at the intended final concentration and begin at half the intended ultimate infusion rate. If the patient tolerates the infusion (e.g., no acidemia, hyperglycemia, or glycosuria) for 6 to 8 hours, the rate can be increased. After an additional period of tolerance, the solution is increased to its final rate. When taking this approach it is essential to supplement with conventional maintenance IV fluids while the total parenteral nutrition (TPN) is being increased. Another approach is to plan for the entire day's nutrients to be placed in a volume of fluids equal to half to two third of the total allowed daily fluid volume. The remaining fluid volume is made up with proprietary crystalloid, maintenance solutions that can be increased or decreased as demanded by the patient's fluid status without affecting the amount of nutrients delivered. Taking this approach also lets the clinician reduce the total fluid intake without sacrificing the prescribed nutritional support. The intolerance to intravenous feeding may be manifest in derangements of minerals, electrolytes, and acid–base status.

SUMMARY

The catabolic response to acute critical illness is proportional to the magnitude, nature, and duration of the stress or injury. Predicting nutritional needs of the critically ill child is difficult. Children with critical illness are not capable of normal growth. Further, calories used for activity are greatly reduced. During periods of critical illness, the utilization of nutrients is markedly inhibited by the hormonal response to stress and the circulating inflammatory mediators. Therefore, one of the most important points for clinicians prescribing nutritional support is to provide calories in a thoughtful manner based on the guidelines given in this chapter and to *avoid excess caloric intake* during the acute phase of illness.

RECOMMENDED READINGS

1. Agus MS, Jaksic T. Nutritional support of the critically ill child. *Curr Opin Pediatr.* 2002;14:470–481.
2. ASPEN Board of Directors and Task Force on Standards for Specialized Nutrition Support for Hospitalized Pediatric Patients. Standards for specialized nutrition support: Hospitalized pediatric patients. *Nutr Clin Pract.* 2005;20:103–116.
3. Heyland DK, Novak F, Drover JW, et al. Should immunonutrition become routine in critically ill patients? A systematic review of the evidence. *JAMA.* 2001;286:944–953.
4. Hotchkiss RS, Karl IE. The pathophysiology and treatment of sepsis. *N Engl J Med.* 2003;348:138–150.
5. Marik PE. Monitoring therapeutic interventions in critically ill septic patients. *Nutr Clin Pract.* 2004;19:423–432.
6. Peter JV, Moran JL, Phillips-Hughes J. A meta-analysis of treatment outcomes of early enteral versus early parenteral nutrition in hospitalized patients. *Crit Care Med.* 2005;33:213–220.
7. Van den Berghe G, Wouters P, Weekers F, et al. Intensive insulin therapy in critically ill patients. *N Engl J Med.* 2001;345:1359–1367.
8. Van den Berghe G. How does blood glucose control with insulin save lives in intensive care? *J Clin Invest.* 2004;114:1187–1195.
9. Wesley JR. Nutrient metabolism in relation to the systemic stress response. In: Fuhrman B, Zimmerman J, eds. *Pediatric critical care.* 2nd ed. St. Louis, MO: Mosby–Year Book; 1998:799–819.

Acute Pancreatitis

66

Ruba K. Azzam   *Miguel Saps*

Pancreatic diseases are relatively uncommon in the pediatric age-group; however, when pancreatitis leads to pediatric intensive care unit (PICU) admission, the consequences can be difficult to manage. Congenital pancreatic anomalies, pancreatic insufficiency, and pancreatitis are the most common causes of exocrine pancreatic diseases in children. Early published series reported an incidence of two to nine cases of acute pancreatitis per institution per year. More recent studies have shown an increasing number of patients in large teaching hospitals, in which 100 or more patients with acute pancreatitis may be seen in a year. Although this increase remains unexplained, it may reflect a change in incidence, alterations in referral patterns, increased frequency of testing, or improved physician awareness.

DEFINITION AND CLASSIFICATION

Acute pancreatitis is an acute inflammatory process within the pancreas that involves localized tissue injury and is occasionally associated with remote effects. It can be classified as mild (interstitial) or severe (necrotizing) according to the extent of the pancreatic injury, involvement of remote systems, presence of major complications requiring prolonged treatment, specific interventions, or an increased mortality. Whereas acute pancreatitis is an *event*, chronic pancreatitis is a *process*. Chronic pancreatitis represents the sequelae of a relapsing or continuing inflammatory process leading to irreversible morphologic changes with loss of normal pancreatic cells and fibrosis.

PATHOGENESIS

Current explanations about the early events leading to acute pancreatitis focus on the uncontrolled intracellular activation of trypsinogen to trypsin. Trypsinogen is usually activated in the duodenum, either by the brush border enzyme enterokinase or by trypsin, and can be potentially autoactivated. A common storage of trypsinogen with other zymogens within the acinar cell may trigger a cascade of events, resulting in the premature activation of trypsinogen. Activated proteolytic enzymes, particularly trypsin, may activate additional enzymes such as elastase and phospholipase. The active enzymes will in turn digest cellular membranes and cause proteolysis, edema, interstitial hemorrhage, vascular damage, parenchymal cell necrosis, coagulation, and fat necrosis of pancreatic and peripancreatic tissues.

ETIOLOGY

Multiple factors can lead to acute pancreatitis (see Table 66.1). A review of 589 cases of pancreatitis in children revealed that the most common etiologies were idiopathic (23%), trauma (22%), structural anomalies (15%), multisystem disease (14%), drugs and toxins (12%), and viral infections (10%). Often, the trauma is blunt and accidental, but child abuse was an important cause in one published series. Pancreatic duct transection, requiring surgical intervention, is a major concern in pancreatitis secondary to trauma. Structural abnormalities increase the risk of pancreatitis. Although pancreatic divisum is the most common of these abnormalities, other pancreatic and common bile duct abnormalities (e.g., choledochal cysts, choledochocele, and partial pancreas divisum) have been reported in children with otherwise unexplained acute pancreatitis. Choi et al. reported gallstones in 16 of 56 cases (29%) with acute pancreatitis.

The incidence of acute pancreatitis associated with severe systemic illnesses and following organ transplant seems to be increasing. Hemolytic uremic syndrome (HUS) is a common systemic disease causing acute pancreatitis in children. The mechanism for pancreatitis in these illnesses is unknown and is likely to be multifactorial. A variety of medications are associated with acute and

TABLE 66.1
CAUSES OF ACUTE PANCREATITIS

Systemic Diseases/Infections

- Viral: mumps, coxsackie B, echovirus, influenza A and B, hepatitis A and B, rubella
- Bacterial: typhoid fever, verocytotoxin-producing *Escherichia coli*, *Mycoplasma*, leptospirosis
- Parasites: malaria, ascariasis
- Inflammatory and vasculitic disorders: collagen vascular diseases, HSP, HUS, Kawasaki disease, IBD
- Sepsis/shock/peritonitis

Mechanical/Structural

- Trauma: blunt injury, child abuse, ERCP
- Perforation: duodenal ulcer
- Anomalies: pancreas divisum, choledochal cyst
- Obstruction: stones, tumors
- Metabolic and toxic factors: hyperlipidemia types I, IV, and V; diabetes mellitus (ketoacidosis); hypercalcemia; uremia; cystic fibrosis; malnutrition (refeeding); organic academia
- Drugs/toxins: valproic acid, thiazides, furosemide, azathioprine, prednisone, L-asparaginase, metronidazole, tetracycline, acetaminophen overdose, heroin

HSP, Henoch-Schönlein purpura; HUS, hemolytic uremic syndrome; IBD, inflammatory bowel disease; ERCP, endoscopic retrograde cholangiopancreatography.

recurrent acute pancreatitis. The mechanism for drug-induced pancreatitis is speculative, and most theories concentrate on the disruption of cellular metabolism by the drugs or their metabolites. The anticonvulsant valproate is the most common medication reported by different series in the literature. This association is believed to be idiosyncratic, and fatal cases have been reported. Other common medications frequently reported in association with pancreatitis are L-asparaginase and prednisone.

Viral infections are the most common cause of infectious acute pancreatitis in North America and Europe. Mumps virus accounted for 39% of the cases of pediatric acute pancreatitis reported in a Scottish study by Haddock. Conversely, in developing countries and tropical regions, acute pancreatitis is often associated with helminth infections such as those caused by *Ascaris lumbricoides*. Metabolic disorders resulting in pancreatitis include cystic fibrosis, hyperlipidemia, and hypercalcemia among others.

Hyperlipidemic pancreatitis is defined by the presence of high triglyceride levels (>1,000 mg per dL) and a lactescent serum in the absence of other etiologies. Pancreatitis and hypertriglyceridemia constitute an association in which the cause and effect remain incompletely understood. Almost all patients with pancreatitis and hypertriglyceridemia have preexisting abnormalities in lipoprotein metabolism and are more prone to recurrent episodes of acute pancreatitis. A few animal studies have shown that hypertriglyceridemia intensifies the course of pancreatitis (both edematous and

necrotizing) and have suggested that it also has a role in the development of respiratory insufficiency. However, the clinical course of hyperlipidemic pancreatitis in humans has been reported to be no different from other forms of pancreatitis.

Pancreatitis has been reported with hypercalcemia of various etiologies. Several theories have been proposed to explain the association of hypercalcemia and hyperparathyroidism with pancreatitis. Calcium is known to accelerate the conversion of trypsinogen to trypsin, thereby possibly promoting the autodigestion of the pancreas. Increased calcium levels within the pancreatic juice may also promote calculus formation and obstruction of the ductules. Acute hypercalcemia increases the permeability of the pancreatic duct, perhaps allowing enzymes to leak and damage the gland. Parathormone may itself have direct toxic effects on the gland as well.

DIAGNOSIS

The diagnosis of acute pancreatitis is based on the constellation of symptoms, including the sudden onset of typical abdominal pain and the elevation of serum levels of pancreatic enzymes (amylase and lipase), with or without visible radiographic changes of the pancreas. The abdominal pain is usually localized to the epigastrium, in the right and left upper quadrant, with the pain radiating through to the back. Although the intensity and duration of pain may be variable, it is usually severe and persists for hours or days. Pain is often associated with nausea and vomiting and is generally aggravated by feeding.

Clinical signs of acute pancreatitis include abdominal guarding, rebound tenderness, and decreased bowel signs. Cullen sign (bluish periumbilical discoloration) and Grey-Turner sign (bluish discoloration in the flanks) may be seen in severe necrotizing pancreatitis. Less common clinical signs encompass fever, tachycardia, hypotension, and jaundice. Rarely, patients exhibit abdominal mass, ascites, respiratory distress, or shock.

Serum amylase and lipase assays remain the standard biochemical tests for the diagnosis of pancreatitis. However, the levels of both enzymes can be elevated in conditions unrelated to pancreatitis, and values may be normal even in the setting of clinical and radiographic evidence of pancreatitis. Levels just above the upper reference may also be secondary to pancreatitis, especially in patients presenting late.

Serum amylase concentration rises within 2 to 12 hours of an episode of acute pancreatitis and remains elevated for 2 to 5 days in uncomplicated cases, whereas serum lipase level rises within 4 to 8 hours, peaks at 24 hours, and returns to normal after 8 to 14 days. The sensitivity of elevated serum amylase (81% to 95%) and lipase (85% to 100%) levels is similar when a computed tomography (CT) scan or an ultrasonography is used to ascertain the clinical diagnosis of acute pancreatitis. The specificity of lipase elevation is

TABLE 66.2

CAUSES OF ELEVATED AMYLASE OR LIPASE

Pancreatic Disease

Acute pancreatitis
Chronic pancreatitis
Complications of pancreatitis: pseudocyst, pancreatic ascites, pancreatic abscess
Pancreatic trauma
Pancreatic carcinoma

Nonpancreatic Disorders

Renal insufficiency: amylase level > lipase level
Salivary gland lesion: mumps, stones, surgery, irradiation sialadenitis
Tumors: carcinoma of lung, breast, ovaries, esophagus
Hepatobiliary diseases: chronic liver disease, cholecystitis, choledocholithiasis
Peritonitis
Perforated or penetrating peptic ulcer
Burns
Macroamylasemia
Drugs: morphine

slightly better than that of amylase. The specificity of these tests is highest when the levels are increased to at least three times the upper limit of normal because lipase determination becomes 100% sensitive and 99% specific while amylase testing becomes 72% sensitive and 99% specific for the diagnosis of pancreatitis. The level of increase of the enzyme levels has no bearing on the severity of pancreatitis.

The limitation in the sensitivity of these tests may result in spuriously normal amylase levels in patients with hypertriglyceridemia in the presence of acute pancreatitis. Amylase and lipase level elevations in the serum and urine may occur in conditions other than pancreatitis (see Table 66.2). Acidemia may result in spurious elevations in serum amylase levels, explaining the marked elevations in serum amylase levels in patients with diabetic ketoacidosis in the absence of acute pancreatitis.

Leukocytosis (15,000 to 20,000 leukocytes per μL) occurs frequently. More severe cases may result in hemoconcentration, with hematocrit values exceeding 50%, secondary to loss of plasma into the retroperitoneal space and peritoneal cavity. Hyperglycemia is common. Multiple factors may be involved in the pathogenesis of this abnormality, including decreased insulin release, increased glucagon release, and increased output of adrenal glucocorticoids and catecholamines. Hypocalcemia is common, and its pathogenesis is not completely understood. Although earlier studies suggested that the response of the parathyroid gland to a decrease in serum calcium level is impaired, subsequent observations have failed to confirm this finding. Intraperitoneal saponification of calcium by fatty acids in areas of fat necrosis occurs occasionally, with large amounts (up to 6.0 g) being dissolved or suspended in

ascitic fluid. Such "soap formation" may also be significant in patients with pancreatitis and mild hypocalcemia, with little or no obvious ascites. Hyperbilirubinemia occurs in approximately 10% of adult patients. However, jaundice is transient, and serum bilirubin levels return to normal in 4 to 7 days. Serum alkaline phosphatase and aspartate aminotransferase (AST) levels are also transiently elevated and are parallel to serum bilirubin values. Markedly elevated serum lactic dehydrogenase (LDH) levels (>500 U per dL) suggest a poor prognosis. Serum albumin level is decreased to 3.0 g per dL in approximately 10% of patients; this sign is associated with more severe pancreatitis and a higher mortality rate. Approximately 25% of patients have hypoxemia (arterial P_{O_2} <60 mm Hg), which may herald the onset of adult respiratory distress syndrome (ARDS). Serum C-reactive protein (CRP) levels peak on the third or fourth day. CRP values >150 mg per L 48 hours after the onset of symptoms are currently accepted as a predictor of the severity of acute pancreatitis in adults. Finally, the electrocardiogram is occasionally abnormal in acute pancreatitis, with ST segment and T-wave abnormalities simulating myocardial ischemia.

Imaging

Conventional radiology is of limited value in the evaluation of acute pancreatitis. Although imaging studies are important to evaluate the course of the disease if complications are suspected, no imaging studies are required to diagnose acute pancreatitis, and the results of these studies can frequently be normal or inconclusive. Abdominal ultrasonography is the most widely used imaging study in patients with suspected acute pancreatitis. The two major sonographic findings include increased pancreatic size and decreased pancreatic echogenicity, with the latter being more reliable. Other important findings are dilated main pancreatic duct, gall stones or biliary sludge, dilated common intrahepatic bile ducts, pancreatic calcifications, choledochal cysts, and cystic or peripancreatic fluid collections. The sensitivity for the diagnosis of acute pancreatitis by ultrasonography ranges from 62% to 95%, with a positive predictive value of 0.93 and a negative predictive value of 0.78. Overlying bowel gas may obscure the pancreas, presenting a technical problem.

Contrast-enhanced (abdominal) computed tomographic (CECT) scan findings are similar to those seen on ultrasonography, except that abnormal attenuation, rather than altered echogenicity, is observed (see Fig. 66.1). Most experts agree that there is no diagnostic utility for CT scan in the early phases of acute pancreatitis. There is experimental evidence indicating that CT scan contrast given early in the course of acute pancreatitis may diminish the already tenuous blood flow to ischemic areas of the pancreas and may thereby extend the area of necrosis. CECT has a sensitivity of 77% to 85% and a specificity of 98% to 100% for establishing a diagnosis of moderately severe pancreatitis,

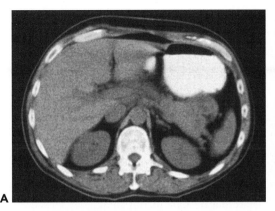 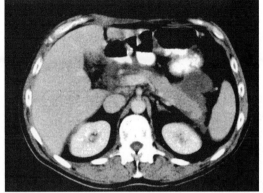

Figure 66.1 Computed tomographic (CT) scan of the pancreas in pancreatitis. **A:** Without contrast. **B:** With intravenous contrast. The absence of contrast enhancement within the pancreatic parenchyma is indicative of necrosis. Noncontrast CT scan cannot differentiate inflammation from necrosis. (From Yamada T, Alpers DH, Laine L, et al., *Atlas of gastroenterology*, 3rd ed. Philadelphia, PA: Lippincott Williams & Wilkins; 2003:506.)

and a sensitivity of 92% to 95% and a specificity of 98% to 100% for diagnosing severe pancreatitis. To exclude complications, a CT scan is usually done several days after the onset of a severe course of acute pancreatitis, when the patient fails to improve.

Diagnostic endoscopic retrograde cholangiopancreatography (ERCP) provides accurate visualization of the ampulla of Vater, bile ducts, and pancreatic ducts. ERCP has greater sensitivity than ultrasonography in the diagnosis of gallstones at the level of the common bile duct and in establishing pancreatic and biliary pathology. ERCP is a technically challenging technique with a considerable index of complications even in an expert's hands. Therefore, the indication of ERCP should be reserved for the evaluation of children with pancreatitis that does not resolve after 1 month, recurrent disease, persistent elevation of the pancreatic enzymes when a structural defect or duct disruption is suspected, and pancreatitis following liver transplantation or that associated with cystic fibrosis. Complications of ERCP include transient pancreatitis, pain, cholangitis, ileus, fever, and perforation. The risk of development of complications is increased in the setting of acute pancreatitis, and, therefore, ERCP is not a routine screening tool for purely diagnostic purposes.

Magnetic resonance cholangiopancreatography (MRCP) is a relatively new imaging modality that provides a fast noninvasive and more economical method of evaluating the pancreatic duct and biliary tree in children. It is able to create projectional images similar in detail and appearance to direct cholangiography, with high resolution of the bile duct and intraductal stones. MRCP may be helpful in defining the ductal abnormalities causing acute pancreatitis, but its utility in pediatric patients has not yet been extensively established. MRCP was able to visualize gallbladder stones in 57 of 62 patients (94%) and correctly predict acute cholecystitis in six of eight patients. It also detected peripancreatic edema and inflammatory changes consistent with acute pancreatitis in 45 of 64 patients (70%). However, MRCP is an exclusively diagnostic technique, whereas ERCP enables the therapy for complications such as bile duct or pancreatic duct strictures through various interventional modalities such as sphincterotomy, endoscopic drainage, and stent placement.

TREATMENT

Supportive therapy, including vigorous hydration, analgesia, correction of glycemia and electrolyte imbalances, and pharmacologic or mechanical support of specific organs constitute the mainstay of therapy. The primary goal is to remove the initiating process whenever possible, but, most commonly, the therapies are targeted at limiting the progression of the disease, relieving pain, restoring homeostasis, and treating complications.

Aggressive intravenous fluid infusions and cardiovascular monitoring are recommended to replace fluid losses and expand the vascular compartment, and to assure cardiovascular stability and prevent the progression of pancreatic necrosis. Pain control for acute pancreatitis should begin with titration of opioids intravenously or should be through a patient-controlled analgesia system. Although meperidine has been preferred historically for analgesia, there is neither clear evidence for reduced spasm of the sphincter of Oddi with meperidine nor scientific evidence to contraindicate the use of morphine in acute pancreatitis. Nasogastric tube placement is indicated to decompress the stomach in case of vomiting or ileus. Patients are initially maintained nothing by mouth (NPO). In the setting of mild acute pancreatitis, it is current practice to begin oral refeeding with clear liquids, slowly advancing to a low-fat/low-protein diet within few days of the onset of pain.

In severe pancreatitis, although the timing of introduction of enteral feedings is still debated, the benefits of enteral versus parenteral nutrition encourage its early introduction. Adult studies showing relapse of symptoms in 20% of patients following the introduction of oral intake led to the belief that enteral nutrition might exacerbate severe acute pancreatitis. The information provided by these and other similar studies resulted in the widespread use of pancreatic rest through the cessation of enteral feeds. Many believe that the delivery of nutrients proximal to the duodenojejunal flexure will cause release of cholecystokinin (CCK), and an exacerbation of the inflammatory process in the pancreas, as a result of stimulation of exocrine pancreatic secretion. A recent randomized study by Eatock et al. revealed no evidence of exacerbation of disease associated with the introduction of nasogastric feeding when compared with the use of the nasojejunal route in adults with severe acute pancreatitis.

A meta-analysis of six adult trials of patients with acute pancreatitis comparing nasojejunal and parenteral feeds, within 48 hours of admission, suggested a considerable benefit for those who were fed enterally. The study concluded that enteral nutrition significantly reduced the risk of infective complications, decreased the likelihood of a surgical intervention to control pancreatic infection, and shortened the length of hospital stay by 3 days. Enteral nutrition is less expensive than parenteral feeding, helps maintain mucosal function, and limits the absorption of endotoxins and cytokines from the gut. Nutritional support should be instituted early, with timely institution of feeding being important to avoid malnutrition. Partial ileus should not be deemed a contraindication to enteral feeding because continuous low-volume infusion is usually well tolerated. An international consensus conference to suggest recommendations for the management of the critically ill adult patients with severe acute pancreatitis has recently recommended the initiation of enteral over parenteral nutrition early in the course of the disease following initial resuscitation, with preference for the jejunal route. The consensus recommended the use of parenteral nutrition only following 5 to 7 days of failed attempts of enteral feeds.

The importance of early initiation of antibiotics is unclear. A study by Nordback et al. on the early introduction of imipenem–cilastatin therapy in patients with acute necrotizing pancreatitis revealed a significant reduction in the need for surgery and in the overall number of major organ complications, and a trend to lower mortality. Several authors recommend the use of prophylactic antibiotics in patients with necrotizing pancreatitis, infected necrosis, or other infectious complications. However, the lack of consistent benefits, methodologic differences across studies, and the significant potential for harm has prompted the critical care consensus group to not recommend the routine use of prophylactic broad-spectrum antibiotics in patients with severe acute pancreatitis with or without necrosis. In the setting of this unresolved controversy, the use of antibiotics in the treatment of patients with severe acute pancreatitis has increased, and cases of emergence of antibiotic resistance have been recently reported.

Although a large number of medications have been used in an attempt to either provide pancreatic rest (e.g., H_2-blockers, atropine, glucagon, somatostatin) or halt the progression of autodigestion (antiproteases such as aprotinin and gabexate), no benefit has been shown in clinical trials. Somatostatin and its synthetic analog, octreotide, reduce exocrine pancreatic secretion in a dose-dependent manner. Except for case reports, there are limited data on its use in children with pancreatitis, and the results of clinical trials in adults are inconsistent.

PROGNOSIS

Because early identification and aggressive treatment of associated organ dysfunction can have a major impact on the outcome, the early assessment of prognosis and severity is important. Acute pancreatitis can lead to local and systemic complications including multiorgan failure and death in some patients, although adverse outcomes do not appear to occur as often in children as in adult patients. Death may occur by several mechanisms, with early causes of death being secondary to cardiovascular collapse and respiratory failure. Patients with severe pancreatitis are at risk for respiratory failure associated with an ARDS-like condition resulting from the leakage of fluid into alveolar spaces and nonspecific inflammatory responses. Late life-threatening complications of acute pancreatitis are related to the infected necrotic pancreatic tissue and multisystem organ failure, although pancreatic necrosis appears to be uncommon in children (0.3%). At the time of admission, it can sometimes be difficult to predict the severity of an attack. A number of severity criteria have been developed including Ranson scores, Glasgow score, the Acute Physiology and Chronic Health Evaluation (APACHE) II score, and the Pediatric score system created by the Midwest Multicenter Pancreatic Study Group. The latter has four initial parameters to be scored at admission.

COMPLICATIONS

The local and systemic complications of acute pancreatitis are listed in Table 66.3. Prolonged, complicated illnesses and significant morbidity and mortality usually mark the clinical course of the minority of patients with acute pancreatitis who develop necrotizing pancreatitis with gross and microscopic destruction of the pancreatic parenchyma. It is within this subgroup that most pancreatic fluid collections arise. These complications include the following:

1. Pancreatic necrosis is characterized by well-marginated zones of nonenhancing parenchyma larger than 3 cm or involving >30% of the pancreas, as visualized by CECT

TABLE 66.3

COMPLICATIONS OF ACUTE PANCREATITIS

Local

- Necrosis
  Sterile or infected
- Pancreatic fluid collections
  Pancreatic abscess
  Pancreatic pseudocyst
  Pancreatic ascites
- Involvement of contiguous organs
- Massive intraperitoneal hemorrhage
- Thrombosis of blood vessels (splenic vein, portal vein)
- Bowel infarction
- Obstructive jaundice

Systemic

- Pulmonary
  Pleural effusion
  Atelectasis
  Pneumonitis
  Adult respiratory distress syndrome
- Cardiovascular
  Hypotension (hypovolemia, hypoalbuminemia)
  Pericardial effusion
  Nonspecific ST-T changes in EKG
- Renal
  Oliguria
  Azotemia
  Acute tubular necrosis
  Renal artery or vein thrombosis
- Gastrointestinal
  Peptic ulcer disease
  Erosive gastritis
  Variceal hemorrhage
- Hematologic
  Disseminated intravascular coagulopathy
- Metabolic
  Hyperglycemia
  Hypertriglyceridemia
  Hypocalcemia
- Central nervous system
  Psychosis
  Fat emboli

EKG, electrocardiogram.

scan. This complication likely occurs in <1% of children compared to <5% in adults.

2. Pseudocyst formation is a well-known complication of acute and chronic pancreatitis and pancreatic trauma and is thought to result from the disruption of the pancreatic duct, with subsequent spilling of the pancreatic fluid into the glandular parenchyma. Although most pseudocysts are not symptomatic, patients may present with persistent or recurrent abdominal pain.

3. Pancreatic abscesses manifest clinically with fever, leukocytosis, persistent abdominal pain, and even frank sepsis. Percutaneous aspiration with resultant bacterial culture growth confirms the diagnosis, with a reported sensitivity of 90% to 100%. Abscesses often can be treated with external drainage and intravenous antibiotics, and surgical drainage is only rarely necessary.

4. Pancreatic ascites and pancreatic pleural effusion are uncommon in children. It was reported to occur in a few infants. It usually occurs as a consequence of the disruption of the main pancreatic duct, often by an internal fistula between the duct and the peritoneal cavity or a leaking pseudocyst. The ascites fluid is rich in amylase, the concentration of which may exceed 20,000 U per L. An internal fistula may develop between the pancreatic duct and the pleural space, leading to the development of pleural effusion. Treatment of the former usually entails paracentesis to keep the peritoneal cavity free of fluid and, therefore, helps seal the leak; the pleural effusion requires thoracentesis. Although the usefulness of octreotide remains controversial, its use has been reported to be beneficial in the resolution of both pancreatic ascites and pleural effusion.

SURGICAL MANAGEMENT

The main indications for surgical intervention are debridement of the infected necrotic pancreatic tissue and cholecystectomy to prevent recurrent gall stone pancreatitis. Surgery in severe pancreatitis is usually deferred for at least 2 weeks to permit the proper demarcation of pancreatic and peripancreatic necrosis to occur so that the risk of bleeding or loss of vital pancreatic tissue can be avoided.

Trypsinogen mutations are responsible for most hereditary pancreatitis. Other hereditary disorders of the exocrine pancreas described in association with pancreatic insufficiency include Shwachman-Diamond syndrome, Johanson-Blizzard syndrome, exocrine pancreatic dysfunction with refractory sideroblastic anemia, pancreatic aplasia/hypoplasia, and isolated pancreatic enzyme deficiencies.

RECOMMENDED READINGS

1. Benifla M, Weizman Z. Acute pancreatitis in childhood: Analysis of literature data. *J Clin Gastroenterol.* 2003;37(2):169–172.
2. Eatock FC, Chong P, Menezes N, et al. A randomized study of early nasogastric versus nasojejunal feeding in severe acute pancreatitis. *Am J Gastroenterol.* 2005;100(2):432–439.
3. Lerner A, Branski D, Lebenthal E. Pancreatic diseases in children. *Pediatr Clin North Am.* 1996;43(1):125–156.
4. Nathens AB, Curtis JR, Beale RJ, et al. Management of the critically ill patient with severe acute pancreatitis. *Crit Care Med.* 2004; 32(12):2524–2536.
5. Whitcomb DC, Lowe M. Pancreatitis: Acute and chronic. In: Kleiman R, Walker WA, Goulet O, eds. *Pediatric gastrointestinal disease.* Ontario, Canada: BC Decker Inc.; 2004.
6. Yadav D, Agarwal N, Pitchumoni CS. A critical evaluation of laboratory tests in acute pancreatitis. *Am J Gastroenterol.* 2002;97(6): 1309–1318.
7. Choi BH, Lim YJ, Yoon CH,et al. Acute pancreatitis associated with biliary disease in children. *J Gastroenterol Hepatol.* 2003;18:915–921.
8. Graham CA, O'Toole SJ, Watson AJ, et al. Pancreatic trauma in Scottish children. *J R Coll Surg Edinb.* 2000;45:223–226.
9. Nordback I, Sand J, Saaristo R, et al. Early treatment with antibiotics reduces the need for surgery in acute necrotizing pancreatitis—a single-center randomized study. *J Gastrointest Surg.* 2001;5:113–118.

Calculations Commonly Used in Critical Care

A

TABLE A.1
TABLE OF CONTENTS

TABLE A.2
ABBREVIATIONS USED IN THE APPENDIX

A	Alveolar	cap	Capillary
D	Dead	cr	Creatinine
E	Expiration	dyn	Dynamic
I	Inspiration	is	Interstitium
P	Pressure	st	Static
Q̇	Net liquid flow	ICP	Intracranial pressure
R	Respiratory quotient	a	Arterial
T	Tidal	d	Distribution
V	Volume	l	Length
Δ	Change	r	Radius
η	Viscosity	t	Time
π	Oncotic pressure	v̄	Mixed venous
σ	Permeability	CO	Cardiac output
atm	Atmosphere	VO	Oxygen consumption
BSA	Body surface area	FIO$_2$	Inspired fraction of oxygen

TABLE A.3
FAHRENHEIT AND CELSIUS TEMPERATURE CONVERSIONS

°C	°F	°C	°F	°C	°F
45	113.0	36	96.8	27	80.6
44	111.2	35	95.0	26	78.8
43	109.4	34	93.2	25	77.0
42	107.6	33	91.4	24	75.2
41	105.8	32	89.6	23	73.4
40	104.0	31	87.8	22	71.6
39	102.2	30	86.0	21	69.8
38	100.4	29	84.2	20	68.0
37	98.6	28	82.4		

TABLE A.4
DOSAGE AND ACTION OF COMMON INTRAVENOUS VASOACTIVE DRUGS

	Dosage	α	β_1	β_2
Dopamine	1–2 μg/kg/min	+	+	0
	2–10 μg/kg/min	++	+++	0
	10–30 μg/kg/min	+++	++	0
Dobutamine	2–30 μg/kg/min	+	+++	++
Norepinephrine	2–80 μg/min	+++	++	+
Epinephrine	1–200 μg/min	++	+++	+++
Isoproterenol	2–10 μg/min	0	+++	+++
Metaraminol	>20 μg/min	++	+	+
Phenylephrine	>30 μg/min	+++	0	0
Amrinone	2–15 μg/kg/min	0	0	0
Phentolamine	1–2 mg/min	—	0	0
Labetolol	>2 mg/min	—	—	—
Esmolol	50–400 μg/kg/min	—	—	—

Each plus sign represents the relative strength of the effect of the drug on the receptor.

TABLE A.5
HEMODYNAMIC CALCULATIONS

Mean Blood Pressure (mm Hg)

$$BP = \frac{\text{Systolic BP} + (2 \times \text{Diastolic BP})}{3}$$
$$= \text{Diastolic BP} + \tfrac{1}{3}(\text{Systolic BP} - \text{Diastolic BP})$$

Normal values: 85–95 mm Hg

The Fick Equation for Cardiac Index (L/min/m^2)

$$CI = \frac{CO}{BSA}$$
$$= \frac{\text{Oxygen consumption}}{\text{Arterial O}_2 \text{ content} - \text{Venous O}_2 \text{ content}}$$
$$= \frac{10 \times \dot{V}_{O_2}(\text{mL/min/m}^2)}{\text{Hgb (g/dL)} \times 1.39}$$
$$\times (\text{Arterial \% saturation} - \text{Venous \% saturation})$$

Normal values: 2.5–4.2 L/min/m^2

Stroke Index (mL/beat/m^2)

$$= \frac{CI \text{ (L/min/m}^2) \times 1000}{\text{Heart rate (beats/min)}}$$

Normal values: 33–47 mL/beat/m^2

Systemic Vascular Resistance (dyne s/cm^{-5})

$$SVR = \frac{80 \times (\text{Arterial BP} - \text{Right atrial BP})}{CO \text{ (L/min)}}$$

Normal values: 770–1500 dyne s/cm^{-5}

Pulmonary Vascular Resistance (dyne s/cm^{-5})

$$PVR = \frac{80 \times (\text{Pulmonary artery BP} - \text{Pulmonary capillary wedge pressure})}{CO \text{ (L/min)}}$$

Normal values: 20–120 dyne s/cm^{-5}

Total Pulmonary Resistance (dyne s/cm^{-5})

$$TPR = \frac{80 \times \text{Pulmonary artery BP}}{CO \text{ (L/min)}}$$

Capillary Fluid Filtration

$$\dot{Q}_f = k(P_{cap} - P_{is}) - k\sigma(\pi_{cap} - \pi_{is})$$

TABLE A.6
NUTRITIONAL CALCULATIONS

Body Mass Index

$$BMI = \frac{\text{Weight (kg)}}{(\text{Height [cm]})^2}$$

Caloric Content of Foods

Food Type	Kcal/g	Range
Carbohydrate	3.4	3.4–4.1
Protein	4.0	3.3–4.7
Fat	9.1	9.1–9.5

Respiratory Quotient

$$= \frac{CO_2 \text{ production (mL/min)}}{O_2 \text{ consumption (mL/min)}}$$
$$= \frac{\dot{V}_{CO_2}}{\dot{V}_{O_2}}$$

Relationship of Fuel Burned to Respiratory Quotient (R)

Fuel	R
Ketones	<0.6
Fat	0.7
Carbohydrate	1.0
Lipogenesis	>1.0

Nitrogen Balance

$$= \text{Nitrogen consumed} - \text{Nitrogen excreted}$$
$$= \frac{\text{Protein calories (kcal/d)}}{25}$$
$$- \text{Urine nitrogen (g/d)} - 5 \text{ (g/d)}$$

Harris-Benedict Equation of Resting Energy Expenditure (kcal/d)

$$\text{Males} = 66 + (13.7 \times \text{Weight [kg]}) + (5 \times \text{Height [cm]})$$
$$- (6.8 \times \text{Age})$$
$$\text{Females} = 655 + (9.6 \times \text{Weight [kg]})$$
$$+ (1.8 \times \text{Height [cm]}) - (4.7 \times \text{Age})$$

Weir Equation (Modified) of Energy Expenditure (kcal/d)

$$= (3.94 \times \dot{V}_{O_2} \text{ [mL/min]}) + (1.11 \times \dot{V}_{CO_2} \text{ [mL/min]})$$

TABLE A.7
TYPICAL INTRAVENOUS DRUG DOSAGES FOR RAPID INTUBATION

Muscle relaxants	
Rocurium	0.6–1.2 mg/kg
Succinylcholine	1 mg/kg
Vecuronium	0.1–0.28 mg/kg
Sedatives	
Thiopental	3–4 mg/kg
Ketamine	1–2 mg/kg
Etomidate	0.3–0.4 mg/kg

TABLE A.8
PULMONARY CALCULATIONS

Tidal Volume

$$V_T = \text{Dead space} + \text{Alveolar space}$$
$$= V_D + V_A$$

Alveolar Gas Equation

$$P\dot{A}O_2 = P_{IO_2} - \frac{P_{aCO_2}}{R}$$
$$= F_{IO_2}(P_{atm} - P_{H_2O}) - \frac{P_{aCO_2}}{R}$$
$$= 150 - \frac{P_{aCO_2}}{R} \text{ (room air, sea level)}$$

Alveolar Arteriolar Gradient

$$= A - A \text{ gradient}$$
$$= P_{AO_2} - P_{aO_2}$$

Normal values (upright): $2.5 + (0.21 \times \text{Age})$

Alveolar Ventilation (L/min)

$$\dot{V}_E = k\frac{\dot{V}_{CO_2}}{P_{aCO_2}}$$
$$= \frac{0.863 \times \dot{V}_{CO_2}(\text{mL/min})}{P_{aCO_2}(1 - V_D/V_T)}$$

Normal values: 4–6 L/min

Bohr Equation of Dead Space

$$\frac{V_D}{V_T} = \frac{P_{aCO_2} - P_{ECO_2}}{P_{aCO_2}}$$

Normal values: 0.2–0.3

Physiologic Dead Space

$$\frac{V_D}{V_T} = \frac{P_{aCO_2} - P_{ECO_2}}{P_{aCO_2}}$$

Normal values: 0.2–0.3

Oxygen Dissolved in Blood (mL/dL)

$$D_{O_2} = 0.003 \text{ (mL } O_2/\text{dL)} \times P_{aO_2} \text{ (mm Hg)}$$

Oxygen Capacity of Hemoglobin (mL O_2/dL)

$$= 1.39 \text{ (mL, } O_2) \times \text{Hgb (g/dL)}$$

Normal values: 17–24 mL/dL

Oxygen Content of Blood (mL/dL)

$$C_{O_2} = D_{O_2} + (1.39 \times \text{Hgb [g/dL]} \times [\% \text{ Hgb saturated with } O_2])$$
$$= D_{O_2} + (1.39 \times \text{Hgb [g/dL]} \times S_{O_2})$$

Normal values: 17.5–23.5 mL/dL

Percentage of Saturation of Hemoglobin with Oxygen

$$S_{O_2} = 100 \times \frac{C_{O_2} - D_{O_2}}{1.39 \times \text{Hgb (g/dL)}}$$

Normal values: >95%

Physiologic Shunt

$$= \dot{Q}_S/\dot{Q}_T$$
$$= \frac{C_{capO_2} - C_{O_2}}{C_{capO_2} - C\bar{v}_{O_2}}$$
$$= \frac{1.39 \times \text{Hgb (g/dL)} + 0.003 \times P_{aO_2} - C_{aO_2}}{1.39 \times \text{Hgb (g/dL)} + 0.003 \times P_{aO_2} - C\bar{v}_{O_2}}$$

Normal values: <5%

Compliance

$$\Delta V/\Delta P \text{ (mL/cm } H_2O)$$

On mechanical ventilation

Static compliance $= C_{st} = \dfrac{V_T}{P_{plateau} - P_{endexp}}$

Dynamic effective compliance $= C_{dyn} = \dfrac{V_T}{P_{peak} - P_{endexp}}$

During spontaneous breathing

Compliance of the lung $= C_L = \dfrac{V_T}{P_{alveolus} - P_{pleura}}$

Compliance of the chest wall $= CW_{cw} = \dfrac{V_T}{P_{pleura} - P_{atm}}$

Compliance of the respiratory system $= C_{rs} = \dfrac{V_T}{P_{alveolus} - P_{atm}}$

Normal values:

C_{st} >60 mL/cm H_2O; C_{dyn} >60 mL/cm H_2O
C_L >200 mL/cm H_2O; C_{rs} >100 mL/cm H_2O

Resistance—Ohm Law

$$\Delta P/\text{flow} = \Delta P/\dot{Q}$$

Normal values: airway resistance of the lung at functional residual capacity (FRC) = 2 cm H_2O/L/s

Work of Breathing

$$W_{thorax} = \int_{t_1}^{t_2} (P_{aw} - P_{atm})\dot{V}\,dt$$
$$W_L = \int_{t_1}^{t_2} (P_{aw} - P_{es})\dot{V}\,dt$$
$$W_{CW} = \int_{t_1}^{t_2} (P_{es} - P_{atm})\dot{V}\,dt$$

Normal values: $W_{thorax} = 0.5$ kg M/min

Laplace Law of Surface Tension of a Sphere

$$P = \frac{2T}{r}$$

Poiseuille Law of Laminar Flow

$$\dot{V} = \frac{P\pi r^4}{8\eta l}$$

TABLE A.9
COMPOSITION AND PROPERTIES OF COMMON INTRAVENOUS SOLUTIONS

Solution	Na$^+$	Cl$^-$	K$^+$	Ca$^+$	Lactate	Kcal/L	mOsm/L
D5W	0	0	0	0	0	170	252
D10W	0	0	0	0	0	240	505
D50W	0	0	0	0	0	1700	2530
1/2 NS	77	77	0	0	0	0	154
NS	154	154	0	0	0	0	308
3% NaCl	513	513	0	0	0	0	1026
Ringer lactate	130	109	4	3	28	0	308
20% Mannitol	0	0	0	0	0	0	1098

NS, normal saline.

TABLE A.10
ELECTROLYTE AND RENAL CALCULATIONS

Anion Gap

$$= [Na^+] - [Cl^-] - [HCO_3^-]$$

Normal values: 9–13 mEq/L

Expected Anion Gap in Hypoalbuminemia

$$= 3 \times (\text{albumin [g/dL]})$$

Calculated Serum Osmolality

$$= 2[Na^+] + \frac{[\text{Glucose}]}{18} + \frac{[\text{BUN}]}{2.8}$$

Normal values: 275–290 mOsm/kg

Osmolar Gap

$$= \text{Serum osmolality measured} - \text{Serum osmolality calculated}$$

Normal values: 0–5 mOsm/kg

Na$^+$ and Glucose

[Na$^+$] decreases 1.6 mEq/L for each 100 mg/dL increase in [glucose]

Ca$^+$ and Albumin

[Ca$^+$] decreases 0.8 mg/dL for each 1.0 g/dL decrease in albumin

Glomerular Filtration Rate

$$\text{GFR Measured} = \text{Creatinine clearance} = \frac{U_{\text{Creat}}V}{P_{\text{Creat}}}$$

$$= \frac{[\text{Creatinine}]_{\text{urine}} \text{ (g/dL)} \times \dfrac{\text{Urine volume (mL/d)}}{1440 \text{ (min/d)}}}{[\text{Creatinine}]_{\text{plasma}} \text{ (mg/dL)}}$$

$$= \text{Estimated for males} = \frac{(140 - \text{Age}) \times (\text{Lean body weight [kg]})}{P_{\text{Creat}} \times 72}$$

Estimated for females $= 0.85 \times \text{Male estimate}$

Normal values: 74–160 mL/min

Water Deficit in Hypernatremia (L)

$$= 0.6 \times (\text{Body weight [kg]}) \times \left(\frac{[Na^+]}{140} - 1\right)$$

Water Excess in Hyponatremia (L)

$$= 0.6 \times (\text{Body weight [kg]}) \times \left(1 - \frac{[Na^+]}{140}\right)$$

Fractional Excretion of Sodium

$$F_E Na = \frac{\text{Excreted Na}^+}{\text{Filtered Na}^+} \times 100$$

$$= \frac{U_{Na^+} \times V}{\text{GFR}} \times [Na^+] \times 100$$

$$= \frac{U_{Na^+}/[Na^+]}{U_{\text{Creat}}/[\text{Creat}]}$$

TABLE A.11
ACID–BASE FORMULAS

Henderson-Hasselbalch Equation

$$pH = pK + \log \frac{[HCO_3^-]}{0.03 \times Paco_2}$$

Henderson Equation for Concentration of H$^+$

$$[H^+] \text{ (nM/L)} = 24 \times \frac{Paco_2}{[HCO_3^-]}$$

Metabolic Acidosis

Bicarbonate deficit (mEq/L) $= 0.5 \times (\text{Body weight [kg]})$
$\times (24 - [HCO_3^-])$
Expected $Pco_2 = 1.5 \times [HCO_3^-] + 8 \pm 2$

Metabolic Alkalosis

Bicarbonate excess $= 0.4 \times (\text{Body weight [kg]})$
$\times ([HCO_3^-] - 24)$

Respiratory Acidosis

$$\text{Acute} = \frac{\Delta H^+}{\Delta Paco_2} = 0.8$$

$$\text{Chronic} = \frac{\Delta H^+}{\Delta Paco_2} = 0.3$$

TABLE A.12
NEUROLOGIC CALCULATIONS

Glasgow Coma Scale (3–15)

$$= \text{Eyes } (1–4) + \text{Motor } (1–6) + \text{Verbal } (1–5)$$

Normal value: 15

Specific Components of the Glasgow Coma Scale

Eye opening	
Spontaneous	4
To speech	3
To pain	2
Nil	1
Motor response	
Obeys commands	6
Localizes	5
Withdraws	4
Exhibits abnormal flexion	3
Exhibits abnormal extension	2
Nil	1
Verbal response	
Oriented	5
Confused, conversant	4
Uses inappropriate words	3
Uses incomprehensible sounds	2
Nil	1

Cerebral Perfusion Pressure (mm Hg)

$$= BP - ICP$$

BODY SURFACE AREA FORMULA AND NOMOGRAM

Body Surface Area

$$BSA = (height\ [cm])^{0.718} \times (weight\ [kg])^{0.427} \times 74.49$$

See Figure A.1 for the nomogram to calculate BSA.

PHARMACOLOGIC CALCULATIONS

Drug Clearance

$$= V_d \times K_{el}$$

Drug Half-life

$$= t^{1/2}$$
$$= \frac{0.693}{K_{el}}$$

Drug Elimination Constant

$$= K_{el}$$
$$= \frac{\ln\left(\frac{[Peak]}{[Trough]}\right)}{t_{peak} - t_{trough}}$$

Drug Loading Dose

$$= V_d \times [Target\ peak]$$

Drug Dosing Interval

$$= \frac{-1}{K_{el}} \times \ln\left(\frac{[Desired\ trough]}{[Desired\ peak]}\right) + Infusion\ time\ hour$$

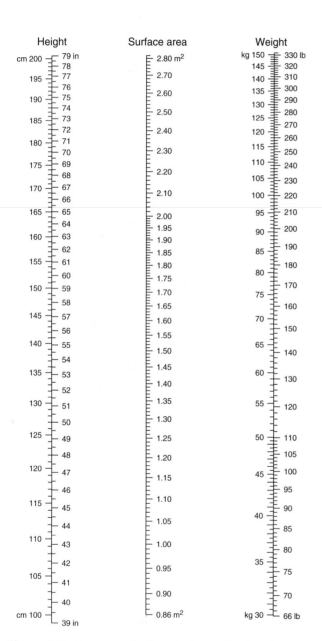

Figure A.1 Nomogram for the calculation of body surface area (BSA) in square meters by height and weight.

TABLE A.15
PEDIATRIC RISK OF MORTALITY III SCORE

Cardiovascular and Neurological Vital Signs

Systolic blood pressure (mm Hg)	Score = 3	Score = 7
Neonate	40–55	<40
Infant	45–65	<45
Child	55–75	<55
Adolescent	65–85	<65
Temperature	**Score = 3**	
	<33°C (91.4°F) or >40°C (104.0°F)	
Mental Status	**Score = 5**	
	Stupor/coma or GCS <8	
Heart Rate (Beats/Min)	**Score = 3**	**Score = 4**
Neonate	215–225	>225
Infant	215–225	>225
Child	185–205	>205
Adolescent	145–155	>155
Pupillary Reflexes	**Score = 7**	**Score = 11**
	One fixed	Both fixed

Acid–Base, Blood Gases

Acidosis (pH or Total CO_2)	Score = 2	Score = 6
pH	7.0–7.28	<7.0
CO_2	5.0–16.9	<5.0
Pco_2 (mm Hg)	**Score = 1**	**Score = 3**
	50–75	>75
Alkalosis: total CO_2 (mmol/L)	**Score = 4**	
	>34	
Pao_2 (mm Hg)	**Score = 3**	**Score = 6**
	42–49	<42

Chemistry Tests

Glucose	Score = 2
	>200 mg/dL or >11 mmol/L
Potassium (mmol/L)	**Score = 3**
	>6.9
Blood Urea Nitrogen	**Score = 3**
Neonate	>11.9 mg/dL or >4.3 mmol/L
All other ages	>14.9 mg/dL or >5.4 mmol/L
Creatinine	**Score = 2**
Neonate	>0.85 mg/dL or >75 μmol/L
Infant	>0.90 mg/dL or >80 μmol/L
Child	>0.90 mg/dL or >80 μmol/L
Adolescent	>0.1.3 mg/dL or >115 μmol/L

Hematology Tests

White Blood Cell Count (Cells/mm^3)	Score = 4		
	<3,000		
Platelet Count (× 10^3 Cells/mm^3)	**Score = 2**	**Score = 4**	**Score = 5**
	100–200	50–99	<50
PT or PTT Please	**Score = 3**		
Neonate	PT >22.0 or PTT >85.0		
All other ages	PT >22.0 or PTT >57.0		

Other factors contributing to mortality risk computation are nonoperative cardiovascular disease, chromosomal anomaly, cancer, pervious pediatric intensive care unit (PICU) admission, pre-ICU cardiopulmonary resuscitation, postoperative acute diabetes (e.g., diabetic ketoacidosis), and admission from inpatient unit.

GCS, Glasgow coma scale; Pco_2, partial pressure of carbon dioxide; Pao_2, arterial partial pressure of oxygen; PT, prothrombin time; PTT, partial prothrombin time.

Pollack MM, Patel KM, Ruttimann UE. PRISM III: An updated pediatric risk of mortality score. *Crit Care Med.* 1996;24:743–752.

Irwin R, Cerra F, Rippe J, eds. *Irwin and Rippe's intensive care medicine.* Philadelphia, PA: Lippincott Williams & Wilkins; 1999.

Index